Drug
Reference for
EMS
Providers

Drug
Reference for
EMS
Providers

Richard K. Beck, BBA, NREMT-P
Program Director
Department of Emergency Medicine
University of Alabama School of Medicine/Huntsville Campus
Huntsville, Alabama

Technical Advisor:
Jill Shelton, Pharm. D.
Clinical Specialist
Huntsville Hospital
Huntsville, Alabama

DELMAR STAFF:

Health Care Publishing Director: William Brottmiller
Executive Editor: Cathy L. Esperti
Acquisitions Editor: Marie Linvill
Development Editor: Deb Flis
Editorial Assistant: Jill Korznat
Executive Marketing Manager: Dawn F. Gerrain
Channel Manager - Career Education: Tara Carter
Executive Production Manager: Karen Leet
Project Editor: Mary Ellen Cox
Production Coordinator: Nina Lontrato
Senior Art/Design Coordinator: Timothy J. Conners

Library of Congress Cataloging-in-Publication Data

Beck, Richard K., 1947-
  Drug reference for EMS providers / Richard K. Beck.
    p. cm.
  Includes index.
  ISBN 0-7668-2677-5 (alk. paper)
  1. Drugs—Handbooks, manuals, etc.   2. Emergency
    medicine—Handbooks, manuals, etc.   I. Title.
  RM301.12.B428 2001
  615'.1—dc21

                                        2001028466

Notice to the Reader

The publisher and the authors do not warrant or guarantee any of the products described herein or perform any independent analysis in connection with any of the product information contained herein. The publisher and the authors do not assume and expressly disclaim any obligation to obtain and include information other than that provided by the manufacturer.

The reader is expressly warned to consider and adopt all safety precautions that might be indicated by the activities described herein and to avoid all potential hazards. By following the instructions contained herein, the reader willingly assumes all risks in connection with such instructions.

The publisher and the authors make no representations or warranties of any kind, including but not limited to the warranties of fitness for a particular purpose or merchantability nor are any such representations implied with respect to the material set forth herein, and the publisher and the authors take no responsibility with respect to such material. The publisher and the authors shall not be liable for any special, consequential, or exemplary damages resulting, in whole or in part, from the reader's use of, or reliance upon, this material.

The authors and publisher have made a conscientious effort to ensure that the drug information and recommended dosages in this book are accurate and in accord with accepted standards at the time of publication. However, pharmacology and therapeutics are rapidly changing sciences, so readers are advised, before administering any drug, to check the package insert provided by the manufacturer for the recommended dose, for any contraindications for administration, and for any added warnings and precautions. This recommendation is especially important for new, infrequently used, or highly toxic drugs.

Table of Contents

Commonly Used Abbreviations and Symbols

aa, A	of each
ABG	arterial blood gas
a.c.	before meals
ACE	angiotensin-converting enzyme
ACLS	advanced cardiac life support
ACS	acute coronary syndrome
ACTH	adrenocorticotropic hormone
ad	to, up to
a.d.	right ear
ADA	adenosine deaminase
ADD	attention deficit disorder
ADH	antidiuretic hormone
ADL	activities of daily living
ad lib	as desired, at pleasure
ADP	adenosine diphosphate
AFB	acid fast bacillus
AHF	antihemophilic factor
AIDS	acquired immune deficiency syndrome
a.l.	left ear
ALL	acute lymphocytic leukemia
ALS	amyotrophic lateral sclerosis
ALT	alanine aminotransferase
a.m., A.M.	morning
AMI	acute myocardial infarction
AML	acute myelogenous leukemia
AMP	adenosine monophosphate
ANA	antinuclear antibody
ANC	absolute neutrophil count
ANS	autonomic nervous system
APTT	activated partial thromboplastin time
aq	water
aq dist.	distilled water
ARBS	angiotensin receptor blockade agents
ARC	AIDS-related complex
ARDS	adult respiratory distress syndrome
ASA	aspirin
ASAP	as soon as possible
ASHD	arteriosclerotic heart disease
AST	aspartate aminotransferase
ATC	around the clock
ATP	adenosine triphosphate
ATS/CDC	American Thoracic Society/Centers for Disease Prevention and Control
ATU	antithrombin unit
ATX	antibiotics

a.u.	each ear, both ears
AV	atrioventricular
b.i.d.	two times per day
b.i.n.	two times per night
BMR	basal metabolic rate
BP	blood pressure
BPD	bronchopulmonary dysplasia
BPH	benign prostatic hypertrophy
BS	blood sugar, bowel sounds
BSA	body surface area
BSE	breast self-exam
BSP	Bromsulphalein
BUN	blood urea nitrogen
C	Celsius/Centigrade
CABG	coronary artery bypass graft
C&DB	cough and deep breathe
CAD	coronary artery disease
caps, Caps	capsule(s)
CBC	complete blood count
CCB	calcium channel blocker
C_{CR}	creatinine clearance
CD_4	helper T_4 lymphocyte cells
CDC	Centers for Disease Control and Prevention
C&DB	cough and deep breathe
CF	cystic fibrosis
CHF	congestive heart failure
CHO	carbohydrate
CLL	chronic lymphocytic leukemia
CLS	capillary leak syndrome
cm	centimeter
CML	chronic myelocytic leukemia
CMV	cytomegalovirus
CN	cranial nerve
CNS	central nervous system
CO	cardiac output
COMT	catechol-o-methyltransferase
COPD	chronic obstructive pulmonary disease
CP	cardiopulmonary
CPAP	continuous positive airway pressure
CPB	cardiopulmonary bypass
CPK	creatine phosphokinase
CPR	cardiopulmonary resuscitation
CRF	chronic renal failure
C&S	culture and sensitivity
CSF	cerebrospinal fluid
CSID	congenital sucrase-isomaltase deficiency
CT	computerized tomography
CTS	carpal tunnel syndrome
CTZ	chemoreceptor trigger zone
CV	cardiovascular
CVA	cerebrovascular accident
CVP	central venous pressure
CXR	chest X ray
dATP	deoxy ATP
DBP	diastolic BP
dc	discontinue

DEA	Drug Enforcement Agency
DI	diabetes insipidus
DIC	disseminated intravascular coagulation
dil.	dilute
dL	deciliter (one-tenth of a liter)
DM	diabetes mellitus
DNA	deoxyribonucleic acid
DOE	dyspnea on exertion
dr.	dram (0.0625 ounce)
DTR	deep tendon reflex
DVT	deep vein thrombosis
EC	enteric-coated
ECB	extracorporeal cardiopulmonary bypass
ECG, EKG	electrocardiogram, electrocardiograph
EDTA	ethylenediaminetetraacetic acid
EEG	electroencephalogram
EENT	eye, ear, nose, and throat
EF	ejection fraction
e.g.	for example
elix	elixir
emuls.	emulsion
ENL	erythema nodosum leprosum
ENT	ear, nose, throat
EPS	electrophysiologic studies, extrapyramidal symptoms
ER	extended release
ESR	erythrocyte sedimentation rate
ESRD	end-stage renal disease
ET	endotracheal
ETOH	alcohol
ext.	extract
F	Fahrenheit, fluoride
FBS	fasting blood sugar
FDA	Food and Drug Administration
FEV	forced expiratory volume
FFP	fresh frozen plasma
FOB	fecal occult blood
FS	finger stick
FSH	follicle-stimulating hormone
F/U	follow-up
FVC	forced vital capacity
g, gm	gram (1,000 mg)
GABA	gamma-aminobutyric acid
G-CSF	granulocyte colony-stimulating factor
GERD	gastroesophageal reflux disease
GFR	glomerular filtration rate
GGT	gamma-glutamyl transferase: *syn.* gamma-glutamyl transpeptidase
GH	growth hormone
gi, GI	gastrointestinal
GnRH	gonadotropin-releasing hormone
GP	glycoprotein
G6PD	glucose-6-phosphate dehydrogenase
gr	grain
gtt	a drop, drops
GU	genitourinary
h, hr	hour

HA, HAL	hyperalimentation
HbAlc	hemoglobin A1c
HCG	human chorionic gonadotropin
HCP	health-care provider
HCV	hepatitis C virus
HDL	high density lipoprotein
HFN	high flow nebulizer
H&H	hematocrit and hemoglobin
HIT	heparin-induced thrombocytopenia
HIV	human immunodeficiency virus
HMG-CoA	3-hydroxy-3-methyl-glutaryl-coenzyme A
HOB	head of bed
HR	heart rate
h.s.	at bedtime
HSE	herpes simplex encephalitis
HSV	herpes simplex virus
5-HT	5-hydroxytryptamine
HTN	hypertension
IA	intra-arterial
IBD	inflammatory bowel disease
IBW	ideal body weight
ICP	intracranial pressure
ICU	intensive care unit
Ig	immunoglobulin
im, IM	intramuscular
IMV	intermittent mandatory ventilation
inh	inhalation
INR	international normalized ratio
I&O	intake and output
IOP	intraocular pressure
IPPB	intermittent positive pressure breathing
ITP	idiopathic thrombocytopenia purpura
IU	international units
iv, IV	intravenous
IVPB	IV piggyback, a secondary IV line
JVD	jugular venous distention
kg	kilogram (2.2 lb)
KVO	keep vein open
l, L	liter (1,000 mL)
L	left
LDH	lactic dehydrogenase
LDL	low density lipoprotein
LFTs	liver function tests
LH	luteinizing hormone
LHRH	luteinizing hormone-releasing hormone
LOC	level of consciousness
LV	left ventricular
LVEF	left ventricular ejection fraction
LVFP	left ventricular function pressure
M	mix
m^2, M^2	square meter
m	meter
MAC	*Mycobacterium avium* complex
MAO	monoamine oxidase
MAP	mean arterial pressure
max	maximum

mcg	microgram
MCH	mean corpuscular hemoglobin
mCi	millicurie
MDI	metered-dose inhaler
mEq	milliequivalent
mg	milligram
MI	myocardial infarction
MIC	minimum inhibitory concentration
min	minute, minim
mist, mixt	mixture
mL	milliliter
mm^3	cubic millimeter
MRI	magnetic resonance imaging
MS	multiple sclerosis
MU	million units
MUGA	multigated radionuclide angiography
NaCl	sodium chloride
ng	nanogram
NG	nasogastric
NGT	nasogastric tube
NIDDM	non-insulin dependent diabetes mellitus
NKA	no known allergies
NKDA	no known drug allergies
noct	at night, during the night
non rep	do not repeat
NPN	nonprotein nitrogen
NPO	nothing by mouth
NR	do not refill (e.g., a prescription)
NSAID	nonsteroidal anti-inflammatory drug
NSR	normal sinus rhythm
NSS	normal saline solution
NYHA	New York Heart Association
N&V	nausea and vomiting
O_2	oxygen
OC	oral contraceptive
o.d.	once a day
O.D.	right eye
OH	orthostatic hypotension
OOB	out of bed
OR	operating room
os	mouth
O.S.	left eye
O_2 sat	oxygen saturation
OTC	over the counter
O.U.	each eye, both eyes
oz	ounce
PA	pulmonary artery
PABA	para-aminobenzoic acid
PAF	paroxysmal atrial fibrillation
PAWP	pulmonary artery wedge pressure
PBI	protein-bound iodine
p.c.	after meals
PCA	patient-controlled analgesia
PCI	percutaneous coronary intervention
PCN	penicillin
PCP	*Pneumocystis carinii* pneumonia

PDE	phosphodiesterase
PE	pulmonary embolus
PEEP	positive end expiratory pressure
per	by, through
PFTs	pulmonary function tests
pH	hydrogen ion concentration
PID	pelvic inflammatory disease
PMH	past medical history
PMI	point of maximal intensity
PMS	premenstrual syndrome
PND	paroxysmal nocturnal dyspnea
po, p.o., PO	by mouth
PPAR	peroxisome proliferator-activated receptor
PPD	purified protein derivative
PR	by rectum
p.r.n., PRN	when needed or necessary
PSA	prostatic specific antigen
PSP	phenolsulfonphthalein
PSVT	paroxysmal supraventricular tachycardia
PT	prothrombin time
PTCA	percutaneous transluminal coronary angioplasty
PTH	parathyroid hormone
PTSD	post traumatic stress disorder
PTT	partial thromboplastin time
PUD	peptic ulcer disease
PUVA	psoralen and ulraviolet A
PVC	premature ventricular contraction; polyvinyl chloride
PVD	peripheral vascular disease
q.d.	every day
q.h.	every hour
q2hr	every two hours
q3hr	every three hours
q4hr	every four hours
q6hr	every six hours
q8hr	every eight hours
qhs	every night
q.i.d.	four times a day
qmo	every month
q.o.d.	every other day
q.s.	as much as needed, quantity sufficient
RA	right atrium; rheumatoid arthritis
RBC	red blood cell
RDA	recommended daily allowance
RDS	respiratory distress syndrome
REM	rapid eye movement
Rept.	let it be repeated
RICE	rest, ice, compression and elevation
RNA	ribonucleic acid
R/O	rule out
ROM	range of motion
ROS	review of systems
RRMS	relapsing-remitting multiple sclerosis
R/T	related to
RV	right ventricular
RUQ	right upper quadrant
Rx	symbol for a prescription

SA	sinoatrial; sustained-action
SAH	subarachnoid hemorrhage
SBE	subacute bacterial endocarditis
SBP	systolic BP
sc, SC, SQ	subcutaneous
SCID	severe combined immunodeficiency disease
SGOT	serum glutamic-oxaloacetic transaminase
SGPT	serum glutamic-pyruvic transaminase
S., Sig.	mark on the label
SI	sacroiliac
SIADH	syndrome inappropriate antidiuretic hormone
SIMV	synchronized intermittent mandatory ventilation
SL	sublingual
SLE	systemic lupus erythematosus
SOB	shortness of breath
sol	solution
sp	spirits
SR	sustained-release
ss	one-half
SSRI	selective serotonin reuptake inhibitor
S&S	signs and symptoms
stat	immediately, first dose
STD	sexually transmitted disease
SV	stroke volume
SVT	supraventricular tachycardia
syr	syrup
t½	halflife
tab	tablet
TB	tuberculosis
TCA	tricyclic antidepressant
TENS	transcutaneous electric nerve stimulation
TIA	transient ischemic attack
TIBC	total iron binding capacity
t.i.d.	three times per day
t.i.n.	three times per night
TKR	total knee replacement
TNF	tumor necrosis factor
T.O.	telephone order
TPN	total parenteral nutrition
TSH	thyroid stimulating hormone
μ	micron
μCi	microcurie
μg	microgram
μm	micrometer
U	unit
U/A	urinalysis
UGI	upper gastrointestinal
ULN	upper limit of normal
ung	ointment
UO	urine output
URI, URTI	upper respiratory infection
US	ultrasound
USP	U. S. Pharmacopeia
ut dict	as directed
UTI	urinary tract infection
UV	ultraviolet

VAD	venous access device
VF	ventricular fibrillation
vin	wine
vit	vitamin
VLDL	very low density lipoprotein
VMA	vanillylmandelic acid
V.O.	verbal order
VS	vital signs
VT	ventricular tachycardia
WBC	white blood cell
XRT	radiation therapy
&	and
>	greater than
<	less than
↑	increased, higher
↓	decreased, lower
-	negative
/	per
%	percent
+	positive
x	times, frequency

Preface

Given the knowledge that the out-of-hospital setting is a different environment than that of the in-hospital setting, coupled with the fact that physicians and nurses have their own respective pharmacology manuals, it is all too clear that the EMS professional needs a manual to address their pharmacologic information as well.

When EMS professionals respond to an emergency, they need to know what medications the patient is taking, for what reason(s), and if there is drug compatibility between the patient's medication and the medication to be given by EMS. *Drug Reference for EMS Providers* is the first comprehensive reference designed to present complete, in-depth profiles for over 850 drugs that EMS professionals may need to use or deal with during the course of treatment. Prescription medications taken at home are also addressed.

Organization

Drug Reference for EMS Providers is organized into four chapters.

- Chapter 1 Patient Medication Assessment emphasizes the importance of health care professionals obtaining a patient medication history. This information can be used to help design a treatment plan for EMS personnel, and alerts personnel at the receiving facility what treatment has been done and what may need to be done upon arrival. Failing to perform a medication assessment may delay treatment, which could lead to serious consequences for the patient. Scenarios are included to reinforce the importance of the medication assessment.

- Chapter 2 The Basics of Pharmacokinetics and Pharmacodynamics provides a review of how drugs travel and respond once in the body. It may be enough to know what drugs a patient is taking, but EMS professionals may also need to know how the drug(s) works once in the body and how the body may respond to the drug(s). Pharmacokinetics and pharmacodynamics reviews drug movement including absorption, solubility, distribution, biotransformation, and excretion. Once the drug reaches its destination, pharmacodynamics explains how a drug's mechanism of action affects the patient.

- Chapter 3 EMS Therapeutic Drug Classifications is organized by drug classification and based on the DOT Paramedic curriculum. Core information that applies to all drugs within the class is discussed.

- Chapter 4 A-Z Listing of Drugs contains drug profiles organized alphabetically by generic and most common trade names. Each profile contains detailed information on each drug's mechanism of action, summary of accepted out-of-hospital indications, contraindications, drug interactions, side effects, dosage, and comprehensive EMS considerations. When appropriate, symptoms and treatment of overdose are discussed as well. The chapter is designed for quick, easy access, and incorporates several features:

1. Drugs are listed by generic and most common trade names.

2. Routes and dosages are clearly delineated and correlated for both adult and pediatric dosages.

3. Life-threatening side effects are listed in **boldface** type.

4. Symptoms and treatment are summarized for appropriate drugs in the ***overdose management*** category.

5. EMS Considerations are presented using criteria for special implications the EMS professional needs to know using drug therapy.

Appendices for quick reference include controlled substances in the United States and Canada, elements of a prescription, pregnancy categories, nomogram for estimating body surface area, easy formulas for IV rate calculation, and tables of weights and measures. A guide to drug compatibility is included on the last page for quick reference.

Acknowledgments

This drug reference was developed from the database for *PDR® Nurse's Drug Handbook™* by George R. Spratto, PhD (Dean and Professor of Pharmacology, School of Pharmacy, West Virginia University, Morgantown, West Virginia) and Adrienne L. Woods, MSN, ARNP, FNP-C (Family Nurse Practitioner, Primary Care, at the Department of Veterans Affairs Medical and Regional Office Center, Wilmington, Delaware).

I would like to thank Doris Smith, former Acquisitions Editor with Delmar/Thomson Learning, for her encouragement. Doris is the person who introduced me to the Delmar/Thomson Learning organization and got me started on this project. In the beginning, Doris made sure that I was going in the right direction. Then, of course, there is Deb Flis. Deb is a great motivator and encourager. She was always available to answer questions, give support and encouragement, and get problems fixed that didn't quite work. If I have the opportunity to work on another Delmar/Thomson Learning project, it would be an honor to work with Deb again. Thanks Deb.

The author and Delmar/Thomson Learning would like to thank the following reviewers:

Mike Kennamer, MPA, EMT-P
Director, Emergency Medical Services
Northeast Alabama Community College
Rainsville, Alabama

Bill Metcalf
Division Chief, EMS and Special Services
North Lake Tahoe Fire Protection District
Incline Village, Nevada

Gerard C. Muench, Jr., MPA, MICP
Director, Office of Emergency Medical Services
New Jersey State Department of Health and Senior Services
Trenton, New Jersey

Matt Myers, EMT-P
EMS Specialist
Fresno, California

USING THE *DRUG REFERENCE FOR EMS PROVIDERS*

Understanding the format of the *Drug Reference for EMS Providers* will help you reference information quickly.

There are four chapters:

Chapter 1 Patient Medication Assessment

Chapter 2 The Basics of Pharmacokinetics and Pharmacodynamics

Chapter 3 EMS Therapeutic Drug Classifications

Chapter 4 A-Z Listing of Drugs

The individual drug entries follow a similar format. All items listed below may not appear in each drug entry, but are represented where appropriate. Each drug entry will follow the following general format:

- GENERIC/nonproprietary name: Drugs are listed in alphabetical order by their generic name.

- PHONETIC PRONUNICATION: Each drug has the phonetic pronunciation of its generic name. For example: atropine sulfate = [AH-troh-peen] or diphenhydramine hydrochloride = [dye-fen-HY-drah-meen].

- PREGNANCY CLASS (FDA Assigned): Each drug has been assigned a use-in-pregnancy rating. For example, procainamide has been assigned a pregnancy category of "C" which states that risk cannot be ruled out.

- TRADE/proprietary name: Drugs are also listed by their trade names— the registered names given by the manufacturers. For example, a trade name for procainamide is Pronestyl.

- CLASSIFICATIONS: Each drug is listed by its pharmacologic class to which the drug has been assigned. For example, procainamide hydrochloride is an antiarrhythmic, class 1A.

- MECHANISM OF ACTION: The drug's mechanism of action describes how the drug produces its desired therapeutic effects. Also included are the therapeutic benefits the drug is expected to achieve. For example, procainamide produces a direct cardiac effect by prolonging the refractory period of the atria and to a lesser extent the bundle of the His-Purkinje system and the ventricles. This is effective in the suppression of ventricular ectopy and arrhythmias.

- ONSET OF ACTION and DURATION OF ACTION: These categories provide information about the rate of drug absorption, distribution, and duration of action. For example, the onset of action for procainamide is approximately 1-5 minutes, and has a therapeutic duration of approximately 3 hours.

- USES: These are the drug's current therapeutic applications. For example, procainamide is used for documented ventricular arrhythmias that may be life threatening in patients where benefits of treatment outweigh the risks.

- CONTRAINDICATIONS: These are conditions for which the drug should not be used. For example, procainamide should not be given to patients experiencing complete AV heart block, torsade de pointes or asymptomatic PVCs.

- PRECAUTIONS: These are situations in which drug use may be dangerous, or when dosage or administration techniques may have to be modified. For example, procainamide should be used with caution in patients who may experience a sudden drop in blood pressure, in CHF patients, or in patients with acute ischemic heart disease.

- ROUTE/DOSAGE: The route describes how the drug is given. For example, IV bolus, IV infusion, IM, PO, etc. The dosage tells how much of the drug should be given. For example, the adult dose of procainamide for ventricular arrhythmias is 20mg/minute for up to 30 minutes, then a maintenance infusion of 2-6mg/minute.

- HOW SUPPLIED: This category lists the various forms available for the drug, and amounts of the drug in each of the dosage forms. For example, procainamide comes supplied in capsules (250mg, 375mg, 500mg) injection (100mg/mL, 500mg/mL) tablets (250mg, 375mg, 500mg) and tablet extended release (250mg, 500mg, 750mg, 1000mg).

- SIDE EFFECTS: This category includes potential drug-related undesired side effects organized by body system. For example, the side effects of procainamide for the cardiovascular system include hypotension, ventricular fibrillation or ventricular asystole, or complete heart block.

- OVERDOSE MANAGEMENT: This category lists the symptoms of drug overdose and the approaches for treatment. For example, some of the symptoms for procainamide overdose include progressive widening of the QRS complex, prolonged QT or PR intervals, lowering of R and T waves and increased AV block. Management for this overdose includes giving IV fluids and/or a vasopressor (dopamine, phenylephrine, or norepinephrine) to treat hypotension or an IV of 1/6 molar sodium lactate to reduce the cardiotoxic effects.

- DRUG INTERACTIONS: This category lists the effects of drugs interacting with one another. Drug interactions may result from such things as additive or inhibitory effects, increased rate of elimination, decreased absorption, receptor site competition or displacement from plasma protein binding sites, and potential lethal/adverse drug interactions. For example, lidocaine has an additive cardio-depressant effect when used with procainamide and succinylcholine has an increased effect on muscle relaxation when used with procainamide.

- EMS CONSIDERATIONS: This category contains guidelines to help the EMS professional apply treatment protocol processes to pharmacotherapeutics to help to ensure safe practice. Special information that may be helpful when referencing drug information is included. Examples of some EMS considerations for procainamide include:

  1. Extended release tablets are not recommended for use in children.

  2. IV use should be reserved for emergency situations.

  3. For IV maintenance infusion, administer with an electronic infusion device.

  4. Discard solutions that are darker than light amber or otherwise colored. Consult pharmacist if unsure.

CHAPTER 1
Patient Medication Assessment

Anyone in medicine knows the importance of a thorough patient assessment. Included in this assessment should be a medication assessment. Information gained from this medication assessment can provide important information, not only for EMS personnel, but for hospital personnel, as well.

Information gained from the medication assessment can be used to design a treatment plan for EMS personnel, and alerts personnel at the receiving facility what treatment was done and what may need to be done upon arrival. Knowing what medications the patient is taking will aid in preventing drug interactions or overdoses, that might occur from administration of drugs in the out-of-hospital setting, as well as at the receiving facility.

If EMS personnel fail to obtain patient medication information while on the scene, the receiving facility will have to begin their own medication assessment, which may delay treatment and could cause serious consequences.

Patient medication information may be obtained in several ways. Usually, the patient is the best source. However, in some cases, the patient may not know what mediations they are taking. They may know why they are taking a medication, but not its name. In other cases, the patient may not know what or why they are taking medications. If the patient is unable to communicate their medication assessment, other sources may include a family member, friend, or a home health aide. Below is an example of a medication assessment:

- *Are you currently taking any medications prescribed by a doctor?*
- *What are the names of the medications?* Some patients may not know the actual names of the drugs they are taking. If this is the case, EMS personnel should also ask: *Do you have some of the medication to show me? We must take it (them) to the hospital.*
- *Why are you taking the medication(s)?* If the patient does not know the name of the medication, he/she may know the reason for taking the drug.
- *When did you last take your medication?*
- *Have you been taking your medication according to the prescribed directions? If not, how have you been taking them?*
- *Are you taking any over-the-counter medications (medications purchased without a prescription at the store)? If so, what are these medications, and when did you last take them?*
- *Are you taking any medications that were prescribed for someone else?*
- *Have you recently completed taking medications? If so, what were they, and why were you taking them?*
- *Have you experienced any side effects or illness from your medications? If so, have you reported these to your doctor?*

Depending on the circumstances, the medication assessment can be

---

bold italic = life threatening side effect

adjusted to address special situations. Additional questions may have to be asked.

It is generally useful to bring any patient medications to the receiving facility with the patient. The most common places patients keep medications include the bathroom, bedroom, and the kitchen (don't forget to look in the refrigerator). To save time, EMS dispatch may have instructed the caller to have any medications ready for EMS when they arrive.

EMS professionals should be familiar with medication labels and the information on them. Figure 1–1 shows the elements of a prescription.

In order to safely communicate the exact elements desired on a prescription, the following items should be addressed:

A. The prescriber: Name, address, phone number, and associated practice/speciality

B. The client: Name, age, address and social security number

C. The prescription itself: Name of the medication (generic or trade); quantity to be dispensed (e.g., tablets or capsules, 1 vial, 1 tube, volume of liquid); the strength of the medication (e.g., 125-mg tablets, 250 mg/5 mL, 80 mg/1 mL, 10%); and directions for use (e.g., 1 tablet po t.i.d.; 2 gtt to each eye q.i.d.; 1 teaspoonful po q 8 hr for 10 days; apply a thin film to lesions b.i.d. for 14 days)

D. Other elements: Date prescription is written, signature of the provider, number of refills; provider number: state license number and Drug Enforcement Agency (DEA) number (when applicable); and brand-product-only indication (when applicable)

A typical prescription is depicted as follows:

A.   **Julia Bryan, MSN, RN, CPNP**
Pediatric Associates
1611 Kirkwood Highway
Wilmington, DE 19805
302-645-8261

Date: July 10, 2001

B. For: **Kathryn Woods, Age 8**
27 East Parkway
Lewes, DE 19958
123-555-1234

C. **Rx**   **Amoxicillin susp. 250 mg/5 mL**
Disp. 150 mL
Sig: 1 teaspoon PO q 8 hr x 10 days

D. Refills: 0

Provider signature
Provider/State license number

Interpretation of prescription: The above prescription is written by Pediatric Nurse Practitioner Julia Bryan for Kathryn Woods and is for amoxicillin suspension. The concentration desired is 250 mg/5 mL. The directions for taking the medication are 1 teaspoon (i.e., 5 mL) by mouth every 8 hr for 10 days. The prescriber wants 150 mL dispensed and there are no refills allowed.

Elements of A Prescription
Figure 1–1

Also be aware that many medication containers have additional secondary labels, which include additional information such as *"swallow whole, DO NOT crush or chew," "take on an empty stomach," "Important: take or use exactly as directed, do not discontinue or skip doses unless directed by your doctor,"* and *"may cause drowsiness."*

MEDICATION ASSESSMENT SCENARIOS

Knowing what medications your patient is taking may provide a basis for determining treatment. Medications may be one of your most useful assessment tools, especially if the patient is unresponsive or incoherent. The following three scenarios illustrate the importance of your medication assessment.

Scenario One

You respond to a 72-year-old male who states he has been feeling weak for the past 4 hours. While performing your initial assessment, you notice some medication containers on the kitchen table. These include Lanoxin, Cardizem, and glyburide. What information do these medications tell you about this patient?

- Lanoxin is the trade name for digoxin, an antiarrhythmic. Digoxin increases both the force and velocity of ventricular contractions, while simultaneously slowing conduction through the AV node of the heart.
- Cardizem is the trade name for diltiazem, a calcium channel blocker that decreases conduction velocity and ventricular rate.
- Glyburide is an oral anti-diabetic agent used to treat type II diabetes.

Knowing what these medications are used for, or having access to a resource to look up the drug uses, tells us that this patient is a diabetic with underlying cardiovascular problems.

Scenario Two

You are called to a 59-year-old female patient who is complaining of dizziness and feeling weak. Her pulse rate is 44 beats/minute and regular. Upon questioning about medications, she tells you that she is on blood pressure medicine, but cannot remember the name. She finds the bottle and the drug name is atenolol. When questioned further, she admits not taking her medicine for "about a couple of days." Further questioning reveals that she had taken 3 tablets to make up for not taking any over the last couple of days.

- Atenolol is a beta-adrenergic blocking agent used for hypertension and angina pectoris due to hypertension.

By taking a multiple dose, this patient is most likely experiencing side effects due to overdosing. Overdosing on prescribed medications is a common problem with patients who forget to take their medications and try and "catch up," or who just do not understand the instructions on the container.

Scenario Three

You respond to a 69-year-old male who states "my heart feels like a runaway train." His pulse rate is 128 beats/minute and regular. During your assessment, you find out that he has chronic obstructive pulmonary disease (COPD) and has just been prescribed Ventolin. The patient used the Ventolin approximately 30 minutes ago, and began feeling his heart racing.

- Ventolin is a trade name for albuterol, a bronchodilator used to treat reversible airway obstruction caused by asthma or COPD. Cardiovascular side effects of albuterol include hypertension, chest pain, and arrhythmias. Unfortunately, the elderly are more prone to develop adverse reactions and side effects.

---

bold italic = life threatening side effect

It is very important for EMS personnel to perform a thorough patient assessment including a medication assessment. Medication interactions are sometimes difficult to assess in the out-of-hospital setting. However, any information gathered will benefit the patient when planning a treatment plan, whether in the out-of-hospital setting or in the hospital.

CHAPTER 2
The Basics of Pharmacokinetics and Pharmacodynamics

Drugs must make a complicated journey through the body before they can produce their desired therapeutic effects. Once a drug is given, it is absorbed into the circulatory system, distributed to its site of action, and finally eliminated from the body. *Pharmacokinetics* is the study of drug absorption, distribution, biotransformation (metabolism), and elimination, with an emphasis on the time it takes for these processes to take place. In other words, pharmacokinetics studies drug movement.

Once a drug reaches its receptors sites (sites of action), certain biochemical and physiologic actions occur, producing the desired pharmacologic effects. These pharmacologic effects are called the drug's mechanism of action. *Pharmacodynamics* is the study of drug actions on the body. Drug pharmacokinetics and pharmacodynamics determine the route, frequency, and dosage of drug administration.

PHARMACOKINETICS

Absorption

Absorption is the passage of a drug from the site of administration (where absorption begins) into the circulatory system. The speed at which a drug is absorbed is very important, because it determines how quickly the drug reaches its target tissue to produce its therapeutic effects. The rate of absorption depends on the following factors:

- Circulatory status. Poor circulation results in slow drug absorption and, therefore, delayed or inadequate therapeutic response. However, drugs that can be given via the IV route bypasses the absorption process. The IV administration technique permits the drug to go directly into the circulation, thereby permitting a faster therapeutic response.
- Solubility. This is the drug's ability to dissolve. The higher a drug's solubility, the faster it enters the bloodstream.
- Body pH. Acidosis delays drug absorption in many cases. For example, acidosis can delay the absorption of epinephrine, thus making it inactive. That is why some patients in cardiac arrest do not respond to epinephrine-inadequate ventilations and/or chest compressions leave them acidotic. However, some drugs can vary significantly in pH. For example, a drug that is acidic will generally absorb better when introduced into the stomach because of the stomach's acidic environment. Also, an alkaline drug will absorb more quickly when introduced into the alkaline environment of the kidneys. Therefore, both a drug's pH and the pH of the environment can affect absorption.
- Concentration. Generally, the higher the percentage of drug in the preparation administered, the faster

the rate of absorption. Approximately 80 percent of drugs used in medicine are formulated to be taken orally. However, the oral route has two drawbacks. First, it is harder to predict and control the final concentration in the circulatory system of an orally administered drug. This unpredictability results from:

1. changes in the rate of absorption, depending on the presence or absence of food in the digestive system
2. the destruction of some of the drug by gastric enzymes

Second, the rate of absorption through the digestive system is slower than the rate from subcutaneous injection and intramuscular injection.

Distribution

Once a drug is administered and absorbed into the circulatory system, it must travel to its site of action before it can be of any benefit. Once in the blood stream, the entire dose does not travel to its targeted tissues. Instead, the drug travels throughout the entire body. As Figure 2–1 illustrates, a certain amount of the drug may become bound to blood proteins (such as hemoglobin, albumen, and globulin). When this occurs, the drug is unavailable for further distribution until it is released from the blood protein. Drugs can also become stored within the body's fatty tissues. Again, until the drug is released from this fatty tissue, it is unavailable for distribution. The amount of drug that binds to blood protein or becomes stored in the body's fatty tissues is termed *bound drug.* Only the drug not bound, termed *free drug,* can be distributed for metabolism and elimination and is available to targeted tissues.

Because drugs are distributed by way of the circulatory system, they generally concentrate in tissues that are well supplied with blood, such as the heart, liver, kidneys, and brain. However, the blood-brain barrier and the blood-cerebrospinal fluid barrier limit delivery of drugs to the brain.

These are tightly packed cell membranes that separate the circulating blood from the brain and cerebrospinal fluid. The blood-brain barrier and the blood-cerebrospinal fluid barrier restrict the movement of some damaging drugs and toxins to the brain and cerebrospinal fluid. Only non-protein-bound, highly lipid-soluble drugs can cross these barriers into the central nervous system. Even these drugs generally enter the brain and spinal fluid at a slower rate than other tissues, because of this extra barrier.

Biotransformation

There are two ways in which the body eliminates a drug: biotransformation and excretion. *Biotransformation* is the chemical alteration of a drug within the body to an active or inactive water-soluble metabolite. A *metabolite* is any product that results from biotransformation. Changing a drug to a water-soluble metabolite makes excretion from the body easier. Most drugs are inactivated as a result of biotransformation. Some drugs, however, become therapeutically active (prodrugs) as a result of biotransformation.

The biotransformation process of a drug to an inactive metabolite begins immediately after drug administration. This actually becomes a race against time. The drug must reach its target site of action at a sufficient therapeutic concentration in the blood before biotransformation converts the drug to an inactive state.

Biotransformation takes place primarily in the liver. However, it can occur in all body cells and tissues. Biotransformation that takes place in the liver is called *hepatic biotransformation.*

If the rate of drug biotransformation is slowed for any reason, cumulative drug effects may occur—in other words, subsequent doses have more effect. Increasing the rate of biotransformation may produce a state of apparent tolerance, in which the drug effect decreases. Generally, when biotransformation is complete, a drug is no longer able to work

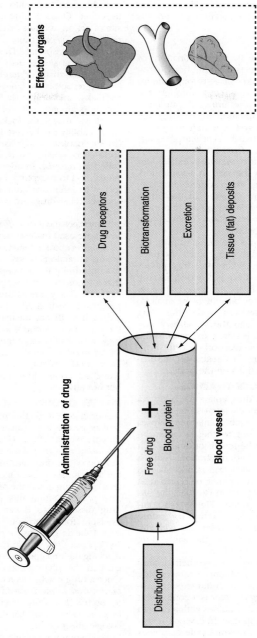

The Pharmacokinetic Phase of Drug Action
Figure 2–1

therapeutically (unless the drug became an active metabolite), and it is excreted.

Excretion

Excretion is the elimination of waste products from the body. Drug excretion takes place through the intestines in the feces, through the kidneys in the urine, through the skin in perspiration, and through the respiratory system in exhaled air.

Volatile (easily evaporated) drugs are excreted from the body through the respiratory system in exhaled air or through the skin in perspiration. Nonvolatile, water-soluble drug metabolites are excreted in the urine. The kidney is the most important site for the excretion of drugs and drug metabolites.

Some drugs are excreted from the body through the alimentary tract. This occurs when the drug passes through the liver, is released into the bile, and is finally eliminated in the feces. When the bile enters the small intestine, however, some the drug travels through the circulatory system until it is finally excreted in the urine. If the reabsorbed drug is in active form, this reabsorption prolongs its actions on the body.

PHARMACODYNAMICS

Unless a drug enters the body via the intravenous, intraosseous, or endotracheal route, some time elapses before the drug reaches its target site of action. The length of time from a drug's first administration until it reaches a concentration necessary to produce a therapeutic response at its target site of action is called the *onset of drug action*. Figure 2–2 compares the onset of action for a drug administered intravenously with the onset of action for the same drug given intramuscularly.

Most drugs produce their desired effects by inhibiting or increasing the action of their targeted receptors. A *drug receptor* is a component of a cell that combines with a drug to initiate a response. In essence, a section of the drug molecule combines with part of the molecular structure on or within a cell to produce a therapeutic effect. Once a drug reaches its site of action, it binds or unites to its receptor so it can cause the desired therapeutic response. This action at the receptor site is also called the drug's *mechanism of action*.

Drug receptors are often referred to as "locks," and drugs that bind to the receptors are generally referred to as the "keys" that fit the locks. A drug's (key's) ability to fit a certain receptor (lock) enables a pharmacologic response to occur. Such a drug is called an *agonist*. In addition, some drugs bind to receptors, but their effect is to inhibit or counteract a response. These drugs are called *antagonists*.

Sometimes the terms *affinity* and *efficacy* are used to describe the nature of drug-receptor interaction. Affinity means attraction; to say that a drug has an affinity for a receptor means that it tends to combine with that receptor. Efficacy means the power to produce a desired effect: to say that a drug has efficacy means that it has the capacity to produce a pharmacologic response when it interacts with its receptor. Drugs that are agonists have both affinity and efficacy, while antagonist drugs have affinity but not efficacy.

PHASES OF DRUG ACTIVITY

A drug goes through four phases of activity before it produces a desired pharmacologic effect (Figure 2–3). The *administration phase* is the introduction of the drug into the body by the appropriate route. Once administered, the drug enters the *pharmaceutical phase*. During this phase, the drug dissolves so it can be made available for absorption. Once dissolved, the drug begins the *pharmacokinetic phase*. Only free drugs capable of reaching their receptors can be said to exist in the pharmacokinetic phase. Once a drug reaches its receptors, the *pharmacodynamic phase* of drug activity occurs. It is only when the drug binds to its receptor that the pharmacologic effect occurs.

The minimum concentration neces-

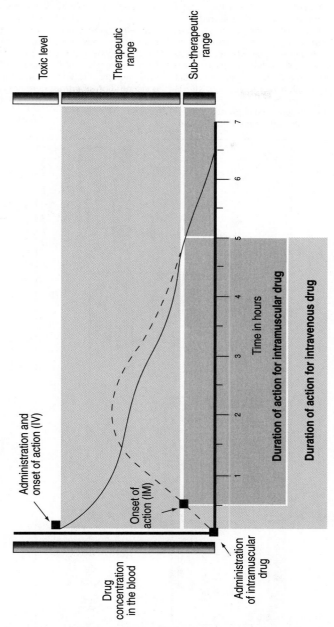

Comparison of Concentration Profile for Intravenous and Intramuscular
Administration of the Same Drug.

Figure 2–2

sary for a drug to produce the desired therapeutic response is referred to as the *minimum therapeutic concentration*. A drug concentration below the minimum therapeutic concentration will not produce an effective response, and drug concentrations that are too high may produce toxic effects or may even be fatal.

Most drugs have a predetermined standard dosage or the dosage is determined by body weight. Dosage guidelines are established to achieve minimum therapeutic concentrations. Any deviation from established dosage guidelines might be harmful. Remember that the goal for drug therapy is to give the minimum concentration of a drug necessary to obtain the desired therapeutic response.

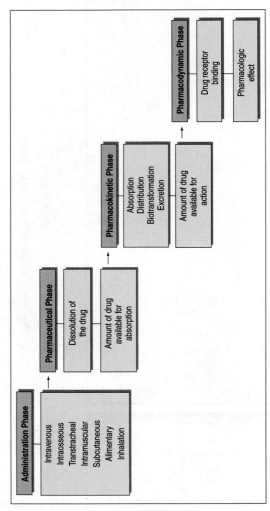

The Phases of Drug Activity
Figure 2–3

CHAPTER THREE
Therapeutic Drug Classifications

ALKYLATING AGENTS

See also the following individual entries:

Busulfan
Chlorambucil
Cyclophosphamide
Lomustine
Melphalan
Streptozocin
Thiotepa

Mechanism of Action: Alkylating agents donate an alkyl group (carbonium ion) to biologically important macromolecules, such as DNA. The molecule is inactivated bringing *cell division* to a halt. This cytotoxic activity affects replication of cancerous cells and other cells, especially in rapidly proliferating tissues, such as the bone marrow, intestinal epithelium, and hair follicles. The toxic effects are usually cell-cycle nonspecific and become apparent when the cell enters the S phase and cell division is blocked at the G_2 phase (premitotic phase), resulting in cells having a double complement of DNA.

Resistance of cancer cells to alkylating agents usually develops slowly and gradually. Resistance seems to be the sum total of several minor adaptations, including decreased permeability of the cells, increased production of noncancer receptors (nucleophilic substances), and increased efficiency of the DNA repair system.

EMS CONSIDERATIONS

See *individual agents* and *Antineoplastic Agents.*

ALPHA-1-ADRENERGIC BLOCKING AGENTS

See also the following individual entries:

Doxazosin mesylate
Prazosin hydrochloride
Tamsulosin hydrochloride
Terazosin

Mechanism of Action: Selectively block postsynaptic alpha-1-adrenergic receptors. Results in dilation of both arterioles and veins leading to a decrease in supine and standing BP. Diastolic BP is affected the most. Prazosin and terazosin do not produce reflex tachycardia. Terazosin also relaxes smooth muscle in the bladder neck and prostate, making it useful to treat BPH. Have many undesirable effects which, although not toxic, limit their use. Always start treatment at low doses and increase gradually.

Uses: Alone or in combination with diuretics or beta-adrenergic blocking agents to treat hypertension. Doxazocin and terazosin are used to treat BPH. *Investigational:* Prazosin is used for refractory CHF, management of Raynaud's vasospasm, and to treat BPH. Doxazosin, along with digoxin and diuretics, is used to treat CHF.

Contraindications: Hypersensitivity to these drugs (i.e., quinazolines).

Precautions: The first few doses may cause postural hypotension and syncope with sudden loss of consciousness. Use with caution in lactation, with impaired hepatic function,

---

bold italic = life threatening side effect

or if receiving drugs known to influence hepatic metabolism. Safety and efficacy have not been established in children.

Side Effects: The following side effects are common to alpha-1-adrenergic blockers. See individual drugs as well. *CV:* Palpitations, postural hypotension, hypotension, tachycardia, chest pain, arrhythmia. *GI:* N&V, dry mouth, diarrhea, constipation, abdominal discomfort or pain, flatulence. *CNS:* Dizziness, depression, decreased libido, sexual dysfunction, nervousness, paresthesia, somnolence, anxiety, insomnia, asthenia, drowsiness. *Musculoskeletal:* Pain in the shoulder, neck, or back; gout, arthritis, joint pain, arthralgia. *Respiratory:* Dyspnea, nasal congestion, sinusitis, bronchitis, **bronchospasm**, cold symptoms, epistaxis, increased cough, flu symptoms, pharyngitis, rhinitis. *Ophthalmic:* Blurred vision, abnormal vision, reddened sclera, conjunctivitis. *GU:* Impotence, urinary frequency, incontinence. *Miscellaneous:* Tinnitus, vertigo, pruritus, sweating, alopecia, lichen planus, headache, edema, weight gain, facial edema, fever.

OD **Overdose Management:** *Symptoms:* Extension of the side effects, especially on BP. *Treatment:* Keep supine to restore BP and normalize heart rate. Shock may be treated with volume expanders or vasopressors; support renal function.

Drug Interactions: Alpha-1 blockers ↓ the antihypertensive effect of clonidine.

Administration/Storage: Take the first dose of prazosin and terazosin at bedtime.

EMS CONSIDERATIONS

See also *Beta-Adrenergic Blocking Agents.*

AMEBICIDES AND TRICHOMONACIDES

See also the following individual entries:

Atovaquone
Erythromycins
Metronidazole
Paromomycin sulfate
Tetracyclines

General Statement: Amebiasis is caused by the protozoan *Entamoeba histolytica. E. histolytica* has two forms: (1) an active motile form known as the trophozoite form and (2) a cystic form that is resistant to destruction and is responsible for the transmission of the disease. The overt manifestations of amebiasis vary, including violent acute dysentery (characterized by sudden development of severe diarrhea, cramps, and passage of bloody, mucoid stools); others have few overt symptoms or are even completely asymptomatic.

Amoebae often migrate from the GI tract to other parts of the body (extraintestinal amebiasis). The spleen, lungs, or liver are frequently affected. The amoebae colonize in these organs and form abscesses that may rupture and thereby serve as infectious foci.

At present, no one drug can cure both intestinal and extraintestinal amebic infestations; thus, combination therapy is used. Often the more effective but toxic agents are used initially for a short period of time, while long-term eradication or prophylaxis is carried out with less toxic agents.

Infestation with the parasite *Trichomonas vaginalis* causes vaginitis. This is treated by various locally applied antitrichomonal agents—often effective amebicides—and also by the oral administration of metronidazole (usually prescribed for both sexual partners to prevent reinfection). Acid douches (vinegar or lactic acid) are a helpful adjunct to treatment.

The incidence of infections by the protozoan, *Giardia lamblia,* is transmitted in the feces. Symptoms include mucous diarrhea, abdominal pain, and weight loss. Drugs of choice are metronidazole and quinacrine.

EMS CONSIDERATIONS

See also *Anti-Infectives.*

AMINOGLYCOSIDES

See also the following individual entries:

Amikacin sulfate
Gentamicin sulfate
Kanamycin sulfate
Neomycin sulfate
Paromomycin sulfate
Tobramycin sulfate

Mechanism of Action: Broad-spectrum antibiotics believed to inhibit protein synthesis by binding irreversibly to ribosomes (30S subunit), thereby interfering with an initiation complex between messenger RNA and the 30S subunit. This leads to production of nonfunctional proteins; polyribosomes are split apart and are unable to synthesize protein. Usually bactericidal due to disruption of the bacterial cytoplasmic membrane. Poorly absorbed from the GI tract; usually administered parenterally (exceptions: some enteric infections of the GI tract and prior to surgery). Also absorbed from the peritoneum, bronchial tree, wounds, denuded skin, and joints. Distributed in the extracellular fluid and cross the placental barrier, but not the blood-brain barrier. Penetration of the CSF is increased when the meninges are inflamed.

Rapidly absorbed after IM injection. **Peak plasma levels, after IM:** Usually ½–2 hr. Measurable levels persist for 8–12 hr after a single administration. **t½:** 2–3 hr (increases sharply in impaired kidney function). Ranges of t½ from 24 to 110 hr have been observed. Excreted mainly unchanged in urine. Resistance develops slowly.

Uses: Are powerful antibiotics that induce serious side effects—**do not use for minor infections**. Gram-negative bacteria causing bone and joint infections, septicemia (including neonatal sepsis), skin and soft tissue infections (including those from burns), respiratory tract infections, postoperative infections, intra-abdominal infections (including per-

itonitis), UTIs. In combination with clindamycin for mixed aerobic-anaerobic infections. Also, see individual drugs.

Used for gram-positive bacteria only when other less toxic drugs are either ineffective or contraindicated. Use in CNS *Pseudomonas* infections such as meningitis or ventriculitis is questionable.

Contraindications: Hypersensitivity to aminoglycosides, long-term therapy (except streptomycin for tuberculosis).

Precautions: Use with extreme caution with impaired renal function or preexisting hearing impairment. Safe use in pregnancy and during lactation not established. Assess premature infants, neonates, and older patients closely; they are particularly sensitive to toxic effects. Considerable cross-allergenicity occurs among the aminoglycosides.

Side Effects: *Ototoxicity:* Both auditory and vestibular damage have been noted. The risk is increased with poor renal function and in the elderly. Auditory symptoms include tinnitus and hearing impairment, while vestibular symptoms include dizziness, nystagmus, vertigo, and ataxia.

Renal Impairment: May be characterized by cylindruria, oliguria, proteinuria, azotemia, hematuria, increase or decrease in frequency of urination; increased BUN, NPN, or creatinine; and increased thirst. *Neurotoxicity:* Neuromuscular blockade, headache, tremor, lethargy, paresthesia, peripheral neuritis (numbness, tingling, or burning of face/mouth), arachnoiditis, encephalopathy, acute organic brain syndrome. CNS depression, characterized by stupor, flaccidity, and rarely, ***coma, and respiratory depression in infants.*** Optic neuritis with blurred vision or loss of vision. *GI:* N&V, diarrhea, increased salivation, anorexia, weight loss. *Allergic:* Rash, urticaria, pruritus, burning, fever, stomatitis, eosinophilia. Rarely, ***agranulocytosis and anaphylaxis.*** Cross-allergy among aminoglycosides has

---

bold italic = life threatening side effect

been observed. *Miscellaneous:* Joint pain, ***laryngeal edema, pulmonary fibrosis,*** superinfection.

OD Overdose Management: *Symptoms:* Extension of side effects. *Treatment:* Undertake hemodialysis (preferred) or peritoneal dialysis.

Drug Interactions

Bumetanide / ↑ Risk of ototoxicity
Capreomycin / ↑ Muscle relaxation
Cephalosporins / ↑ Risk of renal toxicity
Ciprofloxacin HCl / Additive antibacterial activity
Cisplatin / Additive renal toxicity
Colistimethate / ↑ Muscle relaxation
Digoxin / Possible ↑ or ↓ effect of digoxin
Ethacrynic acid / ↑ Risk of ototoxicity
Furosemide / ↑ Risk of ototoxicity
Methoxyflurane / ↑ Risk of renal toxicity
Penicillins / ↓ Effect of aminoglycosides
Polymyxins / ↑ Muscle relaxation
Skeletal muscle relaxants (surgical) / ↑ Muscle relaxation
Vancomycin / Additive ototoxicity and renal toxicity
Vitamin A / ↓ Effect of vitamin A due to ↓ absorption from GI tract

Administration/Storage

1. Check expiration date.
2. Warn if drug being administered stings or causes a burning sensation.
3. During IM administration
• Inject deep into muscle mass to minimize transient pain.
• Use a Z track method for thin, elderly patients.
• Rotate/document injection sites.
4. With IV administration
• Dilute with compatible solution.
• Infuse at the rate ordered to prevent excessive serum concentrations.
5. Administer for only 7–10 days and avoid repeating course of therapy unless a serious infection is present that does not respond to other antibiotics.
6. Administer ATC to maintain therapeutic drug levels.

EMS CONSIDERATIONS

See also *Anti-Infectives.*

AMPHETAMINES AND DERIVATIVES

See also the following individual entries:

> Amphetamine sulfate
> Dextroamphetamine sulfate
> Mazindol
> Methamphetamine hydrochloride
> Phendimetrazine tartrate
> Phenylpropanolamine hydrochloride

Mechanism of Action: Thought to act on the cerebral cortex and reticular activating system (including the medullary, respiratory, and vasomotor centers) by releasing norepinephrine from central adrenergic neurons. High doses cause release of dopamine from the mesolimbic system. The stimulatory effect on the CNS causes an increase in motor activity and mental alertness, a mood-elevating effect, a slight euphoric effect, and an anorexigenic effect. The anorexigenic effect is thought to be produced by direct stimulation of the satiety center in the lateral hypothalamic feeding center of the brain. Peripheral effects are mediated by alpha- and beta-adrenergic receptors and include increases in both systolic and diastolic BP and respiratory stimulation. Readily absorbed from the GI tract and distributed throughout most tissues, with the highest concentrations in the brain and CSF. Duration of anorexia (PO): 3–6 hr. Metabolized in liver and excreted by kidneys. Excreted slowly (5–7 days); cumulative effects may occur with continued administration.

Psychic stimulation is often followed by a rebound effect manifested as fatigue. Tolerance will develop to all drugs of this class. There is a relatively wide margin of safety between the therapeutic and toxic doses of amphetamines. However, both acute and chronic toxicity can occur.

Uses: See individual drugs.

Contraindications: Hyperthyroidism, advanced arteriosclerosis, nephritis, diabetes mellitus, hypertension, narrow-angle glaucoma, angina pectoris, CV disease, and individuals with hypersensitivity to these drugs. Use in emotionally unstable persons susceptible to drug abuse and in agitated states. Psychotic children. Lactation. Appetite suppressants in children less than 12 years of age. Within 14 days of MAO inhibitors.

Precautions: Use with caution in patients suffering from hyperexcitability states; in elderly, debilitated, or asthenic patients; and in patients with psychopathic personality traits or a history of homicidal or suicidal tendencies.

Side Effects: *CNS:* Nervousness, dizziness, depression, headache, insomnia, euphoria, symptoms of excitation. Rarely, psychoses. In children, manifestation of vocal and motor tics and Tourette's syndrome. *GI:* N&V, cramps, diarrhea, dry mouth, constipation, metallic taste, anorexia. *CV:* Arrhythmias, palpitations, dyspnea, pulmonary hypertension, peripheral hyper- or hypotension, precordial pain, fainting. *Dermatologic:* Symptoms of allergy including rash, urticaria, erythema, burning. Pallor. *GU:* Urinary frequency, dysuria. *Ophthalmologic:* Blurred vision, mydriasis. *Hematologic:* **Agranulocytosis,** leukopenia. *Endocrine:* Menstrual irregularities, gynecomastia, impotence, and changes in libido. *Miscellaneous:* Alopecia, increased motor activity, fever, sweating, chills, muscle pain, chest pain.

Long-term use results in psychic dependence, as well as a high degree of tolerance.

OD **Overdose Management:** *Symptoms of Acute Overdose (Toxicity):* Restlessness, irritability, insomnia, tremor, hyperreflexia, rhabdomyolysis, rapid respiration, **hyperpyrexia,** assaultiveness, hallucinations, panic states, sweating, mydriasis, flushing, hyperactivity, confusion, hypertension or hypotension, extrasystoles, tachypnea, fever, delirium, self-injury, arrhythmias, **seizures, coma, circulatory collapse, death. Death usually results from CV collapse or convulsions.** *Symptoms of*

Chronic Toxicity: Chronic use/abuse is characterized by emotional lability, loss of appetite, severe dermatoses, hyperactivity, insomnia, irritability, somnolence, mental impairment, occupational deterioration, a tendency to withdraw from social contact, teeth grinding, continuous chewing, and ulcers of the tongue and lips. Prolonged use of high doses can elicit symptoms of paranoid schizophrenia, including auditory and visual hallucinations and paranoid ideation. *Treatment of Acute Toxicity (Overdosage):*
• Symptomatic treatment. After oral ingestion, induce emesis or perform gastric lavage, followed by use of activated charcoal. Acidification of the urine increases the rate of excretion. Give fluids until urine flow is 3–6 mL/kg/hr; furosemide or mannitol may be beneficial.
• Maintain adequate circulation and respiration.
• Treat CNS stimulation with chlorpromazine and psychotic symptoms with haloperidol. Treat hyperactivity with diazepam or a barbiturate. Reduce stimuli and maintain in a quiet, dim environment. Treat patients who have ingested an overdose of long-acting products for toxicity until all symptoms of overdosage have disappeared.
• IV phentolamine may be used for hypertension, whereas hypotension may be reversed by IV fluids and possibly vasopressors (used with caution).

Drug Interactions
Acetazolamide / ↑ Effect of amphetamine by ↑ renal tubular reabsorption
Ammonium chloride / ↓ Effect of amphetamine by ↓ renal tubular reabsorption
Anesthetics, general / ↑ Risk of cardiac arrhythmias
Antihypertensives / Amphetamines ↓ effect of antihypertensives
Ascorbic acid / ↓ Effect of amphetamine by ↓ renal tubular reabsorption

---

bold italic = life threatening side effect

Furazolidone / ↑ Toxicity of anorexiants due to MAO activity of furazolidone

Guanethidine / ↓ Effect of guanethidine by displacement from its site of action

Haloperidol / ↓ Effect of amphetamine by ↓ uptake of drug at its site of action

Insulin / Amphetamines alter insulin requirements

MAO inhibitors / All peripheral, metabolic, cardiac, and central effects of amphetamine are potentiated for up to 2 weeks after termination of MAO inhibitor therapy (symptoms include hypertensive crisis with possible intracranial hemorrhage, hyperthermia, convulsions, coma); death may occur. ↓ Effect of amphetamine by ↓ uptake of drug into its site of action

Methyldopa / ↓ Hypotensive effect of methyldopa by ↑ sympathomimetic activity

Phenothiazines / ↓ Effect of amphetamine by ↓ uptake of drug at its site of action

Sodium bicarbonate / ↑ Effect of amphetamine by ↑ renal tubular reabsorption

Thiazide diuretics / ↑ Effect of amphetamine by ↑ renal tubular reabsorption

Tricyclic antidepressants / ↓ Effect of amphetamines

Administration/Storage

1. If prescribed to suppress appetite, administer 30 min before anticipated meal time.

2. Use a small initial dose; then increase gradually as necessary.

3. Unless otherwise ordered, give the last dose of the day at least 6 hr before bedtime.

EMS CONSIDERATIONS

None.

ANGIOTENSIN-CONVERTING ENZYME (ACE) INHIBITORS

See also the following individual entries:

Benazepril hydrochloride
Captopril
Enalapril maleate
Fosinopril sodium
Lisinopril
Moexipril hydrochloride
Quinapril hydrochloride
Ramipril
Trandolapril

Mechanism of Action: Believed to act by suppressing the renin-angiotensin-aldosterone system. Renin, synthesized by the kidneys, produces angiotensin I, an inactive decapeptide derived from plasma globulin substrate. Angiotensin I is converted to angiotensin II by ACE. Angiotensin II is a potent vasoconstrictor that also stimulates secretion of aldosterone from the adrenal cortex, resulting in sodium and fluid retention. The ACE inhibitors prevent the conversion of angiotensin I to angiotensin II. This results in a decrease in plasma angiotensin II and subsequently a decrease in peripheral resistance and decreased aldosterone secretion (leading to fluid loss) and therefore a decrease in BP. There may be either no change or an increase in CO. Several weeks of therapy may be required to achieve the maximum effect to reduce BP. Standing and supine BPs are lowered to about the same extent. Are also antihypertensive in low renin hypertensive patients. ACE inhibitors are additive with thiazide diuretics in lowering blood pressure; however, β-blockers and captopril have less than additive effects when used with ACE inhibitors.

Uses: Alone or in combination with other antihypertensive agents (especially thiazide diuretics) for the treatment of hypertension. Some are effective in CHF as adjunctive therapy or to treat LV dysfunction. See also individual drug entries.

Contraindications: History of angioedema due to previous treatment with an ACE inhibitor. Use of fosinopril, ramipril, or trandolapril in lactation.

Precautions: Use during the second and third trimesters of pregnancy can result in injury and even death to the developing fetus. May cause a profound drop in BP following the first dose; initiate therapy under close medical supervision. Use with caution in renal disease (especially renal artery stenosis) as increases in BUN and serum creatinine have occurred. Use with caution in patients with aortic stenosis due to possible decreased coronary perfusion following vasodilator use. Most are used with caution during lactation. Geriatric patients may show a greater sensitivity to the hypotensive effects of ACE inhibitors although these drugs may preserve or improve renal function and reverse LV hypertrophy. For most ACE inhibitors, safety and effectiveness have not been determined in children.

Side Effects: See individual entries. Side effects common to most ACE inhibitors include the following. *GI:* Abdominal pain, N&V, diarrhea, constipation, dry mouth. *CNS:* Sleep disturbances, insomnia, headache, dizziness, fatigue, nervousness, paresthesias. *CV:* Hypotension (especially following the first dose), palpitations, angina pectoris, *MI,* orthostatic hypotension, chest pain. *Hepatic:* Rarely, cholestatic jaundice progressing to ***hepatic necrosis and death.*** *Miscellaneous:* Chronic cough, dyspnea, increased sweating, diaphoresis, pruritus, rash, impotence, syncope, asthenia, arthralgia, myalgia. ***Angioedema*** of the face, lips, tongue, glottis, larynx, extremities, and mucous membranes. ***Anaphylaxis.***

OD   Overdose   Management: *Symptoms:* Hypotension is the most common. *Treatment:* Supportive measures. The treatment of choice to restore BP is volume expansion with an IV infusion of NSS. Certain of the ACE inhibitors (captopril, enalaprilat, lisinopril) may be removed by hemodialysis.

Drug Interactions
Allopurinol / ↑ Risk of hypersensitivity reactions

Anesthetics / ↑ Risk of hypotension if used with anesthetics that also cause hypotension
Antacids / Possible ↓ bioavailability of ACE inhibitors
Capsaicin / Capsaicin may cause or worsen cough associated with ACE inhibitor use
Digoxin / ↑ Plasma digoxin levels
Indomethacin / ↓ Hypotensive effects of ACE inhibitors, especially in low renin or volume-dependent hypertensive patients
Lithium / ↑ Serum lithium levels → ↑ risk of toxicity
Phenothiazines / ↑ Effect of ACE inhibitors
Potassium-sparing diuretics / ↑ Serum potassium levels
Potassium supplements / ↑ Serum potassium levels
Thiazide diuretics / Additive effect to ↓ BP

Administration/Storage: Do not interrupt or discontinue ACE inhibitor therapy without consulting provider.

EMS CONSIDERATIONS
None.

ANTHELMINTICS

See also the following individual entries:

   Albendazole
   Ivermectin
   Mebendazole
   Praziquantel
   Pyrantel pamoate
   Thiabendazole

General   Statement: Helminths (worms) may infect the intestinal lumen or the worm also may migrate to a particular tissue. Treatment of helminth infections is complicated by the fact that a worm may have one or more morphologic stages. Thus, it is important to ensure that therapy rids the body of eggs and larvae, as well as worms. Also, a patient may be infected by more than one type of worm. Factors such as availability and cost of the drug, toxicity, ease of administration, and how long it takes to complete therapy also have a significant impact on successful treatment of helminths. Accurate diagnosis is extremely important before treatment is started because its success depends on selecting the drug best suited for the eradication of a specific infestation. Parasites that infest only the intestinal tract can be eradicated by locally acting drugs. Other parasites enter tissues and must be treated by drugs that are absorbed from the GI tract.

Since many parasitic infestations are transmitted by persons sharing bathroom facilities, the provider may wish to examine all members of the household for parasitic infestation. Treatment is often accompanied or followed by repeated laboratory examinations to determine whether the parasite has been eradicated.

Helminths can be divided into three groups: cestodes (flatworms, tapeworms), nematodes (roundworms), and trematodes (flukes). The following is a brief description of the more common helminths and the drug of choice to treat infections by that particular helminth.

CESTODES (FLATWORMS, TAPEWORMS): The more common tapeworms are the beef tapeworm (*Taenia saginata*), pork tapeworm (*T. solium*), dwarf tapeworm (*Hymenolepis nana*), and fish tapeworm (*Diphyllobothrium latum*). Tapeworm infestations are difficult to eradicate. **Drug treatment:** Praziquantel.

NEMATODES: **1. Filaria (filariasis).** Infections due to *Wuchereria bancrofti, Brugia malayi,* and *B. timori* are transmitted by mosquitoes. Mosquito control is the best means of combating this infestation. Other filarial infections include *Loa loa,* transmitted by the bite of a horsefly, and *Onchocerca volvulus* (onchocerciasis, river blindness), which is transmitted by the bite of a blackfly. **Drug treatment:** Diethylcarbamazine. Suramin sodium (available from Centers for Disease Control) is used to treat onchocerciasis.

2. Hookworm (uncinariasis). Intestinal infection caused by *Ancylostoma duodenale* or *Necator americanus*. **Drug treatment:** Mebendazole or pyrantel pamoate.

3. Pinworm (enterobiasis). Caused by *Enterobius vermicularis.* **Drug treatment:** Mebendazole, pyrantel pamoate, thiabendazole.

4. Roundworm (ascariasis). Caused by *Ascaris lumbricoides.* **Drug treatment:** Mebendazole, pyrantel pamoate.

5. Trichinosis. Caused by *Trichinella spiralis,* these parasites are transmitted by the consumption of raw or inadequately cooked pork. **Drug treatment:** Corticosteroids to control the inflammation caused by systemic infestation; mebendazole, thiabendazole.

6. Threadworm (strongyloidiasis). This parasite (*Strongyloides stercoralis*) infests the upper GI tract. **Drug treatment:** Thiabendazole.

7. Whipworm (trichuriasis). This threadlike parasite (*Trichuris trichiura*) lodges in the mucosa of the cecum. **Drug treatment:** Mebendazole.

TREMATODES: Schistosomiasis (blood flukes or bilharziasis) can be transmitted by *Schistosoma mansoni, S. japonicum, S. haematobium,* and *S. mekongi.* The infection is difficult to eradicate. **Drug treatment:** Praziquantel, oxamniquine (*S. mansoni* only).

Side Effects: N&V, cramps, and diarrhea are common to most.

EMS CONSIDERATIONS

See also *Anti-Infectives.*

ANTIANEMIC DRUGS

See also the following individual entries:

Ferrous fumarate
Ferrous gluconate
Ferrous sulfate
Ferrous sulfate, dried

Mechanism of Action: The normal daily iron intake for males is 12–20 mg and for females is 8–15 mg, although only about 10% (1–2 mg) of this iron is absorbed. Iron is absorbed from the duodenum and upper jejunum by an active mechanism through the mucosal cells where it combines with the protein transferrin. Iron is stored in the body as hemosiderin or aggregated ferritin which is found in reticuloendothelial cells of the liver, spleen, and bone marrow. About two-thirds of total body iron is in the circulating RBCs in hemoglobin. Absorption of the ferrous salt is three times greater than the ferric salt. Absorption is enhanced when stored iron is depleted or when erythropoiesis occurs at an increased rate. Food decreases iron absorption by up to two-thirds. The daily loss of iron thorugh urine, sweat, and sloughing of intestinal mucosal cells is 0.5–1mg in healthy men; in menstruating women, 1–2 mg is the normal daily loss.

General Statement: Anemia is a deficiency in the number of RBCs or in the hemoglobin level in RBCs. The two main types of anemia are (1) iron-deficiency anemias, resulting from greater than normal loss or destruction of blood cells, and (2) megaloblastic anemias, resulting from deficient production of blood cells. Iron deficiency can affect muscle metabolism, heat production, and catecholamine metabolism and can cause behavioral or learning problems in children. The cause of the iron deficiency must be determined before therapy is started.

Uses: Prophylaxis and treatment of iron deficiency and iron-deficiency anemias. Dietary supplement for iron. Optimum therapeutic responses are usually noted within 2–4 weeks. *Investigational:* Patients receiving epoetin therapy (failure to give iron supplements either IV or PO can impair the hematologic response to epoetin).

Contraindications: Hemosiderosis, hemochromatosis, peptic ulcer, regional enteritis, and ulcerative colitis. Hemolytic anemia, pyridoxine-responsive anemia, and cirrhosis of the liver. Use in those with normal iron balance.

Precautions: Allergic reactions may result due to certain products containing tartrazine and some products containing sulfites.

Side Effects: *GI:* Constipation, gastric irritation, nausea, abdominal cramps, anorexia, vomiting, diarrhea, dark-colored stools. These effects may be minimized by administering preparations as a coated tablet. Soluble iron preparations may stain the teeth.

OD **Overdose Management:** *Symptoms:* Symptoms occur in four stages—(1) Lethargy, N&V, abdominal pain, weak and rapid pulse, tarry stools, dehydration, acidosis, hypotension, and *coma* within 1–6 hr. (2) If patient survives, symptoms subside for about 24 hr. (3) Within 24–48 hr symptoms return with *diffuse vascular congestion, shock, pulmonary edema, acidosis, seizures, anuria, hyperthermia, and death.* (4) If patient survives, pyloric or antral stenosis, hepatic cirrhosis, and CNS damage are seen within 2–6 weeks. Toxic reactions are more likely to occur after parenteral administration.*Treatment (Iron Toxicity):*
• General supportive measures.
• Maintain a patent airway, respiration, and circulation.
• Induce vomiting with syrup of ipecac followed by gastric lavage using tepid water or 1%–5% sodium bicarbonate (to convert from ferrous sulfate to ferrous carbonate, which is poorly absorbed and less irritating). Saline cathartics can also be used.
• Deferoxamine is indicated for patients with serum iron levels greater than 300 mg/dL. Deferoxamine is usually given IM, but in severe cases of poisoning it may be given IV. Hydration should be maintained.
• It may be necessary to treat for shock, acidosis, renal failure, and seizures.

Drug Interactions
Antacids, oral / ↓ Absorption of iron from GI tract

Ascorbic acid / Doses of ascorbic acid of 200 mg or more ↑ absorption if iron

Chloramphenicol / ↑ Serum iron levels

Cholestyramine / ↓ Absoprtion of iron from GI tract

Cimetidine / ↓ Absorption of iron from GI tract

Fluoroquinolones / ↓ Absorption of fluoroquinolones from GI tract due to formation of a ferric ion-quinolone complex

Levodopa / ↓ Absorption of levodopa due to formation of chelates with iron salts

Levothyroxine / ↓ Efficacy of levothyroxine

Methyldopa / ↓ Absorption of methyldopa from GI tract

Pancreatic extracts / ↓ Absorption of iron from GI tract

Penicillamine / ↓ Absorption of penicillamine from GI tract due to chelation

Tetracyclines / ↓ Absorption of both tetracyclines and iron from GI tract

Vitamin E / Vitamin E ↓ response to iron therapy

EMS CONSIDERATIONS

Administration/Storage

1. For infants and young children, administer liquid preparation with a dropper. Deposit liquid well back against the cheek.

2. Eggs and milk or coffee and tea consumed with a meal or 1 hr after may significantly inhibit absorption of dietary iron.

3. Ingestion of calcium and iron supplements with food can decrease iron absorption by one-third; iron absorption is not decreased if calcium carbonate is used and taken between meals.

4. Do not crush or chew sustained-release products.

ANTIANGINAL DRUGS— NITRATES/NITRITES

See also Beta-Adrenergic Blocking Agents, Calcium Channel Blocking Drugs, and the following individual entries:

Amyl nitrite
Isosorbide dinitrate
Isosorbide mononitrate, oral
Nitroglycerin IV
Nitroglycerin sublingual
Nitroglycerin sustained release
Nitroglycerin topical ointment
Nitroglycerin transdermal system
Nitroglycerin translingual spray

Mechanism of Action: Nitrates relax vascular smooth muscle by stimulating production of intracellular cyclic guanosine monophosphate. Dilation of postcapillary vessels decreases venous return to the heart due to pooling of blood; thus, LV end-diastolic pressure (preload) is reduced. Relaxation of arterioles results in a decreased systemic vascular resistance and arterial pressure (afterload). The oxygen requirements of the myocardium are reduced and there is more efficient redistribution of blood flow through collateral channels in myocardial tissue. Diastolic, systolic, and mean BP are decreased. Also, elevated central venous and pulmonary capillary wedge pressures, pulmonary vascular resistance, and systemic vascular resistance are reduced. Reflex tachycardia may occur due to the overall decrease in BP. Cardiac index may increase, decrease, or remain the same; those with elevated left ventricular filling pressure and systemic vascular resistance values with a depressed cardiac index are likely to see improvement of the cardiac index. The onset and duration depend on the product and route of administration (sublingual, topical, transdermal, parenteral, oral, and buccal). **Onset:** Less than 1 min for amyl nitrite to 1 to 3 min for IV, sublingual, translingual, and transmucosal nitroglycerin or sublingual isosorbide dinitrate; 20 to 60 min for sustained-release, topical, and transdermal nitroglycerin or oral isosorbide dinitrate or mononitrate; and up to 4 hr for sustained-release isosorbide dinitrate. **Duration of action:** 3 to 5 min for amyl nitrite and IV nitroglycerin; 30 to 60 min for sublingual or translingual nitroglycerin; several hours for transmucosal, sustained-release, or topical nitroglycerin and all isosorbide dinitrate products; and up to 24 hr for transdermal nitroglycerin.

Uses: Treatment and prophylaxis of acute angina pectoris (use sublingual, transmucosal, or translingual nitroglycerin; amyl nitrite). Nitrates are first-line therapy for unstable angina. Prophylaxis of chronic angina pectoris (topical, transdermal, translingual, transmucosal, or oral sustained-release nitroglycerin; isosorbide dinitrate and mononitrate; erythrityl tetranitrate; pentaerythritol tetranitrate). IV nitroglycerin is used to decrease BP in surgical procedures resulting in hypertension, as well as an adjunct in treating hypertension or CHF associated with MI. *Investigational:* Nitroglycerin ointment has been used as an adjunct in treating Raynaud's disease. Also, isosorbide dinitrate with prostaglandin E₁ for peripheral vascular disease. Sublingual and topical nitroglycerin and oral nitrates have been used to decrease cardiac workload in patients with acute MI and in CHF.

Contraindications: Sensitivity to nitrites, which may result in severe hypotensive reactions, MI, or tolerance to nitrites. Severe anemia, cerebral hemorrhage, recent head trauma, postural hypotension, closed angle glaucoma, impaired hepatic function, hypertrophic cardiomyopathy, hypotension, recent MI. PO dosage forms should not be used in patients with GI hypermotility or with malabsorption syndrome. IV nitroglycerin should not be used in patients with hypotension, uncorrected hypovolemia, inadequate cerebral circulation, constrictive pericarditis, increased ICP, or pericardial tamponade.

Precautions: Use with caution during lactation and in glaucoma. Tolerance to the antianginal and vascular effects may occur. Safety and efficacy have not been determined during lactation and in children.

Side Effects: *CNS:* Headaches (most common) which may be severe and persistent, restlessness, dizziness, weakness, apprehension, vertigo, anxiety, insomnia, confusion, nightmares, hypoesthesia, hypokinesia, dyscoordination. *CV:* Postural hypotension (common) with or without paradoxical bradycardia and increased angina, tachycardia, palpitations, syncope, rebound hypertension, crescendo angina, retrosternal discomfort, *CV collapse,* atrial fibrillation, PVCs, *arrhythmias.* *GI:* N&V, dyspepsia, diarrhea, dry mouth, abdominal pain, involuntary passing of feces and urine, tenesmus, tooth disorder. *Dermatologic:* Crusty skin lesions, pruritus, rash, exfoliative dermatitis, cutaneous vasodilation with flushing. *GU:* Urinary frequency, impotence, dysuria. *Respiratory:* URTI, bronchitis, pneumonia. *Allergic:* Itching, wheezing, tracheobronchitis. *Miscellaneous:* Perspiration, muscle twitching, methemoglobinemia, cold sweating, blurred vision, diplopia, *hemolytic anemia,* arthralgia, edema, malaise, neck stiffness, increased appetite, rigors. **Topical use:** Peripheral edema, contact dermatitis.

Tolerance can occur following chronic use. Nitrites convert hemoglobin to methemoglobin, which impairs the oxygen-carrying capacity of the blood, resulting in *anemic hypoxia.* This interaction is dangerous in patients with preexisting anemia.

OD **Overdose Management:** *Symptoms (Toxicity):* Severe toxicity is rarely encountered with therapeutic use. Symptoms include hypotension, flushing, tachycardia, headache, palpitations, vertigo, perspiring skin followed by cold and cyanotic skin, visual disturbances, syncope, nausea, dizziness, diaphoresis, initial hyperpnea, dyspnea and slow breathing, slow pulse, *heart block,* vomiting with the possibility of bloody diarrhea and colic, anorexia, and increased ICP with symptoms of confusion, moderate fever, and paralysis. Tissue hypoxia (due to methemoglobinemia) may result in *cyanosis, metabolic acidosis, coma, seizures, and death due to CV collapse.* Treatment (Toxicity):

---

bold italic = life threatening side effect

- Induction of emesis or gastric lavage followed by activated charcoal (nitrates are usually rapidly absorbed from the stomach). Gastric lavage may be used if the drug has been recently ingested.
- Maintain in a recumbent shock position and keep warm. Give oxygen and artificial respiration if required.
- Monitor methemoglobin levels.
- Elevate legs and administer IV fluids to treat severe hypotension and reflex tachycardia. Phenylephrine or methoxamine may also be helpful.
- Do not use epinephrine and similar drugs as they are ineffective in reversing severe hypotension.

Drug Interactions

Acetylcholine / Effects ↓ when used with nitrates

Alcohol, ethyl / Hypotension and CV collapse due to vasodilator effect of both agents

Antihypertensive drugs / Additive hypotension

Aspirin / ↑ Serum levels and effects of nitrates

Beta-adrenergic blocking drugs / Additive hypotension

Calcium channel blocking drugs / Additive hypotension, including significant orthostatic hypotension

Dihydroergotamine / ↑ Effect of dihydroergotamine due to increased bioavailability or antagonism resulting in ↓ antianginal effects

Heparin / Possible ↓ effect of heparin

Narcotics / Additive hypotensive effect

Phenothiazines / Additive hypotension

Sympathomimetics / ↓ Effect of nitrates; also, nitrates may ↓ effect of sympathomimetics resulting in hypotension

EMS CONSIDERATIONS

Administration/Storage: Store tablets and capsules tightly closed in their original container. Avoid exposure to air, heat, and moisture.

Assessment

1. Note any sensitivity to nitrites.
2. Document location, intensity, duration, extension, and any precipitating factors (i.e., activity, stress) surrounding anginal pain. Use a pain-rating scale to rate pain.
3. Note any changes in ECG.

Interventions

1. Monitor VS. Assess for sensitivity to hypotensive effects of nitrites (N&V, pallor, restlessness, and CV collapse).
2. Monitor for hypotension.

ANTIARRHYTHMIC DRUGS

See also the following individual entries:

> Adenosine
> Amiodarone hydrochloride
> Bretylium tosylate
> Calcium Channel Blocking Drugs
> Digoxin
> Diltiazem hydrochloride
> Disopyramide phosphate
> Flecainide acetate
> Ibutilide fumarate
> Lidocaine hydrochloride
> Moricizine hydrochloride
> Phenytoin
> Phenytoin sodium
> Procainamide hydrochloride
> Propafenone hydrochloride
> Propranolol hydrochloride
> Quinidine bisulfate
> Quinidine gluconate
> Quinidine polygalacturonate
> Quinidine sulfate
> Tocainide hydrochloride
> Verapamil

Mechanism of Action: Examples of cardiac arrhythmias are *premature ventricular beats, ventricular tachycardia, atrial flutter, atrial fibrillation, ventricular fibrillation,* and *atrioventricular heart block.* The various antiarrhythmic drugs are classified according to both their mechanism of action and their effects on the action potential of cardiac cells. Importantly, one drug in a particular class may be more effective and safer in an individual patient. The antiarrhythmic drugs are classified as follows:

1. Group I. Decrease the rate of entry of sodium during cardiac membrane depolarization, decrease the rate of rise of phase O of the cardiac membrane action potential, prolong the effective refractory period of fast-response fibers, and require that a more negative membrane potential be reached before the membrane becomes excitable (and thus can propagate to other membranes). Group I drugs are further listed in subgroups (according to their effects on action potential duration) as follows:

• Group IA: Depress phase O and prolong the duration of the action potential. Examples: Disopyramide, procainamide, and quinidine.

• Group IB: Slightly depress phase O and are thought to shorten the action potential. Examples: Lidocaine, phenytoin, and tocainide.

• Group IC: Slight effect on repolarization but marked depression of phase O of the action potential. Significant slowing of conduction. Examples: Flecainide, indecainide, and propafenone.

NOTE: Moricizine is classified as a group I agent but it has characteristics of agents in groups IA, B, and C.

2. Group II. Competitively block beta-adrenergic receptors and depress phase 4 depolarization. Examples: Acebutolol, esmolol, and propranolol.

3. Group III. Prolong the duration of the membrane action potential (relative refractory period) without changing the phase of depolarization or the resting membrane potential. Examples: Amiodarone, bretylium, and sotalol.

4. Group IV. Verapamil, a calcium channel blocker that slows conduction velocity and increases the refractoriness of the AV node.

Adenosine and digoxin are also used to treat arrhythmias. Adenosine slows conduction time through the AV node and can interrupt the reentry pathways through the AV node. Digoxin causes a decrease in maximal diastolic potential and duration of the action potential; it also increases the slope of phase 4 depolarization.

Precautions: Monitor serum levels of antiarrhythmic drugs since some drugs can cause toxic side effects which can be confused with the purpose for which the drug is used. For example, toxicity from quinidine can result in cardiac arrhythmias. Antiarrhythmic drugs may cause new or worsening of arrhythmias, ranging from an increase in frequency of PVCs to severe ventricular tachycardia, ventricular fibrillation, or tachycardia that is more sustained and rapid. Such situations (called proarrhythmic effect) may make it difficult to distinguish the proarrhythmic effect from the underlying rhythm disorder.

EMS CONSIDERATIONS

Assessment

1. Note drug sensitivity.

2. Assess extent of palpitations, fluttering sensations, chest pains, fainting episodes, or missed beats; obtain ECG with arrhythmia documentation.

3. Assess heart sounds and VS.

Interventions

1. Use a cardiac monitor if administering drugs by IV route. Monitor for rhythm changes; report and document rhythm strips.

2. Monitor BP and pulse. A HR < 50 bpm or > 120 should be avoided.

ANTICOAGULANTS

See also the following:

> Ardeparin sodium
> Dalteparin sodium injection
> Danaparoid sodium
> Enoxaparin injection
> Heparin sodium and Sodium chloride
> Heparin sodium lock flush solution
> Warfarin sodium

---

bold italic = life threatening side effect

Mechanism of Action: Drugs that affect blood coagulation can be divided into three classes: (1) *anticoagulants,* or drugs that prevent or slow blood coagulation; (2) *thrombolytic agents,* which increase the rate at which an existing blood clot dissolves; and (3) *hemostatics,* which prevent or stop internal bleeding. Carefully monitor the dosage of all agents since overdosage can have serious consequences. The major anticoagulants are warfarin, heparin, and low molecular weight heparin derivatives. The following considerations are pertinent to all types. Anticoagulants do not dissolve previously formed clots, but they do forestall their enlargement and prevent new clots from forming.

See also *Nursing Considerations* for individual agents.

Uses: Venous thrombosis, pulmonary embolism, acute coronary occlusions with MIs, and strokes caused by emboli or cerebral thrombi. Prophylactically for rheumatic heart disease, atrial fibrillation, traumatic injuries of blood vessels, vascular surgery, major abdominal, thoracic, and pelvic surgery, prevention of strokes in patients with transient attacks of cerebral ischemia, or other signs of impending stroke.

Heparin is often used concurrently during the therapeutic initiation period. *Investigational (Warfarin):* Reduce risk of postconversion emboli; prophylaxis of recurrent, cerebral thromboembolism; prophylaxis of myocardial reinfarction; treatment of transient ischemic attacks; reduce the risk of thromboembolic complications in patients with certain types of prosthetic heart valves; reduced risk of thrombosis and/or occlusion following coronary bypass surgery.

Contraindications: Hemorrhagic tendencies (including hemophilia), patients with frail or weakened blood vessels, blood dyscrasias, ulcerative lesions of the GI tract (including peptic ulcer), diverticulitis, colitis, SBE, threatened abortion, recent operations on the eye, brain, or spinal cord, regional anesthesia and lumbar block, vitamin K deficiency, leukemia with bleeding tendencies, thrombocytopenic purpura, open wounds or ulcerations, acute nephritis, impaired hepatic or renal function, or severe hypertension. Hepatic and renal dysfunction. In the presence of drainage tubes in any orifice. Alcoholism.

Precautions: Use with caution in menstruation, in pregnant women (because they may cause hypoprothrombinemia in the infant), during lactation, during the postpartum period, and following cerebrovascular accidents. Geriatric patients may be more susceptible to the effects of anticoagulants.

Side Effects: See individual drugs.

EMS CONSIDERATIONS

See also individual agents.

ANTICONVULSANTS

See also the following individual entries:

Acetazolamide
Acetazolamide sodium
Carbamazepine
Clonazepam
Clorazepate dipotassium
Diazepam
Ethosuximide
Felbamate
Fosphenytoin sodium
Gabapentin
Lamotrigine
Levetiracetam
Magnesium sulfate
Methsuximide
Phenobarbital
Phenobarbital sodium
Phensuximide
Phenytoin
Phenytoin sodium extended
Phenytoin sodium parenteral
Phenytoin sodium prompt
Primidone
Tiagabine hydrochloride
Topiramate
Valproic acid

General Statement: Therapeutic agents cannot cure convulsive disorders, but do control seizures without impairing the normal functions of the CNS. This is often accomplished by selective depression of hyperactive areas of the brain responsible for the convulsions. Therefore, these drugs are taken at all times (prophylactically) to prevent the occurrence of the seizures. There are several different types of epileptic disorders; consult the International Classification of Epileptic Seizures. No single drug can control all types of epilepsy; thus, accurate diagnosis is important. Drugs effective against one type of epilepsy may not be effective against another. Therapy begins with a small dose of the drug, which is continuously increased until either the seizures disappear or drug toxicity occurs. If a certain drug decreases the frequency of seizures but does not completely prevent them, another drug can be added to the dosage regimen and administered concomitantly with the first. Failure of therapy most often results from the administration of doses too small to have a therapeutic effect or from failure to use two or more drugs together. With appropriate diagnosis and selection of drugs, four out of five cases of epilepsy can be controlled adequately, but it may take the provider some time to find the best drug or combination of drugs with which to treat the patient.

EMS CONSIDERATIONS
Interventions
1. Monitor VS; observe for S&S of impending seizures.
2. With IV administration, monitor closely for respiratory depression and CV collapse.

ANTIDEPRESSANTS, TRICYCLIC

See also the following individual entries:

Amitriptyline and Perphenazine
Amitriptyline hydrochloride
Amoxapine

Clomipramine hydrochloride
Desipramine hydrochloride
Doxepin hydrochloride
Imipramine hydrochloride
Imipramine pamoate
Nortriptyline hydrochloride
Trimipramine maleate

Mechanism of Action: It is now believed that antidepressant drugs cause adaptive changes in the serotonin and norepinephrine receptor systems, resulting in changes in the sensitivities of both presynaptic and postsynaptic receptor sites. These effects may increase the sensitivity of postsynaptic α-1 adrenergic and serotonin receptors and decrease the sensitivity of presynaptic receptor sites. The overall effect is a reregulation of the abnormal receptorneurotransmitter relationship.

The tricyclic antidepressants are chemically related to the phenothiazines; thus, they exhibit many of the same pharmacologic effects (e.g., anticholinergic, antiserotonin, sedative, antihistaminic, and hypotensive). The TCAs are less effective for depressed patients in the presence of organic brain damage or schizophrenia. Also, they can induce mania; note when given to patients with manic-depressive psychoses. Well absorbed from the GI tract. All have a long serum half-life. Up to 46 days may be required to reach steady plasma levels and maximum therapeutic effects may not be noted for 24 weeks. Because of the long half-life, single daily dosage may suffice. More than 90% bound to plasma protein. Partially metabolized in the liver and excreted primarily in the urine.

General Statement: Drugs with antidepressant effects include the tricyclic antidepressants (TCAs), selective serotonin reuptake inhibitors (SSRIs) i.e., fluoxetine, fluvoxamine, paroxetine, sertraline; and monoamine oxidase inhibitors (MAOIs) i.e., phenelzine, tranylcypromine.

Uses: Endogenous and reactive depressions. Preferred over MAO inhibitors because they are less toxic. See also individual drugs.

Contraindications: Severely impaired liver function. Use during acute recovery phase from MI. Concomitant use with MAO inhibitors.

Precautions: Use with caution during lactation and with epilepsy, CV diseases, glaucoma, BPH, suicidal tendencies, a history of urinary retention, and the elderly. Use during pregnancy only when benefits clearly outweigh risks. Generally not recommended for children less than 12 years of age. Geriatric patients may be more sensitive to the anticholinergic and sedative side effects.

Side Effects: Most frequent side effects are sedation and atropine-like reactions. *CNS:* Confusion, anxiety, restlessness, insomnia, nightmares, hallucinations, delusions, mania or hypomania, headache, dizziness, inability to concentrate, panic reaction, worsening of psychoses, fatigue, weakness. *Anticholinergic:* Dry mouth, blurred vision, mydriasis, constipation, paralytic ileus, urinary retention or difficulty in urination. *GI:* N&V, anorexia, gastric distress, unpleasant taste, stomatitis, glossitis, cramps, increased salivation, black tongue. *CV:* Fainting, tachycardia, hypo- or hypertension, arrhythmias, **heart block,** possibility of palpitations, **MI, stroke.** *Neurologic:* Paresthesias, numbness, incoordination, neuropathies, extrapyramidal symptoms including tardive dyskinesia, dysarthria, seizures. *Dermatologic:* Skin rashes, urticaria, flushing, pruritus, petechiae, photosensitivity, edema. *Endocrine:* Testicular swelling and gynecomastia in males, increase or decrease in libido, impotence, menstrual irregularities and galactorrhea in females, hypo- or hyperglycemia, changes in secretion of ADH. *Miscellaneous:* Sweating, alopecia, nasal congestion, lacrimation, increase in body temperature, chills, urinary frequency including nocturia. Bone marrow depression including thrombocytopenia, leukopenia, **agranulocytosis,** eosinophilia.

High dosage increases the frequency of seizures in epileptic patients and may cause epileptiform attacks in normal subjects.

OD Overdose Management: *Symptoms:* CNS symptoms include agitation, confusion, hallucinations, hyperactive reflexes, choreoathetosis, **seizures, coma.** Anticholinergic symptoms include dilated pupils, dry mouth, flushing, and **hyperpyrexia.** CV toxicity includes depressed myocardial contractility, decreased HR, decreased coronary blood flow, tachycardia, intraventricular block, **complete AV block, re-entry ventricular arrhythmias, PVCs, ventricular tachycardia or fibrillation, sudden cardiac arrest, hypotension, pulmonary edema.** *Treatment:* Admit patient to hospital and monitor ECG closely for 3 to 5 days.

• Empty stomach in alert patients by inducing vomiting followed by gastric lavage and charcoal administration **after insertion of cuffed ET tube.** Maintain respiration and avoid the use of respiratory stimulants.

• Normal or half-normal saline to prevent water intoxication.

• To reverse the CV effects (e.g., hypotension and cardiac dysrhythmias), give hypertonic sodium bicarbonate. The usual dose is 0.52 mEq/kg by IV bolus followed by IV infusion to maintain the blood at pH 7.5. If hypotension is not reversed by bicarbonate, vasopressors (e.g., dopamine) and fluid expansion may be needed. If the cardiac dysrhythmias do not respond to bicarbonate, lidocaine or phenytoin may be used.

• Isoproterenol may be effective in controlling bradyarrhythmias and torsades de pointes ventricular tachycardia. Use propranolol, 0.1 mg/kg IV (up to 0.25 mg by IV bolus), to treat life-threatening ventricular arrhythmias in children.

• Treat shock and metabolic acidosis with IV fluids, oxygen, bicarbonate, and corticosteroids.

• Control hyperpyrexia by external means (ice pack, cool baths, spongings).

• To reduce possibility of convulsions, minimize external stimulation.

If necessary, use diazepam or phenytoin to control convulsions. Avoid barbiturates if MAO inhibitors have been used recently.

Drug Interactions

Acetazolamide / ↑ Effect of tricyclics by ↑ renal tubular reabsorption of the drug

Alcohol, ethyl / Concomitant use may lead to ↑ GI complications and ↓ performance on motor skill tests-death has been reported

Ammonium chloride / ↓ Effect of tricyclics by ↓ renal tubular reabsorption of the drug

Anticholinergic drugs / Additive anticholinergic side effects

Anticoagulants, oral / ↑ Hypoprothrombinemia due to ↓ breakdown by liver

Anticonvulsants / Tricyclics may ↑ incidence of epileptic seizures

Antihistamines / Additive anticholinergic side effects

Ascorbic acid / ↓ Effect of tricyclics by ↓ renal tubular reabsorption of the drug

Barbiturates / Additive depressant effects; also, barbiturates may ↑ breakdown of antidepressants by liver

Benzodiazepines / Tricyclic antidepressants ↑ effect of benzodiazepines

Beta-adrenergic blocking agents / Tricyclic antidepressants ↓ effect of the blocking agents

Charcoal / ↓ Absorption of tricyclic antidepressants → ↓ effectiveness (or toxicity)

Chlordiazepoxide / Concomitant use may cause additive sedative effects and/or additive atropine-like side effects

Cimetidine / ↑ Effect of tricyclics (especially serious anticholinergic symptoms) due to ↓ breakdown by liver

Clonidine / Dangerous ↑ BP and hypertensive crisis

Diazepam / Concomitant use may cause additive sedative effects and/or additive atropine-like side effects

Dicumarol / Tricyclic antidepressants may ↑ the t½ of dicumarol → ↑ anticoagulation effects

Disulfiram / ↑ Levels of tricyclic antidepressant; also, possibility of acute organic brain syndrome

Ephedrine / Tricyclics ↓ effects of ephedrine by preventing uptake at its site of action

Estrogens / Depending on the dose, estrogens may ↑ or ↓ the effects of tricyclics

Ethchlorvynol / Combination may result in transient delirium

Fluoxetine / Fluoxetine ↑ pharmacologic and toxic effects of tricyclic antidepressants (effect may persist for several weeks after fluoxetine is discontinued)

Furazolidone / Toxic psychoses possible

Glutethimide / Additive anticholinergic side effects

Guanethidine / Tricyclics ↓ antihypertensive effect of guanethidine by preventing uptake at its site of action

Haloperidol / ↑ Effect of tricyclics due to ↓ breakdown by liver

Levodopa / ↓ Effect of levodopa due to ↓ absorption

MAO inhibitors / Concomitant use may result in excitation, increase in body temperature, delirium, tremors, and convulsions although combinations have been used successfully

Meperidine / Tricyclics enhance narcotic-induced respiratory depression; also, additive anticholinergic side effects

Methyldopa / Tricyclics may block hypotensive effects of methyldopa

Methylphenidate / ↑ Effect of tricyclics due to ↓ breakdown by liver

Narcotic analgesics / Tricyclics enhance narcotic-induced respiratory depression; also, additive anticholinergic effects

Oral contraceptives / ↑ Plasma levels of tricyclic antidepressants due to ↓ breakdown by liver

---

bold italic = life threatening side effect

Oxazepam / Concomitant use may cause additive sedative effects and/or atropine-like side effects

Phenothiazines / Additive anticholinergic side effects; also, phenothiazines ↑ effects of tricyclics due to ↓ breakdown by liver

Procainamide / Additive cardiac effects

Quinidine / Additive cardiac effects

Reserpine / Tricyclics ↓ hypotensive effect of reserpine

Sodium bicarbonate / ↑ Effect of tricyclics by ↑ renal tubular reabsorption of the drug

Sympathomimetics / Potentiation of sympathomimetic effects→ hypertension or cardiac arrhythmias

Tobacco (smoking) / ↓ Serum levels of tricyclic antidepressants due to ↑ breakdown by liver

Thyroid preparations / Mutually potentiating effects observed

Vasodilators / Additive hypotensive effect

EMS CONSIDERATIONS

None.

ANTIDIABETIC AGENTS: HYPOGLYCEMIC AGENTS

See also *Antidiabetic Agents: Insulins.*

See also the following individual entries:

Acarbose
Chlorpropamide
Glimepiride
Glipizide
Glyburide
Metformin hydrochloride
Miglitol
Pioglitazone hydrochloride
Rosiglitazone maleate
Tolazamide
Tolbutamide
Tolbutamide sodium

General Statement: The American Diabetes Association has developed standards for treating patients with diabetes. If followed, these standards will enable patients to decrease their blood glucose levels closer to normal; this will reduce the risk of complications, including blindness, kidney disease, heart disease, and amputations. The goals of these standards include establishing specific targets for control of blood glucose (usually between 80 and 120 mg/dL before meals and between 100 and 140 mg/dL at bedtime) and increased emphasis on educating patients for self-management of their disease. Targets for BP and lipid levels are also provided. If the guidelines are followed, it is estimated that the risk of development or progression of retinopathy, nephropathy, and neuropathy can be reduced by 50%–75% in patients with insulin-dependent (type I) diabetes. The guidelines suggest the following treatment modalities:

• Frequent monitoring of blood glucose.

• Regular exercise.

• Close attention to meal planning; consult a registered dietitian.

• For type I diabetics, either continuous SC insulin infusion or multiple daily insulin injections; for type II diabetics, consider insulin administration in certain situations, although dietary modification, exercise, and weight reduction are the cornerstone of treatment.

• Instruction in the prevention and treatment of hypoglycemia and other complications (both acute and chronic) of diabetes.

• Development of a process for ongoing support and continuing education for the patient.

• Routine assessment of treatment goals.

Mechanism of Action: Oral hypoglycemic drugs are classified as either first or second generation. *Generation* refers to structural changes in the basic molecule. Second-generation oral hypoglycemic drugs are more lipophilic and, as such, have greater hypoglycemic potency. Also, second-generation drugs are bound to plasma protein by covalent bonds, whereas first-generation drugs are bound to plasma protein by ionic bonds. The implication is that the second-generation drugs are potentially less susceptible to displacement from plasma protein by drugs such as salicylates and oral anticoagulants.

The oral hypoglycemics are believed to act by one or more of the following mechanisms: (1) stimulating insulin release from pancreatic beta cells, possibly due to increased intracellular cyclic AMP; (2) the peripheral tissues become more sensitive to insulin due to an increase in the number of insulin receptors or an increased ability of circulating insulin to combine with receptors; or (3) extrapancreatic effects, including decreased glucagon release and hepatic glucose production. To be effective, the patient must have some ability for endogenous insulin production. Differences in oral hypoglycemic drugs are mainly in their pharmacokinetic properties and duration of action.

Uses: Non-insulin-dependent diabetes mellitus (type II) that does not respond to diet management alone. Concurrent use of insulin and an oral hypoglycemic for type II diabetics who are difficult to control with diet and sulfonylurea therapy alone. One method used is the BIDS system: bedtime insulin (usually NPH) with daytime (morning only or morning and evening) oral hypoglycemic.

Guidelines for oral hypoglycemic therapy include onset of diabetes in patients over 40 years of age, duration of diabetes less than 5 years, absence of ketoacidosis, patient is obese or has normal body weight, fasting serum glucose of 200 mg/dL or less, has a daily insulin requirement of 40 units or less, and hepatic and renal function is normal.

Contraindications: Stress before and during surgery, ketosis, severe trauma, fever, infections, pregnancy, diabetes complicated by recurrent episodes of ketoacidosis or coma; juvenile, growth-onset, insulin-dependent, or brittle diabetes; impaired endocrine, renal, or liver function. Use in diabetics who can be controlled by diet alone. Relapse may occur with the sulfonylureas in undernourished patients. Long-acting products in geriatric patients.

Special Concerns: Use with caution in debilitated and malnourished patients and during lactation since hypoglycemia may occur in the infant. Safety and effectiveness in children have not been established. Geriatric patients may be more sensitive to oral hypoglycemics and hypoglycemia may be more difficult to recognize in these patients. Use of sulfonylureas has been associated with an increased risk of CV mortality compared to treatment with either diet alone or diet plus insulin. There may be loss of blood glucose control if the patient experiences stress such as infection, fever, surgery, or trauma.

Side Effects: Hypoglycemia is the most common side effect. *GI:* Nausea, heartburn, full feeling. *CNS:* Fatigue, dizziness, fever, headache, weakness, malaise, vertigo. *Hepatic:* Cholestatic jaundice, aggravation of hepatic porphyria. *Dermatologic:* Skin rashes, urticaria, erythema, pruritus, eczema, photophobia, morbilliform or maculopapular eruptions, lichenoid reactions, porphyria cutanea tardia. *Hematologic:* Thrombocytopenia, leukopenia, ***agranulocytosis, aplastic anemia,*** pancytopenia, ***hemolytic anemia.*** *Endocrine:* Inappropriate secretion of ADH resulting in excessive water retention, hyponatremia, low serum osmolality, and high urine osmolality. *Miscellaneous:* Paresthesia, tinnitus, resistance to drug action develops in a small percentage of patients.

OD **Overdose Management:** *Symptoms:* Hypoglycemia. The following symptoms of hypoglycemia are listed in their general order of appearance: tingling of lips and tongue, hunger, nausea, decreased cerebral function (lethargy, yawning, confusion, agitation, nervousness), increased sympathetic activity (tachycardia, sweating, tremor), sei-

---

bold italic = life threatening side effect

zures, stupor, coma. *Treatment:* Mild hypoglycemia is treated with PO glucose and adjusting the dose of the drug or meal patterns. Severe hypoglycemia requires hospitalization. Concentrated (50%) dextrose is given by rapid IV and is followed by continuous infusion of 10% dextrose at a rate that will maintain blood glucose above 100 mg/dL. Patient should be monitored for at least 24–48 hr as hypoglycemia may recur (patients with chlorpropamide toxicity should be monitored for 3–5 days due to the long duration of action of this drug).

Drug Interactions

Alcohol / Possible Antabuse-like syndrome, especially flushing of face and SOB. Also, ↓ effect of oral hypoglycemic due to ↑ breakdown by liver

Androgens/anabolic steroids / ↑ Hypoglycemic effect

Anticoagulants, oral / ↑ Effect of oral hypoglycemics by ↓ breakdown by liver and ↓ plasma protein binding

Beta-adrenergic blocking agents / ↓ Hypoglycemic effect; also, symptoms of hypoglycemia may be masked

Charcoal / ↓ Hypoglycemic effect due to ↓ absorption from GI tract

Chloramphenicol / ↑ Effect due to ↓ breakdown by liver and ↓ renal excretion

Cholestyramine / ↓ Hypoglycemic effect

Clofibrate / ↑ Hypoglycemic effect due to ↓ plasma protein binding

Diazoxide / ↓ Effects of both drugs

Digitoxin / ↑ Digitoxin serum levels

Fenfluramine / ↑ Hypoglycemic effect

Fluconazole / ↑ Hypoglycemic effect

Gemfibrozil / ↑ Hypoglycemic effect

Histamine H$_2$ antagonists / ↑ *Hypoglycemic effect due to ↓ breakdown by liver*

Hydantoins / ↓ Effect of sulfonylureas due to ↓ insulin release

Magnesium salts / ↑ Hypoglycemic effect

MAO inhibitors / ↑ Hypoglycemic effect due to ↓ breakdown by liver

Methyldopa / ↑ Hypoglycemic effect due to ↓ breakdown by liver

NSAIDs / ↑ Hypoglycemic effect of oral antidiabetics

Phenylbutazone / ↑ Effect of oral hypoglycemics due to ↓ breakdown by liver, ↓ plasma protein binding, and ↓ renal excretion

Probenecid / ↑ Hypoglycemic effect

Rifampin / ↓ Effect of sulfonylureas due to ↑ breakdown by liver

Salicylates / ↑ Effect of oral hypoglycemics by ↓ plasma protein binding

Sulfinpyrazone / ↑ Hypoglycemic effect

Sulfonamides / ↑ Effect of oral hypoglycemics by ↓ plasma protein binding and ↓ breakdown by liver

Sympathomimetics / ↑ Requirements for sulfonylureas

Thiazides / ↓ Effect of sulfonylureas

Tricyclic antidepressants / ↑ Hypoglycemic effect

Urinary acidifiers / ↑ Hypoglycemic effect due to ↓ renal excretion

Urinary alkalinizers / ↓ Hypoglycemic effect due to ↑ renal excretion

Laboratory Test Considerations: ↑ BUN and serum creatinine.

Route/Dosage —————————

PO. See individual preparations. Adjust dosage according to needs of patient. Exercise, weight loss, and diet are of primary importance in the control of diabetes.

EMS CONSIDERATIONS

None.

ANTIDIABETIC AGENTS: INSULINS

See also *Antidiabetic Agents: Hypoglycemic Agents.*

See also the following individual entries:

   Insulin injection
   Insulin injection concentrated
   Insulin lispro injection
   Insulin zinc suspension (Lente)

Insulin zinc suspension, Extended (Ultralente)

Mechanism of Action: Following combination with insulin receptors on cell plasma membranes, insulin facilitates the transport of glucose into cardiac and skeletal muscle and adipose tissue. It also increases synthesis of glycogen in the liver. Insulin stimulates protein synthesis and lipogenesis and inhibits lipolysis and release of free fatty acids from fat cells.This latter effect prevents or reverses the ketoacidosis sometimes observed in the type I diabetic. Insulin also causes intracellular shifts in magnesium and potassium.

Since insulin is a protein, it is destroyed in the GI tract. Thus, it must be administered SC so that it is readily absorbed into the bloodstream and distributed throughout the extracellular fluid. Metabolized mainly by the liver.

General Statement: Insulin preparations with different times of onset, peak activity, and duration of action have been developed. Such products are prepared by precipitating insulin in the presence of zinc chloride to form zinc insulin crystals and/or by combining insulin with a protein such as protamine. Based on these modifications, insulin products are classified as fast-acting, intermediate-acting, and long-acting. These preparations permit the provider to select the preparation best suited to the life-style of the patient.

RAPID-ACTING INSULIN:Insulin injection (Regular Insulin, Crystalline Zinc Insulin, Unmodified Insulin)

INTERMEDIATE-ACTING INSULIN
1. Isophane insulin suspension (NPH)
2. Insulin zinc suspension (Lente)

LONG-ACTING INSULIN: Insulin zinc suspension extended (Ultralente)

NOTE: Insulin preparations with various times of onset and duration of action are often mixed to obtain optimum control in diabetic patients.

Uses: Human insulins are being used almost exclusively. Replacement therapy in type I diabetes. Diabetic ketoacidosis or diabetic coma (use regular insulin). Insulin is also indicated in type II diabetes when other measures have failed (e.g., diet, exercise, weight reduction) or with surgery, trauma, infection, fever, endocrine dysfunction, pregnancy, gangrene, Raynaud's disease, kidney or liver dysfunction.

Regular insulin is used in IV HA solutions, in IV dextrose to treat severe hyperkalemia, and IV as a provocative test for growth hormone secretion.

Insulin and oral hypoglycemic drugs have been used in type II diabetics who are difficult to control with diet and PO therapy alone.

Contraindications: Hypersensitivity to insulin.

Precautions: Pregnant diabetic patients often manifest decreased insulin requirements during the first half of pregnancy and increased requirements during the latter half. Lactation may decrease insulin requirements.

Side Effects: *Hypoglycemia:* Due to insulin overdose, delayed or decreased food intake, too much exercise in relationship to insulin dose, or when transferring from one preparation to another. Even carefully controlled patients occasionally develop signs of insulin overdosage characterized by one or more of the following: hunger, weakness, fatigue, nervousness, pallor or flushing, profuse sweating, headache, palpitations, numbness of mouth, tingling in the fingers, tremors, blurred and double vision, hypothermia, excess yawning, mental confusion, incoordination, tachycardia, loss of sensitivity, and loss of consciousness. Level of awareness is markedly diminished after an attack.

Symptoms of hypoglycemia may mimic those of psychic disturbances. Severe prolonged hypoglycemia may cause brain damage, and in the elderly, may mimic stroke.

---

bold italic = life threatening side effect

Allergic: Urticaria, angioedema, lymphadenopathy, bullae, anaphylaxis. Occurs mostly following intermittent insulin therapy or IV administration of large doses to insulin-resistant patients. Antihistamines or corticosteroids may be used to treat these symptoms. Patients who are highly allergic to insulin and cannot be treated with oral hypoglycemics may respond to human insulin products.

At site of injection: Swelling, stinging, redness, itching, warmth. These symptoms often disappear with continued use. Lipoatrophy or hypertrophy of subcutaneous fat tissue (minimize by rotating site of injection).

Insulin resistance: Usual cause is obesity. Acute resistance may occur following infections, trauma, surgery, emotional disturbances, or other endocrine disorders.

Ophthalmologic: Blurred vision, transient presbyopia. Occurs mainly during initiation of therapy or in patients who have been uncontrolled for a long period of time.

Hyperglycemic rebound (Somogyi effect): Usually in patients who receive chronic overdosage.

DIFFERENTIATION BETWEEN DIABETIC COMA AND HYPOGLYCEMIC REACTION (INSULIN SHOCK): Coma in diabetes may be caused by uncontrolled diabetes (high sugar content in blood or urine, ketoacidosis) or by too much insulin (insulin shock, hypoglycemia).

Diabetic coma and insulin shock can be differentiated in the following manner:

Drug Interactions

Alcohol, ethyl / ↑ Hypoglycemia → low blood sugar and shock

Anabolic steroids / ↑ Hypoglycemic effect of insulin

Beta-adrenergic blocking agents / ↑ Hypoglycemic effect of insulin

Chlorthalidone / ↓ Hypoglycemic effect of antidiabetics

Clofibrate / ↑ Hypoglycemic effects of insulin

Contraceptives, oral / ↑ Dosage of antidiabetic due to impairment of glucose tolerance

Corticosteroids / ↓ Effect of insulin due to corticosteroid-induced hyperglycemia

Dextrothyroxine / ↓ Effect of insulin due to dextrothyroxine-induced hyperglycemia

Diazoxide / Diazoxide-induced hyperglycemia ↓ diabetic control

Digitalis glycosides / Use with caution, as insulin affects serum potassium levels

Diltiazen / ↓ Effect of insulin

Dobutamine / ↓ Effect of insulin

Epinephrine / ↓ Effect of insulin due to epinephrine-induced hyperglycemia

Estrogens / ↓ Effect of insulin due to impairment of glucose tolerance

Ethacrynic acid / ↓ Hypoglycemic effect of antidiabetics

Fenfluramine / Additive hypoglycemic effects

Furosemide / ↓ Hypoglycemic effect of antidiabetics

Glucagon / Glucagon-induced hyperglycemia ↓ effect of antidiabetics

Guanethidine / ↑ Hypoglycemic effect of insulin

MAO inhibitors / MAO inhibitors ↑ and prolong hypoglycemic effect of antidiabetics

Oxytetracycline / ↑ Effect of insulin

Phenothiazines / ↑ Dosage of antidiabetic due to phenothiazine-induced hyperglycemia

Phenytoin / Phenytoin-induced hyperglycemia ↓ diabetic control

Propranolol / Inhibits rebound of blood glucose after insulin-induced hypoglycemia

Salicylates / ↑ Effect of hypoglycemic effect of insulin

Sulfinpyrazone / ↑ Hypoglycemic effect of insulin

Tetracyclines / May ↑ hypoglycemic effect of insulin

Thiazide diuretics / ↓ Hypoglycemic effect of antidiabetics

Thyroid preparations / ↓ Effect of antidiabetic due to thyroid-induced hyperglycemia

Triamterene / ↓ Hypoglycemic effect of antidiabetic

Hypoglycemia (Insulin Shock)

Onset / Sudden (24–48 hr)

Medication / Excess insulin

Food intake / Probably too little
Overall appearance / Very weak
Skin / Moist and pale
Infection / Absent
Fever / Absent
Mouth / Drooling
Thirst / Absent
Hunger / Occasional
Vomiting / Absent
Abdominal pain / Rare
Respiration / Normal
Breath / Normal
BP / Normal
Pulse / Full and bounding
Vision / Diplopia
Tremor / Frequent
Convulsions / In late stages
Urine sugar / Absent in second specimen
Ketone bodies / Absent in second specimen
Blood sugar / Less than 60 mg/100 mL

Source: Adapted with permission from *The Merck Manual*, 11th ed.

Diabetic coma is usually precipitated by the patient's failure to take insulin. Hypoglycemia is often precipitated by the patient's unpredictable response, excess exertion, stress due to illness or surgery, errors in calculating dosage, or failure to eat.

TREATMENT OF DIABETIC COMA OR SEVERE ACIDOSIS: Administer 30–60 units regular insulin. This is followed by doses of 20 units or more q 30 min. To avoid a hypoglycemic state, 1 g dextrose is administered for each unit of insulin given. Treatment is often supplemented by electrolytes and fluids. Urine samples are collected for analysis, and VS are monitored as ordered.

TREATMENT OF HYPOGLYCEMIA (INSULIN SHOCK): Mild hypoglycemia can be relieved by PO administration of CHO such as orange juice, candy, or a lump of sugar. If comatose, adults may be given 10–30 mL of 50% dextrose solution IV; children should receive 0.5–1 mL/kg of 50% dextrose solution. Epinephrine, hydrocortisone, or glucagon may be used in severe cases to cause an increase in blood glucose.

Hyperglycemia (Diabetic Coma)
Onset / Gradual (days)
Medication / Insufficient insulin
Food intake / Normal or excess
Overall appearance / Extremely ill
Skin / Dry and flushed
Infection / Frequent
Fever / Frequent
Mouth / Dry
Thirst / Intense
Hunger / Absent
Vomiting / Common
Abdominal pain / Frequent
Respiration / Increased, air hunger
Breath / Acetone odor
BP / Low
Pulse / Weak and rapid
Vision / Dim
Tremor / Absent
Convulsions / None
Urine sugar / High
Ketone bodies / High (type I only)
Blood sugar / High

Diet: The dietary control of diabetes is as important as medication with appropriate drugs. The role of the nurse and dietitian in teaching the patient how to eat properly cannot be underestimated. They must teach the patient how to calculate exchange values of various foods. Food lists and food-exchange values published by the American Diabetes Association and the American Dietetic Association are valuable teaching aids.

Diabetic patients should adhere to a regular meal schedule. The frequency of meals and the overall caloric intake vary with the type of drug taken and individual patient needs. Close attention to meal frequency and meal planning is imperative and a registered dietitian should be consulted. Diabetic children may be on a less restricted diet, adjusting the insulin dosage according to blood and urine glucose readings. Children with negative urine glucose tend to become hypoglycemic rapidly with exercise or decrease in appetite, and many providers allow for glucose spilling.

bold italic = life threatening side effect

EMS CONSIDERATIONS

Assessment

1. Assess for S&S of hyperglycemia: thirst, polydypsia, polyuria, drowsiness, blurred vision, loss of appetite, fruity ordor to the breath, and flushed dry skin. Note state of consciousness.

2. Assess for S&S of hypoglycemia: drowsiness, chills, confusion, anxiety, cold sweats, cool pale skin, excessive hunger, nausea, headache, irritability, shakiness, rapid pulse, and unusual weakness or tiredness.

ANTIEMETICS

See also the following individual entries:

Dimenhydrinate
Diphenhydramine hydrochloride
Dronabinol
Granisetron hydrochloride
Hydroxyzine hydrochloride
Hydroxyzine pamoate
Meclizine hydrochloride
Ondansetron hydrochloride
Phosphorated carbohydrate
    solution
Prochlorperazine
Prochlorperazine edisylate
Prochlorperazine maleate
Scopolamine hydrobromide
Trimethobenzamide
    hydrochloride

General Statement: Nausea and vomiting can be caused by a variety of conditions, such as infections, drugs, radiation, motion, organic disease, or psychologic factors. The underlying cause of the symptoms must be elicited before emesis is corrected. Many drugs used for other conditions, such as the antihistamines, phenothiazines, barbiturates, and scopolamine, have antiemetic properties and can be used. However, CNS depression make their routine use undesirable.

Drug Interactions: Because of their antiemetic and antinauseant activity, the antiemetics may mask overdosage caused by other drugs.

EMS CONSIDERATIONS

None.

ANTIHISTAMINES (H₁ BLOCKERS)

See also the following individual entries:

Astemizole
Brompheniramine maleate
Cetirizine hydrochloride
Chlorpheniramine maleate
Cyproheptadine hydrochloride
Dexchlorpheniramine maleate
Dimenhydrinate
Diphenhydramine hydrochloride
Emedastine difumarate
Fexofenadine hydrochloride
Levocabastine hydrochloride
Loratidine
Meclizine hydrochloride
Olopatadine hydrochloride
Promethazine hydrochloride
Tripelennamine hydrochloride

Mechanism of Action: Compete with histamine at H_1 histamine receptors (competitive inhibition), thus preventing or reversing the effects of histamine. First-generation antihistamines bind to central and peripheral H_1 receptors and can cause CNS depression or stimulation. Second-generation antihistamines are selective for peripheral H_1 receptors and cause less sedation. Antihistamines do not prevent the release of histamine, antibody production, or antigen-antibody interactions. Antihistamines prevent or reduce increased capillary permeability (i.e., decrease edema, itching) and bronchospasms. Allergic reactions unrelated to histamine release are not affected by antihistamines. Certain of the first-generation antihistamines also have anticholinergic, antiemetic, antipruritic, or antiserotonin effects. Patients unresponsive to a certain antihistamine may regain sensitivity by switching to a different antihistamine.

From a chemical point of view, the antihistamines can be divided into the following classes.

FIRST GENERATION:

1. **Ethylenediamine Derivatives.** Moderate sedative effects; almost no anticholinergic or antiemetic activity. Frequently cause GI distress. Example: Tripelennamine.

2. **Ethanolamine Derivatives.** Moderate to high sedative, anticholinergic, and antiemetic effects. Low incidence of GI side effects. Examples: Clemastine, diphenhydramine.

3. **Alkylamines.** Among the most potent antihistamines. Minimal sedation, moderate anticholinergic effects, and no antiemetic effects. Paradoxical excitation may also occur. Examples: Brompheniramine, chlorpheniramine, dexchlorpheniramine.

4. **Phenothiazines.** High antihistaminic, sedative, and anticholinergic effects; very high antiemetic effect. Example: Promethazine.

5. **Phthalazinone.** High antihistaminic effect; low to no sedative and anticholinergic effects; no antiemetic effect. Example: Azelastine.

6. **Piperazine.** High antihistaminic, sedative, and antiemetic effects; moderate anticholinergic effects. Example: Hydroxyzine.

7. **Piperidines.** Moderate antihistaminic and anticholinergic effects; low to moderate sedation; no antiemetic effects. Examples: Azatadine, cyproheptadine, phenindamine.

SECOND GENERATION:

1. **Piperazine.** Moderate to high antihistamine effect; low to no sedation or anticholinergic effects; no antiemetic activity. Example: Cetirizine.

2. **Piperidines.** Moderate to high antihistamine activity; low to no sedation and anticholinergic activity; no antiemetic action. Examples: Astemizole, fexofenadine, loratidine, terfenadine.

The kinetics of most first-generation antihistamines are similar. **Onset:** 15–30 min; **peak:** 1–2 hr; **duration:** 4–6 hr (piperidines have a longer duration). Many antihistamines are available as timed-release preparations. Most first-generation antihista-mines are metabolized by the liver and excreted in the urine. The pharmacokinetics of the second-generation antihistamines vary; consult individual drugs.

Uses: PO: Treatment of vasomotor, perennial, or seasonal allergic rhinitis and allergic conjunctivitis. Treatment of angioedema, urticarial transfusion reactions, urticaria, pruritus. Atopic dermatitis, contact dermatitis, pruritus ani, pruritus vulvae, insect bites. Sneezing and rhinorrhea due to the common cold. Treatment of anaphylaxis, parkinsonism, drug-induced extrapyramidal reactions, vertigo. Prophylaxis and treatment of motion sickness, including N&V. Nighttime sleep aid.

Parenteral: Relief of allergic reactions due to blood or plasma. As an adjunct to epinephrine in treating anaphylaxis. Uncomplication allergic conditions when PO therapy is not possible.

Contraindications: *First-generation antihistamines.* Hypersensitivity to the drug, narrow-angle glaucoma, symptomatic prostatic hypertrophy, stenosing peptic ulcer, and pyloroduodenal or bladder neck obstruction. Use with MAO inhibitors. Pregnancy or possibility thereof (some agents), lactation, premature and newborn infants. The phenothiazine-type antihistamines are contraindicated in CNS depression from any cause, bone marrow depression, jaundice, dehydrated or acutely ill children, and in comatose patients. Use to treat lower respiratory tract symptoms such as asthma.

Second-generation antihistamines. Hypersensitivity. Astemizole and terfenadine use in significant hepatic dysfunction and concomitant use with clarithromycin, erythromycin, itraconazole, ketoconazole, quinine, and troleandomycin due to the possibility of serious CV effects (including torsades de pointes, prolongation of the QT interval, other ventricular arrhythmias, cardiac arrest, and death). Also terfenadine use with cisapride,

---

bold italic = life threatening side effect

HIV protease inhibitors, mibefradil, serotonin reuptake inhibitors, sparfloxacin, and zileuton.

Precautions: Administer with caution to patients with convulsive disorders and in respiratory disease. Excess dosage may cause hallucinations, convulsions, and death in infants and children. Use in geriatric patients may result in dizziness, excessive sedation, syncope, toxic confusional states, and hypotension.

Side Effects: *CNS:* Sedation ranging from mild drowsiness to deep sleep. Dizziness, incoordination, faintness, fatigue, confusion, lassitude, restlessnesss, excitation, nervousness, tremor, **tonic-clonic seizures,** headache, irritability, insomnia, euphoria, paresthesias, oculogyric crisis, torticollis, catatonic-like states, hallucinations, disorientation, tongue protrusion (usually with IV use or overdosage), disturbing dreams, nightmares, pseudoschizophrenia, weakness, diplopia, vertigo, hysteria, neuritis, paradoxical excitation, epileptiform seizures in patients with focal lesions. Extrapyramidal reactions include opisthotonus, dystonia, akathisia, dyskinesia, and parkinsonism. *CV:* Postural hypotension, palpitations, bradycardia, tachycardia, reflex tachycardia, extrasystoles, increased or decreased BP, ECG changes (including blunting of T waves and prolongation of the Q-T interval), **cardiac arrest.** *GI:* Epigastric distress, anorexia, increased appetite and weight gain, N&V, diarrhea, constipation, change in bowel habits, stomatitis. *GU:* Urinary frequency, dysuria, urinary retention, gynecomastia, inhibition of ejaculation, decreased libido, impotence, early menses, induction of lactation. *Hematologic:* Hypoplastic anemia, **aplastic anemia, hemolytic anemia,** thrombocytopenia, leukopenia, pancytopenia, **agranulocytosis,** thrombocytopenic purpura. *Respiratory:* Thickening of bronchial secretions, wheezing, nasal stuffiness, chest tightness, sore throat, **respiratory depression;** dry mouth, nose, and throat. *Ophthalmic:* Blurred vision, diplopia. *Miscellaneous:* Tinnitus, photosensitivity, acute labyrinthitis, obstructive jaundice, erythema, high or prolonged glucose tolerance curves, glycosuria, elevated spinal fluid proteins, increased plasma cholesterol, increased perspiration, chills; tingling, heaviness, and weakness of the hands.

Topical use: Prolonged use may result in local irritation and allergic contact dermatitis.

OD **Overdose Management:** *Symptoms (Acute Toxicity):* Although antihistamines have a wide therapeutic range, overdosage can nevertheless be fatal. Children are particularly susceptible. Early toxic effects may be seen within 30–120 min and include drowsiness, dizziness, blurred vision, tinnitus, ataxia, and hypotension. Symptoms range from CNS depression (sedation, **coma,** decreased mental alertness) to *CV collapse* and CNS stimulation (insomnia, hallucinations, tremors, or *seizures*). Also, *profound hypotension, respiratory depression, coma, and death* may occur. Anticholinergic effects include flushing, dry mouth, hypotension, fever, *hyperthermia* (especially in children), and fixed, dilated pupils. Body temperature may be as high as 107°F. In children, symptoms include hallucinations, toxic psychosis, delirium tremens, ataxia, incoordination, muscle twitching, excitement, athetosis, *hyperthermia, seizures,* and hyperreflexia followed by postictal depression and *cardiorespiratory arrest.* *Treatment:*

• Treat symptoms and provide supportive care.

• Vomiting is induced with syrup of ipecac (do not use for phenothiazine overdosage) followed by activated charcoal and a cathartic. If vomiting has not been induced within 3 hr of ingestion, gastric lavage can be undertaken.

• Hypotension can be treated with a vasopressor such as norepinephrine, dopamine, or phenylephrine (do not use epinephrine).

• For convulsions, use only short-acting depressants (e.g., diazepam). IV physostigmine can be used to treat centrally mediated convulsions.

- Ice packs and a cool sponge bath are effective in reducing fever in children.
- Severe cases of overdose can be treated by hemoperfusion.

Drug Interactions

Alcohol, ethyl / See *CNS depressants*

Antidepressants, tricyclic / Additive anticholinergic side effects

CNS depressants, antianxiety agents, barbiturates, narcotics, phenothiazines, procarbazine, sedative-hypnotics / Potentiation or addition of CNS depressant effects. Concomitant use may lead to drowsiness, lethargy, stupor, respiratory depression, coma, and possibly death

Heparin / Antihistamines may ↓ the anticoagulant effects

MAO inhibitors / Intensification and prolongation of anticholinergic side effects; use with phenothiazine antihistamine → hypotension and extrapyramidal reactions

NOTE: Also see *Drug Interactions* for *Phenothiazines.*

EMS CONSIDERATIONS

None.

ANTIHYPERLIPIDEMIC AGENTS—HMG-COA REDUCTASE INHIBITORS

See also the following individual entries:

Atorvastatin calcium
Cerivastatin sodium
Fluvastatin sodium
Lovastatin
Pravastatin sodium
Simvastatin

Mechanism of Action: The HMG-CoA reductase inhibitors competitively inhibit HMG-CoA reductase; this enzyme catalyzes the early rate-limiting step in the synthesis of cholesterol. HMG-CoA reductase inhibitors increase HDL cholesterol and decrease LDL cholesterol, VLDL cholesterol, and plasma triglycerides. The mechanism to lower LDL choles-

terol may be due to both a decrease in VLDL cholesterol levels and induction of the LDL receptor, leading to reduced production or increased catabolism of LDL cholesterol. The maximum therapeutic response is seen in 4–6 weeks.

General Statement: The National Cholesterol Education Program Expert Panel on Detection, Evaluation, and Treatment of High Blood Cholesterol in Adults has developed guidelines for the treatment of high cholesterol and LDL in adults. Cholesterol levels less than 200 mg/dL are desirable. Cholesterol levels between 200 and 239 mg/dL are considered borderline-high while levels greater than 240 mg/dL are considered high. With respect to LDL, levels less than 130 mg/dL are considered desirable while levels between 130 and 159 md/dL are considered borderline-high and levels greater than 160 mg/dL are considered high. Depending on the levels of cholesterol and LDL and the number of risk factors present for CAD, the provider will develop a treatment regimen.

Uses: Adjunct to diet to decrease elevated total LDL and cholesterol in patients with primary hypercholesterolemia (types IIa and IIb) when the response to diet and other nondrug approaches has not been adequate. See also individual drugs.

Contraindications: Active liver disease or unexplained persistent elevated liver function tests. Pregnancy, lactation. Use in children.

Precautions: Use with caution in those who ingest large quantities of alcohol or who have a history of liver disease. May cause photosensitivity. Safety and efficacy have not been established in children less than 18 years of age.

Side Effects: The following side effects are common to most HMG-CoA reductase inhibitors. Also see individual drugs. *GI:* N&V, diarrhea, constipation, abdominal cramps or pain, flatulence, dyspepsia, heartburn. *CNS:* Headache, dizziness, dysfunction of certain cranial nerves (e.g., alteration of taste, facial paresis, impairment of extraocular movement), tremor, vertigo, memory loss, paresthesia, anxiety, insomnia, depression. *Musculoskeletal:* Localized pain, myalgia, muscle cramps or pain, myopathy, rhabdomyolysis, arthralgia. *Respiratory:* URI, rhinitis, cough. *Ophthalmic:* Progression of cataracts (lens opacities), ophthalmoplegia. *Hypersensitivity:* **Anaphylaxis, angioedema,** vasculitis, purpura, thrombocytopenia, leukopenia, **hemolytic anemia,** lupus erythematosus-like syndrome, polymyalgia rheumatica, positive ANA, ESR increase, arthritis, arthralgia, eosinophilia, urticaria, photosensitivity, fever, chills, flushing, malaise, dyspnea, **toxic dermal necrolysis, Stevens-Johnson syndrome.** *Miscellaneous:* Rash, pruritus, cardiac chest pain, fatigue, influenza, alopecia, edema, dryness of skin and mucous membranes, changes to hair and nails, skin discoloration.

Drug Interactions: See also individual drugs.

Cyclosporine / Possibility of myopathy or severe rhabdomyolysis
Digoxin / Slight ↑ in digoxin levels
Gemfibrozil / Possibility of severe myopathy or rhabdomyolysis
Itraconazole / ↑ Levels of HMG-CoA inhibitors
Nicotinic acid / Possibility of myopathy or severe rhabdomyolysis
Propranolol / ↓ Antihyperlipidemic activity
Warfarin / ↑ Anticoagulant effect of warfarin.

EMS CONSIDERATIONS

None.

ANTIHYPERTENSIVE AGENTS

See also the following drug classes and individual drugs:

Agents Acting Directly on Vascular Smooth Muscle

Diazoxide IV

Hydralazine hydrochloride
Nitroprusside sodium

Alpha-1-Adrenergic Blocking Agents

Doxazosin mesylate
Prazosin hydrochloride
Terazosin

Angiotensin-II Receptor Blockers

Candesartan cilexetil
Irbesartan
Losartan potassium
Valsartan

Angiotensin-Converting Enzyme Inhibitors

Benazepril hydrochloride
Captopril
Enalapril maleate
Eprosartan mesylate
Fosinopril sodium
Lisinopril
Moexipril hydrochloride
Quinapril hydrochloride
Ramipril
Trandolapril

Beta-Adrenergic Blocking Agents

Calcium Channel Blocking Agents

Amlodipine
Bepridil hydrochloride
Diltiazem hydrochloride
Felodipine
Isradipine
Nicardipine hydrochloride
Nifedipine
Nimodipine
Nisoldipine
Verapamil

Centrally-Acting Agents

Clonidine hydrochloride
Guanabenz acetate
Guanfacine hydrochloride
Methyldopa
Methyldopate hydrochloride

Combination Drugs Used for Hypertension

Amiloride and
    Hydrochlorothiazide
Amlodipine and Benazepril
    hydrochloride
Bisoprolol fumarate and
    Hydrochlorothiazide
Enalapril maleate and
    Hydrochlorothiazide

Fosinopril sodium
Lisinopril and
    Hydrochlorothiazide
Losartan potassium and
    Hydrochlorothiazide
Methyldopa and
    Hydrochlorothiazide
Propranolol and
    Hydrochlorothiazide
Spironolactone and
    Hydrochlorothiazide
Triamterene and
    Hydrochlorothiazide

Miscellaneous Agents

Carvedilol
Epoprostenol sodium
Labetalol hydrochloride
Minoxidil, oral

Peripherally-Acting Agents

Guanadrel sulfate
Guanethidine monosulfate
Phentolamine mesylate

General Statement: The Sixth Report of the Joint National Committee on Prevention, Detection, Evaluation and Treatment of High Blood Pressure classifies BP for adults aged 18 and over as follows: Optimal as <120/<80 mm Hg, Normal as <130/<85 mm Hg, High Normal as 130–139/85–89 mm Hg, Stage 1 Hypertension as 140–159/90–99 mm Hg, Stage 2 Hypertension as 160–179/100–109 mm Hg, and Stage 3 Hypertension as 180 or greater/110 or greater mm Hg. Drug therapy is recommended depending on the BP and whether certain risk factors (e.g., smoking, dyslipidemia, diabetes, age, gender, target organ damage, clinical CV disease) are present. Life-style modification is an important component of treating hypertension, including weight reduction, reduction of sodium intake, regular exercise, cessation of smoking, and moderate alcohol intake.

The goal of antihypertensive therapy is a BP of <140/90 mm Hg, except in hypertensive diabetics where the goal is <135/85 mm Hg and those with renal insufficiency where the goal is <130/85 mm Hg. Generally speaking, the primary agents for initial monotherapy to treat uncomplicated hypertension are diuretics and beta blockers. Alternative drugs include ACE inhibitors, alpha-1 blockers, alpha-beta blocker, and calcium antagonists.

EMS CONSIDERATIONS

None.

ANTI-INFECTIVE DRUGS

See also the following individual drugs and drug classes:

Amebicides and Trichomonacides
Aminoglycosides
4-Aminoquinolines
Anthelmintics
Antimalarials
Antiviral Drugs
Aztreonam for injection
Bacitracin
Becaplermin
Butenafine hydrochloride
Cephalosporins
Chloramphenicol
Clindamycin
Erythromycins
Fluoroquinolones
Fosfomycin tromethamine
Gatifloxacin
Imipenem-Cilastatin sodium
Loracarbef
Macrolides
Meropenem
Mupirocin
Penicillins
Pentamidine isethionate
Spectinomycin hydrochloride
Sulfonamides
Tetracyclines
Trimetrexate glucuronate
Trovafloxacin mesylate
    Alatrofloxacin mesylate
Vancomycin hydrochloride

Mechanism of Action: The mechanism of action of the anti-infectives varies. The following modes of action have been identified.* Note the considerable overlap among these mechanisms:

1. Inhibition of synthesis of or activa-

tion of enzymes that disrupt bacterial cell walls leading to loss of viability and possibly cell lysis (e.g., penicillins, cephalosporins, cycloserine, bacitracin, vancomycin, miconazole, ketoconazole, clotrimazole).

2. Direct effect on the microbial cell membrane to affect permeability and leading to leakage of intracellular components (e.g., polymyxin, colistimethate, nystatin, amphotericin).

3. Effect on the function of 30S and 50S bacterial ribosomes to cause a reversible inhibition of protein synthesis (e.g., chloramphenicol, tetracyclines, erythromycin, clindamycin).

4. Bind to the 30S ribosomal subunit that alters protein synthesis and leads to cell death (e.g., aminoglycosides).

5. Effect on nucleic acid metabolism which inhibits DNA-dependent RNA polymerase (e.g., rifampin) or inhibition of gyrase (e.g., fluoroquinolones).

6. Antimetabolites that block specific metabolic steps essential to the life of the microorganism (e.g., trimethoprim, sulfonamides).

7. Bind to viral enzymes that are essential for DNA synthesis leading to a halt of viral replication (e.g., acyclovir, ganciclovir, vidarabine, zidovudine).

General Statement

The following general guidelines apply to the use of most anti-infective drugs:

1. Anti-infective drugs can be divided into those that are *bacteriostatic,* that is, arrest the multiplication and further development of the infectious agent, or *bactericidal,* that is, kill and thus eradicate all living microorganisms. Both time of administration and length of therapy may be affected by this difference.

2. Some anti-infectives halt the growth of or eradicate many different microorganisms and are termed *broad-spectrum antibiotics.* Others affect only certain specific organisms and are termed *narrow-spectrum antibiotics.*

3. Some of the anti-infectives elicit a hypersensitivity reaction in some persons. Penicillins cause more severe and more frequent hypersensitivity reactions than any other drug.

4. Because of differences in susceptibility of infectious agents to anti-infectives, the sensitivity of the microorganism to the drug ordered should be determined before treatment is initiated. Several sensitivity tests are commonly used for this purpose.

5. Certain anti-infective agents have marked side effects, some of the more serious of which are neurotoxicity, including ototoxicity, and nephrotoxicity. Care must be taken not to administer two anti-infectives with similar side effects concomitantly, or to administer these drugs to patients in whom the side effects might be damaging (e.g., a nephrotoxic drug to a patient suffering from kidney disease). The choice of anti-infective also depends on its distribution in the body (i.e., whether it passes the blood-brain barrier).

6. Anti-infective drugs can also eradicate the normal intestinal flora necessary for proper digestion, synthesis of vitamin K, and control of fungi that may gain access to the GI tract (superinfection).

Uses: See individual drugs. The choice of the anti-infective depends on the nature of the illness to be treated, the sensitivity of the infecting agent, and the patient's previous experience with the drug. Hypersensitivity and allergic reactions may preclude the use of the agent of choice.

Contraindications: Hypersensitivity or allergies to the drug.

Side Effects: The antibiotics and anti-infective agents have few direct toxic effects. Kidney and liver damage,

---

*Chambers, H.F., Sande, M.A.: Antimicrobial agents. In *Goodman and Gilman's The Pharmacological Basis of Therapeutics,* 9th ed. Edited by Hardman, J.G., Limbud, L.E., New York, McGraw-Hill, 1996, p. 1029.

deafness, and blood dyscrasias are occasionally observed.

The following undesirable manifestations, however, occur frequently:
1. Suppresion of the normal flora of the body, which in turn keeps certain pathogenic microorganisms, such as *Candida albicans, Proteus,* or *Pseudomonas,* from causing infections. If the flora is altered, *superinfections* (monilial vaginitis, enteritis, UTIs), which necessitate the discontinuation of therapy or the use of other antibiotics, can result.
2. Incomplete eradication of an infectious organism. Casual use of antiinfectives favors the emergence of *resistant* strains insensitive to a particular drug.

To minimize the chances for the development of resistant strains, antiinfectives are usually given at specified doses for a prescribed length of time after acute symptoms have subsided.

OD Overdose Management: *Treatment:* Discontinue the drug and treat symptomatically. Supportive measures should be instituted as needed. Hemodialysis may be used although its effectiveness is questionable, depending on the drug and the status of the patient (i.e., more effective in impaired renal function).

EMS CONSIDERATIONS

None.

ANTIMALARIAL DRUGS, 4-AMINOQUINOLINES

See also the following individual entries:

Chloroquine hydrochloride
Chloroquine phosphate
Hydroxychloroquine sulfate

Mechanism of Action: Several mechanisms have been proposed for the action of 4-aminoquinolines. These include (a) an active chloroquine-concentrating mechanism in the acid vesicles of the parasite causing inhibition of growth, (b) release of aggregates of ferriprotoporphyrin IX from erythrocytes in the parasite causing membrane damage and erythrocyte or parasite lysis, (c) interference with hemoglobin digestion by the parasite, and (d) interference with synthesis of nucleoprotein by the parasite. The drugs are active against the erythrocytic forms of *Plasmodium vivax* and *P. malariae* as well as most strains of *P. falciparum.* The aminoquinolines are rapidly and almost completely absorbed from the GI tract and are widely distributed throughout the body. **Peak serum levels:** 1–6 hr. Very slowly excreted; presence of drug has been demonstrated in the bloodstream weeks and even months after the drug has been discontinued. Up to 70% may be excreted unchanged. Urinary excretion is increased by acidifying the urine; excretion is slowed by alkalinization.

Uses: Treatment or prophylaxis of acute attacks of malaria caused by *Plasmodium falciparum, P. vivax, P. ovale,* and *P. malariae.* Will cause a radical cure of vivax and malariae malaria if combined with primaquine. Effective only against the erythrocytic stages and therefore will not prevent infections. However, complete cure of infections due to sensitive strains of falciparum malaria is possible.

Extraintestinal amebiasis caused by *Entamoeba histolytica.* Discoid or lupus erythematosus, scleroderma, pemphigus, lichen planus, polymyositis, sarcoidosis, porphyria cutanea tarda.

Contraindications: Hypersensitivity. Changes in retinal or visual field. Lactation. Use in psoriasis or porphyria only if benefits clearly outweigh risks. Concomitantly with gold or phenylbutazone or in patients receiving drugs that depress blood-forming elements of bone marrow.

Precautions: Use with extreme caution in the presence of hepatic, severe

---

bold italic = life threatening side effect

GI, neurologic, and blood disorders. Infants and children are sensitive to the effects of 4-aminoquinolines. Certain strains of *P. falciparum* are resistant to 4-aminoquinolines.

Side Effects: *GI:* N&V, diarrhea, cramps, anorexia, epigastric distress, stomatitis, dry mouth. *CNS:* Headache, fatigue, nervousness, anxiety, irritability, agitation, apathy, confusion, personality changes, depression, psychoses, **seizures.** *CV:* Hypotension, ECG changes (inversion or depression of T wave, widening of QRS complex). *Dermatologic:* Pruritus, changes in pigment of skin and mucous membranes, dermatoses, bleaching of hair. *Hematologic:* Neutropenia, **aplastic anemia,** thrombocytopenia, **agranulocytosis.** *Ocular:* Retinopathy that may be permanent and may lead to blindness. Blurred vision, difficulty in focusing or in accommodation; chronic use may lead to corneal deposits or keratopathy. *Miscellaneous:* Peripheral neuritis, ototoxicity, neuromyopathy manifested by muscle weakness.

OD **Overdose Management:** *Symptoms:* Headache, drowsiness, visual disturbances, *CV collapse, seizures followed by sudden and early respiratory and cardiac arrest.* Infants and children have manifested respiratory depression, *CV collapse, shock, seizures, and death following overdoses of parenteral chloroquine.* ECG changes include nodal rhythm, atrial standstill, prolonged intraventricular conduction, and bradycardia, which lead to *ventricular fibrillation or arrest. Treatment:* Undertake gastric lavage or emesis followed by activated charcoal. Seizures should be controlled prior to gastric lavage. Seizures due to anoxia can be treated by oxygen, mechanical ventilation, or vasopressors (in shock with hypotension). Tracheostomy or tracheal intubation may be required. Forced fluids and acidification of the urine may hasten excretion. Peritoneal dialysis and exchange transfusions may also help.

Drug Interactions
Acidifying agents, urinary (ammonium chloride, etc.) / ↑ Urinary excretion of antimalarial and thus ↓ its effectiveness
Alkalinizing agents, urinary (bicarbonate, etc.) / ↓ Excretion of antimalarial and thus ↑ amount of drug in system
Antipsoriatics / 4-Aminoquinolines inhibit antipsoriatic drugs
MAO inhibitors / ↑ Toxicity of 4-Aminoquinolines due to ↓ breakdown in liver

EMS CONSIDERATIONS

See also *Anti-Infectives.*

ANTINEOPLASTIC AGENTS

See also the following individual entries:

Altretamine
Bicalutamide
Bleomycin sulfate
Busulfan
Capecitabine
Chlorambucil
Cyclophosphamide
Diethylstilbestrol diphosphate
Estramustine phosphate sodium
Etoposide
Exemestane
Fluorouracil
Flutamide
Goserelin acetate
Hydroxyurea
Interferon Alfa-2a Recombinant
Interferon Alfa-2b Recombinant
Letrozole
Leuprolide acetate
Levamisole hydrochloride
Lomustine
Megestrol acetate
Melphalan
Mercaptopurine
Methotrexate
Methotrexate sodium
Mitotane
Nilutamide
Octreotide acetate
Plicamycin
Porfimer sodium
Procarbazine hydrochloride
Rituximab
Streptozocin

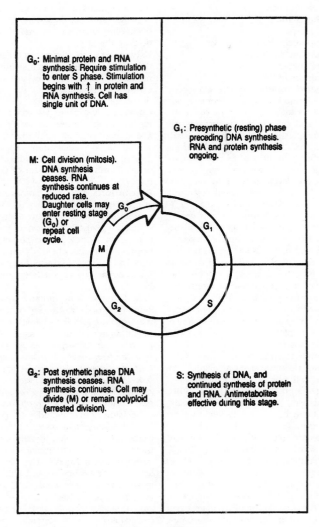

Figure 1   Cell stages

Strontium-89 chloride
Tamoxifen
Temozolomide
Teniposide
Testolactone
Thioguanine
Thiotepa
Topotecan hydrochloride
Toremifene citrate
Trastuzumab
Valrubicin

General Statement: The choice of the chemotherapeutic agent(s) depends both on the cell type of the tumor and on its site of growth. All antineoplastic agents are cytotoxic (i.e., cell poisons) and therefore interfere with normal as well as neoplastic cells. However, neoplastic cells are more active and multiply more rapidly than normal cells and are thus more affected by the antineoplastic agents. Normal, rapidly growing tissue cells, such as those of the bone marrow, the GI mucosal epithelium, and hair follicles, are particularly susceptible to antineoplastic agents. The margin between the dose of antineoplastic drug needed to destroy the neoplastic cells and that needed to cause bone marrow damage, for example, is narrow. Since WBCs or platelets show the effect of an overdose more rapidly than do erythrocytes, the platelet and WBC counts are often used as a guide to dosage. If a blood or marrow test indicates a precipitous fall in the WBC or platelet count, the antineoplastic agent may have to be discontinued or the dosage modified significantly. Drugs are frequently withheld when the WBC count falls below 2,000/mm^3 and the platelet count falls below 100,000/mm^3. With the advent of granulocyte colony-stimulating factors, providers may now utilize this to support large dosing on an aggressive cancer, thus preventing postponement of therapy until recovery of the patient's hematologic parameters. Sometimes the effect of the antineoplastic drugs on the bone marrow is cumulative, with the depression of WBCs and platelets occurring weeks or months after initiation of therapy.

GI tract toxicity is manifested by development of oral ulcers, intestinal bleeding, nausea, vomiting, loss of appetite, and diarrhea. Finally, alopecia often results from antineoplastic drug therapy.

Uses: Most of the drugs discussed in this section are used exclusively for neoplastic disease. A few are used on an experimental basis for some of the rheumatic diseases.

Contraindications: Hypersensitivity to drug. Some antineoplastic agents may be contraindicated for a period of 4 weeks after radiation therapy or chemotherapy with similar drugs. During first trimester of pregnancy.

Precautions: Use with caution, and at reduced dosages, in patients with preexisting bone marrow depression, malignant infiltration of bone marrow or kidney, liver dysfunction, or previous recent chemotherapy usage. The safe use of these drugs during pregnancy has not been established.

Side Effects: *Bone marrow depression* (leukopenia, thrombocytopenia, **agranulocytosis,** anemia) is the major danger of antineoplastic therapy. *Bone marrow depression can sometimes be irreversible. It is mandatory that the patient have frequent total blood counts and periodic bone marrow examinations. Precipitous falls must be reported to a physician.* Other side effects include: *GI:* N&V (may be severe), anorexia, diarrhea (may be hemorrhagic), stomatitis, mucositis, enteritis, abdominal cramps, intestinal ulcers. *Hepatic:* Hepatic toxicity including jaundice and changes in liver enzymes. *Dermatologic:* Dermatitis, erythema, various dermatoses including maculopapular rash, alopecia (reversible), pruritus, staining of vein path with some drugs, urticaria, cheilosis. *Immunologic:* Immunosuppression with increased susceptibility to viral, bacterial, or fungal infections. *CNS:* Depression, lethargy, confusion, dizziness, headache, fatigue, malaise, fever, weakness. *GU: **Acute renal failure,*** reproductive abnormalities including amenorrhea and azoospermia. *NOTE:* Alkylating agents, in particular, may be both carcinogenic and mutagenic.

EMS CONSIDERATIONS

None.

ANTIPARKINSON AGENTS

See also the following individual entries:

Amantadine hydrochloride
Benztropine mesylate
Biperiden hydrochloride
Bromocriptine mesylate
Carbidopa
Carbidopa/Levodopa
Diphenhydramine hydrochloride
Entacapone
Levodopa
Pergolide mesylate
Pramipexole
Ropinirole hydrochloride
Tolcapone
Trihexyphenidyl hydrochloride

General Statement: Parkinson's disease is a progressive disorder of the nervous system, affecting mostly people over the age of 50. Parkinsonism is a frequent side effect of certain antipsychotic drugs, including prochlorperazine, chlorpromazine, and reserpine. Drug-induced symptoms usually disappear when the responsible agent is discontinued. The cause of Parkinson's disease is unknown; however, it is associated with a depletion of the neurotransmitter dopamine in the nervous system. Administration of levodopa—the precursor of dopamine—relieves symptoms in 75%–80% of the patients. Most of the newer antiparkinson drugs must be given with levodopa. Anticholinergic agents also have a beneficial effect by reducing tremors and rigidity and improving mobility, muscular coordination, and motor performance. They are often administered together with levodopa. Cer-

tain antihistamines, notably diphenhydramine (Benadryl), are also useful in the treatment of parkinsonism. Patients suffering from Parkinson's disease need emotional support and encouragement because the debilitating nature of the disorder often causes depression. Comprehensive treatment also includes physical therapy.

EMS CONSIDERATIONS

None.

ANTIPSYCHOTIC AGENTS, PHENOTHIAZINES

See also the following individual entries:

Chlorpromazine hydrochloride
Fluphenazine decanoate
Fluphenazine enanthate
Fluphenazine hydrochloride
Mesoridazine besylate
Perphenazine
Prochlorperazine
Prochlorperazine edisylate
Prochlorperazine maleate
Promazine hydrochloride
Thioridazine hydrochloride
Trifluoperazine
Triflupromazine hydrochloride

Mechanism of Action: It has been postulated that excess amounts of dopamine in certain areas of the CNS cause psychoses. Phenothiazines are thought to act by blocking postsynaptic mesolimbic dopamine receptors, leading to a reduction in psychotic symptoms. Phenothiazines block both D_1 and D_2 dopamine receptors. The antiemetic effects are thought to be due to inhibition or blockade of dopamine (D_2) receptors in the chemoreceptor trigger zone in the medulla as well as by peripheral blockade of the vagus nerve in the GI tract. Relief of anxiety is manifested as a result of an indirect decrease in arousal and increased filtering of internal stimuli to the brain stem reticular system. Alpha-adrenergic blockade produces sedation. Phenothiazines also raise pain threshold and produce amnesia due to suppression of sensory impulses. In addition, these drugs produce anticholinergic and antihistaminic effects and depress the release of hypothalamic and hypophyseal hormones. Peripheral effects include anticholinergic and alpha-adrenergic blocking properties.

Peak plasma levels: 2–4 hr after PO administration. Widely distributed throughout the body. **t½ (average):** 10–20 hr. Most metabolized in the liver and excreted by the kidney.

General Statement: Antipsychotic drugs do not cure mental illness, but they calm the intractable patient, relieve the despondency of the severely depressed, activate the immobile and withdrawn, and make some more accessible to psychotherapy.

Most phenothiazines induce some sedation, especially during the initial phase of the treatment. Medicated patients can, however, be easily roused. In this manner, the phenothiazines differ markedly from the narcotic analgesics and sedative hypnotics. However, phenothiazines potentiate the analgesic properties of opiates and prolong the action of CNS depressant drugs. These drugs also cause sedation, decrease spontaneous motor activity, and many lower BP.

According to their detailed chemical structure, the phenothiazines belong to three subgroups:
1. **Aliphatic compounds.** Moderate to high sedative, anticholinergic, and orthostatic hypotensive effects. Moderate extrapyramidal symptoms. Often the first choice for patients in acute excitatory states. Examples: Chlorpromazine, promazine, trifluopromazine.
2. **Piperazine compounds.** Act most selectively on the subcortical sites. Low to moderate sedative effects; low anticholinergic and orthostatic hypotensive effects; high incidence of extrapyramidal symptoms. Greatest antiemetic effects because they specifically depress the CTZ of the vomiting center. Examples: Fluphenazine, perphenazine, prochlorperazine, trifluoperazine.
3. **Piperidine compounds.** Low incidence of extrapyramidal effects; high sedative and anticholinergic effects; low to moderate orthostatic hypotensive effect. Examples: Mesoridazine, thioridazine.

Uses: Psychoses, especially if excessive psychomotor activity manifested. Involutional, toxic, or senile psychoses. Used in combination with MAO inhibitors in depressed patients manifesting anxiety, agitation, or panic (use with caution). With lithium in acute manic phase of manic-depressive illness. As an adjunct in alcohol withdrawal to reduce anxiety, tension, depression, nausea, and/or vomiting. For severe behavioral problems in children, manifested by hyperexcitable and/or combative behavior; also, for short-term use in hyperactive children who exhibit excess motor activity and conduct disorders.

Prophylaxis and control of severe N&V due to cancer chemotherapy, radiation therapy, postoperatively. Intractable hiccoughs, intermittent porphyria, tetanus (as adjunct). As preoperative and/or postoperative medications. Some phenothiazines are antipruritics. See also individual drugs.

Contraindications: Severe CNS depression, coma, patients with subcortical brain damage, bone marrow depression, lactation. In patients with a history of seizures and in those on anticonvulsant drugs. Geriatric or debilitated patients, hepatic or renal disease, CV disorders, glaucoma, prostatic hypertrophy. Contraindicated in children with chickenpox, CNS infections, measles, gastroenteritis, dehydration due to increased risk of extrapyramidal symptoms.

Precautions: Use with caution in patients exposed to extreme heat or cold and in those with asthma, emphysema, or acute respiratory tract infections. Use during pregnancy only when benefits outweigh risks.

Children may be more sensitive to the neuromuscular or extrapyramidal effects (especially dystonias); those especially at risk include children with chickenpox, CNS infections, measles, dehydration, or gastroenteritis. Thus, generally, phenothiazines are not recommended for use in children less than 12 years of age. Geriatric patients often manifest higher plasma levels due to decreases in lean body mass, total body water, and albumin and an increase in total body fat. Also, geriatric patients may be more likely to manifest orthostatic hypotension, anticholinergic effects, sedative effects, and extrapyramidal side effects.

Side Effects: *CNS:* Depression, drowsiness, dizziness, lethargy, fatigue. Extrapyramidal effects, Parkinson-like symptoms including shuffling gait or tic-like movements of head and face, tardive dyskinesia (see what follows), akathisia, dystonia. *Seizures,* especially in patients with a history thereof. *Neuroleptic malignant syndrome (rare).* *CV:* Orthostatic hypotension, increase or decrease in BP, tachycardia, fainting. *GI:* Dry mouth, anorexia, constipation, paralytic ileus, diarrhea. *Endocrine:* Breast engorgement, galactorrhea, gynecomastia, increased appetite, weight gain, hyper- or hypoglycemia, glycosuria. Delayed ejaculation, increased or decreased libido. *GU:* Menstrual irregularities, loss of bladder control, urinary difficulty. *Dermatologic:* Photosensitivity, pruritus, erythema, eczema, exfoliative dermatitis, pigment changes in skin (long-term use of high doses). *Hematologic: Aplastic anemia,* leukopenia, *agranulocytosis,* eosinophilia, thrombocytopenia. *Ophthalmologic:* Deposition of fine particulate matter in lens and cornea leading to blurred vision, changes in vision. *Respiratory: Laryngospasm, bronchospasm, laryngeal edema,* breathing difficulties. *Miscellaneous:* Fever, muscle stiffness, decreased sweating, muscle spasm of face, neck, or back, obstructive jaundice, nasal congestion, pale skin, mydriasis, systemic lupus-like syndrome.

Tardive dyskinesia has been observed with all classes of antipsychotic drugs, although the precise cause is not known. The syndrome is most commonly seen in older patients, especially women, and in individuals with organic brain syndrome. It is often aggravated or precipitated by the sudden discontinuance of antipsychotic drugs and may persist indefinitely after the drug is discontinued. Early signs of tardive dyskinesia include fine vermicular movements of the tongue and grimacing or tic-like movements of the head and neck. Although there is no known cure for the syndrome, it may not progress if the dosage of the drug is slowly reduced. Also, a few drug-free days may unmask the symptoms of tardive dyskinesia and help in early diagnosis.

OD **Overdose Management:** *Symptoms:* CNS depression including deep sleep and *coma,* hypotension, extrapyramidal symptoms, agitation, restlessness, seizures, hypothermia, *hyperthermia,* autonomic symptoms, *cardiac arrhythmias,* ECG changes. *Treatment:* Emetics are not to be used as they are of little value and may cause a dystonic reaction of the head or neck that may result in aspiration of vomitus.

• Hypotension: Volume replacement; norepinephrine or phenylephrine may be used (do not use epinephrine).

• Ventricular arrhythmias: phenytoin, 1 mg/kg IV, not to exceed 50 mg/min; may be repeated q 5 min up to 10 mg/kg.

• Seizures or hyperactivity: Diazepam or pentobarbital.

• Extrapyramidal symptoms: Antiparkinson drugs, diphenhydramine, barbiturates.

Drug Interactions

Alcohol, ethyl / Potentiation or addition of CNS depressant effects. Concomitant use may lead to drowsi-

---

bold italic = life threatening side effect

ness, lethargy, stupor, respiratory collapse, coma, or death

Aluminum salts (antacids) / ↓ Absorption from GI tract

Amphetamine / ↓ Effect of amphetamine by ↓ uptake of drug to the site of action

Anesthetics, general / See *Alcohol*

Antacids, oral / ↓ Effect of phenothiazines due to ↓ absorption from GI tract

Antianxiety drugs / See *Alcohol*

Anticholinergic drugs / Additive anticholinergic side effects and/or ↓ antipsychotic effect

Antidepressants, tricyclic / Additive anticholinergic side effects; also, ↑ TCA serum levels

Barbiturate anesthetics / ↑ Chance of tremor, involuntary muscle activity, and hypotension

Barbiturates / See *Alcohol;* also, barbiturates may ↓ effect due to ↑ breakdown by liver

Bromocriptine / Phenothiazines ↓ effect

Charcoal / ↓ Effect of phenothiazines due to ↓ absorption from GI tract

CNS depressants / See *Alcohol;* also, ↓ effect of phenothiazines due to ↑ breakdown by liver

Colistimethate / Additive respiratory depression

Diazoxide / Additive hyperglycemic effect

Guanethidine / ↓ Effect of guanethidine by ↓ uptake of drug at the site of action

Hydantoins / ↑ Risk of hydantoin toxicity

Lithium carbonate / ↑ Risk of extrapyramidal symptoms, disorientation, or unconsciousness

MAO inhibitors / ↑ Effect of phenothiazines due to ↓ breakdown by liver

Meperidine / ↑ Risk of hypotension and sedation

Metrizamide / ↑ Risk of seizures during subarachnoid administration of metrizamide

Narcotics / See *Alcohol*

Phenytoin / ↑ or ↓ Serum levels of phenytoin

Pimozide / Additive effect on QT interval; do not use together

Propranolol / ↑ Plasma levels of both drugs

Sedative-hypnotics, nonbarbiturate / See *Alcohol*

EMS CONSIDERATIONS

None.

ANTITHYROID DRUGS

See also the following individual entries:

Methimazole
Propylthiouracil

Mechanism of Action: These drugs inhibit (partially or completely) the production of thyroid hormones by the thyroid gland by preventing the incorporation of iodide into tyrosine and coupling of iodotyrosines. They do not affect release or activity of preformed hormone; thus, it may take several weeks for the therapeutic effect to become established.

Uses: Hyperthyroidism; prior to surgery or radiotherapy. Adjunct in treatment of thyrotoxicosis or thyroid storm. Propylthiouracil is also used to reduce mortality due to alcoholic liver disease.

Contraindications: Lactation (may cause hypothyroidism in the infant).

Precautions: Use with caution in the presence of CV disease. PT should be monitored during therapy as propylthiouracil may cause hypoprothrombinemia and bleeding.

Side Effects: *Hematologic: **Agranulocytosis,*** thrombocytopenia, granulocytopenia, hypoprothrombinemia, ***aplastic anemia,*** leukopenia. *GI:* N&V, taste loss, epigastric pain, sialadenopathy. *CNS:* Headache, paresthesia, drowsiness, vertigo, depression, CNS stimulation. *Dermatologic:* Skin rash, urticaria, alopecia, skin pigmentation, pruritus, exfoliative dermatitis, erythema nodosum. *Miscellaneous:* Jaundice, arthralgia, myalgia, neuritis, edema, lymphadenopathy, vasculitis, lupus-like syndrome, drug fever, periarteritis, hepatitis, nephritis, interstitial pneumonitis, insulin autoimmune syndrome resulting in hypoglycemic coma.

OD **Overdose Management:** *Symptoms:* N&V, headache, fever, pruritus, epigastric distress, arthralgia, pancytopenia, *agranulocytosis* (most serious). Rarely, exfoliative dermatitis, hepatitis, neuropathies, CNS stimulation or depression. *Treatment:* Maintain a patent airway and support ventilation and perfusion. Very carefully monitor and maintain VS, blood gases, and serum electrolytes. Monitor bone marrow function.

EMS CONSIDERATIONS

None.

ANTIVIRAL DRUGS

See also the following individual entries:

Abacavir sulfate
Acyclovir (Acycloguanosine)
Amantadine hydrochloride
Delavirdine mesylate
Didanosine (ddI, Dideoxyinosine)
Efavirenz
Famciclovir
Ganciclovir sodium
Idoxuridine (IDU)
Indinavir sulfate
Lamivudine
Lamivudine and Zidovudine
Nelfinavir mesylate
Nevirapine
Oseltamivir phosphate
Penciclovir
Ribavirin
Rimantidine hydrochloride
Ritonavir
Saquinavir mesylate
Stavudine
Trifluridine
Valacyclovir hydrochloride
Vidarabine
Zanamivir
Zalcitabine
Zidovudine (Azidothymidine, AZT)

Mechanism of Action: To maintain their growth and reproduce, viruses must enter living cells. Thus, it is difficult to find a drug that is specific for the virus and that does not interfere with the function of the host cell. However, there are enzymes and replicative mechanisms that are unique to viruses and an increasing number of drugs with specific antiviral activity have been developed. The antiviral drugs currently marketed act by one of the following mechanisms:

1. Inhibition of enzymes required for DNA synthesis. Example: Idoxuridine.

2. Inhibition of viral nucleic acid synthesis by interacting directly with herpes virus DNA polymerase or HIV reverse transcriptase. Example: Foscarnet.

3. Inhibition of viral DNA or protein synthesis. Examples: Acyclovir, cidofovir, famciclovir, fomivirsen, ganciclovir, penciclovir, trifluridine, valacyclovir, vidarabine.

4. Prevent penetration of the virus into cells by inhibiting uncoating of the RNA virus. Examples: Amantadine, rimantadine.

5. Protease inhibitors resulting in release of immature, noninfectious viral particles. Examples: Indinavir, nelfinavir, ritonavir, saquinavir.

6. Reverse transcriptase inhibitors (nucleoside and non-nucleoside) resulting in inhibition of replication of the virus. Examples of nucleoside inhibitors: Abacavir, didanosine, lamivudine, stavudine, zalcitabine, zidovudine. Examples of non-nucleoside inhibitors: Efavirenz, delavirdine, nevirapine. It is often necessary to combine two antiviral drugs that have the same or different mechanisms of action in order to treat HIV infections and to minimize development of resistant viruses. For example, regimens of choice include two nucleosides and one protease inhibitor or two nucleosides and one non-nucleoside.

---

bold italic = life threatening side effect

See *General Nursing Considerations For All Anti-Infectives.*

EMS CONSIDERATIONS

See *Anti-Infectives.*

BARBITURATES

See also the following individual entries:

Pentobarbital
Pentobarbital sodium
Phenobarbital
Phenobarbital sodium
Secobarbital sodium

Mechanism of Action: Barbiturates produce all levels of CNS depression, ranging from mild depression (sedation) following low doses to hypnotic (sleep-inducing) effects, and even coma and death, as dosage is increased. Certain barbiturates are also effective anticonvulsants. The depressant and anticonvulsant effects may be related to their ability to increase and/or mimic the inhibitory activity of the neurotransmitter GABA on nerve synapses. Importantly, barbiturates are not analgesics and therefore should not be given to patients for the purpose of ameliorating pain. Sodium salts are readily absorbed after PO, rectal, or parenteral administration. They are distributed throughout all tissues, cross the placental barrier, and appear in breast milk. The main difference between the various barbiturates is in the onset of action, which ranges from 10 to 15 min for pentobarbital and secobarbital and 60 or more minutes for phenobarbital. Metabolized almost completely in the liver (except for phenobarbital) and are excreted in the urine.

Uses: Preanesthetic medication. Sedation, hypnotic, anticonvulsant (phenobarbital) and for the control of acute convulsive conditions (only phenobarbital, mephobarbital), as in epilepsy, tetanus, meningitis, eclampsia, and toxic reactions to local anesthetics or strychnine. The benzodiazepines have replaced barbiturates for the treatment of many conditions, especially daytime sedation. See also information on individual drugs.

Contraindications: Hypersensitivity to barbiturates, severe trauma, pulmonary disease when dyspnea or obstruction is present, edema, uncontrolled diabetes, history of porphyria, and impaired liver function and for patients in whom they produce an excitatory response. Also, patients who have been addicted previously to sedative-hypnotics.

Precautions: Use with caution during lactation and in patients with CNS depression, hypotension, marked asthenia (characteristic of Addison's disease, hypoadrenalism, and severe myxedema), porphyria, fever, anemia, hemorrhagic shock, cardiac, hepatic or renal damage, and a history of alcoholism in suicidal patients. Geriatric patients usually manifest increased sensitivity to barbiturates, as evidenced by confusion, excitement, mental depression, and hypothermia. When given in the presence of pain, restlessness, excitement, and delirium may result. Intra-arterial use may cause symptoms from transient pain to gangrene; SC use produces tissue irritation, including tenderness and redness to necrosis.

Side Effects: *CNS:* Sleepiness, drowsiness, agitation, confusion, hyperkinesia, ataxia, CNS depression, nightmares, nervousness, psychiatric disturbances, hallucinations, insomnia, anxiety, dizziness, headache, abnormal thinking, vertigo, lethargy, hangover, excitement, appearance of being inebriated. Irritability and hyperactivity in children. *Musculoskeletal:* Localized or diffuse myalgic, neuralgic, or arthritic pain, especially in psychoneurotic patients. Pain is often most intense in the morning and is frequently located in the neck, shoulder girdle, and arms. *Respiratory:* Hypoventilation, **apnea, respiratory depression.** *CV:* Bradycardia, hypotension, syncope, **circulatory collapse.** *GI:* N&V, constipation, liver damage (especially with chronic use of phenobarbital). *Allergic:* Skin rashes, **angioedema,** exfoliative dermatitis (including

Stevens-Johnson syndrome and toxic epidermal necrolysis). Allergic reactions are most common in patients who have asthma, urticaria, angioedema, and similar conditions. Symptoms include localized swelling (especially of the lips, cheeks, or eyelids) and erythematous dermatitis).

After SC use: Tissue necrosis, pain, tenderness, redness, permanent neurologic damage if injected near peripheral nerves.

After IV use. CV: Circulatory depression, thrombophlebitis, *peripheral vascular collapse, seizures with cardiorespiratory arrest, myocardial depression, cardiac arrhythmias. Respiratory: Apnea, laryngospasm, bronchospasm,* dyspnea, rhinitis, sneezing, coughing. *CNS:* Emergence delirium, headache, anxiety, prolonged somnolence and recovery, restlessness, *seizures. GI:* N&V, abdominal pain, diarrhea, cramping. *Hypersensitivity: Acute allergic reactions, including erythema, pruritus, anaphylaxis.* Miscellaneous: Pain or nerve injury at injection site, salivation, hiccups, skin rashes, shivering, skeletal muscle hyperactivity, *immune hemolytic anemia with renal failure,* and radial nerve palsy.

After IM use: Pain at injection site.

Barbiturates can induce physical and psychologic dependence if high doses are used regularly for long periods of time. Withdrawal symptoms usually begin after 12–16 hr of abstinence. Manifestations of withdrawal include anxiety, weakness, N&V, muscle cramps, delirium, and even *tonic-clonic seizures.*

OD Overdose Management: *Symptoms (Acute Toxicity):* Characterized by cortical and *respiratory depression; anoxia; peripheral vascular collapse;* feeble, rapid pulse; pulmonary edema; decreased body temperature; clammy, cyanotic skin; depressed reflexes; stupor; and *coma.* After initial constriction the pupils become dilated. *Death results from respiratory failure or arrest followed by cardiac arrest. Symptoms (Chronic Toxicity):* Prolonged use of barbiturates at high doses may lead to

physical and psychologic dependence, as well as tolerance. Doses of 600–800 mg daily for 8 weeks may lead to physical dependence. The addict usually ingests 1.5 g/day. Addicts prefer short-acting barbiturates. Symptoms of dependence are similar to those associated with chronic alcoholism, and withdrawal symptoms are equally severe. Withdrawal symptoms usually last for 5–10 days and are terminated by a long sleep. *Treatment (Acute Toxicity):*

• Maintenance of an adequate airway, oxygen intake, and carbon dioxide removal are essential.

• After PO ingestion, gastric lavage or gastric aspiration may delay absorption. Emesis should not be induced once the symptoms of overdosage are manifested, as the patient may aspirate the vomitus into the lungs. Also, if the dose of barbiturate is high enough, the vomiting center in the brain may be depressed.

• Absorption following SC or IM administration of the drug may be delayed by the use of ice packs or tourniquets.

• Maintain renal function.

• Removal of the drug by peritoneal dialysis or an artificial kidney should be carried out.

• Supportive physiologic methods have proven superior to use of analeptics.

Treatment (Chronic Toxicity): Cautious withdrawal of the hospitalized addict over a 2–4-week period. A stabilizing dose of 200–300 mg of a short-acting barbiturate is administered q 6 hr. The dose is then reduced by 100 mg/day until the stabilizing dose is reduced by one-half. The patient is then maintained on this dose for 2–3 days before further reduction. The same procedure is repeated when the initial stabilizing dose has been reduced by three-quarters. If a mixed spike and slow activity appear on the EEG, or if insomnia, anxiety, tremor, or weakness is observed, the dosage is maintained at a constant level or in-

---

bold italic = life threatening side effect

creased slightly until symptoms disappear.

Drug Interactions

GENERAL CONSIDERATIONS

1. Barbiturates stimulate the activity of enzymes responsible for the metabolism of a large number of other drugs by a process known as *enzyme induction*. As a result, when barbiturates are given to patients receiving such drugs, their therapeutic effectiveness is markedly reduced or even abolished.

2. The CNS depressant effect of the barbiturates is potentiated by many drugs. Concomitant administration may result in coma or fatal CNS depression. Barbiturate dosage should either be reduced or eliminated when other CNS drugs are given.

3. Barbiturates also potentiate the toxic effects of many other agents.

Acetaminophen / ↑ Risk of hepatotoxicity when used with large or chronic doses of barbiturates

Alcohol / Potentiation or addition of CNS depressant effects. Concomitant use may lead to drowsiness, lethargy, stupor, respiratory collapse, coma, or death

Anesthetics, general / See *Alcohol*

Anorexiants / ↓ Effect of anorexiants due to opposite activities

Antianxiety drugs / See *Alcohol*

Anticoagulants, oral / ↓ Effect of anticoagulants due to ↓ absorption from GI tract and ↑ breakdown by liver

Antidepressants, tricyclic / ↓ Effect of antidepressants due to ↑ breakdown by liver

Antidiabetic agents / Prolong the effects of barbiturates

Antihistamines / See *Alcohol*

Beta-adrenergic agents / ↓ Beta blockade due to ↑ breakdown by the liver

Carbamazepine / ↓ Serum carbazepine levels may occur

Charcoal / ↓ Absorption of barbiturates from the GI tract

Chloramphenicol / ↑ Effect of barbiturates by ↓ breakdown by the liver and ↓ effect of chloramphenicol by ↑ breakdown by liver

Clonazepam / Barbiturates may ↑ excretion of clonazepam → loss of efficacy

CNS depressants / See *Alcohol*

Corticosteroids / ↓ Effect of corticosteroids due to ↑ breakdown by liver

Digitoxin / ↓ Effect of digitoxin due to ↑ breakdown by liver

Doxorubicin / ↓ Effect of doxorubicin due to ↑ excretion

Doxycycline / ↓ Effect of doxycycline due to ↑ breakdown by liver (effect may last up to 2 weeks after barbiturates are discontinued)

Estrogens / ↓ Effect of estrogen due to ↑ breakdown by liver

Felodipine / ↓ Plasma levels of felodipine → ↓ effect

Fenoprofen / ↓ Bioavailability of fenoprofen

Furosemide / ↑ Risk or intensity of orthostatic hypotension

Griseofulvin / ↓ Effect of griseofulvin due to ↓ absorption from GI tract

Haloperidol / ↓ Effect of haloperidol due to ↑ breakdown by liver

MAO inhibitors / ↑ Effect of barbiturates due to ↓ breakdown by liver

Meperidine / CNS depressant effects may be prolonged

Methadone / ↓ Effect of methadone

Methoxyflurane / ↑ Kidney toxicity due to ↑ breakdown of methoxyflurane by liver to toxic metabolites

Metronidazole / ↓ Effect of metronidazole

Narcotic analgesics / See *Alcohol*

Oral contraceptives / ↓ Effect of contraceptives due to ↑ breakdown by liver

Phenothiazines / ↓ Effect of phenothiazines due to ↑ breakdown by liver; also see *Alcohol*

Phenylbutazone / ↓ Elimination t½ of phenylbutazone

Phenytoin / Effect variable and unpredictable; monitor carefully

Probenecid / Anesthesia with thiobarbiturates may be ↑ or achieved at lower doses

Procarbazine / ↑ Effect of barbiturates

Quinidine / ↓ Effect of quinidine due to ↑ breakdown by liver

Rifampin / ↓ Effect of barbiturates due to ↑ breakdown by liver

Sedative-hypnotics, nonbarbiturate / See *Alcohol*

Sulfisoxazole / Sulfisoxazole may ↑ the anesthetic effects of thiobarbiturates

Theophyllines / ↓ Effect of theophyllines due to ↑ breakdown by liver

Valproic acid / ↑ Effect of barbiturates due to ↓ breakdown by liver

Verapamil / ↑ Excretion of verapamil → ↓ effect

Vitamin D / Barbiturates may ↑ requirements for vitamin D due to ↑ breakdown by the liver

EMS CONSIDERATIONS

None.

BETA-ADRENERGIC BLOCKING AGENTS

See also Alpha-1-Adrenergic Blocking Agents and the following individual agents:

Acebutolol hydrochloride
Atenolol
Betaxolol hydrochloride
Bisoprolol fumarate
Carteolol hydrochloride
Esmolol hydrochloride
Levobunolol hydrochloride
Metipranolol hydrochloride
Metoprolol succinate
Metoprolol tartrate
Nadolol
Penbutolol sulfate
Pindolol
Propranolol hydrochloride
Sotalol hydrochloride
Timolol maleate

Mechanism of Action: Combine reversibly with beta-adrenergic receptors to block the response to sympathetic nerve impulses, circulating catecholamines, or adrenergic drugs. Beta-adrenergic receptors are classified as beta-1 (predominantly in the cardiac muscle) and beta-2 (mainly in the bronchi and vascular musculature). Blockade of beta-1 receptors decreases HR, myocardial contractility, and CO; in addition, AV conduction is slowed. These effects lead to a decrease in BP, as well as a reversal of cardiac arrhythmias. Blockade of beta-2 receptors increases airway resistance in the bronchioles and inhibits the vasodilating effects of catecholamines on peripheral blood vessels. The various beta-blocking agents differ in their ability to block beta-1 and beta-2 receptors (see individual drugs); also, certain of these agents have intrinsic sympathomimetic action.

Certain of these drugs (betaxolol, carteolol, levobunolol, metipranolol, and timolol) are used for glaucoma. Act by reducing production of aqueous humor; metipranolol and timolol may also increase outflow of aqueous humor. Drugs have little or no effect on the pupil size or on accommodation.

Uses: See individual drugs.

Contraindications: Sinus bradycardia, second- and third-degree AV block, cardiogenic shock, CHF unless secondary to tachyarrhythmia treatable with beta blockers, overt cardiac failure. Most are contraindicated in chronic bronchitis, bronchial asthma or history thereof, bronchospasm, emphysema, severe COPD.

Precautions: Use with caution in diabetes, thyrotoxicosis, cerebrovascular insufficiency, and impaired hepatic and renal function. Withdrawing beta blockers before major surgery is controversial. Safe use during pregnancy and lactation and in children has not been established. May be absorbed systemically when used for glaucoma; thus, there is the potential for an additive effect with beta blockers used systemically. Certain of the products for use in glaucoma contain sulfites, which may result in an allergic reaction. Also, see individual agents.

Side Effects: *CV:* Bradycardia, hypotension (especially following IV use), CHF, cold extremities, claudication, worsening of angina, strokes, edema, syncope, arrhythmias, chest pain, peripheral ischemia, flushing, SOB, sinoatrial block, pulmonary edema, vasodilation, increased HR, palpitations, conduction disturbances, **first-, second-, and third-degree heart block,** worsening of AV block, thrombosis of renal or mesenteric arteries, precipitation or worsening of Raynaud's phenomenon. Sudden withdrawal of large doses may cause angina, ventricular tachycardia, **fatal MI, sudden death,** or **circulatory collapse.** *GI:* N&V, diarrhea, flatulence, dry mouth, constipation, anorexia, cramps, bloating, gastric pain, dyspepsia, distortion of taste, weight gain or loss, retroperitoneal fibrosis, ischemic colitis. *Hepatic:* Hepatomegaly, acute pancreatitis, elevated liver enzymes, liver damage (especially with chronic use of phenobarbital). *Respiratory:* Asthma-like symptoms, **bronchospasms, bronchial obstruction, laryngospasm with respiratory distress,** wheeziness, worsening of chronic obstructive lung disease, dyspnea, cough, nasal stuffiness, rhinitis, pharyngitis, rales. *CNS:* Dizziness, fatigue, lethargy, vivid dreams, depression, hallucinations, delirium, psychoses, paresthesias, insomnia, nervousness, nightmares, headache, vertigo, disorientation of time and place, hypoesthesia or hyperesthesia, decreased concentration, short-term memory loss, change in behavior, emotional lability, slurred speech, lightheadedness. In the elderly, paranoia, disorientation, and combativeness have occurred. *Hematologic:* **Agranulocytosis,** thrombocytopenia. *Allergic:* Fever, sore throat, respiratory distress, rash, pharyngitis, **laryngospasm, anaphylaxis.** *Skin:* Pruritus, rashes, increased skin pigmentation, sweating, dry skin, alopecia, skin irritation, psoriasis (reversible). *Musculoskeletal:* Joint and muscle pain, arthritis, arthralgia, back pain, muscle cramps, muscle weakness when used in patients with myasthenic symptoms. *GU:* Impotence, decreased libido, dysuria, UTI, nocturia, urinary retention or frequency, pollakiuria. *Ophthalmic:* Visual disturbances, eye irritation, dry or burning eyes, blurred vision, conjunctivitis. When used ophthalmically: keratitis, blepharoptosis, diplopia, ptosis, and visual disturbances including refractive changes. *Other:* Hyperglycemia or hypoglycemia, lupus-like syndrome, Peyronie's disease, tinnitus, increase in symptoms of myasthenia gravis, facial swelling, decreased exercise tolerance, rigors, speech disorders. *Systemic effects due to ophthalmic beta-1 and beta-2 blockers:* Headache, depression, arrhythmia, heart block, CVA, syncope, CHF, palpitation, cerebral ischemia, nausea, localized and generalized rash, bronchospasm (especially in those with preexisting bronchospastic disease), respiratory failure, masked symptoms of hypoglycemia in insulin-dependent diabetics, keratitis, visual disturbances (including refractive changes), blepharoptosis, ptosis, diplopia.

OD **Overdose Management:** *Symptoms:* CV symptoms include bradycardia, hypotension, CHF, **cardiogenic shock,** intraventricular conduction disturbances, **AV block, pulmonary edema, asystole,** and tachycardia. Also, overdosage of pindolol may cause hypertension and overdosage of propranolol may result in systemic vascular resistance. CNS symptoms include respiratory depression, decreased consciousness, **coma, and seizures.** Miscellaneous symptoms include **bronchospasm** (especially in patients with obstructive pulmonary disease), hyperkalemia, and hypoglycemia. *Treatment:*
• To improve blood supply to the brain, place patient in a supine position and raise the legs.
• Measure blood glucose and serum potassium. Monitor BP and ECG continuously.
• Provide general supportive treatment such as inducing emesis or gastric lavage and artificial respiration.
• *Seizures:* Give IV diazepam or phenytoin.

• *Excessive bradycardia:* If hypotensive, give atropine, 0.6 mg; if no response, give q 3 min for a total of 2–3 mg. Cautious administration of isoproterenol may be tried. Also, glucagon, 5–10 mg rapidly over 30 sec, followed by continuous IV infusion of 5 mg/hr may reverse bradycardia. Transvenous cardiac pacing may be needed for refractory cases.

• *Cardiac failure:* Digitalis, diuretic, and oxygen; if failure is refractory, IV aminophylline or glucagon may be helpful.

• *Hypotension:* Place patient in Trendelenburg position. IV fluids unless pulmonary edema is present; also vasopressors such as norepinephrine (may be drug of choice), dobutamine, dopamine with monitoring of BP. If refractory, glucagon may be helpful. In intractable cardiogenic shock, intra-aortic balloon insertion may be required.

• *Premature ventricular contractions:* Lidocaine or phenytoin. Disopyramide, quinidine, and procainamide should be avoided as they depress myocardial function further.

• *Bronchospasms:* Give a beta-2-adrenergic agonist, epinephrine, or theophylline.

• *Heart block, second or third degree:* Isoproterenol or transvenous cardiac pacing.

Drug Interactions

Anesthetics, general / Additive depression of myocardium

Anticholinergic agents / Counteract bradycardia produced by beta-adrenergic blockers

Antihypertensives / Additive hypotensive effect

Ophthalmic beta blockers / Additive systemic beta-blocking effects if used with oral beta blockers

Chlorpromazine / Additive beta-adrenergic blocking action

Cimetidine / ↑ Effect of beta blockers due to ↓ breakdown by liver

Clonidine / Paradoxical hypertension; also, ↑ severity of rebound hypertension

Disopyramide / ↑ Effect of both drugs

Epinephrine / Beta blockers prevent beta-adrenergic action of epinephrine but not alpha-adrenergic action → ↑ systolic and diastolic BP and ↓ HR

Furosemide / ↑ Beta-adrenergic blockade

Hydralazine / ↑ Beta-adrenergic blockade

Indomethacin / ↓ Effect of beta blockers possibly due to inhibition of prostaglandin synthesis

Insulin / Beta blockers ↑ hypoglycemic effect of insulin

Lidocaine / ↑ Effect of lidocaine due to ↓ breakdown by liver

Methyldopa / Possible ↑ BP to alpha-adrenergic effect

NSAIDs / ↓ Effect of beta blockers, possibly due to inhibition of prostaglandin synthesis

Oral contraceptives / ↑ Effect of beta blockers due to ↓ breakdown by liver

Phenformin / ↑ Hypoglycemia

Phenobarbital / ↓ Effect of beta blockers due to ↑ breakdown by liver

Phenothiazines / ↑ Effect of both drugs

Phenytoin / Additive depression of myocardium; also phenytoin ↓ effect of beta blockers due to ↑ breakdown by liver

Prazosin / ↑ First-dose effect of prazosin (acute postural hypotension)

Reserpine / Additive hypotensive effect

Rifampin / ↓ Effect of beta blockers due to ↑ breakdown by liver

Ritodrine / Beta blockers ↓ effect of ritodrine

Salicylates / ↓ Effect of beta blockers, possibly due to inhibition of prostaglandin synthesis

Succinylcholine / Beta blockers ↑ effects of succinylcholine

Sympathomimetics / Reverse effects of beta blockers

Theophylline / Beta blockers reverse the effect of theophylline; also, beta

---

bold italic = life threatening side effect

blockers ↓ renal clearance of theophylline

Tubocurarine / Beta blockers ↑ effects of tubocurarine

Verapamil / Possible side effects since both drugs ↓ myocardial contractility or AV conduction; bradycardia and asystole when beta blockers are used ophthalmically

EMS CONSIDERATIONS

Interventions

1. Monitor HR and BP; obtain written parameters for medication administration (e.g., hold for SBP < 90 or HR < 50).

2. When assessing respirations note rate and quality; may cause dyspnea and bronchospasm.

3. With diabetics watch for symptoms of hypoglycemia, such as hypotension or tachycardia; most mask these signs.

4. During IV administration, monitor EKG (may slow AV conduction and increase PR interval) and activities closely until drug effects evident.

CALCIUM CHANNEL BLOCKING AGENTS

See also the following individual entries:

Amlodipine
Bepridil hydrochloride
Diltiazem hydrochloride
Felodipine
Isradipine
Nicardipine hydrochloride
Nifedipine
Nimodipine
Nisoldipine
Verapamil

Mechanism of Action: For contraction of cardiac and smooth muscle to occur, extracellular calcium must move into the cell through openings called *calcium channels*. The calcium channel blocking agents (also called *slow channel blockers* or *calcium antagonists*) inhibit the influx of calcium through the cell membrane, resulting in a depression of automaticity and conduction velocity in both smooth and cardiac muscle. This leads to a depression of contraction in these tissues. Drugs in this class have different degrees of selectivity on vascular smooth muscle, myocardium, and conduction and pacemaker tissues. In the myocardium, these drugs dilate coronary vessels in both normal and ischemic tissues and inhibit spasms of coronary arteries. They also decrease total peripheral resistance, thus reducing energy and oxygen requirements of the heart. Also effective against certain cardiac arrhythmias by slowing AV conduction and prolonging repolarization. In addition, they depress the amplitude, rate of depolarization, and conduction in atria.

Uses: See individual drugs.

Contraindications: Sick sinus syndrome, second- or third-degree AV block (except with a functioning pacemaker). Use of bepridil, diltiazem, or verapamil for hypotension (<90 mm Hg systolic pressure). Lactation.

Precautions: Abrupt withdrawal may result in increased frequency and duration of chest pain. Hypertensive patients treated with calcium channel blockers have a higher risk of heart attack than patients treated with diuretics or beta-adrenergic blockers. May also be an increased risk of heart attacks in diabetics (only nisoldipine studied). Safety and effectiveness of bepridil, diltiazem, felodipine, and isradipine have not been established in children.

Side Effects: Side effects vary from one calcium channel blocker to another; refer to individual drugs.

OD Overdose Management: *Symptoms:* Nausea, weakness, drowsiness, dizziness, slurred speech, confusion, marked and prolonged hypotension, bradycardia, junctional rhythms, *second- or third-degree block. Treatment:*

• Treatment is supportive. Monitor cardiac and respiratory function.

• If patient is seen soon after ingestion, emetics or gastric lavage should be considered followed by cathartics.

• *Hypotension:* IV calcium, dopamine, isoproterenol, metaraminol, norepinephrine. Also, provide IV fluids. Place patient in Trendelenburg position.

• *Ventricular tachycardia:* IV procainamide or lidocaine; also, cardioversion may be necessary. Also, provide slow-drip IV fluids.

• *Bradycardia, asystole, AV block:* IV atropine sulfate (0.6–1 mg), calcium gluconate (10% solution), isoproterenol, norepinephrine; also, cardiac pacing may be indicated. Provide slow-drip IV fluids.

Drug Interactions
Beta-adrenergic blocking agents / Beta blockers may cause depression of myocardial contractility and AV conduction
Cimetidine / ↑ Effect of calcium channel blockers due to ↓ first-pass metabolism
Fentanyl / Severe hypotension or increased fluid volume requirements
Ranitidine / ↑ Effect of calcium channel blockers due to ↓ first-pass metabolism

EMS CONSIDERATIONS
None.

CALCIUM SALTS

See also the following individual entries:

Calcium carbonate
Calcium chloride
Calcium citrate
Calcium glubionate
Calcium gluceptate
Calcium gluconate
Calcium lactate

Mechanism of Action: Calcium is essential for maintaining normal function of nerves, muscles, the skeletal system, and permeability of cell membranes and capillaries. The normal serum calcium concentration is 9–10.4 mg/dL (4.5–5.2 mEq/L). Hypocalcemia is characterized by muscular fibrillation, twitching, skel-etal muscle spasms, leg cramps, tetanic spasms, cardiac arrhythmias, smooth muscle hyperexcitability, mental depression, and anxiety states. Excessive, chronic hypocalcemia is characterized by brittle, defective nails, poor dentition, and brittle hair. Calcium is well absorbed from the upper GI tract. However, severe low-calcium tetany is best treated by IV administration of calcium gluconate. The presence of vitamin D is necessary for maximum calcium utilization. The hormone of the parathyroid gland is necessary for the regulation of the calcium level.

Uses: IV: Acute hypocalcemic tetany secondary to renal failure, hypoparathyroidism, premature delivery, maternal diabetes mellitus in infants, and poisoning due to magnesium, oxalic acid, radiophosphorus, carbon tetrachloride, fluoride, phosphate, strontium, and radium. To treat depletion of electrolytes. Also during cardiac resuscitation when epinephrine or isoproterenol has not improved myocardial contraction (may also be given into the ventricular cavity for this purpose). To reverse cardiotoxicity or hyperkalemia. **IM or IV:** Reduce spasms in renal, biliary, intestinal, or lead colic. To relieve muscle cramps due to insect bites and to decrease capillary permeability in various sensitivity reactions. **PO:** Osteoporosis, osteomalacia, chronic hypoparathyroidism, rickets, latent tetany, hypocalcemia secondary to use of anticonvulsant drugs. Myasthenia gravis, Eaton-Lambert syndrome, supplement for pregnant, postmenopausal, or nursing women. Also, prophylactically for primary osteoporosis. *Investigational:* As an infusion to diagnose Zollinger-Ellison syndrome and medullary thyroid carcinoma. To antagonize neuromuscular blockade due to aminoglycosides.

Contraindications: Digitalized patients, sarcoidosis, renal or cardiac disease, ventricular fibrillation. Cancer patients with bone metastases. Renal

---

bold italic = life threatening side effect

calculi, hypophosphatemia, hypercalcemia.

Precautions: Calcium requirements decrease in geriatric patients; thus, dose may have to be adjusted. Also, low levels of active vitamin D metabolites may impair calcium absorption in older patients. Use with caution in cor pulmonale, respiratory acidosis, renal disease or failure, ventricular fibrillation, hypercalcemia.

Side Effects: Following PO use: GI irritation, constipation. **Following IV use:** Venous irritation, tingling sensation, feeling of oppression or heat, chalky taste. Rapid IV administration may result in vasodilation, decreased BP and HR, *cardiac arrhythmias,* syncope, or *cardiac arrest.* **Following IM use:** Burning feeling, necrosis, tissue sloughing, cellulitis, soft tissue calcification. *NOTE:* If calcium is injected into the myocardium rather than into the ventricle, *laceration of coronary arteries, cardiac tamponade, pneumothorax, and ventricular fibrillation* may occur. *Symptoms due to excess calcium (hypercalcemia):* Lassitude, fatigue, GI symptoms (anorexia, N&V, abdominal pain, dry mouth, thirst), polyuria, depression of nervous and neuromuscular function (emotional disturbances, confusion, skeletal muscle weakness, and constipation), confusion, delirium, stupor, *coma,* impairment of renal function (polyuria, polydipsia, and azotemia), renal calculi, arrhythmias, and bradycardia.

OD **Overdose Management:** *Symptoms:* Systemic overloading from parenteral administration can result in an acute hypercalcemic syndrome with symptoms including markedly increased plasma calcium levels, lethargy, intractable N&V, weakness, *coma, and sudden death. Treatment:* Discontinue therapy and lower serum calcium levels by giving an IV infusion of sodium chloride plus a potent diuretic such as furosemide. Consider hemodialysis.

Drug Interactions
Atenolol / ↓ Effect of atenolol due to ↓ bioavailability and plasma levels

Cephalocin / Incompatible with calcium salts
Corticosteroids / Interfere with absorption of calcium from GI tract
Digitalis / ↑ Digitalis arrhythmias and toxicity. Death has resulted from combination of digitalis and IV calcium salts
Iron salts / ↓ Absorption of iron from the GI tract
Milk / Excess of either may cause hypercalcemia, renal insufficiency with azotemia, alkalosis, and ocular lesions
Norfloxacin / ↓ Bioavailability of norfloxacin
Sodium polystyrene sulfonate / Metabolic alkalosis and ↓ binding of resin to potassium in patients with renal impairment
Tetracyclines / ↓ Effect of tetracyclines due to ↓ absorption from GI tract
Thiazide diuretics / Hypercalcemia due to thiazide-induced renal tubular reabsorption of calcium and bone release of calcium
Verapamil / Calcium antagonizes the effect of verapamil
Vitamin D / Enhances intestinal absorption of dietary calcium

EMS CONSIDERATIONS
None.

CARDIAC GLYCOSIDES

See also:

Digoxin

Mechanism of Action: Cardiac glycosides increase the force and velocity of myocardial contraction (positive inotropic effect) by increasing the refractory period of the AV node and increasing total peripheral resistance. This effect is due to inhibition of sodium/potassium–ATPase in the sarcolemmal membrane, which alters excitation–contraction coupling. Inhibiting sodium, potassium–ATPase, results in an increase of calcium influx and an increased release of free calcium ions within the myocardial cells, which then potentiate the contractility of cardiac muscle fibers. The digitalis glycosides also decrease the rate of conduction and increase the refractory period of the AV node due to an increase in parasympathetic tone and a decrease in sympathetic tone. Clinical effects are not seen until steady-state plasma levels are reached. The initial dose of digitalis glycosides is larger (loading dose) and is traditionally referred to as the *digitalizing dose;* subsequent doses are referred to as *maintenance doses.*

Uses: All types of CHF, including that due to venous congestion, edema, dyspnea, orthopnea, and cardiac arrhythmia. Control of rapid ventricular contraction rate in patients with atrial fibrillation or flutter. Slow HR in sinus tachycardia due to CHF. Supraventricular tachycardia. Prophylaxis and treatment of recurrent paroxysmal atrial tachycardia with paroxysmal AV junctional rhythm. Cardiogenic shock (value not established).

Contraindications: Ventricular fibrillation or tachycardia (unless congestive failure supervenes after protracted episode not due to digitalis), in presence of digitalis toxicity, hypersensitivity to cardiac glycosides, beriberi heart disease, certain cases of hypersensitive carotid sinus syndrome.

Precautions: Use with caution in patients with ischemic heart disease, acute myocarditis, hypertrophic subaortic stenosis, hypoxic or myxedemic states, Adams-Stokes or carotid sinus syndromes, cardiac amyloidosis, or cyanotic heart and lung disease, including emphysema and partial heart block. Those with carditis associated with rheumatic fever or viral myocarditis are especially sensitive to digoxin-induced disturbances in rhythm. Electric pacemakers may sensitize the myocardium to cardiac glycosides. Also use with caution and at reduced dosage in elderly, debilitated patients, pregnant women and nursing mothers, and newborn, term, or premature infants who have immature renal and hepatic function

and in reduced renal and/or hepatic function.

Side Effects: Cardiac glycosides are extremely toxic and have caused death even in patients who have received the drugs for long periods of time. There is a narrow margin of safety between an effective therapeutic dose and a toxic dose. Overdosage caused by the cumulative effects of the drug is a constant danger in therapy with cardiac glycosides. Digitalis toxicity is characterized by a wide variety of symptoms, which are hard to differentiate from those of the cardiac disease itself.

CV: Changes in the rate, rhythm, and irritability of the heart and the mechanism of the heartbeat. Extrasystoles, bigeminal pulse, coupled rhythm, ectopic beat, and other forms of arrhythmias have been noted. ***Death most often results from ventricular fibrillation.*** Cardiac glycosides should be discontinued in adults when pulse rate falls below 60 beats/min. All cardiac changes are best detected by the ECG, which is also most useful in patients suffering from intoxication. ***Acute hemorrhage.*** *GI:* Anorexia, N&V, excessive salivation, epigastric distress, abdominal pain, diarrhea, bowel necrosis. Patients on digitalis therapy may experience two vomiting stages. The first is an early sign of toxicity and is a direct effect of digitalis on the GI tract. Late vomiting indicates stimulation of the vomiting center of the brain, which occurs after the heart muscle has been saturated with digitalis. *CNS:* Headaches, fatigue, lassitude, irritability, malaise, muscle weakness, insomnia, stupor. Psychotomimetic effects (especially in elderly or arteriosclerotic patients or neonates) including disorientation, confusion, depression, aphasia, delirium, hallucinations, and, rarely, ***convulsions.*** *Neuromuscular:* Neurologic pain involving the lower third of the face and lumbar areas, paresthesia. *Visual disturbances:* Blurred vision, flickering dots, white halos, borders

---

bold italic = life threatening side effect

around dark objects, diplopia, amblyopia, color perception changes. *Hypersensitivity (5–7 days after starting therapy):* Skin reactions (urticaria, fever, pruritus, facial and **angioneurotic edema**). *Other:* Chest pain, coldness of extremities.

OD **Overdose Management:** The relationship of cardiac glycoside levels to symptoms of toxicity varies significantly from patient to patient; thus, it is not possible to identify glycoside levels that would define toxicity accurately. *Symptoms (Toxicity): GI:* Anorexia, N&V, diarrhea, abdominal discomfort, or pain. *CNS:* Blurred, yellow, or green vision and halo effect; headache, weakness, drowsiness, mental depression, apathy, restlessness, disorientation, confusion, **seizures,** EEG abnormalities, delirium, hallucinations, neuralgia, psychosis. *CV:* Ventricular tachycardia, unifocal or multiform PVCs (especially in bigeminal or trigeminal patterns), paroxysmal and nonparoxysmal nodal rhythms, AV dissociation, accelerated junctional rhythm, excessive slowing of the pulse, *AV block (may proceed to complete block),* atrial fibrillation, *ventricular fibrillation (most common cause of death).* Children: Visual disturbances, headache, weakness, apathy, and psychosis occur but may be difficult to recognize. *CV:* Conduction disturbances, supraventricular tachyarrhythmias (e.g., *AV block*), atrial tachycardia with or without block, nodal tachycardia, unifocal or multiform ventricular premature contractions, ventricular tachycardia, sinus bradycardia (especially in infants). *Treatment in Adults:*

• Discontinue drug and admit to the intensive care area for continuous monitoring of ECG.

• If serum potassium is below normal, potassium chloride should be administered in divided PO doses totaling 3–6 g (40–80 mEq). Potassium should not be used when severe or complete heart block is due to digitalis and not related to tachycardia.

• *Atropine:* A dose of 0.01 mg/kg IV to treat severe sinus bradycardia or slow ventricular rate due to secondary AV block.

• *Cholestyramine, colestipol, activated charcoal:* To bind digitalis in the intestine, thus preventing enterohepatic recirculation.

• *Digoxin immune FAB:* See drug entry. Given in approximate equimolar quantities as digoxin, it reverses S&S of toxicity, often with improvement seen within 30 min.

• *Lidocaine:* A dose of 1 mg/kg given over 5 min followed by an infusion of 15–50 mcg/kg/min to maintain normal cardiac rhythm.

• *Phenytoin:* For atrial or ventricular arrhythmias unresponsive to potassium, can give a dose of 0.5 mg/kg at a rate not exceeding 50 mg/min (given at 1–2 hr intervals). The maximum dose should not exceed 10 mg/kg/day.

• *Countershock:* A direct-current countershock can be used *only as a last resort*. If required, therapy should be initiated at low voltage levels.

Treatment in Children: Give potassium in divided doses totaling 1–1.5 mEq/kg (if correction of arrhythmia is urgent, a dose of 0.5 mEq/kg/hr can be used) with careful monitoring of the ECG. The potassium IV solution should be dilute to avoid local irritation although IV fluid overload must be avoided. Digoxin immune FAB may also be used.

Digoxin is not removed effectively by dialysis, by exchange transfusion, or during cardiopulmonary bypass as most of the drug is found in tissues rather than the circulating blood. Digitoxin is not effectively removed by either peritoneal or hemodialysis due to its high degree of plasma protein binding.

Drug Interactions: One of the most serious side effects of digitalis-type drugs is hypokalemia (lowering of serum potassium levels). This may lead to cardiac arrhythmias, muscle weakness, hypotension, and respiratory distress. Other agents causing hypokalemia reinforce this effect and increase the chance of digitalis toxicity. Such reactions may occur in patients who have been on digitalis maintenance for a long time.

Albuterol / ↑ Skeletal muscle binding of digoxin

Amiloride / ↓ Inotropic effects of digoxin

Aminoglycosides / ↓ Effect of digitalis glycosides due to ↓ absorption from GI tract

Aminosalicylic acid / ↓ Effect of digitalis glycosides due to ↓ absorption from GI tract

Amphotericin B / ↑ K depletion caused by digitalis; ↑ risk of digitalis toxicity

Antacids / ↓ Effect of digitalis glycosides due to ↓ absorption from GI tract

Beta blockers / Complete heart block possible

Calcium preparations / Cardiac arrhythmias if parenteral calcium given with digitalis

Chlorthalidone / ↑ K and Mg loss with ↑ chance of digitalis toxicity

Cholestyramine / Binds digitoxin in the intestine and ↓ its absorption

Colestipol / Binds digitoxin in the intestine and ↓ its absorption

Ephedrine / ↑ Chance of cardiac arrhythmias

Epinephrine / ↑ Chance of cardiac arrhythmias

Ethacrynic acid / ↑ K and Mg loss with ↑ chance of digitalis toxicity

Furosemide / ↑ K and Mg loss with ↑ chance of digitalis toxicity

Glucose infusions / Large infusions of glucose may cause ↓ in serum potassium and ↑ chance of digitalis toxicity

Hypoglycemic drugs / ↓ Effect of digitalis glycosides due to ↑ breakdown by liver

Methimazole / ↑ Chance of toxic effects of digitalis

Metoclopramide / ↓ Effect of digitalis glycosides by ↓ absorption from GI tract

Muscle relaxants, nondepolarizing / ↑ Risk of cardiac arrhythmias

Propranolol / Potentiates digitalis-induced bradycardia

Reserpine / ↑ Chance of cardiac arrhythmias

Spironolactone / Either ↑ or ↓ toxic effects of digitalis glycosides

Succinylcholine / ↑ Chance of cardiac arrhythmias

Sulfasalazine / ↓ Effect of digitalis glycosides by ↓ absorption from GI tract

Sympathomimetics / ↑ Chance of cardiac arrhythmias

Thiazides / ↑ K and Mg loss with ↑ chance of digitalis toxicity

Thioamines / ↑ Effect and toxicity of cardiac glycosides

Thyroid / ↓ Effectiveness of digitalis glycosides

Triamterene / ↑ Pharmacologic effects of digoxin

EMS CONSIDERATIONS
Assessment
1. Obtain ECG; note rhythm/rate.
2. Document cardiopulmonary findings; note presence of S3, JVD, HJR, HR above 100 bpm, rales, peripheral edema, DOE, PND,.
Interventions
1. Observe monitor for bradycardia and/or arrhythmias.
• Document adult HR below 50 bpm or if an arrhythmia (irregular pulse) occurs.

CEPHALOSPORINS

See also the following individual entries:

Cefaclor
Cefadroxil monohydrate
Cefazolin sodium
Cefdinir
Cefepime hydrochloride
Cefixime oral
Cefoperazone sodium
Cefotaxime sodium
Cefotetan disodium
Cefoxitin sodium
Cefpodoxime proxetil
Cefprozil
Ceftazidime
Ceftibuten
Ceftizoxime sodium

bold italic = life threatening side effect

Ceftriaxone sodium
Cefuroxime axetil
Cefuroxime sodium
Cephalexin hydrochloride monohydrate
Cephalexin monohydrate
Cephapirin sodium
Cephradine
Loracarbef

Mechanism of Action: The cephalosporins interfere with a final step in the formation of the bacterial cell wall (inhibition of mucopeptide biosynthesis), resulting in unstable cell membranes that undergo lysis (same mechanism of actions as penicillins). Also, cell division and growth are inhibited. The cephalosporins are most effective against young, rapidly dividing organisms and are considered bactericidal. Cephalosporins are widely distributed to most tissues and fluids. First- and second-generation drugs do not enter the CSF well but third-generation drugs enter inflamed meninges readily. Rapidly excreted by the kidneys.

General Statement: Cephalosporins are broad-spectrum antibiotics classified as first-, second-, and third-generation drugs. The difference among generations is based on pharmacokinetics and antibacterial spectra. Generally, third-generation cephalosporins have more activity against gram-negative organisms and resistant organisms and less activity against gram-positive organisms than first-generation drugs. Third-generation cephalosporins are also stable against beta-lactamases. Cephalosporins can be destroyed by cephalosporinase.

See also *General Nursing Considerations for All Anti-Infectives.*

Uses: See individual drugs. A listing of the drugs in each generation follows:

First-Generation Cephalosporins: Cefadroxil, cefazolin, cephalexin, cephapirin, cephradine.

Second-Generation Cephalosporins: Cefaclor, cefmetazole, cefonicid, cefotetan, cefoxitin, cefprozil, cefuroxime, and loracarbef.

Third-Generation Cephalosporins: Cefdinir, cefepime, cefixime, cefoperazone, cefotaxime, cefpodoxime, ceftazidime, ceftibuten, ceftizoxime, ceftriaxone.

Contraindications: Hypersensitivity to cephalosporins or related antibiotics.

Precautions: Safe use in pregnancy and lactation has not been established (pregnancy category: B). Use with caution in the presence of impaired renal or hepatic function, together with other nephrotoxic drugs, and in patients over 50 years of age. Perform C_{cr} on all patients with impaired renal function who receive cephalosporins. If hypersensitive to penicillin, may occasionally cross-react to cephalosporins.

Side Effects: *GI:* N&V, diarrhea, abdominal cramps or pain, dyspepsia, glossitis, heartburn, sore mouth or tongue, dysgeusia, anorexia, flatulence, cholestasis. Pseudomembranous colitis. *Allergic:* Urticaria, rashes (maculopapular, morbilliform, or erythematous), pruritus (including anal and genital areas), fever, chills, erythema, *angioedema,* serum sickness, joint pain, exfoliative dermatitis, chest tightness, myalgia, erythema multiforme, edema, itching, numbness, chills, *Stevens-Johnson syndrome, anaphylaxis. NOTE:* Cross-allergy may be manifested between cephalosporins and penicillins. *Hematologic:* Leukopenia, leukocytosis, lymphocytosis, neutropenia (transient), eosinophilia, thrombocytopenia, thrombocythemia, *agranulocytosis,* granulocytopenia, bone marrow depression, *hemolytic anemia,* pancytopenia, decreased platelet function, *aplastic anemia,* hypoprothrombinemia (may lead to bleeding), thrombocytosis (transient). *CNS:* Headache, malaise, fatigue, vertigo, dizziness, lethargy, confusion, paresthesia, precipitation of *seizures* (especially in patients with impaired renal function). *Hepatic:* Hepatomegaly, hepatitis. Intrathecal use may result in hallucinations, nystagmus, or *seizures. Miscellaneous:* Superinfection including oral candidiasis and enterococcal infections, hypotension, sweating, flushing, dyspnea, interstitial pneumonitis.

IV or IM use may result in local swelling, inflammation, cellulitis, paresthesia, burning, phlebitis, thrombophlebitis. IM use may also cause pain and induration, tenderness, increased temperature. Sterile abscesses have been observed following SC use. Nephrotoxicity (↑ BUN with and without ↑ serum creatinine) may occur in patients over 50 and in young children.

OD **Overdose Management:** *Symptoms:* Parenteral use of large doses of cephalosporins may cause seizures, especially in patients with impaired renal function. *Treatment:* If seizures occur, discontinue the drug immediately and give anticonvulsant drugs. Hemodialysis may also be effective.

Drug Interactions
Alcohol / Antabuse-like reaction if used with cefazolin, cefmetazole, cefoperazone, or cefotetan
Aminoglycosides / ↑ Risk of renal toxicity with certain cephalosporins
Antacids / ↓ Plasma levels of cefaclor, cefdinir, or cefpodoxime
Anticoagulants / ↑ Hypoprothrombinemic effects if used with cefazolin, cefmetazole, cefoperazone, or cefotetan
Colistimethate / ↑ Risk of renal toxicity
Colistin / ↑ Risk of renal toxicity
Ethacrynic acid / ↑ Risk of renal toxicity
Furosemide / ↑ Risk of renal toxicity
H_2 antagonists / ↓ *Plasma levels of cefpodoxime or cefuroxime*
Polymyxin B / ↑ Risk of renal toxicity
Probenecid / ↑ Effect of cephalosporins by ↓ excretion by kidneys
Vancomycin / ↑ Risk of renal toxicity

EMS CONSIDERATIONS

See also *Anti-Infectives*.

CHOLINERGIC BLOCKING AGENTS

Atropine sulfate
Benztropine mesylate
Biperiden hydrochloride
Dicyclomine hydrochloride
Ipratropium bromide
Propantheline bromide
Scopolamine hydrobromide
Scopolamine transdermal
    therapeutic system
Trihexyphenidyl hydrochloride

Mechanism of Action: Cholinergic blocking agents prevent the neurotransmitter acetylcholine from combining with receptors on the postganglionic parasympathetic nerve terminal (muscarinic site). Effects include reduction of smooth muscle spasms, blockade of vagal impulses to the heart, decreased secretions (e.g., gastric, salivation, bronchial mucus, sweat glands), production of mydriasis and cycloplegia, and various CNS effects. In therapeutic doses, these drugs have little effect on transmission of nerve impulses across ganglia (nicotinic sites) or at the neuromuscular junction. Several anticholinergic drugs abolish or reduce the S&S of Parkinson's disease, such as tremors and rigidity, and result in some improvement in mobility, muscular coordination, and motor performance. These effects may be due to blockade of the effects of acetylcholine in the CNS.

Uses: See individual drugs.

Contraindications: Glaucoma, adhesions between iris and lens of the eye, tachycardia, myocardial ischemia, unstable CV state in acute hemorrhage, partial obstruction of the GI and biliary tracts, prostatic hypertrophy, renal disease, myasthenia gravis, hepatic disease, paralytic ileus, pyloroduodenal stenosis, pyloric obstruction, intestinal atony, ulcerative colitis, obstructive uropathy. Cardiac patients, especially when there is danger of tachycardia; older persons suffering from atherosclerosis or mental impairment. Lactation.

---

bold italic = life threatening side effect

Precautions: Use with caution in pregnancy. Infants and young children are more susceptible to the toxic side effects of anticholinergic drugs. Use in children when the ambient temperature is high may cause a rapid increase in body temperature due to suppression of sweat glands. Geriatric patients are particularly likely to manifest anticholinergic side effects and CNS effects, including agitation, confusion, drowsiness, excitement, glaucoma, and impaired memory. Use with caution in hyperthyroidism, CHF, cardiac arrhythmias, hypertension, Down syndrome, asthma, spastic paralysis, blonde individuals, allergies, and chronic lung disease.

Side Effects: These are desirable in some conditions and undesirable in others. Thus, the anticholinergics have an antisalivary effect that is useful in parkinsonism. This same effect is unpleasant when the drug is used for spastic conditions of the GI tract. Most side effects are dose-related and decrease when dosage decreases. *GI:* N&V, dry mouth, dysphagia, constipation, heartburn, change in taste perception, bloated feeling, paralytic ileus. *CNS:* Dizziness, drowsiness, nervousness, disorientation, headache, weakness, insomnia, fever (especially in children). Large doses may produce CNS stimulation including tremor and restlessness. Anticholinergic psychoses: ataxia, euphoria, confusion, disorientation, loss of short-term memory, decreased anxiety, fatigue, insomnia, hallucinations, dysarthria, agitation. *CV:* Palpitations. *GU:* Urinary retention or hesitancy, impotence. *Ophthalmologic:* Blurred vision, dilated pupils, photophobia, cycloplegia, precipitation of acute glaucoma. *Allergic:* Urticaria, skin rashes, ***anaphylaxis.*** *Other:* Flushing, decreased sweating, nasal congestion, suppression of glandular secretions including lactation. Heat prostration (fever and heat stroke) in presence of high environmental temperatures due to decreased sweating.

OD **Overdose Management:** *Symptoms* *("Belladonna Poison-*

ing"): Infants and children are especially susceptible to the toxic effects of atropine and scopolamine. Poisoning (dose-dependent) is characterized by the following symptoms: dry mouth, burning sensation of the mouth, difficulty in swallowing and speaking, blurred vision, photophobia, rash, tachycardia, increased respiration, ***increased body temperature*** (up to 109°F, 42.7°C), restlessness, irritability, confusion, muscle incoordination, dilated pupils, hot dry skin, ***respiratory depression and paralysis,*** tremors, ***seizures,*** hallucinations, and ***death.*** *Treatment ("Belladonna Poisoning"):*

• Gastric lavage or induction of vomiting followed by activated charcoal. General supportive measures.

• Anticholinergic effects can be reversed by physostigmine (Eserine), 1–3 mg IV (effectiveness uncertain; thus use other agents if possible). Neostigmine methylsulfate, 0.5–2 mg IV, repeated as necessary.

• If there is excitation, diazepam, a short-acting barbiturate, IV sodium thiopental (2% solution), or chloral hydrate (100–200 mL of a 2% solution by rectal infusion) may be given.

• For fever, cool baths may be used. Keep patient in a darkened room if photophobia is manifested.

• Artificial respiration should be instituted if there is paralysis of respiratory muscles.

Drug Interactions

Amantadine / Additive anticholinergic side effects

Antacids / ↓ Absorption of anticholinergics from GI tract

Antidepressants, tricyclic / Additive anticholinergic side effects

Antihistamines / Additive anticholinergic side effects

Atenolol / Anticholinergics ↑ effects of atenolol

Benzodiazepines / Additive anticholinergic side effects

Corticosteroids / Additive ↑ intraocular pressure

Cyclopropane / ↑ Chance of ventricular arrhythmias

Digoxin / ↑ Effect of digoxin due to ↑ absorption from GI tract

Disopyramide / Potentiation of anti-cholinergic side effects

Guanethidine / Reversal of inhibition of gastric acid secretion caused by anticholinergics

Haloperidol / Additive ↑ intraocular pressure

Histamine / Reversal of inhibition of gastric acid secretion caused by anticholinergics

Levodopa / Possible ↓ effect of levodopa due to ↑ breakdown of levodopa in stomach (due to delayed gastric emptying time)

MAO inhibitors / ↑ Effect of anticholinergics due to ↓ breakdown by liver

Meperidine / Additive anticholinergic side effects

Methylphenidate / Potentiation of anticholinergic side effects

Metoclopramide / Anticholinergics block action of metoclopramide

Nitrates, nitrites / Potentiation of anticholinergic side effects

Nitrofurantoin / ↑ Bioavailability of nitrofurantoin

Orphenadrine / Additive anticholinergic side effects

Phenothiazines / Additive anticholinergic side effects; also, effects of phenothiazines may ↓

Primidone / Potentiation of anticholinergic side effects

Procainamide / Additive anticholinergic side effects

Quinidine / Additive anticholinergic side effects

Reserpine / Reversal of inhibition of gastric acid secretion caused by anticholinergics

Sympathomimetics / ↑ Bronchial relaxation

Thiazide diuretics / ↑ Bioavailability of thiazide diuretics

Thioxanthines / Potentiation of anticholinergic side effects

EMS CONSIDERATIONS

Assessment: Monitor VS and ECG. Assess for any hemodynamic changes and intraventricular conduction blocks.

CORTICOSTEROIDS

See also the following individual entries:

Beclomethasone dipropionate
Betamethasone
Betamethasone dipropionate
Betamethasone sodium
  phosphate
Betamethasone sodium
  phosphate and Betamethasone
  acetate
Betamethasone valerate
Budesonide
Corticotropin injection
Corticotropin repository injection
Cortisone acetate
Dexamethasone
Dexamethasone acetate
Dexamethasone sodium
  phosphate
Fludrocortisone acetate
Flunisolide
Fluticasone propionate
Hydrocortisone
Hydrocortisone acetate
Hydrocortisone butyrate
Hydrocortisone cypionate
Hydrocortisone sodium
  phosphate
Hydrocortisone sodium succinate
Hydrocortisone valerate
Loteprednol etabonate
Methylprednisolone
Methylprednisolone acetate
Methylprednisolone sodium
  succinate
Mometasone furoate
  monohydrate
Prednisolone
Prednisolone acetate
Prednisolone acetate and
  Prednisolone sodium
  phosphate
Prednisolone sodium phosphate
Prednisolone tebutate
Prednisone
Rimexolone
Triamcinolone
Triamcinolone acetonide
Triamcinolone diacetate
Triamcinolone hexacetonide

Mechanism of Action: The hormones of the adrenal gland influence many metabolic pathways and all organ systems and are essential for survival. These processes include carbohydrate metabolism (e.g., glycogen deposition in the liver and conversion of glycogen to glucose), protein metabolism (e.g., gluconeogenesis, protein catabolism), fat metabolism (e.g., deposition of fatty tissue), and water and electrolyte balance (e.g., fluid retention, excretion of potassium, calcium, and phosphorus).

According to their chemical structure and chief physiologic effect, the corticosteroids fall into two subgroups, which have considerable functional overlap. First are those, like cortisone and hydrocortisone, that mainly regulate the metabolic pathways involving protein, carbohydrate, and fat. This group is often referred to as *glucocorticoids*. In the second group are those, like aldosterone and desoxycorticosterone, that are more specifically involved in electrolyte and water balance. These are often referred to as *mineralocorticoids*. Hormones, such as cortisone and hydrocortisone, although classified as glucocorticoids, possess significant mineralocorticoid activity. Therapeutically, a distinction must be made between physiologic doses used for replacement therapy and pharmacologic doses used to treat inflammatory and other disease states.

The hormones have a marked anti-inflammatory effect because of their ability to inhibit prostaglandin synthesis. These agents also inhibit accumulation of macrophages and leukocytes at sites of inflammation as well as inhibit phagocytosis and lysosomal enzyme release. They aid the organism in coping with various stressful situations (trauma, severe illness). The immunosuppressant effect is thought to be due to a reduction of the number of T lymphocytes, monocytes, and eosinophils. Corticosteroids also decrease binding of immunoglobulin to receptors on the cell surface and inhibit the synthesis and/or release of interleukins which, in turn, decrease T-lymphocyte blastogenesis and reduce the primary immune response.

Uses: When used for anti-inflammatory or immunosuppressant therapy, the corticosteroid should possess minimal mineralocorticoid activity. Therapy with glucocorticoids is not curative and in many situations should be considered as adjunctive rather than primary therapy. The following list is not inclusive but provides examples of the physiologic and pharmacologic uses of corticosteroids.

1. **Replacement therapy.** Acute and chronic adrenal insufficiency, including Addison's disease. For replacement therapy, drugs must possess both glucocorticoid and mineralocorticoid effects.

2. **Rheumatic disorders,** including rheumatoid arthritis (including juveniles), other types of arthritis, ankylosing spondylitis, acute and subacute bursitis.

3. **Collagen diseases,** including SLE.

4. **Allergic diseases,** including control of severe allergic conditions as serum sickness, drug hypersensitivity reactions, anaphylaxis.

5. **Respiratory diseases,** including prophylaxis and treatment of bronchial asthma (and status asthmaticus), seasonal or perennial rhinitis.

6. **Ocular diseases,** including severe acute and chronic allergic and inflammatory conditions. Corneal injury.

7. **Dermatologic diseases,** including angioedema or urticaria, contact dermatitis, atopic dermatitis, severe erythema multiforme (Stevens-Johnson syndrome).

8. **Diseases of the intestinal tract,** including chronic ulcerative colitis, regional enteritis.

9. **Nervous system,** including acute exacerbations of multiple sclerosis, optic neuritis.

10. **Malignancies,** including leukemias and lymphomas in adults and acute leukemia in children.

11. **Nephrotic syndrome,** includ-

ing that due to lupus erythematosus or of the idiopathic type.

12. **Hematologic diseases,** including acquired hemolytic anemia, RBC anemia, idiopathic and secondary thrombocytopenic purpura in adults, congenital hypoplastic anemia.

13. **Intra-articular or soft tissue administration,** including acute episodes of synovitis osteoarthritis, rheumatoid arthritis, acute gouty arthritis, bursitis.

14. **Intralesional administration,** including keloids, psoriatic plaques, discoid lupus erythematosus.

Lotions are considered best for weeping eruptions, especially in areas subject to chafing (axilla, feet, and groin). Creams are suitable for most inflammations; ointments are preferred for dry, scaly lesions.

Contraindications: Suspected infection as these drugs may mask infections. Also peptic ulcer, psychoses, acute glomerulonephritis, herpes simplex infections of the eye, vaccinia or varicella, the exanthematous diseases, Cushing's syndrome, active tuberculosis, myasthenia gravis. Recent intestinal anastomoses, CHF or other cardiac disease, hypertension, systemic fungal infections, open-angle glaucoma. Also, hyperlipidemia, hyperthyroidism or hypothyroidism, osteoporosis, myasthenia gravis, tuberculosis. Lactation (if high doses are used). Inhalation products to relieve acute bronchospasms.

Topically in the eye for dendritic keratitis, vaccinia, chickenpox, other viral disease that may involve the conjunctiva or cornea, and tuberculosis and fungal or acute purulent infections of the eye. Topically in the ear in aural fungal infections and perforated eardrum. Topically in tuberculosis of the skin, herpes simplex, vaccinia, varicella, and infectious conditions in the absence of anti-infective agents.

Inhalation products for relief of acute bronchospasms, primary treatment of status asthmaticus, or other acute episodes of asthma.

Precautions: Use with caution in diabetes mellitus, hypertension, chronic nephritis, thrombophlebitis, convulsive disorders, infectious diseases, renal or hepatic insufficiency, pregnancy. Chronic use may inhibit the growth and development of children or adolescents. Pediatric patients are also at greater risk for developing cataracts, osteoporosis, avascular necrosis of the femoral heads, and glaucoma. Geriatric patients are more likely to develop hypertension and osteoporosis (especially postmenopausal women). Use inhalation products with caution in children less than 6 years of age.

Side Effects: Small physiologic doses given as replacement therapy or short-term high-dosage therapy during emergencies rarely cause side effects. Prolonged therapy may cause a Cushing-like syndrome with atrophy of the adrenal cortex and subsequent adrenocortical insufficiency. A steroid withdrawal syndrome may occur following prolonged use; symptoms include anorexia, N&V, lethargy, headache, fever, joint pain, desquamation, myalgia, weight loss, hypotension.

SYSTEMIC: *Fluid and electrolyte:* Edema, hypokalemic alkalosis, hypokalemia, hypocalcemia, hypotension or shock-like reaction, hypertension, CHF. *Musculoskeletal:* Muscle wasting, muscle pain or weakness, osteoporosis, spontaneous fractures including vertebral compression fractures and fractures of long bones, tendon rupture, aseptic necrosis of femoral and humeral heads. *GI:* N&V, anorexia or increased appetite, diarrhea or constipation, abdominal distention, pancreatitis, gastric irritation, ulcerative esophagitis. ***Development or exacerbation of peptic ulcers with the possibility of perforation and hemorrhage; perforation of the small and large bowel,*** especially in inflammatory bowel disease. *Endocrine:* Cushing's syndrome (e.g., central obesity, moonface, buffalo hump, enlargement of supraclavicular fat

---

bold italic = life threatening side effect

pads), amenorrhea, postmenopausal bleeding, menstrual irregularities, decreased glucose tolerance, hyperglycemia, glycosuria, increased insulin or sulfonylurea requirement in diabetics, development of diabetes mellitus, negative nitrogen balance due to protein catabolism, suppression of growth in children, secondary adrenocortical and pituitary unresponsiveness (especially during periods of stress). *CNS/Neurologic:* Headache, vertigo, insomnia, restlessness, increased motor activity, ischemic neuropathy, EEG abnormalities, ***seizures,*** pseudotumor cerebri. Also, euphoria, mood swings, depression, anxiety, personality changes, psychoses. *CV:* Thromboembolism, thrombophlebitis, ECG changes (due to potassium deficiency), fat embolism, necrotizing angiitis, cardiac arrhythmias, ***myocardial rupture following recent MI,*** syncopal episodes. *Dermatologic:* Impaired wound healing, skin atrophy and thinning, petechiae, ecchymoses, erythema, purpura, striae, hirsutism, urticaria, ***angioneurotic edema,*** acneiform eruptions, allergic dermatitis, lupus erythematosus-like lesions, suppression of skin test reactions, perineal irritation. *Ophthalmic:* Glaucoma, posterior subcapsular cataracts, increased intraocular pressure, exophthalmos. *Miscellaneous:* Hypercholesterolemia, atherosclerosis, aggravation or masking of infections, leukocytosis, increased or decreased motility and number of spermatozoa. **In children:** Suppression of linear growth; reversible pseudo-brain tumor syndrome characterized by papilledema, oculomotor or abducens nerve paralysis, visual loss, or headache.

PARENTERAL USE: Sterile abscesses, Charcot-like arthropathy, subcutaneous and cutaneous atrophy, burning or tingling (especially in the perineal area following IV use), scarring, inflammation, paresthesia, induration, hyperpigmentation or hypopigmentation, blindness when used intralesionally around the face and head (rare), transient or delayed pain or soreness, nystagmus, ataxia, muscle twitching, hiccoughs, ***anaphylaxis with or without circulatory collapse, cardiac arrest, bronchospasm,*** arachnoiditis after intrathecal use, foreign body granulomatous reactions.

INTRA-ARTICULAR: Postinjection flare, Charcot-like arthropathy, tendon rupture, skin atrophy, facial flushing, osteonecrosis. Due to reduction in inflammation and pain, patients may overuse the joint.

INTRASPINAL: Aseptic, bacterial, chemical, cryptococcal, or tubercular meningitis; adhesive arachnoiditis, conus medullaris syndrome.

INTRAOCULAR: Increased ocular pressure, thereby inducing or aggravating simple glaucoma. Stinging, burning, dendritic keratitis (herpes simplex), corneal perforation (especially when the drugs are used for diseases that cause corneal thinning). Posterior subcapsular cataracts, especially in children. Exophthalmos, secondary fungal or viral eye infections.

TOPICAL USE: When used over large areas, when the skin is broken, or with occlusive dressings, may cause atrophy of the epidermis, drying of the skin, or atrophy of the dermal collagen. When used on the face, diffuse thinning and homogenization of the collagen, epidermal thinning, and striae formation. Occasionally, sensitization reaction may occur, which necessitates discontinuation of the drug.

OD **Overdose Management:** *Symptoms (Continued Use of Large Doses)—Cushing's Syndrome:* Acne, hypertension, moonface, striae, hirsutism, central obesity, ecchymoses, myopathy, sexual dysfunction, osteoporosis, diabetes, hyperlipidemia, increased susceptibility to infection, peptic ulcer, electrolyte and fluid imbalance. Acute toxicity or death is rare. *Treatment of Chronic Overdose:* Gradually taper the dose of the steroid and frequently monitor lab tests. During periods of stress, steroid supplementation is necessary. Dose should be reduced to the lowest one that will control the symptoms (or discontinue the steroid completely). Recovery of normal adrenal and pituitary function may take up to 9 months. Large, acute overdoses may be treated with gastric lavage, emesis, and general supportive measures.

Drug Interactions

Acetaminophen / ↑ Risk of hepatotoxicity due to ↑ rate of formation of hepatotoxic acetaminophen metabolite

Alcohol / ↑ Risk of GI ulceration or hemorrhage

Amphotericin B / Corticosteroids ↑ K depletion caused by amphotericin B

Aminoglutethimide / ↓ Adrenal response to corticotropin

Anabolic steroids / ↑ Risk of edema

Antacids / ↓ Effect of corticosteroids due to ↓ absorption from GI tract

Antibiotics, broad-spectrum / Concomitant use may result in emergence of resistant strains, leading to severe infection

Anticholinergics / Combination ↑ intraocular pressure; will aggravate glaucoma

Anticoagulants, oral / ↓ Effect of anticoagulants by ↓ hypoprothrombinemia; also ↑ risk of hemorrhage due to vascular effects of corticosteroids

Anticholinesterases / Corticosteroids may ↓ effect of anticholinesterases when used in myasthenia gravis

Antidiabetic agents / Hyperglycemic effect of corticosteroids may necessitate an ↑ dose of antidiabetic agent

Asparaginase / ↑ Hyperglycemic effect of asparaginase and the risk of neuropathy and disturbances in erythropoiesis

Barbiturates / ↓ Effect of corticosteroids due to ↑ breakdown by liver

Bumetanide / Enhanced potassium loss due to potassium-losing properties of both drugs

Carbonic anhydrase inhibitors / Corticosteroids ↑ K depletion caused by carbonic anhydrase inhibitors

Cholestyramine / ↓ Effect of corticosteroids due to ↓ absorption from GI tract

Colestipol / ↓ Effect of corticosteroids due to ↓ absorption from GI tract

Contraceptives, oral / Estrogen ↑ anti-inflammatory effect of hydrocortisone by ↓ breakdown by liver

Cyclophosphoramide / ↑ Effect of cyclophosphoramide due to ↓ breakdown by liver

Cyclosporine / ↑ Effect of both drugs due to ↓ breakdown by liver

Digitalis glycosides / ↑ Chance of digitalis toxicity (arrhythmias) due to hypokalemia

Ephedrine / ↓ Effect of corticosteroids due to ↑ breakdown by liver

Estrogens / ↑ Anti-inflammatory effect of hydrocortisone by ↓ breakdown by liver

Ethacrynic acid / Enhanced potassium loss due to potassium-losing properties of both drugs

Folic acid / Requirements may ↑

Furosemide / Enhanced potassium loss due to potassium-losing properties of both drugs

Heparin / Ulcerogenic effects of corticosteroids may ↑ risk of hemorrhage

Immunosuppressant drugs / ↑ Risk of infection

Indomethacin / ↑ Chance of GI ulceration

Insulin / Hyperglycemic effect of corticosteroids may necessitate ↑ dose of antidiabetic agent

Isoniazid / ↓ Effect of isoniazid due to ↑ breakdown by liver and ↑ excretion

Ketoconazole / ↓ Effect of corticosteroids due to ↑ rate of clearance

Mexiletine / ↓ Effect of mexiletine due to ↑ breakdown by liver

Mitotane / ↓ Response of adrenal gland to corticotropin

Muscle relaxants, nondepolarizing / ↓ Effect of muscle relaxants

Neuromuscular blocking agents / ↑ Risk of prolonged respiratory depression or paralysis

---

bold italic = life threatening side effect

NSAIDs / ↑ Risk of GI hemorrhage or ulceration

Phenobarbital / ↓ Effect of corticosteroids due to ↑ breakdown by liver

Phenytoin / ↓ Effect of corticosteroids due to ↑ breakdown by liver

Potassium supplements / ↓ Plasma levels of potassium

Rifampin / ↓ Effect of corticosteroids due to ↑ breakdown by liver

Ritodrine / ↑ Risk of maternal edema

Salicylates / Both are ulcerogenic; also, corticosteroids may ↓ blood salicylate levels

Somatrem, Somatropin / Glucocorticoids may inhibit effect of somatrem

Streptozocin / ↑ Risk of hyperglycemia

Theophyllines / Corticosteroids ↑ effect of theophyllines

Thiazide diuretics / Enhanced potassium loss due to potassium-losing properties of both drugs

Tricyclic antidepressants / ↑ Risk of mental disturbances

Vitamin A / Topical vitamin A can reverse impaired wound healing in patients receiving corticosteroids

EMS CONSIDERATIONS

None.

DIURETICS, LOOP

See also the following individual entries:

Bumetanide
Ethacrynate sodium
Ethacrynic acid
Furosemide
Torsemide

Mechanism of Action: Loop diuretics inhibit reabsorption of sodium and chloride in the proximal and distal tubules and the loop of Henle. Metabolized in the liver and excreted primarily through the urine. Significantly bound to plasma protein.
Uses: See individual drugs.
Contraindications: Hypersensitivity to loop diruetics or to sulfonylureas. In hepatic coma or severe electro-

lyte depletion (until condition improves or is corrected). Lactation.
Precautions: Sudden alterations of electrolytes in hepatic cirrhosis and ascites may precipitate hepatic encephalopathy and coma. SLE may be activated or worsened. Ototoxicity is most common with rapid injection, in severe renal impairment, with doses several times the usual dose, and with concurrent use of other ototoxic drugs. The risk of hospitalization is doubled in geriatric patients who take diuretics and NSAIDs. Safety and efficacy of most loop diuretics have not been determined in children or infants.
Side Effects: See individual drugs. Excessive diuresis may cause dehydration with the possibility of ***circulatory collapse and vascular thrombosis or embolism.*** Ototoxicity including tinnitus, hearing impairment, deafness (usually reversible), and vertigo with a sense of fullness are possible. Electrolyte imbalance, especially in patients with restricted salt intake. Photosensitivity. Changes include hypokalemia, hypomagnesemia, and hypocalcemia.
OD **Overdose Management:** *Symptoms:* Acute profound water loss, volume and electrolyte depletion, dehydration, decreased blood volume, and ***circulatory collapse with possibility of fascicular thrombosis and embolism.*** *Treatment:* Replace fluid and electrolyte loss. Carefully monitor urine and plasma electrolyte levels. Emesis and gastric lavage may be useful. Supportive measures may include oxygen or artificial respiration.
Drug Interactions
Aminoglycosides / ↑ Ototoxicity with hearing loss
Anticoagulants / ↑ Anticoagulant activity
Chloral hydrate / Transient diaphoresis, hot flashes, hypertension, tachycardia, weakness and nausea
Cisplatin / Additive ototoxicity
Digitalis glycosides / ↑ Risk of arrhythmias due to diuretic-induced electrolyte disturbances
Lithium / ↑ Plasma levels of lithium → toxicity

Muscle relaxants, nondepolarizing / Effect of muscle relaxants may be either ↑ or ↓, depending on the dose of diuretic

Nonsteroidal anti-inflammatory drugs / ↓ Effect of loop diuretics

Probenecid / ↓ Effect of loop diuretics

Salicylates / Diuretic effect may be ↓ in patients with cirrhosis and ascites

Sulfonylureas/ Loop diuretics may ↓ glucose tolerance

Theophyllines / Action of theophyllines may be ↑ or ↓

Thiazide diuretics / Additive effects with loop diuretics → profound diuresis and serious electrolyte abnormalities

EMS CONSIDERATIONS

See also *Diuretics, Thiazides.*

DIURETICS, THIAZIDES

See also the following individual entries:

Chlorothiazide
Chlorothiazide sodium
Chlorthalidone
Hydrochlorothiazide
Indapamide

Mechanism of Action: Thiazides promote diuresis by decreasing the rate at which sodium and chloride are reabsorbed by the distal renal tubules of the kidney. By increasing the excretion of sodium and chloride, they force excretion of additional water. They also increase the excretion of potassium and, to a lesser extent, bicarbonate, as well as decrease the excretion of calcium and uric acid. Sodium and chloride are excreted in approximately equal amounts. Thiazides do not affect the glomerular filtration rate. Thiazides also have an antihypertensive effect which is attributed to direct dilation of the arterioles, as well as to a reduction in the total fluid volume of the body and altered sodium balance. The thi-

azide diuretics are related chemically to the sulfonamides. Although devoid of anti-infective activity, the thiazides can cause the same hypersensitivity reactions as the sulfonamides. A large fraction is excreted unchanged in urine.

Uses: Edema, CHF, hypertension, pregnancy, and premenstrual tension. Thiazides are used for edema due to CHF, nephrosis, nephritis, renal failure, PMS, hepatic cirrhosis, corticosteroid or estrogen therapy. Hypertension. *Investigational:* Thiazides are used alone or in combination with allopurinol (or amiloride) for prophylaxis of calcium nephrolithiasis. Nephrogenic diabetes insipidus.

Contraindications: Hypersensitivity to drug, anuria, renal decompensation. Impaired renal function and advanced hepatic cirrhosis. Do not use indiscriminately in patients with edema and toxemia of pregnancy, even though they may be therapeutically useful, because the thiazides may have adverse effects on the newborn (thrombocytopenia and jaundice).

Precautions: Geriatric patients may manifest an increased risk of hypotension and changes in electrolyte levels. The risk of hospitalization is doubled in geriatric patients who take diuretics and NSAIDs. Administer with caution to debilitated patients or to those with a history of hepatic coma or precoma, gout, diabetes mellitus, or during pregnancy and lactation. Particular care must be exercised when thiazides are administered concomitantly with drugs that also cause potassium loss, such as digitalis, corticosteroids, and some estrogens. Patients with advanced heart failure, renal disease, or hepatic cirrhosis are most likely to develop hypokalemia. May activate or worsen SLE.

Side Effects: The following side effects may be observed with most thiazides. See also individual drugs. *Electrolyte imbalance:* Hypokalemia (most frequent) characterized by

---

bold italic = life threatening side effect

cardiac arrhythmias. Hyponatremia characterized by weakness, lethargy, epigastric distress, N&V. Hypokalemic alkalosis. *GI:* Anorexia, epigastric distress or irritation, N&V, cramping, bloating, abdominal pain, diarrhea, constipation, jaundice, pancreatitis. *CNS:* Dizziness, lightheadedness, headache, vertigo, xanthopsia, paresthesias, weakness, insomnia, restlessness. *CV:* Orthostatic hypotension, MIs in elderly patients with advanced arteriosclerosis, especially if the patient is also receiving therapy with other antihypertensive agents. *Hematologic:* **Agranulocytosis, aplastic or hypoplastic anemia, hemolytic anemia,** leukopenia, thrombocytopenia. *Dermatologic:* Purpura, photosensitivity, photosensitivity dermatitis, rash, urticaria, necrotizing angiitis, vasculitis, cutaneous vasculitis. *Metabolic:* neutropenia, hemolytic anemia. *Endocrine:* Hyperglycemia, glycosuria, hyperuricemia. *Miscellaneous:* Blurred vision, impotence, reduced libido, fever, muscle cramps, muscle spasm, respiratory distress.

OD Overdose Management: *Symptoms:* Symptoms of plasma volume depletion, including orthostatic hypotension, dizziness, drowsiness, syncope, electrolyte abnormalities, hemoconcentration, hemodynamic changes. Signs of potassium depletion, including confusion, dizziness, muscle weakness, and GI disturbances. Also, N&V, GI irritation, GI hypermotility, CNS effects, cardiac abnormalities, **seizures, hypotension, decreased respiration, and coma.** *Treatment:*

• Induce emesis or perform gastric lavage followed by activated charcoal. Undertake measures to prevent aspiration.

• Electrolyte balance, hydration, respiration, CV, and renal function must be maintained. Cathartics should be avoided, as use may enhance fluid loss.

• Although GI effects are usually of short duration, treatment may be required.

Drug Interactions
Allopurinol / ↑ Risk of hypersensitivity reactions to allopurinol
Amphotericin B / Enhanced loss of electrolytes, especially potassium
Anesthetics / Thiazides may ↑ effects of anesthetics
Anticholinergic agents / ↑ Effect of thiazides due to ↑ amount absorbed from GI tract
Anticoagulants, oral / Anticoagulant effects may be decreased
Antidiabetic agents / Thiazides antagonize hypoglycemic effect of antidiabetic agents
Antigout agents / Thiazides may ↑ uric acid levels; thus, ↑ dose of antigout drug may be necessary
Antihypertensive agents / Thiazides potentiate the effect of antihypertensive agents
Antineoplastic agents / Thiazides may prolong leukopenia induced by antineoplastic agents
Calcium salts / Hypercalcemia due to renal tubular reabsorption or bone release may be ↑ by exogenous calcium
Cholestyramine / ↓ Effect of thiazides due to ↓ absorption from GI tract
Colestipol / ↓ Effect of thiazides due to ↓ absorption from GI tract
Corticosteroids / Enhanced potassium loss due to potassium-losing properties of both drugs
Diazoxide / Enhanced hypotensive effect. Also, ↑ hyperglycemic response
Digitalis glycosides / Thiazides produce ↑ potassium and magnesium loss with ↑ chance of digitalis-induced arrhythmias
Ethanol / Additive orthostatic hypotension
Fenfluramine / ↑ Antihypertensive effect of thiazides
Furosemide / Profound diuresis and electrolyte loss
Guanethidine / Additive hypotensive effect
Indomethacin / ↓ Effect of thiazides, possibly by inhibition of prostaglandins

Insulin / ↓ Effect due to thiazide-induced hyperglycemia

Lithium / ↑ Risk of lithium toxicity due to ↓ renal excretion; may be used together but use should be carefully monitored

Loop diuretics / Additive effect to cause profound diuresis and serious electrolyte losses

Methenamine / ↓ Effect of thiazides due to alkalinization of urine by methenamine

Methyldopa / ↑ Risk of hemolytic anemia (rare)

Muscle relaxants, nondepolarizing / ↑ Effect of muscle relaxants due to hypokalemia

Norepinephrine / Thiazides ↓ arterial response to norepinephrine

Quinidine / ↑ Effect of quinidine due to ↑ renal tubular reabsorption

Reserpine / Additive hypotensive effect

Sulfonamides / ↑ Effect of thiazides due to ↓ plasma protein binding

Sulfonylureas / ↓ Effect due to thiazide-induced hyperglycemia

Tetracyclines / ↑ Risk of azotemia

Tubocurarine / ↑ Muscle relaxation and ↑ hypokalemia

Vasopressors (sympathomimetics) / Thiazides ↓ responsiveness of arterioles to vasopressors

Vitamin D / ↑ Effect of vitamin D due to thiazide-induced hypercalcemia

EMS CONSIDERATIONS

None.

ESTROGENS

See also the following individual entries:

Mechanism of Action: The three primary estrogens in the human female are estradiol 17–β, estrone, and estriol, which are steroids. Nonsteroidal estrogens include diethylstilbestrol. Estrogens combine with receptors in the cytoplasm of the cell, resulting in an increase in protein synthesis. For example, estrogens are required for development of secondary sex characteristics, development and maintenance of the female genital system and breasts. They also produce effects in the pituitary and hypothalamus. In adult women, estrogens participate in bone maintenance by aiding the deposition of calcium in the protein matrix of bones. They increase elastic elements in the skin, tend to cause sodium and fluid retention, and produce an anabolic effect by enhancing the turnover of dietary nitrogen and other elements into protein. Furthermore, they tend to keep plasma cholesterol at relatively low levels. Natural estrogens have a significant first-pass effect; thus, they are given parenterally. Synthetic derivatives can be given PO and are rapidly absorbed, distributed, and excreted. Estrogens are metabolized in the liver and excreted in urine (major portion) and feces. When given transdermally, the skin metabolizes estradiol only to a small extent.

Uses: Uses include hormone replacement therapy in postmenopausal women and as a component of combination oral contraceptives. See individual drugs. Estrogens are used both systemically and vaginally.

Contraindications: Breast cancer, except in those patients being treated for metastatic disease. Cancer of the genital tract and other estrogen-dependent neoplasms. Undiagnosed abnormal genital bleeding. History of thrombophlebitis, thrombosis, or thromboembolic disorders associated with previous estrogen use (except when used to treat breast or prostatic cancer). Known or suspected pregnancy. Prolonged therapy in women who plan to become pregnant. Use during lactation. May be contraindicated in patients with blood dyscrasias, hepatic disease, or thyroid dysfunction.

Precautions: Use with caution, if at all, in those with asthma, epilepsy, migraine, cardiac failure, renal insufficiency, diseases involving calcium or phosphorous metabolism, or a family history of mammary or genital tract cancer. Increased risk of endometrial carcinoma in postmenopausal women. Safety and effectiveness have not been determined in children and should be used with caution in adolescents in whom bone growth is incomplete.

Side Effects: Systemic use. Side effects to estrogens are dose dependent. *CV:* Potentially, the most serious side effects involve the CV system. ***Thromboembolism,*** thrombophlebitis, ***MI, pulmonary embolism,*** retinal thrombosis, ***mesenteric thrombosis, subarachnoid hemorrhage, postsurgical thromboembolism.*** Hypertension, edema, ***stroke.*** *GI:* N&V, abdominal cramps, bloating, cholestatic jaundice, colitis, acute pancreatitis, changes in appetite. *Dermatologic:* Most common are chloasma or melasma. Also, erythema multiforme, erythema nodosum, hemorrhagic eruptions, urticaria, dermatitis, photosensitivity. *Hepatic:* Cholestatic jaundice, aggravation of porphyria, benign (most common) or malignant liver tumors. *GU:* Breakthrough bleeding, spotting, changes in amount and/or duration of menstrual flow, amenorrhea during and after use, dysmenorrhea, premenstrual-like syndrome, change in cervical eversion and degree of cervical secretion, cystitis-like syndrome, hemolytic uremic syndrome, endometrial cystic hyperplasia, increased incidence of *Candida* vaginitis. *CNS:* Mental depression, dizziness, changes in libido, chorea, headache, aggravation of migraine headaches, fatigue, nervousness, ***convulsions.*** *Ocular:* Steepening of corneal curvature resulting in intolerance of contact lenses. Optic neuritis or retinal thrombosis, resulting in sudden or gradual, partial or com-

plete loss of vision, double vision, papilledema. *Hematologic:* Increase in prothrombin and blood coagulation factors VII, VIII, IX, and X. Decrease in antithrombin III. *Local:* Pain at injection site, sterile abscesses, postinjection flare, redness and irritation at site of application of transdermal system. *Miscellaneous:* Breast tenderness, enlargement, or secretions. Increased risk of gallbladder disease (with high doses). Premature closure of epiphyses in children. Increased frequency of benign or malignant tumors of the cervix, uterus, vagina, and other organs. Weight gain. Increased risk of congenital abnormalities. Hypercalcemia in patients with metastatic breast carcinoma. In males, estrogens may cause gynecomastia, loss of libido, decreased spermatogenesis, testicular atrophy, and feminization. Prolonged use of high doses may inhibit the function of the anterior pituitary. Estrogen therapy affects many laboratory tests. **Vaginal use.** *GU:* Vaginal bleeding, vaginal discharge, endometrial withdrawal bleeding, serious bleeding in ovariectomized women with endometriosis. *Miscellaneous:* Breast tenderness.

Drug Interactions

Anticoagulants, oral / ↓ Anticoagulant response by ↑ activity of certain clotting factors

Anticonvulsants / Estrogen-induced fluid retention may precipitate seizures. Also, contraceptive steroids ↑ effect of anticonvulsants by ↓ breakdown in liver and ↓ plasma protein binding

Antidiabetic agents / Estrogens may impair glucose tolerance and thus change requirements for antidiabetic agent

Barbiturates / ↓ Effect of estrogen by ↑ breakdown by liver

Corticosteroids / ↑ Pharmacologic and toxicologic effects of corticosteroids

Phenytoin / See *Anticonvulsants*

Rifampin / ↓ Effect of estrogen due to ↑ breakdown by liver

Succinylcholine / Estrogens may ↑ effects of succinylcholine

Tricyclic antidepressants / Possible ↑ effects of tricyclic antidepressants

EMS CONSIDERATIONS

None.

FLUOROQUINOLONES

See also the following individual entries:

Ciprofloxacin hydrochloride
Enoxacin
Levofloxacin
Lomefloxacin hydrochloride
Norfloxacin
Ofloxacin
Sparfloxacin
Trovafloxacin mesylate
Alatrofloxacin mesylate

Mechanism of Action: Synthetic, broad-spectrum antibacterial agents. The fluorine molecule confers increased activity against gram-negative organisms as well as broadens the spectrum against gram-positive organisms. Are bactericidal agents by interfering with DNA gyrase, an enzyme needed for the synthesis of bacterial DNA. Food may delay the absorption of ciprofloxacin, lomefloxacin, and norfloxacin. Ciprofloxacin, levofloxacin, ofloxacin, and trovafloxacin may be given IV; all fluoroquinolones may be given PO.

See also *General Nursing Considerations for All Anti-Infectives.*
Uses: See individual drugs. Used for a large number of gram-positive and gram-negative infections.
Contraindications: Hypersensitivity to the quinolone group of antibiotics, including cinoxacin and nalidixic acid. Lactation. Use in children less than 18 years of age.
Precautions: Use lower doses in impaired renal function. There may be differences in CNS toxicity between the various fluoroquinolones. Use may increase the risk of Achilles and other tendon inflammation and rupture.

Side Effects: See individual drugs. The following side effects are common to each of the fluoroquinolone antibiotics. *GI:* N&V, diarrhea, abdominal pain or discomfort, dry or painful mouth, heartburn, dyspepsia, flatulence, constipation, pseudomembranous colitis. *CNS:* Headache, dizziness, malaise, lethargy, fatigue, drowsiness, somnolence, depression, insomnia, *seizures,* paresthesia. *Dermatologic:* Rash, photosensitivity, pruritus (except for ciprofloxacin). *Hypersensitivity reactions:* Facial or **pharyngeal edema,** dyspnea, urticaria, itching, tingling, loss of consciousness, **CV collapse.** *Other:* Visual disturbances and ophthalmologic abnormalities, hearing loss, superinfection, phototoxicity, eosinophilia, crystalluria, Achilles and other tendon inflammation and rupture. Fluoroquinolones, except norfloxacin, may also cause vaginitis, syncope, chills, and edema.
OD Overdose Management: *Symptoms:* Extension of side effects. *Treatment:* For acute overdose, vomiting should be induced or gastric lavage performed. The patient should be carefully observed and, if necessary, symptomatic and supportive treatment given. Hydration should be maintained.
Drug Interactions
Antacids / ↓ Serum levels of fluoroquinolones due to ↓ absorption from the GI tract
Anticoagulants / ↑ Effect of anticoagulant
Antineoplastic agents / ↓ Serum levels of fluoroquinolones
Cimetidine / ↓ Elimination of fluoroquinolones
Cyclosporine / ↑ Risk of nephrotoxicity
Didanosine / ↓ Serum levels of fluoroquinolones due to ↓ absorption from the GI tract
Iron salts / ↓ Serum levels of fluoroquinolones due to ↓ absorption from the GI tract

Probenecid / ↑ Serum levels of fluoroquinolones due to ↓ renal clearance

Sucralfate / ↓ Serum levels of fluoroquinolones due to ↓ absorption from the GI tract

Theophylline / ↑ Plasma levels and ↑ toxicity of theophylline due to ↓ clearance

Zinc salts / ↓ Serum levels of fluoroquinolones due to ↓ absorption from the GI tract

EMS CONSIDERATIONS

See also *Anti-Infectives*.

HISTAMINE H₂ ANTAGONISTS

See also the following individual entries:

Cimetidine
Famotidine
Nizatidine
Ranitidine bismuth citrate
Ranitidine hydrochloride

Mechanism of Action: Histamine H_2 antagonists are competitive blockers of histamine. As such they inhibit all phases of gastric acid secretion including that caused by histamine, gastrin, and muscarinic agents. Both fasting and nocturnal acid secretion are inhibited. In addition, the volume and hydrogen ion concentration of gastric juice are decreased. Cimetidine, famotidine, and ranitidine have no effect on gastric emptying; cimetidine and famitidine have no effect on lower esophageal pressure. Fasting or postprandial serum gastrin is not affected by famotidine, nizatidine, or ranitidine. Cimetidine is known to affect the cytochrome P-450 drug metabolizing system for other drugs. Ranitidine also affects the P-450 enzyme system, but its effect on elimination of other drugs is not significant. Neither famotidine nor nizatidine affects the P-450 enzyme system.

Uses: See individual drugs. Also, these drugs are used as part of combination therapy to treat *Helicobact-*

er pylori–associated duodenal ulcer and maintenance therapy after healing of the active ulcer.

Contraindications: Hypersensitivity. Use of cimetidine, famotidine, and nizatidine during lactation.

Precautions: Use with caution in impaired hepatic and renal function. Symptomatic response to these drugs does not preclude gastric malignancy. Use ranitidine with caution during lactation. Safety and effectiveness have not been established for use in children. Use of cimetidine in children less than 16 years of age unless benefits outweigh risks.

Side Effects: The following side effects are common to all or most of the H_2-histamine antagonists. See individual drugs for complete listing. *GI:* N&V, abdominal discomfort, diarrhea, constipation, hepatocellular effects. *CNS:* Headache, fatigue, somnolence, dizziness, confusion, hallucinations, insomnia. *Dermatologic:* Rash, urticaria, pruritus, alopecia (rare), erythema multiforme (rare). *Hematologic:* Rarely, thrombocytopenia, agranulocytosis, granulocytopenia. *Other:* Gynecomastia, impotence, loss of libido, arthralgia, bronchospasm, transient pain at injection site, cardiac arrhythmias following rapid IV use (rare), arthralgia (rare), ***anaphylaxis*** (rare).

OD **Overdose Management:** *Symptoms:* No experience is available for deliberate overdose. *Treatment:* Induce vomiting or perform gastric lavage to remove any unabsorbed drug. Monitor the patient and undertake supportive therapy.

EMS CONSIDERATIONS

See *Antidiabetic Agents: Insulins*.

LAXATIVES

See also the following individual entries:

Docusate calcium
Docusate potassium
Docusate sodium
Lactulose

Magnesium sulfate

Psyllium hydrophilic muciloid

Mechanism of Action: Laxatives act locally, either by stimulating the smooth muscles of the bowel or by changing the bulk or consistency of the stools. Laxatives can be divided into five categories.

1. *Stimulant laxatives:* Substances that chemically stimulate the smooth muscles of the bowel to increase contractions. Examples: Bisacodyl, cascara, danthron, and senna.

2. *Saline laxatives:* Substances that increase the bulk of the stools by retaining water. Examples: Magnesium salts and sodium phosphate.

3. *Bulk-forming laxatives:* Nondigestible substances that pass through the stomach and then increase the bulk of the stools. Examples: Methylcellulose and psyllium.

4. *Emollient and lubricant laxatives:* Agents that soften hardened feces and facilitate their passage through the lower intestine. Examples: Docusate and mineral oil.

5. *Miscellaneous:* Includes glycerin suppositories and lactulose.

Uses: See individual agents. Short-term treatment of constipation. Prophylaxis in patients who should not strain during defecation, i.e., following anorectal surgery or after MI (fecal softeners or lubricant laxatives). To evacuate the colon for rectal and bowel examinations (certain lubricant, saline, and stimulant laxatives). In conjunction with surgery or anthelmintic therapy. The underlying cause of constipation should be determined since a marked change in bowel habits may be a symptom of a pathologic condition.

Contraindications: Severe abdominal pain that *might* be caused by appendicitis, enteritis, ulcerative colitis, diverticulitis, intestinal obstruction. Laxative use in these conditions may cause rupture of the abdomen or intestinal hemorrhage. Undiagnosed abdominal pain. Children under the age of 2. Castor oil is contraindicated

during pregnancy as the irritant effects may result in premature labor.

Side Effects: *GI:* Excess activity of the colon resulting in nausea, diarrhea, griping, or vomiting. Perianal irritation, bloating, flatulence. *Electrolyte Balance:* Dehydration, disturbance of the electrolyte balance. *Miscellaneous:* Dizziness, fainting, weakness, sweating, palpitations.

Bulk laxatives: Obstruction in the esophagus, stomach, small intestine, or rectum. *Stimulant laxatives:* Chronic abuse may lead to malfunctioning colon. *Mineral Oil:* Large doses may cause anal seepage resulting in itching, irritation, hemorrhoids, and perianal discomfort.

Chronic use of laxatives may cause laxative dependency and result in chronic constipation and other intestinal disorders because the patient may start to depend on the psychologic effect and physical stimulus of the drug rather than on the body's own natural reflexes.

Drug Interactions

Anticoagulants, oral / ↓ Absorption of vitamin K from GI tract induced by laxatives may ↑ effects of anticoagulants and result in bleeding

Digitalis / Cathartics may ↓ absorption of digitalis

Tetracyclines / Laxatives containing Al, Ca, or Mg may ↓ effect of tetracyclines due to ↓ absorption from GI tract

EMS CONSIDERATIONS

None.

NARCOTIC ANALGESICS

See also the following individual entries:

Buprenorphine hydrochloride
Butorphanol tartrate
Codeine phosphate
Codeine sulfate
Dezocine
Fentanyl citrate

Fentanyl transdermal system
Fiorinal
Fiorinal with Codeine
Hydrocodone bitartrate and
  Acetaminophen
Hydromorphone hydrochloride
Levomethadyl acetate
  hydrochloride
Meperidine hydrochloride
Methadone hydrochloride
Morphine hydrochloride
Morphine sulfate
Nalbuphine hydrochloride
Oxycodone hydrochloride
Oxymorphone hydrochloride
Paregoric
Pentazocine hydrochloride with
  Naloxone hydrochloride
Pentazocine lactate
Percocet
Propoxyphene hydrochloride
Propoxyphene napsylate
Remifentanil hydrochloride
Sufentanil
Tramadol hydrochloride
Tylenol with Codeine

Mechanism of Action: Narcotic analgesics are classified as agonists, mixed agonist-antagonists, or partial agonists depending on their activity at opiate receptors.The narcotic analgesics attach to specific receptors located in the CNS (cortex, brain stem, and spinal cord) resulting in various CNS effects. The mechanism is believed to involve decreased permeability of the cell membrane to sodium, which results in diminished transmission of pain impulses. Five categories of opioid receptors have been identified: mu, kappa, sigma, delta, and epsilon. Narcotic analgesics are believed to exert their activity at mu, kappa, and sigma receptors. Mu receptors are thought to mediate supraspinal analgesia, euphoria, and respiratory and physical depression. Pentazocine-like spinal analgesia, miosis, and sedation are mediated by kappa receptors while sigma receptors mediate dysphoria, hallucinations, as well as respiratory and vasomotor stimulation (caused by drugs with antagonist activity). In addition to an alteration of pain perception (analgesia), the drugs, especially at higher doses, induce euphoria, drowsiness, changes in mood, mental clouding, and deep sleep.

The narcotic analgesics also depress respiration. Death by overdosage is almost always the result of respiratory arrest. These drugs cause nausea and emesis due to direct stimulation of the CTZ. They depress the cough reflex, and small doses of narcotic analgesics (e.g., codeine) are found in certain antitussive products. Little effect on BP when the patient is in a supine position. Most narcotics decrease the capacity of the patient to respond to stress. Morphine and other narcotic analgesics induce peripheral vasodilation, which may result in hypotension. Many narcotic analgesics constrict the pupil, a sign of dependence with such drugs. They also decrease peristaltic motility causing constipation. The constipating effects (e.g., Paregoric) are sometimes used therapeutically in diarrhea. The narcotic analgesics also increase the pressure within the biliary tract. See also individual agents.

Uses: See individual drugs. Generally are used to treat pain due to various causes (e.g., MI, carcinoma, surgery, burns, postpartum), as preanesthetic medication, as adjuncts to anesthesia, acute vascular occlusion, diarrhea, and coughs. Methadone is used for heroin withdrawal and maintenance.

Contraindications: Asthma, emphysema, kyphoscoliosis, severe obesity, convulsive states as in epilepsy, delirium tremens, tetanus and strychnine poisoning, diabetic acidosis, myxedema, Addison's disease, hepatic cirrhosis, and children under 6 months.

Precautions: Use with caution in patients with head injury or after head surgery because of morphine's capacity to elevate ICP and mask the pupillary response. Use with caution in the elderly, in the debilitated, in young children, in individuals with increased ICP, in obstetrics, and with patients in shock or during acute alcoholic intoxication.

Use morphine with extreme caution in pulmonary heart disease (cor pulmonale). Deaths following ordinary therapeutic doses have been reported. Use cautiously in prostatic hypertrophy, because it may precipitate acute urinary retention. Use cautiously in patients with reduced blood volume, such as in hemorrhaging patients who are more susceptible to the hypotensive effects of morphine.

Since the drugs depress the respiratory center, give early in labor, at least 2 hr before delivery, to reduce the danger of respiratory depression in the newborn. When given before surgery, give at least 1–2 hr preoperatively so that the danger of maximum depression of respiratory function will have passed before anesthesia is initiated. These drugs may need to be withheld prior to diagnostic procedures so that the physician can use pain to locate dysfunction.

Side Effects: *Respiratory:* **Respiratory depression, apnea.** *CNS:* Dizziness, lightheadedness, sedation, lethargy, headache, euphoria, mental clouding, fainting. Idiosyncratic effects including excitement, restlessness, tremors, delirium, insomnia. *GI:* N&V, vomiting, constipation, increased pressure in biliary tract, dry mouth, anorexia. *CV:* Flushing, changes in HR and BP, circulatory collapse. *Allergic:* Skin rashes including pruritus and urticaria. Sweating, **laryngospasm,** edema. *Miscellaneous:* Urinary retention, oliguria, reduced libido, changes in body temperature. Narcotics cross the placental barrier and depress respiration of the fetus or newborn.

DEPENDENCE AND TOLERANCE: All drugs of this group are addictive. Psychologic and physical dependence and tolerance develop even when patients use clinical doses. Tolerance is characterized by the fact that the patient requires shorter periods of time between doses or larger doses for relief of pain. Tolerance usually develops faster when the narcotic analgesic is administered regularly and when the dose is large.

OD **Overdose Management:** *Symptoms (Acute Toxicity):* Severe toxicity is characterized by **profound respiratory depression, apnea, deep sleep, stupor or coma, circulatory collapse, seizures, cardiopulmonary arrest, and death.** Less severe toxicity results in symptoms including CNS depression, miosis, respiratory depression, deep sleep, flaccidity of skeletal muscles, hypotension, bradycardia, hypothermia, pulmonary edema, pneumonia, shock. The respiratory rate may be as low as 2–4 breaths/min. The patient may be cyanotic. Urine output is decreased, the skin feels clammy, and body temperature decreases. If death occurs, it almost always results from **respiratory depression.** *Symptoms (Chronic Toxicity):* The problem of chronic dependence on narcotics occurs not only as a result of "street" use but is also found often among those who have easy access to narcotics (physicians, nurses, pharmacists). All the principal narcotic analgesics (morphine, opium, heroin, codeine, meperidine, and others) have, at times, been used for nontherapeutic purposes.

The nurse must be aware of the problem and be able to recognize signs of chronic dependence. These are constricted pupils, GI effects (constipation), skin infections, needle scars, abscesses, and itching, especially on the anterior surfaces of the body, where the patient may inject the drug.

Withdrawal signs appear after drug is withheld for 4–12 hr. They are characterized by intense craving for the drug, insomnia, yawning, sneezing, vomiting, diarrhea, tremors, sweating, mental depression, muscular aches and pains, chills, and anxiety. Although the symptoms of narcotic withdrawal are uncomfort-

---

bold italic = life threatening side effect

able, they are rarely life-threatening. This is in contrast to the withdrawal syndrome from depressants, where the life of the individual may be endangered because of the possibility of tonic-clonic seizures.

Treatment (Acute Overdose): Initial treatment is aimed at combating progressive respiratory depression by maintaining a patent airway and by artificial respiration. Gastric lavage and induced emesis are indicated in case of oral poisoning. The narcotic antagonist naloxone (Narcan), 0.4 mg IV, is effective in the treatment of acute overdosage. Respiratory stimulants (e.g., caffeine) should not be used to treat depression from the narcotic overdosage.

Drug Interactions

Alcohol, ethyl / Potentiation or addition of CNS depressant effects; concomitant use may lead to drowsiness, lethargy, stupor, respiratory collapse, coma, or death

Anesthetics, general / See *Alcohol*

Antianxiety drugs / See *Alcohol*

Antidepressants, tricyclic / ↑ Narcotic-induced respiratory depression

Antihistamines / See *Alcohol*

Barbiturates / See *Alcohol*

Cimetidine / ↑ CNS toxicity (e.g., disorientation, confusion, respiratory depression, apnea, seizures) with narcotics

CNS depressants / See *Alcohol*

MAO inhibitors / Possible potentiation of either MAO inhibitor (excitation, hypertension) or narcotic (hypotension, coma) effects; death has resulted

Methotrimeprazine / Potentiation of CNS depression

Phenothiazines / See *Alcohol*

Sedative-hypnotics, nonbarbiturate / See *Alcohol*

Skeletal muscle relaxants (surgical) / ↑ Respiratory depression and ↑ muscle relaxation

EMS CONSIDERATIONS

Assessment

1. Obtain baseline VS; generally, if the respiratory rate < 12/min or the SBP < 90 mm Hg, a narcotic should not be administered unless there is ventilatory support or specific written guidelines, with parameters for administration.

2. Note weight, age, and general body size. Too large a dosage for the patient's weight and age can result in serious side effects.

Interventions

• Monitor VS and mental status. During parenteral therapy:

• Monitor for respiratory depression.

• Monitor for hypotension.

• If HR below 60 beats/min in the adult or 110 beats/min in an infant, withhold and report.

• Observe for decrease in BP, deep sleep, or constricted pupils.

NARCOTIC ANTAGONISTS

See also the following individual entries:

Nalmefene hydrochloride
Naloxone hydrochloride
Naltrexone

Mechanism of Action: Narcotic antagonists competitively block the action of narcotic analgesics by displacing previously given narcotics from their receptor sites or by preventing narcotics from attaching to the opiate receptors, thereby preventing access by the analgesic. Not effective in reversing the respiratory depression induced by barbiturates, anesthetics, or other nonnarcotic agents. These drugs almost immediately induce withdrawal symptoms in narcotic addicts and are sometimes used to unmask dependence.

EMS CONSIDERATIONS

Assessment

1. Determine etiology of respiratory depression. Narcotic antagonists do not relieve the toxicity of nonnarcotic CNS depressants.

2. Note mental status and VS.

Interventions

1. Note agent being reversed. If narcotic is long acting or sustained re-

lease, repeated doses will be required in order to continue to counteract drug effects. Monitor VS and respirations closely after duration of action of antagonist; additional doses may be necessary.

2. Observe for appearance of withdrawal symptoms characterized by restlessness, crying out due to sudden loss of pain control, lacrimation, rhinorrhea, yawning, perspiration, vomiting, diarrhea, sweating, writhing, anxiety, pain, chills, and an intense craving for the drug.

3. Observe for symptoms of airway obstruction.

NEUROMUSCULAR BLOCKING AGENTS

See also the following individual entries:

Pancuronium bromide
Pipecuronium bromide
Rapacuronium bromide
Rocuronium bromide
Succinylcholine chloride
Tubocurarine chloride
Vecuronium bromide

Mechanism of Action: These drugs are categorized as competitive (nondepolarizing) and depolarizing agents, both of which act peripherally. Competitive agents include all of the above listed drugs *except* succinylcholine. They compete with acetylcholine for the receptor site in the muscle cells. The depolarizing agent—succinylcholine—initially excites skeletal muscle and then prevents the muscle from contracting by prolonging the time during which the receptors at the end plate cannot respond to acetylcholine (depolarization during refractory time).

The muscle paralysis caused by the neuromuscular blocking agents is sequentialin the following order: heaviness of eyelids, difficulty in swallowing and talking, diplopia, progressive weakening of the extremities and neck, followed by relaxation of the trunk and spine. The diaphragm (respiratory paralysis) is affected last. The drugs do not affect consciousness, and their use, in the absence of adequate levels of general anesthesia, may be frightening to the patient. After IV infusion, flaccid paralysis occurs within a few minutes with maximum effects within about 6 min. Maximal effects last 35–60 min and effective muscle paralysis may last for 25–90 min with complete recovery taking several hours. There is a narrow margin of safety between a therapeutically effective dose causing muscle relaxation and a toxic dose causing respiratory paralysis. **The neuromuscular blocking agents are always administered initially by a physician.** The nurse must be prepared to maintain and monitor respiration until the effect of the drug subsides.

Uses: See individual agents. General uses include as an adjunct to general anesthesia to cause muscle relaxation; to reduce the intensity of skeletal muscle contractions in either drug-induced or electrically induced convulsions; to assist in the management of mechanical ventilation.

Contraindications: Allergy or hypersensitivity to any of these drugs.

Precautions: Use with caution in myasthenia gravis; renal, hepatic, endocrine, or pulmonary impairment; respiratory depression; during lactation; and in elderly, pediatric, or debilitated patients. The action may be altered in patients by electrolyte imbalances (especially hyperkalemia), some carcinomas, body temperature, dehydration, renal disease, and in those taking digitalis.

Side Effects: *Respiratory paralysis. Severe and prolonged muscle relaxation. CV:* Cardiac arrhythmias, bradycardia, hypotension, cardiac arrest. These side effects are more frequent in neonates and premature infants. *GI:* Excessive salivation during light anesthesia. *Miscellaneous: Bronchospasms, hyperthermia,* hypersensitivity (rare). See also individual agents.

---

bold italic = life threatening side effect

OD Overdose Management: *Symptoms:* Decreased respiratory reserve, extended skeletal muscle weakness, prolonged apnea, low tidal volume, sudden release of histamine, **CV collapse.** *Treatment:* There are no known antidotes.

• Use a peripheral nerve stimulator to monitor and assess patient's response to the neuromuscular blocking medication.

• Have anticholinesterase drugs, such as edrophonium, pyridostigmine, or neostigmine available to counteract respiratory depression due to paralysis of skeletal muscles. These drugs increase the body's production of acetylcholine. To minimize the muscarinic cholinergic side effects, give atropine.

• Correct BP, electrolyte imbalance, or circulating blood volume by fluid and electrolyte therapy. Vasopressors can be used to correct hypotension due to ganglionic blockade.

Drug Interactions: The following drug interactions are for nondepolarizing skeletal muscle relaxants. See also succinylcholine.

Aminoglycoside antibiotics / Additive muscle relaxation, including prolonged respiratory depression

Amphotericin B / ↑ Muscle relaxation

Anesthetics, inhalation / Additive muscle relaxation

Carbamazepine / ↓ Duration or effect of muscle relaxants

Clindamycin / Additive muscle relaxation, including prolonged respiratory depression

Colistin / ↑ Muscle relaxation

Corticosteroids / ↓ Effect of muscle relaxants

Furosemide / ↑ or ↓ Effect of skeletal muscle relaxants (may be dose-related)

Hydantoins / ↓ Duration or effect of muscle relaxants

Ketamine / ↑ Muscle relaxation, including prolonged respiratory depression

Lincomycin / ↑ Muscle relaxation, including prolonged respiratory depression

Lithium / ↑ Recovery time of muscle relaxants → prolonged respiratory depression

Magnesium salts / ↑ Muscle relaxation, including prolonged respiratory depression

Methotrimeprazine / ↑ Muscle relaxation

Narcotic analgesics / ↑ Respiratory depression and ↑ muscle relaxation

Nitrates / ↑ Muscle relaxation, including prolonged respiratory depression

Phenothiazines / ↑ Muscle relaxation

Pipercillin / ↑ Muscle relaxation, including prolonged respiratory depression

Polymyxin B / ↑ Muscle relaxation

Procainamide / ↑ Muscle relaxation

Procaine / ↑ Muscle relaxation by ↓ plasma protein binding

Quinidine / ↑ Muscle relaxation

Ranitidine / Significant ↓ effect of muscle relaxants

Theophyllines / Reversal of effects of muscle relaxant (dose-dependent)

Thiazide diuretics / ↑ Muscle relaxation due to hypokalemia

Verapamil / ↑ Muscle relaxation, including prolonged respiratory depression

EMS CONSIDERATIONS
Assessment
1. Monitor ECG.
2. Note initial selective paralysis in the following sequence: levator muscles of the eyelids, mastication muscles, limb muscles, abdominal muscles, glottis muscles, intercostal muscles, and the diaphragm muscles; neuromuscular recovery occurs in the reverse order.
Interventions
1. Administer in a closely monitored environment and generally only when intubated.
2. Monitor VS frequently and pulmonary status continuously.
3. Observe for excessive bronchial secretions or respiratory wheezing; suction to maintain patent airway.
4. Consciousness and pain thresholds are not affected by neuromuscu-

lar blocking agents; patients can still hear, feel, and see while receiving these agents. Avoid discussions that should not be overheard. Adequate anesthesia and analgesics should be administered for pain or fear with procedures.

NONSTEROIDAL ANTI-INFLAMMATORY DRUGS

See also the following individual entries:

Auranofin
Aurothioglucose
Celecoxib
Diclofenac potassium
Diclofenac sodium
Diclofenac sodium/Misoprostol
Diflunisal
Etodolac
Fenoprofen calcium
Flurbiprofen
Flurbiprofen sodium
Gold sodium thiomalate
Ibuprofen
Indomethacin
Indomethacin sodium trihydrate
Ketoprofen
Ketorolac tromethamine
Meclofenamate sodium
Mefenamic acid
Nabumetone
Naproxen
Naproxen sodium
Oxaprozin
Piroxicam
Rofecoxib
Sulindac
Suprofen
Tolmetin sodium

Mechanism of Action: The anti-inflammatory effect is likely due to inhibition of the enzyme cyclooxygenase, resulting in decreased prostaglandin synthesis. Effective in reducing joint swelling, pain, and morning stiffness, as well as in increasing mobility in individuals with inflammatory disease. They do not alter the course of the disease, however. Their anti-inflammatory activity is comparable to that of aspirin. The analgesic activity is due, in part, to relief of inflammation. Also, the drugs may inhibit lipoxygenase, inhibit synthesis of leukotrienes, inhibit release of lysosomal enzymes, and inhibit neutrophil aggregation. Rheumatoid factor production may also be inhibited. The antipyretic action occurs by decreasing prostaglandin synthesis in the hypothalamus, resulting in an increase in peripheral blood flow and heat loss as well as promoting sweating. NSAIDs also inhibit miosis induced by prostaglandins during the course of cataract surgery; thus, these drugs are useful for a number of ophthalmic inflammatory conditions.

The NSAIDs differ from one another with respect to their rate of absorption, length of action, anti-inflammatory activity, and effect on the GI mucosa. Most are rapidly and completely absorbed from the GI tract; food delays the rate, but not the total amount, of drug absorbed. These drugs are metabolized in the kidney and are excreted through the urine, mainly as metabolites.

Uses: See individual drugs. Generally are used to treat inflammatory disease, including rheumatoid arthritis, osteoarthritis, ankylosing spondylitis, gout, and other musculoskeletal diseases. Treatment of nonrheumatic inflammatory conditions including bursitis, acute painful shoulder, synovitis, tendinitis, or tenosynovitis. Mild to moderate pain including primary dysmenorrhea, episiotomy pain, strains and sprains, postextraction dental pain. Primary dysmenorrhea. Ophthalmically to inhibit intraoperative miosis, for postoperative inflammation after cataract surgery, and for relief of ocular itching due to seasonal allergic conjunctivitis.

Contraindications: Most for children under 14 years of age. Lactation. Individuals in whom aspirin, NSAIDs, or iodides have caused hypersensitivity, including acute asthma, rhinitis, urticaria, nasal polyps,

---

bold italic = life threatening side effect

bronchospasm, angioedema or other symptoms of allergy or anaphylaxis. **Precautions:** Patients intolerant to one of the NSAIDs may be intolerant to others in this group. Use with caution in patients with a history of GI disease, reduced renal function, in geriatric patients, in patients with intrinsic coagulation defects or those on anticoagulant therapy, in compromised cardiac function, in hypertension, in conditions predisposing to fluid retention, and in the presence of existing controlled infection. The risk of hospitalization is doubled in geriatric patients taking NSAIDs and diuretics. The safety and efficacy of most NSAIDs have not been determined in children or in functional class IV rheumatoid arthritis (i.e., patients incapacitated, bedridden, or confined to a wheelchair).

Side Effects: *GI (most common):* Peptic or duodenal ulceration and GI bleeding, intestinal ulceration with obstruction and stenosis, reactivation of preexisting ulcers. Heartburn, dyspepsia, N&V, anorexia, diarrhea, constipation, increased or decreased appetite, indigestion, stomatitis, epigastric pain, abdominal cramps or pain, gastroenteritis, paralytic ileus, salivation, dry mouth, glossitis, pyrosis, icterus, rectal irritation, gingival ulcer, occult blood in stool, hematemesis, gastritis, proctitis, eructation, sore or dry mucous membranes, ulcerative colitis, rectal bleeding, melena, *perforation and hemorrhage of esophagus, stomach, duodenum, small or large intestine. CNS:* Dizziness, drowsiness, vertigo, headaches, nervousness, migraine, anxiety, mental confusion, aggravation of parkinsonism and epilepsy, lightheadedness, paresthesia, peripheral neuropathy, akathisia, excitation, tremor, *seizures,* myalgia, asthenia, malaise, insomnia, fatigue, drowsiness, confusion, emotional lability, depression, inability to concentrate, psychoses, hallucinations, depersonalization, amnesia, *coma,* syncope. *CV:* CHF, hypotension, hypertension, arrhythmias, peripheral edema and fluid retention, vasodilation, exacer-

bation of angiitis, palpitations, tachycardia, chest pain, sinus bradycardia, peripheral vascular disease, peripheral edema. *Respiratory: Bronchospasm, laryngeal edema,* rhinitis, dyspnea, pharyngitis, hemoptysis, SOB, eosinophilic pneumonitis. *Hematologic:* Bone marrow depression, neutropenia, leukopenia, pancytopenia, eosinophila, thrombocytopenia, granulocytopenia, *agranulocytosis, aplastic anemia, hemolytic anemia,* decreased H&H, hypocoagulability, epistaxis. *Ophthalmologic:* Amblyopia, visual disturbances, corneal deposits, retinal hemorrhage, scotomata, retinal pigmentation changes or degeneration, blurred vision, photophobia, diplopia, iritis, loss of color vision (reversible), optic neuritis, cataracts, swollen, dry, or irritated eyes. *Dermatologic:* Pruritus, skin eruptions, sweating, erythema, eczema, hyperpigmentation, ecchymoses, petechiae, rashes, urticaria, purpura, onycholysis, vesiculobullous eruptions, cutaneous vasculitis, *toxic epidermal necrolysis, angioneurotic edema,* erythema nodosum, *Stevens-Johnson syndrome,* exfoliative dermatitis, photosensitivity, alopecia, skin irritation, peeling, erythema multiforme, desquamation, skin discoloration. *GU:* Menometrorrhagia, menorrhagia, impotence, menstrual disorders, hematuria, cystitis, azotemia, nocturia, proteinuria, UTIs, polyuria, dysuria, urinary frequency, oliguria, pyuria, anuria, renal insufficiency, nephrosis, nephrotic syndrome, glomerular and interstitial nephritis, urinary casts, acute renal failure in patients with impaired renal function, renal papillary necrosis *Metabolic:* Hyperglycemia, hypoglycemia, glycosuria, hyperkalemia, hyponatremia, diabetes mellitus. *Other:* Tinnitus, hearing loss or disturbances, ear pain, deafness, metallic or bitter taste in mouth, thirst, chills, fever, flushing, jaundice, sweating, breast changes, gynecomastia, muscle cramps, dyspnea, involuntary muscle movements, muscle weakness, facial edema, pain, serum sickness, aseptic meningitis, hypersensitivity reactions including asthma, acute respiratory distress, *shock-like syndrome, angioedema,* angiitis, dyspnea, *anaphylaxis.*

Following ophthalmic use: Transient burning and stinging upon installation, ocular irritation.

OD **Overdose Management:** *Symptoms:* CNS symptoms include dizziness, drowsiness, mental confusion, lethargy, disorientation, intense headache, paresthesia, and *seizures.* GI symptoms include N&V, gastric irritation, and abdominal pain. Miscellaneous symptoms include tinnitus, sweating, blurred vision, increased serum creatinine and BUN, and acute renal failure. *Treatment:* There are no antidotes; treatment includes general supportive measures. Since the drugs are acidic, it may be beneficial to alkalinize the urine and induce diuresis to hasten excretion.

Drug Interactions:

Anticoagulants / Concomitant use results in ↑ PT

Aspirin / ↓ Effect of NSAIDs due to ↓ blood levels; also, ↑ risk of adverse GI effects

Beta-adrenergic blocking agents / ↓ Antihypertensive effect of blocking agents

Cimetidine / ↑ or ↓ Plasma levels of NSAIDs

Cyclosporine / ↑ Risk of nephrotoxicity

Lithium / ↑ Serum lithium levels

Loop diuretics / ↓ Effect of loop diuretics

Methotrexate / ↑ Risk of methotrexate toxicity (i.e., bone marrow suppression, nephrotoxicity, stomatitis)

Phenobarbital / ↓ Effect of NSAIDs due to ↑ breakdown by liver

Phenytoin / ↑ Effect of phenytoin due to ↓ plasma protein binding

Probenecid / ↑ Effect of NSAIDs due to ↑ plasma levels

Salicylates / Plasma levels of NSAIDs may be ↓ ; also, ↑ risk of GI side effects

Sulfonamides / ↑ Effect of sulfonamides due to ↓ plasma protein binding

Sulfonylureas / ↑ Effect of sulfonylureas due to ↓ plasma protein binding

EMS CONSIDERATIONS
None.

OPHTHALMIC CHOLINERGIC (MIOTIC) AGENTS

See also the following individual entries:

Ketotifen fumaratePemirolast potassium
Physostigmine salicylate
Physostigmine sulfate
Pilocarpine hydrochloride
Pilocarpine ocular therapeutic system

Mechanism of Action: The ophthalmic cholinergic drugs fall into two classes: direct-acting (carbachol, pilocarpine) and indirect-acting (demecarium, echothiophate, isofluorphate, neostigmine, physostigmine), which inhibit the enzyme acetylcholinesterase. In the treatment of glaucoma, the drugs lead to an accumulation of acetylcholine, which stimulates the ciliary muscles and increases contraction of the iris sphincter muscle. This opens the angle of the eye and results in increased outflow of aqueous humor and consequently in a decrease of intraocular pressure. This effect is of particular importance in narrow-angle glaucoma. The drugs also cause spasms of accommodation.

Uses: See individual drugs.

Contraindications: *Direct-acting drugs:* Inflammatory eye disease (iritis), asthma, hypertension. *Indirect-acting drugs:* Same as for *direct-acting drugs,* as well as acute-angle glaucoma, history of retinal detachment, ocular hypotension accompanied by intraocular inflammatory processes, intestinal or urinary obstruction, peptic ulcer, epilepsy, parkinsonism, spastic GI conditions,

---

bold italic = life threatening side effect

vasomotor instability, severe bradycardia or hypotension, and recent MIs. Lactation.

Side Effects: *Local:* Painful contraction of ciliary muscle, pain in eye, blurred vision, spasms of accommodation, darkened vision, failure to accommodate to darkness, twitching, headaches, painful brow. Most of these symptoms lessen with prolonged usage. Iris cysts and retinal detachment (indirect-acting drugs only).

Systemic: Systemic absorption of drug may cause nausea, GI discomfort, diarrhea, hypotension, bronchial constriction, and increased salivation.

EMS CONSIDERATIONS

None.

ORAL CONTRACEPTIVES: ESTROGEN-PROGESTERONE COMBINATIONS

Mechanism of Action: The combination oral contraceptives act by inhibiting ovulation due to an inhibition (through negative-feedback mechanism) of LH and FSH, which are required for development of ova. These products also alter the cervical mucus so that it is not conducive to sperm penetration, render the endometrium less suitable for implantation of the blastocyst should fertilization occur, and inhibit enzymes required by sperm to enter the ovum.

The estrogen used in combination oral contraceptives is either ethinyl estradiol or mestranol. Mestranol is demethylated to ethinyl estradiol in the liver. **t½:** 6–20 hr. The progestin used in combination oral contraceptives is either desogestrel, ethynodiol diacetate, levonorgestrel, norethindrone, norethindrone acetate, norgestimate, or norgestrel.

The progestin-only products do not consistently inhibit ovulation.

However, these products also alter the cervical mucus and render the endometrium unsuitable for implantation. These products contain either norethindrone or norgestrel. This method of contraception is less reliable than combination therapy.

Although oral contraceptives may be associated with serious side effects, a number of noncontraceptive health benefits have been confirmed. These include increased regularity of the menstrual cycle, decreased incidence of dysmenorrhea, decreased blood loss, decreased incidence of functional ovarian cysts and ectopic pregnancies, and decreased incidence of diseases such as fibroadenomas, fibrocystic disease, acute pelvic inflammatory disease, endometrial cancer, and ovarian cancer.

General Statement: There are three types of combination (i.e., both an estrogen and progestin in each tablet) oral contraceptives: (1) monophasic—contain the same amount of estrogen and progestin in each tablet; (2) biphasic—contain the same amount of estrogen in each tablet but the progestin content is lower for the first part of the cycle and higher for the last part of the cycle; (3) triphasic—the estrogen content may be the same or may vary throughout the medication cycle; the progestin content may be the same or varies, depending on the part of the cycle. The purpose of the biphasic and triphasic products is to provide hormones in a manner similar to that occurring physiologically. This is said to decrease breakthrough bleeding during the medication cycle. The other type of oral contraceptive is the progestin-only ("mini-pill") product, which contains a small amount of a progestin in each tablet.

Also available is an emergency contraceptive kit (Preven) containing just four tablets of ethinyl estradiol and levonorgestrel. It is intended to be used after unprotected intercourse.

Uses: Contraception, prevent pregnancy after unprotected intercourse, menstrual irregularities, menopausal symptoms. High doses are used for endometriosis and hypermenorrhea. *Investigational:* High doses of Ovral (ethinyl estradiol and norgestrel) have been used as a postcoital contraceptive.

Contraindications: Thrombophlebitis, history of deep-vein thrombophlebitis, thromboembolic disorders, cerebral vascular disease, CAD, MI, current or past angina, known or suspected breast cancer or estrogen-dependent neoplasm, endometrial carcinoma, hepatic adenoma or carcinoma, undiagnosed abnormal genital bleeding, known or suspected pregnancy, cholestatic jaundice of pregnancy. Smoking.

Precautions: Cigarette smoking increases the risk of cardiovascular side effects from use of oral contraceptives. Low estrogen-containing oral contraceptives do not increase the risk of stroke in women. Use with caution in patients with a history of hypertension, preexisting renal disease, hypertension-related diseases during pregnancy, familial tendency to hypertension or its consequences, a history of excessive weight gain or fluid retention during the menstrual cycle; these individuals are more likely to develop elevated BP. Use with caution in patients with asthma, epilepsy, migraine, diabetes, metabolic bone disease, renal or cardiac disease, and a history of mental depression. Use with drugs (e.g., barbiturates, hydantoins, rifampin) that increase the hepatic metabolism of oral contraceptives may result in breakthrough bleeding and an increased risk of pregnancy. Use combination products during lactation only if absolutely necessary; progestin-only products do not appear to have any adverse effects on breastfeeding performance or on the health, growth, or development of the infant.

Side Effects: The oral contraceptives have wide-ranging effects.

These are particularly important, since the drugs may be given for several years to healthy women. Many authorities have voiced concern about the long-term safety of these agents. Some advise discontinuing therapy after 18–24 months of continuous use. The majority of side effects of oral contraceptives are due to the estrogen component. *CV: **MI, thrombophlebitis, venous thrombosis with or without embolism, pulmonary embolism, coronary thrombosis, cerebral thrombosis, arterial thromboembolism, mesenteric thrombosis, thrombotic and hemorrhagic strokes, postsurgical thromboembolism, subarachnoid hemorrhage,** elevated BP, hypertension. CNS:* Onset or exacerbation of migraine headaches, depression. *GI:* N&V, bloating, abdominal cramps. *Ophthalmic:* Optic neuritis, retinal thrombosis, steepening of the corneal curvature, contact lens intolerance. *Hepatic: **Benign and malignant hepatic adenomas,** focal nodular hyperplasia, **hepatocellular carcinoma,** gallbladder disease, cholestatic jaundice. GU:* Breakthrough bleeding, spotting, amenorrhea, change in menstrual flow, change in cervical erosion and cervical secretions, ***invasive cervical cancer,*** bleeding irregularities (more common with progestin-only products), vaginal candidiasis, ***ectopic pregnancies in contraceptive failures,*** breast tenderness, breast enlargement. *Miscellaneous:* Acute intermittent porphyria, photosensitivity, congenital anomalies, melasma, skin rash, edema, increase or decrease in weight, decreased carbohydrate tolerance, increased incidence of cervical *Chlamydia trachomatis,* decrease in the quantity and quality of breast milk.

Drug Interactions

Acetaminophen / ↓ Effect of acetaminophen due to ↑ breakdown by liver

Anticoagulants, oral / ↓ Effect of anticoagulants by ↑ levels of certain clotting factors (however, an ↑ eff-

---

bold italic = life threatening side effect

Table 1   Combination Oral Contraceptive Preparations and Hormone Replacement Combinations Available in the United States

Trade Name	Estrogen	Progestin
	MONOPHASIC	
Alesse 21-Day and 28-Day	Ethinyl estradiol (20 mcg)	Levonorgestrel (0.1 mg)
Apri	Ethinyl estradiol (30 mcg)	Desogestrel (0.15 mg)
Brevicon 21-Day and 28-Day	Ethinyl estradiol (35 mcg)	Norethindrone (0.5 mg)
Demulen 1/35–21 and 1/35–28	Ethinyl estradiol (35 mcg)	Ethynodiol diacetate (1 mg)
Demulen 1/50–21 and 1/50–28	Ethinyl estradiol (50 mcg)	Ethynodiol diacetate (1 mg)
Desogen (28 day)	Ethinyl estradiol (30 mcg)	Desogestrel (0.15 mg)
Levlen 21 and 28	Ethinyl estradiol (30 mcg)	Levonorgestrel (0.15 mg)
Levlite 21 and 28	Ethinyl estradiol (20 mcg)	Levonorgestrel (0.1 mg)
Levora 0.15/30–21 and -28	Ethinyl estradiol (30 mcg)	Levonorgestrel (0.15 mg)
Loestrin 21 1/20	Ethinyl estradiol (20 mcg)	Norethindrone acetate (1 mg)
Loestrin 21 1.5/30	Ethinyl estradiol (30 mcg)	Norethindrone acetate (1.5 mg)
Loestrin Fe 1/20 (28 day)	Ethinyl estradiol (20 mcg)	Norethindrone acetate (1 mg)
Loestrin Fe 1.5/30 (28 day)	Ethinyl estradiol (30 mcg)	Norethindrone acetate (1.5 mg)
Lo/Ovral-21 and -28	Ethinyl estradiol (30 mcg)	Norgestrel (0.3 mg)
Modicon 21 and 28	Ethinyl estradiol (35 mcg)	Norethindrone (0.5 mg)
Necon 0.5/35–21 Day and 28 Day	Ethinyl estradiol (35 mcg)	Norethindrone (0.5 mg)
Necon 1/35–21 Day and 28 Day	Ethinyl estradiol (35 mcg)	Norethindrone (1 mg)
Necon 1/50–21 Day and 28 Day	Mestranol (50 mcg)	Norethindrone (1 mg)
Nelova 0.5/35E 21 Day and 28 Day	Ethinyl estradiol (35 mcg)	Norethindrone (0.5 mg)
Nelova 1/35E 21 Day and 28 Day	Ethinyl estradiol (35 mcg)	Norethindrone (1 mg)
Nelova 1/50M 21 Day and 28 Day	Mestranol (50 mcg)	Norethindrone (1 mg)
Nordette-21 and -28	Ethinyl estradiol (30 mcg)	Levonorgestrel (0.15 mg)
Norinyl 1 + 35 21-Day and 28-Day	Ethinyl estradiol (35 mcg)	Norethindrone (1 mg)
Norinyl 1 + 50 21-Day and 28-Day	Mestranol (50 mcg)	Norethindrone (1 mg)

Trade Name	Estrogen	Progestin
	MONOPHASIC	
Ortho-Cept 21 Day and 28 Day	Ethinyl estradiol (30 mcg)	Desogestrel (0.15 mg)
Ortho-Cyclen-21 and -28	Ethinyl estradiol (35 mcg)	Norgestimate (0.25 mg)
Ortho Novum 1/35–21 and –28	Ethinyl estradiol (35 mcg)	Norethindrone (1 mg)
Ortho Novum 1/50–21 and –28	Mestranol (50 mcg)	Norethindrone (1 mg)
Ovcon-35 21 Day and 28 Day	Ethinyl estradiol (35 mcg)	Norethindrone (0.4 mg)
Ovcon-50 21 Day and 28 Day	Ethinyl estradiol (50 mcg)	Norethindrone (1 mg)
Ovral 28 Day	Ethinyl estradiol (50 mcg)	Norgestrel (0.5 mg)
Zovia 1/35E-21 and -28	Ethinyl estradiol (35 mcg)	Ethynodiol diacetate (1 mg)
Zovia 1/50E-21 and -28	Ethinyl estradiol (50 mcg)	Ethynodiol diacetate (1 mg)
	BIPHASIC	
Jenest-28	Ethinyl estradiol (35 mcg in each tablet)	Norethindrone (10 tablets of 0.5 mg followed by 11 tablets of 1 mg)
Mircette	Ethinyl estradiol (20 mcg for Days 1 - 21; 10 mcg for Days 24 - 28)	Desogestrel (0.15 mg for Days 1 - 21)
Necon 10/11 21 Day and 28 Day	Ethinyl estradiol (35 mcg in each tablet)	Norethindrone (10 tablets of 0.5 mg followed by 11 tablets of 1 mg)
Nelova 10/11–21 and –28	Ethinyl estradiol (35 mcg in each tablet)	Norethindrone (10 tablets of 0.5 mg followed by 11 tablets of 1 mg)
Ortho-Novum 10/11–21 and –28	Ethinyl estradiol (35 mcg in each tablet)	Norethindrone (10 tablets of 0.5 mg followed by 11 tablets of 1 mg)
	TRIPHASIC	
Estrostep 21 and Estrostep Fe	Ethinyl estradiol (20 mcg for 5 days, 30 mcg for 7 days, and 35 mcg for 9 days)	Norethindrone (1 mg in each tablet)

Table 1 *(continued)*

Trade Name	Estrogen	Progestin
	TRIPHASIC	
Ortho-Novum 7/7/7 (21 or 28 days)	Ethinyl estradiol (35 mcg in each tablet)	Norethindrone (0.5 mg the first 7 days, 0.75 the next 7 days, and 1 mg the last 7 days)
Ortho-Tri-Cyclen (21 or 28 days)	Ethinyl estradiol (35 mcg in each tablet)	Norgestimate (0.18 mg the first 7 days, 0.215 mg the next 7 days, and 0.25 mg the last seven days)
Tri-Levlen 21 or 28 Days	First 6 days: Ethinyl estradiol (30 mcg)	Levonorgestrel (0.05 mg)
Tri-Levlen 28 Day	Next 5 days: Ethinyl estradiol (40 mcg)	Levonorgestrel (0.075 mg)
	Last 10 days: Ethinyl estradiol (30 mcg)	Levonorgestrel (0.125 mg)
Tri-Norinyl (21 or 28 day)	Ethinyl estradiol (35 mcg in each tablet)	Norethindrone (0.5 mg the first 7 days, 1 mg the next 9 days, and 0.5 mg the last 5 days)
Triphasil 21 or 28 day	First 6 days: Ethinyl estradiol (30 mcg)	Levonorgestrel (0.05 mg)
	Next 5 days: Ethinyl estradiol (40 mcg)	Levonorgestrel (0.075 mg)
	Last 10 days: Ethinyl estradiol (30 mcg)	Levonorgestrel (0.125 mg)
Trivora-28 day	First 6 days: Ethinyl estradiol (30 mcg)	Levonorgestrel (0.05 mg)
	Next 5 days: Ethinyl estradiol (40 mcg)	Levonorgestrel (0.075 mg)
	Last 10 days: Ethinyl estradiol (30 mcg)	Levonorgestrel (0.125 mg)
EMERGENCY CONTRACEPTIVE KIT		
Plan B	No estrogen	Levonorgestrel (0.75 mg)
A total of 2 tablets containing levonorgestrel.		
Preven	Ethinyl estradiol (50 mcg)	Levonorgestrel (0.25 mg)
A total of four tablets containing the above hormones		

All combination oral contraceptives and hormone replacement combinations are Rx and Pregnancy category: X.

ect of anticoagulants has also been noted in some patients)

Antidepressants, tricyclic / ↑ Effect of antidepressants due to ↓ breakdown by liver

Benzodiazepines / ↑ or ↓ Effect of benzodiazepines due to changes in breakdown by liver

Beta-adrenergic blockers / ↑ Effect of beta blockers due to ↓ breakdown by liver

Carbamazepine / ↓ Effect of oral contraceptives due to ↑ breakdown by liver

Corticosteroids / ↑ Effect of corticosteroids due to ↓ breakdown by liver

Erythromycins / ↓ Effect of oral contraceptives due to altered enterohepatic absorption

Griseofulvin / May ↓ effect of oral contraceptives due to ↑ breakdown

Hypoglycemics / Oral contraceptives ↓ effect of hypoglycemics due to their effect on carbohydrate metabolism

Insulin / Oral contraceptives may ↑ insulin requirements

Penicillins, oral / ↓ Effect of oral contraceptives due to altered enterohepatic absorption

Phenobarbital / ↓ Effect of oral contraceptives due to ↑ breakdown by liver

Phenytoin / ↓ Effect of oral contraceptives due to ↑ breakdown by liver

Rifampin / ↓ Effect of contraceptives due to ↑ breakdown by liver

Tetracyclines / ↓ Effect of contraceptives due to altered enterohepatic absorption

Theophyllines / ↑ Effect of theophyllines due to ↓ breakdown by liver

Troleandomycin / ↑ Chance of jaundice

EMS CONSIDERATIONS

See also *Estrogens,* and *Progesterone and Progestins.*

PENICILLINS

See also the following individual entries:

Amoxicillin
Amoxicillin and Potassium clavulanate
Ampicillin oral
Ampicillin sodium parenteral
Ampicillin sodium/Sulbactam sodium
Bacampicillin hydrochloride
Carbenicillin indanyl sodium
Cloxacillin sodium
Dicloxacillin sodium
Mezlocillin sodium
Nafcillin sodium
Oxacillin sodium
Penicillin G sodium for injection
Penicillin G benzathine and procaine combined, intramuscular
Penicillin G benzathine, intramuscular
Penicillin G potassium for injection
Penicillin G procaine, intramuscular
Penicillin V potassium
Piperacillin sodium
Piperacillin sodium and Tazobactam sodium
Ticarcillin disodium
Ticarcillin disodium and Clavulanate potassium

Mechanism of Action: The bactericidal action of penicillins depends on their ability to bind penicillin-binding proteins (PBP-1 and PBP-3) in the cytoplasmic membranes of bacteria, thus inhibiting cell wall synthesis. Some penicillins act by acylation of membrane-bound transpeptidase enzymes, thereby preventing cross-linkage of peptidoglycan chains, which are necessary for bacterial cell wall strength and rigidity. Cell division and growth are inhibited and often lysis and elongation of susceptible bacteria occur. Penicillin is most effective against young, rapidly dividing organisms and has little effect on mature resting cells. Depending on the concentration of the drug at the site of infection and the susceptibility of the infectious microorganism, penicillin is either bacteriostatic or bactericidal. Penicillins are distributed through-

---

bold italic = life threatening side effect

out most of the body and pass the placental barrier. They also pass into synovial, pleural, pericardial, peritoneal, ascitic, and spinal fluids. Although normal meninges and the eyes are relatively impermeable to penicillins, they are better absorbed by inflamed meninges and eyes. **Peak serum levels, after PO:** 1 hr. **t½:** 30–110 min; protein binding: 20%–98% (see individual agents). Excreted largely unchanged by the urine as a result of glomerular filtration and active tubular secretion.

General Statement: Penicillins may be classifed as: (1) Natural: Penicillin G, Penicillin V. (2) Aminopenicillins: Amoxicillin, Amoxicillin/potassium clavulanate, Ampicillin, Ampicillin/sulbactam, Bacampicillin. (3) Penicillinase-resistant: Cloxacillin, Dicloxacillin, Nafcillin, Oxacillin. (4) Extended spectrum: Carbenicillin, Mezlocillin, Piperacillin, Piperacillin/tazobactam sodium, Ticarcillin, Ticarcillin/potassium clavulanate.

Uses: See individual drugs. Effective against a variety of gram-positive, gram-negative, and anaerobic organisms.

Contraindications: Hypersensitivity to penicillins, imipenem, β–lactamase inhibitors, and cephalosporins. PO use of penicillins during the acute stages of empyema, bacteremia, pneumonia, meningitis, pericarditis, and purulent or septic arthritis. Use with a history of amoxicillin/clavulanate–associated cholestatic jaundice or hepatic dysfunction. Lactation.

Precautions: Use of penicillins during lactation may lead to sensitization, diarrhea, candidiasis, and skin rash in the infant. Use with caution in patients with a history of asthma, hay fever, or urticaria. Patients with cystic fibrosis have a higher incidence of side effects with broad spectrum penicillins. Safety and effectiveness of carbenicillin, piperacillin, and the beta-lactamase inhibitor/penicillin combinations (e.g., amoxicillin/potassium clavulanate, ticarcillin/ potassium clavulanate) have not been determined in children less than 12 years of age. The incidence of resistant strains of staphylococci to penicillinase-resistant penicillins is increasing. Use of prolonged therapy may lead to superinfection (i.e., bacterial or fungal overgrowth of nonsusceptible organisms). Cystic fibrosis patients have a higher incidence of side effects if given extended spectrum penicillins.

Side Effects: Penicillins are potent sensitizing agents; it is estimated that up to 10% of the US population is allergic to the antibiotic. Hypersensitivity reactions are reported to be on the increase in pediatric populations. Sensitivity reactions may be immediate (within 20 min) or delayed (as long as several days or weeks after initiation of therapy). *Allergic:* Skin rashes (including maculopapular and exanthematous), exfoliative dermatitis, erythema multiforme (rarely, **Stevens-Johnson syndrome**), hives, pruritus, wheezing, **anaphylaxis,** fever, eosinophilia, hypersensitivity myocarditis, **angioedema,** serum sickness, **laryngeal edema, laryngospasm, prostration, angioneurotic edema, bronchospasm, hypotension, vascular collapse, death.** *GI:* Diarrhea (may be severe), abdominal cramps or pain, N&V, bloating, flatulence, increased thirst, bitter/unpleasant taste, glossitis, gastritis, stomatitis, dry mouth, sore mouth or tongue, furry tongue, black "hairy" tongue, bloody diarrhea, rectal bleeding, enterocolitis, pseudomembranous colitis. *CNS:* Dizziness, insomnia, hyperactivity, fatigue, prolonged muscle relaxation. Neurotoxicity including lethargy, neuromuscular irritability, **seizures,** hallucinations following large IV doses (especially in patients with renal failure). *Hematologic:* Thrombocytopenia, leukopenia, **agranulocytosis,** anemia, thrombocytopenic purpura, **hemolytic anemia,** granulocytopenia, neutropenia, bone marrow depression. *Renal:* Oliguria, hematuria, hyaline casts, proteinuria, pyuria (all symptoms of interstitial nephritis), nephropathy. Electrolyte imbalance following IV use. *Miscellaneous:* Hepatotoxicity (cholestatic jaundice), superinfection, swelling of face and ankles, anorexia, hyperthermia, transient hepatitis, vaginitis, itchy eyes. IM injection may cause pain and induration at the injection site, ecchymosis, and hematomas. IV use may cause vein irritation, deep vein thrombosis, and thrombophlebitis.

OD **Overdose Management:** *Symptoms:* Neuromuscular hyperexcitability, convulsive seizures. Massive IV doses may cause agitation, asterixis, hallucinations, confusion, stupor, multifocal myoclonus, seizures, coma, hyperkalemia, and encephalopathy. *Treatment (Severe Allergic or Anaphylactic Reactions):* Administer epinephrine (0.3–0.5 mL of a 1:1,000 solution SC or IM, or 0.2–0.3 mL diluted in 10 mL saline, given slowly by IV). Corticosteroids should be on hand. In those instances where penicillin is the drug of choice, the physician may decide to use it even though the patient is allergic, adding a medication to the regimen to control the allergic response.

Drug Interactions
Aminoglycosides / Penicillins ↓ effect of aminoglycosides, although they are used together
Antacids / ↓ Effect of penicillins due to ↓ absorption from GI tract
Antibiotics, Chloramphenicol, Erythromycins, Tetracyclines / ↓ Effect of penicillins, although synergism has also been seen
Anticoagulants / ↑ Bleeding risk by prolonging bleeding time if used with parenteral penicillins
Aspirin / ↑ Effect of penicillins by ↓ plasma protein binding
Chloramphenicol / Either ↑ or ↓ effects
Erythromycins / Either ↑ or ↓ effects
Heparin / ↑ Risk of bleeding following parenteral penicillins
Oral contraceptives / ↓ Effect of oral contraceptives
Probenecid / ↑ Effect of penicillins by ↓ excretion
Tetracyclines / ↓ Effect of penicillins

EMS CONSIDERATIONS
See also *Anti-Infectives.*

PROGESTERONE AND PROGESTINS

See also the following individual entries:

  Levonorgestrel implants
  Medroxyprogesterone acetate
  Megestrol acetate
  Oral Contraceptives
  Progesterone gel

Mechanism of Action: Progesterone is the primary endogenous progestin. Progesterone inhibits, through positive feedback, the secretion of pituitary gonadotropins; in turn, this prevents follicular maturation and ovulation or alternatively promotes it for the "primed" follicle. It is required to prepare the endometrium for implantation of the embryo. Once implanted, progesterone is required to maintain pregnancy. Progestins inhibit spontaneous uterine contractions; certain progestins may cause androgenic or anabolic effects. Progestins given PO are rapidly absorbed and quickly metabolized in the liver. **Peak levels, after PO:** 1–2 hr. **t½, after PO:** 2–3 hr during the first 6 hr after ingestion; thereafter, 8–9 hr. **After IM,** effective levels can be maintained for 3–6 months with a **t½** of about 10 weeks. **t½, elimination, gel:** 5–20 min. A major portion is excreted in the urine with a small amount in the bile and feces.

Uses: Abnormal uterine bleeding, primary or secondary amenorrhea (used with an estrogen), endometriosis. Alone or with an estrogen for contraception. May also be used in combination with an estrogen for endometriosis and hypermenorrhea. Certain types of cancer. AIDS wasting syndrome (megestrol acetate). Infertility (progesterone gel). *NOTE:* Not to be used to prevent habitual abortion or to treat threatened abortion. *In-*

---

bold italic = life threatening side effect

vestigational: Medroxyprogesterone has been used to treat menopausal symptoms.

Contraindications: Carcinoma of the breast or genital organs, thromboembolic disease, thrombophlebitis, vaginal bleeding of unknown origin, impaired liver function, cerebral hemorrhage or those with a history of such, missed abortion, as a diagnostic test for pregnancy. Pregnancy, especially during the first 4 months.

Precautions: Use with caution in case of asthma, epilepsy, depression, migraine, and cardiac or renal dysfunction.

Side Effects: See also individual drugs. Occasionally noted with short-term dosage, frequently observed with prolonged high dosage. *CNS:* Depression, insomnia, somnolence. *GU:* Breakthrough bleeding, spotting, amenorrhea, changes in amount and/or duration of menstrual flow, changes in cervical secretions and cervical erosion, breast tenderness or secretions. *Dermatologic:* Allergic rashes with and without pruritus, acne, melasma, chloasma, photosensitivity, local reactions at the site of injection. *Note:* Progesterone is especially irritating at the site of injection, especially aqueous products. *Miscellaneous:* Weight gain or loss, cholestatic jaundice, masculinization of the female fetus, nausea, edema, precipitation of acute intermittent porphyria, pyrexia, hirsutism.

EMS CONSIDERATIONS

None.

SKELETAL MUSCLE RELAXANTS, CENTRALLY ACTING

See also the following individual entries:

Baclofen
Carisoprodol
Chlorzoxazone
Cyclobenzaprine hydrochloride
Dantrolene sodium
Diazepam

Methocarbamol
Tizanidine

Mechanism of Action: These drugs decrease muscle tone and involuntary movement. Many relieve anxiety and tension as well. Although the precise mechanism of action is unknown, most of these agents depress spinal polysynaptic reflexes. Their beneficial effects may also be attributable to their antianxiety activity. Several of the drugs in this group also manifest analgesic properties.

Uses: Musculoskeletal and neurologic disorders associated with muscle spasms, hyperreflexia, and hypertonia, including parkinsonism, tetanus, tension headaches, acute muscle spasms caused by trauma, and inflammation (e.g., low back syndrome, sprains, arthritis, bursitis). They also may be useful in the management of cerebral palsy and multiple sclerosis.

Side Effects: See individual drugs.

OD Overdose Management: *Symptoms:* Often extensions of the side effects. Stupor, ***coma, shock-like syndrome, respiratory depression,*** loss of muscle tone, and impaired deep tendon reflexes may also occur. *Treatment:* Symptomatic. Emesis or gastric lavage (followed by activated charcoal). If necessary, artificial respiration, oxygen administration, pressor agents, and IV fluids may be used. It may be possible to increase the rate of excretion of selected drugs by diuretics (including mannitol), peritoneal dialysis, or hemodialysis.

Drug Interactions: Centrally acting muscle relaxants may increase the sedative and respiratory depressant effects of CNS depressants (e.g., alcohol, barbiturates, sedatives and hypnotics, and antianxiety agents).

EMS CONSIDERATIONS

None.

SUCCINIMIDE ANTICONVULSANTS

See also the following individual entries:

Ethosuximide
Methsuximide
Phensuximide

Mechanism of Action: Suppress the paroxysmal 3-cycle/sec spike and wave activity that is associated with lapses of consciousness seen in absence seizures. Act by depressing the motor cortex and by raising the threshold of the CNS to convulsive stimuli. Rapidly absorbed from the GI tract.

Uses: Primarily absence seizures (petit mal). May be given concomitantly with other anticonvulsants if other types of epilepsy are manifested with absence seizures.

Contraindications: Hypersensitivity to succinimides.

Precautions: Safe use during pregnancy has not been established. Use with caution in patients with abnormal liver and kidney function.

Side Effects: *CNS:* Drowsiness, ataxia, dizziness, headaches, euphoria, lethargy, fatigue, insomnia, irritability, nervousness, dream-like state, hyperactivity. Psychiatric or psychologic aberrations such as mental slowing, hypochondriasis, sleep disturbances, inability to concentrate, depression, night terrors, instability, confusion, aggressiveness. Rarely, auditory hallucinations, paranoid psychosis, increased libido, suicidal behavior. *GI:* N&V, hiccoughs, anorexia, diarrhea, gastric distress, weight loss, abdominal and epigastric pain, cramps, constipation. *Hematologic:* Leukopenia, granulocytopenia, eosinophilia, *agranulocytosis,* pancytopenia with or without bone marrow suppression, monocytosis. *Dermatologic:* Pruritus, urticaria, erythema multiforme, lupus erythematosus, *Stevens-Johnson syndrome,* pruritic erythematous rashes, skin eruptions, alopecia, hirsutism, photophobia. *GU:* Urinary frequency, vaginal bleeding, renal damage, microscopic hematuria. *Miscellaneous:* Blurred vision, muscle weakness, hyperemia, hypertrophy of gums, swollen tongue, myopia, periorbital edema.

OD **Overdose Management:** *Symptoms (Acute Overdose):* Confusion, sleepiness, slow shallow respiration, N&V, *CNS depression with coma and respiratory depression,* hypotension, cyanosis, hyper- or hypothermia, absence of reflexes, unsteadiness, flaccid muscles. *Symptoms (Chronic Overdose):* Ataxia, dizziness, drowsiness, confusion, depression, proteinuria, skin rashes, hangover, irritability, poor judgment, N&V, muscle weakness, periorbital edema, hepatic dysfunction, *fatal bone marrow aplasia, delayed onset of coma,* nephrosis, hematuria, casts. *Treatment:* General supportive measures. Charcoal hemoperfusion may be helpful.

Drug Interactions: Succinimides may ↑ effects of hydantoins by ↓ breakdown by the liver.

EMS CONSIDERATIONS

See also *Anticonvulsants.*

SULFONAMIDES

See also the following individual entries:

Mafenide acetate
Pediazole
Sulfacetamide sodium
Sulfadiazine
Sulfamethoxazole
Sulfasalazine
Sulfisoxazole
Sulfisoxazole diolamine
Trimethoprim and
   Sulfamethoxazole

Mechanism of Action: Structurally related to PABA and, as such, competitively inhibit the enzyme dihydropteroate synthetase, which is responsible for incorporating PABA into dihydrofolic acid. Thus, the synthesis of dihydrofolic acid is inhibited, resulting in a decrease in tetrahydrofolic acid, which is required for synthesis of DNA, purines, and thymidine. Are bacteriostatic. Readily absorbed from the GI tract. Distributed throughout all tissues, including the CSF, where

---

bold italic = life threatening side effect

concentrations attain 50%–80% of those found in the blood. Metabolized in the liver and primarily excreted by the kidneys. Small amounts are found in the feces, bile, breast milk, and other secretions. **Uses: PO, Parenteral.** See individual drugs. Uses include urinary tract infections, chancroid, meningitis caused by *Hemophilus influenzae*, meningococcal meningitis, rheumatic fever, nocardiosis, trachoma, with pyrimethamine for toxoplasmosis, with quinine sulfate and pyrimethamine for chloroquine-resistant *Plasmodium falciparum*, and with penicillin for otitis media.

Ophthalmic. Conjunctivitis, corneal ulcer, and other superficial ocular infections due to susceptible organisms. Adjunct to systemic sulfonamides to treat trachoma.

Vaginal. Sulfanilamide is used to treat *Candida albicans* vulvovaginitis only.

Contraindications: Hypersensitivity reactions to sulfonamides and chemically related drugs (e.g., thiazides, sulfonylureas, loop diuretics, carbonic anhydrase inhibitors, local anesthetics, PABA-containing sunscreens). Use in infants less than 2 years of age, except with pyrimethamine to treat congenital toxoplasmosis. Use at term during pregnancy. Use in premature infants who are nursing or those with hyperbilirubinemia or G6PD deficiency. Group A beta-hemolytic streptococcal infections.

Precautions: Use with caution, and in reduced dosage, in patients with impaired liver or renal function, intestinal or urinary tract obstructions, blood dyscrasias, allergies, asthma, and hereditary G6PD deficiency. Use with caution if exposed to sunlight or ultraviolet light as photosensitivity may occur. Superinfection is a possibility. Use ophthalmic products with caution in patients with dry eye. Safety and efficacy of ophthalmic use in children have not been determined.

Side Effects: Systemic. *GI:* N&V, diarrhea, abdominal pain, glossitis, stomatitis, anorexia, pseudomembranous enterocolitis, pancreatitis, hepatitis, *hepatocellular necrosis*. *Allergic:* Rash, pruritus, photosensitivity, erythema nodosum or multiforme, generalized skin eruptions, *Stevens-Johnson syndrome*, conjunctivitis, rhinitis, balanitis. Serum sickness, urticaria, pruritus, exfoliative dermatitis, *anaphylaxis, toxic epidermal necrolysis* with or without corneal damage, periorbital edema, conjunctival and scleral injection, allergic myocarditis, decreased pulmonary function with eosinophila, disseminated lupus erythematosus, periarteritis nodosa, arteritis. *CNS:* Headaches, mental depression, *seizures*, hallucinations, vertigo, insomnia, apathy, ataxia, drowsiness, restlessness. *Renal:* Crystalluria, toxic nephrosis with oliguria and anuria, elevated creatinine. *Hematologic: Aplastic anemia*, leukopenia, neutropenia, *agranulocytosis*, thrombocytopenia, hemolytic anemia, methemoglobinemia, purpura, hypoprothrombinemia. *Neurologic:* Peripheral neuropathy, polyneuritis, neuritis, optic neuritis. *Miscellaneous:* Jaundice, tinnitus, arthralgia, superinfection, hearing loss, drug fever, pyrexia, chills, lupus erythematosus phenomenon, transient myopia.

By killing the intestinal flora, the sulfonamides also reduce the bacterial synthesis of vitamin K. This may result in *hemorrhage*. Administration of vitamin K to patients on long-term sulfonamide therapy is recommended.

Ophthalmic Use. Headache, browache. Blurred vision, eye irritation, itching, transient epithelial keratitis, reactive hyperemia, conjunctival edema, burning and transient stinging. Rarely, *Stevens-Johnson syndrome*, exfoliative dermatitis, *toxic epidermal necrolysis*, photosensitivity, fever, skin rash, GI disturbances, and bone marrow depression.

OD **Overdose Management:** *Symptoms:* N&V, anorexia, colic, dizziness, drowsiness, headache, unconsciousness, vertigo, toxic fever. More serious manifestations include *acute hemolytic anemia, agranulocytosis*, acidosis, maculopapular dermatitis, hepatic jaundice, sensitivity reactions, toxic neuritis, **death** (several days after the first dose). *Treatment:* Immediately discontinue the drug.

• Induce emesis or perform gastric lavage, especially if large doses were taken.

• To hasten excretion, alkalinize the urine and force fluids (if kidney function is normal). If there is renal blockage due to sulfonamide crystals, catheterization of the ureters may be needed.

• In the event of agranulocytosis, antibiotic therapy is needed to combat infection.

• To treat severe anemia or thrombocytopenia, blood or platelet transfusions are required.

Drug Interactions

Anticoagulants, oral / ↑ Effect of anticoagulants due to ↓ plasma protein binding

Antidiabetics, oral / ↑ Hypoglycemic effect due to ↓ plasma protein binding

Cyclosporine / ↓ Effect of cyclosporine and ↑ nephrotoxicity

Diuretics, thiazide / ↑ Risk of thrombocytopenia with purpura

Indomethacin / ↑ Effect of sulfonamides due to ↓ plasma protein binding

Methenamine / ↑ Chance of sulfonamide crystalluria due to acid urine

Methotrexate / ↑ Risk of methotrexate-induced bone marrow suppression

Phenytoin / ↑ Effect of phenytoin due to ↓ breakdown in liver

Probenecid / ↑ Effect of sulfonamides due to ↓ plasma protein binding

Salicylates / ↑ Effect of sulfonamides due to ↓ plasma protein binding

Silver products / Incompatible with ophthalmic products

Uricosuric agents / Potentiation of uricosuric action

EMS CONSIDERATIONS

See also *Anti-Infectives.*

SYMPATHOMIMETIC DRUGS

See also the following individual entries:

Albuterol
Bitolterol mesylate
Brimonidine tartrate
Dobutamine hydrochloride
Dopamine hydrochloride
Ephedrine sulfate
Epinephrine
Epinephrine bitartrate
Epinephrine borate
Epinephrine hydrochloride
Isoetharine hydrochloride
Isoproterenol hydrochloride
Isoproterenol sulfate
Levalbuterol hydrochloride
Levarterenol bitartrate
Mephentermine sulfate
Metaproterenol sulfate
Metaraminol bitartrate
Phenylephrine hydrochloride
Phenylpropanolamine
    hydrochloride
Pirbuterol acetate
Pseudoephedrine hydrochloride
Pseudoephedrine sulfate
Salmeterol xinafoate
Terbutaline sulfate

Mechanism of Action: Adrenergic drugs act: (1) by mimicking the action of norepinephrine or epinephrine by combining with alpha and/or beta receptors (directly acting sympathomimetics) or (2) by causing or regulating the release of the natural neurohormones from their storage sites at the nerve terminals (indirectly acting sympathomimetics). Some drugs exhibit a combination of both effects.

Adrenergic stimulation of receptors will manifest the following general effects:

Alpha-1-adrenergic: / Vasoconstriction, decongestion, constriction of the pupil of the eye, contraction of splenic capsule, contraction of the trigone-sphincter muscle of the urinary bladder.

Alpha-2-adrenergic: / Presynaptic to regulate amount of transmitter released; decrease tone, motility, and secretory activity of the GI tract (possibly involved in hypersecretory response also); decrease insulin secretion.

Beta-1-adrenergic: / Myocardial contraction (inotropic), regulation of heartbeat (chronotropic), improved impulse conduction, ↑ lipolysis.

Beta-2-adrenergic: / Peripheral vasodilation, bronchial dilation; ↓ tone, motility, and secretory activity of the GI tract; ↑ renin secretion.

Uses: See individual drugs.

Contraindications: Tachycardia due to arrhythmias; tachycardia or heart block caused by digitalis toxicity.

Precautions: Use with caution in hyperthyroidism, diabetes, prostatic hypertrophy, seizures, degenerative heart disease, especially in geriatric patients or those with asthma, emphysema, or psychoneuroses. Also, use with caution in patients with coronary insufficiency, CAD, ischemic heart disease, CHF, cardiac arrhythmias, hypertension, or history of stroke. Asthma patients who rely heavily on inhaled beta-2-agonist bronchodilators may increase their chances of death. Thus, use to "rescue" patients but do not prescribe for regular long-term use. Beta-2 agonists may inhibit uterine contractions.

Side Effects: See individual drugs; side effects common to most sympathomimetics are listed. *CV:* Tachycardia, arrhythmias, palpitations, BP changes, anginal pain, precordial pain, pallor, skipped beats, chest tightness, hypertension. *GI:* N&V, heartburn, anorexia, altered taste or bad taste, GI distress, dry mouth, diarrhea. *CNS:* Restlessness, anxiety, tension, insomnia, hyperkinesis, drowsiness, weakness, vertigo, irritability, dizziness, headache, tremors, general CNS stimulation, nervousness, shakiness, hyperactivity. *Respiratory:* Cough, dyspnea, dry

throat, pharyngitis, **_paradoxical bronchospasm,_** irritation. *Other:* Flushing, sweating, **_allergic reactions_**.

OD **Overdose Management:** *Symptoms:* Following inhalation: Exaggeration of side effects resulting in anginal pain, hypertension, hypokalemia, **_seizures._** Following systemic use: CV symptoms include bradycardia, tachycardia, palpitations, extrasystoles, **_heart block,_** elevated BP, chest pain, hypokalemia. CNS symptoms include anxiety, insomnia, tremor, delirium, **_convulsions, collapse, and coma._** Also, fever, chills, cold perspiration, N&V, mydriasis, and blanching of the skin. *Treatment:*

• For overdosage due to inhalation: General supportive measures with sedatives given for restlessness. Use metoprolol or atenolol cautiously as they may induce an asthmatic attack in patients with asthma.

• For systemic overdosage: Discontinue or decrease dose. General supportive measures. For overdose due to PO agents, emesis, gastric lavage, or charcoal may be helpful. In severe cases, propranolol may be used but this may cause airway obstruction. Phentolamine may be given to block strong alpha-adrenergic effects.

Drug Interactions

Beta-adrenergic blocking agents / Inhibit adrenergic stimulation of the heart and bronchial tree; cause bronchial constriction; hypertension, asthma, not relieved by adrenergic agents

Ammonium chloride / ↓ Effect of sympathomimetics due to ↑ excretion by kidney

Anesthetics / Halogenated anesthetics sensitize heart to adrenergics—causes cardiac arrhythmias

Anticholinergics / Concomitant use aggravates glaucoma

Antidiabetics / Hyperglycemic effect of epinephrine may necessitate ↑ dosage of insulin or oral hypoglycemic agents

Corticosteroids / Chronic use with sympathomimetics may result in or aggravate glaucoma; aerosols containing sympathomimetics and corticosteroids may be lethal in asthmatic children

Digitalis glycosides / Combination may cause cardiac arrhythmias

Furazolidone / Furazolidone ↑ effects of mixed-acting sympathomimetics

Guanethidine / Direct-acting sympathomimetics ↑ effects of guanethidine, while indirect-acting sympathomimetics ↓ effects of guanethidine; also reversal of hypotensive effects of guanethidine

Lithium / ↓ Pressor effect of direct-acting sympathomimetics

MAO inhibitors / All effects of sympathomimetics are potentiated; symptoms include hypertensive crisis with possible intracranial hemorrhage, hyperthermia, convulsions, coma; death may occur

Methyldopa / ↑ Pressor response

Methylphenidate / Potentiates pressor effect of sympathomimetics; combination hazardous in glaucoma

Oxytocics / ↑ Chance of severe hypertension

Phenothiazines / ↑ Risk of cardiac arrhythmias

Reserpine / ↑ Risk of hypertension following use of direct-acting sympathomimetics and ↓ effect of indirect-acting sympathomimetics

Sodium bicarbonate / ↑ Effect of sympathomimetics due to ↓ excretion by kidney

Theophylline / Enhanced toxicity (especially cardiotoxicity); also ↓ theophylline levels

Thyroxine / Potentiation of pressor response of sympathomimetics

Tricyclic antidepressants / ↑ Effect of direct-acting sympathomimetics and ↓ effect of indirect-acting sympathomimetics

EMS CONSIDERATIONS

Assessment: Obtain baseline data and hemodynamic status including ECG, VS.

SPECIAL EMS CONSIDERATIONS FOR ADRENERGIC BRONCHODILATORS

Assessment

1. Monitor VS to assess CV response.

2. Note characteristics of cough and sputum production.

Interventions

1. With status asthmaticus, continue to provide oxygen and ventilating assistance even though the symptoms appear to be relieved by the bronchodilator.

2. To prevent depression of respiratory effort, administer oxygen based on patient's clinical symptoms and ABGs or O_2 saturations.

TETRACYCLINES

See also the following individual entries:

> Doxycycline calcium
> Doxycycline hyclate
> Doxycycline monohydrate
> Tetracycline

Mechanism of Action: Tetracyclines inhibit protein synthesis by microorganisms by binding to the ribosomal 50S subunit, thereby interfering with protein synthesis. They block the binding of aminoacyl transfer RNA to the messenger RNA complex. Cell wall synthesis is not inhibited. Are mostly bacteriostatic and are effective only against multiplying bacteria. Well absorbed from the stomach and upper small intestine. Well distributed throughout all tissues and fluids and diffuse through noninflamed meninges and the placental barrier. Are deposited in the fetal skeleton and calcifying teeth. **t½:** 7–18.6 hr (see individual agents); increased in the presence of renal impairment. They bind to serum protein (range: 20%–93%; see individual agents). Concentrated in the liver in the bile; excreted mostly unchanged in the urine and feces.

Uses: See individual drugs. Used mainly for infections caused by *Rickettsia, Chlamydia,* and *Mycoplasma.* Due to development of resistance, tetracyclines are usually not used for infections by common gram-negative or gram-positive organisms. Atypical pneumonia caused by *Mycoplasma pneumoniae*. Adjunct in the treatment of trachoma.

As an alternative to penicillin for uncomplicated gonorrhea or disseminated gonococcal infections, especially with penicillin allergy. Acute pelvic inflammatory disease. Useful as an alternative to penicillin for early syphilis.

Although not generally used for gram-positive infections, may be beneficial in anthrax, *Listeria* infections, and actinomycosis. Have also been used in conjunction with quinine sulfate for chloroquine-resistant *Plasmodium falciparum* malaria and as an intracavitary injection to control pleural or pericardial effusions caused by metastatic carcinoma. As an adjunct to amebicides in acute intestinal amebiasis. Used PO to treat uncomplicated endocervical, rectal, or urethral *Chlamydia* infections.

Topical uses include skin granulomas caused by *Mycobacterium marinum;* ophthalmic bacterial infections causing blepharitis, conjunctivitis, or keratitis; and as an adjunct in the treatment of ophthalmic chlamydial infections such as trachoma or inclusion conjunctivitis. As an alternative to silver nitrate for prophylaxis of neonatal gonococcal ophthalmia. Vaginitis. Severe acne.

Contraindications: Hypersensitivity. Use during tooth development stage (last trimester of pregnancy, neonatal period, during breast-feeding, and during childhood up to 8 years) because tetracyclines interfere with enamel formation and dental pigmentation. Never administer intrathecally.

Precautions: Use with caution and at reduced dosage in patients with impaired kidney function.

Side Effects: *GI* (most common): N&V, thirst, diarrhea, anorexia, sore throat, flatulence, epigastric distress, bulky loose stools. Less commonly, stomatitis, dysphagia, black hairy tongue, glossitis, or inflammatory lesions of the anogenital area. Rarely, pseudomembranous colitis. PO dosage forms may cause esophageal ulcers, especially in patients with esophageal obstructive element or hiatal hernia. *Allergic* (rare): Urticaria, pericarditis, polyarthralgia, fever, rash, pulmonary infiltrates with eosinophilia, **angioneurotic edema,** worsening of SLE, **anaphylaxis,** purpura. *Skin:* Photosensitivity, maculopapular and erythematous rashes, exfoliative dermatitis (rare), onycholysis, discoloration of nails. *CNS:* Dizziness, lightheadedness, unsteadiness, paresthesias. *Hematologic:* Eosinophilia, **hemolytic anemia,** neutropenia, thrombocytopenia, thrombocytopenic purpura. *Hepatic:* Fatty liver, increases in liver enzymes; rarely, hepatotoxicity, hepatitis, hepatic cholestasis. *Miscellaneous:* Candidal superinfections including oral and vaginal candidiasis, discoloration of infants' and children's teeth, bone lesions, delayed bone growth, abnormal pigmentation of the conjunctiva, pseudotumor cerebri in adults and bulging fontanels in infants.

IV administration may cause thrombophlebitis; IM injections are painful and may cause induration at the injection site.

Use of deteriorated tetracyclines may result in Fanconi-like syndrome characterized by N&V, acidosis, proteinuria, glycosuria, aminoaciduria, polydipsia, polyuria, hypokalemia.

Drug Interactions

Aluminum salts / ↓ Effect of tetracyclines due to ↓ absorption from GI tract

Antacids, oral / ↓ Effect of tetracyclines due to ↓ absorption from GI tract

Anticoagulants, oral / IV tetracyclines ↑ hypoprothrombinemia

Bismuth salts / ↓ Effect of tetracyclines due to ↓ absorption from GI tract

Bumetanide / ↑ Risk of kidney toxicity

Calcium salts / ↓ Effect of tetracyclines due to ↓ absorption from GI tract

Cimetidine / ↓ Effect of tetracyclines due to ↓ absorption from GI tract

Contraceptives, oral / ↓ Effect of oral contraceptives

Digoxin / Tetracyclines ↑ bioavailability of digoxin

Diuretics, thiazide / ↑ Risk of kidney toxicity

Ethacrynic acid / ↑ Risk of kidney toxicity

Furosemide / ↑ Risk of kidney toxicity

Insulin / Tetracyclines may ↓ insulin requirement

Iron preparations / ↓ Effect of tetracyclines due to ↓ absorption from GI tract

Lithium / Either ↑ or ↓ levels of lithium

Magnesium salts / ↓ Effect of tetracyclines due to ↓ absorption from GI tract

Methoxyflurane / ↑ Risk of kidney toxicity

Penicillins / Tetracyclines may mask bactericidal effect of penicillins

Sodium bicarbonate / ↓ Effect of tetracyclines due to ↓ absorption from GI tract

Zinc salts / ↓ Effect of tetracyclines due to ↓ absorption from GI tract

EMS CONSIDERATIONS

See also *Anti-Infectives.*

THEOPHYLLINE DERIVATIVES

See also the following individual entries:

Aminophylline
Theophylline

Mechanism of Action: Theophyllines stimulate the CNS, directly relax the smooth muscles of the bronchi and pulmonary blood vessels (relieve bronchospasms), produce diuresis, inhibit uterine contractions, stimulate gastric acid secretion, and increase the rate and force of contraction of the heart. The bronchodilator activity is due to direct relaxation of the bronchiolar smooth muscle and pulmonary blood vessels, which relieves bronchospasm. Although the exact mechanism is not known, theophyllines may act by altering the calcium levels of smooth muscle, blocking adenosine receptors, inhibiting the effect of prostaglandins on smooth muscle, and inhibiting the release of slow-reacting substance of anaphylaxis and histamine. Aminophylline releases free theophylline in vivo. Response to the drugs is highly individualized. Theophylline is well absorbed from uncoated plain tablets and PO liquids. *Theophylline salts:* **Onset:** 1–5 hr, depending on route and formulation. **Therapeutic plasma levels:** 10–20 mcg/mL. **$t^1/2$:** 3–15 hr in nonsmoking adults, 4–5 hr in adult heavy smokers, 1–9 hr in children, and 20–30 hr for premature neonates. An increased $t^1/2$ may be seen in individuals with CHF, alcoholism, liver dysfunction, or respiratory infections. Because of great variations in the rate of absorption (due to dosage form, food, dose level) as well as its extremely narrow therapeutic range, theophylline therapy is best monitored by determination of the serum levels. If these determinations cannot be obtained, saliva (contains 60% of corresponding theophylline serum levels) determinations can be used. Eighty-five percent to 90% metabolized in the liver and various metabolites, including the active 3-methylxanthine. Theophylline is metabolized partially to caffeine in the neonate. The premature neonate excretes 50% unchanged theophylline and may accumulate the caffeine metabolite. Excretion is through the kidneys (about 10% unchanged in adults).

Uses: Prophylaxis and treatment of bronchial asthma. Reversible bronchospasms associated with chronic bronchitis, emphysema, and COPD. *Investigational:* Treatment of neonatal apnea and Cheyne-Stokes respiration.

---

bold italic = life threatening side effect

Contraindications: Hypersensitivity to any xanthine, peptic ulcer, seizure disorders (unless on medication), hypotension, CAD, angina pectoris.

Precautions: Use during lactation may result in irritability, insomnia, and fretfulness in the infant. Use with caution in premature infants due to the possible accumulation of caffeine. Xanthines are not usually tolerated by small children because of excessive CNS stimulation. Geriatric patients may manifest an increased risk of toxicity. Use with caution in the presence of gastritis, alcoholism, acute cardiac diseases, hypoxemia, severe renal and hepatic disease, severe hypertension, severe myocardial damage, hyperthyroidism, glaucoma.

Side Effects: Side effects are uncommon at serum theophylline levels less than 20 mcg/mL. At levels greater than 20 mcg/mL, 75% of individuals experience side effects including N&V, diarrhea, irritability, insomnia, and headache. At levels of 35 mcg/mL or greater, individuals may manifest *cardiac arrhythmias,* hypotension, tachycardia, hyperglycemia, *seizures, brain damage, or death. GI:* N&V, diarrhea, anorexia, epigastric pain, hematemesis, dyspepsia, rectal irritation (following use of suppositories), rectal bleeding, gastroesophageal reflux during sleep or while recumbent (theophylline). *CNS:* Headache, insomnia, irritability, fever, dizziness, lightheadedness, vertigo, reflex hyperexcitability, *seizures,* depression, speech abnormalities, alternating periods of mutism and hyperactivity, *brain damage, death. CV:* Hypotension, *life-threatening ventricular arrhythmias,* palpitations, tachycardia, *peripheral vascular collapse,* extrasystoles. *Renal:* Proteinuria, excretion of erythrocytes and renal tubular cells, dehydration due to diuresis, urinary retention (men with prostatic hypertrophy). *Other:* Tachypnea, *respiratory arrest,* fever, flushing, hyperglycemia, antidiuretic hormone syndrome, leukocytosis, rash, alopecia.

NOTE: Aminophylline given by rapid IV may produce hypotension, flushing, palpitations, precordial pain, headache, dizziness, or hyperventilation. Also, the ethylenediamine in aminophylline may cause allergic reactions, including urticaria and skin rashes.

OD Overdose Management: *Symptoms:* Agitation, headache, nervousness, insomnia, tachycardia, extrasystoles, anorexia, N&V, fasciculations, tachypnea, *tonic-clonic seizures.* The first signs of toxicity may be seizures or ventricular arrhythmias. Toxicity is usually associated with parenteral administration but can be observed after PO administration, especially in children. *Treatment:*

• Have ipecac syrup, gastric lavage equipment, and cathartics available to treat overdose if the patient is conscious and not having seizures. Otherwise a mechanical ventilator, oxygen, diazepam, and IV fluids may be necessary for the treatment of overdosage.

• For postseizure coma, maintain an airway and oxygenate the patient. To remove the drug, perform only gastric lavage and give the cathartic and activated charcoal by a large-bore gastric lavage tube. Charcoal hemoperfusion may be necessary.

• Treat atrial arrhythmias with verapamil and treat ventricular arrhythmias with lidocaine or procainamide.

• Use IV fluids to treat acid-base imbalance, hypotension, and dehydration. Hypotension may also be treated with vasopressors.

• To treat hyperpyrexia, use a tepid water sponge bath or a hypothermic blanket.

• Treat apnea with artificial respiration.

• Monitor serum levels of theophylline until they fall below 20 mcg/mL as secondary rises of theophylline may occur, especially with sustained-release products.

Drug Interactions

Allopurinol / ↑ Theophylline levels

Aminogluthethimide / ↓ Theophylline levels

Barbiturates / ↓ Theophylline levels

Benzodiazepines / Sedative effect may be antagonized by theophylline

Beta-adrenergic agonists / Additive effects

Beta-adrenergic blocking agents / ↑ Theophylline levels

Calcium channel blocking drugs / ↑ Theophylline levels

Carbamazepine / Either ↑ or ↓ theophylline levels

Charcoal / ↓ Theophylline levels

Cimetidine / ↑ Theophylline levels

Ciprofloxacin / ↑ Plasma levels of theophylline with ↑ possibility of side effects

Corticosteroids / ↑ Theophylline levels

Digitalis / Theophylline ↑ toxicity of digitalis

Disulfiram / ↑ Theophylline levels

Ephedrine and other sympathomimetics / ↑ Theophylline levels

Erythromycin / ↑ Effect of theophylline due to ↓ breakdown by liver

Ethacrynic acid / Either ↑ or ↓ theophylline levels

Furosemide / Either ↑ or ↓ theophylline levels

Halothane / ↑ Risk of cardiac arrhythmias

Interferon / ↑ Theophylline levels

Isoniazid / Either ↑ or ↓ theophylline levels

Ketamine / Seizures of the extensor-type

Ketoconazole / ↓ Theophylline levels

Lithium / ↓ Effect of lithium due to ↑ rate of excretion

Loop diuretics / ↓ Theophylline levels

Mexiletine / ↑ Theophylline levels

Muscle relaxants, nondepolarizing / Theophylline ↓ effect of these drugs

Oral contraceptives / ↑ Effect of theophyllines due to ↓ breakdown by liver

Phenytoin / ↓ Theophylline levels

Propofol / Theophyllines ↓ sedative effect of propofol

Quinolones / ↑ Theophylline levels

Reserpine / ↑ Risk of tachycardia

Rifampin / ↓ Theophylline levels

Sulfinpyrazone / ↓ Theophylline levels

Sympathomimetics / ↓ Theophylline levels

Tetracyclines / ↑ Risk of theophylline toxicity

Thiabendazole / ↑ Theophylline levels

Thyroid hormones / ↓ Theophylline levels in hypothyroid patients

Tobacco smoking / ↓ Effect of theophylline due to ↑ breakdown by liver

Troleandomycin / ↑ Effect of theophylline due to ↓ breakdown by liver

Verapamil / ↑ Effect of theophylline

Administration/Storage: Dilute drugs and maintain proper infusion rates to minimize problems of overdosage.

EMS CONSIDERATIONS

Assessment: Assess lung fields closely. Note characteristics of sputum and cough; assess CXR, ABGs, and PFTs.

Interventions: Observe for S&S of toxicity such as nausea, anorexia, insomnia, irritability, hyperexcitability, or cardiac arrhythmias; monitor serum levels.

TRANQUILIZERS/ANTI-MANIC DRUGS/HYPNOTICS

See also the following individual entries:

Alprazolam
Barbiturates
Buspirone hydrochloride
Chlordiazepoxide
Clorazepate dipotassium
Diazepam
Estazolam
Flurazepam hydrochloride

---

bold italic = life threatening side effect

Hydroxyzine hydrochloride
Hydroxyzine pamoate
Lithium carbonate
Lithium citrate
Lorazepam
Meprobamate
Midazolam hydrochloride
Oxazepam
Temazepam
Triazolam
Zolpidem tartrate

Mechanism of Action: Benzodiazepines are the major antianxiety agents. They are thought to affect the limbic system and reticular formation to reduce anxiety by increasing or facilitating the inhibitory neurotransmitter activity of GABA. Two benzodiazepine receptor subtypes have been identified in the brain–BZ_1 and BZ_2. Receptor subtype BZ_1 is believed to be associated with sleep mechanisms, whereas receptor subtype BZ_2 is associated with memory, motor, sensory, and cognitive function. When used for 3–4 weeks for sleep, certain benzodiazepines may cause REM rebound when discontinued. Meprobamate and the benzodiazepines also possess varying degrees of anticonvulsant activity, skeletal muscle relaxation, and the ability to alleviate tension. The benzodiazepines generally have long half-lives (1–8 days); thus cumulative effects can occur. Several of the benzodiazepines are metabolized to active metabolites in the liver, which prolongs their duration of action. Benzodiazepines are widely distributed throughout the body. Approximately 70%–99% of an administered dose is bound to plasma protein. Metabolites of benzodiazepines are excreted through the kidneys. All tranquilizers have the ability to cause psychologic and physical dependence.

Contraindications: Hypersensitivity, acute narrow-angle glaucoma, psychoses, primary depressive disorder, psychiatric disorders in which anxiety is not a signficiant symptom.

Precautions: Use with caution in impaired hepatic or renal function and in the geriatric or debilitated patient. Use during lactation may cause sedation, weight loss, and possibly feeding difficulties in the infant. Geriatric patients may be more sensitive to the effects of benzodiazepines; symptoms may include oversedation, dizziness, confusion, or ataxia. When used for insomnia, rebound sleep disorders may occur following abrupt withdrawal of certain benzodiazepines.

Side Effects: *CNS:* Drowsiness, fatigue, confusion, ataxia, sedation, dizziness, vertigo, depression, apathy, lightheadedness, delirium, headache, lethargy, disorientation, hypoactivity, crying, anterograde amnesia, slurred speech, stupor, **coma,** fainting, difficulty in concentration, euphoria, nervousness, irritability, akathisia, hypotonia, vivid dreams, "glassy-eyed," hysteria, **suicide attempt,** psychosis. Paradoxical excitement manifested by anxiety, acute hyperexcitability, increased muscle spasticity, insomnia, hallucinations, sleep disturbances, rage, and stimulation. *GI:* Increased appetite, constipation, diarrhea, anorexia, N&V, weight gain or loss, dry mouth, bitter or metallic taste, increased salivation, coated tongue, sore gums, difficulty in swallowing, gastritis, fecal incontinence. *Respiratory:* **Respiratory depression and sleep apnea,** especially in patients with compromised respiratory function. *Dermatologic:* Urticaria, rash, pruritus, alopecia, hirsutism, dermatitis, edema of ankles and face. *Endocrine:* Increased or decreased libido, gynecomastia, menstrual irregularities. *GU:* Difficulty in urination, urinary retention, incontinence, dysuria, enuresis. *CV:* Hypertension, hypotension, bradycardia, tachycardia, palpitations, edema, **CV collapse.** *Hematologic:* Anemia, **agranulocytosis,** leukopenia, eosinophilia, thrombocytopenia. *Ophthalmologic:* Diplopia, conjunctivitis, nystagmus, blurred vision. *Miscellaneous:* Joint pain, lymphadenopathy, muscle cramps, paresthesia, dehydration, lupus-like symptoms, sweating, SOB, flushing, hiccoughs, fever, hepatic dysfunction. *Following*

IM use: Redness, pain, burning. *Following IV use:* Thrombosis and phlebitis at site.

OD **Overdose Management:** *Symptoms:* Severe drowsiness, confusion with reduced or absent reflexes, tremors, slurred speech, staggering, hypotension, SOB, labored breathing, ***respiratory depression,*** impaired coordination, ***seizures,*** weakness, slow HR, ***coma.*** *NOTE:* Geriatric patients, debilitated patients, young children, and patients with liver disease are more sensitive to the CNS effects of benzodiazepines. *Treatment:* Supportive therapy. In the event of an overdose of a benzodizepine, have a benzodiazepine antagonist (flumazenil) readily available. Gastric lavage, provided that an ET tube with an inflated cuff is used to prevent aspiration of vomitus. Emesis only if drug ingestion was recent and patient is fully conscious. Activated charcoal and saline cathartic may be given after emesis or lavage. Maintain adequate respiratory function. Reverse hypotension by IV fluids, norepinephrine, or metaraminol. **Do not** treat excitation with barbiturates.

Drug Interactions

Alcohol / Potentiation or addition of CNS depressant effects. Concomitant use may lead to drowsiness, lethargy, stupor, respiratory collapse, coma, or death
Anesthetics, general / See *Alcohol*
Antacids / ↓ Rate of absorption of benzodiazepines
Antidepressants, tricyclic / Concomitant use with benzodiazepines may cause additive sedative effect and/or atropine-like side effects
Antihistamines / See *Alcohol*
Barbiturates / See *Alcohol*
Cimetidine / ↑ Effect of benzodiazepines by ↓ breakdown in liver
CNS depressants / See *Alcohol*
Digoxin / Benzodiazepines ↑ effect of digoxin by ↑ serum levels
Disulfiram / ↑ Effect of benzodiazepines by ↓ breakdown in liver
Erythromycin / ↑ Effect of benzodiazepines by ↓ breakdown in liver

Fluoxetine / ↑ Effect of benzodiazepines due to ↓ breakdown in liver
Isoniazid / ↑ Effect of benzodiazepines due to ↓ breakdown in liver
Ketoconazole / ↑ Effect of benzodiazepines due to ↓ breakdown in liver
Levodopa / Effect may be ↓ by benzodiazepines
Metoprolol / ↑ Effect of benzodiazepines due to ↓ breakdown in liver
Narcotics / See *Alcohol*
Neuromuscular blocking agents / Benzodiazepines may ↑, ↓, or have no effect on the action of neuromuscular blocking agents
Oral contraceptives / ↑ Effect of benzodiazepines due to ↓ breakdown in liver; or, ↑ rate of clearance of benzodiazepines that undergo glucuronidation (e.g., lorazepam, oxazepam)
Phenothiazines / See *Alcohol*
Phenytoin / Concomitant use with benzodiazepines may cause ↑ effect of phenytoin due to ↓ breakdown by liver
Probenecid / ↑ Effect of selected benzodiazepines due to ↓ breakdown by liver
Propoxyphene / ↑ Effect of benzodiazepines due to ↓ breakdown by liver
Propranolol / ↑ Effect of benzodiazepines due to ↓ breakdown by liver
Ranitidine / May ↓ absorption of benzodiazepines from the GI tract
Rifampin / ↓ Effect of benzodiazepines due to ↑ breakdown by liver
Sedative-hypnotics, nonbarbiturate / See *Alcohol*
Theophyllines / ↓ Sedative effect of benzodiazepines
Valproic acid / ↑ Effect of benzodiazepines due to ↓ breakdown by liver

EMS CONSIDERATIONS

Interventions

1. Monitor BP before and after IV dose of antianxiety medication.
2. Administer the lowest possible effective dose, especially if elderly or debilitated.

---

bold italic = life threatening side effect

Table 2   Common Diseases, General Recommended Immunization Schedule, and Length of Immunity

DISEASE	IMMUNIZATION SCHEDULE	LENGTH OF IMMUNITY
Cholera	Two doses 1 week to 1 month apart	6 months
Diphtheria	Given as DPT; four doses at ages 2, 4, 6, and 15–18 months	10 years
Haemophilus influenzae (Hib)	Four doses at ages 2, 4, 6, and 15 months	Unknown
Hepatitis B	Three doses: at birth (or initial dose), 1 month later, and 6 months after second dose	Unknown
Influenza	One dose (or two doses of split virus if under 13 years)	1–3 years
Lyme Disease	Three doses at ages 15–70 years old; at 0, 1, and 12 months; plan 3rd dose just before tick season	1 yr; yearly booster
Measles	Given as MMR at ages 12–15 months and 4–6 yearsLifetime	Lifetime
Meningococcal meningitis	One dose (antibody response requires 5 days); antibiotic prophylaxis (Rifampin 600 mg or 10 mg/kg q 12 hr for four doses should be given to all contacts per exposure)	?Lifetime; not consistently effective in those <2 years of age
Mumps	Given as MMR at ages 12–15 months and 4–6 years	Lifetime
Pertussis	Given as DPT; four doses at ages 2, 4, 6, and 15–18 months	10 years
Pneumococcus	One dose (0.5 mL)	Approx. 5–10 years
Poliomyelitis	Four doses at ages 2, 4, and 6 months, then at age 4–6 years	Lifetime
Rabies	Postexposure: five doses on days 0, 3, 7, 14, and 28 with the rabies immune globulin; pre-exposure: two doses 1 week apart, third dose 2–3 weeks later	Approx. 2 years
Rubella	Given as MMR at ages 12–15 months and 4–6 years	Lifetime

Smallpox	One dose; this disease has been eradicated and vaccine is used only with military personnel and lab workers using pox viruses	3 years
Tetanus	Given initially as DPT; four doses at ages 2, 4, 6, and 15–18 months	10 years; a tetanus booster is required q 10 years
VZV (varicellazoster virus; chicken pox)	One dose (0.5 mL) age 12 months to 12 years; two injections of 0.5 mL 4–8 weeks apart in age 13 and older	?Lifetime
Yellow fever	One dose	10 years

Table 3   Active Childhood Immunization Schedule

	#1	#2	#3	#4
DPT	2 months	4 months	6 months	15–18 months
OPV	2 months	4 months	6 months	4–6 years
Hib	2 months	4 months	6 months	15–18 months
MMR	12 months	4 years		
Hep B	birth or initial dose	1 month after first dose	6 months or more after second dose	

Table 4   Active Adult Immunization Schedule

Tetanus	Tetanus booster every 10 years; with injury obtain one in 5 yrs
Pneumococcus	Every 5-10 years
Influenza	Every year
Lyme	Yearly booster in endemic areas after series completed

VACCINES

General Statement: Vaccines have played an important role in the health and life span of our population. They have been in use over 200 years, but since World War II, once the importance of disease prevention became evident, research into the area of vaccine development exploded.

Use of a vaccine (or actually contracting the disease) usually renders one temporary or permanent resistance to an infectious disease. Vaccines and toxoids promote the type of antibody production one would see if they had experienced the natural infection. This active immunization involves the direct administration of antigens to the host to cause them to produce the desired antibodies and cell-mediated immunity. These agents may consist of live attenuated agents or killed (inactivated) agents. Immunizations confer resistance without actually producing disease.

Passive immunization occurs when immunologic agents are administered. Immunoglobulins and antivenins only offer passive short-term immunity and are usually administered for a specific exposure.

Aggressive pediatric immunization programs have helped reduce preventable infections and death in children worldwide. This focus should continue and be expanded to the adult population, many of whom have missed the natural infection and their past immunizations. A careful immunization history should be documented for every patient, regardless of age. When in doubt or if unknown if had infection or immunization, appropriate titers may be drawn. Table 2 lists some of the more common diseases, the general recommended schedule to confer immunization, and the length of immunity conferred; Table 3 outlines the active childhood immunization schedule.

EMS CONSIDERATIONS

None.

VITAMINS

General Statement: Vitamins are essential, carbon-containing, noncaloric substances that are required for normal metabolism. They are produced by living materials such as plants and animals and they are generally obtained from the diet. Vitamin D is synthesized in the diet to a limited extent and Vitamin B–12 is synthesized in the intestinal tract by bacterial flora.

Vitamins are essential for promoting growth, health, and life. They are necessary for the metabolic processes responsible for transforming foods into tissue or energy. Vitamins are also involved in the formation and maintenance of blood cells, chemicals supporting the nervous system, hormones, and genetic materials. Vitamins do not provide energy because they contain no calories. Yet, some do help convert the calories in fats, carbohydrates, and proteins into usable body energy.

Disease states caused by severe nutritional deficiencies prompted the discovery of vitamins because scientists were able to reverse the signs and symptoms of these disease states with vitamins. Severe deficiencies include scurvy, rickets, pellagra, pernicious anemia, xerophthalmia, beriberi, osteomalacia, infantile hemolytic anemia, and hemorrhagic diseases of the newborn. Moderate vitamin deficiencies may also produce symptoms of impaired health.

Environmental factors and genetic predisposition may influence individual requirements for specific vitamins. Disease processes, growth, hormone balance, and drugs may also alter the dietary requirements and function of vitamins.

Many deficiency states can be traced to special circumstances such as pernicious anemia after gastrectomy; pellagra in corn–eating populations, and scurvy in the elderly subsisting on soft foods (e.g., eggs, bread, milk) while neglecting citrus fruits. Generally, although not common in the United States, vitamin deficiency usually involves multiple rather than single deficiencies and usually can be attributed to poor lifestyle choices and poor dietary habits with an inadequate intake of many nutrients, including all vitamins.

There are two categories of vitamins: fat soluble and water soluble. Fat soluble viatmins A, D, E, and K are found in the fat or oil of foods and require digestible fat and bile salts for absorption in the small intestine. The water-soluble vitamins, C and B complex (B-1, B-2, niacin, B-6, folic acid, B-12, pantothenic acid, and biotin) are found in the watery portion of foods and are well absorbed by the GI tract. They are easily lost through overcooking and do not require fat for absorption. Water soluble vitamins mix easily in the blood, are excreted by the kidneys, and only small amounts are stored in the tissues, so regular daily intake is essential. Fat soluble vitamins are stored in the body after binding to specific plasma globulins in fat parts of the body.

Recommended Dietary Allowances (RDAs) are the recommended human vitamin and mineral intake requirements. These were developed by the Food and Nutrition Board, National Research Council of the National Academy of Sciences and have evolved over the past 50 years and are updated every 5 years. They are based on age, height, weight, and gender. These are only estimates of nutrient needs; each patient and the surrounding factors warrant individualized evaluation when replacement is being considered.

EMS CONSIDERATIONS

None.

Table 5   Common Vitamin Requirements

Vitamin	RDA	Physiologic Effects Essential for:
A (retinol, retinaldehyde, retonic acid)	1400-6000 IU	Growth & development epithelial tissue maintenance; reproduction prevents night blindness
B complex:		
B-1 (thiamine)	0.3-1.5 mg	Energy metabolism: normal nerve function
B-2 (riboflavin)	0.4-1.8 mg	Reactions in energy cycle that produce ATP; oxidation of amino acids and hydroxy acids; oxidation of purines
B-3 Niacin (nicotinic acid, nicotinamide)	5-19 mg	Synthesis of fatty acids and cholesterol; blocks FFA; conversion of phenylalanine to tyrosine
B-6 (pyridoxine, pyridoxal, pyridoxamine)	0.3-2.5 mg	Amino acid metabolism; glycogenolysis, RBC/Hb synthesis; formation of neurotransmitters; formation of antibodies
Folacin (folic acid, pteroylglutamic acid)	50-800 mcg	DNA synthesis, formation of RBCs in bone marrow with cyanocobalamine

Table 5   *(continued)*

Vitamin	RDA	Physiologic Effects Essential for:
Pantothenic acid (calcium pantothenate, dexpanthenol)	10 mg	Synthesis of sterols, steroid hormones, porphyrins; synthesis and degradation of fatty acids; oxidative metabolism of carbohydrates, gluconeogenesis
B-12 (cyanocobalamin, hydroxocobalamin, extrinsic factor)	0.3–4.0 mcg	DNA synthesis in bone marrow; RBC production with folacin; nerve tissue maintenance
B-7 (Biotin)	No recommendation	Synthesis of fatty acids, generation of tricarboxylic acid cycle; formation of purines Coenzyme in CHO metabolism
C (ascorbic acid, ascorbate)	60 mg	Formation of collagen; conversion of cholesterol to bile acids; protects A and E and polyunsaturated fats from excessive oxidation; absorption and utilization of iron; converts folacin to folinic acid; some role in clotting, adrenocortical hormones, and resistance to cancer and infections
D (calcitriol, cholecalciferol, dihydrotachysterol, ergocalciferol, viosterol)	400 IU	Intestinal absorption and metabolism of calcium and phosphorus as well as renal reabsorption; release of calcium from bone and resorption
E (tocopherol)	4–15 IU	May oppose destruction of Vit. A and fats by oxygen fragments called free radicals; antioxidant; may affect production of prostaglandins which regulate a variety of body processes
K (menadione, phytonadione)	No recommendation	Formation of prothrombin and other clotting proteins by the liver; blood coagulation

Table 6   Vitamins and Uses

Vitamin	Effect	Uses
A (retinoic acid)	Reduces formation of comedones; keratin production suppression	Acne, psoriasis, ichthyosis, Darier's disease xerophthalmia, intestinal infections, prevents night blindness
Niacin	Reduction of blood cholesterol and triglycerides blocks FFA release	Hypercholesterolemia, hyperbetalipoproteinemia
D (dihydrotachysterol)	Maintains calcium and phosphorus levels in bone and blood	Hypoparathyroidism: increase intestinal absorption of calcium
C	Reduces urine pH; converts methemoglobin to hemoglobin	Idiopathic methemoglobin; recurrent UTIs in high risk clients aids in iron absorption
E	Reduces endogenous peroxidases	Hemolytic anemia in premature infants protects cell membranes from oxidation
K	Increases liver production of thrombin	Warfarin toxicity essential for blood coagulation

Table 7   Vitamin Deficiency States

Vitamin	Deficiency	Signs & Symptoms
A	Xerophthalmia	Progressive eye changes: night blindness to xerosis of conjunctiva and cornea with scarring
	Keratomalacia	Degeneration of epithelial cells with hardening and shrinking
B-6	Beriberi	Fatigue, weight loss, weakness, irritability; headaches, insomnia, peripheral neuropathy, CHF, cardiomyopathy
Niacin	Pellagra	Depression, anorexia, beefy red glossitis, cheilosis, dermatitis
B-12	Pernicious anemia	Macrocytic, megaloblastic anemia; progressive neuropathy R/T demyelination
C	Scurvy	Joint pain, growth retardation, anemia, poor wound healing with increased susceptibility to infection; petechial hemorrhages
D	Rickets (child) Osteomalacia (adult)	Demineralization of bones and teeth with bone pain and skeletal muscle deformities

Table 7   Vitamin Deficiency States   *(continued)*

Vitamin	Deficiency	Signs & Symptoms
E	Hemolytic anemia in low birth weight infants	Macrocytic anemia; increased hemolysis of RBC's and increased capillarity fragility
K	Hemorrhagic disease in newborns	Increase tendency to hemorrhage

CHAPTER FOUR
A–Z Listing of Drugs

Abacavir sulfate
(uh-BACK-ah-veer)
Pregnancy Class: C
Ziagen (Rx)
Classification: Antiviral, antiretroviral drug

Uses: In combination with other antiretroviral drugs to treat HIV-1 infection. Do not add as a single agent when antiretroviral regimens are changed due to loss of virologic response.
Precautions: Fatal hypersensitivity reactions are possible (See *Side Effects*). Efficacy for long-term suppression of HIV RNA or disease progression have not been determined. Abacavir is not a cure for HIV infection; patients may continue to show illnesses associated with HIV infection, including opportunistic infections. The drug has not been shown to reduce the risk of transmission of HIV to others through sexual contact or blood.

Route/Dosage
• **Oral Solution, Tablets**
Treat HIV-1 infection.
Adults: 300 mg b.i.d. with other antiretroviral drugs. **Pediatric, 3 months to 16 years:** 8 mg/kg b.i.d., not to exceed 30 mg b.i.d., in combination with other antiretroviral drugs.
How Supplied: *Oral Solution:* 20 mg/mL; *Tablets:* 300 mg
Side Effects: *Hypersensitivity:* Fever, skin rash, fatigue, N&V, diarrhea, abdominal pain, malaise, lethargy, myalgia, arthralgia, edema, SOB, paresthesia, lymphadenopathy, conjunctivitis, mouth ulcerations, maculopapular or urticarial rash *life-threatening hypotension, liver failure, renal failure, death*. *GI:* N&V, diarrhea, loss of appetite, pancreatitis. *Miscellaneous:* Severe hepatomegaly with steatosis (may be fatal), insomnia, other sleep disorders, headache, fever, skin rashes.
Drug Interactions: Ethanol ↓ excretion of abacavir → ↑ exposure.

EMS CONSIDERATIONS
See also *Antiviral Drugs.*

Acarbose
(ah-KAR-bohs)
Pregnancy Class: B
Precose (Rx)
Classification: Antidiabetic agent

Uses: Used alone, with diet control, to decrease blood glucose in type 2 diabetes mellitus. Also, used with a sulfonylurea when diet plus either acarbose or a sulfonylurea alone do not control blood glucose adequately.
Contraindications: Diabetic ketoacidosis, cirrhosis, inflammatory bowel disease, colonic ulceration, partial intestinal obstruction or predisposition to intestinal obstruction, chronic intestinal diseases associated with marked disorders of digestion or absorption, conditions that may deteriorate as a result of increased gas formation in the intestine. In significant renal dysfunction. Severe, persistent bradycardia. Lactation.
Precautions: Safety and efficacy have not been determined in children. Acarbose does not cause hypo-

glycemia; however, sulfonylureas and insulin can lower blood glucose sufficiently to cause symptoms or even life-threatening hypoglycemia.

Route/Dosage
• **Tablets**

Type 2 diabetes mellitus.
Individualized, depending on effectiveness and tolerance. **Initial:** 25 mg (one-half of a 50-mg tablet) t.i.d. with the first bite of each main meal. **Maintenance:** After the initial dose of 25 mg t.i.d., the dose can be increased to 50 mg t.i.d. Some may benefit from 100 mg t.i.d. The dosage can be adjusted at 4- to 8-week intervals. **Recommended maximum daily dose:** 50 mg t.i.d. for patients weighing less than 60 kg and 100 mg t.i.d. for those weighing more than 60 kg.

How Supplied: *Tablet:* 25 mg, 50 mg, 100 mg

Side Effects: *GI:* Abdominal pain, diarrhea, flatulence. GI side effects may be severe and be confused with paralytic ileus.

OD **Overdose Management:** *Symptoms:* Flatulence, diarrhea, abdominal discomfort. *Treatment:* Reduce dose; symptoms will subside.

Drug Interactions
Charcoal / ↓ Effect of acarbose
Digestive enzymes / ↓ Effect of acarbose
Digoxin / ↓ Serum digoxin levels
Insulin / ↑ Hypoglycemia which may cause severe hypoglycemia
Sulfonylureas / ↑ Hypoglycemia which may cause severe hypoglycemia

EMS CONSIDERATIONS
None.

Acebutolol hydrochloride
(ays-BYOU-toe-lohl)
Pregnancy Class: B
Sectral (Rx)
Classification: Beta-adrenergic blocking agent

Mechanism of Action: Predominantly beta-1 blocking activity but will inhibit beta-2 receptors at higher doses. Some intrinsic sympathomimetic activity.
Duration of Action: 24-30 hr.
Uses: Hypertension (either alone or with other antihypertensive agents such as thiazide diuretics). Premature ventricular contractions.
Contraindications: Severe, persistent bradycardia.
Precautions: Dosage not established in children.

Route/Dosage
• **Capsules**
Hypertension.
Initial: 400 mg/day (although 200 mg b.i.d. may be needed for optimum control; **then,** 400–800 mg/day (range: 200–1,200 mg/day).
Premature ventricular contractions.
Initial: 200 mg b.i.d.; **then,** increase dose gradually to reach 600–1,200 mg/day.
Dosage should not exceed 800 mg/day in geriatric patients. In those with impaired kidney or liver function, decrease dose by 50% when C_{CR} is 50 mL/min/1.73 m² and by 75% when it is less than 25 mL/min/1.73 m².
How Supplied: *Capsule:* 200 mg, 400 mg

EMS CONSIDERATIONS

See also *Beta-Adrenergic Blocking Agents.*

Acetaminophen (Apap, Paracetamol)
(ah-SEAT-ah-MIN-oh-fen)
Caplets: Arthritis Foundation Pain Reliever Aspirin Free, Aspirin Free Pain Relief, Aspirin Free Anacid Maximum Strength, Genapap Extra Strength, Genebs Extra Strength Caplets, Panadol, Panadol Junior Strength Caplets, Panadol Junior Strength, Tapanol Extra Strength, Tylenol Arthritis Extended Relief, Tylenol Caplets,
Capsules: Dapacin, Deda Cap, **Elixir:** Aceta, Genapap Children's, Mapap Children's, Oraphen-PD, Ridenol, Silapap Children's, Tylenol Children's,
Gelcaps: Aspirin Free Anacid Maximum Strength, Tapanol Extra

Strength, Tylenol Extra Strength, **Oral Liquid/Syrup:** Halenol Children's, Panadol Children's, Tylenol Extra Strength, **Oral Solution:** Acetaminophen Drops, Apacet, Genapap Infants' Drops, Mapap Infant Drops, Panadol Infants' Drops, Silapap Infants, Tempra 1, Tylenol Infants' Drops, Uni-Ace, **Oral Suspension:** Tylenol Children's Suspension, Tylenol Infants' Suspension, **Sprinkle Capsules:** Feverall Children's, Feverall Junior Strength, **Suppositories:** Acephen, Acetaminophen Uniserts, Children's Feverall, Infant's Feverall, Junior Strength Feverall, Neopap, **Tablets:** Aceta, Aspirin Free Pain Relief, Aspirin Free Anacin Maximum Strength, Fem-Etts, Genapap, Genapap Extra Strength, Genebs, Genebs Extra Strength, Mapap Extra Strength, Maranox, Meda Tab, Panadol, Redutemp, Tapanol Regular Strength, Tapanol Extra Strength, Tempra, Tylenol Regular Strength, Tylenol Extra Strength, Tylenol Junior Strength, **Tablets Chewable:** Apacet, Children's Genapap, Children's Panadol, Children's Tylenol, Tempra 3, Tylenol Chewable Tablets Fruit.**(OTC)** Classification: Nonnarcotic analgesic, para-aminophenol type

Mechanism of Action: Decreases fever by an effect on the hypothalamus leading to sweating and vasodilation. It also inhibits the effect of pyrogens on the hypothalamic heat-regulating centers. May cause analgesia by inhibiting CNS prostaglandin synthesis; however, due to minimal effects on peripheral prostaglandin synthesis, acetaminophen has no anti-inflammatory or uricosuric effects. Does not cause any anticoagulant effect or ulceration of the GI tract. Antipyretic and analgesic effects are comparable to those of aspirin.

Uses: Control of pain due to headache, earache, dysmenorrhea, arthralgia, myalgia, musculoskeletal pain, arthritis, immunizations, teething, tonsillectomy. To reduce fever in bacterial or viral infections. As a substitute for aspirin in upper GI disease, aspirin allergy, bleeding disorders, patients on anticoagulant thera-

py, and gouty arthritis. *Investigational:* In children receiving diptheria-pertussis-tetanus vaccination to decrease incidence of fever and pain at injection site.

Contraindications: Renal insufficiency, anemia. Patients with cardiac or pulmonary disease are more susceptible to toxic effects of acetaminophen.

Precautions: May have to be used with caution in pregnancy. Heavy drinking and fasting may be risk factors or acetaminophen toxicity, especially if larger than recommended doses of acetaminophen are used. As little as twice the recommended dosage, over time, can lead to serious liver damage.

Route/Dosage

• **Caplets, Capsules, Chewable Tablets, Gelcaps, Elixir, Oral Liquid, Oral Solution, Oral Suspension, Sprinkle Capsules, Syrup, Tablets**
Analgesic, antipyretic.
Adults: 325–650 mg q 4 hr; doses up to 1 g q.i.d. may be used. Daily dosage should not exceed 4 g. **Pediatric:** Doses given 4–5 times/day. **Up to 3 months:** 40 mg/dose; **4–11 months:** 80 mg/dose; **1–2 years:** 120 mg/dose; **2–3 years:** 160 mg/dose; **4–5 years:** 240 mg/dose; **6–8 years:** 320 mg/dose; **9–10 years:** 400 mg/dose; **11 years:** 480 mg/dose. **12–14 years:** 640 mg/dose. **Over 14 years:** 650 mg/dose. *Alternative pediatric dose:* 10–15 mg/kg q 4 hr.

• **Extended Relief Caplets**
Analgesic, antipyretic.
Adults: 2 caplets (1,300 mg) q 8 hr.

• **Suppositories**
Analgesic, antipyretic.
Adults: 650 mg q 4 hr, not to exceed 4 g/day for up to 10 days. Patients on long-term therapy should not exceed 2.6 g/day. **Pediatric, 3–11 months:** 80 mg q 6 hr. **1–3 years:** 80 mg q 4 hr; **3–6 years:** 120–125 mg q 4–6 hr, with no more than 720 mg in 24 hr. **6–12 years:** 325 mg q 4–6 hr

with no more than 2.6 g in 24 hr. Dosage should be given as needed while symptoms persist.

BUFFERED

Analgesic, antipyretic.

Adult, usual: 1 or 2 three-quarter capfuls are placed into an empty glass; add half a glass of cool water. May be taken while fizzing or after settling. Can be repeated q 4 hr as required or directed by provider.

How Supplied: Acetominophen: *Capsule:* 80 mg, 160 mg, 325 mg, 500 mg, 650 mg; *Chew tablet:* 80 mg, 160 mg; *Elixir:* 120 mg/5 mL, 160 mg/5 mL; *Liquid:* 160 mg/5 mL, 325 mg/5 mL, 500 mg/15 mL, 500 mg/5 mL; *Powder for reconstitution:* 950 mg; *Solution:* 80 mg/0.8 mL, 120 mg/2.5 mL, 160 mg/mL; *Suppository:* 80 mg, 120 mg, 325 mg, 650 mg; *Suspension:* 160 mg/5 mL, 80 mg/0.8 mL; *Tablet:* 160 mg, 325 mg, 500 mg, 648 mg, 650 mg; *Tablet, Extended Release:* 650 mg. Acetaminophen, buffered: *Granule, effervescent*

Side Effects: Few when taken in usual therapeutic doses. Chronic and even acute toxicity can develop after long symptom-free usage. *Hematologic:* Methemoglobinemia, **hemolytic anemia,** neutropenia, thrombocytopenia, pancytopenia, leukopenia. *Allergic:* Urticarial and erythematous skin reactions, skin eruptions, fever. *Miscellaneous:* CNS stimulation, hypoglycemic coma, jaundice, drowsiness, glossitis.

OD Overdose Management: *Symptoms:* May be no early specific symptoms. Within first 24 hr: N&V, diaphoresis, anorexia, drowsiness, confusion, liver tenderness, cardiac arrhythmias, low BP, jaundice, acute hepatic and renal failure. Within 24–48 hr, increased AST, ALT, bilirubrin, prothrombin levels. After 72–96 hr, peak hepatotoxicity with death possible due to liver necrosis. *Treatment:* Initially, induction of emesis, gastric lavage, activated charcoal. Oral *N*-acetylcysteine is said to reduce or prevent hepatic damage by inactivating acetaminophen metabolites, which cause liver toxicity.

Drug Interactions

Alcohol, ethyl / Chronic use of alcohol ↑ toxicity of larger therapeutic doses of acetaminophen

Barbiturates / ↑ Potential of hepatotoxicity due to ↑ breakdown of acetaminophen by liver

Carbamazepine / ↑ Potential of hepatotoxicity due to ↑ breakdown of acetaminophen by liver

Charcoal, activated / ↓ Absorption of acetaminophen when given as soon as possible after overdose

Diuretics, loop / ↓ Effect of diuretic due to ↓ renal prostaglandin excretion and ↓ plasma renin activity

Hydantoins (including Phenytoin) / ↑ Potential of hepatotoxicity due to ↑ breakdown of acetaminophen by liver

Isoniazid / ↑ Potential of hepatotoxicity due to ↑ breakdown of acetaminophen by liver

Lamotrigene / ↓ Serum lamotrigene levels → ↓ effect

Oral contraceptives / ↑ Breakdown of acetaminophen by liver → ↓ t½

Propranolol / ↑ Effect due to ↓ breakdown by liver

Rifampin / ↑ Potential of hepatotoxicity due to ↑ breakdown of acetaminophen by liver

Sulfinpyrazone / ↑ Potential of hepatotoxicity due to ↑ breakdown of acetaminophen by liver

AZT / ↓ Effect of AZT due to ↑ nonhepatic or renal clearance

EMS CONSIDERATIONS

None.

Acetazolamide
Acetazolamide sodium

(ah-set-ah-ZOE-la-myd)
Pregnancy Class: C
Dazamide, Diamox, Diamox Sequels
Classification: Anticonvulsant, carbonic anhydrase inhibitor

Mechanism of Action: Sulfonamide derivative possessing carbonic anhydrase inhibitor activity. As an anticonvulsant, beneficial effects may be due to inhibition of carbonic anhydrase in the CNS, which increases carbon dioxide tension resulting in a decrease in neuronal conduction. Systemic acidosis may also be involved. As a diuretic, the drug inhibits carbonic anhydrase in the kidney, which decreases formation of bicarbonate and hydrogen ions from carbon dioxide, thus reducing the availability of these ions for active transport. Acetazolamide also reduces intraocular pressure.

Onset of Action: Tablets: 60-90 minutes; **Peak:** 1-4 hr, **Sustained-release capsules:** 2 hr; **Peak:** 3-6 hr, **Injection (IV):** 2 min.; **Peak:**15 min.

Duration of Action: Tablets: 8-12 hrs., **Sustained-release capsules:**18-24 hrs., **Injection (IV):** 4-5 hrs.

Uses: Adjunct in the treatment of edema due to congestive heart failure or drug-induced edema. Absence (petit mal) and unlocalized seizures. Open-angle, secondary, or acute-angle closure glaucoma when delay of surgery is desired to lower intraocular pressure. Prophylaxis or treatment of acute mountain sickness in climbers attempting a rapid ascent or in those who are susceptible to mountain sickness even with gradual ascent.

Contraindications: Low serum sodium and potassium levels. Renal and hepatic dysfunction. Hyperchloremic acidosis, adrenal insufficiency, suprarenal gland failure, hypersensitivity to thiazide diuretics, cirrhosis. Chronic use in presence of noncongestive angle-closure glaucoma.

Precautions: Use with caution in the presence of mild acidosis and advanced pulmonary disease and during lactation. Increasing the dose does not increase effectiveness and may increase the risk of drowsiness or paresthesia. Safety and efficacy have not been established in children.

Route/Dosage ────────
• **Extended-Release   Capsules, Tablets, IV**
   Epilepsy.
Adults/children: 8–30 mg/kg/day in divided doses. Optimum daily

dosage: 375–1,000 mg (doses higher than 1,000 mg do not increase therapeutic effect).
   Adjunct to other anticonvulsants.
Initial: 250 mg/day; dose can be increased up to 1,000 mg/day in divided doses if necessary.
   Glaucoma, simple open-angle.
Adults: 250–1,000 mg/day in divided doses. Doses greater than 1 g/day do not increase the effect.
   Glaucoma, closed-angle prior to surgery or secondary.
Adults, short-term therapy: 250 mg q 4 hr or 250 mg b.i.d. **Adults, acute therapy:** 500 mg followed by 125–250 mg q 4 hr using tablets. For extended-release capsules, give 500 mg b.i.d. in the morning and evening. IV therapy may be used for rapid decrease in intraocular pressure. **Pediatric:** 5–10 mg/kg/dose IM or IV q 6 hr or 10–15 mg/kg/day in divided doses q 6–8 hr using tablets.
   Acute mountain sickness.
Adults: 250 mg b.i.d.–q.i.d. (500 mg 1–2 times/day of extended-release capsules). During rapid ascent, 1 g/day is recommended.
   Diuresis in CHF.
Adults, initial: 250–375 mg (5 mg/kg) once daily in the morning. If the patient stops losing edema fluid after an initial response, the dose should not be increased; rather, medication should be skipped for a day to allow the kidney to recover. The best diuretic effect occurs when the drug is given on alternate days or for 2 days alternative with a day of rest.
   Drug-induced edema.
Adults: 250–375 mg once daily for 1 or 2 days. The drug is most effective if given every other day or for 2 days followed by a day of rest. **Children:** 5 mg/kg/dose PO or IV once daily in the morning.
How   Supplied: Acetazolamide: *Capsule, Extended Release:* 500 mg; *Tablet:* 125 mg, 250 mg. Acetazolamide sodium: *Powder for injection:* 500 mg

---

bold italic = life threatening side effect

Side Effects: *GI:* Anorexia, N&V, melena, constipation, alteration in taste, diarrhea. *GU:* Hematuria, glycosuria, urinary frequency, renal colic, renal calculi, crystalluria, polyuria, phosphaturia, decreased or absent libido, impotence. *CNS:* **Seizures,** weakness, malaise, fatigue, nervousness, drowsiness, depression, dizziness, disorientation, confusion, ataxia, tremor, headache, tinnitus, flaccid paralysis, lassitude, paresthesia of the extremities. *Hematologic:* **Bone marrow depression,** thrombocytopenic purpura, thrombocytopenia, **hemolytic anemia,** leukopenia, pancytopenia, agranulocytosis. *Dermatologic:* Pruritus, urticaria, skin rashes, erythema multiforme, **Stevens-Johnson syndrome, toxic epidermal necrolysis,** photosensitivity. *Other:* Weight loss, fever, acidosis, electrolyte imbalance, transient myopia, hepatic insufficiency. *NOTE:* Side effects similar to those produced by sulfonamides may also occur.

OD Overdose Management: *Symptoms:* Drowsiness, anorexia, N&V, dizziness, ataxia, tremor, paresthesias, tinnitus. *Treatment:* Emesis or gastric lavage. Hyperchloremic acidosis may respond to bicarbonate. Administration of potassium may also be necessary. Observe carefully and give supportive treatment.

Drug Interactions: Also see *Diuretics.*
Amphetamine / ↑ Effect of amphetamine by ↑ renal tubular reabsorption
Cyclosporine / ↑ Levels of cyclosporine → possible nephrotoxicity and neurotoxicity
Diflunisal / Significant ↓ in intraocular pressure with ↑ side effects
Ephedrine / ↑ Effect of ephedrine by ↑ renal tubular reabsorption
Lithium carbonate / ↓ Effect of lithium by ↑ renal excretion
Methotrexate / ↓ Effect of methotrexate due to ↑ renal excretion
Primidone / ↓ Effect of primidone due to ↓ GI absorption
Pseudoephedrine / ↑ Effect of pseudoephedrine by ↑ renal tubular reabsorption
Quinidine / ↑ Effect of quinidine by ↑ renal tubular reabsorption
Salicylates / Accumulation and toxicity of acetazolamide (including CNS depression and metabolic acidosis). Also, acidosis due to acetazolamide may ↑ CNS penetration of salicylates

EMS CONSIDERATIONS

See also *Anticonvulsants.*
Administration/Storage
IV 1. IV administration is preferred; IM administration is painful due to alkalinity of solution.
2. For parenteral use, reconstitute each 500-mg vial with at least 5 mL of sterile water for injection.
3. For direct IV use, administer over at least 1 min. For intermittent IV use, further dilute in dextrose or saline solution.

Acetylcysteine
(ah-see-til-SIS-tay-een)
Pregnancy Class: B
Mucomyst, Mucosil, Parvolex (Rx)
Classification: Mucolytic

Mechanism of Action: Reduces the viscosity of purulent and nonpurulent pulmonary secretions and facilitates their removal by splitting disulfide bonds.
Onset of Action: Inhalation: Within 1 min. **by direct instillation:** Immediate. **Time to peak effect:** 5-10 min.
Uses: Adjunct in the treatment of acute and chronic bronchitis, emphysema, tuberculosis, pneumonia, bronchiectasis, atelectasis. Routine care of patients with tracheostomy, pulmonary complications after thoracic or CV surgery, or in posttraumatic chest conditions. Pulmonary complications of cystic fibrosis. Diagnostic bronchial asthma. Antidote in acetaminophen poisoning to reduce hepatotoxicity. *Investigational:* As an ophthalmic solution for dry eye.
Contraindications: Sensitivity to drug.
Precautions: Use with caution during lactation, in the elderly, and in patients with asthma.

Route/Dosage

- **10% or 20% Solution: Nebulization, Direct Application, or Direct Intratracheal Instillation**

Nebulization into face mask, tracheostomy, mouth piece.
1–10 mL of 20% solution or 2–10 mL of 10% solution 3–4 times/day.

Closed tent or croupette.
Up to 300 mL of 10% or 20% solution/treatment.

Direct instillation into tracheostomy.
1–2 mL of 10%–20% solution q 1–4 hr.

Percutaneous intratracheal catheter.
1–2 mL of 20% solution or 2–4 mL of 10% solution q 1–4 hr by syringe attached to catheter.

Instillation to particular portion of bronchopulmonary tree using small plastic catheter into the trachea.
2–5 mL of 20% solution instilled into the trachea by means of a syringe connected to a catheter.

Diagnostic procedures.
2–3 doses of 1–2 mL of 20% or 2–4 mL of 10% solution by nebulization or intratracheal instillation before the procedure.

Acetaminophen overdose.
Given PO, initial: 140 mg/kg; **then,** 70 mg/kg q 4 hr for a total of 17 doses.

How Supplied: *Solution:* 10%, 20%

Side Effects: *Respiratory:* Increased incidence of bronchospasm in patients with asthma. Increased amount of liquefied bronchial secretions, which must be removed by suction if cough is inadequate. Bronchial and tracheal irritation, tightness in chest, bronchoconstriction. *GI:* N&V, stomatitis. *Other:* Rashes, fever, drowsiness, rhinorrhea.

Drug Interactions: Acetylcysteine is incompatible with antibiotics and should be administered separately.

EMS CONSIDERATIONS

None.

Acetylsalicylic acid (ASA, Aspirin)

(ah-SEE-till-sal-ih-SILL-ick AH-sid)

Pregnancy Class: C

Aspergum, Aspirin, Aspirin Regimen Bayer 81 mg with Calcium, Bayer Children's Aspirin, Easprin, Ecotrin Caplets and Tablets, Ecotrin Maximum Strength Caplets and Tablets, Empirin, Excedrin Geltabs and Tablets, Halfprin, 8-Hour Bayer Timed-Release Caplets and Tablets, Norwich Extra Strength, St. Joseph Adult Chewable Aspirin, Therapy Bayer Caplets, ZOR-prin. **Buffered:** Alka-Seltzer with Aspirin, Alka-Seltzer with Aspirin (flavored), Alka-Seltzer Extra Strength with Aspirin, Arthritis Pain Formula, Ascriptin Regular Strength, Ascriptin A/D, Bayer Buffered Aspirin, Bufferin, Buffex, Cama Arthritis Pain Reliever, Magnaprin, Magnaprin Arthritis Strength Captabs, Tri-Buffered Bufferin Caplets and Tablets.

Classification: Nonnarcotic analgesic, antipyretic, anti-inflammatory agent

---

Mechanism of Action: Exhibits antipyretic, anti-inflammatory, and analgesic effects. The antipyretic effect is due to an action on the hypothalamus, resulting in heat loss by vasodilation of peripheral blood vessels and promoting sweating. Prostaglandins have been implicated in the inflammatory process, as well as in mediation of pain. Thus, if levels are decreased, the inflammatory reaction may subside.The anti-inflammatory effects are probably mediated through inhibition of cyclo-oxygenase, which results in a decrease in prostaglandin synthesis and other mediators of the pain response. The mechanism of action for the analgesic effects of aspirin is not known fully but is partly attributable to improvement of the inflammatory condition. Aspirin also produces inhibition of platelet aggregation by decreasing the synthesis of endoperoxides and thromboxanes—substances that mediate platelet aggregation.

Uses: Analgesic: Pain arising from integumental structures, myalgias,

---

A

neuralgias, arthralgias, headache, dysmenorrhea, and similar types of pain. Antipyretic. **Anti-Inflammatory:** Arthritis, osteoarthritis, SLE, acute rheumatic fever, gout, and many other conditions. Mucocutaneous lymph node syndrome (Kawasaki disease). Reduce the risk of recurrent transient ischemic attacks and strokes in men. Decrease risk of death from nonfatal MI in patients who have a history of infarction or who manifest unstable angina; aortocoronary bypass surgery. Gout. May be effective in less severe postoperative and postpartum pain; pain secondary to trauma and cancer. *Investigational:* Chronic use to prevent cataract formation; low doses to prevent toxemia of pregnancy; in pregnant women with inadequate uteroplacental blood flow. Reduce colon cancer mortality (low doses). Low doses of aspirin and warfarin to reduce the risk of a second heart attack. **Contraindications:** Hypersensitivity to salicylates. Patients with asthma, hay fever, or nasal polyps have a higher incidence of hypersensitivity reactions. Severe anemia, history of blood coagulation defects, in conjunction with anticoagulant therapy. Salicylates can cause congestive failure when taken in the large doses used for rheumatic diseases. Vitamin K deficiency; 1 week before and after surgery. In pregnancy, especially the last trimester as the drug may cause problems in the newborn child or complications during delivery. In children or teenagers with chickenpox or flu due to possibility of development of Reye's syndrome.

Controlled-release aspirin is not recommended for use as an antipyretic or short-term analgesic because adequate blood levels may not be reached. Also, controlled-release products are not recommended for children less than 12 years of age and in children with fever accompanied by dehydration.

Precautions: Use with caution during lactation and in the presence of gastric or prptic ulcers, in mild diabetes, erosive gastritis, bleeding tendencies, in cardiac disease, and in liver or kidney disease. Aspirin products now carry the following labeling: "It is especially important not to use aspirin during the last three months of pregnancy unless specifically directed to do so by a doctor because it may cause problems in the newborn child or complications during delivery."

Route/Dosage ─────────

• **Gum, Chewable Tablets, Coated Tablets, Effervescent Tablets, Enteric-Coated Tablets, Suppositories, Tablets, Timed (Controlled) Release Tablets**

Analgesic, antipyretic.

Adults: 325–500 mg q 3 hr, 325–600 mg q 4 hr, or 650–1,000 mg q 6 hr. As an alternative, the adult chewable tablet (81 mg each) may be used in doses of 4–8 tablets q 4 hr as needed. **Pediatric:** 65 mg/kg/day (alternate dose: 1.5 g/m²/day) in divided doses q 4–6 hr, not to exceed 3.6 g/day. Alternatively, the following dosage regimen can be used: **Pediatric, 2–3 years:** 162 mg q 4 hr as needed; **4–5 years:** 243 mg q 4 hr as needed; **6–8 years:** 320–325 mg q 4 hr as needed; **9–10 years:** 405 mg q 4 hr as needed; **11 years:** 486 mg q 4 hr as needed; **12–14 years:** 648 mg q 4 hr.

Arthritis, rheumatic diseases.

Adults: 3.2–6 g/day in divided doses.

Juvenile rheumatoid arthritis.

60–110 mg/kg/day (alternate dose: 3 g/m²) in divided doses q 6–8 hr. When initiating therapy at 60 mg/kg/day, dose may be increased by 20 mg/kg/day after 5–7 days and by 10 mg/kg/day after another 5–7 days.

Acute rheumatic fever.

Adults, initial: 5–8 g/day. **Pediatric, initial,** 100 mg/kg/day (3 g/m²/day) for 2 weeks; **then,** decrease to 75 mg/kg/day for 4–6 weeks.

TIAs in men.

Adults: 650 mg b.i.d. or 325 mg q.i.d. A dose of 300 mg/day may be as effective and with fewer side effects.

Prophylaxis of MI.

A

Adults: 300 or 325 mg/day (both solid PO dosage forms–regular and buffered as well as buffered aspirin in solution). The adult chewable tablets be also be used.

Kawasaki disease.

Adults: 80–180 mg/kg/day during the febrile period. After the fever resolves, the dose may be adjusted to 10 mg/kg/day.

NOTE: Doses as low as 80–100 mg/day are being studied for use in unstable angina, MI, and aortocoronary bypass surgery. Aspirin Regimen Bayer 81 mg with Calcium contains 250 mg calcium carbonate (10% of RDA) and 81 mg of acetylsalicylic acid for individuals who require aspirin to prevent recurrent heart attacks and strokes.

How Supplied: *Chew tablet:* 80 mg, 81 mg; *Enteric coated tablet:* 81 mg, 162 mg, 324 mg, 325 mg, 500 mg, 650 mg, 975 mg; *Gum:* 227 mg; *Suppository:* 60 mg, 120 mg, 125 mg, 200 mg, 300 mg, 325 mg, 600 mg, 650 mg; *Tablet:* 81 mg, 324 mg, 325 mg, 486 mg, 500 mg, 650 mg; *Tablet, Extended Release:* 650 mg, 800 mg

Side Effects: The toxic effects of the salicylates are dose-related. *GI:* Dyspepsia, heartburn, anorexia, nausea, occult blood loss, epigastric discomfort, *massive GI bleeding, potentiation of peptic ulcer. Allergic: Bronchospasm, asthma-like symptoms, anaphylaxis,* skin rashes, angioedema, urticaria, rhinitis, nasal polyps. *Hematologic:* Prolongation of bleeding time, thrombocytopenia, leukopenia, purpura, shortened erythrocyte survival time, decreased plasma iron levels. *Miscellaneous:* Thirst, fever, dimness of vision.

NOTE: Use of aspirin in children and teenagers with flu or chickenpox may result in the development of *Reye's syndrome.* Also, dehydrated, febrile children are more prone to salicylate intoxication.

OD Overdose Management: *Symptoms of Mild Salicylate Toxicity (Salicylism): GI:* N&V, diarrhea, thirst. *CNS:* Tinnitus (most common), dizziness,

difficulty in hearing, mental confusion, lassitude. *Miscellaneous:* Flushing, sweating, tachycardia. Symptoms of salicylism may be observed with doses used for inflammatory disease or rheumatic fever. *Symptoms of Severe Salicylate Poisoning: CNS:* Excitement, confusion, disorientation, irritability, hallucinations, lethargy, stupor, *coma, respiratory failure, seizures. Metabolic:* Respiratory alkalosis (initially), respiratory acidosis and metabolic acidosis, dehydration. *GI:* N&V. *Hematologic:* Platelet dysfunction, hypoprothrombinemia, increased capillary fragility. *Miscellaneous: Hyperthermia, hemorrhage, CV collapse, renal failure,* hyperventilation, pulmonary edema, tetany, hypoglycemia (late). *Treatment (Toxicity):*

1. If the patient has had repeated administration of large doses of salicylates, document and report evidence of hyperventilation or complaints of auditory or visual disturbances (symptoms of salicylism).

2. Severe salicylate poisoning, whether due to overdose or accumulation, will have an exaggerated effect on the CNS and the metabolic system:

• Patients may develop a salicylate jag characterized by garrulous behavior. They may act as if they were inebriated.

• Convulsions and coma may follow.

3. When working with febrile children or the elderly who have been treated with aspirin, maintain adequate fluid intake. These patients are more susceptible to salicylate intoxication if they are dehydrated.

4. The following treatment approaches may be considered for treatment of *acute salicylate toxicity:*

• Initially induce vomiting or perform gastric lavage followed by activated charcoal (most effective if given within 2 hr of ingestion).

• Monitor salicylate levels and acid-base and fluid and electrolyte balance. If required, administer IV solutions of dextrose, saline, potassium,

---

bold italic = life threatening side effect

and sodium bicarbonate as well as vitamin K.
- Seizures may be treated with diazepam.
- Treat hyperthermia if present.
- Alkaline diuresis will enhance renal excretion. Hemodialysis is effective but should be reserved for severe poisonings.
- If necessary, administer oxygen and artificial ventilation

Drug Interactions

Acetazolamide / ↑ CNS toxicity of salicylates; also, ↑ excretion of salicylic acid if urine kept alkaline

Alcohol, ethyl / ↑ Chance of GI bleeding caused by salicylates

Alteplase, recombinant / ↑ Risk of bleeding

PAS / Possible ↑ effect of PAS due to ↓ excretion by kidney or ↓ plasma protein binding

Ammonium chloride / ↑ Effect of salicylates by ↑ renal tubular reabsorption

ACE inhibitors / ↓ Effect of ACE inhibitors possibly due to prostaglandin inhibition

Antacids / ↓ Salicylate levels in plasma due to ↑ rate of renal excretion

Anticoagulants, oral / ↑ Effect of anticoagulant by ↓ plasma protein binding and plasma prothrombin

Antirheumatics / Both are ulcerogenic and may cause ↑ GI bleeding

Ascorbic acid / ↑ Effect of salicylates by ↑ renal tubular reabsorption

Beta-adrenergic blocking agents / Salicylates ↓ action of beta-blockers, possibly due to prostaglandin inhibition

Charcoal, activated / ↓ Absorption of salicylates from GI tract

Corticosteroids / Both are ulcerogenic; also, corticosteroids may ↓ blood salicylate levels by ↑ breakdown by liver and ↑ excretion

Dipyridamole / Additive anticoagulant effects

Furosemide / ↑ Chance of salicylate toxicity due to ↓ renal excretion; also, salicylates may ↓ effect of furosemide in patients with impaired renal function or cirrhosis with ascites

Heparin / Inhibition of platelet adhesiveness by aspirin may result in bleeding tendencies

Hypoglycemics, oral / ↑ Hypoglycemia due to ↓ plasma protein binding and ↓ excretion

Indomethacin / Both are ulcerogenic and may cause ↑ GI bleeding

Insulin / Salicylates ↑ hypoglycemic effect of insulin

Methionine / ↑ Effect of salicylates by ↑ renal tubular reabsorption

Methotrexate / ↑ Effect of methotrexate by ↓ plasma protein binding; also, salicylates block renal excretion of methotrexate

Nitroglycerin / Combination may result in unexpected hypotension

Nizatidine / ↑ Serum levels of salicylates

NSAIDs / Additive ulcerogenic effects; also, aspirin may ↓ serum levels of NSAIDs

Phenylbutazone / Combination may produce hyperuricemia

Phenytoin / ↑ Effect of phenytoin by ↓ plasma protein binding

Probenecid / Salicylates inhibit uricosuric activity of probenecid

Sodium bicarbonate / ↓ Effect of salicylates by ↑ rate of excretion

Spironolactone / Aspirin ↓ diuretic effect of spironolactone

Sulfinpyrazone / Salicylates inhibit uricosuric activity of sulfinpyrazone

Sulfonamides / ↑ Effect of sulfonamides by ↑ blood levels of salicylates

Valproic acid / ↑ Effect of valproic acid due to ↓ plasma protein binding

---

EMS CONSIDERATIONS

None.

Acitretin
(ah-sih-TREH-tin)
Pregnancy Class: X
Soriatane **(Rx)**
Classification: Antipsoriasis product.

Mechanism of Action: Retinoic acid derivative that is the main metabolite of etretinate. Mechanism is not known. Absorption optimal when given with food.

Uses: Severe psoriasis, including erythrodermic and generalized pustular types. *Investigational:* Darier's disease, palmoplantar pustulosis, lichen planus, children with lamellar ichthyosis, non-bullous and bullous ichthyosiform erythroderma, Sjögren-Larsson syndrome, lichen sclerosus et atrophicus of the vulva and palmoplantar lichen nitidus.

Contraindications: Use during pregnancy or in those who intend to become pregnant during therapy or at any time for at least 3 years following discontinuation of therapy. Use by females who may not use reliable contraception during treatment or for at least 3 years following treatment. Use of ethanol in women either during treatment or for 2 months after cessation of treatment. Lactation.

Precautions: Use with caution in patients with severely impaired liver or kidney function. Safety and efficacy have not been determined in children.

Route/Dosage ——————————
• **Capsules**
Psoriasis.
Must individualize dosage. **Initial:** 25 or 50 mg/day given as a single dose with main meal. **Maintenance:** 25 to 50 mg/day.

How Supplied: *Capsules:* 10 mg, 25 mg

Side Effects: *Dermatologic:* Alopecia, skin peeling, dry skin, nail disorder, pruritus, erythematous rash, hyperesthesia, paresthesia, paronychia, skin atrophy, sticky skin, abnormal skin odor, abnormal hair texture, bullous eruption, cold/clammy skin, dermatitis, increased sweating, infection, psoriasis-like rash, purpura, pyogenic granuloma, rash, seborrhea, skin fissures, skin ulceration, sunburn. *CNS:* Rigors, headache, pain, depression, insomnia, somnolence. *GI:* Abdominal pain, nausea, diarrhea, tongue disorder, altered taste, hepatotoxicity. *Ophthalmic:* Xerophthalmia, blurred vision, abnormal vision, blepharitis, irritation, conjunctivitis, corneal epithelial abnormality, decreased night vision, blindness, eye abnormality, eye pain, photophobia. *Musculoskeletal:* Arthralgia, spinal hyperostosis, arthritis, arthrosis, back pain, hypertonia, myalgia, osteodynia, peripheral joint hyperostosis. *Mucous membranes:* Cheilitis, rhinitis, epistaxis, dry mouth, gingival bleeding, gingivitis, increased salivation, stomatitis, thirst, ulcerative stomatitis. *Body as a whole:* Anorexia, edema, fatigue, hot flashes, increased appetite, flushing, sinusitis. *Otic:* Earache, tinnitus.

Drug Interactions
Ethanol / Possible formation of etretinate which has a longer half-life than acitretin
Glyburide / Enhanced clearance of blood glucose
Methotrexate / ↑ Risk of hepatotoxicity
Oral contraceptives, "minipill" / Acitretin interferes with the contraceptive effect

EMS CONSIDERATIONS
None.

Acyclovir (Acycloguanosine)
Acyclovir: (ay-SYE-kloh-veer)Acycloguanosine: (sy-SYE-kloh-GWON-oh-seen)
Pregnancy Class: C
Zovirax **(Rx)**
Classification: Antiviral anti-infective

Mechanism of Action: A synthetic acyclic purine nucleoside analog converted by HSV-infected cells to acyclovir triphosphate, which interferes with HSV DNA polymerase, thereby inhibiting DNA replication. Food does not affect absorption. Reduce dosage in patients with impaired renal function.

Onset of Action: Peak levels after PO: 1.5-2 hr.

Uses: PO. Initial and recurrent genital herpes in immunocompromised and nonimmunocompromised patients. Prophylaxis of frequently recurrent genital herpes infections in nonimmunocompromised patients. Treatment of chickenpox in children ranging from 2 to 18 years of age. Acute treatment of herpes zoster (shingles).

Parenteral. Initial therapy for severe genital herpes in patients who are not immunocompromised; initial and recurrent mucosal and cutaneous HSV-1 and HSV-2 infections in immunocompromised individuals. Varicella zoster infections (shingles) in immunocompromised patients. HSE in patients over 6 months of age. Neonatal herpes simplex infections.

Topical. To decrease healing time and duration of viral shedding in initial herpes genitalis. Limited non-life-threatening mucocutaneous HSV infections in immunocompromised patients. No beneficial effect in recurrent herpes genitalis or in herpes labialis in nonimmunocompromised patients.

Investigational: Cytomegalovirus and HSV infection following bone marrow or renal transplantation; herpes simplex ocular infections; herpes simplex proctitis; herpes simplex labialis; herpes simplex whitlow; herpes zoster encephalitis; disseminated primary eczema herpeticum; herpes simplex–associated erythema multiforme; infectious mononucleosis; and varicella pneumonia.

Contraindications: Hypersensitivity to formulation. Use in the eye. Use to prevent recurrent HSV infections.

Precautions: Use with caution during lactation or with concomitant intrathecal methotrexate or interferon. Safety and effecacy of PO form not established in children less that 2 years of age. Use of oral acyclovir does not eliminate latent HSV and is not a cure.

Route/Dosage ⸻
• **Capsules, Suspension, Tablets**
Initial genital herpes.
200 mg q 4 hr, 5 times/day for 10 days.
Chronic genital herpes.

400 mg b.i.d., 200 mg t.i.d., or 200 mg 5 times/day for up to 12 months.
Intermittent therapy for genital herpes.
200 mg q 4 hr, 5 times/day for 5 days. Start therapy at the first symptom/sign of recurrence.
Herpes zoster, acute treatment.
800 mg q 4 hr, 5 times/day for 7–10 days.
Chickenpox.
20 mg/kg (of the suspension) q.i.d. for 5 days. A single dose should not exceed 800 mg. Begin therapy at the earliest sign/symptom.
• **IV Infusion**
Mucosal and cutaneous herpes simplex in immunocompromised patients.
Adults: 5 mg/kg infused at a constant rate over 1 hr, q 8 hr (15 mg/kg/day) for 7 days. **Children less than 12 years of age:** 250 mg/m^2 infused at a constant rate over 1 hr, q 8 hr for 7 days.
Varicella-zoster infections (shingles) in immunocompromised patients.
Adults: 10 mg/kg infused at a constant rate over 1 hr, q 8 hr for 7 days (not to exceed 500 mg/m^2 q 8 hr). **Children less than 12 years of age:** 500 mg/m^2 infused at a constant rate over at least 1 hr, q 8 hr for 7 days.
Herpes simplex encephalitis.
Adults: 10 mg/kg infused at a constant rate over at least 1 hr, q 8 hr for 10 days. **Children less than 12 years of age and greater than 6 months of age:** 500 mg/m^2 infused at a constant rate over at least 1 hr, q 8 hr for 10 days.
• **Topical (5% Ointment)**
Adults and children: Lesion should be covered with sufficient amount of ointment (0.5-in. ribbon/4 in.^{2} of surface area) q 3 hr, 6 times/day for 7 days. Initiate treatment as soon as possible after onset of symptoms.
How Supplied: *Capsule:* 200 mg; *Injection:* 5 mg/mL, 25 mg/mL, 50 mg/ml; *Ointment:* 5%; *Powder for injection:* 500 mg, 1000 mg; *Suspension:* 200 mg/5 mL; *Tablet:* 400 mg, 800 mg

Side Effects: PO. *Short-term treatment of herpes simplex. GI:* N&V, diarrhea, anorexia, sore throat, taste of drug. *CNS:* Headache, dizziness, fatigue. *Miscellaneous:* Edema, skin rashes, leg pain, inguinal adenopathy.

Long-term treatment of herpes simplex. GI: Nausea, diarrhea. *CNS:* Headache. *Other:* Skin rash, asthenia, paresthesia.

Treatment of herpes zoster. GI: N&V, diarrhea, constipation. *CNS:* Headache, malaise.

Treatment of chickenpox. GI: Vomiting, diarrhea, abdominal pain, flatulence. *Dermatologic:* Rash.

Parenteral (frequency greater than 1%). *At injection site:* Phlebitis, inflammation. *GI:* N&V. *CNS:* Encephalopathic changes, including lethargy, obtundation, tremors, agitation, confusion, hallucination, *seizures, coma* , jitters, headache. *Miscellaneous:* Skin rashes, urticaria, itching, transient elevation of serum creatinine or BUN (most often following rapid IV infusion), elevation of transaminases, *fatal renal failure, fatal thrombotic thrombocytopenic purpura or hemolytic uremic syndrome in immunocompromised patients.*

Topical. Transient burning, stinging, pain. Pruritus, rash, vulvitis, local edema. *NOTE:* All of these effects have also been reported with the use of a placebo preparation.

OD Overdose Management: *Symptoms:* Increased BUN and serum creatinine, *renal failure following parenteral overdose. Treatment:* Hemodialysis (peritoneal dialysis is less effective).

Drug Interactions
Probenecid / ↑ Bioavailability and half-life of acyclovir → ↑ effect
Zidovudine / Severe lethargy and drowsiness

EMS CONSIDERATIONS

See also *Antiviral Drugs.*

Adapalene
(ah-DAP-ah-leen)
Pregnancy Class: C

Defferin **(Rx)**
Classification: Topical acne product

Mechanism of Action: Binds to specific retinoic acid receptors which may normalize the differentiation of follicular epithelial cells resulting in decreased microcomedone formation.

Uses: Topical treatment of acne vulgaris.

Contraindications: Hypersensitivity to adapalene or any components of the vehicle gel. Use in sunburn until fully recovered.

Precautions: Use with caution in those who normally have high levels of sun exposure or in those more sensitive to the sun. Use with caution with medicated or abrasive soaps and cleaners, with soaps and cosmetics that have strong drying effect, and with products that have high concentrations of alcohol, stringents, spices, or lime. Also use particular caution with products containing sulfur, resorcinol, or salicylic acid. Use with caution during lactation. Safety and efficacy have not been determined in children less than 12 years of age.

Route/Dosage
• **Topical Gel**
Treatment of acne vulgaris.
Adults and children over 12 years of age: Apply a thin film once a day to affected areas after washing in the evening prior to retiring.
How Supplied: Gel: 0.1%; *Topical Solution:* 0.1%.
Side Effects: *Dermatologic:* Erythema, scaling, dryness, pruritus, burning, pruritus or burning immediately after application, skin irritation, stinging sunburn, acne flares.

EMS CONSIDERATIONS
None.

Adenosine
(ah-DEN-oh-seen)
Pregnancy Class: C
Adenocard, Adenoscan **(Rx)**
Classification: Antiarrhythmic

---

bold italic = life threatening side effect

Mechanism of Action: Found naturally in all cells of the body. It slows conduction time through the AV node, interrupts the reentry pathways through the AV node, and restores normal sinus rhythm in paroxysmal supraventricular Competitively antagonized by caffeine, theophylline, and dipyridamole.

Onset of Action: after IV: 34 sec.

Duration of Action: 1-2 min.

Uses: Conversion of sinus rhythm of paroxysmal SVT (including that associated with accessory bypass tracts). The phosphate salt is used for symptomatic relief of complications with stasis dermatitis in varicose veins. *Investigational:* With thallium-201 tomography in noninvasive assessment of patients with suspected CAD who cannot exercise adequately prior to being stress-tested. Adenosine is not effective in converting rhythms other than paroxysmal SVT. The phosphate salt has been used to treat herpes infections and to increase blood flow to brain tumors and in porphyria cutanea tarda.

Contraindications: Second- or third-degree AV block or sick sinus syndrome (except in patients with a functioning artificial pacemaker), atrial flutter, atrial fibrillation, ventricular tachycardia. History of MI or cerebral hemorrhage.

Precautions: At time of conversion to normal sinus rhythm, new rhythms (PVC, atrial premature contractions, sinus bradycardia, skipped beats, varying degrees of AV block, sinus tachycardia) lasting a few seconds may occur. Use with caution in patients with asthma. Safety and efficacy as a diagnostic agent havae not been determined in patients less than 18 years of age.

Route/Dosage ———————

• **Rapid IV Bolus Only**
Antiarrhythmic.

Initial: 6 mg over 1–2 sec. If the first dose does not reverse the SVT within 1–2 min, 12 mg should be given as a rapid IV bolus. The 12-mg dose may be repeated a second time, if necessary. Doses greater than 12 mg are not recommended.

• **IV Infusion Only**
Diagnostic aid.

Adults: 140 mcg/kg/min infused over 6 min (total dose of 0.84 mg/kg).

• **IM Only**
Varicose veins.

Initial: 25–50 mg 1–2 times daily until symptoms subside. **Maintenance:** 25 mg 2 or 3 times weekly.

How Supplied: *Injection:* 3 mg/mL

Side Effects: *CV:* Short lasting first-, second-, or *third-degree heart block; cardiac arrest,* sustained ventricular tachycardia, sinus bradycardia, ST-segment depression, sinus exit block, sinus pause, arrhythmias, T-wave changes, hypertension. prolonged asystole, Nonfatal MI, transient increase in BP, *ventricular fibrillation.* Facial flushing (common), chest pain, sweating, palpitations, hypotension (may be significant). *CNS:* Lightheadedness, dizziness, numbness, headache, blurred vision, apprehension, paresthesia, drowsiness, emotional instability, tremors, nervousness. *GI:* Nausea, metallic taste, tightness in throat. *Respiratory:* SOB or dyspnea (common), urge to breathe deeply, chest pressure or discomfort, cough, hyperventilation, nasal congestion. *GU:* Urinary urgency, vaginal pressure. *Miscellaneous:* Pressure in head, burning sensation, neck and back pain, weakness, blurred vision, dry mouth, ear discomfort, pressure in groin, scotomas, tongue discomfort, discomfort (tingling, heaviness) in upper extremities, discomfort in throat, neck, or jaw.

Drug Interactions

Carbamazepine / ↑ Degree of heart block

Caffeine / Competitively antagonizes effect of adenosine

Digitalis / Possibility of ventricular fibrillation (rare)

Dipyridamole / ↑ Effect of adenosine

Theophylline / Competitively antagonizes effect of adenosine

EMS CONSIDERATIONS

See also *Antiarrhythmic Agents.*

Administration/Storage
IV 1. Drug can be stored at room temperature; crystallization may result if the drug is refrigerated. If crystals form, dissolve by warming to room temperature. The solution must be clear when administered.
2. Administer directly into a vein. If it is to be given into an IV line, introduce the drug in the most proximal line and follow with a rapid saline flush.

Albendazole
(al-BEN-dah-zohl)
Pregnancy Class: C
Albenza (Rx)
Classification: Anthelmintic

Mechanism of Action: Acts by inhibiting tubular polymerization, resulting in the loss of cytoplasmic microtubules and inability of the cell to function. Poorly absorbed from the GI tract; enhance absorption by ingesting a meal containing at least 40 g of fat. Rapidly converted to albendazole sulfoxide, the active metabolite. **Peak plasma levels, sulfoxide:** 2–5 hr. **t½, terminal, of sulfoxide:** 8–12 hr. Further metabolized to other metabolites with excretion through the bile, accounting for a portion of elimination.
Uses: Treatment of parenchymal neurocysticercosis due to *Taenia solium*. Treatment of cystic hydatid disease of the liver, lung, and peritoneum caused by the larval form of the dog tapeworm, Echinococcus granulosus.
Contraindications: Hypersensitivity to benzimidazole compounds.

Route/Dosage
• **Tablets**
Hydatid disease.
Those weighing 60 kg or more: 400 mg b.i.d. with meals for a 28-day cycle followed by a 14-day albendazole-free interval, for a total of three cycles. **Those weighing less than 60 kg:** 15 mg/kg/day given in divided doses b.i.d. with meals, up to a maximum of 800 mg/day, using the same duration as for those weighing 60 kg or more.
Neurocysticercosis.
Those weighing 60 kg or more: 400 mg b.i.d. with meals for 8 to 30 days. **Those weighing less than 60 kg:** 15 mg/kg/day given in divided doses b.i.d. with meals, up to a maximum dose of 800 mg/day, for 8 to 30 days.
How Supplied: *Tablet:* 200 mg
Side Effects: *GI:* N&V, abdominal pain. *CNS:* Headache, dizziness, vertigo, increased ICP, meningeal signs. *Hematologic:* Leukopenia, granulocytopenia, pancytopenia, agranulocytosis, thrombocytopenia (rare). *Dermatologic:* Reversible alopecia, rash, urticaria. *Miscellaneous:* Fever, allergic reactions, acute renal failure.
Drug Interactions
Cimetidine / ↑ Levels of albendazole sulfoxide in bile and cystic fluid in hydatid cyst patients
Dexamethasone / Possible ↑ plasma levels of albendazole sulfoxide
Praziquantel / ↑ Plasma levels of albendazole sulfoxide

EMS CONSIDERATIONS
Administration/Storage: Patients being treated for neurocysticercosis should receive corticosteroid and anticonvulsant therapy as needed. Consider PO or IV steroids for the first week of treatment to prevent cerebral hypertensive episodes.
Assessment
1. Document indications for therapy as length of therapy is based on condition requiring treatment.
2. Obtain negative pregnancy test, baseline cultures, and neurologic assessment.
3. Determine baseline CBC and check every 2 weeks during each 28-day cycle.
4. Obtain LFTs and monitor for significant enzyme elevations which may necessitate interruption of drug therapy until return to baseline.
5. Assess for retinal lesions with cysticercosis. The need for anticysticeral

---

therapy should be weighed against the possibility of retinal damage due to albendazole-induced changes to the retinal lesion.

Interventions

1. Anticipate coadministration of PO or IV corticosteroids during the first week of therapy to prevent cerebral hypertensive episodes.

2. Monitor neurologic status carefully. Administer steroids and anticonvulsants with neurocysticerosis.

Albuterol (Salbutamol)

(al-BYOU-ter-ohl)

Pregnancy Class: C

Proventil, Proventil HFA-3M, Proventil Repetabs, Ventolin, Ventolin Rotacaps, Volmax **(Rx)**

Classification: Direct-acting adrenergic (sympathomimetic) agent

Mechanism of Action: Stimulates beta-2 receptors of the bronchi, leading to bronchodilation.

Onset of Action: PO: 15-30 min. **Inhalation:** 5-15 min. **Peak effect PO:** 2-3 hr., **Inhalation:** 60-90 min (after 2 inhalations).

Duration of Action: PO: 8 hr (up to 12 hr for extended-release); **Inhalation:** 3-6 hr.

Uses: Bronchial asthma; bronchospasm due to bronchitis or emphysema; bronchitis; reversible obstructive pulmonary disease in those 4 years of age and older; exercise-induced bronchospasm. Prophylaxis of bronchial asthma or bronchospasms. Parenteral for treatment of status asthmaticus. *Investigational:* Nebulized albuterol may be useful as an adjunct to treat serious acute hyperkalemia in hemodialysis patients.

Contraindications: Aerosol for prevention of exercise-induced bronchospasm is not recommended for children less than 12 years of age. Use during lactation.

Precautions: Dosage has not been established for the syrup in children less than 2 years of age, for tablets in children less than 6 years of age, and for extended-release tablets in children less than 12 years of age. Albuterol may delay preterm labor.

Do not use tablets in children less than 12 years of age.

Route/Dosage

• **Metered Dose Inhaler**

Bronchodilation.

Adults and children over 12 years of age: 180 mcg (2 inhalations) q 4–6 hr (Ventolin aerosol may be used in children over 4 years of age). In some patients 1 inhalation (90 mcg) q 4 hr may be sufficient.

Prophylaxis of exercise-induced bronchospasm.

Adults and children over 12 years of age: 180 mcg (2 inhalations) 15 min before exercise.

• **Solution for Inhalation**

Bronchodilation.

Adults and children over 12 years of age: 2.5 mg t.i.d.–q.i.d. by nebulization (dilute 0.5 mL of the 0.5% solution with 2.5 mL sterile NSS and deliver over 5–15 min).

• **Capsule for Inhalation**

Bronchodilation.

Adults and children over 4 years of age: 200 mcg q 4–6 hr using a Rotahaler inhalation device. In some patients, 400 mcg q 4–6 hr may be required.

Prophylaxis of exercise-induced bronchospasm.

Adults and children over 12 years: 200 mcg 15 min before exercise using a Rotahaler inhalation device.

• **Syrup**

Bronchodilation.

Adults and children over 14 years of age: 2–4 mg t.i.d.–q.i.d., up to a maximum of 8 mg q.i.d. **Children, 6–14 years, initial:** 2 mg (base) t.i.d.–q.i.d.; **then,** increase as necessary to a maximum of 24 mg/day in divided doses. **Children, 2–6 years, initial:** 0.1 mg/kg t.i.d.; **then,** increase as necessary up to 0.2 mg/kg, not to exceed 4 mg t.i.d.

• **Tablets**

Bronchodilation.

Adults and children over 12 years of age, initial: 2–4 mg (of the base) t.i.d.–q.i.d.; **then,** increase dose as needed up to a maximum of 8 mg t.i.d.–q.i.d. In geriatric patients or those sensitive to beta agonists, start with 2 mg t.i.d.–q.i.d. and then increase dose gradually, if needed, to a maximum of 8 mg t.i.d.–q.i.d. **Children, 6–12 years of age, usual, initial:** 2 mg t.i.d.–q.i.d.; **then,** if necessary, increase the dose in a stepwise fashion to a maximum of 24 mg/day in divided doses.

* **Extended-Release Tablets**
  Bronchodilation.

Adults and children over 12 years of age: 4 or 8 mg (of the base) q 12 hr up to a maximum of 32 mg/day. Patients on regular-release albuterol can be switched to the Repetabs in that a 4-mg extended-release tablet q 12 hr is equivalent to a regular 2-mg tablet q 6 hr.

How Supplied: *Metered dose inhaler:* 0.09 mg/inh; *Capsule:* 200 mcg; *Solution:* 0.083%, 0.5%; *Syrup:* 2 mg/5 mL; *Tablet:* 2 mg, 4 mg; *Tablet, Extended Release:* 4 mg, 8 mg

Side Effects: GI: Diarrhea, dry mouth, increased appetite, epigastric pain.CNS: CNS stimulation, malaise, emotional lability, fatigue, lightheadedness, nightmares, disturbed sleep, aggressive behavior, irritability.Respiratory: Bronchitis, epistaxis, hoarseness (especially in children), nasal congestion, increase in sputum.Hypersensitivity (may be immediate): Urticaria, angioedema, rash, bronchospasm. Miscellaneous: Muscle cramps, pallor, teeth discoloration, conjunctivitis, dilated pupils, difficulty in urination, muscle spasm, voice changes, oropharyngeal edema.

OD Overdose Management: *Symptoms:* Seizures, anginal pain, hypertension, hypokalemia, tachycardia (rate may increase to 200 beats/min).

See *Sympathomimetic Drugs.*

EMS CONSIDERATIONS

See also *Sympathomimetic Drugs.*

Alendronate sodium
(ay-LEN-droh-nayt)
Pregnancy Class: C

Fosamax **(Rx)**
Classification: Bone growth regulator (biphosphonate)

Mechanism of Action: Binds to bone hydroxyapatite and inhibits osteoclast activity, thereby preventing bone resorption. Appears to reduce fracture risk and reverse the progression of osteoporosis. Does not inhibit bone mineralization.

Uses: Prevention and treatment of osteoporosis in postmenopausal women. Paget's disease of bone in those with alkaline phosphatase at least two times the upper limit of normal or for those who are symptomatic or at risk for future complications from the disease.

Contraindications: In hypocalcemia. Severe renal insufficiency (C_{CR} less than 35 mL/min). Use of hormone replacement therapy with alendronate for osteoporosis in postmenopausal women. Lactation.

Precautions: Use with caution in those with upper GI problems, such as dysphagia, symptomatic esophageal diseases, gastritis, duodenitis, or ulcers. Safety and effectiveness have not been determined in children or for use in male osteoporosis.

Route/Dosage

* **Tablets**
  Prevention of osteoporosis in postmenopausal women.

5 mg once a day in the morning ½ hr before the first food, beverage, or medication of the day with 6–8 oz of plain water.

Treatment of osteoporosis or prevention of fractures in postmenopausal women with osteoporosis.

10 mg once a day in the morning ½ hr before the first food, beverage, or medication of the day with 6–8 oz of plain water. Safety of treatment for more than 4 years has not been determined.

Paget's disease of bone.

40 mg once a day for 6 months taken as for osteoporosis.

How Supplied: *Tablet:* 5 mg, 10 mg, 40 mg

---

bold italic = life threatening side effect

A

Side Effects: *GI:* Flatulence, acid regurgitation, esophageal ulcer, dysphagia, abdominal distention, gastritis, abdominal pain, constipation, diarrhea, dyspepsia, N&V. *Miscellaneous:* Musculoskeletal pain, pain, headache, taste perversion, rash and erythema (rare), back pain, glaucoma, accidental injury, edema, flu–like symptoms.

OD Overdose Management: *Symptoms:* Hypocalcemia, hypophosphatemia, upset stomach, heartburn, esophagitis, gastritis, ulcer. *Treatment:* Administration of milk or antacids to bind the drug should be considered.

Drug Interactions

Antacids / ↓ Absorption of alendronate

Aspirin / ↑ Risk of upper GI side effects

Calcium supplements / ↓ Absorption of alendronate

Ranitidine / ↑ Bioavailability of alendronate (significance not known)

EMS CONSIDERATIONS

None.

Alitretinoin
(al-eh-TRET-ih-noh-in)
Pregnancy Class: D
Panretin Gel
Classification: Retinoid

Mechanism of Action: Retinoid binds to and activates all known intracellular retinoid receptor subtypes. Upon activation, the receptors regulate the expression of genes that control cellular differentiation and proliferation in both healthy and cancerous cells. Inhibits growth of Kaposi's sarcoma cells in vitro.

Uses: Treat cutaneous lesions in AIDS-related Kaposi's sarcoma.

Contraindications: Hypersensitivity to retinoids. Use when systemic treatment of Kaposi's sarcoma is needed (i.e., 10 new sarcoma lesions in the prior month, symptomatic lymphedema, symptomatic pulmonary Kaposi's sarcoma, symptomatic visceral involvement). Lactation.

Precautions: Safety and efficacy have not been determined in children or in patients 65 years of age or older.

Route/Dosage
• **Gel**
  Kaposi's sarcoma cutaneous lesions.
Initial: Apply b.i.d. Can increase frequency of application to t.i.d. or q.i.d., according to individual lesion tolerance.

How Supplied: Gel: 0.1%

Side Effects: *Dermatologic:* Rash (erythema, scaling, irritation, redness, dermatitis), pain, burning pain, pruritus, exfoliative dermatitis, paresthesia, edema, inflammation, vesiculation, skin disorder (excoriation, cracking, scabbing, crusting, drainage, eschar, fissure, oozing).

Drug Interactions: Increased toxicity when combined with (DEET) N,N-diethyl-m-toluamide, a common component of insect repellents.

EMS CONSIDERATIONS
Administration/Storage
1. A reponse may be seen within 2 weeks. However, most patients require 4–8 weeks of treatment; some require 14 or more weeks of treatment before beneficial effects are noted.
2. Continue application as long as the patient is getting benefit.
3. Application frequency can be reduced if application site toxicity occurs. Discontinue for a few days if severe irritation occurs.

Allopurino
(al-oh-PYOUR-ih-nohl)
Pregnancy Class: C
Zyloprim **(Rx)**
Classification: Antigout agent

Mechanism of Action: Allopurinol and its major metabolite, oxipurinol, are potent inhibitors of xanthine oxidase, an enzyme involved in the synthesis of uric acid, without disrupting the biosynthesis of essential purine. This results in decreased levels of uric acid. The drug also increases reutilization of xanthine and hypoxanthine for synthesis of nucleotide and nucleic acid synthesis by acting on the enzyme hypoxanthineguanine phosphoribosyltransferase. The resultant increases in nucleotides cause a negative feedback to inhibit synthesis of purines and a decrease in uric acid levels.

Onset of Action: Maximum therapeutic effect: 1-3 weeks.

Uses: Primary or secondary gout (acute attacks, tophi, joint destruction, nephropathy, uric acid lithiasis). Patients with leukemia, lymphoma, or other malignancies in whom drug therapy causes elevations of serum and urinary uric acid. Recurrent calcium oxalate calculi where daily uric acid excretion exceed 800 mg/day in males and 750 mg/day in females. *Investigational:* Mixed with methylcellulose as a mouthwash to prevent stomatitis following fluorouracil administration. Reduce the granulocyte suppressant effect of fluorouracil. Prevent ischemic reperfusion tissue damage. Reduce the incidence of perioperative mortality and postoperative arrhythmias in coronary artery bypass surgery. Reduce the rates of *Helicobacter pylori*-induced duodenal ulcers and treatment of hematemesis from NSAID-induced erosive esophagitis. Alleviate pain due to acute pancreatitis. Treatment of American cutaneous leishmaniasis and against *Trypanosoma cruzi*. Treat Chagas' disease. As an alternative in epileptic seizures refractory to standard therapy.

Contraindications: Hypersensitivity to drug. Patients with idiopathic hemochromatosis or relatives of patients suffering from this condition. Children except as an adjunct in treatment of neoplastic disease. Severe skin reactions on previous exposure. To treat asymptomatic hyperuricemia.

Precautions: Use with caution during lactation and in patients with liver or renal disease. In children use has been limited to rare inborn errors of pruine metabolism or hyperuricemia

as a result of malignancy or cancer therapy.

Route/Dosage
- **Tablets**
  Gout/hyperuricemia.
  Adults: 200–600 mg/day, depending on severity (minimum effective dose: 100–200 mg/day). Maximum daily dose should not exceed 800 mg.
  Prevention of uric acid nephropathy during treatment of neoplasms.
  Adults: 600–800 mg/day for 2–3 days (with high fluid intake).
  Prophylaxis of acute gout.
  Initial: 100 mg/day; increase by 100 mg at weekly intervals until serum uric acid level of 6 mg/100 mL or less is reached.
  Hyperuricemia associated with malignancy.
  Pediatric, 6–10 years of age: 300 mg/day either as a single dose of 100 mg t.i.d.; **under 6 years of age:** 150 mg/day in three divided doses.
  Recurrent calcium oxalate calculi. 200–300 mg/day in one or more doses (dose may be adjusted according to urinary levels of uric acid).
  To ameliorate granulocyte suppressant effect of fluorouracil. 600 mg/day.
  Reduce perioperative mortality and postoperative arrhythmias in coronary artery bypass surgery. 300 mg 12 hr and 1 hr before surgery.
  Reduce relapse rates of H. pylori-*induced duodenal ulcers; treat hematemesis from NSAID-induced erosive gastritis.* 50 mg q.i.d.
  Alleviate pain due to acute pancreatitis. 50 mg q.i.d.
  Treat American cutaneous leishmaniasis and T. cruzi. 20 mg/kg for 15 days.
  Treat Chagas' disease. 600–900 mg/day for 60 days.
  Alternative to treat epileptic seizures refractory to standard therapy. 300 mg/day, except use 150 mg/day in those less than 20 kg.

---

bold italic = life threatening side effect

- **Mouthwash**
    Prevent fluorouracil-induced stomatitis.
    20 mg in 3% methylcellulose (1 mg/mL).

How Supplied: *Tablet:* 100 mg, 300 mg

Side Effects: *Dermatologic* (most frequent): Pruritic maculopapular skin rash (may be accompanied by fever and malaise). Vesicular bullous dermatitis, eczematoid dermatitis, pruritus, urticaria, onycholysis, purpura, lichen planus, **Stevens-Johnson syndrome, toxic epidermal necrolysis.** Skin rash has been accompanied by hypertension and cataract development. *Allergy:* Fever, chills, leukopenia, eosinophilia, arthralgia, skin rash, pruritus, N&V, nephritis. *GI:* N&V, diarrhea, gastritis, dyspepsia, abdominal pain (intermittent). *Hematologic:* Leukopenia, eosinophilia, thrombocytopenia, leukocytosis. *Hepatic:* Hepatomegaly, cholestatic jaundice, **hepatic necrosis,** granulomatous hepatitis. *Neurologic:* Headache, peripheral neuropathy, paresthesia, somnolence, neuritis. *CV:* Necrotizing angiitis, hypersensitivity vasculitis. *Miscellaneous:* Ecchymosis, epistaxis, taste loss, arthralgia, acute attacks of gout, fever, myopathy, renal failure, uremia, alopecia.

Drug Interactions
ACE inhibitors / ↑ Risk of hypersensitivity reactions
Aluminum salts / ↓ Effect of allopurinol
Ampicillin / ↑ Risk of ampicillin-induced skin rashes
Anticoagulants, oral / ↑ Effect of anticoagulant due to ↓ breakdown by liver
Azathioprine / ↑ Effect of azathioprine due to ↓ breakdown by liver
Cyclophosphamide / ↑ Risk of bleeding or infection due to ↑ myelosuppressive effects of cyclophosphamide
Iron preparations / Allopurinol ↑ hepatic iron concentrations
Mercaptopurine / ↑ Effect of mercaptopurine due to ↓ breakdown by liver

Theophylline / Allopurinol ↑ plasma theophylline levels → possible toxicity
Thiazide diuretics / ↑ Risk of hypersensitivity reactions to allopurinol
Uricosuric agents / ↓ Effect of oxipurinol due to ↑ rate of excretion

EMS CONSIDERATIONS

None.

Alprazolam
(al-PRAYZ-oh-lam)
Pregnancy Class: D
Xanax **(C-IV) (Rx)**
Classification: Antianxiety agent

Mechanism of Action: See Tranquilizers/Antimanic Drugs/Hypnotics
Uses: Anxiety. Anxiety associated with depression with or without agoraphobia. *Investigational:* Agoraphobia with social phobia, depression, PMS.
Contraindications: Use with itraconazole or ketoconazole.

Route/Dosage
- **Tablets**
    Anxiety disorder.
Adults, initial: 0.25–0.5 mg t.i.d.; **then,** titrate to needs of patient, with total daily dosage not to exceed 4 mg. **In elderly or debilitated: initial;** 0.25 mg b.i.d.–t.i.d.; **then,** adjust dosage to needs of patient.
    Antipanic agent.
Adults: 0.5 mg t.i.d.; increase dose as needed up to a maximum of 10 mg/day.
    Agoraphobia with social phobia.
Adults: 2–8 mg/day.
    PMS.
0.25 mg t.i.d.
How Supplied: *Tablet:* 0.25 mg, 0.5 mg, 1 mg, 2 mg

EMS CONSIDERATIONS

See also *Tranquilizers/Antimanic Drugs/Hypnotics.*

Alteplase, recombinant
(AL-teh-playz)
Pregnancy Class: C

Activase **(Rx)**
Classification: Thrombolytic agent
(tissue plasminogen activator)

Mechanism of Action: Alteplase, a tissue plasminogen activator, is synthesized by a human melanoma cell line using recombinant DNA technology. This enzyme binds to fibrin in a thrombus, causing a conversion of plasminogen to plasmin. This conversion results in local fibrinolysis and a decrease in circulating fibrinogen.

Onset of Action: t½ initial: 4 min; **final:** 35 min (elimination phase).

Uses: Improvement of ventricular function following acute MI, including reducing the incidence of CHF and decreasing mortality. Treat acute ischemic stroke, after intracranial hemorrhage has been excluded by CT scan or other diagnostic imaging. Acute pulmonary thromboembolism. *Investigational:* Unstable angina pectoris.

Contraindications: *Acute MI or pulmonary embolism:* Active internal bleeding, history of CVA, within 2 months of intracranial or intraspinal surgery or trauma, intracranial neoplasm, AV malformation or aneurysm, bleeding diathesis, severe uncontrolled hypertension.

Acute ischemic stroke: Symptoms of intracranial hemorrhage on pretreatment evaluation, suspected subarachnoid hemorrhage, recent intracranial surgery or serious head trauma, recent previous stroke, history of intracranial hemorrhage, uncontrolled hypertension (above 185 mm Hg systolic or above 110 Hg diastolic) at time of treatment, active internal bleeding, seizure at onset of stroke, intracranial neoplasm, AV malformation or aneurysm, bleeding diathesis.

Precautions: Use with caution in the presence of recent GI or GU bleeding (within 10 days), subacute bacterial endocarditis, acute pericarditis, significant liver dysfunction, concomitant use of oral anticoagulants, diabetic hemorrhagic retinopathy, septic thrombophlebitis or occluded arteriovenous cannula (at infected site), lactation, mitral stenosis with atrial fibrillation. Since fibrin will be lysed during therapy, careful attention should be given to potential bleeding sites such as sites of catheter insertion and needle puncture sites. Use with caution within 10 days of major surgery (e.g., obstetrics, coronary artery bypass) and in patients over 75 years of age. Safety and efficacy have not been established in children. NOTE: Doses greater than 150 mg have been associated with an increase in intracranial bleeding.

Route/Dosage

• **IV Infusion Only**
AMI, accelerated infusion.
Weight >67 kg: 100 mg as a 15-mg IV bolus, followed by 50 mg infused over the next 30 min and then 35 mg infused over the next 60 min. **Weight <67 kg:** 15 mg IV bolus, followed by 0.75 mg/kg infused over the next 30 min (not to exceed 50 mg) and then 0.50 mg/kg infused over the next 60 min (not to exceed 35 mg). The safety and efficacy of this regimen have only been evaluated using heparin and aspirin concomitantly.
AMI, 3-hr infusion.
100 mg total dose subdivided as follows: 60 mg (34.8 million IU) the first hour with 6–10 mg given in a bolus over the first 1–2 min and the remaining 50-54 mg given over the hour; 20 mg (11.6 million IU) over the second hour and 20 mg (11.6 million IU) given over the third hour. **Patients less than 65 kg:** 1.25 mg/kg given over 3 hr, with 60% given the first hour with 6%–10% given by direct IV injection within the first 1–2 min; 20% is given the second hour and 20% during the third hour. Doses of 150 mg have caused an increase in intracranial bleeding.
Pulmonary embolism.
100 mg over 2 hr; heparin therapy should be instituted near the end of or right after the alteplase infusion

---

bold italic = life threatening side effect

when the partial thromboplastin or thrombin time returns to twice that of normal or less.

Acute ischemic stroke.

0.9 mg/kg (maximum of 90 mg) infused over 60 min with 10% of the total dose given as an initial IV bolus over 1 min. Doses greater than 0.9 mg/kg may cause an increased incidence of intracranial hemorrhage. Use with aspirin and heparin during the first 24 hr after onset of symptoms has not been investigated.

How Supplied: *Powder for injection:* 50 mg, 100 mg

Side Effects: *Bleeding tendencies: Internal bleeding* (including the GI and GU tracts and intracranial or retroperitoneal site). Superficial bleeding (e.g., gums, sites of recent surgery, venous cutdowns, arterial punctures). Ecchymosis, epistaxis. *CV:* Bradycardia, hypotension, cardiogenic shock, arrhythmias, *heart failure, cardiac arrest, cardiac tamponade, myocardial rupture,* recurrent ischemia, reinfarction, mitral regurgitation, pericardial effusion, pericarditis, venous thrombosis and embolism, electromechanical dissociation. *Allergic:* Rash, *laryngeal edema, anaphylaxis. GI:* N&V. *Miscellaneous:* Fever, urticaria, pulmonary edema, cerebral edema.

Due to accelerated infusion: Strokes, hemorrhagic stroke, nonfatal stroke. Incidence increases with age.

OD **Overdose Management:** *Symptoms:* Bleeding disorders. *Treatment:* Discontinue therapy immediately as well as any concomitant heparin therapy.

Drug Interactions

Abciximab / ↑ Risk of bleeding
Acetylsalicylic acid / ↑ Risk of bleeding
Dipyridamole / ↑ Risk of bleeding
Heparin / ↑ Risk of bleeding, especially at arterial puncture sites

---

EMS CONSIDERATIONS

Administration/Storage

IV 1. Initiate alteplase therapy as soon as possible after onset of symptoms and within 3 hr after the onset of stroke symptoms.

2. Reconstitute with only sterile water for injection without preservatives immediately prior to use. The reconstituted preparation contains 1 mg/mL and is a colorless to pale yellow transparent solution.

3. Using an 18-gauge needle, direct the stream of sterile water for injection into the lyophilized cake. Leave the product undisturbed for several minutes to allow dissipation of any large bubbles.

4. If necessary, the reconstituted solution may be further diluted immediately prior to use in an equal volume of 0.9% NaCl injection or 5% dextrose injection to yield a concentration of 0.5 mg/mL. Dilute by gentle swirling or slow inversion.

Interventions

1. Observe in a closely monitored environment; obtain VS and review and document monitor strips.

2. Anticipate and assess for reperfusion reactions such as:

• Reperfusion arrhythmias usually of short duration. These may include accelerated idioventricular rhythm and sinus bradycardia.

• Reduction of chest pain

• Return of the elevated ST segment to near baseline levels

• Smaller Q waves

3. Check all access sites for any evidence of bleeding.

4. In the event of any uncontrolled bleeding, terminate the alteplase and heparin infusions and report immediately.

5. Monitor neurologic status and record findings q 15–30 min during infusion.

Altretamine (Hexylmethmelamine)

(all-TRET-ah-meen)
Pregnancy Class: D
Hexalen**(Rx)**
Classification: Antineoplastic, miscellaneous

Mechanism of Action: The mechanism of action is unknown.

Onset of Action: Peak plasma levels:0.5-3 hr. **t½**4.7-10.2 hr.

Uses: Used alone in the palliative treatment of persistent or recurrent ovarian cancer after first-line cisplatin- or alkylating agent-based combination therapy.

Contraindications: Preexisting bone marrow depression or severe neurologic toxicity, although the drug has been used safely in patients with preexisting cisplatin neuropathies. Lactation.

Precautions: Safety and effectiveness have not been determined in children. High daily doses may result in gradual onset of N&V.

Route/Dosage ─────────────
• **Capsules**
Ovarian cancer.
260 mg/m²/day given either for 14 or 21 consecutive days in a 28-day cycle. The total daily dose is given as four divided doses PO after meals and at bedtime.

How Supplied: *Capsule:* 50 mg

Side Effects: *GI:* N&V (most common). *Neurologic:* Peripheral sensory neuropathy, fatigue, anorexia, seizures. *CNS:* Mood disorders, disorders of consciousness, ataxia, dizziness, vertigo. *Hematologic:* Leukopenia, thrombocytopenia, anemia. *Miscellaneous: **Hepatic toxicity,*** skin rash, pruritus, alopecia.

Drug Interactions: Use with MAO inhibitors may cause severe orthostatic hypotension, especially in patients over the age of 60 years.

EMS CONSIDERATIONS

See also *Antineoplastic Agents.*

─────────────

Amantadine hydrochloride
(ah-MAN-tah-deen)
Pregnancy Class: C
Symadine, Symmetrel **(Rx)**
Classification: Antiviral and antiparkinson agent

Mechanism of Action: Amantadine is believed to prevent penetration of the virus into cells, possibly by inhibiting uncoating of the RNA virus.

The reaction appears to be virus specific for influenza A but not host specific. It may also prevent the release of infectious viral nucleic acid into the host cell. The drug reduces symptoms of viral infections if given within 24–48 hr after onset of illness. For the treatment of parkinsonism, amantadine may increase the release of dopamine from dopaminergic nerve terminals in the substantia nigra of parkinson patients, resulting in an increase in dopamine levels in dopaminergic synapses. The drug decreases extrapyramidal symptoms, including akinesia, rigidity, tremors, excessive salivation, gait disturbances, and total functional disability.

Onset of Action: 48 hr.

Uses: Influenza A viral infections of the respiratory tract (prophylaxis and treatment of high-risk patients with immunodeficiency, CV, metabolic, neuromuscular, or pulmonary disease). Symptomatic treatment of idiopathic parkinsonism and parkinsonism syndrome resulting from encephalitis, carbon monoxide intoxication, drugs, or cerebral arteriosclerosis. Favorable results have been obtained in about 50% of the patients. Improvements can last for up to 30 months, although some patients report that the effect of the drug wears off in 1–3 months. A rest period or an increased dosage may reestablish effectiveness. For parkinsonism, amantadine hydrochloride is usually used concomitantly with other agents, such as levodopa and anticholinergic agents.

Amantadine is recommended for prophylaxis in the following situations:

• Short-term prophylaxis during the course of a presumed outbreak of influenza A

• Adjunct to late immunization in high-risk patients

• To reduce disruption of medical care and to decrease spread of virus in high-risk patients when influenza A virus outbreaks occur

─────────────

bold italic = life threatening side effect

• To supplement vaccination protection in patients with impaired immune responses

• As chemoprophylaxis during flu season for those high-risk patients for whom influenza vaccine is contraindicated due to anaphylactic response to egg protein or prior severe reactions associated with flu vaccination

Contraindications: Hypersensitivity to drug.

Precautions: Use with caution in patients with liver and renal disease, history of epilepsy, CHF, peripheral edema, orthostatic hypotension, recurrent eczematoid detmatitis, or severe psychosis, in patients taking CNS stimulant drugs, to those exposed to rubella, and to nursing mothers. Safe use in lactating mothers and children less than 1 year has not been established.

Route/Dosage ——————
• **Capsules, Syrup**
  Antiviral.
  Adults: 200 mg/day as a single or divided dose. **Children, 1–9 years:** 4.4–8.8 mg/kg/day up to a maximum of 150 mg/day in one or two divided doses (use syrup); **9–12 years:** 100 mg b.i.d.
  Prophylactic treatment.
Institute before or immediately after exposure and continue for 10–21 days if used concurrently with vaccine or for 90 days without vaccine.
  Symptomatic management.
Initiate as soon as possible and continue for 24–48 hr after disappearance of symptoms. Decrease dose in renal impairment (see package insert). Reduce dose to 100 mg/day for persons with active seizure disorders due to the increased risk of seizure frequency using daily doses of 200 mg.
  Parkinsonism.
  Use as sole agent, usual: 100 mg b.i.d., up to 400 mg/day in divided doses, if necesssary. **Use with other antiparkinson drugs:** 100 mg 1–2 times/day.
  Drug-induced   extrapyramidal symptoms.

100 mg b.i.d. (up to 300 mg/day may be required in some). Reduce dose in impaired renal function.

How Supplied: *Capsule:* 100 mg; *Syrup:* 50 mg/5 mL; *Tablet:* 100 mg

Side Effects: *GI:* N&V, constipation, anorexia, xerostomia. *CNS:* Depression, psychosis, **convulsions,** hallucinations, lightheadedness, confusion, ataxia, irritability, anxiety, headache, dizziness, fatigue, insomnia. *CV:* **CHF,** orthostatic hypotension, peripheral edema. *Miscellaneous:* Urinary retention, leukopenia, neutropenia, mottling of skin of the extremities due to poor peripheral circulation (livedo reticularis), skin rashes, visual problems, slurred speech, oculogyric episodes, dyspnea, weakness, eczematoid dermatitis.

OD Overdose Management: *Symptoms:* Anorexia, N&V, CNS effects. *Treatment:* Gastric lavage or induction of emesis followed by supportive measures. Ensure that patient is well hydrated; give IV fluids if necessary. To treat CNS toxicity: IV physostigmine, 1–2 mg given q 1–2 hr in adults or 0.5 mg at 5–10-min intervals (maximum of 2 mg/hr) in children. Sedatives and anticonvulsants may be given if needed; antiarrhythmics and vasopressors may also be required.

Drug Interactions
Anticholinergics / Additive anticholinergic effects (including hallucinations, confusion), especially with trihexyphenidyl and benztropine
CNS stimulants / May ↑ CNS and psychic effects of amantadine; use cautiously together
Hydrochlorothiazide/triamterene combination / ↓ Urinary excretion of amantadine → ↑ plasma levels
Levodopa / Potentiated by amantadine

EMS CONSIDERATIONS

See also *Antiviral Drugs.*

————*COMBINATION DRUG*————

Amiloride and Hydrochlorothiazide
(ah-MILL-oh-ryd, hy-droh-klor-oh-THIGH-ah-zyd)

Pregnancy Class: C
Moduretic(Rx)
Classification: Antihypertensive

Uses: Hypertension or CHF, especially when hypokalemia occurs. Used alone or with other antihypertensive drugs, such as beta-adrenergic blocking drugs and methyldopa.

Precautions: Use with caution during lactation. Geriatric patients may be more sensitive to the hypotensive and electrolyte effects of this combination; also, age-related decreases in renal function may require a decrease in dosage.

Route/Dosage
• **Tablets**
  All uses.
Initial: 1 tablet/day; **then,** dosage may be increased to 2 tablets/day.
How Supplied: *Diuretic, potassium-sparing:*Amiloride HCL, 5 mg. *Antihypertensive/diuretic:* Hydrochlorothiazide, 50 mg.

EMS CONSIDERATIONS

See also *Amiloride* and *Hydrochlorothiazide.*

Amiloride hydrochloride
(ah-MILL-oh-ryd)
Pregnancy Class: B
Midamor(Rx)
Classification: Diuretic, potassium-sparing

Mechanism of Action: Acts on the distal tubule to inhibit Na^+, K^+-ATPase, thereby inhibiting sodium exchange for potassium; this results in increased secretion of sodium and water and conservation of potassium. In the proximal tubule, amiloride inhibits the Na^+/H^+ exchange mechanism. Has weak diuretic and antihypertensive activity.
Onset of Action: 2 hr. **Peak effect:** 6-10 hr.
Duration of Action: 24 hr.t½6-9 hr.
Uses: Adjunct with thiazides or loop diuretics in the treatment of hypertension or edema due to CHF, hepatic cirrhosis, and nephrotic syndrome

to help restore normal serum potassium or prevent hypokalemia. Prophylaxis of hypokalemia in patients who would be at risk if hypokalemia developed (e.g., digitalized patients or patients with significant cardiac arrhythmias). *Investigational:* To reduce lithium-induced polyuria. Aerosolized amiloride may slow the progression of pulmonary function reduction in adults with cystic fibrosis.
Contraindications: Hyperkalemia (>5.5 mEq potassium/L). In patients receiving other potassium-sparing diuretics or potassium supplements. Impaired renal function. Diabetes mellitus. Use during lactation.
Precautions: Use with caution in metabolic or respiratory acidosis; during lactation. Geriatric patients may have a greater risk of developing hyperkalemia. Safety and efficacy have not been determined in children.

Route/Dosage
• **Tablets**
  As single agent or with other diuretics.
Adults, initial: 5 mg/day; 10 mg/day may be necessary in some patients. Doses as high as 20 mg/day may be used, if needed, with careful monitoring of electrolytes.
  Reduce lithium-induced polyuria.
10–20 mg/day.
  Slow progression of pulmonary function reduction in cystic fibrosis.
Adults: Drug is dissolved in 0.3% saline and delivered by nebulizer.
How Supplied: *Tablet:* 5 mg
Side Effects: *Electrolyte:* Hyperkalemia, hyponatremia, and hypochloremia if used with other diuretics. *CNS:* Headache, dizziness, encephalopathy, tremors, paresthesias, mental confusion, insomnia, decreased libido, depression, sleepiness, vertigo, nervousness. *GI:* Nausea, anorexia, vomiting, diarrhea, changes in appetite, gas and abdominal pain, dry mouth, flatulence, abdominal fullness, GI bleeding, GI disturbance, thirst, dyspepsia, heartburn, jaun-

---

bold italic = life threatening side effect

dice, constipation, activation of preexisting peptic ulcer. *Respiratory:* Dyspnea, cough, SOB. *Musculoskeletal:* Weakness; muscle cramps; fatigue; joint, chest and back pain; neck or shoulder ache; pain in extremities. *GU:* Impotence, polyuria, dysuria, bladder spasms, urinary frequency. *CV:* Angina, palpitations, *arrhythmias,* orthostatic hypotension. *Hematologic: Aplastic anemia,* neutropenia. *Dermatologic:* Skin rash, itching, pruritus, alopecia. *Miscellaneous:* Visual disturbances, nasal congestion, tinnitus, increased intraocular pressure, abnormal liver function.

OD **Overdose Management:** *Symptoms:* Electrolyte imbalance, *dehydration. Treatment:* Induce emesis or gastric lavage. Treat hyperkalemia by IV sodium bicarbonate or oral or parenteral glucose with a rapid-acting insulin. Sodium polystyrene sulfonate, oral or by enema, may also be used.

Drug Interactions
ACE inhibitors / ↑ Risk of significant hyperkalemia
Digoxin / Possible ↑ renal clearance and ↓ nonrenal clearance of digoxin. Possible ↑ inotropic effect of digoxin
Lithium / ↓ Renal excretion of lithium → ↑ chance of toxicity
NSAIDs / ↓ Therapeutic effect of amiloride
Potassium products / Hyperkalemia with possibility of cardiac arrhythmias or cardiac arrest
Spironolactone, Triamterene / Hyperkalemia, hyponatremia, hypochloremia

EMS CONSIDERATIONS

See also *Diuretics.*

Aminophylline
(am-in-OFF-ih-lin)
Pregnancy Class: C
Aminophyllin, Truphyllin**(Rx)**
Classification: Bronchodilator

Mechanism of Action: Contains 79% theophylline.
Uses: Additional: Neonatal apnea, respiratory stimulant in Cheyne-

Stokes respiration. Parenteral form has been used for biliary colic and as a cardiac stimulant, a diuretic, and an adjunct in treating CHF, although such uses have been replaced by more effective drugs.
Precautions: Use with caution when aminophylline and sodium chloride are used with corticosteroids or in patients with edema.

Route/Dosage
• **Oral Solution, Tablets**
Bronchodilator, acute attacks, in patients not currently on theophylline therapy.
Adults and children up to 16 years of age, loading dose: Equivalent of 5–6 mg of anhydrous theophylline/kg.
Bronchodilator, acute attacks, in patients currently receiving theophylline.
Adults and children up to 16 years of age: If possible, a serum theophylline level should be obtained first. Then, base loading dose on the premise that each 0.5 mg theophylline/kg lean body weight will result in a 0.5–1.6-mcg/mL increase in serum theophylline levels. If immediate therapy is needed and a serum level cannot be obtained, a single dose of the equivalent of 2.5 mg/kg of anhydrous theophylline can be given.
Maintenance in acute attack, based on equivalent of anhydrous theophylline.
Young adult smokers: 4 mg/kg q 6 hr; **healthy, nonsmoking adults:** 3 mg/kg q 8 hr; **geriatric patients or patients with cor pulmonale:** 2 mg/kg q 8 hr; **patients with CHF or liver failure:** 2 mg/kg q 8–12 hr. **Pediatric, 12–16 years:** 3 mg/kg q 6 hr; **9–12 years:** 4 mg/kg q 6 hr; **1–9 years:** 5 mg/kg q 6 hr; **6–12 months:** Use the formula: dose (mg/kg q 8 hr) = (0.05) (age in weeks) + 1.25; **up to 6 months:** Use the formula: dose (mg/kg q 8 hr) = (0.07) (age in weeks) + 1.7.
Chronic therapy, based on equivalent of anhydrous theophylline.

Adults, initial: 6–8 mg/kg up to a maximum of 400 mg/day in three to four divided doses at 6–8-hr intervals; **then,** dose can be increased in 25% increments at 2–3 day intervals up to a maximum of 13 mg/kg or 900 mg/day, whichever is less. **Pediatric, initial:** 16 mg/kg up to a maximum of 400 mg/day in three to four divided doses at 6–8 hr intervals; **then,** dose may be increased in 25% increments at 2–3 day intervals up to the following maximum doses (without measuring serum theophylline): **16 years and older:** 13 mg/kg or 900 mg/day, whichever is less; **12–16 years:** 18 mg/kg/day; **9–12 years:** 20 mg/kg/day; **1–9 years:** 24 mg/kg/day; **up to 12 months,** Use the following formula: dose (mg/kg/day) = (0.3) (age in weeks) + 8.0.

• **Enteric-Coated Tablets**

Bronchodilator, chronic therapy, based on equivalent of anhydrous theophylline.

Adults, initial: 6–8 mg/kg up to a maximum of 400 mg/day in three to four divided doses at 6–8-hr intervals; **then,** dose may be increased, if needed and tolerated, by increments of 25% at 2–3 day intervals up to a maximum of 13 mg/kg/day or 900 mg/day, whichever is less, without measuring serum theophylline. **Pediatric, over 12 years of age, initial:** 4 mg/kg q 8–12 hr; **then,** dose may be increased by 2–3 mg/kg/day at 3-day intervals up to the following maximum doses (without measuring serum levels): **16 years and older:** 13 mg/kg/day or 900 mg/day, whichever is less; **12–16 years:** 18 mg/kg/day.

• **Enema**

For use as a bronchodilator for loading doses and for maintenance in acute attacks, see doses for oral solution and tablets.

• **IV Infusion**

Bronchodilator, acute attacks, for patients not currently on theophylline.

Adults and children up to 16 years, loading dose based on anhy- **drous theophylline:** 5 mg/kg given over a period of 20 min.

Bronchodilator, acute attack, for patients currently on theophylline.

Adults and children up to 16 years, loading dose based on anhydrous theophylline: If possible, a serum theophylline level should be obtained first. Then, base loading dose on the premise that each 0.5 mg theophylline/kg lean body weight will result in a 0.5–1.6 mcg/mL increase in serum theophylline levels. If immediate therapy is needed and a serum level cannot be obtained, a single dose of the equivalent of 2.5 mg/kg of anhydrous theophylline can be given.

Maintenance for acute attacks, based on equivalent of anhydrous theophylline.

Young adult smokers: 0.7 mg/kg/hr; **nonsmoking, healthy adults:** 0.43 mg/kg/hr; **geriatric patients or patients with cor pulmonale:** 0.26 mg/kg/hr; **patients with CHF or liver failure:** 0.2 mg/kg/hr. **Pediatric, 12–16 years, nonsmokers:** 0.5 mg/kg/hr; **9–12 years,** 0.7 mg/kg/hr; **1–9 years,** 0.8 mg/kg/hr; **up to 1 year,** Based on the following formula: dose (mg/kg/hr) = (0.008) (age in weeks) + 0.21.

How Supplied: *Injection:* 25 mg/mL; *Oral Solution:* 105 mg/5 mL; *Suppository:* 250 mg, 500 mg; *Tablet:* 100 mg, 200 mg

Side Effects: The ethylenediamine in the product may cause exfoliative dermatitis or urticaria.

EMS CONSIDERATIONS

See also *Theophylline Derivatives.*
Administration/Storage
1. IM injection is not recommended due to severe, persistent pain at the site of injection.
IV 2. To avoid hypotension, administer IV doses at a rate not to exceed 25 mg/min.
3. Use only the 25 mg/mL injection (which should be further diluted) for IV administration. Use an infusion

A

pump or device to regulate infusion rates.

Assessment

1. Monitor VS closely during IV administration; may cause a transitory lowering of BP. If evident, adjust the drug dosage and rate of flow.

2. Monitor patients with a history of CAD for chest pain and ECG changes.

Amiodarone hydrochloride

(am-ee-OH-dah-rohn)
Pregnancy Class: D
Pacerone**(Rx)**
Classification: Antiarrhythmic, class III

Mechanism of Action: Blocks sodium channels at rapid pacing frequencies, causing an increase in the duration of the myocardial cell action potential and refractory period, as well as alpha- and beta-adrenergic blockade. The drug decreases sinus rate, increases PR and QT intervals, results in development of U waves, and changes T-wave contour. After IV use, amiodarone relaxes vascular smooth muscle, reduces peripheral vascular resistance (afterload), and increases cardiac index slightly. Effects may persist for several weeks or months after therapy is terminated.

Onset of Action: Maximum plasma levels: 3-7 hr after single dose. **Onset:** Several days up to 1-3 weeks.

Duration of Action: Several weeks or months after therapy is terminated.

Uses: Oral. Use should be reserved for life-threatening ventricular arrhythmias unresponsive to other therapy, such as recurrent ventricular fibrillation and recurrent, hemodynamically unstable ventricular tachycardia.

IV. Initial treatment and prophylaxis of frequently recurring ventricular fibrillation and hemodynamically unstable ventricular tachycardia in patients refractory to other therapy. Ventricular tachycardia/ventricular fibrillation patients unable to take PO medication. *Investigational:* Refractory sustained or paroxysmal atrial fibrillation, paroxysmal SVT,

symptomatic atrial flutter. Also, low doses in CHF with decreased LV ejection fraction, exercise tolerance and ventricular arrhythmias.

Contraindications: Parenteral or PO use: Marked sinus bradycardia due to severe sinus node dysfunction, second- or third-degree AV block, syncope caused by bradycardia (except when used with a pacemaker). Cardiogenic shock (parenteral use only). Lactation.

Precautions: Safety and effectiveness in children have not been determined. The drug may be more sensitive in geriatric patients, especially in thyroid dysfunction. Carefully monitor the IV product in geriatric patients and in those with severe left ventricular dysfunction.

Route/Dosage —————

Due to the drug's side effects, unusual pharmacokinetic properties, and difficult dosing schedule, administer amiodarone in a hospital only by physicians trained in treating life-threatening arrhythmias. Loading doses are required to ensure a reasonable onset of action.

• **IV Infusion**

Life-threatening ventricular arrhythmias.

Loading dose, rapid: 150 mg over the first 10 minutes (15 mg/min). **Then, slow loading dose:** 360 mg over the next 6 hr (1 mg/min). **Maintenance dose:** 540 mg over the remaining 18 hr (0.5 mg/min). After the first 24 hr, continue maintenance infusion rate of 0.5 mg/min (720 mg/24 hr). This may be continued with monitoring for 2 to 3 weeks.

Once arrhythmias have been suppressed, the patient may be switched to PO amiodarone. The following is intended only as a guideline for PO amiodarone dosage after IV infusion. **IV infusion less than 1 week:** Initial daily dose of PO amiodarone, 800–1,600 mg. **IV infusion from 1 to 3 weeks:** Initial daily dose of PO amiodarone, 600–800 mg. **IV infusion longer than 3 weeks:** Initial daily dose of PO amiodarone, 400 mg.

• **Tablets**

Life-threatening ventricular arrhythmias.
Loading dose: 800–1,600 mg/day for 1–3 weeks (or until initial response occurs); **then,** reduce dose to 600–800 mg/day for 1 month. **Maintenance dose:** 400 mg/day (as low as 200 mg/day or as high as 600 mg/day may be needed in some patients).

Refractory sustained or paroxysmal atrial fibrillation, paroxysmal SVT.
Initial: 600–800 mg/day for 7 to 10 days; **then,** 200–400 mg/day.

LV ejection fraction, exercise tolerance, ventricular arrhythmias with CHF.
200 mg/day.

How Supplied: *Injection:* 50 mg/mL; *Tablet:* 200 mg

Side Effects: Adverse reactions, some potentially fatal, are common with doses greater than 400 mg/day. *Pulmonary:* Pulmonary infiltrates or fibrosis, interstitial/alveolar pneumonitis, hypersensitivity pneumonitis, alveolitis, pulmonary inflammation or fibrosis, ***ARDS (after parenteral use),*** lung edema, cough and progressive dyspnea. Oral use may cause a clinical syndrome of cough and progressive dyspnea accompanied by functional, radiographic, gallium scan, and pathologic data indicating pulmonary toxicity. *CV:* ***Worsening of arrhythmias, paroxysmal ventricular tachycardia,*** proarrhythmias, symptomatic bradycardia, sinus arrest, SA node dysfunction, ***CHF,*** edema, hypotension (especially with IV use), ***cardiac conduction abnormalities, coagulation abnormalities, cardiac arrest (after IV use).*** IV use may result in atrial fibrillation, nodal arrhythmia, prolonged QT interval, and sinus bradycardia. *Hepatic:* Abnormal liver function tests, nonspecific hepatic disorders, cholestatic hepatitis, cirrhosis, hepatitis. *CNS:* Malaise, tremor, lack of coordination, fatigue, ataxia, paresthesias, peripheral neuropathy, abnormal involuntary movements, sleep disturbances, dizziness, insom-

nia, headache, decreased libido, abnormal gait. *GI:* N&V, constipation, anorexia, abdominal pain, abnormal taste and smell, abnormal salivation. *Ophthalmologic:* Ophthalmic abnormalities, including optic neuropathy and/or optic neuritis (may progress to permanent blindness). Papilledema, corneal degeneration, photosensitivity, eye discomfort, scotoma, lens opacities, macular degeneration. Corneal microdeposits (asymptomatic) in patients on therapy for 6 months or more, photophobia, dry eyes, visual disturbances, blurred vision, halos. *Dermatologic:* Photosensitivity, solar dermatitis, blue discoloration of skin, rash, alopecia, spontaneous ecchymosis, flushing. *Miscellaneous:* Hypothyroidism or hyperthyroidism, vasculitis, flushing, pseudotumor cerebri, epididymitis, thrombocytopenia, angioedema. IV use may cause abnormal kidney function, Stevens-Johnson syndrome, respiratory syndrome, and ***shock.***

OD Overdose Management: *Symptoms:* Bradycardia, hypotension, ***disorders of cardiac rhythm, cardiogenic shock,*** AV block, hepatoxicity. *Treatment:* Use supportive treatment. Monitor cardiac rhythm and BP. Use a beta-adrenergic agonist or a pacemaker to treat bradycardia; treat hypotension due to insufficient tissue perfusion with a vasopressor or positive inotropic agents. Cholestyramine may hasten the reversal of side effects by increasing elimination. Drug is not dialyzable.

Drug Interactions
Anticoagulants / ↑ Anticoagulant effect → bleeding disorders
Beta-adrenergic blocking agents / ↑ Chance of bradycardia and hypotension
Calcium channel blockers / ↑ Risk of AV block with verapamil or diltiazem or hypotension with all calcium channel blockers
Cholestyramine / ↑ Elimination of amiodarone → ↓ serum levels and half-ife

Cimetidine / ↑ Serum levels of amiodarone

Cyclosporine / ↑ Levels of plasma cyclosporine → elevated creatinine levels (even with ↓ doses of cyclosporine)

Dextromethorphan / Chronic use of PO amiodarone (> 2 weeks) impairs metabolism of dextromethorphan

Digoxin / ↑ Serum digoxin levels → toxicity

Disopyramide / ↑ QT prolongation → possible arrhythmias

Fentanyl / Possibility of hypotension, bradycardia, ↓ CO

Flecainide / ↑ Plasma levels of flecainide

Methotrexate / Chronic use of PO amiodarone (> 2 weeks) impairs metabolism of methotrexate

Procainamide / ↑ Serum procainamide levels → toxicity

Phenytoin / ↑ Serum phenytoin levels → toxicity; also, ↓ levels of amiodarone

Quinidine / Serum quinidine toxicity, including fatal cardiac arrhythmias

Ritonavir / ↑ Levels of amiodarone → ↑ risk of amiodarone toxicity

Theophylline / ↑ Serum theophylline levels → toxicity (effects may not be seen for 1 week and may last for a prolonged period after drug is discontinued)

EMS CONSIDERATIONS

See also *Antiarrhythmic Agents.*

IV **Administration/Storage** For the first rapid loading dose, add 3 mL amiodarone IV (150 mg) to 100 mL D5W for a concentration of 1.5 mg/mL; infuse at a rate of 100 mL/10 min. For the slower loading dose, add 18 mL amiodarone IV (900 mg) to 500 mL of D5W for a concentration of 1.8 mg/mL.

Assessment: Obtain ECG and document rhythm strips; note EPS findings. During administration, observe ECG for increased PR and QRS intervals, increased arrhythmias, and HR below 60 bpm.

Amitriptyline and Perphenazine

(ah-me-TRIP-tih-leen, per-FEN-ah-zeen)

Triavil 2-10, 2-25, 4-10, 4-25, and 4-50 **(Rx)**

Classification: Antidepressant

Uses: Depression with moderate to severe anxiety and/or agitation. Depression and anxiety in patients with chronic physical disease. Also schizophrenic patients with symptoms of depression.

Contraindications: Use during pregnancy. CNS depression due to drugs. In presence of bone marrow depression. Concomitant use with MAO inhibitors. During acute recovery phase from MI. Use in children.

Route/Dosage

• **Tablets**
Antidepressant.

Adults, initial: One tablet of Triavil 2–25 or 4–25 t.i.d.–q.i.d. or 1 tablet of Triavil 4–50 b.i.d. Schizophrenic patients should receive an initial dose of 2 tablets of Triavil 4–50 t.i.d., with a fourth dose at bedtime, if necessary. Initial dosage for geriatric or adolescent patients in whom anxiety dominates is Triavil 4–10 t.i.d.–q.i.d., with dosage adjusted as required. **Maintenance:** One tablet Triavil 2–25 or 4–25 b.i.d.–q.i.d. or 1 tablet Triavil 4–50 b.i.d.

How Supplied: See also information on individual components.

Antidepressant: Amitriptyline HCl, 10, 25, or 50 mg. *Antipsychotic:* Perphenazine, 2 or 4 mg.

There are five different strengths of Triavil: Triavil 2–10, Triavil 2–25, Triavil 4–10, Triavil 4–25, and Triavil 4–50. *NOTE:* The first number refers to the number of milligrams of perphenazine and the second number refers to the number of milligrams of amitriptyline.

EMS CONSIDERATIONS

None.

Amitriptyline hydrochloride

(ah-me-TRIP-tih-leen)
Pregnancy Class: C
Elavil**(Rx)**
Classification: Antidepressant, tricyclic

Mechanism of Action: Amitriptyline is metabolized to an active metabolite, nortriptyline. Has significant anticholinergic and sedative effects with moderate orthostatic hypotension. Very high ability to block serotonin uptake and moderate activity with respect to norepinephrine uptake.

Onset of Action: Up to 1 month may be required for beneficial effects to be manifested.

Uses: Relief of symptoms of depression, including depression accompanied by anxiety and insomnia. Chronic pain due to cancer or other pain syndromes. Prophylaxis of cluster and migraine headaches. *Investigational:* Pathologic laughing and crying secondary to forebrain disease, bulimia nervosa, antiulcer agent, enuresis.

Contraindications: Use in children less than 12 years of age.

Route/Dosage
- **Tablets**
   Antidepressant.

Adults (outpatients): 75 mg/day in divided doses; may be increased to 150 mg/day. *Alternate dosage:* **Initial,** 50–100 mg at bedtime; **then,** increase by 25–50 mg, if necessary, up to 150 mg/day. **Hospitalized patients: initial,** 100 mg/day; may be increased to 200–300 mg/day. **Maintenance: usual,** 40–100 mg/day (may be given as a single dose at bedtime). **Adolescent and geriatric:** 10 mg t.i.d. and 20 mg at bedtime up to a maximum of 100 mg/day. **Pediatric, 6–12 years:** 10–30 mg (1–5 mg/kg) daily in two divided doses.

   Chronic pain.
50–100 mg/day.
   Enuresis.

Pediatric, over 6 years: 10 mg/day as a single dose at bedtime; dose may be increased up to a maximum of 25 mg. **Less than 6 years:** 10 mg/day as a single dose at bedtime.
- **IM Only**
   Antidepressant.
Adults: 20–30 mg q.i.d.; switch to **PO** therapy as soon as possible.
How Supplied: *Injection:* 10 mg/mL; *Tablet:* 10 mg, 25 mg, 50 mg, 75 mg, 100 mg, 150 mg

EMS CONSIDERATIONS

See also *Antidepressants, Tricyclic.*

Amlexanox

(am-LEX-an-ox)
Pregnancy Class: B
Aphthasol **(Rx)**
Classification: Aphthous ulcer product.

Mechanism of Action: Mechanism not known.
Uses: Treat aphthous ulcers in those with normal immune systems.
Precautions: Use caution during lactation. Safety and eficacy in children have not been determined.

Route/Dosage
- **Paste**
   Aphthous ulcers.
Squeeze about 0.25 inch of paste onto fingertip and, with gentle pressure, dab onto each mouth ulcer. Apply following oral hygiene after breakfast, lunch, dinner, and at bedtime. Start as soon as possible after symptoms of aphthous ulcer noted and continue until ulcer heals.
How Supplied: *Paste:* 5%
Side Effects: Transient pain, burning, or stinging at application site. Contact mucositis, nausea, diarrhea.

EMS CONSIDERATIONS

None.

Amlodipine

(am-LOH-dih-peen)
Pregnancy Class: C

---

bold italic = life threatening side effect

Norvasc **(Rx)**
Classification: Antihypertensive, antianginal (calcium channel blocking agent)

Mechanism of Action: Increases myocardial contractility although this effect may be counteracted by reflex activity. CO is increased and there is a pronounced decrease in peripheral vascular resistance.
Onset of Action: Peak plasma levels:6-12 hr. **t½, elemination:**30-50 hr.
Uses: Hypertension alone or in combination with other antihypertensives. Chronic stable angina alone or in combination with other antianginal drugs. Confirmed or suspected Prinzmetal's or variant angina alone or in combination with other antianginal drugs.
Precautions: Use with caution in patients with CHF and in those with impaired hepatic function or reduced hepatic function or reduced hepatic blood flow. Safety and efficacy have not been determined in children.

Route/Dosage
• **Tablets**
  Hypertension.
Adults, usual, individualized: 5 mg/day, up to a maximum of 10 mg/day. Titrate the dose over 7–14 days.
  Chronic stable or vasospastic angina.
Adults: 5–10 mg, using the lower dose for elderly patients and those with hepatic insufficiency. Most patients require 10 mg.
How Supplied: *Tablet:* 2.5 mg, 5 mg, 10 mg
Side Effects: *CNS:* Headache, fatigue, lethargy, somnolence, dizziness, lightheadedness, sleep disturbances, depression, amnesia, psychosis, hallucinations, paresthesia, asthenia, insomnia, abnormal dreams, malaise, anxiety, tremor, hand tremor, hypoesthesia, vertigo, depersonalization, migraine, apathy, agitation, amnesia. *GI:* Nausea, abdominal discomfort, cramps, dyspepsia, diarrhea, constipation, vomiting, dry mouth, thirst, flatulence, dysphagia, loose stools. *CV:* Peripheral edema, palpitations, hypotension, syncope, bradycardia, unspecified arrhythmias, tachycardia, ventricular extrasystoles, peripheral ischemia, **cardiac failure,** pulse irregularity, increased risk of MI. *Dermatologic:* Dermatitis, rash, pruritus, urticaria, photosensitivity, petechiae, ecchymosis, purpura, bruising, hematoma, cold/clammy skin, skin discoloration, dry skin. *Musculoskeletal:* Muscle cramps, pain, or inflammation; joint stiffness or pain, arthritis, twitching, ataxia, hypertonia. *GU:* Polyuria, dysuria, urinary frequency, nocturia, sexual difficulties. *Respiratory:* Nasal or chest congestion, sinusitis, rhinitis, SOB, dyspnea, wheezing, cough, chest pain. *Ophthalmologic:* Diplopia, abnormal vision, conjunctivitis, eye pain, abnormal visual accommodation, xerophthalmia. *Miscellaneous:* Tinnitus, flushing, sweating, weight gain, epistaxis, anorexia, increased appetite, taste perversion, parosmia.

EMS CONSIDERATIONS

See also *Calcium Channel Blocking Agents.*

————COMBINATION DRUG————
Amlodipine and Benazepril hydrochloride
(am-LOH-dih-peen, beh-NAYZ-eh-prill)
Pregnancy Class: C (first trimester), D (second and third trimesters)
Lotrel **(Rx)**
Classification: Antihypertensive

Mechanism of Action: The incidence of edema is significantly reduced with this combination product.
Onset of Action: Peak plasma levels, amlodipine: 6-12 hr.
Duration of Action: Elimination t½, benazeprilat: 10-11 hr; **elimination t½, amlodipine:**2 days.
Uses: Treatment of hypertension. Therapy with this combination is suggested when the patient either has failed to achieve the desired antihypertensive effect with either

drug alone or has demonstrated inability to achieve an adequate antihypertensive effect with amlodipine without developing edema.
Contraindications: Initial treatment of hypertension. Hypersensitivity to amlodipine or benazepril. Lactation.
Precautions: Discontinue ACE inhibitors as soon as pregnancy is determined. The addition of benazepril to amlodipine should not be expected to provide additional antihypertensice effects in African-Americans, although there will be less edema. Use with caution in those with severe renal disease, in CHF, and in severe hepatic impairment. Safety and efficacy have not been determined in children.

Route/Dosage
• **Capsules**
Hypertension.
One 2.5/10 mg, 5/10 mg, or 5/20 mg capsule once daily. In those with severe renal impairment, the recommended initial dose of benazepril is 5 mg (Lotrel is not recommended in these patients). In small, elderly, frail, or hepatically impaired patients, the recommended initial dose of amlodipine (either as monotherapy or in combination) is 2.5 mg.
How Supplied: Lotrel 2.5/10: *Calcium channel blocking agent:* Amlodipine, 2.5 mg. *ACE inhibitor:* Benazepril hydrochloride, 10 mg. Lotrel 5/10 and Lotrel 5/20 contain 5 mg of amlodipine and either 10 or 20 mg of benazepril hydrochloride.
Side Effects: See individual drugs. Side effects include angioedema, cough, headache, and edema.

EMS CONSIDERATIONS

Also see *Antihypertensive Agents, Amlodipine,* and *Benazepril hydrochloride.*

Amoxapine
(ah-MOX-ah-peen)
Pregnancy Class: C

Asendin**(Rx)**
Classification: Antidepressant, tricyclic

Mechanism of Action: In addition to its effect on monoamines, this drug also blocks dopamine receptors. Significant anticholinergic effects, moderate sedation, and slight orthostatic hypotensive effect.
Onset of Action: Peak blood levels: 90 min.
Uses: Endogenous and reactive depression. Antianxiety agent.
Contraindications: Avoid high dose levels in patients with a history of convulsive seizures. During acute recovery period after MI.
Precautions: Safe use in children under 16 years of age and during lactation not established.

Route/Dosage
• **Tablets**
Antidepressant.
Adults, individualized, initial: 50 mg t.i.d. Can be increased to 100 mg t.i.d. during first week. Do not use doses greater than 300 mg/day unless this dose has been ineffective for at least 14 days. **Maintenance:** 300 mg as a single dose at bedtime. **Hospitalized patients:** Up to 150 mg q.i.d. **Geriatric, initial:** 25 mg b.i.d.–t.i.d. If necessary, increase to 50 mg b.i.d.–t.i.d. after first week. **Maintenance:** Up to 300 mg/day at bedtime.
How Supplied: *Tablet:* 25 mg, 50 mg, 100 mg, 150 mg
Side Effects: Additional: Tardive dyskinesia. **Overdosage may cause seizures (common), neuroleptic malignant syndrome,** testicular swelling, impairment of sexual function, and breast enlargement in males and females. Also, renal failure may be seen 2-5 days after overdosage.

EMS CONSIDERATIONS
See also *Antidepressants, Tricyclic.*

---

bold italic = life threatening side effect

A

Amoxicillin (amoxycillin)

(ah-mox-ih-SILL-in)

Amoxil, Amoxil Pediatric Drops, Tri-mox, Trimox Pediatric Drops, Wymox **(Rx)** NOTE:All products are amoxicillin trihydrate.

Classification: Antibiotic, penicillin

Mechanism of Action: Semisynthetic broad-spectrum penicillin closely related to ampicillin.

Uses: Gram-positive streptococcal infections including *Streptococcus faecalis, S. pneumoniae,* and non-penicillinase-producing staphylococci. Gram-negative infections due to *Hemophilus influenzae, Proteus mirabilis, Escherichia coli,* and *Neisseria gonorrhoeae.* In combination with omeprazole and clarithromycin to treat duodenal ulcers by eradicating *Helicobacter pylori.*

Precautions: Safe use during pregnancy has not been established.

Route/Dosage

• **Capsules, Oral Suspension, Chewable Tablets**

Susceptible infections of ear, nose, throat, GU tract, skin and soft tissues.

Adults and children over 20 kg: 250–500 mg q 8 hr; alternatively, 500 mg or 875 mg q 12 hr. **Children under 20 kg:** 20–40 (or more) mg/kg/day in three equal doses. The pediatric dose should not exceed the maximum adult dose.

Infections of the lower respiratory tract.

Adults and children over 20 kg: 500 mg q 8 hr. **Children under 20 kg:** 40 mg/kg/day in divided doses q 8 hr.

Prophylaxis of bacterial endocarditis: dental, oral, or pper respiratory tract procedures in those at risk.

Adults: 2 g (50 mg/kg for children) PO 1 hr prior to procedure.

Prophylaxis of bacterial endocarditis: GU or GI procedures.

Adults, standard regimen: 2 g ampicillin plus 1.5 mg/kg gentamicin not to exceed 80 mg, either IM or IV, 30 min prior to procedure, followed by 1.5 g amoxicillin. **Children, standard regimen:** 50 mg/kg ampicillin plus 2 mg/kg gentamicin 30 min prior to procedure, followed by 25 mg/kg amoxcillin.. **Adults, moderate risk:** 2 g PO 1 hr prior to procedure. **Children, moderate risk:** 50 mg/kg PO 1 hr pior to procedure. **Adults, alternate low-risk regimen:** 3 g 1 hr before procedure, followed by 1.5 g 6 hr after the initial dose.

Treat duodenal ulcers due to H. pylori.

A ten day course of therapy consisting of amoxicillin, 1,000 mg b.i.d.; omeprazole, 20 mg b.i.d.; and, clarithromycin, 500 mg b.i.d.

Gonococcal infections,uncomplicated urethral, endocervical, or rectal infections.

Adults: 3 g as a single PO dose. **Children, over 2 years (prepubertal):** 50 mg/kg amoxicillin combined with 25 mg/kg probenecid as a single dose.

Chlamydia trachomatis during pregnancy (as an alternative to erythromycin).

0.5 g t.i.d. for 7 days.

How Supplied: *Capsule:* 250 mg, 500 mg; *Chew tablet:* 125 mg, 250 mg; *Powder for oral suspension:* 50 mg/mL, 125 mg/5 mL, 250 mg/5 mL; *Tablet:* 500 mg, 875 mg

EMS CONSIDERATIONS

See also *Anti-infectives* and *Penicillins.*

Amoxicillin and Potassium clavulanate

(ah-mox-ih-SILL-in, poh-TASS-ee-um klav-you-LAN-ayt)

Pregnancy Class: B

Augmentin **(Rx)**

Classification: Antibiotic, penicillin

Mechanism of Action: *For details, see amoxicillin.* Potassium clavulanate inactivates lactamase enzymes, which are responsible for resistance to penicillins. Effective against microorganisms that have manifested resistance to amoxicillin.

Onset of Action: Peak serum levels: 1-2 hr. **t½:** 1hr.

Uses: For beta-lactamase-producing strains of the following organisms: Lower respiratory tract infections, otitis media, and sinusitis caused by *Hemophilus influenzae* and *Moraxella catarrhalis*; Skin and skin structure infections caused by *Staphylococcus aureus, Escherichia coli,* and *Klebsiella*; UTI caused by *E. coli, Klebsiella,* and *Enterobacter.* *Note:* Mixed infections caused by organisms susceptible to ampicillin and organisms susceptible to amoxicillin/potassium clavulanate should not require an additional antibiotic.

Route/Dosage
• **Oral Suspension, Chewable Tablets, Tablets**
Susceptible infections.
Adults, usual: One 500-mg tablet q 12 hr or one 250-mg tablet q 8 hr. Adults unable to take tablets can be given the 125-mg/5 mL or the 250-mg/5 mL suspension in place of the 500-mg tablet or the 200-mg/5 mL or 400-mg/5 mL suspension can be given in place of the 875-mg tablet. **Children less than 3 months old:** 30 mg/kg/day amoxicillin in divided doses q 12 hr. Use of the 125-mg/5 mL suspension is recommended. **Children over 3 months old:** 25 mg/kg/day amoxicillin in divided doses q 12 hr or 20 mg/kg/day in divided doses q 8 hr.
Respiratory tract and severe infections.
Adults: One 875-mg tablet q 12 hr or one 500-mg tablet q 8 hr. **Children over 3 months old:** 45 mg/kg/day of amoxicillin in divided doses q 12 hr or 40 mg/kg/day amoxicillin in divided doses q 8 hr (these doses are used in children for otitis media, lower respiratory tract infections, or sinusitis). Treatment duration for otitis media is 10 days.
How Supplied: Each '250' Tablet contains: 250 mg amoxicillin and 125 mg potassium clavulanate. Each '500' Tablet contains 500 mg amoxicillin and 125 mg potassium clavulanate.

Each '875' tablet contains: 875 mg amoxicillin, 125 mg potassium clavulanate

Each '125' Chewable Tablet contains 125 mg amoxicillin and 31.25 mg potassium clavulanate. Each 200 Chewable Tablet contains 200 mg amoxicillin and 28.5 mg potassium clavulanate. Each '250' Chewable Tablet contains 250 mg amoxicillin and 62.5 mg potassium clavulanate.

Each 400 Chewable Tablet contains 400 mg amoxicillin and 57 mg potassium clavulanate.

Each 5 mL of the '125' Powder for Oral Suspension contains 125 mg amoxicillin and 31.25 mg potassium clavulanate. Each 5 mL of the 200 Powder for Oral Suspension contains 200 mg amoxicillin and 28.5 mg potassium clavulanate. Each 5 mL of the '250' Powder for Oral Suspension contains 250 mg amoxicillin and 62.5 mg potassium clavulanate. Each 5 mL of the 400 Powder or the 400 Powder for Oral Suspension contains 400 mg amoxicillin and 57 mg potassium clavulanate.

EMS CONSIDERATIONS

See also *Anti-Infectives* and *Penicillins.*

Amphetamine sulfate
(am-FET-ah-meen)
Pregnancy Class: C
Adderall, **(C-II) (Rx)**
Classification: CNS stimulant

Onset of Action: Peak effects:2-3 hr.
Duration of Action: 4-24 hr.
Uses: Attention deficit hyperactivity disorder in children, narcolepsy. Adderall contains dextroamphetamine sulfate, dextroamphetamine saccharate, amphetamine sulfate, and amphetamine aspartate and is used in children aged three years and older who have attention deficit hyperactivity disorder or narcolepsy.
Precautions: Use in children less than 3 years of age for attention deficit disorders and in children less

than 6 years of age for narcolepsy. Not recommended as an appetite suppressant.

Route/Dosage
• **Tablets**
  Narcolepsy.
  Adults: 5–20 mg 1–3 times/day. **Children over 12 years, initial:** 5 mg b.i.d.; increase in increments of 10 mg/day at weekly intervals until optimum dose is reached. **Children, 6–12 years, initial:** 2.5 mg b.i.d.; increase in increments of 5 mg at weekly intervals until optimum dose is reached (maximum is 60 mg/day).
  Attention deficit disorders in children.
  3–6 years, initial: 2.5 mg/day; increase by 2.5 mg/day at weekly intervals until optimum dose is achieved (usual range 0.1–0.5 mg/kg/dose each morning). **6 years and older, initial:** 5 mg 1–2 times/day; increase in increments of 5 mg/week until optimum dose is achieved (rarely over 40 mg/day). The dose of Adderall is 5–30 mg per day.
  How Supplied: *Tablet:* 5 mg, 10 mg. *Adderall:* 5 mg, 10 mg, 20 mg, 30 mg.

EMS CONSIDERATIONS

See also *Amphetamines and Derivatives.*

Amphotericin B (Deoxycholate)
(am-foe-TER-ih-sin)
Pregnancy Class: B
Fungizone Intravenous **(Rx)**
Classification: Antibiotic, antifungal

Mechanism of Action: This antibiotic is produced by *Streptomyces nodosus;* it is fungistatic or fungicidal depending on the concentration of the drug in body fluids and the susceptibility of the fungus. Amphotericin B binds to specific chemical structures—sterols—of the fungal cellular membrane, increasing cellular permeability and promoting loss of potassium and other substances. Liposomal encapsulation or incorporation in a lipid complex can significantly affect the functional properties of the drug compared with those of the unencapsulated or non-lipid-associated drug. The liposomal amphotericin B product causes less nephrotoxicity. Amphotericin B is used either IV or topically.

Uses: The drug is toxic and should be used only for patients under close medical supervision with progressive or potentially fatal fungal infections. **Systemic Amphotericin B deoxycholate:** Disseminated North American blastomycosis, cryptococcosis, and other systemic fungal infections, including coccidioidomycosis, histoplasmosis, aspergillosis, sporotrichosis, disseminated candidiasis, and monilial overgrowth resulting from oral antibiotic therapy. Zygomycosis, including mucormycosis due to *Mucor, Rhizopus,* and *Absidia* species. Infections due to susceptible species of *Conidiobolus* and *Basidiobolus.* Secondary therapy to treat American mucocutaneous leishmaniasis.

Lipid-based Amphotericin B: The lipid complex (Abelcet) is used in those refractory to amphotericin B deoxycholate or where renal impairment or unacceptable toxicity precludes use of the deoxycholate product for treatment of invasive fungal infections. The cholesteryl product (Amphotec) is used to treat invasive aspergillosis infections. The liposomal product (AmBisome) is used to treat infections caused by *Aspergillus, Candida,* or *Cryptococcus* species, as well as for empirical treatment in febrile, neutropenic patients with presumed fungal infections.

Investigational: Prophylaxis of fungal infections in patients with bone marrow transplantation. Treatment of primary amoebic meningoencephalitis due to *Naegleria fowleri.* Subconjunctival or intravitreal injection in ocular aspergillosis. As a bladder irrigation for candidal cystitis. Chemoprophylaxis by low dose IV, intranasal, or nebulized administration in immunocompromised patients at risk of aspergillosis. Intrathecally in those with severe meningitis unresponsive to IV deoxycholate therapy. Intra-articularly or IM for coccidiodal arthritis.

Topical: Cutaneous and mucocutaneous infections of *Candida (Monilia)* infections, especially in children, adults, and AIDS patients with thrush.

Contraindications: Hypersensitivity to drug unless the condition is life-threatening and amenable only to amphotericin B therapy. Use to treat common forms of fungal diseases showing only positive skin or serologic tests. Use to treat noninvasive forms of fungal disease such as oral thrush, vaginal candidiasis, and esophageal candidiasis in patients with normal neutrophil counts. Lactation.

Precautions: The bone marrow depressant effects may result in increased incidence of microbial infection, delayed healing, and gingival bleeding. Although used in children, safety and efficacy have not been determined. Use with caution in patients receiving leukocyte transfusions.

Route/Dosage ——————
• **Amphotericin B deoxycholate, IV**
Test dose by slow IV infusion.
1 mg in 20 mL of 5% dextrose injection should be infused over 20 to 30 min to determine tolerance.
Severe and rapidly progressing fungal infection.
Initial: 0.3 mg/kg over 2 to 6 hr.
Note: In impaired cardiorenal function or if a severe reaction to the test dose, therapy should be initiated with smaller daily doses (e.g., 5–10 mg). Depending on the status of the patient, the dose may be increased gradually by 5–10 mg/day to a final daily dose of 0.5–0.7 mg/kg. The total daily dose should not exceed 1.5 mg/kg.
Sporotrichosis.

0.5 mg/kg/day, up to 2.5 g total dose.
Aspergillosis.
1–1.5 mg/kg/day for a total dose of 3.6 g.
Rhinocerebral phycomyosis.
0.25–0.3 mg/kg/day, up to 1–1.5 mg/kg/day, for a total dose of 3 to 4 g.
Prophylaxis of fungal infections in bone marrow transplants.
0.1 mg/kg/day.
Blastomyces, Histoplasmosis.
0.5–0.6 mg/kg/day for 4 to 12 weeks.
Candidiasis, Coccidioidomycosis.
0.5–1 mg/kg/day for 4 to 12 weeks.
Cryptococcus.
0.5–0.7 mg/kg/day for 4 to 12 weeks.
Mucormycosis.
1–1.5 mg/kg/day for 4 to 12 weeks.
Leishmaniasis.
0.5 mg/kg/day given on alternate days for 14 doses (not recommended as primary therapy).
Paracoccidioidomycosis.
0.4–0.5 mg/kg/day by slow IV infusion for 4 to 12 weeks.
• **Amphotericin B Deoxycholate Suspension**
Oral candidiasis.
Swish the suspension in the mouth and then swallow.
• **Liposomal Amphotericin B (Ambisome)**
All uses.
Adults and children, initial: 3–5 mg/kg/day prepared as a 1 to 2 mg/mL infusion and given initially over 120 min; infusion time may be reduced to 60 min if well tolerated or increased if patient experiences discomfort. Infusion concentrations of 0.2 to 0.5 mg/mL may be used for infants and small children. An in-line membrane filter of 1 micron or more mean pore diameter may be used. When used to treat leishmaniasis, give 3 mg/kg/day on days 1 through 5, 14 and 21 to immunocompetent patients; a repeat course may be given. Give 4 mg/kg/day on days 1

——————————
bold italic = life threatening side effect

through 5, 10, 17, 24, 31, and 38 to immunosuppressed patients.

• **Amphotericin B cholesteryl (Amphotec)**

All uses.

Initial: Give a test dose of 1.6–8.3 mg/10 mL infused over 15 to 30 min. **Recommended dose:** 3–4 mg/kg/day prepared as a 0.6 mg/mL (range of 0.16–0.83 mg/mL) infusion delivered at a rate of 1 mg/kg/hr without an in-line filter.

• **Amphotericin B lipid complex (Abelcet)**

All uses.

5 mg/kg/day prepared as a 1 mg/mL infusion and delivered at a rate of 2.5 mg/kg/hr. For pediatric patients and those with CV disease, the drug may be diluted to a final concentration of 2 mg/mL. Do not use an in-line filter. If the infusion time exceeds 2 hr, mix by shaking the infusion bag q 2 hr.

• **Intrathecal**

Coccidioidal or cryptococcal meningitis.

Initial: 0.025 mg; **then,** increase gradually up to 0.25–1 mg q 48 to 72 hr, up to a maximum total dose of 15 mg.

• **Bladder Irritation**

Candidal cystitis.

50 mcg/mL solution instilled periodically or continuously for 5 to 10 days.

• **Topical (Lotion, Cream, Ointment—Each 3%)**

Apply liberally to affected areas b.i.d.–q.i.d. Depending on the type of lesion, up to 4 weeks of therapy may be necessary.

How Supplied: *Cream:* 3%; *Lotion:* 3%; *Powder for injection:* 50 mg, 100 mg; *Suspension for injection:* 100 mg/20 mL

Side Effects: After topical use. Irritation, pruritus, dry skin. Redness, itching, or burning especially in skin folds. **After IV use.** Most common are listed. *General toxic reaction:* Fever sometimes with shaking chills usually within 15 to 20 min after treatment, headache, anorexia, malaise, generalized pain (including muscle and joint pain). *GI:* N&V,

dyspepsia, diarrhea, cramping, epigastric pain, abdominal pain, melena, stomatitis, anorexia. *CNS:* Confusion, headache, depression, abnormal thinking, insomnia. *CV:* Hypotension, hypertension, tachycardia, tachypnea, arrhythmias. *Dermatologic:* Rash, pruritus, maculopapular rash. *GU:* Hematuria, decreased renal function, renal tubular acidosis, nephrocalcinosis, azotemia, hypokalemia, hyposthenuria. *Respiratory: Respiratory failure,* respiratory disorder, pneumonia, dyspnea, hypoxia, epistaxis, increased cough, lung disorder, hemoptysis, hyperventilation, apnea, pleural effusion, rhinitis. *Hematologic:* Normochromic, normocytic anemia; increased PT, anemia, coagulation disorder. *Metabolic:* Bilirubinemia, acidosis, hypovolemia. *At site of injection:* Venous pain at injection site with phlebitis and thrombophlebitis. *Miscellaneous:* Weight loss, *multiple organ failure,* infection, sweating, pain, chest pain, back pain, *sepsis,* facial edema, mucous membrane disorder, asthenia, peripheral edema, eye hemorrhage, blood product transfusion reaction, chills. **After intrathecal use:** Blurred vision, changes in vision, difficulty in urination, numbness, tingling, pain, or weakness.

OD Overdose Management: *Symptoms:* Cardiopulmonary arrest. *Treatment:* Discontinue therapy, monitor clinical status, and provide supportive therapy.

Drug Interactions

Aminoglycosides / Additive nephrotoxicity and/or ototoxicity

Antineoplastic drugs / ↑ Risk for renal toxicity, bronchospasm, and hypotension

Corticosteroids, Corticotropin / ↑ Potassium depletion caused by amphotericin B → cardiac dysfunction

Cyclosporine / ↑ Renal toxicity

Digitalis glycosides / ↑ Potassium depletion caused by amphotericin B → ↑ incidence of digitalis toxicity

Flucytosine / ↑ Risk of flucytosine toxicity due to ↑ cellular uptake or ↓ renal excretion

Nephrotoxic drugs / ↑ Risk of neph-rotoxicity

Skeletal muscle relaxants, surgical (e.g., succinylcholine, *d*-tubocu-rarine) / ↑ Muscle relaxation due to amphotericin B–induced hypokale-mia

Tacrolimus / ↑ Serum creatinine levels

Thiazides / ↑ Electrolyte depletion, especially potassium

AZT / ↑ Risk of myelotoxicity and nephrotoxicity

EMS CONSIDERATIONS

See also *Anti-Infectives.*
Interventions
1. Premedicate with antipyretics, antihistamines, corticosteroids, and/or antiemetic drugs to reduce side effects. Rashes, fevers, and chills may occur with this therapy.
2. Infuse slowly, monitoring VS every 15–30 min during first dose; interrupt for adverse effects.
3. Anticipate hypokalemia with digoxin therapy. Observe for toxicity and muscle weakness.

Ampicillin oral

(am-pih-SILL-in)
Pregnancy Class: B
Omnipen, Principen, Totacillin**(Rx)**
Classification: Antibiotic, penicillin

Mechanism of Action: Synthetic, broad-spectrum antibiotic suitable for gram-negative bacteria.

Uses: Infections of respiratory, GI, and GU tracts caused by *Shigella, Salmonella, Escherichia coli, Hemophilus influenzae, Proteus* strains, *Neisseria gonorrhoeae, N. meningitis,* and *Enterococcus.* Also, otitis media in children, bronchitis, rat-bite fever, and whooping cough. Penicillin G-sensitive staphylococci, streptococci, pneumococci.

Route/Dosage ─────────
• **Ampicillin: Capsules, Oral Suspension; Ampicillin Sodium: IV, IM**

Respiratory tract and soft tissue infections.

PO: 20 kg or more: 250 mg q 6 hr; **less than 20 kg:** 50 mg/kg/day in equally divided doses q 6–8 hr. **IV, IM: 40 kg or more:** 250–500 mg q 6 hr; **less than 40 kg:** 25–50 mg/kg/day in equally divided doses q 6–8 hr.

Bacterial meningitis.
Adults and children: 150–200 mg/kg/day in divided doses q 3 to 4 hr. Initially give IV drip, followed by IM q 3 to 4 hr.

Bacterial endocarditis prophylaxis (dental, oral, or upper respiratory tract procedures).
Patients at moderate risk or those unable to take PO medications: **Adults, IM, IV:** 2 g 30 min prior to procedure; **children:** 50 mg/kg, 30 min prior to procedure. Patients at high risk: **Adults, IM, IV:** 2 g ampicillin plus gentamicin, 1.5 mg/kg, given 30 min before procedure followed in 6 hr by ampicillin, 1 g IM or IV, or amoxicillin, 1 g PO. **Children, IM, IV:** Ampicillin, 50 mg/kg, plus gentamicin, 1.5 mg/kg, 30 min prior to procedure followed in 6 hr by ampicillin, 25 mg/kg IM or IV, or amoxicillin, 25 mg/kg PO.

Septicemia.
Adults/children: 150–200 mg/kg/day, IV for first 3 days, then IM q 3–4 hr.

GI and GU infections, other than N. gonorrhea.
Adults/children, more than 20 kg: 500 mg PO q 6 hr. Use larger doses, if needed, for severe or chronic infections. **Children, less than 20 kg:** 100 mg/kg/day q 6 hr.

N. gonorrhea infections.
PO: Single dose of 3.5 g given together with probenecid, 1 g. **Parenteral, Adults/children over 40 kg:** 500 mg IV or IM q 6 hr. **Children, less than 40 kg:** 50 mg/kg/day IV or IM in equally divided doses q 6 to 8 hr.

Urethritis in males caused by N. gonorrhea.
Parenteral, males over 40 kg: Two 500 mg doses IV or IM at an interval of 8 to 12 hr. Repeat treatment

---

bold italic = life threatening side effect

if necessary. In complicated gonorrheal urethritis, prolonged and intensive therapy is recommended.

• **Ampicillin with Probenecid: Oral Suspension**

Urethral, endocervical, or rectal infections due to N. gonorrhoeae.

Adults: 3.5 g ampicillin and 1 g probenecid as a single dose.

Prophylaxis of infection in rape victims.

3.5 g with 1 g probenecid.

How Supplied: The Powder for Oral Suspension of Ampicillin with Probenecid contains 3.5 g ampicillin and 1 g probenecid per bottle. Ampicillin oral: *Capsule:* 250 mg, 500 mg; *Powder for reconstitution:* 125 mg/5 mL, 250 mg/5 mL. Ampicillin with Probenecid: See Content. Ampicillin sodium parenteral: *Powder for injection:* 125 mg, 250 mg, 500 mg, 1 g, 2 g, 10 g

EMS CONSIDERATIONS

See also *Anti-Infectives* and *Penicillins.*

————COMBINATION DRUG————
Ampicillin sodium/ Sulbactam sodium
(am-pih-SILL-in/sull-BACK-tam)
Pregnancy Class: B
Unasyn**(Rx)**
Classification: Antibiotic, penicillin

Mechanism of Action: For details, see *Ampicillin oral.* Sulbactam is present in this product because it irreversibly inhibits beta-lactamases, thus ensuring activity of ampicillin against beta-lactamase-producing microorganisms. Thus, sulbactam broadens the antibiotic spectrum of ampicillin to those bacteria normally resistant to it. **Onset of Action: Peak serum levels, after IV infusion:** 15 min.**t½, both drugs:** about 1 hr.

Uses: Infections caused by beta-lactamase-producing strains of the following: (a) skin and skin structure infections caused by *Staphylococcus aureus, Escherichia coli, Klebsiella* species (including *K. pneumoniae*), *Proteus mirabilis, Bacteroides fragilis, Enterobacter* species, and *Acinetobacter calcoaceticus;* (b) intra-abdominal infections caused by *E. coli, Klebsiella* species (including *K. pneumoniae*), *Bacteroides* (including *B. fragilis* and *Enterobacter)* (c) gynecologic infections caused by *E. coli* and *Bacteroides* (including *B. fragilis*). *NOTE:* Mixed infections caused by ampicillin-susceptible organisms and beta-lactamase-producing organisms are susceptible to this product; thus, additional antibiotics do not have to be used.

Precautions: Safety and efficacy in children 1 year of age and older have not been established for intra-abdominal infections or for IM administration.

Route/Dosage ————
• **IV, IM**

Adults: 1 g ampicillin/0.5 g sulbactam to 2 g ampicillin/1 g sulbactam q 6 hr, not to exceed 4 g sulbactam daily. Doses must be decreased in renal impairment. **Children, over 40 kg:** Use adult doses; total sulbactam dose should not exceed 4 g/day. **Children, one year and older but less than 40 kg:** 200 mg ampicillin/kg/day and 100 mg sulbactam/kg/day in divided doses q 6 hr.

How Supplied: The Powder for Injection contains either 1 g ampicillin sodium and 0.5 g sulbactam sodium, 2 g ampicillin sodium and 1 g sulbactam sodium, or 10 g ampicillin and 5 g sulbactam sodium.

Side Effects: *At site of injection:* Pain and thrombophlebitis. *GI:* Diarrhea, N&V, flatulence, abdominal distention, glossitis. *CNS:* Fatigue, malaise, headache. *GU:* Dysuria, urinary retention. *Miscellaneous:* Itching, chest pain, edema, facial swelling, erythema, chills, tightness in throat, epistaxis, substernal pain, mucosal bleeding, candidiasis.

OD **Overdose Management:** *Symptoms:* **Neurologic symptoms, including convulsions.** *Treatment:* Both ampicillin and sulbactam may be removed by hemodialysis.

EMS CONSIDERATIONS

See also *Anti-Infectives* and *Penicillins.*

Amprenavir

(am-PREH-naah-vir)
Pregnancy Class: C
Agenerase **(Rx)**
Classification: Antiviral drug, protease inhibitor

Mechanism of Action: Inhibitor of HIV-1 protease. Binds to the active site of HIV-1 protease, thus preventing the processing of viral gag and gag-pol polyprotein precursors. Results in formation of immature noninfectious viral particles.

Uses: In combination with other antiretroviral drugs for the treatment of HIV-1 infections.

Contraindications: Use with astemizole, bepridil, cisapride, dihydroergotamine, ergotamine, midazolam, rifampin, and triazolam. Lactation.

Precautions: Use with caution in those with impaired hepatic function and in the elderly. Safety and efficacy have not been determined in children less than 4 years of age. Use with caution in combination with sildenafil. Amprenavir is a sulfonamide; thus, there is potential for cross-sensitivity between drugs in the sulfonamide class. Possibility of resistance/cross-resistance among protease inhibitors.

Route/Dosage

• **Capsules**

HIV-1 infection.

Adults and adolescents, aged 13–16 years old: 1200 mg (eight 150 mg capsules) b.i.d. in combination with other antiretroviral drugs. **Children, 4–12 years old or aged 13–16 years old with weight less than 50 kg:** 20 mg/kg b.i.d. or 15 mg/kg t.i.d., up to a maximum of 2400 mg daily in combination with other antiretroviral drugs.

Give capsules at a dose of 450 mg b.i.d. to patients with a Child-Pugh score from 5–8; give capsules at a dose of 300 mg b.i.d. to those with a Child-Pugh score from 9–12.

• **Oral Solution**

HIV-1 infection.

Children, 4–12 years old or aged 13–16 years old with weight less than 50 kg: 22.5 mg/kg (1.5 mL/kg) b.i.d. or 17 mg/kg (1.1 mL/kg) t.i.d., up to a maximum of of 2800 mg daily in combination with other antiretroviral drugs.

Note: Capsules and Oral Solution are **not** interchangeable on a mg per mg basis.

How Supplied: *Capsules:* 50 mg, 150 mg; *Oral Solution:* 15 mg/mL

Side Effects: *GI:* N&V, diarrhea, abdominal pain, taste disorders. *CNS:* Depression, mood disorders. *Dermatologic:* Maculopapular rash, pruritus, oral/perioral paresthesia, peripheral paresthesia, **Stevens-Johnson syndrome.** *Metabolic:* New onset diabetes mellitus, exacerbation of pre-existing diabetes mellitus, hyperglycemia, diabetic ketoacidosis. *Miscellaneous:* Spontaneous bleeding in patients with hemophilia A and B. Redistribution/accumulation of body fat, including central obesity, dorsocervical fat enlargement, peripheral wasting, breast enlargement, "cushinoid" appearance.

Drug Interactions

Amiodarone / Serious or life-threatening interactions; monitor levels

Antacids / ↓ Amprenavir absorption

Bepridil / Possible serious or life-threatening effects; do not use together

Carbamazepine / ↓ Amprenavir levels R/T ↑ liver metabolism; also, possible ↑ carbamazepine plasma levels

Cimetidine / ↑ Plasma amprenavir levels

Cisapride / Possible serious or life-threatening effects; do not use together

Clarithromycin / Possible ↑ plasma amprenavir levels and ↓ plasma clarithromycin levels

Clozapine / ↑ Plasma clozapine levels

Dapsone / ↑ Plasma dapsone levels

Delavirdine / ↑ Amprenavir serum levels

Efavirenz / ↓ Amprenavir serum levels

Ergot alkaloids / Possible serious or life-threatening effects; do not use together

Erythromycin / Possible ↑ plasma amprenavir levels and ↓ plasma erythromycin levels

HMG-CoA reductase inhibitors / ↑ Serum levels of HMG-CoA reductase inhibitors → ↑ activity or toxicity

Indinavir / ↑ Plasma amprenavir levels and ↓ plasma indinavir levels

Itraconazole / Possible ↑ plasma levels of both drugs

Ketoconazole / Possible ↑ plasma levels of both drugs

Lidocaine / Serious or life-threatening interactions; monitor levels

Loratidine / ↑ Plasma loratidine levels

Midazolam / Possible serious or life-threatening effects; do not use together

Nelfinavir / Possible ↓ plasma amprenavir levels and ↑ plasma nelfinair levels

Nevirapine / ↓ Amprenavir serum levels

Oral contraceptives / ↓ Effectiveness of oral contraceptives; use alternate contraceptive measures

Phenobarbital / ↓ Amprenavir levels R/T ↑ liver metabolism

Phenytoin / ↓ Amprenavir levels R/T ↑ liver metabolism

Pimozide / ↑ Plasma pimozide levels

Quinidine / Serious or life-threatening interactions; monitor levels

Rifabutin / ↓ Amprenavir levels and significant ↑ rifabutin levels; reduce dose of rifabutin to at least one-half

Rifampin / ↓ (by 90%) Amprenavir plasma levels

Ritonavir / ↑ Amprenavir plasma levels

Saquinavir / Possible ↑ saquinavir plasma levels and ↓ amprenavir plasma levels

Sildenafil / ↑ Risk of sildenafil side effects, including hypotension, visual changes, and priapism

Triazolam / Possible serious or life-threatening effects; do not use together

Tricyclic antidepressants / Serious or life-threatening interactions; monitor levels

Warfarin / Possible ↑ Plasma warfarin levels; monitor INR if used together

Zidovudine / ↑ Amprenavir and zidovudine plasma levels

EMS CONSIDERATIONS

None.

Amrinone lactate

(AM-rih-nohn)
Pregnancy Class: C
Inocor**(Rx)**
Classification: Cardiac inotropic agent

Mechanism of Action: Causes an increase in CO by increasing the force of contraction of the heart, probably by inhibiting cyclic AMP phosphodiesterase, thereby increasing cellular levels of c-AMP. It reduces afterload and preload by directly relaxing vascular smooth muscle.

Onset of Action: Time to peak effect:10 min.**t½, after rapid IV**3.6 hr;**after IV infusion:**5.8 hr.

Duration of Action: 30 min-2 hr, depending on the dose.

Uses: Congestive heart failure (short-term therapy in patients unresponsive to digitalis, diuretics, and/or vasodilators). Can be used in digitalized patients.

Contraindications: Hypersensitivity to amrinone or bisulfites. Severe aortic or pulmonary valvular disease in lieu of surgery. Acute MI.

Precautions: Safety and efficacy not established in children. Use with caution during lactation.

Route/Dosage ———
• **IV**
CHF.

Initial: 0.75 mg/kg as a bolus given slowly over 2–3 min; may be repeated after 30 min if necessary. **Maintenance, IV infusion:** 5–10 mcg/kg/min. Do not exceed a daily dose of 10

mg/kg, although up to 18 mg/kg/ day has been used in some patients for short periods.

How Supplied: *Injection:* 5 mg/mL

Side Effects: *GI:* N&V, abdominal pain, anorexia. *CV:* Hypotension, *supraventricular and ventricular arrhythmias.* *Allergic:* Pericarditis, pleuritis, ascites, allergic reaction to sodium bisulfite present in the product. *Other:* Thrombocytopenia, *hepatotoxicity,* fever, chest pain, burning at site of injection.

OD Overdose Management: *Symptoms:* Hypotension. *Treatment:* Reduce or discontinue drug administration and begin general supportive measures.

Drug Interactions: Excessive hypotension when used with disopyramide.

EMS CONSIDERATIONS

Administration/Storage

IV 1. Administer undiluted or diluted in 0.9% or 0.45% saline to a concentration of 1–3 mg/mL.

2. Do not dilute with solutions containing dextrose (glucose) prior to injection.

3. Administer loading dose over 2–3 min; may be repeated in 30 min.

4. Solutions should be clear yellow.

Amyl nitrite
(AM-il)

Pregnancy Class: X

Amyl Nitrite Aspirols, Amy Nitrite Vaporole**(Rx)**

Classification: Coronary vasodilator, antidote for cyanide poisoning

Mechanism of Action: Believed to act by reducing systemic and PA pressure (afterload) and by decreasing CO due to peripheral vasodilation. Vascular relaxation occurs due to stimulation of intracellular cyclic guanosine monophosphate. As an antidote to cyanide poisoning, amyl nitrite promotes formation of methemoglobin which combines with cyanide to form the nontoxic cyanmethemoglobin.

Onset of Action: Inhalation: 30 sec.

Duration of Action: 3–5 min. About 33% is excreted through the kidneys.

Uses: Prophylaxis or relief of acute attacks of angina pectoris; acute cyanide poisoning. *Investigational:* Diagnostic aid to assess reserve cardiac function.

Contraindications: Lactation.

Precautions: Use in children has not been studied. Hypotensive effects are more likely to occur in geriatric patients.

Route/Dosage
* **Inhalation**
  Angina pectoris.

Usual: 0.3 mL (1 container crushed). Usually, 1–6 inhalations from one container produces relief. Dosage may be repeated after 3–5 min.

  Antidote for cyanide poisoning.

Administer for 30–60 sec q 5 min until patient is conscious; is then repeated at longer intervals for up to 24 hr.

How Supplied: *Solution*

EMS CONSIDERATIONS

See also *Antianginal Drugs - Nitrates/Nitrites.*

Administration/Storage

1. Administer only by inhalation.

2. Protect containers from light, store at 15°C–30°C (59°F–86°F).

3. *Amyl nitrite vapors are highly flammable. Do not use near flame or intense heat.*

Anagrelide hydrochloride
(an-AG-greh-lyd)

Pregnancy Class: C

Agrylin**(Rx)**

Classification: Antiplatelet drug

Mechanism of Action: May act to reduce platelets by decreasing megakaryocyte hypermaturation. Does not cause significant changes in white cell counts or coagulation parameters. Inhibits platelet aggregation at higher doses than needed to reduce platelet count.

---

bold italic = life threatening side effect

Uses: Reduce platelet count in essential thrombocythemia.

Contraindications: Lactation.

Precautions: Use with caution in known or suspected heart disease and in impaired rneal or hepatic function. Safety and efficacy have not been determined in those less than 16 years of age.

Route/Dosage
- **Capsules**

  Essential thrombocythemia.

  Initial: 0.5 mg q.i.d. or 1 mg b.i.d. Maintain for one week or more. **Then,** adjust to lowest effective dose to maintain platelet count less than 600,000/mcL. Can increase the dose by 0.5 mg or less/day in any 1 week. **Maximum dose:** 10 mg/day or 2.5 mg in single dose. Most respond at a dose of 1.5 to 3 mg/day.

How Supplied: *Capsules:* 0.5 mg

Side Effects: *CV:* CHF, palpitations, chest pain, tachycardia, arrhythmias, angina, postural hypotension, hypertension, cardiovascular disease, vasodilation, migraine, syncope, *MI, cardiomyopathy, complete heart block, fibrillation, CVA, pericarditis, hemorrhage, heart failure,* cardiomegaly, atrial fibrillation. *GI:* Diarrhea, abdominal pain, pancreatitis, gastric/duodenal ulcers, N&V, flatulence, anorexia, constipation, GI distress, *GI hemorrhage,* gastritis, melena, aphthous stomatitis, eructations. *Respiratory:* Rhinitis, epistaxis, respiratory disease, sinusitis, pneumonia, bronchitis, asthma, pulmonary infiltrate, *pulmonary fibrosis, pulmonary hypertension,* dyspnea. *CNS:* Headache, *seizures,* dizziness, paresthesia, depression, somnolence, confusion, insomnia, nervousness, amnesia. *Musculoskeletal:* Arthralgia, myalgia, leg cramps. *Dermatologic:* Pruritus, skin disease, alopecia, rash, urticaria. *Hematologic:* Anemia, thrombocytopenia, ecchymosis, lymphadenoma. *Body as a whole:* Fever, flu symptoms, chills, photosensitivity, dehydration, malaise, asthenia, edema, pain. *Ophthalmic:* Amblyopia, abnormal vision, visual field abnormality, diplopia. *Miscellaneous:* Back pain, tinnitus.

OD Overdose Management: *Symptoms:* Thrombocytopenia. *Treatment:* Close clinical monitoring. Decrease or stop dose until platelet count returns to within the normal range.

EMS CONSIDERATIONS

None.

Anistreplase

(an-ih-STREP-layz)

Pregnancy Class: C

Eminase**(Rx)**

Classification: Thrombolytic enzyme

Mechanism of Action: Prepared by acylating human plasma derived from lys-plasminogen and purified streptokinase derived from group C beta-hemolytic streptococci. When prepared, anistreplase is an inactive derivative of a fibrinolytic enzyme although the compound can still bind to fibrin. Anistreplase is activated by deacylation and subsequent release of the anisoyl group in the blood stream. The production of plasmin from plasminogen occurs in both the blood stream and the thrombus leading to thrombolysis. Lyses thrombi obstructing coronary arteries and reduces the size of infarcts.

Onset of Action: $t^{1}/_{2}$:70-120 min.

Uses: Management of AMI in adults, resulting in improvement of ventricular function and reduction of mortality. Treatment should be initiated as soon as possible after the onset of symptoms of AMI.

Contraindications: Use in active internal bleeding; within 2 months of intracranial or intraspinal surgery; recent trauma, including cardiopulmonary resuscitation; history of CVA; intracranial neoplasm; arteriovenous malformation or aneurysm; known bleeding diathesis; severe, uncontrolled hypertension; severe allergic reactions to streptokinase.

Precautions: Use with caution in nursing mothers. Safety and effectiveness have not been determined in children.*NOTE:*The risks of anistreplase therapy may be increased in the following conditions; thus, benefit versus risk must be assessed prior to use. Within 10 days of major surgery (e.g., CABG, obstetric delivery, organ biopsy, previous puncture of noncompressible vessels); cerebrovascular disease; within 10 days of GI or GU bleeding; within 10 days of trauma including cardiopulmonary resuscitation; SBP > 180 mm Hg or DBP > 110 mm Hg; likelihood of left heart thrombus (e.g., mitral stenosis with atrial fibrillation); SBE; acute pericarditis; hemostatic defects including those secondary to severe hepatic or renal disease; pregnancy; patients older than 75 years of age; diabetic hemorrhagic retinopathy or other hemorrhagic ophthalmic conditions; septic thrombophlebitis or occluded arteriovenous cannula at seriously infected site; patients on oral anticoagulant therapy; any condition which bleeding constitutes a significant hazard or would be difficult to manage due to its location.

Route/Dosage
IV only: 30 units over 2–5 min into an IV line or vein as soon as possible after onset of symptoms.
How Supplied: *Powder for injection:* 30 U
Side Effects: *Bleeding:* Including at the puncture site (most common), nonpuncture site hematoma, hematuria, hemoptysis, ***GI hemorrhage, intracranial bleeding,*** gum/mouth hemorrhage, epistaxis, anemia, eye hemorrhage. *CV:* ***Arrhythmias,*** conduction disorders, hypotension; ***cardiac rupture,*** chest pain, emboli (causal relationship to use of anistreplase unknown). *Allergic:* ***Anaphylaxis, bronchospasm,*** angioedema, urticaria, itching, flushing, rashes, eosinophilia, delayed purpuric rash which may be associated with arthralgia, ankle edema, mild hematuria, GI symptoms, and proteinuria. *GI:* N&V. *Hematologic:* Thrombocytopenia. *CNS:* Agitation, dizziness, paresthesia, tremor, vertigo. *Respiratory:* Dyspnea, lung edema. *Miscellaneous:* Chills, fever, headache, shock.

Drug Interactions: Increased risk of bleeding or hemorrhage if used with heparin, oral anticoagulants, vitamin K antagonists, aspirin, or dipyridamole.

EMS CONSIDERATIONS
See also *Alteplase, Recombinant.*
Administration/Storage
IV 1. To reconstitute slowly add 5 mL of sterile water for injection. To minimize foaming, gently roll the vial after directing the stream of sterile water against the side of the vial. Do not shake the vial.
2. The reconstituted solution should be colorless to pale yellow without particulate matter or discoloration.
3. Do not further dilute the reconstituted solution before administration.
4. Do not add the reconstituted solution to any infusion fluids and no other medications should be added to the vial or syringe.
5. Discard solution if not administered within 30 min of reconstitution.
Assessment
1. Note any history and/or evidence of excessive bleeding.
2. Take a full drug history, noting any aspirin, anticoagulant, or vitamin K antagonist use.

Antihemophilic factor (AHF, Factor VIII)
(an-tie-hee-moh-FILL-ick)
Pregnancy Class: C
Alphanate, Antihemophillic Factor (Porcine) Hyate:C, Bioclate, Helixate, Hemofil M, Humate-P, Koate-HP, Kogenate, Monoclate-P, Profilate HP, Recombinate **(Rx)**
Classification: Hemostatic, systemic

Mechanism of Action: Antihemophilic factor either is isolated from pooled normal human blood or is derived from monoclonal antibodies. The potency and purity of preparation vary but each lot is standardized. Details on the package should be noted. Plasma protein (factor VIII) accelerates abnormally slow

A

transformation of prothrombin to thrombin.

Onset of Action: t½: 9-15 hr. One AHF unit is the activity found in 1 mL of normal pooled human plasma.

Uses: Control of bleeding in patients suffering from hemophilia A (factor VIII deficiency and acquired factor VIII inhibitors). These products temporarily replace the missing clotting factor in order to correct or prevent bleeding episodes or to perform surgery. AHF is safe and effective for use in children of all ages, including neonates.

Contraindications: Use of monoclonal antibody-derived AHF in patients hypersensitive to bovine, hamster, or mouse protein.

Precautions: Since AHF is prepared from human plasma, there is a risk of transmitting hepatitis or AIDS. However, the products are carefully prepared and tested.

Route/Dosage ⎯⎯⎯⎯⎯⎯⎯
• **IV Only**

Individualized, depending on severity of bleeding, degree of deficiency, body weight, and presence of inhibitors of factor VIII. *NOTE:* AHF levels may rise 2% for every unit of AHF per kilogram administered. The following formula provides a guide for dosage calculation :Expected Factor VIII increase (in % of normal):AHF/IU administered × 2 ÷ body weight (in kg) Dosages given are only guidelines.

Prophylaxis of spontaneous hemorrhage.
Increase AHF levels to about 5% of normal; 30% of normal is the minimum required for hemostasis following surgery and trauma. A single dose of 10 IU/kg (increases of approximately 20%) may be sufficient for mild superficial bleeds or early hemorrhages. Smaller doses may be sufficient for early hemarthrosis.

Mild hemorrhage.
Single infusion to achieve AHF levels of at least 30%. Dosage should not be repeated.

Minor surgery, moderate hemorrhage.

AHF levels should be raised to 30%–50% of normal. **Initial:** 15–25 IU/kg; **maintenance, if necessary:** 10–15 IU/kg q 8–12 hr.

Severe hemorrhage.
Increase AHF levels to 80%–100% of normal. **Initial:** 40–50 IU/kg; **maintenance:** 20–25 IU/kg q 8–12 hr.

Major surgery.
Raise AHF levels to 80%–100% of normal. Administer 1 hr before surgery; one-half the priming dose may be given 5 hr after the first dose. AHF levels should be maintained at 30% of normal for at least 10–14 days.

Dental extraction.
Factor VIII level should be increased to 50% immediately before the procedure.

How Supplied: *Powder for injection*

Side Effects: *CNS:* Headache, somnolence, lethargy, fatigue, dizziness. *CV:* Increased bleeding tendency, flushing, slight hypotension, acute hemolytic anemia, hyperfibrinogenemia. *Allergic:* Nausea, fever, hives, chills, urticaria, wheezing, hypotension, chest tightness, stinging at infusion site, hypotension, ***anaphylaxis.*** *Miscellaneous:* Sore throat, cold feet, taste perversion, nonspecific rash.

Antibodies may form to the mouse protein found in AHF derived from monoclonal antibodies. Approximately 10% of patients develop inhibitors to Factor VIII, which leads to a significantly decreased response. Antihemophilic factor contains traces of blood group A and B isohemagglutins. These may cause ***intravascular hemolysis*** in patients with types A, B, or AB blood.

Both hepatitis and AIDS may be transmitted from AHF prepared from human plasma.

EMS CONSIDERATIONS

None.

Ardeparin sodium
(ar-dee-PAH-rin)

Pregnancy Class: C
Normiflo (Rx)
Classification: Anticoagulant, low molecular weight heparin

Mechanism of Action: Binds to and accelerates activity of antithrombin III, thus inhibiting thrombosis by inactivating Factor Xa and thrombin. Also inhibits thrombin by binding to heparin cofactor II. At usual doses, no effect on PT; APTT may not be affected or may be slightly prolonged.

Uses: Prevention of deep vein thrombosis following knee replacement surgery.

Contraindications: Use with active major bleeding, hypersensitivity to drug or to pork products, thrombocytopenia associated with a positive *in vitro* test for anti-platelet antibodies in the presence of ardeparin. IM or IV use.

Precautions: Use with caution during lactation, in hypersensitivity to methylparaben or propylparaben, in those with bleeding diathesis, recent GI bleeding, thrombocytopeniz or platelet defects, severe liver disease, hypertensive or diabetic retinopathy, in those undergoing invasive procedures (especially if they are receiving other drugs that interfere with hemostasis), or in severe renal failure. Use with extreme caution in those with a history of heparin-induced thrombocytopenia or in which there is an increase risk of hemorrhage (e.g., bacterial endocarditis, congenital or acquired bleeding disorders, active ulceration or angiodysplastic GI disease, severe uncontrolled hypertension, hemorrhagic stroke, soon after brain, spinal, or ophthalmologic surgery; or, with concomitant treatment with platelet inhibitors). Product contains metasulfite which may cause an allergic reaction in some. Safety and efficacy have not been determined in children.

Route/Dosage ——————
• **SC**
Prophylaxis of deep vein thrombosis during knee replacement surgery.

Adults: 50 anti-Xa U/kg q 12 hr. Begin treatment evening of day of surgery or following morning and continue for up to 14 days or until patient is fully ambulatory, whichever is shorter.

How Supplied: *Injection:* 5,000 U/0.5 mL; 10,000 U/0.5 mL

Side Effects: *Bleeding events:* Intraoperative bleeding, postoperative surgical site or nonsurgical site hematoma or hemorrhage, bleeding requiring an invasive procedure; ecchymosis, *GI hemorrhage,* hematemesis, hematuria, melena, petechiae, *rectal hemorrhage, retroperitoneal hemorrhage, CVA,* abnormal stools. *GI:* N&V, constipation. *Allergic reaction:* Maculopapular rash, vesiculobullous rash, urticaria. *CNS:* Confusion, dizziness, headache, insomnia. *Miscellaneous:* Fever, pruritus, anemia, thrombocytopenia, arthralgia, chest pain, dyspnea, reactions at injection site (edema, hypersensitivity, inflammation, pain), peripheral edema.

OD **Overdose Management:** *Symptoms:* Bleeding at the surgical site or at venipuncture sites. Epistaxis, hematuria, blood in stools, easy bruising, petechiae. *Treatment:* Most bleeding can be controlled by discontinuing drug, applying pressure to site, and replacing volume and hemostatic blood elements as needed. If above is ineffective, can give protamine sulfate (1 mg protamine sulfate neutralizes about 100 anti-Xa units of ardeparin). If bleeding persists about 2 hr after protamine sulfate, draw blood and determine residual anti-Xa levels. Additional protamine sulfate can be given if clinically important bleeding persists or if anti-Xa levels are higher than desired.

Drug Interactions: Additive anticoagulant effects if given with other anticoagulants or platelet inhibitors (e.g., aspirin, NSAIDs).

EMS CONSIDERATIONS
None.

---

bold italic = life threatening side effect

Astemizole
(ah-STEM-ih-zohl)
Pregnancy Class: C
Hismanil **(Rx)**
Classification: Antihistamine, miscellaneous

Mechanism of Action: Low to no sedative, antiemetic, or anticholinergic effects. Absorption decreased up to 60% when taken with food.
Onset of Action: 2-3 days.
Duration of Action: Up to several weeks.
Uses: Allergic rhinitis, urticaria.
Contraindications: Impaired hepatic function. Concomitant use with erythromycin, clarithromycin, itraconazole, ketoconazole, mibefradil, quinine, and troleandomycin.
Precautions: Dose should not exceed 10 mg/day.

Route/Dosage
• **Tablets**
Adults and children over 12 years: 10 mg once daily. **Children, 6–12 years:** 5 mg daily; **children, less than 6 years:** 0.2 mg/kg/day.
How Supplied: *Tablet:* 10 mg
Side Effects: Serious CV side effects, including death, cardiac arrest, QT interval prolongation, torsades de points and other ventricular arrhythmias have been observed in patients exceeding the recommended dose of astemizole. Severe hepatic impairment. Syncope may precede severe arrhythmias. Overdose may be observed with doses as low as 20-30 mg/day.
Drug Interactions
Clarithromycin / Possible serious CV effects, including death, cardiac arrest, torsades de pointes, and other ventricular arrhythmias (including QT interval prolongation).
Erythromycin / Possible serious CV effects, including death, cardiac arrest, torsades de pointes, and other ventricular arrhythmias (including QT interval prolongation).
Itraconazole / Possible serious CV effects, including death, cardiac arrest, torsades de pointes, and other ventricular arrhythmias (including QT interval prolongation).
Ketoconazole / Possible serious CV effects, including death, cardiac arrest, torsades de pointes, and other ventricular arrhythmias (including QT interval prolongation).
Miconazole / Possible serious CV effects, including death, cardiac arrest, torsades de pointes, and other ventricular arrhythmias (including QT interval prolongation).
Mibefradil / Possible serious CV effects, including death, cardiac arrest, torsades de pointes, and other ventricular arrhythmias (including QT interval prolongation).
Protease inhibitors (indinavir, nelfinavir, ritonavir, saquinavir) / Inhibition of metabolism of astemizole
Quinine / Possible serious CV effects, including death, cardiac arrest, torsades de pointes, and other ventricular arrhythmias (including QT interval prolongation).
Serotonin reuptake inhibitors (fluoxetine, fluvoxamine, nefazodone, paroxetin, sertraline) / Inhibition of metabolism of astemizole
Troleandomycin / Possible serious CV effects, including death, cardiac arrest, torsades de pointes, and other ventricular arrhythmias (including QT interval prolongation).
Zileuton / Inhibition of metabolism of astemizole

EMS CONSIDERATIONS

See also *Antihistamines.*

Atenolol
(ah-TEN-oh-lohl)
Pregnancy Class: C
Tenormin **(Rx)**
Classification: Beta-adrenergic blocking agent

Mechanism of Action: Predominantly beta-1 blocking activity. Has no membrane stabilizing activity or intrinsic sympathomimetic activity.
Uses: Hypertension (either alone or with other antihypertensives such as thiazide diuretics). Angina pectoris due to hypertension, coronary atherosclerosis, and AMI. *Investigational:* Prophylaxis of migraine, alcohol

withdrawal syndrome, situational anxiety, ventricular arrhythmias, prophylactically to reduce incidence of supraventricular arrhythmias in coronary artery bypass surgery.

Precautions: Dosage not established in children.

Route/Dosage
• **Tablets**

Hypertension.

Initial: 50 mg/day, either alone or with diuretics; if response is inadequate, 100 mg/day. Doses higher than 100 mg/day will not produce further beneficial effects. Maximum effects usually seen within 1–2 weeks.

Angina.

Initial: 50 mg/day; if maximum response is not seen in 1 week, increase dose to 100 mg/day (some patients require 200 mg/day).

Alcohol withdrawal syndrome.

50–100 mg/day.

Prophylaxis of migraine.

50–100 mg/day.

Ventricular arrhythmias.

50–100 mg/day.

Prior to coronary artery bypass surgery.

50 mg/day started 72 hr prior to surgery.

Adjust dosage in cases of renal failure to 50 mg/day if creatinine clearance is 15–35 mL/min/1.73 m² and to 50 mg every other day if creatinine clearance is less than 15 mL/min/1.73 m².

• **IV**

Acute myocardial infarction.

Initial: 5 mg over 5 min followed by a second 5-mg dose 10 min later. Begin treatment as soon as possible after patient arrives at the hospital. In patients who tolerate the full 10-mg dose, give a 50-mg tablet 10 min after the last IV dose followed by another 50-mg dose 12 hr later. **Then,** 100 mg/day or 50 mg b.i.d. for 6–9 days (or until discharge from the hospital).

How Supplied: *Injection:* 0.5 mg/mL; *Tablet:* 25 mg, 50 mg, 100 mg

EMS CONSIDERATIONS

See also *Beta-Adrenergic Blocking Agents.*

A

Atorvastatin calcium
(ah-TORE-vah-stah-tin)
Pregnancy Class: X
Lipitor **(Rx)**
Classification: Antihyperlipidemic, HMG–CoA reductase inhibitor

---

Uses: Adjunct to diet to reduce elevated total and LDL cholesterol levels in primary hypercholesterolemia (Types IIa and IIb) when the response to diet and other nondrug measures alone have been inadequate. With changes in diet in patients with high triglyceride or fat levels. Treat dysbetalipoproteinemia in those with inadequate response to diet changes.

Contraindications: Active liver disease or unexplained persistently high liver function tests. Pregnancy, lactation.

Precautions: Safety and efficacy have not been determined in children less than 18 years of age.

Route/Dosage
• **Tablets**

Hyperlipidemia.

Initial: 10 mg/day; **then,** a dose range of 10–80 mg/day may be used.
How Supplied: *Tablets:* 10 mg, 20 mg, 40 mg

Side Effects: See also *Antihyperlipidemic Agents—HMG-CoA Reductase Inhibitors. GI:* Altered liver function tests (usually within the first 3 months of therapy), flatulence, dyspepsia. *CNS:* Headache. *Musculoskeletal:* Myalgia. *Miscellaneous:* Infection, rash, pruritus, allergy.

Drug Interactions

Antacids / ↓ Atorvastatin plasma levels

Colestipol / ↓ Plasma levels of atorvastatin

Erythromycin / ↑ Plasma levels of atorvastatin; possibility of severe myopathy or rhabdomyolysis

---

bold italic = life threatening side effect

A

Oral contraceptives / ↑ Plasma levels of norethindrone and ethinyl estradiol

EMS CONSIDERATIONS

See also *Antihyperlipidemic Agents—HMG—CoA Reductase Inhibitors*.

Atovaquone
(ah-TOV-ah-kwohn)
Pregnancy Class: C
Mepron **(Rx)**
Classification: Antiprotozoal agent

Mechanism of Action: The mechanism of action of atovaquone against *Pneumocystis carinii* is not known. However, in *Plasmodium*, appears to act by inhibiting electron transport resulting in inhibition of nucleic acid and ATP synthesis. The bioavailability of the drug is increased twofold when taken with food.

Uses: Acute oral treatment of mild to moderate *P. carinii* in patients who are intolerant to trimethoprim-sulfamethoxazole. Has not been evaluated as an agent for prophylaxis of *P. carinii*. Not effective for concurrent pulmonary diseases such as bacterial, viral, or fungal pneumonia or in mycobacterial diseases.

Contraindications: Hypersensitivity to atovaquone or any components of the formulation; potentially life-threatening allergic reactions are possible.

Precautions: Use with caution during lactation and in elderly patients. There are no efficacy studies in children. GI disorders may limit absorption of atovaquone.

Route/Dosage ———————————
• **Suspension**
Adults: 750 mg (5 mL) given with food b.i.d. for 21 days (total daily dose: 1,500 mg).
How Supplied: *Suspension:* 750 mg/5 mL

Side Effects: Since many patients taking atovaquone have complications of HIV disease, it is often difficult to distinguish side effects caused by atovaquone from symptoms caused by the underlying medical condition. *Dermatologic:* Rash (including maculopapular), pruritus. *GI:* Nausea, diarrhea, vomiting, abdominal pain, constipation, dyspepsia, taste perversion. *CNS:* Headache, fever, insomnia, dizziness, anxiety, anorexia. *Respiratory:* Cough, sinusitis, rhinitis. *Hematologic:* Anemia, neutropenia. *Miscellaneous:* Asthenia, oral monilia, pain, sweating, hypoglycemia, hypotension, hyperglycemia, hyponatremia.

Drug Interactions: Since atovaquone is highly bound to plasma proteins (>99.9%), caution should be exercised when giving the drug with other highly plasma protein-bound drugs with narrow therapeutic indices as competition for binding may occur.

EMS CONSIDERATIONS

None.

Atropine sulfate
(AH-troh-peen)
Pregnancy Class: C
Atropari, Atropine-1 Ophthalmic, Atropine Sulfate Ophthalmic, Atropine Care Ophthalmic, Atropisol Ophthalmic, Isopto Atropine Ophthalmic **(Rx)**
Classification: Cholinergic blocking agent

Mechanism of Action: Atropine blocks the action of acetylcholine on postganglionic cholinergic receptors in smooth muscle, cardiac muscle, exocrine glands, urinary bladder, and the AV and SA nodes in the heart. Ophthalmologically, atropine blocks the effect of acetylcholine on the sphincter muscle of the iris and the accommodative muscle of the ciliary body. This results in dilation of the pupil (mydriasis) and paralysis of the muscles required to accommodate for close vision (cycloplegia).
Onset of Action: Peak effect:*Mydriasis,*30-40 min; *cycloplegia,*1-3 hr.
Recovery: Up to 12 days.
Duration of Action: PO:4-6 hr.
Uses: PO: Adjunct in peptic ulcer treatment. Irritable bowel syndrome. Adjunct in treatment of spastic disorders of the biliary tract. Urologic dis-

orders, urinary incontinence. During anesthesia to control salivation and bronchial secretions. Has been used for parkinsonism but more effective drugs are available.

Parenteral: Antiarrhythmic, adjunct in GI radiography. Prophylaxis of arrhythmias induced by succinylcholine or surgical procedures. Reduce sinus bradycardia (severe) and syncope in hyperactive carotid sinus reflex. Prophylaxis and treatment of toxicity due to cholinesterase inhibitors, including organophosphate pesticides. Treatment of curariform block. As a preanesthetic or in dentistry to decrease secretions.

Ophthalmologic: Cycloplegic refraction or pupillary dilation in acute inflammatory conditions of the iris and uveal tract. *Investigational:* Treatment and prophylaxis of posterior synechiae; pre- and postoperative mydriasis; treatment of malignant glaucoma.

Contraindications: *Ophthalmic use:* Infants less than 3 months of age, primary glaucoma or a tendency toward glaucoma, adhesions between the iris and the lens, geriatric patients and others where undiagnosed glaucoma or excessive pressure in the eye may be present, in children who have had a previous severe systemic reaction to atropine. **Precautions:** Use with caution in infants, small children, geriatric patients, diabetes, hypo- or hyperthyroidism, narrow anterior chamber angle, individuals with Down syndrome.

Route/Dosage
• **Tablets**
Anticholinergic or antispasmodic.
Adults: 0.3–1.2 mg q 4–6 hr. **Pediatric, over 41 kg:** same as adult; **29.5–41 kg:** 0.4 mg q 4–6 hr; **18.2–29.5 kg:** 0.3 mg q 4–6 hr; **10.9–18.2 kg:** 0.2 mg q 4–6 hr; **7.3–10.9 kg:** 0.15 mg q 4–6 hr; **3.2–7.3 kg:** 0.1 mg q 4–6 hr.

Prophylaxis of respiratory tract secretions and excess salivation during anesthesia.

Adults: 2 mg.
Parkinsonism.
Adults: 0.1–0.25 mg q.i.d.
• **IM, IV, SC**
Anticholinergic.
Adults, IM, IV, SC: 0.4–0.6 mg q 4–6 hr. **Pediatric, SC:** 0.01 mg/kg, not to exceed 0.4 mg (or 0.3 mg/m²).
To reverse curariform blockade.
Adults, IV: 0.6–1.2 mg given at the same time or a few minutes before 0.5–2 mg neostigmine methylsulfate (use separate syringes).
Treatment of toxicity from cholinesterase inhibitors.
Adults, IV, initial: 2–4 mg; **then,** 2 mg repeated q 5–10 min until muscarinic symptoms disappear and signs of atropine toxicity begin to appear. **Pediatric, IM, IV, initial:** 1 mg; **then,** 0.5–1 mg q 5–10 min until muscarinic symptoms disappear and signs of atropine toxicity appear.
Treatment of mushroom poisoning due to muscarine.
Adults, IM, IV: 1–2 mg q hr until respiratory effects decrease.
Treatment of organophosphate poisoning.
Adults, IM, IV, initial: 1–2 mg; **then,** repeat in 20–30 min (as soon as cyanosis has disappeared). Dosage may be continued for up to 2 days until symptoms improve.
Arrhythmias.
Pediatric, IV: 0.01–0.03 mg/kg.
Prophylaxis of respiratory tract secretions, excessive salivation, succinylcholine- or surgical procedure-induced arrhythmias.
Pediatric, up to 3 kg, SC: 0.1 mg; **7–9 kg:** 0.2 mg; **12–16 kg:** 0.3 mg; **20–27 kg:** 0.4 mg; **32 kg:** 0.5 mg; **41 kg:** 0.6 mg.
• **Ophthalmic Solution**
Uveitis.
Adults: 1–2 gtt instilled into the eye(s) up to q.i.d. **Children:** 1–2 gtt of the 0.5% solution into the eye(s) up to t.i.d.
Refraction.
Adults: 1–2 gtt of the 1% solution into the eye(s) 1 hr before refracting. **Children:** 1–2 gtt of the 0.5% solution

---

bold italic = life threatening side effect

into the eye(s) b.i.d. for 1–3 days before refraction.

• **Ophthalmic Ointment**
Instill a small amount into the conjunctival sac up to t.i.d.
How Supplied: *Injection:* 0.05 mg/mL, 0.1 mg/mL, 0.4 mg/mL, 0.5 mg/mL, 0.8 mg/mL, 1 mg/mL; *Ophthalmic Ointment:* 1%; *Ophthalmic Solution:* 0.5%, 1%; Tablet: 0.4 mg
Side Effects: *Ophthalmologic:*Blurred vision, stinging, increased intraocular pressure, contact dermatitis. Long-term use may cause irritation, photophobia, eczematoid dermatitis, conjunctivitis, hyperemia, or edema.
OD Overdose Management: *Treatment of Ocular Overdose:* Eyes should be flushed with water or normal saline. A topical miotic may be necessary.

EMS CONSIDERATIONS

See also *Cholinergic Blocking Agents.*
Assessment: Obtain VS and ECG; monitor C-P status during IV therapy.

Auranofin
(or-AN-oh-fin)
Pregnancy Class: C
Ridaura**(Rx)**
Classification: Antiarthritic, oral gold compound

Mechanism of Action: Auranofin is a gold-containing (29%) compound for PO administration. It has fewer side effects than injectable gold products. Although the mechanism is not known, auranofin will improve symptoms of rheumatoid arthritis; it is most effective in the early stages of active synovitis and may act by inhibiting sulfhydryl systems. Other possible mechanisms include inhibition of phagocytic activity of macrophages and polymorphonuclear leukocytes, alteration of biosynthesis of collagen, and alteration of the immune response. Gold will not reverse damage to joints caused by disease.
Onset of Action: Plasma t½ of auranofin gold: 26 days.**Onset:** 3-4 months (up to 6 months in certain patients).

Uses: Adults and children with rheumatoid arthritis that have not responded to other drugs. Up to 6 months may be required for beneficial effects to occur. Auranofin should be part of a total treatment regimen for rheumatoid arthritis, including nondrug treatments.
Contraindications: History of gold-induced disorders including necrotizing enterocolitis, pulmonary fibrosis, exfoliative dermatitis, bone marrow aplasia, or other hematologic severe disorders. Use during lactation.
Precautions: Use with extreme caution in renal or hepatic disease, skin rashes, marked hypertension, compromised cerebral or CV circulation, or history of bone marrow depression (e.g., agranulocytopenia anemia).Gold dermatitis may be aggravated by exposure to sunlight. Although used in children, a recommended dosage has not been established. Tolerance to gold is often decreased in geriatric patients.

Route/Dosage
• **Capsules**
Rheumatoid arthritis.
Adults, initial: Either 6 mg/day or 3 mg b.i.d. If response is unsatisfactory after 6 months, increase to 3 mg t.i.d. If response is still inadequate after 3 additional months, discontinue the drug. Dosages greater than 9 mg/day are not recommended.
Children, initial: 0.1 mg/kg/day; **maintenance:** 0.15 mg/kg/day, not to exceed 0.2 mg/kg/day.
Transfer from injectable gold.
Discontinue injectable gold and begin auranofin at a dose of 6 mg/day.
How Supplied: *Capsule:* 3 mg
Side Effects: *GI:* N&V, diarrhea (common), abdominal pain, metallic taste, stomatitis, glossitis, gingivitis, anorexia, constipation, flatulence, dyspepsia, dysgeusia, melena. Rarely, dysphagia, *GI bleeding, ulcerative enterocolitis. Dermatologic:* Skin rashes, pruritus, alopecia, urticaria, angioedema, actinic rash. *Hematologic:* Leukopenia, anemia, thrombocytopenia (with or without purpura),

neutropenia, agranulocytosis, eosinophilia, pancytopenia, hypoplastic anemia, *aplastic anemia,* pure red cell aplasia. *Renal:* Proteinuria, hematuria. *Hepatic:* Jaundice (with or without cholestasis, hepatitis with jaundice, *toxic hepatitis,* intrahepatic cholestasis. *Other:* Conjunctivitis, cholestatic jaundice, fever, interstitial pneumonia and fibrosis, peripheral neuropathy.

OD **Overdose Management:** *Symptoms:* Rapid appearance of hematuria, proteinuria, thrombocytopenia, granulocytopenia. Also, N&V, diarrhea, fever, urticaria, papulovesicular lesions, urticaria, exfoliative dermatitis, pruritus. *Treatment:* Discontinue promptly and give dimercaprol. Supportive therapy should be provided for renal and hematologic symptoms. Treat moderately severe skin and mucous membrane symptoms with topical corticosteroids, oral antihistamines, and anesthetic lotions. Treat severe stomatitis or dermatitis with prednisone, 10–40 mg daily. Treat serious renal, hematologic, pulmonary, and enterocolitic complications with prednisone, 40–100 mg daily in divided doses. The duration of treatment varies, depending on the severity of symptoms and the response to steroids. In acute overdosage, induce emesis or perform gastric lavage immediately.

EMS CONSIDERATIONS

None.

Aurothioglucose
(or-oh-thigh-oh-GLOO-kohz)
Pregnancy Class: C
Solganol **(Rx)**
Classification: Antiarthritic

Mechanism of Action: The gold content of aurothioglucose is 50%.
Onset of Action: Time to peak effect: 4-6 hr.

Route/Dosage
• **IM Only**
Rheumatoid arthritis.

Adults: *Week 1:* 10 mg; *weeks 2 and 3:* 25 mg; **then,** 25–50 (maximum) mg/week until a total of 0.8–1 g has been administered. If patient tolerates the dose and has improved, 50 mg may be given q 3–4 weeks for several months. **Pediatric, 6–12 years:** *Week 1:* 2.5 mg; *weeks 2 and 3:* 6.25 mg; **then,** 12.5 mg/week until a total dose of 200–250 mg has been administered. **Maintenance:** 6.25–12.5 mg q 3–4 weeks.

How Supplied: *Injection:* 50 mg/mL

Side Effects: *GI:* N&V, anorexia, abdominal cramps, metallic taste, gastritis, *ulcerative enterocolitis,* colitis. *Dermatologic:* Dermatitis (papular, vesicular, exfoliative), rash, urticaria, angioedema, chrysiasis. *Renal:* Nephrotic syndrome, glomerulonephritis with proteinuria and hematuria, acute renal failure secondary to acute tubular necrosis, acute nephritis, degeneration of proximal tubular epithelium. *Hematologic:* **Granulocytopenia, panmyelopathy, hemorrhagic diathesis.** *Respiratory:* Inflammation of upper respiratory tract, pharyngitis, tracheitis, bold bronchitis, interstitial pneumonitis, fibrosis. *CNS:* Confusion, hallucinations, *seizures.* *Mucous membranes:* Stomatitis, diffuse glossitis, gingivitis. *Reactions of the nitroid type:* Anaphylactoid symptoms, flushing, fainting, dizziness, sweating, N&V, malaise, headache, weakness. *Ophthalmologic:* Iritis, corneal ulcers, gold deposits in ocular tissues. *Miscellaneous:* Vaginitis.

OD **Overdose Management:** *Treatment:* Discontinue and give dimercaprol. Provide supportive therapy for renal and hematologic symptoms. In acute overdose, induce emesis or gastric lavage immediately.

EMS CONSIDERATIONS

For additional information regarding aurothioglucose, see *Gold Sodium Thiomalate.*

---

bold italic = life threatening side effect

A

Azathioprine

(ay-zah-THIGH-oh-preen)
Pregnancy Class: D
Imuran**(Rx)**
Classification: Immunosuppressant

Mechanism of Action: Antimetabolite that is quickly split to form mercaptopurine. To be effective, the drug must be given during the induction period of the antibody response. The precise mechanism in depressing the immune response is unknown, but it suppresses cell-mediated hypersensitivities and alters antibody production. Inhibits synthesis of DNA, RNA, and proteins and may interfere with meiosis and cellular metabolism. The mechanism for its effect on autoimmune diseases is not known.

Onset of Action: 6-8 weeks for rheumatoid arthritis.

Uses: As an adjunct to prevent rejection in renal homotransplantation. In adult patients meeting criteria for classic or definite rheumatoid arthritis as defined by the American Rheumatism Association. Restrict use to patients with severe, active, and erosive disease that is not responsive to conventional therapy. *Investigational:* Chronic ulcerative colitis, generalized myasthenia gravis, to control the progression of Behçet's syndrome (especially eye disease), Crohn's disease (low doses).

Contraindications: Treatment of rheumatoid arthritis in pregnancy or in patients previously treated with alkylating agents. Pregnancy and lactation.

Precautions: Hematologic toxicity is dose-related and may occur late in the course of therapy; may be more severe in renal transplant patients undergoind rejection. Although used in children, safety and efficacy have not been established.

Route/Dosage

• **Tablets, IV**
  Use in renal homotransplantation.
Adults and children, initial: 3–5 mg/kg (120 mg/m^2), 1–3 days before

or on the day of transplantation; **maintenance:** 1–3 mg/kg (45 mg/m^2) daily.

Rheumatoid arthritis, SLE.
Adults and children, tablets, initial: 1 mg/kg (50–100 mg); **then,** increase dose by 0.5 mg/kg/day after 6–8 weeks and thereafter q 4 weeks, up to maximum of 2.5 mg/kg/day; **maintenance:** lowest effective dose. Dosage should be reduced in patients with renal dysfunction.

Myasthenia gravis.
2–3 mg/kg/day. However, side effects occur in more than 35% of patients.

To control progression of Behçet's syndrome.
2.5 mg/kg/day.

To treat Crohn's disease.
75–100 mg/day.

How Supplied: *Powder For Injection:* 100 mg; *Tablet:* 50 mg

Side Effects: *Hematologic:* Leukopenia, thrombocytopenia, macrocytic anemia, *severe bone marrow depression,* selective erythrocyte aplasia. *GI:* N&V, diarrhea, abdominal pain, steatorrhea. *CNS:* Fever, malaise. *Other: Increased risk of carcinoma,* severe infections (fungal, viral, bacterial, and protozoal), and *hepatotoxicity* are major side effects. Also, skin rashes, alopecia, myalgias, increase in liver enzymes, hypotension, negative nitrogen balance.

OD **Overdose Management:** *Symptoms:* Large doses may result in *bone marrow hypoplasia,* bleeding, infection, and death. *Treatment:* Approximately 45% can be removed from the body following 8 hr of hemodialysis.

Drug Interactions

ACE inhibitors / ↑ Risk of severe leukopenia

Allopurinol / ↑ Pharmacologic effect of azathioprine due to ↓ breakdown in liver

Anticoagulants / ↓ Effect of anticoagulants

Corticosteroids / With azathioprine, it may cause muscle wasting after prolonged therapy

Cyclosporine / ↑ Plasma levels of cyclosporine

Methotrexate / ↑ Plasma levels of the active metabolite, 6-mercaptopurine

Tubocurarine / Azathioprine ↓ effect of tubocurarine and other nondepolarizing neuromuscular blocking agents

EMS CONSIDERATIONS

None.

Azelaic acid
(ah-zih-LAY-ic ah-SID)
Pregnancy Class: B
Azelex**(Rx)**
Classification: Antiacne drug

Mechanism of Action: The precise mechanism of action in treating acne is not known, but the drug possesses antimicrobial activity against *Propionibacterium acnes* and *Staphylococcus epidermidis*. Causes a decrease in the thickness of the stratum corneum, a reduction in the number and size of keratohyalin granules, and a reduction in the amount and distribution of filaggrin in epidermal layers. After application, the drug penetrates to the stratum corneum, epidermis, and dermis.

Uses: Treatment of mild to moderate inflammatory acne vulgaris.
Contraindications: Ophthalmic use.

Precautions: Use with caution during lactation. Safety and efficacy have not been determined in children less than 12 years of age.

Route/Dosage
• **Cream**
Acne vulgaris.
Gently but thoroughly massage a thin film into the affected areas b.i.d., in the morning and evening, after the skin is thoroughly washed and patted dry.
How Supplied: *Cream:* 20%
Side Effects: *Dermatologic:* Pruritus, burning, stinging, tingling, erythema, dryness, rash, peeling, irritation, dermatitis, contact dermatitis, vitiligo depigmentation, small depigmented

spots, hypertrichosis, reddening (sign of keratosis pilaris), exacerbation of recurrent herpes labialis (rare). *Miscellaneous:* **Worsening of asthma, allergic reactions.**

EMS CONSIDERATIONS

None.

Azithromycin
(az-sith-roh-MY-sin)
Pregnancy Class: B
Zithromax**(Rx)**
Classification: Antibiotic, macrolide

Mechanism of Action: A macrolide antibiotic derived from erythromycin. The drug acts by binding to the P site of the 50S ribosomal subunit and may inhibit RNA-dependent protein synthesis by stimulating the dissociation of peptidyl t-RNA from ribosomes. Food increases the absorption of azithromycin.
Onset of Action: Time to reach maximum concentration: 2.2 hr. **t½, terminal:** 68 hr.
Uses: Adults: Acute bacterial exacerbations of COPD due to *Hemophilus influenzae, Moraxella catarrhalis,* or *Streptococcus pneumoniae.* Required initial IV therapy in community-acquired pneumonia due to *S. pneumoniae, Chlamydia pneumoniae, Mycoplasma pneumoniae, H. influenzae, M. catarrhalis, Legionella pneumophila,* and *Staphylococcus aureus.* Those who can take PO therapy in community-acquired pneumonia due to *C. pneumoniae, M. pneumoniae, S. pneumoniae, or H. influenzae.* PO for genital ulcer disease in men due to *Haemophilus ducreyi.* Initial IV therapy in pelvic inflammatory disease due to *Chlamydia trachomatis, Neisseria gonorrhoeae,* or *Mycoplasma hominis.* As an alternative to first-line therapy to treat streptococcal pharyngitis or tonsillitis due to *Streptococcus pyogenes.* PO for uncomplicated skin and skin structure infections due to *S. aureus, Staphyloccus pyogenes,* or *Streptococcus agalactiae.* Abscesses

usually require surgical drainage. PO for urethritis and cervicitis due to *C. trachomatis* or *N. gonorrhoeae*.

Children: PO for acute otitis media due to *H. influenzae, M. catarrhalis,* or *S. pneumoniae* in children over 6 months of age. PO for community-acquired pneumonia due to *C. pneumoniae, H. influenzae, M. pneumoniae,* or *S. pneumoniae* in children over 6 months of age. Pharyngitis/tonsillitis due to *S. pyogenes* in children over 2 years of age who cannot use first-line therapy.

Investigational: Uncomplicated gonococcal pharyngitis of the cervix, urethra, and rectum caused by *N. gonorrhoeae*. Gonococcal phayrngitis due to *N. gonorrhoeae*. Chlamydial infections due to *C. trachomatis*.

Contraindications: Hypersensitivity to azithromycin, any macrolide antibiotic, or erythromycin. In patients who are not eligible for outpatient PO therapy (e.g., known or suspected bacteremia, immunodeficiency, functional asplenia, nosocomially acquired infections, geriatric or debilitated patients). Use with astemizole, cisapride, or pimozide.

Route/Dosage ————————
• **Suspension, Tablets**
Adults: Mild to moderate acute bacterial exacerbations of COPD, mild community-acquired pneumonia, second-line therapy for pharyngitis/tonsillitis; uncomplicated skin and skin structure infections.
Adults and children over 16 years of age: 500 mg as a single dose on day 1 followed by 250 mg once daily on days 2–5 for a total dose of 1.5 g.

Nongonococcal urethritis and cervicitis due to C. trachomatis *or genital ulcer disease due to* H. ducreyi.

1 g given as a single dose.

Gonococcal urethritis/cervicitis due to N. gonnorheae.

2 g given as a single dose.

Uncomplicated gonococcal infections due to N. gonorrhoeae.

1 g given as a single dose plus a single dose of 400 mg PO cefixime, 125 mg IM ceftriaxone, 500 mg PO ciprofloxacine, or 400 mg PO ofloxacin.

Gonococcal pharyngitis.

1 g given as a single dose plus a single dose of 125 mg IM ceftriaxone, 500 mg ciprofloxacin, or 400 mg ofloxacin.

Chlamydial infections caused by C. trachomatis.

1 g given as a single dose.
• **Oral Suspension**
Pediatric: Otitis media or community-acquired pneumonia.

10 mg/kg (not to exceed 500 mg) on day 1, followed by 5 mg/kg (not to exceed 250 mg/day) on days 2 through 5.

Pediatric: Pharyngitis/tonsillitis.

12 mg/kg once daily for 5 days, not to exceed 500 mg/day.

Chlamydial infections in children caused by C. trachomatis.

Children 45 kg or more and less than 8 years of age or over 8 years of age: 1 g given as a single dose.
• **IV**
Community-acquired pneumonia.

500 mg IV as a single daily dose for at least 2 days followed by a single daily dose of 500 mg PO to complete a 7- to 10-day course of therapy.

Pelvic inflammatory disease.

500 mg IV as a single daily dose for 1 or 2 days followed by a single daily dose of 250 mg PO to complete a 7-day course of therapy.

How Supplied: *Powder for Injection:* 500 mg; *Powder for Oral Suspension:* 100 mg/5mL, 200 mg/5mL, 1 gm/packet; *Tablet:* 250 mg, 600 mg

Side Effects: *GI:* N&V, diarrhea, loose stools, abdominal pain, dyspepsia, anorexia, gastritis, flatulence, melena, mucositis, oral moniliasis, taste perversion, cholestatic jaundice, pseudomembranous colitis. In children, gastritis, constipation, and anorexia have also been noted. *CNS:* Dizziness, headache, somnolence, fatigue, vertigo. In children, hyperkinesia, agitation, nervousness, insomnia, fever, and malaise have also been noted. *CV:* Chest pain, palpitations, ***ventricular arrhythmias (in-***

cluding ventricular tachycardia and torsades de pointes in patients with prolonged QT intervals observed with other macrolides). GU: Monilia, nephritis, vaginitis. *Allergic:* Angioedema, photosensitivity, rash, **anaphylaxis.** *Hematologic:* Leukopenia, neutropenia, decreased platelet count. *Miscellaneous:* Superinfection, bronchospasm, local IV site reactions. In children, pruritus, urticaria, conjunctivitis, and chest pain have been noted.

Drug Interactions: See also *Drug Interactions* for *Erythromycins.*
Aluminum- and magnesium-containing antacids / ↓ Peak serum levels of azithromycin but not the total amount absorbed
Cyclosporine / ↑ Serum levels of cyclosporine due to ↓ metabolism → ↑ risk of nephrotoxicity and neurotoxicity
HMG-CoA reductase inhibitors / ↑ Risk of severe myopathy or rhabdomyolysis
Phenytoin / ↑ Serum levels of phenytoin due to ↓ metabolism
Pimozide / Possibility of sudden death

EMS CONSIDERATIONS

See also *Erythromycins.*

Aztreonam for injection
(as-TREE-oh-nam)
Pregnancy Class: B
Azactam for injection**(Rx)**
Classification: Monobactam antibiotic

Mechanism of Action: Synthetic monobactam antibiotic. It is bactericidal against gram-negative aerobic pathogens. Acts by inhibiting cell wall synthesis due to a high affinity of the drug for penicillin binding protein 3; this results in cell lysis and death.
Onset of Action: Time to peak levels: 0.6-1.3 hr. t½:1.5-2 hr.
Uses: Complicated and uncomplicated urinary tract infections (including pyelonephritis and cystitis) due to *Escherichia coli, Klebsiella pneu-*moniae, Proteus mirabilis, Pseudomonas aeruginosa, Enterobacter cloacae, Klebsiella oxytoca, Citrobacter* species, and *Serratia marcescens.* Lower respiratory tract infections (including bronchitis and pneumonia) due to *E. coli, K. pneumoniae, P. aeruginosa, Hemophilus influenzae, P. mirabilis, Enterobacter* species, and *S. marcescens.* Septicemia due to *E. coli, K. pneumoniae, P. aeruginosa, P. mirabilis, S. marcescens* and *Enterobacter* species. Skin and skin structure infections (including postoperative wounds, ulcers, and burns) caused by *E. coli, P. mirabilis, S. marcescens, Enterobacter* species, *P. aeruginosa, K. pneumoniae,* and *Citrobacter* species. Intraabdominal infections (including peritonitis) due to *E. coli, Klebsiella* species including *K. pneumoniae, Enterobacter* species including *E. cloacae, P. aeruginosa, Citrobacter* species including *C. freundii,* and *Serratia* species including *S. marcescens.* Gynecologic infections (including endometritis and pelvic cellulitis) due to *E. coli, K. pneumoniae, P. mirabilis,* and *Enterobacter* species including *E. cloacae.* As an adjunct to surgery to manage infections caused by susceptible organisms. As an alternative to spectinomycin in patients with acute uncomplicated gonorrhea who are resistant to penicillin. Concomitant initial therapy with other anti-infective drugs and aztreonam in seriously ill patients is recommended before the causative organism is known and who are at risk for an infection due to gram-positive aerobic pathogens.
Contraindications: Allergy to aztreonam. Lactation.
Precautions: Safety and effectiveness have not been determined in children and infants. Use with caution in patients allergic to penicillins or cephalosporins and in those with impaired hepatic or renal function.

Route/Dosage —————
• **IM, IV**

---

bold italic = life threatening side effect

B

Urinary tract infections.
Adults: 0.5–1 g q 8–12 hr, not to exceed 8 g/day. **Children:** 30 mg/kg q 6–8 hr.
Moderate to severe systemic infections.
1–2 g q 8–12 hr, not to exceed 8 g/day.
Severe systemic or life-threatening infections.
2 g q 6–8 hr, not to exceed 8 g/day.
P. aeruginosa infections in children.
50 mg/kg q 4–6 hr.
NOTE: Dose must be reduced in patients with impaired renal function.
How Supplied: *Injection:* 1 g/50 mL, 2 g/50 mL; *Powder for injection:* 500 mg, 1 g, 2 g
Side Effects: *GI:* N&V, diarrhea, abdominal cramps, mouth ulcers, numb tongue, halitosis, pseudomembranous colitis, *Clostridium difficile*-associated diarrhea or GI bleeding. *CNS:* Confusion, **seizures,** vertigo, headache, paresthesia, insomnia, dizziness. *Hematologic:* Anemia, neutropenia, thrombocytopenia, leukocytosis, thrombocytosis, pancytopenia, eosinophilia. *Dermat-*

ologic: Rash, purpura, erythema multiforme, urticaria, petechiae, pruritus, diaphoresis, exfoliative dermatitis, ***toxic epidermal necrolysis.*** *CV:* Hypotension, transient ECG changes, flushing. *Following parenteral use:* Phlebitis and thrombophlebitis after IV use; discomfort and swelling at the injection site after IM use. *Allergic:* ***Anaphylaxis,*** angioedema, bronchospasm. *Miscellaneous:* Superinfection, weakness, fever, malaise, hepatitis, jaundice, muscle aches, tinnitus, diplopia, nasal congestion, altered taste, sneezing, vaginal candidiasis, vaginitis, breast tenderness, chest pain, numb tongue, wheezing.
OD **Overdose Management:** *Treatment:* Hemodialysis or peritoneal dialysis to reduce serum levels.
Drug Interactions
Aminoglycosides / ↑ Risk of nephrotoxicity and ototoxicity
Cefoxitin / Inhibition of activity of aztreonam
Imipenem / Inhibition of activity of aztreonam

EMS CONSIDERATIONS

See also *Anti-Infectives.*

B

Baclofen

(BAK-low-fen)
Pregnancy Class: C
Lioresal(Rx)
Classification: Skeletal muscle relaxant, centrally acting

Mechanism of Action: Related chemically to GABA, an inhibitory neurotransmitter. May act by combining with the $GABA_B$ receptor subtype. It increases threshold for excitation of primary afferent nerves and decreases the release of excitatory amino acids from presynaptic sites. May also act at certain brain sites. Has CNS depressant effects.
Onset of Action: Peak serum levels, PO: 2-3 hr. **t½, PO:** 3-4 hr. **Onset after intrathecal bolus:** 30-60 min; **peak effect after intrathecal**

bolus: 4 hr; **Onset after intrathecal continuous infusion:** 6-8 hr; **peak effect after intrathecal continuous infusion:** 24-48 hr.
Uses: PO. Multiple sclerosis (flexor spasms, pain, clonus, and muscular rigidity) and diseases and injuries of the spinal cord associated with spasticity. Not effective for the treatment of cerebral palsy, stroke, parkinsonism, or rheumatic disorders. *Investigational:* Trigeminal neuralgia, tardive dyskinesia, intractable hiccoughs.
Intrathecal. Severe spasticity of spinal cord of cerebral origin in patients unresponsive to PO baclofen therapy or who have intolerable CNS side effects. *Investigational:* Reduce spasticity in children with cerebral palsy.

Contraindications: Hypersensitivity. PO used to treat rheumatic disorders, spasm resulting from Parkinson's disease, stroke, cerebral palsy. Intrathecal product for IV, IM, SC, or epidural use.

Precautions: Use during lactation only if potential benefit outweighs the potential risk. Safe use of the oral product for children under 12 years of age and of the intrathecal product for children under 4 years of age has not been established. Use with caution in impaired renal function, in those with psychotic disorders, schizophrenia, or confusional states as worsening of these conditions has occurred following PO use. Geriatric patients may be at higher risk for developing CNS toxicity, including mental depression, confusion, hallucinations, and significant sedation. Due to serious, life-threatening side effects after intrathecal use, physicians must be trained and educated in chronic intrathecal infusion therapy. Abrup drug withdrawal may cause hallucinations and seizures.

Route/Dosage
- **Tablets**
  Muscle relaxant, spasticity.
Adults, initial: 5 mg t.i.d. for 3 days; **then,** 10 mg t.i.d. for 3 days, 15 mg t.i.d. for 3 days, and 20 mg t.i.d. Additional increases in dose may be required but should not exceed 20 mg q.i.d. Maximum daily dose for spasticity should not exceed 260 mg. **Children (treatment of spasticity), initial:** 10–15 mg/kg/day in 3 divided doses. Titrate to a maximum of 40 mg/day if less than 8 years of age and to a maximum of 80 mg/day if more than 8 years of age.
  Trigeminal neuralgia.
50–60 mg/day.
  Tardive dyskinesia.
40 mg/day used in combination with neuroleptics.
- **Intrathecal**
  Initial screening bolus.
50 mcg/mL given into the intrathecal space by barbotage over a period of not less than 1 min. The patient is ob-

served for 4–8 hr for a positive response consisting of a decrease in muscle tone, frequency, and/or severity of muscle spasms. If the response is not adequate, a second bolus dose of 75 mcg/1.5 mL, 24 hr after the first bolus dose, can be given with the patient observed for 4–8 hr. If the response is still inadequate, a final bolus screening dose of 100 mcg/2 mL can be given 24 hr later.
  Postimplant dose titration.
To determine the initial daily dose of baclofen following the implant for intrathecal use, the screening dose that gave a positive response should be doubled and given over a 24-hr period. However, if the effectiveness of the bolus dose lasted for more than 12 hr, the daily dose should be the same as the screening dose but delivered over a period of 24 hr. After the first 24 hr, the dose can be increased slowly by 10%–30% increments only once each 24 hr until the desired effect is reached.
  Maintenance therapy.
The maintenance dose may need to be adjusted during the first few months of intrathecal therapy. The daily dose may be increased by 10% to no more than 40% daily. If side effects occur, the daily dose may be decreased by 10%–20%. Daily doses for long-term continuous infusion have ranged from 12 to 1,500 mcg (usual maintenance is 300-800 mcg/day). The lowest dose producing optimal control should be used.
  Reduce spasticity of cerebral palsy in children.
25, 50, or 100 mcg.
How Supplied: *Kit:* 0.05 mg/mL, 0.5 mg/mL, 2 mg/mL; *Tablet:* 10 mg, 20 mg
Side Effects: PO. *CNS:* Drowsiness, dizziness, lightheadedness, weakness, lethargy, fatigue, confusion, headaches, insomnia, euphoria, excitement, depression, paresthesia, muscle pain, coordination disorder, tremor, ridigity, dystonia, ataxia, strabismus, dysarthria. Hallucinations following abrupt withdrawal. *CV:* Hypotension.

---

bold italic = life threatening side effect

Rarely, chest pain, syncope, palpitations. *GI:* N&V, constipation, dry mouth, anorexia, taste disorder, abdominal pain, diarrhea. *GU:* Urinary frequency, enuresis, urinary retention, dysuria, impotence, inability to ejaculate, nocturia. *Ophthalmic:* Nystagmus, miosis, mydriasis, diplopia. *Miscellaneous:* Rash, pruritus, ankle edema, increased perspiration, weight gain, dyspnea, nasal congestion.

Intrathecal, spasticity of spinal origin. *CNS:* Dizziness, somnolence, paresthesia, headache, **convulsion,** confusion, speech disorder, coma, **death,** insomnia, anxiety, depression, hallucinations. *GI:* N&V, constipation, dry mouth, diarrhea, anorexia. *GU:* Urinary retention, impotence, urinary incontinence, urinary frequency. *CV:* Hypotension, hypertension. *Miscellaneous:* Accidental injury, asthenia, amblyopia, pain, peripheral edema, dyspnea, hypoventilation, fever, urticaria, anorexia, diplopia, dysautonomia.

Intrathecal, spasticity of cerebral origin. *CNS:* Somnolence, headache, **convulsion,** dizziness, paresthesia, abnormal thinking, agitation, coma, speech disorder, tremor. *GI:* N&V, increased salivation, constipation, dry mouth. *GU:* Urinary retention, urinary incontinence, impaired urination. *Miscellaneous:* Hypertonia, hypoventilation, hypotension, back pain, pain, pruritus, peripheral edema, asthenia, chills, pneumonia.

OD **Overdose Management:** *Symptoms:* Symptoms after PO use include vomiting, drowsiness, muscular hypotonia, muscle twitching, accommodation disorders, respiratory depression, seizures, coma. Symptoms after intrathecal use include drowsiness, dizziness, lightheadedness, somnolence, respiratory depression, rostral progression of hypotonia, **seizures, loss of consciousness leading to coma (for up to 24 hr).** *Treatment:*
1. After PO use:
• Induce vomiting (only if the patient is alert and conscious) followed by gastric lavage.

• If the patient is not alert and conscious, undertake only gastric lavage making sure the airway is secured with a cuffed ET tube.
• Maintain an adequate airway.
• Atropine may be used to improve HR, BP, ventilation, and core body temperature.
2. After intrathecal use:
• The residual solution is to be removed from the pump as soon as possible.
• Intubate the patient with respiratory depression until the drug is eliminated.
• IV physostigmine (total dose of 1–2 mg given over 5–10 min) may be tried, with caution.
• Consideration can also be given to withdrawing 30–60 mL of CSF to decrease baclofen levels (provided that lumbar puncture is not contraindicated).

Drug Interactions
CNS depressants / Additive CNS depression
MAO Inhibitors / ↑ CNS depression and hypotension
Ticyclic antidepressants / Muscle hypotonia

EMS CONSIDERATIONS

See also *Skeletal Muscle Relaxants, Centrally Acting.*
Administration/Storage
IV 1. To reconstitute, add 5 mL of sterile water for injection to the powder vial (20 mg/5 mL). Shake gently to dissolve.
2. After reconstitution, the solution should be colorless and clear to opalescent. If particulate matter is present or the solution is colored, do not use.
3. Dilute the reconstituted solution (20 mg in 5 mL) to a volume of 50 mL with NSS or D5W and infuse over 20–30 min.
4. Do not add or infuse other drugs simultaneously through the same IV line.
5. Use the reconstituted solution immediately. If not used immediately, store at 2°C–8°C (36°F–46°F) for 24 hr or at room temperature for 4 hr. Discard if not used within 24 hr.

Assessment

1. Drug is used in conjunction with cyclosporine and corticosteroids.

2. Given as 2 doses: infuse the first dose 2 hr prior to transplant surgery and then give the 2nd dose 4 days after transplantation.

3. Assess carefully for any evidence of infection. Monitor labs and serum drug levels.

Becaplermin

(beh-KAP-ler-min)

Pregnancy Class: Pregnancy Class: C

Regranex**(Rx)**

Classification: Topical wound healing drug

Mechanism of Action: Topical recombinant human platelet-derived growth factor. Promotes chemotactic recruitment and proliferation of cells involved in wound repair and enhances formation of granulation tissue. **Uses:** As adjunct to good ulcer care practices to treat lower extremity diabetic neuropathic ulcers that extend into SC tissue or beyond and have adequate blood supply. Use for diabetic neuropathic ulcers that do not extend through dermis into SC tissue or ischemic ulcers has not been studied.

Contraindications: Known neoplasms at application site. Use in wounds that close by primary intention.

Precautions: Effect on exposed joints, tendons, ligaments, and bone has not been established. Use with other topical drugs has not been studied. Use with caution during lactation. Safety and efficacy have not been determined in children less than 16 years of age.

Route/Dosage

• **Gel, 0.01%**

Lower extremity diabetic neuropathic ulcers.

Dose depends on size of ulcer area. To determine length of gel to be applied, measure greatest length of ulcer by greatest width of ulcer in either inches or centimeters. To calculate length of gel in inches:

7.5 g or 15 g tube: length x width x 0.6

2 g tube: length x width x 1.3

Generally, each square inch of ulcer surface will require about $2/3$ inch from 7.5 g or 15 g tube and about $1\frac{1}{4}$ inches from 2 g tube.

To calculate length of gel in centimeters:

7.5 g or 15 g tube: length x width divided by 4

2 g tube: length x width divided by 2

Generally, each square centimeter of ulcer surface will require about 0.25 cm of gel from 7.5 or 15 g tube or about 0.5 cm of gel from 2 g tube. Calculate amount to be applied at weekly or biweekly intervals depending on rate of change in ulcer area.

How Supplied: *Gel:* 0.01%

Side Effects: *General:* Infection, cellulitis, osteomyelitis, erythematous rashes.

EMS CONSIDERATIONS

Administration/Storage

1. Squeeze calculated length of gel onto a clean measuring surface (e.g., wax paper). Gel is transferred from clean measuring surface using an application aid and then spread over entire ulcer area. This should yield thin continuous layer of about $1/16$ inch thickness.

2. Cover site with saline moistened dressing and leave in place about 12 hr.

3. Remove dressing after 12 hr and rinse ulcer with saline or water to remove residual gel. Cover again with second moist dressing without gel for remainder of day.

4. Apply once daily until complete ulcer healing has occurred.

5. If ulcer does not decrease in size by about 30% after 10 weeks of therapy or complete healing has not occurred in 20 weeks, reassess treatment.

6. Refrigerate gel but do not freeze.

---

bold italic = life threatening side effect

Do not use gel after expiration date at bottom of tube.

Assessment

1. Document onset, duration, size, and characteristics of area requiring treatment. May record initial wound assessment with photographs.

2. Assess area to ensure it is free from infection, cellulitis, rash, and osteomyelitis.

3. Ensure patient is enrolled in active wound management program with ongoing debridement, relief of pressure (e.g., wheel chair, wedge shoe), systemic management of infections, and moist dressings changed bid.

Beclomethasone dipropionate

(be-kloh-METH-ah-zohn)

Pregnancy Class: C

Beclovent, Vanceril, Vanceril DS**(Rx)** **Intrannasal:**Beconase AQ Nasal, Beconase Inhalation, Vancenase AQ 84 mcg Double Strength, Vancenase AQ Forte, Vancenase AQ Nasal, Vancenase Nasal Inhaler**(Rx)**

Classification: Glucocorticoid

Mechanism of Action: Rapidly inactivated, thereby resulting in few systemic effects.

Uses: Relief of symptoms of seasonal or perennial rhinitis in patients not responsive to more conventional therapy, to prevent recurrence of nasal polyps following surgical removal, and to treat allergic or nonallergic (vasomotor) rhinitis (spray formulations). Inhalation therapy for chronic use in bronchial asthma. In glucocorticoid-dependent patients, beclomethasone often permits a decrease in the dosage of the systemic agent. Withdrawal of systemic corticosteroids must be done gradually.

Contraindications: Status asthmaticus, acute episodes of asthma, hypersensitivity to drug or aerosol ingredients.

Precautions: Safe use during lactation and in children under 6 years of age not established.

Route/Dosage

- **Metered Dose Inhaler**
  Asthma.

Beclovent. **Adults:** 2 inhalations (total of 84 mcg beclomethasone) t.i.d.–q.i.d. In some patients, 4 inhalations (168 mcg) b.i.d. have been effective. Do not exceed 20 inhalations (840 mcg) daily. **Pediatric, 6–12 years:** 1–2 inhalations (42–84 mcg) t.i.d.–q.i.d. In some, 4 inhalations (168 mcg) b.i.d. have been effective. Do not to exceed 10 inhalations (420 mcg) daily. Dosage has not been determined in children less than 6 years of age.

Vanceril. **Adults:** 2 inhalations (total of 168 mcg) b.i.d. In those with severe asthma, start with 6–8 inhalations/day and adjust dose downward as determined by patient response. Do not exceed 10 inhalations (840 mcg) daily. **Children, 6–12 years:** 2 inhalations (168 mcg) b.i.d. Do not exceed 5 inhalations (420 mcg) daily. Dosage has not been determined in children less than 6 years of age.

NOTE: Vanceril DS can be used once daily for treatment of asthma.

In patients also receiving systemic glucocorticosteroids, beclomethasone should be started when patient's condition is relatively stable.

- **Nasal Aerosol or Spray**
  Allergic or nonallergic rhinitis, Prophylaxis of nasal polyps.

Adults and children over 12 years: 1 inhalation (42 mcg) in each nostril b.i.d.–q.i.d. (i.e., total daily dose: 168–336 mcg). If no response after 3 weeks, discontinue therapy. **Maintenance, usual:** 1 inhalation in each nostril t.i.d. (252 mcg/day). For nasal polyps, treatment may be required for several weeks or more before a therapeutic effect can be assessed fully. Two sprays of the double-strength product (Vancenase AQ 84 mcg Double Strength) are administered once daily.

Vancenase AQ Forte may be used once daily for treatment of rhinitis.

How Supplied: *Metered dose inhaler:* 0.042 mg/inh, 0.084 mg/inh; *Nasal Spray:* 0.042 mg/inh, 0.084 mg/inh

Side Effects: *Intranasal:* Headache, pharyngitis, coughing, epistaxis, nasal burning, pain, conjunctivitis, myalgia, tinnitus. Rarely, ulceration of the nasal mucosa and nasal septum perforation.

EMS CONSIDERATIONS

See also *Corticosteroids.*

Benazepril hydrochloride
(beh-NAYZ-eh-prill)
Pregnancy Class: D
Lotensin(Rx)
Classification: Antihypertensive, ACE inhibitor

Mechanism of Action: Both supine and standing BPs are reduced with mild-to-moderate hypertension and no compensatory tachycardia.
Onset of Action: 1 hr.
Duration of Action: 24 hr.**Peak reduction in BP:**2-4 hr after dosing.
Peak effect with chronic therapy:1-2 weeks.
Uses: Alone or in combination with thiazide diuretics to treat hypertension.
Contraindications: Hypersensitivity to benazepril or any other ACE inhibitor.
Precautions: Use with caution during lactation. Safety and effectiveness have not been determined in children.

Route/Dosage
• **Tablets**
Patients not receiving a diuretic.
Initial: 10 mg once daily; **maintenance:** 20–40 mg/day given as a single dose or in two equally divided doses. Total daily doses greater than 80 mg have not been evaluated.
Patients receiving a diuretic.
Initial: 5 mg/day.
$C_{CR} < 30$ mL/min/1.73 m². *The recommended starting dose is 5 mg/day;* **maintenance:** *titrate dose upward until BP is controlled or to a maximum total daily dose of 40 mg.*
How Supplied: *Tablet:* 5 mg, 10 mg, 20 mg, 40 mg

Side Effects: *CNS:* Headache, dizziness, fatigue, anxiety, insomnia, drowsiness, nervousness. *GI:* N&V, constipation, abdominal pain, gastritis, melena, pancreatitis. *CV:* Symptomatic *hypotension,* postural hypotension, syncope, angina pectoris, palpitations, peripheral edema, ECG changes. *Dermatologic:* Flushing, photosensitivity, pruritus, rash, diaphoresis. *GU:* Decreased libido, impotence, UTI. *Respiratory:* Cough, asthma, bronchitis, dyspnea, sinusitis, bronchospasm. *Neuromuscular:* Paresthesias, arthralgia, arthritis, asthenia, myalgia. *Hematologic:* Occasionally, eosinophilia, leukopenia, neutropenia, decreased hemoglobin. *Miscellaneous:* Angioedema, which may be associated with involvement of the tongue, glottis, or larynx; hypertonia; proteinuria; hyponatremia; infection.
Drug Interactions
Diuretics / Excessive ↓ in BP
Lithium / ↑ Serum lithium levels with ↑ risk of lithium toxicity
Potassium-sparing diuretics, potassium supplements / ↑ Risk of hyperkalemia

EMS CONSIDERATIONS

See also *Angiotensin-Converting Enzyme Inhibitors,* and *Antihypertensive Agents.*

Benzonatate
(ben-ZOH-nah-tayt)
Pregnancy Class: Pregnancy Class: C
Tessalon Perles(Rx)
Classification: Antitussive, nonnarcotic

Mechanism of Action: Acts peripherally by anesthetizing stretch receptors in the respiratory passages, lungs, and pleura, thus depressing the cough reflex at its source. No effect on the respiratory center in the doses recommended.
Onset of Action: 15-20 min.
Duration of Action: 3-8 hr.
Uses: Symptomatic relief of cough.

---

bold italic = life threatening side effect

Contraindications: Sensitivity to benzonatate or related drugs such as procaine and tetracaine.

Precautions: Use with caution during lactation. Safety and efficacy have not been determine in children less than 10 years of age.

Route/Dosage
• **Capsules (Perles)**
Antitussive.
Adults and children over 10 years of age: 100 mg t.i.d., up to a maximum of 600 mg/day.
How Supplied: *Perles:* 100 mg.

Side Effects: *Hypersensitivity reactions: Bronchospasm, laryngospasm, CV collapse. GI:* Nausea, GI upset, constipation. *CNS:* Sedation, headache, dizziness, mental confusion, visual hallucinations. *Dermatologic:* Pruritus, skin eruptions. *Miscellaneous:* Nasal congestion, sensation of burning in the eyes, "chilly" sensation, numbness of the chest.

OD **Overdose Management:** *Symptoms:* Oropharyngeal anesthesia if capsules are chewed or dissolved in the mouth. CNS stimulation, including restlessness, tremors, and clonic convulsions followed by profound CNS depression. *Treatment:* Evacuate gastric contents followed by copious amounts of activated charcoal slurry. Due to depressed cough and gag reflexes, efforts may be needed to protect against aspiration of gastric contents and orally administered substances. Treat convulsions with a short-acting IV barbiturate. Do not use CNS stimulants. Support of respiration and CV-renal function.

EMS CONSIDERATIONS
Assessment
1. Document indications for therapy, onset, duration, and characteristics of symptoms.
2. Note any sensitivity to benzonatate or tetracaine.
3. Not for use during pregnancy.

Benztropine mesylate
(BENS-troh-peen)
Pregnancy Class: C

Cogentin**(Rx)**
Classification: Synthetic anticholinergic, antiparkinson agent

Mechanism of Action: Synthetic anticholinergic possessing antihistamine and local anesthetic properties. Low incidence of side effects.
Onset of Action: PO: 1-2 hr; **IM, IV:** within a few minutes. Effects are cumulative; is long-acting (24 hr).
Full effects: 2-3 days.
Uses: Adjunct in the treatment of parkinsonism (all types). To reduce severity of extrapyramidal effects in phenothiazine or other antipsychotic drug therapy (not effective in tardive dyskinesia).
Contraindications: Use in children under 3 years of age.
Precautions: Geriatric and emaciated patients cannot tolerate large doses. Certain drug-induced extrapyramidal symptoms may not respond to benztropine.

Route/Dosage
• **Tablets**
Parkinsonism.
Adults: 1–2 mg/day (range: 0.5–6 mg/day).
Idiopathic parkinsonism.
Adults, initial: 0.5–1 mg/day, increased gradually to 4–6 mg/day, if necessary.
Postencephalitic parkinsonism.
Adults: 2 mg/day in one or more doses.
Drug-induced extrapyramidal effects.
Adults: 1–4 mg 1–2 times/day.
• **IM, IV (Rarely)**
Acute dystonic reactions.
Adults, initial: 1–2 mg; **then,** 1–2 mg PO b.i.d. usually prevents recurrence. Patients can rarely tolerate full dosage.
How Supplied: *Injection:* 1 mg/mL; *Tablet:* 0.5 mg, 1 mg, 2 mg

EMS CONSIDERATIONS
See also *Cholinergic Blocking Agents.*

Bepridil hydrochloride
(BEH-prih-dill)
Pregnancy Class: C

Vascor**(Rx)**
Classification: Antianginal, calcium channel blocking drug

Mechanism of Action: Inhibits the transmembrane influx of calcium ions into cardiac and vascular smooth muscle. Increases the effective refractory period of the atria, AV node, His-Purkinje fibers, and ventricles. Dilates peripheral arterioles and reduces total peripheral resistance; reduces HR and arterial pressure at rest and at a given level of exercise.
Onset of Action: 60 min. **Time to peak plasma levels:** 2-3 hr.
Uses: Chronic stable angina (classic effort-associated angina) in patients who have failed to respond to other antianginal medications or who are intolerant to such medications. May be used alone or with beta blockers or nitrates. An additive effect occurs if used with propranolol.
Contraindications: Patients with a history of serious ventricular arrhythmias, sick sinus syndrome, second- or third-degree heart block (except in the presence of a functioning ventricular pacemaker), hypotension (less than 90 mm Hg systolic), uncompensated cardiac insufficiency, congenital QT interval prolongation, and in those taking other drugs that prolong the QT interval (e.g., quinidine, procainamide, tricyclic antidepressants). Use in patients with MI during the previous 3 months. Lactation.
Precautions: Safety and effectiveness have not been determined in children. Use with caution in patients with CHF, left bundle block, sinus bradycardia (less than 50 beats/min), serious hepatic or renal disorders. New arrhythmias can be induced. Geriatric patients may require more frequent monitoring.

Route/Dosage
• **Tablets**
  Chronic stable angina.
Adults, initial: 200 mg once daily; after 10 days the dosage may be adjusted upward depending on the re-

sponse of the patient (e.g., ability to perform ADL, QT interval, HR, frequency and severity of angina).
Maintenance: 300 mg/day, not to exceed 400 mg/day. The minimum effective dose is 200 mg.
How Supplied: *Tablet:* 200 mg, 300 mg
Side Effects: *CV: Induction of new serious arrhythmias such as torsades de pointes type ventricular tachycardia, prolongation of QTc and QT interval, increased PVC rates, new sustained VT and VT/VF,* sinus tachycardia, sinus bradycardia, hypertension vasodilation, palpitations. *GI:* Nausea (common), dyspepsia, GI distress, diarrhea, dry mouth, anorexia, abdominal pain, constipation, flatulence, gastritis, increased appetite. *CNS:* Nervousness, dizziness, drowsiness, insomnia, depression, vertigo, akathisia, anxiousness, tremor, hand tremor, syncope, paresthesia. *Respiratory:* Cough, pharyngitis, rhinitis, dyspnea, respiratory infection. *Body as a whole:* Asthenia, headache, flu syndrome, fever, pain, superinfection. *Dermatologic:* Rash, skin irritation, sweating. *Miscellaneous:* Tinnitus, arthritis, blurred vision, taste change, loss of libido, impotence, agranulocytosis.
Drug Interactions
Cardiac glycosides / Exaggeration of the depression of AV nodal conduction
Digoxin / Possible ↑ serum digoxin levels
Potassium-wasting diuretics / Hypokalemia, which causes an ↑ risk of serious ventricular arrhythmias
Procainamide / ↑ Risk of serious side effects due to exaggerated prolongation of the QT interval
Quinidine / ↑ Risk of serious side effects due to exaggerated prolongation of the QT interval
Tricyclic antidepressants / ↑ Risk of serious side effects due to exaggerated prolongation of the QT interval

EMS CONSIDERATIONS

See also *Calcium Channel Blocking Agents.*

---

bold italic = life threatening side effect

Betamethasone

(bay-tah-METH-ah-zohn)
Celestone, Celestone Phosphate, Celestone Soluspan, Cel-U-Jec, Diprosone, Valisone, Valisone Reduced Strength, Valnac**(Rx)**
Classification: Glucocorticoid

Mechanism of Action: Causes low degree of sodium and water retention, as well as potassium depletion. The injectable form contains both rapid-acting and repository forms of betamethasone (mixture of betamethasone sodium phosphate and betamethasone acetate). Long-acting.

Contraindications: Not recommended for replacement therapy in any acute or chronic adrenal cortical insufficiency because it does not have strong sodium-retaining effects.

Precautions: Safe use during pregnancy and lacatation has not been established.

Route/Dosage

BETAMETHASONE

• **Syrup, Tablets**
0.6–7.2 mg/day.

BETAMETHASONE SODIUM PHOSPHATE

• **IV, Intra-articular, Intralesional, Soft Tissue Injection**
Initial: up to 9 mg/day; **then,** adjust dosage at minimal level to reduce symptoms.

BETAMETHASONE SODIUM PHOSPHATE AND BETAMETHASONE ACETATE (contains 3 mg/mL each of the acetate and sodium phosphate)

• **IM**
Initial: 0.5–9 mg/day (dose ranges are ⅓–½ the PO dose given q 12 hr.)

• **Intra-articular, Intrabursal, Intradermal, Intralesional**

Bursitis, peritendinitis, tenosynovitis.
1 mL.

Rheumatoid arthritis and osteoarthritis.
0.25–2 mL, depending on size of the joint.

Foot disorders, bursitis.
0.25–0.5 mL under heloma durum or heloma molle; 0.5 mL under calcaneal spur or over hallux rigidus or digiti quinti varus. Tenosynovitis or periostitis of cuboid: 0.5 mL.

Acute gouty arthritis.
0.5–1 mL.

• **Intradermal**
0.2 mL/cm² not to exceed 1 mL/week.

BETAMETHASONE DIPROPIONATE, BETA-METHASONE VALERATE

• **Topical Aerosol, Cream, Lotion, Ointment**
Apply sparingly to affected areas and rub in lightly.

How Supplied: Betamethasone: *Syrup:* 0.6 mg/5 mL; *Tablet:* 0.6 mg. Betamethasone dipropionate: *Cream:* 0.05%; *Lotion:* 0.05%; *Ointment:* 0.05%; *Spray:* 0.1%. Betamethasone sodium phosphate: *Injection:* 3 mg/mL, 4 mg/mL. Betamethasone sodium phosphate and betamethasone acetate: *Injection:* 3 mg/mL. Betamethasone valerate: *Cream:* 0.1%; *Lotion:* 0.1%; *Ointment:* 0.1%

EMS CONSIDERATIONS

See also *Corticosteroids*.

Betaxolol hydrochloride

(beh-TAX-oh-lohl)
Pregnancy Class: C
Betoptic, Betoptic S, Kerlone**(Rx)**
Classification: Beta-adrenergic blocking agent

Mechanism of Action: Inhibits beta-1-adrenergic receptors although beta-2 receptors will be inhibited at high doses. Has some membrane stabilizing activity but no intrinsic sympathomimetic activity. Low lipid solubility. Reduces the production of aqueous humor, thus, reducing intraocular pressure. No effect on pupil size or accommodation.

Onset of Action: t½:14-22 hr.

Uses: PO: Hypertension, alone or with other antihypertensive agents (especially diuretics). **Ophthalmic:** Ocular hypertension and chronic open-angle glaucoma (used alone or in combination with other antiglaucoma drugs).

Precautions: Use with caution during lactation. Safety and effectiveness have not been determined in children. Geriatric patients are at greater risk of developing bradycardia.

Route/Dosage
- **Tablets**
    Hypertension.
Initial: 10 mg once daily either alone or with a diuretic. If the desired effect is not reached, the dose can be increased to 20 mg although doses higher than 20 mg will not increase the therapeutic effect. In geriatric patients the initial dose should be 5 mg/day.
- **Ophthalmic Solution, Suspension**
Adults: 1–2 gtt b.i.d. If used to replace another drug, continue the drug being used and add 1 gtt of betaxolol b.i.d. The previous drug should be discontinued the following day. If transferring from several antiglaucoma drugs being used together, adjust one drug at a time at intervals of not less than 1 week. The agents being used can be continued and add 1 gtt betaxolol b.i.d. The next day, another agent should be discontinued. The remaining antiglaucoma drug dosage can be decreased or discontinued depending on the response of the patient.
How Supplied: *Ophthalmic Solution:* 0.5%; *Ophthalmic Suspension:* 0.25%; *Tablet:* 10 mg, 20 mg

EMS CONSIDERATIONS

See also *Beta-Adrenergic Blocking Agents.*

Bethanechol chloride
(beh-THAN-eh-kohl)
Pregnancy Class: C
Duvoid, Urecholine **(Rx)**
Classification: Cholinergic (parasympathomimetic), direct-acting

Mechanism of Action: Directly stimulates cholinergic receptors, primarily muscarinic type. This results in stimulation of gastric motility, increases gastric tone, and stimulates the detrusor muscle of the urinary bladder. Produces a slight transient fall of DBP, accompanied by minor reflex tachycardia. Is resistant to hydrolysis by acetylcholinesterase, which increases its duration of action.
Onset of Action: PO: 30-90 min; **maximum:** 60-90 min; **SC:** 5-15 min; **maximum:** 15-30 min.
Duration of Action: PO: 1 hr (large doses up to 6 hr). **SC:** 2hr.
Uses: Postpartum or postoperative urinary retention, neurogenic atony of the bladder with urinary retention. *Investigational:* Reflux esophagitis in adults and gastroesophageal reflux in infants and children.
Contraindications: Hypotension, hypertension, CAD, coronary occlusion, AV conduction defects, vasomotor instability, pronounced bradycardia, peptic ulcer, bronchial asthma (latent or active), hyperthyroidism, parkinsonism, epilepsy, obstruction of the bladder or bladder neck, if the strength or integrity of the GI or bladder wall is questionable, peritonitis, GI spastic disease, acute inflammatory lesions of the GI tract, when increased muscular activity of the GI tract or urinary bladder might be harmful (e.g., following recent urinary bladder surgery), GI resection and anastomosis, GI obstruction, marked vagotonia. Lactation. Not to be used IM or IV.
Precautions: Safety and effectiveness have not been determined in children.

Route/Dosage
- **Tablets**
    Urinary retention.
Adults, usual: 10–50 mg t.i.d.–q.i.d. The minimum effective dose can be determined by giving 5–10 mg initially and repeating this dose q 1–2 hr until a satisfactory response is observed or a maximum of 50 mg has been given.
    Treat reflux esophagitis in adults.
25 mg q.i.d.
    Gastroesophageal reflex in infants and children.
3 mg/m^2/dose t.i.d.
- **SC**
    Urinary retention.

Adults, usual: 5 mg t.i.d.–q.i.d. The minimum effective dose is determined by giving 2.5 mg initially and repeating this dose at 15–30-min intervals to a maximum of four doses or until a satisfactory response is obtained.

Diagnosis of reflux esophagitis in adults.
Two 50-mcg/kg doses 15 min apart.

How Supplied: *Injection:* 5 mg/mL; *Tablet:* 5 mg, 10 mg, 25 mg, 50 mg

Side Effects: Serious side effects are uncommon with PO dosage but more common following SC use. *GI:* Nausea, diarrhea, salivation, GI upset, involuntary defecation, cramps, colic, belching, rumbling/gurgling of stomach. *CV:* Hypotension with reflex tachycardia, vasomotor response. *CNS:* Headache, malaise. *Other:* Flushing, sensation of heat about the face, sweating, urinary urgency, attacks of asthma, bronchial constriction, miosis, lacrimation.

OD **Overdose Management:** *Symptoms:* Early signs include N&V, abdominal discomfort, salivation, sweating, flushing. *Treatment:* Atropine, 0.6 mg SC for adults; a dose of 0.01 mg/kg atropine SC (up to a maximum of 0.4 mg) is recommended for infants and children up to 12 years of age. IV atropine may be used in emergency situations.

Drug Interactions
Cholinergic inhibitors / Additive cholinergic effects
Ganglionic blocking agents / Critical hypotensive response preceded by severe abdominal symptoms
Procainamide / Antagonism of cholinergic effects
Quinidine / Antagonism of cholinergic effects

EMS CONSIDERATIONS

None.

Bicalutamide
(buy-kah-LOO-tah-myd)
Pregnancy Class: X
Casodex (Rx)
Classification: Antineoplastic, antiandrogen

Mechanism of Action: A nonsteroidal antiandrogen that competitively inhibits the action of androgens by binding to androgen receptors in the cytosol in target tissues. Food does not affect the rate or amount absorbed.

Uses: In combination therapy with a leutinizing hormone-releasing hormone analog for the treatment of advanced prostate cancer.

Contraindications: Pregnancy.

Precautions: Use with caution in patients with moderate to severe hepatic impairment and during lactation. Safety and efficacy have not been established in children.

Route/Dosage
• **Tablets**
Prostatic carcinoma.
50 mg (1 tablet) once daily (morning or evening) in combination with an LHRH analog with or without food.

How Supplied: *Tablet:* 50 mg

Side Effects: *GI:* Constipation, N&V, diarrhea, anorexia, dyspepsia, rectal hemorrhage, dry mouth, melena. *CNS:* Dizziness, paresthesia, insomnia, anxiety, depression, decreased libido, hypertonia, confusion, neuropathy, somnolence, nervousness. *GU:* Gynecomastia, nocturia, hematuria, UTI, impotence, urinary incontinence, urinary frequency, impaired urination, dysuria, urinary retention, urinary urgency. *CV:* Hot flashes (most common), hypertension, angina pectoris, CHF. *Metabolic:* Peripheral edema, hyperglycemia, weight loss or gain, dehydration, gout. *Musculoskeletal:* Myasthenia, arthritis, myalgia, leg cramps, pathologic fracture. *Respiratory:* Dyspnea, increased cough, pharyngitis, bronchitis, pneumonia, rhinitis, lung disorder. *Dermatologic:* Rash, sweating, dry skin, pruritus, alopecia. *Hematologic:* Anemia, hypochromic and iron deficiency anemia. *Body as a whole:* General pain, back pain, asthenia, pelvic pain, abdominal pain, chest pain, flu syndrome, edema, neoplasm, fever, neck pain, chills, ***sepsis***. *Miscellaneous:* Infection, bone pain, headache, breast pain, diabetes mellitus.

Drug Interactions: Bicalutamide may displace coumarin anticoagulants from their protein-binding sites, resulting in an increased anticoagulant effect.

EMS CONSIDERATIONS

See also *Antineoplastic Agents.*

Biperiden hydrochloride
(bye-PER-ih-den)
Pregnancy Class: C
Akineton Hydrochloride **(Rx)**
Classification: Synthetic anticholinergic, antiparkinson agent

Mechanism of Action: Synthetic anticholinergic. Tremor may increase as spasticity is relieved. Slight respiratory and CV effects. Tolerance may develop.
Onset of Action: Time to peak levels: 60–90 min. **t½:** About 18–24 hr.
Uses: Parkinsonism, especially of the postencephalitic, arteriosclerotic, and idiopathic types. Drug-induced (e.g., phenothiazines) extrapyramidal manifestations.
Contraindications: Children under 3 years of age.
Precautions: Use with caution in older children.

Route/Dosage —————————
• **Tablets**
  Parkinsonism.
Adults: 2 mg t.i.d.–q.i.d., to a maximum of 16 mg/day.
  Drug-induced extrapyramidal effects.
Adults: 2 mg 1–3 times/day. Maximum daily dose: 16 mg.
Adults: 2 mg; repeat q 30 min until symptoms improve, but not more than four doses daily. **Pediatric:** 0.04 mg/kg (1.2 mg/m²); repeat q 30 min until symptoms improve, but not more than four doses daily.
How Supplied: *Tablet:* 2 mg.
Side Effects: Muscle weakness, inability to move certain muscles.

EMS CONSIDERATIONS

See also *Antiparkinson Drugs* and *Cholinergic Blocking Agents.*

Bismuth subsalicylate/ Metronidazole/ Tetracycline hydrochloride
(BIS-muth, meh-troh-NYE-dah-zohl, teh-trah-SYE-kleen)
Pregnancy Class: B (Metronidazole), D (Tetracycline)
Helidac **(Rx)**
Classification: Agent to treat *Helicobacter pylori* infections

Mechanism of Action: The information to follow was derived from each drug being given alone and not in the combination in this product.
Onset of Action: Peak plasma levels, metronidazole: 1-2 hr; **t½, elimination:** 8 hr.
Uses: In combination with an H_2 antagonist to treat active duodenal ulcer associated with *H. pylori* infection.
Contraindications: Use during pregnancy or lactation, in children, or in renal or hepatic impairment. Hypersensitivity to bismuth subsalicylate, metronidazole or other imidazole derivatives, and any tetracycline derivatives. Use in those allergic to aspirin or salicylates. Children and teenagers who have or who are recovering from chicken pox or the flu should not take bismuth subsalicylate due to the possibility of Reye's syndrome. Tetracyclines should not be used during tooth development in children (i.e., last half of pregnancy, infancy, and childhood to 8 years of age) due to the possibility of permanent tooth discoloration.
Precautions: Use with caution in elderly patients and in patients with evidence or history of blood dyscrasias. Safety and efficacy have not been determined in children.

Route/Dosage —————————
• **Tablets (Bismuth Subsalicylate, Metronidazole) and Capsules (Tetracycline Hydrochloride)**
  Treatment of H. pylori.
Each dose includes two pink, round chewable tablets (525 mg bismuth

subsalicylate), one white tablet (250 mg metronidazole), and one pale orange and white capsule (500 mg tetracycline hydrochloride). Each dose is taken q.i.d. with meals and at bedtime for 14 days. *NOTE:* Concomitant therapy with an H₂ antagonist is also required.

How Supplied: *Patient Pak. Capsule:* Tetracycline hydrochloride, 500 mg; *Tablets:* Bismuth subsalicylate, 262.4 mg; Metronidzole, 250 mg.

Side Effects: See also *Metronidazole* and *Tetracyclines* for specific side effects for these drugs. The following side effects were noted when the three drugs were given concomitantly. *GI:* N&V, diarrhea, abdominal pain, melena, anal discomfort, anorexia, constipation. *CNS:* Dizziness, paresthesia, insomnia. *Miscellaneous:* Asthenia, pain, upper respiratory infection.

Excessive doses of bismuth subsalicylate may cause neurotoxicity, which is reversible if therapy is terminated. Large doses of metronidazole have been associated with seizures and peripheral neuropathy (characterized by numbness or paresthesia of an extremity). Metronidazole may exacerbate candidiasis. Tetracycline use may cause superinfection, benign intracranial hypertension (pseudotumor cerebri), and photosensitivity.

Drug Interactions: See also *Metronidazole,* and *Tetracyclines.* There may be a decrease in absorption of tetracycline due to the presence of bismuth or calcium carbonate (an excipient in bismuth subsalicylate tablets).

EMS CONSIDERATIONS

See also *Metronidazole,* and *Tetracycline hydrochloride.*
Administration/Storage
1. Bismuth subsalicylate may cause darkening of the tongue and black stools, do not confuse with melena.
2. The bismuth subsalicylate tablets should be chewed and swallowed. Take Metronidazole and tetracycline whole with 8 oz of water.
3. Ingest adequate fluids, especially with the bedtime dose, in order to decrease the risk of esophageal irritation and ulceration.
4. If a dose is missed, it can be made up by continuing the normal dosage schedule until the medication is gone. Double doses are not to be taken. Report if more than four doses are missed.

Assessment
1. Note clinical presentation and characteristics of symptoms, including onset and duration.
2. Document any allergy to aspirin or salicylates.
3. Determine women of child-bearing age are not pregnant. Do not use in children under age 8.
4. Obtain CBC, liver and renal function studies; note dysfunction.
5. Document serum and/or endoscopic confirmation of organism.
6. Note H₂ agent prescribed; therapy requires an H₂ antagonist.

Bisoprolol fumarate
(BUY-soh-proh-lol)
Pregnancy Class: C
Zibeta **(Rx)**
Classification: Beta-adrenergic blocking agent

Mechanism of Action: Inhibits beta-1-adrenergic receptors and, at higher doses, beta-2 receptors. No intrinsic sympathomimetic activity and no membrane-stabilizing activity.
Onset of Action: t½: 9-12 hr.
Uses: Hypertension alone or in combination with other antihypertensive agents. *Investigational:* Angina pectoris, SVTs, PVCs.
Precautions: Use with catuion during lactation. Safety and efficacy have not been determined in children. Since bisoprolol is selective for beta-1 receptors, it may be used with caution in patients with bronchospastic disease who do not repond to, or who cannot tolerate, other antihypertensive therapy.

Route/Dosage —————
• **Tablets**
Antihypertensive.
Dose must be individualized. **Adults, initial:** 5 mg once daily (in some pa-

tients, 2.5 mg/day may be appropriate). **Maintenance:** If the 5-mg dose is inadequate, the dose may be increased to 10 mg/day and then, if needed, to 20 mg once daily. In patients with impaired renal or hepatic function, the initial daily dose should be 2.5 mg with caution used in titrating the dose upward.

How Supplied: *Tablet:* 5 mg, 10 mg

EMS CONSIDERATIONS

See also *Beta-Adrenergic Blocking Agents.*

————*COMBINATION DRUG*————

Bisoprolol fumarate and Hydrochlorothiazide

(BUY-soh-proh-lol, high-droh-klor-oh-THIGH-ah-zyd)
Pregnancy Class: C
Ziac **(Rx)**
Classification: Antihypertensive

Uses: First-line therapy in mild to moderate hypertension.
Contraindications: Use in bronchospastic pulmonary disease, cardiogenic shock, overt CHF, second- or third-degree AV block, marked sinus bradycardia, anuria, hypersensitivity to either drug or to other sulfonamide-derived drugs, during lactation.
Precautions: Use with caution in patients with peripheral vascular disease, impaired renal or hepatic function, and progressive liver disease and in patients also receiving myocardial depressants or inhibitors of AV conduction such as verapamil, diltiazem, and disopyramide. Elderly patients may be more sensitive to the effects of this drug product. Safety and effectiveness have not been determined in children.

Route/Dosage ————————
• **Tablets**
  Antihypertensive.
Adults, initial: One 2.5/6.25-mg tablet given once daily. If needed, the dose may be increased q 14 days to a maximum of two 10/6.25-mg tablets given once daily.

How Supplied: *Beta-adrenergic blocking agent:* Bisoprolol fumarate: 2.5, 5, or 10 mg. *Diuretic/antihypertensive:* Hydrochlorothiazide: 6.25 mg in all tablets.
Side Effects: See individual drugs. Most commonly, dizziness and fatigue. At higher doses, bisoprolol inhibits beta-2-adrenergic receptors located in bronchial and vascular muscle.

Drug Interactions
Antihypertensives / Additive effect to decrease BP
Cyclopropane / Additive depression of myocardium
Trichloroethylene / Additive depression of myocardium

EMS CONSIDERATIONS

See also *Bisoprolol fumarate* and *Hydrochlorothiazide.*

Bitolterol mesylate

(bye-TOHL-ter-ohl)
Pregnancy Class: C
Tornalate Aerosol **(Rx)**
Classification: Bronchodilator

Mechanism of Action: Bitolterol is a prodrug in that it is converted by esterases in the body to the active colterol. Colterol combines with beta-2-adrenergic receptors, producing dilation of bronchioles. Minimal beta-1-adrenergic activity.
Onset of Action: Following inhalation: 3-4 min. **Time to peak effect:** 30-60 min.
Duration of Action: 5-8 hr.
Uses: Prophylaxis and treatment of bronchial asthma and bronchospasms. Treatment of bronchitis, emphysema, bronchiectasis, and COPD. May be used with theophylline and/or steroids.
Precautions: Safety has not been established for use during lactation and in children less than 12 years of age. Use with caution in ischemic heart disease, hypertension, hyperthyroidism, diabetes mellitus, cardiac arrhythmias, seizure disorders, or in those who respond unusually to

beta-adrenergic agonists. There may be decreased effectiveness in steroid-dependent asthmatic patients. Hypersensitivity reactions may occur.

Route/Dosage
• **Metered Dose Inhaler**
  Bronchodilation.

Adults and children over 12 years: 2 inhalations at an interval of 1–3 min q 8 hr (if necessary, a third inhalation may be taken). The dose should not exceed 3 inhalations q 6 hr or 2 inhalations q 4 hr.
  Prophylaxis of bronchospasm.

Adults and children over 12 years: 2 inhalations q 8 hr.

How Supplied: *Metered dose inhaler:* 0.37 mg/inh; *Solution:* 0.2%

Side Effects: Additional Side Effects: *CNS:* Hyperactivity, hyperkinesia, lightheadedness. *CV:* Premature ventricular contractions. *Other:* Throat irritation.

Drug Interactions: Additive effects with other beta-adrenergic bronchodilators.

EMS CONSIDERATIONS

See also *Sympathomimetic Drugs.*

Bretylium tosylate
(breh-TILL-ee-um TOZ-ill-ayt)
Pregnancy Class: C
Bretylol **(Rx)**
Classification: Antiarrhythmic, class III

Mechanism of Action: Inhibits catecholamine release at nerve endings by decreasing excitability of the nerve terminal. Initially there is a release of norepinephrine, which may cause tachycardia and a rise in BP; this is followed by a blockade of release of catecholamines. Also increases the duration of the action potential and the effective refractory period, which may assist in reversing arrhythmias.

Onset of Action: Peak plasma concentration and effect: 1 hr after IM injection. Antifibrillatory effect within a few minutes after IV use. Suppression of ventricular tachycardia and ventricular arrhythmias takes 20-120 min, whereas suppression of PVCs does not occur for 6-9 hr.

Duration of Action: 6-8 hr.

Uses: Life-threatening ventricular arrhythmias that have failed to respond to other antiarrhythmics. Prophylaxis and treatment of ventricular fibrillation. For short-term use only. *Investigational:* Second-line drug (after lidocaine) for advanced cardiac life support during CPR.

Contraindications: Severe aortic stenosis, severe pulmonary hypertension.

Precautions: Safety and efficacy in children have not been established. Dosage adjustment is required in patients with impaired renal function.

Route/Dosage
• **IV**
  Ventricular fibrillation, hemodynamically unstable ventricular tachycardia.

Adults: 5 mg/kg of undiluted solution given rapidly. Can increase to 10 mg/kg if ventricular fibrillation persists; repeat as needed. **Maintenance, IV infusion:** 1–2 mg/min; or, 5–10 mg/kg q 6 hr of diluted drug infused over more than 8 min. **Children:** 5 mg/kg/dose IV followed by 10 mg/kg at 15–30-min intervals for a maximum total dose of 30 mg/kg; **maintenance:** 5–10 mg/kg q 6 hr.
  Other ventricular arrhythmias.

• **IV Infusion**
5–10 mg/kg of diluted solution over more than 8 min. **Maintenance:** 5–10 mg/kg q 6 hr over a period of 8 min or more or 1–2 mg/min by continuous IV infusion. **Children:** 5–10 mg/kg/dose q 6 hr.

• **IM**
  Other ventricular arrhythmias.

Adults: 5–10 mg/kg of undiluted solution followed, if necessary, by the same dose at 1–2-hr intervals; **then,** give same dosage q 6–8 hr.

How Supplied: *Injection:* 50 mg/mL

Side Effects: *CV:* Hypotension (including postural hypotension), transient hypertension, increased frequency of PVCs, bradycardia, precipitation of anginal attacks, initial increase in arrhythmias, sensation of substernal pressure. *GI:* N&V (especially after rapid IV administration), diarrhea, abdominal pain, hiccoughs. *CNS:* Vertigo, dizziness, lightheadedness, syncope, anxiety, paranoid psychosis, confusion, mood swings. *Miscellaneous:* Renal dysfunction, flushing, hyperthermia, SOB, nasal stuffiness, diaphoresis, conjunctivitis, erythematous macular rash, lethargy, generalized tenderness.

OD **Overdose Management:** *Symptoms:* Marked hypertension followed by hypotension. *Treatment:* Treat hypertension with nitroprusside or another short-acting IV antihypertensive. Treat hypotension with appropriate fluid therapy and pressor agents such as norepinephrine or dopamine.

Drug Interactions

Digitoxin, Digoxin / Bretylium may aggravate digitalis toxicity due to initial release of norepinephrine

Procainamide, Quinidine / Concomitant use with bretylium ↓ inotropic effect of bretylium and ↑ hypotension

EMS CONSIDERATIONS

See also *Antiarrhythmic Agents.*
Administration/Storage
1. For IM injection, use drug undiluted.
2. Rotate injection sites so that no more than 5 mL of drug is given at any site.
3. Keep supine during therapy or closely observe for postural hypotension.
IV 4. For IV infusion, bretylium is compatible with D5W, 0.9% NaCl.
5. For direct IV, administer undiluted over 15–30 sec; may repeat in 15–30 min if symptoms persist. May further dilute 500 mg in 50 mL and infuse over 10–30 min.
Interventions
1. Monitor VS and rhythm strips as dose is titrated on patient response.
2. To reduce N&V, administer IV slowly over 10 min while supine. Once infusion complete remain supine until the BP has stabilized.

3. Bretylium often causes a fall in supine BP within 1 hr of IV administration. If SBP < 75 mm Hg, anticipate need for pressor agents.

B

Brinzolamide ophthalmic suspension

(brin-ZOH-lah-myd)
Pregnancy Class: C
Azopt **(Rx)**
Classification: Antiglaucoma drug

Mechanism of Action: Inhibits carbonic hydrase in the ciliary processes of the eye, thus decreasing aqueous humor production and reducing intraocular pressure (IOP). Is absorbed into the systemic circulation following ocular use.

Uses: Treatment of elevated IOP in ocular hypertension or open-angle glaucoma.

Contraindications: Use in those with severe renal impairment (C_{CR} less than 30 mL/min). Concomitant use with oral carbonic anhydrase inhibitors. Lactation.

Precautions: Is a sulfonamide; thus, similar side effects can occur. Use with caution in hepatic impairment. Safety and efficacy have not been determined in children.

Route/Dosage
• **Ophthalmic suspension**
  Increased intraocular pressure.
  1 gtt in the affected eye(s) t.i.d.
How Supplied: *Ophthalmic Suspension:* 1%

Side Effects: *Ophthalmic:* Blurred vision following dosing, blepharitis, dry eye, foreign body sensation, hyperemia, ocular discharge, ocular discomfort, ocular keratitis, ocular pain, ocular pruritus, rhinitis, conjunctivitis, diplopia, eye fatigue, keratoconjunctivitis, keratopathy, lid margin crusting or sticky sensation, tearing, hypertonia. *GI:* Bitter, sour, or unusual taste; nausea, diarrhea, dry mouth, dyspepsia. *CNS:* Headache, dizziness. *Miscellaneous:* Dermatitis, allergic reactions, alopecia, chest

---

bold italic = life threatening side effect

pain, dyspnea, kidney pain, pharyngitis, urticaria.

Drug Interactions: Possible additive effects with oral carbonic anhydrase inhibitors.

EMS CONSIDERATIONS

None.

Bromocriptine mesylate

(broh-moh-KRIP-teen)
Pregnancy Class: B
Parlodel **(Rx)**
Classification: Prolactin secretion inhibitor; antiparkinson agent

Mechanism of Action: Nonhormonal agent that inhibits the release of the hormone prolactin by the pituitary. Use only when prolactin production by pituitary tumors has been ruled out. Effect in parkinsonism is due to a direct stimulating effect on dopamine type 2 receptors in the corpus striatum. Use for parkinsonism may allow the dose of levodopa to be decreased, thus decreasing the incidence of severe side effects following long-term levodopa therapy.

Onset of Action: Lower prolactin: 2 hr. **antiparkinson:** 30-90 min; **decreased growth hormone:** 1-2 hr.

Duration of Action: Lower prolactin: 24 hr (after a single dose); **decrease growth hormone:** 4-8 hr.

Uses: Short-term treatment of amenorrhea with or without galactorrhea, infertilitiy, or hypogonadism. Alone or as an adjunct in the treatment of acromegaly. As adjunctive therapy with levodopa in the treatment of idiopathic or postencephalitic Parkinson's disease. May provide additional benefit in patients who are taking optimal doses of levodopa, in those who are developing tolerance to levodopa therapy, or in those who are manifesting levodopa "end of dose failure." Patients unresponsive to levodopa are not good candidates for bromocriptine therapy. No longer recommended to suppress postpartum lactation. *Investigational:* Hyperprolactinemia due to pituitary adenoma, neuroleptic malignant syndrome, co-caine dependence, cyclical mastalgia.

Contraindications: Sensitivity to ergot alkaloids. Pregnancy, lactation, children under 15 years of age. Peripheral vascular disease, ischemic heart disease.

Precautions: Geriatric patients may manifest more CNS effects. Use with caution in liver or kidney disease.

Route/Dosage ───────────

• **Capsules, Tablets**
  For hyperprolactinemic conditions.
Adults, initial: 0.5–2.5 mg/day with meals; **then,** increase dose by 2.5 mg q 3–7 days until optimum response observed (usual: 5–7.5 mg/day; range: 2.5–15 mg/day). For amenorrhea/galactorrhea, do not use for more than 6 months. Side effects may be reduced by temporarily decreasing the dose to ½ tablet 2–3 times/day.
  Parkinsonism.
Initial: 1.25 mg (½ tablet) b.i.d. with meals while maintaining dose of levodopa, if possible. Dosage may be increased q 14–28 days by 2.5 mg/day with meals. The usual dosage range is 10–40 mg/day. Any decrease in dosage should be done gradually in 2.5-mg decrements.
  Acromegaly.
Initial: 1.25–2.5 mg for 3 days with food and on retiring; **then,** increased by 1.25–2.5 mg q 3–7 days until optimum response observed. Usual optimum therapeutic range: 20–30 mg/day, not to exceed 100 mg/day. Patients should be reevaluated monthly and dosage adjusted accordingly.
  Hyperprolactinemia associated with pituitary adenomas.
Maintenance: 0.625–10 mg/day for 6 to 52 months.

How Supplied: *Capsule:* 5 mg; *Tablet:* 2.5 mg

Side Effects: The type and incidence of side effects depend on the use of the drug. *When used for hyperprolactinemia. GI:* N&V, abdominal cramps, diarrhea, constipation. *CNS:* Headache, dizziness, fatigue, drowsiness, lightheadedness, psychoses. *Other:* Nasal congestion, hypotension, CSF rhinorrhea.

When used for acromegaly. GI: N&V, anorexia, dry mouth, dyspepsia, indigestion, GI bleeding. *CNS:* Dizziness, syncope, drowsiness, tiredness, headache, lightheadedness, lassitude, vertigo, sluggishness, paranoia, insomnia, heavy headedness, decreased sleep requirement, delusional psychosis, visual hallucinations. *CV:* Orthostatic hypotension, digital vasospasm, Raynaud's syndrome; rarely, arrhythmias, ventricular tachycardia, bradycardia, vasovagal attack. *Respiratory:* Nasal stuffiness, SOB. *Other:* Potentiation of effects of alcohol, hair loss, paresthesia, tingling of ears, muscle cramps, facial pallor, reduced tolerance to cold.

When used for parkinsonism. GI: N&V, abdominal discomfort, constipation, anorexia, dry mouth, dysphagia. *CNS:* Confusion, hallucinations, fainting, drowsiness, dizziness, insomnia, depression, vertigo, anxiety, fatigue, headache, lethargy, nightmares. *GU:* Urinary incontinence, urinary retention, urinary frequency. *Other:* Abnormal involuntary movements, asthenia, visual disturbances, ataxia, hypotension, SOB, edema of feet and ankles, blepharospasm, erythromelalgia, skin mottling, nasal stuffiness, paresthesia, skin rash.

Drug Interactions
Alcohol / ↑ Chance of GI toxicity; alcohol intolerance
Antihypertensives / Additive ↓ BP
Butyrophenones / ↓ Effect of bromocriptine because butyrophenones are dopamine antagonists
Diuretics / Should be avoided during bromocriptine therapy
Erythromycins / ↑ Levels of bromocriptine → ↑ pharmacologic and toxic effects
Phenothiazines / ↓ Effect of bromocriptine because phenothiazines are dopamine antagonists
Sympathomimetics / ↑ Side effects of bromocriptine, including ventricular tachycardia and cardiac dysfunction

EMS CONSIDERATIONS
None.

Brompheniramine maleate
(brohm-fen-EAR-ah-meen)
Pregnancy Class: B
Brombay, Chlorphed, Conjec-B, Cophene-B, Diamine T.D., Dimetane Extentabs, Dimetane-Ten, Histaject Modified, Nasahist B, ND Stat Revised, Oraminic II, Sinusol-B, Veltane (Rx; Dimetane and Dimetane Extentabs are OTC)
Classification: Antihistamine, alkylamine type

Mechanism of Action: Fewer sedative effects.
Onset of Action: Time to peak effect: 3-9 hr.
Duration of Action: 4-25 hr.
Uses: Allergic rhinitis (oral). Parenterally to treat allergic reactions to blood or plasma; adjunct to treat anaphylaxis; uncomplicated allergic conditions when PO therapy is not possible or is contraindicated.
Contraindications: Use in neonates.
Precautions: Geriatric patients may be more sensitive to the usual adult dose.

Route/Dosage ————
• **Liqui-Gels**
Allergic rhinitis.
Adults and children over 12 years: 4 mg q 4–6 hr, not to exceed 24 mg/day.
• **IM, IV, SC**
Adults: usual, 10 mg (range: 5–20 mg) b.i.d. (maximum daily dose: 40 mg); **pediatric, under 12 years:** 0.5 mg/kg/day (15 mg/m²/day) divided into three or four doses.
How Supplied: *Capsule:* 4 mg; *Elixir:* 2 mg/5 mL; *Injection:* 10 mg/mL; *Tablet:* 4 mg; *Tablet, Extended Release:* 12 mg

EMS CONSIDERATIONS
See also *Antihistamines.*

---

bold italic = life threatening side effect

Budesonide

(byou-DES-oh-nyd)
Pregnancy Class: C
Pulmicort Turbuhaler, Rhinocort, Rhinocort Aquaor **(Rx)**
Classification: Corticosteroid

Mechanism of Action: Exerts a direct local anti-inflammatory effect with minimal systemic effects when used intranasally. Exceeding the recommended dose may result in suppression of hypothalamic-pituitary-adrenal function.
Onset of Action: t½: 2-3 hr.

Uses: Treat symptoms of seasonal or perennial allergic rhinitis in both adults and children. Also, nonallergic perennial rhinitis in adults. The Turbuhaler is used for maintenance and prophylaxis of asthma in adults and children 6 years of age and older; also for those requiring oral corticosteroid therapy for asthma.

Contraindications: Hypersensitivity to the drug. Untreated localized nasal mucosa infections. Lactation. Use in children less than 6 years of age or for acute or life-threatening asthma attacks, including status asthmaticus.

Precautions: Use with caution in patients already on alternate day corticosteroids (e.g., prednisone), in patients with active or quiescent tuberculosis infections of the respiratory tract, or in untreated fungal, bacterial, or systemic viral infections or ocular herpes simplex. Use with caution in patients with recent nasal septal ulcers, recurrent epistaxis, nasal surgery, or trauma. Exposure to chicken pox or measles should be avoided.

Route/Dosage

• **Inhalation Aerosol**
Seasonal or perennial rhinitis.
Adults and children 6 years of age and older, initial: 256 mcg/day given as either 2 sprays in each nostril in the morning and evening or 4 sprays in each nostril in the morning. Doses greater than 256 mcg/day are not recommended. **Maintenance:** Reduce initial dose to the smallest amount necessary to control symptoms; decrease dose q 2–4 weeks as long as desired effect is maintained. If symptoms return, the dose may be increased briefly to the initial dose.

• **Pulmicort Turbuhaler**
Prevention or treatment of asthma.
Adults: 200–400 mcg b.i.d. **Children, over 6 years of age:** 200 mcg b.i.d. 200 mcg released with each actuation actually delivers about 160 mcg to the patient.

How Supplied: *Inhalation Powder:* 200 mcg/inh

Side Effects: *Respiratory:* Nasopharyngeal irritation, nasal irritation, pharyngitis, increased cough, hoarseness, nasal pain, burning, stinging, dryness, epistaxis, bloody mucus, rebound congestion, **bronchial asthma,** occasional sneezing attacks (especially in children), rhinorrhea, reduced sense of smell, throat discomfort, ulceration of the nasal mucosa, sore throat, dyspnea, localized infections of nose and pharynx with *Candida albicans,* wheezing (rare). *CNS:* Lightheadedness, headache, nervousness. *GI:* Nausea, loss of sense of taste, bad taste in mouth, dry mouth, dyspepsia. *Miscellaneous:* Watery eyes, **immediate and delayed hypersensitivity reactions,** moniliasis, facial edema, rash, pruritus, herpes simplex, alopecia, arthralgia, myalgia, contact dermatitis (rare).

OD **Overdose Management:** *Symptoms:* Symptoms of hypercorticism, including menstrual irregularities, acneiform lesions, and cushingoid features (all are rarely seen, however). *Treatment:* Discontinue the drug slowly using procedures that are acceptable for discontinuing oral corticosteroids.

EMS CONSIDERATIONS

See also *Corticosteroids.*

Bumetanide

(byou-MET-ah-nyd)
Pregnancy Class: C
Bumex **(Rx)**
Classification: Loop diuretic

Mechanism of Action: Inhibits reabsorption of both sodium and chloride in the proximal tubule as well as the ascending loop of Henle.
Onset of Action: PO: 30-60 min.
Peak effect, PO: 1-2 hr. **IV:** Several minutes. **Peak effect, IV:** 15-30 min.
Duration of Action: PO: 4-6 hr. **IV:** 3.5-4 hr.
Uses: Edema associated with CHF, nephrotic syndrome, hepatic disease. Adjunct to treat acute pulmonary edema. Especially useful in patients refractory to other diuretics. *Investigational:* Treatment of adult nocturia. Not effective in males with prostatic hypertrophy.
Contraindications: Anuria. Hepatic coma or severe electrolyte depletion until the condition is improved or corrected. Hypersensitivity to the drug. Lactation.
Precautions: Safety and efficacy in children under 18 have not been established. Geriatric patients may be more sensitive to the hypotensive and electrolyte effects and are at greater risk in developing thromboembolic problems and circulatory collapse. SLE may be activated or make worse. Patients allergic to sulfonamides may show cross sensitivity to bumetanide. Sudden changes in electrolyte balance may cause hepatic encephalopathy and coma in patients with hepatic cirrhosis and ascites.

Route/Dosage ────────────
• **Tablets**
Adults: 0.5–2 mg once daily; if response is inadequate, a second or third dose may be given at 4–5-hr intervals up to a maximum of 10 mg/day.
• **IV, IM**
Adults: 0.5–1 mg; if response is inadequate, a second or third dose may be given at 2–3-hr intervals up to a maximum of 10 mg/day. Initiate PO dosing as soon as possible.
How Supplied: *Injection:* 0.25 mg/mL; *Tablet:* 0.5 mg, 1 mg, 2 mg
Side Effects: *Electrolyte and fluid changes:* Excess water loss, *dehydra-*

tion, electrolyte depletion including hypokalemia, hypochloremia, hyponatremia; hypovolemia, thromboembolism, *circulatory collapse. Otic:* Tinnitus, reversible and irreversible hearing impairment, deafness, vertigo (with a sense of fullness in the ears).
CV: Reduction in blood volume may cause circulatory collapse and vascular thrombosis and embolism, especially in geriatric patients. Hypotension, ECG changes, chest pain. *CNS:* Asterixis, encephalopathy with preexisting liver disease, vertigo, headache, dizziness. *GI:* Upset stomach, dry mouth, N&V, diarrhea, GI pain. *GU:* Premature ejaculation, difficulty maintaining erection, renal failure. *Musculoskeletal:* Arthritic pain, weakness, muscle cramps, fatigue. *Hematologic:* Agranulocytosis, thrombocytopenia. *Allergic:* Pruritus, urticaria, rashes. *Miscellaneous:* Sweating, hyperventilation, rash, nipple tenderness, photosensitivity, pain following parenteral use.
OD **Overdose Management:** *Symptoms: Profound loss of water, electrolyte depletion, dehydration, decreased blood volume, circulatory collapse (possibility of vascular thrombosis and embolism).* Symptoms of electrolyte depletion include: anorexia, cramps, weakness, dizziness, vomiting, and mental confusion. *Treatment:* Replace electrolyte and fluid losses and monitor urinary electrolyte levels as well as serum electrolytes. Emesis or gastric lavage. Oxygen or artificial respiration may be necessary. General supportive measures.

EMS CONSIDERATIONS
See also *Diuretics, Loop.*

Buprenorphine hydrochloride
(byou-pren-OR-feen)
Pregnancy Class: C
Buprenex **(C-V) (Rx)**
Classification: Narcotic agonist/antagonist

Mechanism of Action: Semisynthetic opiate possessing both narcot-

B

ic agonist and antagonist activity. It has limited activity at the mu receptor. Is about equipotent with naloxone as a narcotic antagonist.

Onset of Action: IM: 15 min. **Peak effect:** 1 hr. May also be given IV with shorter onset and peak effect.

Duration of Action: 6 hr.

Uses: Moderate to severe pain.

Precautions: Use during lactation only if benefits outweigh risks. Use in children less than 2 years of age has not been established. Use with caution in patients with compromised respiratory function, in head injuries, in impairment of liver or renal function, Addison's disease, prostatic hypertrophy, biliary tract dysfunction, urethral stricture, myxedema, and hypothyroidism. Administration to individuals physically dependent on narcotics may result in precipetation of a withdrawal syndrome.

Route/Dosage
• **IM, Slow IV**
    Analgesia.

Over 13 years of age: 0.3 mg q 6 hr. Up to 0.6 mg may be given; doses greater than 0.6 mg not recommended. **Children, 2–12 years of age:** 2–6 mcg/kg q 4–6 hr. Do not give single doses greater than 6 mcg/kg.

How Supplied: *Injection:* Equivalent to 0.3 mg/mL buprenorphine

Side Effects: *CNS:* Sedation, dizziness, confusion, headache, euphoria, slurred speech, depression, paresthesia, psychosis, malaise, hallucinations, coma, dysphoria, agitation, seizures. *GI:* N&V, constipation, dyspepsia, loss of appetite, dry mouth. *Ophthalmologic:* Miosis, blurred vision, double vision, conjunctivitis. *CV:* Hypotension, bradycardia, tachycardia, Wenckebach block. *Respiratory:* Decreased respiratory rate, cyanosis, dyspepsia. *Dermatologic:* Sweating, rash, pruritus, flushing. *Other:* Urinary retention, chills, tinnitus.

Drug Interactions: Additive CNS depression with alcohol, general anesthetics, antianxiety agents, sedative-hypnotics, phenothiazines, and other narcotic analgesics.

EMS CONSIDERATIONS

See also *Narcotic Analgestics.*

Bupropion hydrochloride
(byou-PROH-pee-on)
Pregnancy Class: B
Wellbutrin, Wellbutrin SR, Zyban **(Rx)**
Classification: Antidepressant, miscellaneous

Mechanism of Action: Bupropion is an antidepressant whose mechanism of action is not known; the drug does not inhibit MAO and it only weakly blocks neuronal uptake of epinephrine, serotonin, and dopamine. Exerts moderate anticholinergic and sedative effects, but only slight orthostatic hypotension.

Onset of Action: Peak plasma levels: 2-3 hr. **t½:** 8-24 hr.

Uses: Short-term (6 weeks or less) treatment of depression. Aid to stop smoking (may be combined with a nicotine transdermal system).

Contraindications: Seizure disorders; presence or history of bulimia or anorexia nervosa due to the higher incidence of seizures in such patients. Concomitant use of an MAO inhibitor. Wellbutrin, Wellbutrin SR, and Zyban all contain bupropion; do not use together.

Precautions: Use with caution in patients with a history of seizures, cranial trauma, with drugs that lower the seizure threshold, and other situations that might cause seizures (e.g., abrupt cessation of a benzodiazepine). Use with caution and in lower doses in patients with liver or kidney disease and in those with a recent history of MI or unstable heart disease. Assess benefits versus risks during lactation. Safety and efficacy have not been established in patients less than 18 years of age.

Route/Dosage
• **Tablets**
    Antidepressant.

Adults, initial: 100 mg in the morning and evening for the first 3 days; **then,** 100 mg t.i.d., given in the morning, midday, and in the evening (6 hr should elapse between doses). If no response is observed after 4 weeks or longer, the dose may be increased to 450 mg/day with individual doses not to exceed 150 mg. Doses higher than 450 mg should not be administered. The sustained-release dosage form may be used for twice-daily dosing. **Maintenance:** Lowest dose to control depression.

Smoking deterrent.

Begin dosing at 150 mg/day for the first 3 days followed by 150 mg b.i.d. Eight hours or more should elapse between successive doses.

How Supplied: *Tablet:* 75 mg, 100 mg; *Tablet Extended Release:* 100 mg, 150 mg

Side Effects: Listed are side effects with an incidence of 0.1% or greater. *CNS:* Insomnia, abnormal dreams, dizziness, disturbed concentration, nervousness, tremor, dysphoria, somnolence, agitation, abnormal thinking, depression, irritability, CNS stimulation, confusion, decreased memory, depersonalization, emotional lability, hostility, hyperkinesia, hypertonia, hypesthesia, paresthesia, suicidal ideation, vertigo. *GI:* Nausea, dry mouth, constipation, diarrhea, anorexia, mouth ulcer, thirst, increased appetite, dyspepsia, flatulence, vomiting, abnormal liver function, bruxism, dysphagia, gastric reflux, gingivitis, glossitis, jaundice, stomatitis. *CV:* Palpitations, hypertension, flushing, migraine, postural hypotension, hot flashes, **stroke,** tachycardia, vasodilation. *Body as a whole:* Abdominal pain, accidental injury, neck pain, chest pain, facial edema, asthenia, fever, headache, back pain, chills, inguinal hernia, musculoskeletal chest pain, pain, photosensitivity. *Dermatologic:* Rash, pruritus, urticaria, dry skin, sweating, acne, dry skin. *Musculoskeletal:* Arthralgia, myalgia, leg cramps. *Respiratory:* Rhinitis, bronchitis, increased cough, pharyngitis, sinusitis, epistaxis, dyspnea. *GU:* Urinary frequency, impotence, polyuria, urinary urgency. *Ophthalmic:* Amblyopia, abnormal accommoda-

tion, dry eye. *Miscellaneous:* Taste perversion, tinnitus, ecchymosis, edema, increased weight, peripheral edema.

OD Overdose Management: *Symptoms:* Seizures, hallucinations, loss of consciousness, tachycardia, multiple uncontrolled seizures, bradycardia, fever, muscle rigidity, hypotension, rhabdomyolysis, stupor, coma, respiratory failure, cardiac failure and cardiac arrest prior to death. *Treatment:* Patient should be hospitalized. If conscious, syrup of ipecac is given to induce vomiting followed by activated charcoal q 6 hr during the first 12 hr after ingestion. Monitor both ECG and EEG for 48 hr; fluid intake must be adequate. If the patient is in a stupor, is comatose, or is convulsing, gastric lavage may be undertaken provided intubation of the airway has been performed. Seizures may be treated with IV benzodiazepines and other supportive procedures.

Drug Interactions

Alcohol / Alcohol ↓ seizure threshold; use with bupropion may precipitate seizures

Amantadine / Psychotic reactions

Carbamazepine / ↑ Bupropion metabolism → ↓ plasma levels

Cimetidine / Cimetidine inhibits the metabolism of bupropion

Fluoxetine / Panic symptoms and psychotic reactions

Levodopa / ↑ Risk of side effects

MAO inhibitors / Acute toxicity to bupropion may ↑ , especially if used with phenelzine

Phenobarbital / ↑ Bupropion metabolism → ↓ plasma levels

Phenytoin / ↑ Bupropion metabolism → ↓ plasma levels

Retonavir / ↑ Risk of bupropion toxicity

EMS CONSIDERATIONS

None.

Buspirone hydrochloride
(byou-SPYE-rohn)
Pregnancy Class: B

---

bold italic = life threatening side effect

BuSpar **(Rx)**
Classification: Nonbenzodiazepine antianxiety agent

Mechanism of Action: The mechanism of action is unknown. Not chemically related to the benzodiazepines; no anticonvulsant, muscle relaxant properties, or significant sedation has been observed. Binds to serotonin (5-HT$_{1A}$) and dopamine (D$_2$) receptors in the CNS; it is thus possible that dopamine-mediated neurologic disorders may occur. These include dystonia, Parkinson-like symptoms, akathisia, and tardive dyskinesia.

Onset of Action: 40-90 min after a single PO dose of 20 mg. **t½:** 2-3 hr.

Uses: Anxiety disorders, short-term use to relieve symptoms of anxiety due to motor tension, apprehension, autonomic hyperactivity, or hyperattentiveness.

Contraindications: Psychoses, severe liver or kidney impairment, lactation. Not usually indicated for treatment of anxiety and tension due to stress of everyday living.

Precautions: Safety and efficacy in children less than 18 years of age not established. A decrease in dose may be necessary in geriatric patients due to age-related impairment of renal function.

Route/Dosage
• **Tablets**
Adults: 5 mg t.i.d. Dosage may be increased in increments of 5 mg/day q 2–3 days to achieve optimum effects; the total daily dose should not exceed 60 mg. BuSpar is available in a 15-mg tablet that is scored in 5-mg increments and notched in 7.5-mg increments so patients can take the drug b.i.d. rather than t.i.d.

How Supplied: *Tablet:* 5 mg, 10 mg, 15 mg

Side Effects: *CNS:* Dizziness, drowsiness, insomnia, fatigue, nervousness, excitement, dream disturbances, dysphoria, noise intolerance, euphoria, depersonalization, akathisia, hallucinations, suicidal ideation, seizures, decreased concentration, confusion, anger or hostility, depression. *CV:* Nonspecific chest pain, hypotension, palpitations, tachycardia, syncope, hypertension. *GI:* N&V, diarrhea, constipation, abdominal distress, dry mouth, altered taste, increased appetite, irritable colon. *Ophthalmologic:* Redness and itching of eyes, conjunctivitis, photophobia, eye pain. *Dermatologic:* Skin rash, pruritus, dry skin, edema of face, acne, easy bruising, flushing. *Neurologic:* Paresthesia, tremor, numbness, incoordination. *GU:* Urinary hesitancy or frequency, enuresis, amenorrhea, pelvic inflammatory disease. *Miscellaneous:* Tinnitus, sore throat, nasal congestion, altered smell, muscle aches or pains, skin rash, headache, sweating, hyperventilation, SOB, hair loss, galactorrhea, decreased or increased libido, delayed ejaculation.

OD **Overdose Management:** *Symptoms:* Dizziness, drowsiness, N&V, gastric distress, miosis. *Treatment:* Immediate gastric lavage; general symptomatic and supportive measures.

Drug Interactions: Use with MAO inhibitors may cause an increase in BP.

EMS CONSIDERATIONS

None.

Busulfan

(byou-SUL-fan)
Pregnancy Class: D
Myleran (Abbreviation: Bus) **(Rx)**
Classification: Antineoplastic, alkylating agent

Mechanism of Action: Busulfan is cell cycle-phase nonspecific and acts predominately against cells of the granulocytic type; thought to act by alkylating cellular thiol groups. Cross-linking of nucleoproteins occurs. May cause severe bone marrow depression. Leukocyte count drops during the second or third week. Thus, close medical supervision, including weekly laboratory tests, is mandatory. Resistance may develop and is thought to be due to the altered transport into the cell and/or increased intracellular inactivation.

Increased appetite and sense of well-being may occur a few days after therapy is started. Sometimes administered with allopurinol to prevent symptoms of clinical gout.
Onset of Action: PO: 0.5-2 hr. **t½:** 2.5 hr.
Uses: Chronic myelogenous leukemia (granulocytic, myelocytic, myeloid). Less effective in individuals with chronic myelogenous leukemia who lack the Philadelphia (Ph[1]) chromosome. Not effective in individuals where the disease is in the "blastic" phase.
Contraindications: Use during lactation only if benefits outweigh risks.

Route/Dosage ─────────────
• **Tablets**
Individualized according to leukocyte count.
  Chronic myelocytic leukemia.
Adults, remission, induction, usual dose: 4–8 mg/day until leukocyte count falls below 15,000/mm³; **maintenance:** 1–3 mg/day. Discontinue therapy if there is a precipitous fall in leukocyte count. **Children, induction:** 0.06–0.12 mg/kg or 1.8 mg/m² daily; **maintenance:** dosage is titrated to maintain a leukocyte count of 20,000/mm³.
How Supplied: *Tablet:* 2 mg
Side Effects: *Hematologic: Pancytopenia, severe bone marrow hypoplasia,* anemia, leukopenia, thrombocytopenia. *Pulmonary: Bronchopulmonary dysplasia with interstitial pulmonary fibrosis.* *Ophthalmologic:* Cataracts after prolonged use. *Dermatologic:* Hyperpigmentation, especially in patients with a dark complexion; also, urticaria, erythema multiforme, erythema nodosum, alopecia, porphyria cutanea tarda, excessive dryness and fragility of the skin with anhidrosis, dryness of the oral mucous membranes, cheilosis. *Metabolic:* Syndrome resembling adrenal insufficiency, including symptoms of weakness, severe fatigue, weight loss, anorexia, N&V, and melanoderma (especially after

prolonged use). Also, hyperuricemia and hyperuricosuria in patients with chronic myelogenous leukemia. *Miscellaneous:* Cellular dysplasia in various organs, including lymph nodes, pancreas, thyroid, adrenal glands, bone marrow, and liver. Also, gynecomastia, seizures after high doses, cataracts after prolonged use, *hepatotoxicity,* cholestatic jaundice, myasthenia gravis, sterility, *endocardial fibrosis,* and suppression of ovarian function.

OD Overdose Management: *Symptoms: Bone marrow toxicity, CNS stimulation with convulsions and death on the first day. Treatment:* If ingestion is recent, gastric lavage or induction of vomiting followed by activated charcoal. Hematologic status must be monitored.
Drug Interactions
Cyclophosphamide / Cardiac tamponade in patients with thalessemia (rare)
Thioguanine / ↑ Risk of esophageal varices with abnormal LFTs

EMS CONSIDERATIONS

See also *Antineoplastic Agents* and *Alkylating Agents.*

Butalbital and Acetaminophen

(byou-TAL-bih-tall, ah-SEAT-ah-MIN-oh-fen)
Pregnancy Class: C
Axocet **(Rx)**
Classification: Sedative, analgesic

Uses: Treatment of tension headaches.
Contraindications: Hypersensitivity to butalbital or acetaminophen. Patients with porphyria.
Precautions: Use with caution as butalbital is habit-forming and has the potential to be abused. Use with caution in geriatric or debilitated patients, those with severe renal or hepatic dysfunction, and patients with acute abdominal conditions. Safety and efficacy have not been deter-

─────────────────────────────────
bold italic = life threatening side effect

mined in children less than 12 years of age.

Route/Dosage ─────────────
• **Capsules**
Treatment of tension headaches.
1 capsule q 4 hr, not to exceed 6 capsules daily.
How Supplied: Each capsule contains: *Sedative/hypnotic:* Butalbital, 50 mg, and *analgesic:* acetaminophen, 650 mg.
Side Effects: See also *Sedative-hypnotics* and *Acetaminophen*. The most frequently reported side effects are drowsiness, lightheadedness, sedation, dizziness, SOB, N&V, abdominal pain, and an intoxicated feeling.
Drug Interactions
CNS depressants (including alcohol, general anesthetics, narcotic analgesics, sedative-hypnotics, tranquilizers) / Additive CNS depression
MAO inhibitors / MAO inhibitors ↑ the CNS effects of butalbital

EMS CONSIDERATIONS

See also *Pentobarbital Sodium* and *Acetaminophen*.

Butenafine hydrochloride
(byou-TEN-ah-feen)
Pregnancy Class: B
Mentax **(Rx)**
Classification: Antifungal drug

Mechanism of Action: Acts by inhibiting epoxidation of squalene, thus blocking the synthesis of ergosterol, an essential component of fungal cell membranes. Depending on the concentration and the fungal species, the drug may be fungicidal. Although applied topically, some of the drug is absorbed into the general circulation.
Uses: Treatment of interdigital tinea pedia (athlete's foot) due to *Epidermophyton floccosum*, *Trichophyton mentagrophytes*, or *T. rubrum*.
Precautions: Use with caution during lactation and in patients sensitive to allylamine antifungal drugs as the drugs may be corss-reactive. Safety and efficacy have not been deter-

mined in children less than 12 years of age.

Route/Dosage ─────────────
• **Cream, 1%**
Athlete's foot.
Apply the cream to cover the affected area and immediate surrounding skin once daily for 4 weeks. Review the diagnosis if no beneficial effects are noted after the treatment period.
How Supplied: *Cream:* 1%
Side Effects: *Dermatologic:* Contact dermatitis, burning or stinging, worsening of the condition, erythema, irritation, itching.

EMS CONSIDERATIONS

See also *Anti-Infectives*.

Butoconazole nitrate
(byou-toe-KON-ah-zohl)
Pregnancy Class: C
Femstat 1 **(Rx)**, Femstat 3 **(OTC)**
Classification: Antifungal agent

Mechanism of Action: By permeating chitin in the fungal cell wall, butoconazole increases membrane permeability to intracellular substances, leading to reduced osmotic resistance and viability of the fungus.
Uses: Vulvovaginal fungal infections caused by *Candida* species.
Contraindications: Use during first trimester of pregnancy.
Precautions: Pediatric dosage has not been established. Use with caution during lactation.

Route/Dosage ─────────────
• **Vaginal Cream (2%)**
During pregnancy, second and third trimesters only.
One full applicator (about 5 g) of the cream intravaginally at bedtime for 6 days.
Nonpregnant.
One full applicator (about 5 g) intravaginally at bedtime for 3 days (if necessary, may be used for up to 6 days). *NOTE:* Vaginal infections may also be treated by one dose of butoconazole.
How Supplied: *Vaginal cream:* 2%

Side Effects: *GU:* Vaginal burning, vulvar burning or itching, discharge; soreness, swelling, and itching of the fingers.

EMS CONSIDERATIONS

None.

Butorphanol tartrate

(byou-TOR-fah-nohl)
Pregnancy Class: C
Stadol, Stadol NS **(C-IV) (Rx)**
Classification: Narcotic agonist/antagonist

Mechanism of Action: Has both narcotic agonist and antagonist properties. Analgesic potency is said to be up to 7 times that of morphine and 30–40 times that of meperidine. Overdosage responds to naloxone. After IV use, CV effects include increased PA pressure, pulmonary wedge pressure, LV end-diastolic pressure, system arterial pressure, pulmonary vascular resistance, and increased cardiac work load. The drug has about 1/40 the narcotic antagonist activity as naloxone. A metered-dose nasal spray is now available.

Onset of Action: IM: 10-15 min; **IV:** rapid; **nasal:** within 15 min. **Peak analgesia, IM, IV:** 30-60 min; **nasal:** 1-2 hr. **t½, IM:** 2.1-8.8 hr; **nasal:** 2.9-9.2 hr.

Duration of Action: IM, IV: 3-4 hr; **nasal:** 1-2 hr.

Uses: Parenteral and nasal: Moderate to severe pain, especially after surgery. **Parenteral:** Preoperative medication (as part of balanced anesthesia). Pain during labor. **Nasal:** Treatment of migraine headaches.

Contraindications: Use of the nasal form during labor or delivery.

Precautions: Safe use during pregnancy, during labor or premature infants, or in children under 18 years of age not established. Use with extreme caution in patients with AMI, vnetricular dysfunction, and coronary sinufficiency (morphine or meperidine are preferred). Use in patients physically dependent on narcotics will result in precipitation of a withdrawal syndrome. Geriatric patients may abe more sensitive to side effects, especially dizziness.

Route/Dosage
- **IM**
  Analgesia.
  Adults, usual: 2 mg q 3–4 hr, as necessary; **range:** 1–4 mg q 3–4 hr. Single doses should not exceed 4 mg.
  Preoperative/preanesthetic.
  Adults: 2 mg 60–90 min before surgery. Individualize dosage.
  Labor.
  Adults: 1–2 mg if at full term and during early labor. May be repeated after 4 hr.
- **IV**
  Analgesia.
  Adults, usual: 1 mg q 3–4 hr; **range:** 0.5–2 mg q 3–4 hr. **Not recommended for use in children.**
  Balanced anesthesia.
  Adults: 2 mg just before induction or 0.5–1 mg in increments during anesthesia. The increment may be up to 0.06 mg/kg, depending on drugs previously given. Total dose range: less than 4 mg to less than 12.5 mg.
  Labor.
  Adults: 1–2 mg if at full term and during early labor. May be repeated after 4 hr.
- **Nasal Spray**
  Analgesia.
  Adults: 1 spray (1 mg) in one nostril. If pain relief is not reached within 60–90 min, an additional 1 mg may be given. The two-dose sequence may be repeated in 3–4 hr if necessary. In severe pain, 2 mg (1 spray in each nostril) may be given initially followed in 3–4 hr by additional 2-mg doses if needed. **Geriatric patients, initial:** 1 mg; wait 90–120 min before determining if a second 1-mg dose is required.

How Supplied: *Injection:* 1 mg/mL, 2 mg/mL; *Spray:* 10 mg/mL

Side Effects: Additional: The most common side effects are somnolence, dizziness, N&V. The nasal product commonly causes nasal congestion and insomnia.

Drug Interactions: Additional: Barbiturate anesthetics may increase respiratory and CNS depression of butorphanol.

EMS CONSIDERATIONS

See also *Narcotic Analgesics*.

Administration/Storage

1. Give geriatric patients one-half the usual dose at twice the usual interval.

2. Have naloxone available for treatment of overdose.

IV 3. If administered by direct IV infusion, may give undiluted. Administer at a rate of 2 mg or less over 3–5-min.

Assessment: Monitor VS and CNS status during therapy.

C

Cabergoline

(cah-BER-goh-leen)
Pregnancy Class: B
Dostinex **(Rx)**
Classification: Drug to treat hyperprolactinemia

Mechanism of Action: Synthetic ergot derivative that is a dopamine receptor agonist at D_2 receptors. Secretion of prolactin occurs through the release of dopamine from tuberofundibular neurons. Inhibits basal and metoclopramide-induced prolactin secretion.

Uses: Treatment of hyperprolactinemia, either idiopathic or due to pituitary adenomas. *Investigational:* Shrink tumors in patients with microprolactinoma or macroprolactinoma. Parkinson's disease. Normalize androgen levels and improve menstrual cyclicity in polycystic ovary syndrome.

Contraindications: Uncontrolled hypertension or in pregnancy-induced hypertension (i.e., preeclampsia, eclampsia). Hypersensitivity to ergot alkaloids. Lactation. Not to be used to inhibit or suppress physiologic lactation.

Precautions: Use with caution in those with impaired hepatic function or with other drug that lower BP. Safety and efficacy have not been determined in children.

Route/Dosage
• **Tablets**
Hyperprolactinemia.

Adults, initial: 0.5 mg twice a week. Dose may be increased by 0.25 mg twice weekly to less than or equal to 1 mg twice a week, depending on the serum prolactin level. Do not increase dose more often than every 4 weeks.

Parkinson's disease.
Adults: 7.5 mg/day.

Improve menstrual cyclicity in polycystic ovary syndrome.
Adults: 0.5 mg/week.

How Supplied: *Tablets:* 0.5 mg.

Side Effects: *GI:* N&V, constipation, abdominal pain, dyspepsia, dry mouth, diarrhea, flatulence, throat irritation, toothache, anorexia, weight loss or gain. *CNS:* Headache, dizziness, somnolence, vertigo, paresthesia, depression, nervousness, anxiety, insomnia. *CV:* Postural hypotension, hypotension, palpitations. *GU:* Breast pain, dysmenorrhea, increased libido. *Body as a whole:* Asthenia, fatigue, syncope, flu-like symptoms, malaise, periorbital edema, peripheral edema, hot flashes. *Miscellaneous:* Nasal stuffiness, abnormal vision, acne, epistaxis, pruritus.

OD Overdose Management: *Symptoms:* Nasal congestion, syncope, hallucinations. *Treatment:* Support BP, if necessary.

Drug Interactions
Antihypertensive drugs / Additive hypotension
Butyrophenones / ↓ Effects of cabergoline

Metoclopramide / Effects of cabergoline

Phenothiazines / Effects of cabergoline

Thioxanthenes / Effects of cabergoline

EMS CONSIDERATIONS

None.

Calcipotriene (Calcipotriol)

(kal-SIH-poh-tren)
Pregnancy Class: C
Dovonex **(Rx)**
Classification: Topical antipsoriatic

Mechanism of Action: Synthetic vitamin D_3 analog. Vitamin D_3 receptors are located in skin cells known as keratinocytes. Abnormal growth and production of keratinocytes cause the scaly red patches of psoriasis. Calcipotriene regulates production and development of these skin cells.

Uses: *Cream, Ointment:* Treatment of moderate plaque psoriasis. *Solution:* Control moderately severe scalp psoriasis.

Contraindications: Demonstrated hypercalcemia or evidence of vitamin D toxicity. Use on the face; oral, ophthalmic, intravaginal use.

Precautions: Side effects are more common in geriatric patients. Use with caution during lactation. Safety and efficacy for use of topical calcipotriene in dermatoses other than psoriasis have not been studied. Safety and efficacy have not been determined in children. Children have a higher ratio of skin surface to body mass; thus, children are at a greater risk than adults of systemic side effects following use of topical medication.

Route/Dosage
• **Ointment, Cream, Solution (each 0.005%)**
Treatment of psoriasis.
A thin layer is applied to the affected skin b.i.d. and rubbed in gently and completely.

How Supplied: *Cream:* 0.005%; *Ointment:* 0.005%; *Solution:* 0.005%

Side Effects: *Topical:* Most commonly burning, itching, skin irritation. Also, erythema, dry skin, peeling, rash, worsening of psoriasis, dermatitis, skin atrophy, hyperpigmentation, hypercalcemia, folliculitis. Irritation of lesions and surrounding uninvolved skin. *Systemic:* Transient, rapidly reversible hypercalcemia.

OD Overdose Management: *Symptoms:* Hypercalcemia and other systemic effects. *Treatment:* Discontinue use of the medication until normal calcium levels are restored.

EMS CONSIDERATIONS

Calcitonin-human Calcitonin-salmon

(kal-sih-TOH-nin)
Pregnancy Class: C
Calcitonin-human **(Rx)** Calcitonin-salmon (Calcimar, Miacalcin, Osteocalcin, Salmonine) **(Rx)**
Classification: Calcium regulator

Mechanism of Action: Calcitonins are polypeptide hormones produced in mammals by the parafollicular cells of the thyroid gland. Calcitonin isolated from salmon has the same therapeutic effect as the human hormone, except for a greater potency per milligram and a somewhat longer duration of action. Calcitonin-human is a synthetic product that has the same sequence of amino acids as the naturally occurring calcitonin found in human beings. Ineffective when administered PO. Beneficial in Paget's disease of bone by reducing the rate of turnover of bone; the drug acts to both block initial bone resorption, decreasing alkaline phosphatase levels in the serum, and urinary hydroxyproline excretion. Its effectiveness in treating osteoporosis or hypercalcemia is due to decreased serum calcium levels from direct inhibition of bone resorption. Use of the nasal spray for osteoporosis results

---

bold italic = life threatening side effect

in significant increases in bone mass density within 6 months.

Uses: Injection: Prevention of progressive loss of bone mass in postmenopausal osteoporosis in women who are more than 5 years past menopause and who have low bone mass compared with women before menopause. Also, for women who cannot or will not take estrogens. Moderate to severe Paget's disease characterized by polyostotic involvement with elevated serum alkaline phosphatase and urinary hydroxyproline excretion. With other therapies for early treatment of hypercalcemic emergencies. *NOTE:* Calcitonin human is now an orphan drug. **Nasal:** Postmenopausal osteoporosis (see above for injection).

Contraindications: Allergy to calcitonin-salmon or its gelatin diluent.

Precautions: Use with caution during lactation. Safe use in children not established.

Route/Dosage

CALCITONIN-HUMAN

• **SC**

Paget's disease.

Adults, initial: 0.5 mg/day; **then,** depending on severity of disease, dosage may range from 0.5 mg 2–3 times/week to 0.25 mg/day.

CALCITONIN-SALMON

• **IM, SC**

Paget's disease.

Adults, initial: 100 IU/day; **maintenance, usual:** 50 IU/day, every other day, or 3 times/week.

Hypercalcemia.

Adults, initial: 4 IU/kg q 12 hr; **then,** increase the dose, if necessary after 1 or 2 days (i.e., if unsatisfactory response), to 8 IU/kg q 12 hr up to a maximum of 8 IU/kg q 6 hr. If the volume to be injected exceeds 2 mL by the SC route, the dose should be given IM with multiple sites used.

Postmenopausal osteoporosis.

Adults: 100 IU/day given with calcium carbonate (1.5 g/day) and vitamin D (400 units/day).

• **Nasal Spray**

Adults: 200 IU/day, alternating nostrils daily given with calcium carbonate (1.5 g/day) and vitamin D (400 units/day).

How Supplied: Calcitonin-salmon: *Injection:* 200 IU/mL; *Nasal Spray:* 200 IU/inh

Side Effects: Side effects listed are for calcitonin-salmon. *GI:* N&V, anorexia, epigastric discomfort, salty taste, flatulence, increased appetite, gastritis, diarrhea, dry mouth, abdominal pain, dyspepsia, constipation. *CNS:* Dizziness, paresthesia, insomnia, anxiety, vertigo, migraine, neuralgia, agitation, depression (rare). *CV:* Hypertension, tachycardia, palpitation, bundle branch block, *MI, CVA, thrombophlebitis,* angina pectoris (rare). *Respiratory:* Sinusitis, URTI, pharyngitis, bronchitis, pneumonia, coughing, dyspnea, taste perversion, parosmia, *bronchospasm. Musculoskeletal:* Arthrosis, arthritis, polymyalgia rheumatica, stiffness, myalgia. *Dermatologic:* Inflammatory reactions at the injection site, flushing of face or hands, pruritus of ear lobes, edema of feet, skin rash, skin ulceration, eczema, alopecia, increased sweating. *Endocrine:* Goiter, hyperthyroidism. *Ophthalmic:* Abnormal lacrimation, conjunctivitis, eye pain, blurred vision, vitreous floater. *Otic:* Tinnitus, hearing loss, earache. *Hematologic:* Lymphadenopathy, anemia, infection. *Metabolic:* Mild tetanic symptoms, asymptomatic mild hypercalcemia, cholelithiasis, thirst, hepatitis, weight increase. *Miscellaneous:* Flu-like symptoms, fatigue, nocturia, feverish sensation. Use of the nasal spray may cause rhinitis, nasal irritation, redness, nasal sores, back pain, arthralgia, epistaxis, and headache.

OD **Overdose Management:** *Symptoms:* N&V.

EMS CONSIDERATIONS

Calcium carbonate

(KAL-see-um KAR-bon-ayt)

Alka-Mints, Amitone, Antacid Tablets, Cal Carb-HD, Calci-Chew, Calciday-667, Calci-Mix, Calcium 600, Cal-Plus, Caltrate 600, Caltrate Jr., Children's Mylanta Upset Stomach Relief, Chooz, Dicarbosil, Equilet, Extra

Strength Antacid, Extra Strength Tums, Florical, Gencalc 600, Maalox Antacid Caplets, Mallamint, Mylanta Lozenges, Nephra-Calci, Os-Cal 500, Os-Cal 500 Chewable, Oysco 500 Chewable, Oyst-Cal 500, Oystercal 500, Oyster Shell Calciuim-500, Tums, Tums Ultra **(OTC)**
Classification: Calcium salt

Uses: Mild hypocalcemia, antacid, antihyperphosphatemic.

Precautions: Dosage not established in children.

Route/Dosage —————————
• **Chewable Tablets, Tablets, Suspension, Gum, Lozenges, Wafers**
Adults: 0.5–1.5 g, as needed.
• **Capsules, Suspension, Tablets, Chewable Tablets**
Hypocalcemia, nutritional supplement.
Adults: 1.25–1.5 g 1–3 times/day with or after meals.
Antihyperphosphatemic.
Adults: 5–13 g/day in divided doses with meals.
NOTE: The preparation contains 40% elemental calcium and 400 mg elemental calcium/g (20 mEq/g).
• **Florical**
1 capsule or tablet daily (also contains 8.3 mg sodium fluoride per capsule or tablet).
• **Children's Mylanta Upset Stomach Relief Chewable Tablets or Liquid**
Upset stomach in children.
1 tablet or 5 mL for children weighing 24–47 pounds (or those aged 2–5 years) and 2 tablets or 10 mL for children weighing 48–95 pounds (or those aged 6–11).
How Supplied: *Capsule:* 500 mg, 600 mg, 900 mg, 1250 mg; *Chew Tablet:* 300 mg, 500 mg, 600 mg, 650 mg; *Lozenge/Troche:* 240 mg; *Suspension:* 500 mg/5 mL; *Tablet:* 10 mg, 250 mg, 375 mg, 420 mg, 500 mg, 600 mg, 625 mg, 650 mg, 750 mg, 1,000 mg, 1,250 mg; *Tablet, Extended Release:* 500 mg

EMS CONSIDERATIONS

See also *Calcium Salts* and *Antacids*.

Calcium chloride
(KAL-see-um KLOH-ryd)
Pregnancy Class: C
(Rx)
Classification: Calcium salt

Uses: Mild hypocalcemia due to neonatal tetany, tetany due to parathyroid deficiency or vitamin D deficiency, and alkalosis. Prophylaxis of hypocalcemia during exchange transfusions. Intestinal malabsorption. Treat effects of serious hyperkalemia as measured by ECG. Cardiac resuscitation after open heart surgery when epinephrine fails to improve weak or ineffective myocardial contractions. Adjunct to treat insect bites or stings to relieve muscle cramping. Depression due to magnesium overdosage. Acute symptoms of lead colic. Rickets, osteomalacia. Reverse symptoms of verapamil overdosage.

Contraindications: Use to treat hypocalcemia of renal insufficiency.

Precautions: Use usually restricted in children due to significant irritation and possible tissue necrosis and sloughing caused by IV calcium chloride.

Route/Dosage —————————
• **IV Only**
Hypocalcemia, replenish electrolytes.
Adults: 0.5–1 g q 1–3 days (given at a rate not to exceed 13.6–27.3 mg/min). **Pediatric:** 25 mg/kg (0.2 mL/kg up to 1–10 mL/kg) given slowly.
Magnesium intoxication.
0.5 g promptly; observe for recovery before other doses given.
Cardiac resuscitation.
0.5–1 g IV or 0.2–0.8 g injected into the ventricular cavity as a single dose. **Pediatric:** 0.2 mL/kg.
Hyperkalemia.
Sufficient amount to return ECG to normal.
NOTE: The preparation contains 27.2% calcium and 272 mg calcium/g (13.6 mEq/g).
How Supplied: *Injection:* 100 mg/mL

Side Effects: Additional: Peripheral vasodilation with moderate decreses in BP. Extravasation can cause severe necrosis, sloughing, or abscess formation following IM or SC use.

EMS CONSIDERATIONS

See also *Calcium Salts.*
Administration/Storage
1. Never administer IM.
IV 2. May administer undiluted by IV push.

Calcium citrate
(KAL-see-um ClH-trayt)
Citracal, Citracal Liquitab **(OTC)**
Classification: Calcium salt

Route/Dosage
• **Tablets, Syrup, Effervescent Tablets**
Hypocalcemia.
Adults: 0.9–1.9 g t.i.d.–q.i.d. after meals.
Nutritional supplement.
3.8–7.1 g/day in three to four divided doses.
NOTE: Contains 21.1% elemental calcium and 211 mg calcium/g (10.5 mEq/g).
How Supplied: *Capsule:* 150 mg, 800 mg; *Syrup; Tablet:* 200 mg, 250 mg, 950 mg, 1150 mg

EMS CONSIDERATIONS

See also *Calcium Salts.*

Calcium glubionate
(KAL-see-um glue-BYE-oh-nayt)
Pregnancy Class: C
Neo-Calglucon, Calcium-Sandoz **(OTC)**
Classification: Calcium salt

Uses: Hypocalcemia, calcium deficiency, tetany of newborn, hypoparathyroidism, pseudohypoparathyroidism, osteoporosis, rickets, osteomalacia.

Route/Dosage
• **Syrup, Tablets**
Dietary supplement.
Adults and children over 4 years: 15 mL t.i.d.–q.i.d. **Pediatric (under 4**

years): 10 mL t.i.d. **Infants:** 5 mL 5 times/day.
Tetany of newborn.
On the basis of laboratory tests, usually 50–150 mg/kg/day in three or more divided doses.
Other calcium deficiencies.
Adults: 15–45 mL 1–3 times/day.
NOTE: The preparation contains 115 mg calcium ion/5 mL.
How Supplied: *Syrup; Tablet*

EMS CONSIDERATIONS

See also *Calcium Salts.*

Calcium gluceptate
(KAL-see-um GLUE-cep-tayt)
Pregnancy Class: C
(Rx)
Classification: Calcium salt

Uses: Mild hypocalcemia due to neonatal tetany, tetany due to parathyroid deficiency or vitamin D deficiency, and alkalosis. Prophylaxis of hypocalcemia during exchange transfusions. Intestinal malabsorption. To replenish electrolytes. Antihypermagnesemic.
Precautions: Give only IM to infants and children in emergency situations when the IV route is not possible.

Route/Dosage
• **IM**
Hypocalcemia.
Adults and children: 0.44–1.1 g.
• **IV**
Hypocalcemia.
Adults: 1.1–4.4 g given slowly at a rate not exceeding 36 mg calcium ion/min (2 mL/min). **Pediatric, IV:** 0.44–1.1 g; give as a single dose at a rate not to exceed 36 mg calcium ion/min.
Antihypermagnesemic.
Adults: 1.2–2.4 g given slowly at a rate not to exceed 36 mg calcium ion/min.
Exchange transfusions in newborns.
0.11 g after every 100 mL blood exchanged.

NOTE: The elemental calcium content is 8.2% and there is 82 mg calcium/g (4.1 mEq/g).
How Supplied: *Injection:* 220 mg /mL

EMS CONSIDERATIONS

See also *Calcium Salts.*

Calcium gluconate

(KAL-see-um GLUE-koh-nayt)
Kalcinate (Rx, injection; OTC tablets)
Classification: Calcium salt

Uses: Mild hypocalcemia due to neonatal tetany, tetany due to parathyroid deficiency or vitamin D deficiency, and alkalosis. Prophylaxis of hypocalcemia during exchange transfusions. Intestinal malabsorption. Adjunct to treat insect bites or stings to relieve muscle cramping. Depression due to magnesium overdosage. Acute symptoms of lead colic. Rickets, osteomalacia. Reverse symptoms of verapamil overdosage. Decrease capillary permeability in allergic conditions, nonthrombocytopenic purpura, and exudative dermatoses (e.g., dermatitis herpetiformis). Pruritus due to certain drugs. Hyperkalemia to antagonize cardiac toxicity (as long as patient is not receiving digitalis).
Contraindications: IM, intramyocardial, or SC use due to severe tissue necrosis, sloughing, and abscess formation.

Route/Dosage ─────────────
• **Chewable Tablets, Tablets**
Treatment of hypocalcemia.
Adults: 8.8–16.5 g/day in divided doses; **pediatric:** 0.5–0.72 g/kg/day in divided doses.
Nutritional supplement.
Adults: 8.8–16.5 g/day in divided doses.
• **IV Only**
Treatment of hypocalcemia.
Adults: 2.3–9.3 mEq (5–20 mL of the 10% solution) as needed (range: 4.65–70 mEq/day). **Children:** 2.3 mEq/kg/day (or 56 mEq/m²/day) given well diluted and slowly in divid-

ed doses. **Infants:** No more than 0.93 mEq (2 mL of the 10% solution).
Emergency elevation of serum calcium.
Adults: 7–14 mEq (15–30.1 mL). **Children:** 1–7 mEq (2.2–15 mL). **Infants:** Less than 1 mEq (2.2 mL). Depending on patient response, the dose may be repeated q 1–3 days.
Hypocalcemic tetany.
Children: 0.5–0.7 mEq/kg (1.1–1.5 mL/kg) t.i.d.–q.i.d. until tetany is controlled. **Infants:** 2.4 mEq/kg/day (5.2 mL/kg/day) in divided doses.
Hyperkalemia with cardiac toxicity.
2.25–14 mEq (4.8–30.1 mL) while monitoring the ECG. If needed, the dose can be repeated after 1–2 min.
Magnesium intoxication.
Initial: 4.5–9 mEq (9.7–19.4 mL). Subsequent dosage based on patient response.
Exchange transfusion.
Adults: 1.35 mEq (2.9 mL) concurrent with each 100 mL citrated blood. **Neonates:** 0.45 mEq (1 mL)/100 mL citrated blood.
• **IM**
Hypocalcemic tetany.
Adults: 4.5–16 mEq (9.7–34.4 mL) until a therapeutic response is noted.
Magnesium intoxication.
If IV administration is not possible: 2–5 mEq (4.3–10.8 mL) in divided doses as needed.
NOTE: The preparation contains 9% calcium and 90 mg calcium/g (4.5 mEq/g).
How Supplied: *Chew tablet:* 650 mg; *Injection:* 100 mg /mL; *Tablet:* 486 mg, 500 mg, 650 mg, 975 mg

EMS CONSIDERATIONS

See also *Calcium Salts.*
Administration/Storage
1. If a precipitate is noted in the syringe, do not use.
2. If a precipitate is noted in the vials or ampules, heat to 80°C (146°F) in a dry heat oven for 1 hr to dissolve. Shake vigorously and allow to cool to room temperature. Do not use if precipitate remains.

IV 3. IV rate should not exceed 0.5–2 mL/min.

4. Give by intermittent IV infusion at a rate not exceeding 200 mg (19.5 mg calcium ion)/min. Can also be given by continuous IV infusion.

Calcium lactate
(KAL-see-um LACK-tayt)
(OTC)
Classification: Calcium salt

Uses: Latent hypocalcemic tetany, hyperphosphatemia.

Route/Dosage
• **Tablets**
Treatment of hypocalcemia.
Adults: 7.7 g/day in divided doses with meals. **Pediatric:** 0.34–0.5 g/kg/day in divided doses.

NOTE: The preparation contains 13% calcium and 130 mg calcium/g (6.5 mEq/g).

How Supplied: *Tablet:* 325 mg, 500 mg, 650 mg

EMS CONSIDERATIONS

See also *Calcium Salts*.

Candesartan cilexetil
(KAN-deh-SAR-tan)
Pregnancy Class: Pregnancy Class: C (first trimester), D (second and third trimesters)
Atacand **(Rx)**
Classification: Antihypertensive, angiotensin II receptor blocker

Mechanism of Action: Prevents the binding of angiotensin II to the AT_1 receptor, resulting in blockade of the vasoconstrictor and aldosterone-secreting effects of angiotensin II.
Uses: Alone or in combination with other drugs to treat hypertension.
Contraindications: Lactation.
Precautions: Fetal and neonatal morbidity and death are possible if given to pregnant women. Safety and efficacy have not been determined in children less than 18 years of age.

Route/Dosage
• **Tablets**

Hypertension, monotherapy.
Adults, usual initial: 16 mg once daily in those not volume depleted. Can be given once or twice daily in doses from 8 to 32 mg.
How Supplied: *Tablets:* 4 mg, 8 mg, 16 mg, 32 mg
Side Effects: *GI:* N&V, abdominal pain, diarrhea, dyspepsia, gastroenteritis. *CNS:* Headache, dizziness, paresthesia, vertigo, anxiety, depression, somnolence. *CV:* Tachycardia, palpitation; rarely, angina pectoris, MI. *Body as a whole:* Fatigue, asthenia, fever, peripheral edema. *Respiratory:* URTI, pharyngitis, rhinitis, bronchitis, coughing, dyspnea, sinusitis, epistaxis. *GU:* Impaired renal function, hematuria. *Dermatologic:* Rash, increased sweating. *Miscellaneous:* Backpain, chest pain, arthralgia, myalgia, angioedema.

EMS CONSIDERATIONS
Administration/Storage
1. Maximum BP reduction is reached within 4 to 6 weeks.
2. Initiate dosage under close supervision in those with possible depletion of intravascular volume. Consider giving a lower dose.
3. Can be given with or without food.
4. If BP is not controlled by candesartan alone, a diuretic may be added.
Assessment
1. Note onset and duration of disease, other agents trialed and the outcome.
2. Assess lytes, renal and LFTs.
3. Ensure adequate hydration, especially with diuretic therapy in renal dysfunction.

Capecitabine
(cap-SITE-ah-bean)
Pregnancy Class: Pregnancy Class: D
Xeloda **(Rx)**
Classification: Antineoplastic, antimetabolite

Mechanism of Action: An oral prodrug of 5'-deoxy-5-fluorouridine (5'DFUR) that is converted to 5-fluorouracil (5-FU). 5-FU is metabolized to

5-fluoro-2-deoxyuridine monophosphate (FdUMP) and 5-fluorouridine triphosphate (FUTP) which cause cell injury in two ways. First, FdUMP and the folate cofactor, N^{5-10}-methylenetetrahydrofolate, bind to thymidylate synthase to form a covalently bound ternary complex which inhibits the formation of thymidylate from uracil. Thymidylate is essential for the synthesis of DNA so a deficiency inhibits cell division. Secondly, nuclear transcriptional enzymes can mistakenly incorporate FUTP in place of uridine triphosphate during RNA synthesis; this interferes with RNA processing and protein synthesis.

Uses: Metastatic breast cancer in those resistant to both paclitaxel and an anthracycline-containing chemotherapy regimen or resistant to paclitaxel and for whom further anthracycline therapy is not indicated (e.g., those who have received cumulative doses of 400 mg/m² of doxorubicin or doxorubicin equivalents).

Contraindications: Lactation.

Precautions: Use with caution in impaired renal function and in the elderly. Those over 80 years may experience a greater incidence of GI side effects. Safety and efficacy in children less than 18 years of age have not been determined.

Route/Dosage
• **Tablets**
Metastatic breast cancer.
2,500 mg/m²/day in two divided doses about 12 hr apart at the end of a meal for 2 weeks. Follow by a 1-week rest period (i.e., 3-week cycles).

How Supplied: *Tablets:* 150 mg, 500 mg

Side Effects: *GI:* Diarrhea (may be severe), N&V, stomatitis, abdominal pain, constipation, dyspepsia, intestinal obstruction, rectal bleeding, *GI hemorrhage,* esophagitis, gastritis, colitis, duodenitis, haematemesis, *necrotizing enterocolitis,* oral/ GI/esophageal candidiasis, gastroenteritis. *CV:* Cardiotoxicity (*MI,* angina, dysrhyth-mias, ECG changes, *cardiogenic shock, sudden death*), angina pectoris, *cardiomyopathy,* hypotension, hypertension, venous phlebitis, thrombophlebitis, DVT, lymphedema, *pulmonary embolism, CVA.* *Hematologic:* Neutropenia (grade 3 or 4), thrombocytopenia, decreased hemoglobin, anemia, lymphopenia, coagulation disorder, idiopathic thrombocytopenia, pancytopenia, *sepsis.* *Dermatologic:* Hand-and-foot syndrome, dermatitis, nail disorder, increased sweating, photosensitivity, radiation recall syndrome. *Neurological:* Paresthesia, fatigue, headache, dizziness, insomnia. *CNS:* Ataxia, encephalopathy, decreased level of consciousness, loss of consciousness, confusion. *Metabolic:* Anorexia, dehydration, cachexia, hypertriglyceridemia. *Respiratory:* Dyspnea, epistaxis, bronchospasm, respiratory distress, URTI, bronchitis, pneumonia, bronchopneumonia, laryngitis. *Musculoskeletal:* Myalgia, pain in limb, bone pain, joint stiffness. *GU:* Nocturia, UTI. *Hepatic:* Hepatic fibrosis, cholestatic hepatitis, hepatitis. *Miscellaneous:* Hyperbilirubinemia (grade 3 or 4), eye irritation, pyrexia, edema, chest pain, drug hypersensitivity.

OD Overdose Management: *Symptoms:* N&V, diarrhea, GI irritation and bleeding, bone marrow suppression. *Treatment:* Supportive medical interventions, dose interruption, adjust dose.

Drug Interactions
Antacids / ↑ Absorption of capecitabine
Leucovorin / ↑ 5-FU levels → ↑ toxicity; deaths from severe enterocolitis, diarrhea, and dehydration seen in elderly patients receiving both drugs

EMS CONSIDERATIONS

Administration/Storage: If the dose has to be reduced due to toxicity, do not increase at a later time.

Assessment
1. Assess for CAD, any sensitivitiy to

---

bold italic = life threatening side effect

5-FU, and other therapies/agents trialed/failed.

2. Monitor weights, CBC, renal and LFTs.

3. Administer cautiously with impaired liver/renal function and in the elderly.

Capsaicin

(kap-SAY-ih-sin)

Zostrix, Zostrix-HP **(Rx)**

Classification: Topical analgesic

Mechanism of Action: Derived from natural sources from plants of the Solanaceae family. Believed the drug depletes and prevents the reaccumulation of substance P, thought to be the main mediator of pain impulses from the periphery to the CNS.

Uses: Temporary relief of pain due to rheumatoid arthritis and osteoarthritis. Pain following herpes zoster (shingles), painful diabetic neuropathy. *Investigational:* Possible use in psoriasis, vitiligo, intractable pruritus, reflex sympathetic dystrophy, postmastectomy, vulvar vestibulitis, apocrine chromhidrosis, and postamputation and postmastectomy neuroma.

Precautions: For external use only.

Route/Dosage

• **Cream or Lotion, 0.025% or 0.075%**

Adults and children over 2 years of age: Apply to affected area no more than 3–4 times/day.

How Supplied: *Cream, Lotion:* 0.025%, 0.075%, 0.25%,

Side Effects: *Skin:* Transient burning following application, stinging, erythema. *Respiratory:* Cough, respiratory irritation.

EMS CONSIDERATIONS

None.

Captopril

(KAP-toe-prill)

Pregnancy Class: C (first trimester); D (second and third trimesters)

Capoten **(Rx)**

Classification: Antihypertensive, inhibitor of angiotensin synthesis

Onset of Action: 60-90 min. **Time to peak effect:** 60-90 min.

Duration of Action: 6-12 hr.

Uses: Antihypertensive, alone or in combination with other antihypertensive drugs, especially thiazide diuretics. In combination with diuretics and digitalis in treatment of CHF not responding to conventional therapy. To improve survival following MI in clinically stable patients with LV dysfunction manifested as an ejection fraction of 40% or less. Treatment of diabetic nephropathy (proteinuria > 500 mg/day) in those with type I insulin-dependent diabetes and retinopathy. *Investigational:* Rheumatoid arthritis, hypertensive crisis, neonatal and childhood hypertension, hypertension related to scleroderma renal crisis, diagnosis of anatomic renal artery stenosis, diagnosis of primary aldosteronism, Raynaud's syndrome, diagnosis of renovascular hypertension, enhance sensitivity and specificity of renal scintigraphy, idiopathic edema, and Bartter's syndrome.

Contraindications: Use with a history of angioedema related to previous use of ACE inhibitors.

Precautions: Use with caution in cases of impaired renal function and during lactation. Use in children only if other antihypertensive therapy has proven ineffective in controlling BP. May cause a profound drop in BP following the first dose or if used with diuretics.

Route/Dosage

• **Tablets**

Hypertension.

Adults, initial: 25 mg b.i.d.–t.i.d. If unsatisfactory response after 1–2 weeks, increase to 50 mg b.i.d.–t.i.d.; if still unsatisfactory after another 1–2 weeks, thiazide diuretic should be added (e.g., hydrochlorothiazide, 25 mg/day). Dosage may be increased to 100–150 mg b.i.d.–t.i.d., not to exceed 450 mg/day.

Accelerated or malignant hypertension.

Stop current medication (except for the diuretic) and initiate captopril at a dose of 25 mg b.i.d.–t.i.d. The dose may be increased q 24 hr until a satisfactory response is obtained or the maximum dose reached. Furosemide may be indicated.

Heart failure.
Initial: 25 mg t.i.d.; **then,** if necessary, increase dose to 50 mg t.i.d. and evaluate response; **maintenance:** 50–100 mg t.i.d., not to exceed 450 mg/day.

NOTE: For adults, an initial dose of 6.25–12.5 mg (0.15 mg/kg t.i.d. in children) should be given b.i.d.–t.i.d. to patients who are sodium- and water-depleted due to diuretics, who will continue to be on diuretic therapy, and who have renal impairment.

Left ventricular dysfunction after MI.
Therapy may be started as early as 3 days after the MI. **Initial dose:** 6.25 mg; **then,** begin 12.5 mg t.i.d. and increase to 25 mg t.i.d. over the next several days. The target dose is 50 mg t.i.d. over the next several weeks. Other treatments for MI may be used concomitantly (e.g., aspirin, beta blockers, thrombolytic drugs).

Diabetic nephropathy.
25 mg t.i.d. for chronic use. Other antihypertensive drugs (e.g., beta blockers, centrally-acting drugs, diuretics, vasodilators) may be used with captopril if additional drug therapy is needed to reduce BP.

Hypertensive crisis.
Initial: 25 mg; **then,** 100 mg 90–120 min later; 200–300 mg/day for 2–5 days (then adjust dose). Sublingual captopril, 25 mg, has also been used successfully.

Rheumatoid arthritis.
75–150 mg/day in divided doses.

NOTE: For all uses, doses should be reduced in patients with renal impairment.

Severe childhood hypertension.
Initial: 0.3 mg/kg titrated to 6 mg or less given in 2 to 3 divided doses.
How Supplied: *Tablet:* 12.5 mg, 25 mg, 50 mg, 100 mg

Side Effects: *Dermatologic:* Rash (usually maculopapular) with pruritus and occasionally fever, eosinophilia, and arthralgia. Alopecia, erythema multiforme, photosensitivity, exfoliative dermatitis, ***Stevens-Johnson syndrome,*** reversible pemphigoid-like lesions, bullous pemphigus, onycholysis, flushing, pallor, scalded mouth sensation. *GI:* N&V, anorexia, constipation or diarrhea, gastric irritation, abdominal pain, dysgeusia, peptic ulcers, aphthous ulcers, dyspepsia, dry mouth, glossitis, pancreatitis. *Hepatic:* Jaundice, cholestasis, hepatitis. *CNS:* Headache, dizziness, insomnia, malaise, fatigue, paresthesias, confusion, depression, nervousness, ataxia, somnolence. *CV:* Hypotension, angina, ***MI,*** Raynaud's phenomenon, chest pain, palpitations, tachycardia, ***CVA, CHF, cardiac arrest,*** orthostatic hypotension, rhythm disturbances, cerebrovascular insufficiency. *Renal:* Renal insufficiency or failure, proteinuria, urinary frequency, oliguria, polyuria, nephrotic syndrome, interstitial nephritis. *Respiratory:* ***Bronchospasm,*** cough, dyspnea, asthma, ***pulmonary embolism, pulmonary infarction.*** *Hematologic:* Agranulocytosis, neutropenia, thrombocytopenia, pancytopenia, ***aplastic or hemolytic anemia.*** *Other:* Decrease or loss of taste perception with weight loss (reversible), angioedema, asthenia, syncope, fever, myalgia, arthralgia, vasculitis, blurred vision, impotence, hyperkalemia, hyponatremia, myasthenia, gynecomastia, rhinitis, eosinophilic pneumonitis.

OD Overdose Management: *Symptoms:* Hypotension with a systolic BP of <80 mm Hg a possibility. *Treatment:* Volume expansion with NSS (IV) is the treatment of choice to restore BP.

EMS CONSIDERATIONS

None.

Carbamazepine
(kar-bah-MAYZ-eh-peen)
Pregnancy Class: C

---

bold italic = life threatening side effect

Tegretol, Tegretol Chewtabs, Tegretol CR, Tegretol XR **(Rx)**
Classification: Anticonvulsant, miscellaneous

Mechanism of Action: Chemically similar to the cyclic antidepressants. It also manifests antimanic, antineuralgic, antidiuretic, anticholinergic, antiarrhythmic, and antipsychotic effects. The anticonvulsant action is not known but may involve depressing activity in the nucleus ventralis anterior of the thalamus, resulting in a reduction of polysynaptic responses and blocking posttetanic potentiation. Due to the potentially serious blood dyscrasias, a benefit-to-risk evaluation should be undertaken before the drug is instituted.

Uses: Partial seizures with complex symptoms (psychomotor, temporal lobe). Tonic-clonic seizures, diseases with mixed seizure patterns or other partial or generalized seizures. Carbamazepine is often a drug of choice due to its low incidence of side effects. For children with epilepsy who are less than 6 years of age for the treatment of partial seizures, generalized tonic-clonic seizures, and mixed seizure patterns and for treating trigeminal neuralgia. To treat pain associated with tic douloureux (trigeminal neuralgia) and glossopharyngeal neuralgia. *Investigational:* Bipolar disorders, unipolar depression, schizoaffective illness, resistant schizophrenia, dyscontrol syndrome associated with limbic system dysfunction, intermittent explosive disorder, PTSD, atypical psychosis. Management of alcohol, cocaine, and benzodiazepine withdrawal symptoms. Restless leg syndrome, nonneuritic pain syndromes, neurogenic or central diabetes insipidus, hereditary and nonhereditary chorea in children.

Contraindications: History of bone marrow depression. Hypersensitivity to drug or tricyclic antidepressants. Lactation. In patients taking MAO inhibitors, discontinue for 14 days before taking carbamazepine. Use for relief of general aches and pains.

Precautions: Safety and effectiveness have not been established in children less than 6 years of age. Use with caution in glaucome and in hepatic, renal, CV disease, and a history of hematologic reaction. Use with caution in patients with mixed seizure disorder that includes atypical absence seizures (carbamazepine is not effective and may be associated with an increased frequency of generalized convulsions). Use in geriatric patients may cause an increased incidence of confusion, agitation, AV heart block, syndrome of inappropriate antidiuretic hormone, and bradycardia.

Route/Dosage ————————————

• **Oral Suspension, Extended Release Capsules, Tablets, Chewable Tablets, Extended-Release Tablets**

Anticonvulsant.

Adults and children over 12 years, initial: 200 mg b.i.d. on day 1 (100 mg q.i.d. of suspension). Increase by 200 mg/day or less at weekly intervals until best response is attained. Divide total dose and administer q 6–8 hr; the extended-release tablets may be used for twice-daily dosing instead of dosing 3 or 4 times a day. **Maximum dose, children 12–15 years:** 1,000 mg/day; **adults and children over 15 years:** 1,200 mg/day. **Maintenance:** decrease dose gradually to minimum effective level, usually 800–1,200 mg/day. **Children, 6–12 years: initial,** 100 mg b.i.d. on day 1 (50 mg q.i.d. of suspension); **then,** increase slowly, at weekly intervals, by 100 mg/day or less; dose is divided and given q 6–8 hr. Daily dose should not exceed 1,000 mg. **Maintenance:** 400–800 mg/day. **Children, less than 6 years:** 10–20 mg/kg/day in two to three divided doses (4 times/day with suspension); dose can be increased slowly in weekly increments to maintenance levels of 35 mg/kg/day (not to exceed 400 mg/day).

Trigeminal neuralgia.

Initial: 100 mg b.i.d. on day 1 (50 mg q.i.d. of suspension); increase by no more than 200 mg/day, using increments of 100 mg q 12 hr as needed, up to maximum of 1,200 mg/day. **Maintenance: Usual:** 400–800 mg/day (range: 200–1,200 mg/day). Attempt discontinuation of drug at least 1 time q 3 months.

Manage alcohol withdrawal.
200 mg q.i.d., up to 1,000 mg/day.
Manage cocaine or benzodiazepine withdrawal.
200 mg b.i.d., up to 800 mg/day.
Restless legs syndrome.
100–300 mg at bedtime.
Hereditary or nonhereditary chorea in children.
15–25 mg/kg/day.
Neurogenic or central diabetes.
200 mg b.i.d.–t.i.d.

How Supplied: *Capsule, Extended Release:* 200 mg, 300 mg; *Chew Tablet:* 100 mg; *Suspension:* 100 mg/5 mL; *Tablet:* 200 mg; *Tablet, Extended Release:* 100 mg, 200 mg, 400 mg

Side Effects: *GI:* N&V (common), diarrhea, constipation, gastric distress, abdominal pain, anorexia, glossitis, stomatitis, dryness of mouth and pharynx. *Hematologic:* **Aplastic anemia,** leukopenia, eosinophilia, thrombocytopenia, **agranulocytosis,** leukocytosis, pancytopenia, **bone marrow depression.** *CNS:* Dizziness, drowsiness, disturbances of coordination, headache, fatigue, confusion, speech disturbances, visual hallucinations, depression with agitation, talkativeness, hyperacusis, abnormal involuntary movements, behavioral changes in children. *CV:* CHF, aggravation of hypertension, hypotension, syncope and collapse, edema, recurrence of or primary thrombophlebitis, aggravation of CAD, paralysis and other symptoms of cerebral arterial insufficiency, thromboembolism, **arrhythmias (including AV block).** *GU:* Urinary frequency, acute urinary retention, oliguria with hypertension, impotence, renal failure, azotemia, albuminuria, glycosuria, increased BUN, microscopic deposits in urine. *Pulmo-*

nary: Pulmonary hypersensitivity characterized by fever, dyspnea, pneumonitis, or pneumonia. *Dermatologic:* Pruritus, urticaria, photosensitivity, exfoliative dermatitis, erythematous rashes, alterations in pigmentation, alopecia, sweating, purpura, toxic epidermal necrolysis (Lyell's syndrome), **Stevens-Johnson syndrome,** aggravation of disseminated lupus erythematosus, alopecia, erythema nodosum or multiforme. *Ophthalmologic:* Nystagmus, double vision, blurred vision, oculomotor disturbances, conjunctivitis; scattered, punctate cortical lens opacities. *Hepatic:* Abnormal liver function tests, cholestatic or hepatocellular jaundice, hepatitis, acute intermittent porphyria. *Other:* Peripheral neuritis, paresthesias, tinnitus, fever, chills, joint and muscle aches and leg cramps, adenopathy or lymphadenopathy, inappropriate ADH secretion syndrome, frank water intoxication with hyponatremia and confusion.

OD Overdose Management: *Symptoms:* First appear after 1 to 3 hours. Neuromuscular disturbances are the most common. *Pulmonary:* Irregular breathing, **respiratory depression.** *CV:* Tachycardia, hypo- or hypertension, conduction disorders, **shock.** *CNS:* Seizures (especially in small children), impaired consciousness (deep coma possible), **motor restlessness,** muscle twitching or tremors, athetoid movements, ataxia, drowsiness, dizziness, nystagmus, mydriasis, psychomotor disturbances, hyperreflexia followed by hyporeflexia, opisthotonos, dysmetria, dizziness, EEG may show dysrhythmias. *GI:* N&V. *GU:* Anuria, oliguria, urinary retention. *Treatment:* Stomach should be irrigated completely even if more than 4 hr has elapsed following drug ingestion, especially if alcohol has been ingested. Activated charcoal, 50–100 g initially, using a NGT (dose of 12.5 or more g/hr until patient is symptom free). Diazepam or phenobarbital may be used to treat seizures (although they may aggravate respirato-

bold italic = life threatening side effect

ry depression, hypotension, and coma). Respiration, ECG, BP, body temperature, pupillary reflexes, and kidney and bladder function should be monitored for several days.

If significant bone marrow depression occurs, the drug should be discontinued and daily CBC, platelet and reticulocyte counts determined. Perform bone marrow aspiration and trephine biopsy immediately and repeat often enough to monitor recovery.

Drug Interactions
Acetaminophen / ↑ Breakdown of acetaminophen → ↓ effect and ↑ risk of hepatotoxicity
Bupropion / ↓ Effect of bupropion due to ↑ breakdown by liver
Charcoal / ↓ Effect of carbamazepine due to ↓ absorption from GI tract
Cimetidine / ↑ Effect of carbamazepine due to ↓ breakdown by liver
Contraceptives, oral / ↓ Effect of contraceptives due to ↑ breakdown by liver
Cyclosporine / ↓ Effect of cyclosporoine due to ↑ breakdown by liver
Danazol / ↑ Effect of carbamazepine due to ↓ breakdown by liver
Diltiazem / ↑ Effect of carbamazepine due to ↓ breakdown by liver
Doxycycline / ↓ Effect of doxycycline due to ↑ breakdown by liver
Erythromycin / ↑ Effect of carbamazepine due to ↓ breakdown by liver
Felbamate / Possible ↓ serum levels of either drug
Felodipine / ↓ Effect of felodipine
Fluoxetine / ↑ Carbamazepine levels → possible toxicity
Fluvoxamine / ↑ Carbamazepine levels → possible toxicity
Haloperidol / ↓ Effect of haloperidol due to ↑ breakdown by liver
Isoniazid / ↑ Effect of carbamazepine due to ↓ breakdown by liver; also, carbamazepine may ↑ risk of isoniazid-induced hepatotoxicity
Lamotrigene / ↓ Effect of lamotrigene; also, ↑ levels of active metabolite of carbamazepine
Lithium / ↑ CNS toxicity

Macrolide antibiotics (e.g., Clarithromycin, Troleandomycin) / Effect of carbamazepine due to breakdown by liver
Muscle relaxants, nondepolarizing / Resistance to or reversal of the neuromuscular blocking effects of these drugs
Phenobarbital / ↓ Effect of carbamazepine due to ↑ breakdown by liver
Phenytoin / ↓ Effect of carbamazepine due to ↑ breakdown by liver; also, phenytoin levels may ↑ or ↓
Primidone / ↓ Effect of carbamazepine due to ↑ breakdown by liver
Propoxyphene / ↑ Effect of carbamazepine due to ↓ breakdown by liver
Ticlopidine / ↑ Effect of carbamazepine due to ↓ breakdown by liver
Tricyclic antidepressants / ↓ Effect of tricyclic antidepressants due to ↑ breakdown by liver; also, ↓ levels of tricyclic antidepressants
Valproic acid / ↓ Effect of valproic acid due to ↑ breakdown by liver; half-life of carbamazepine may be ↑
Vasopressin / ↑ Effect of vasopressin
Verapamil / ↑ Effect of carbamazepine due to ↓ breakdown by liver
Warfarin sodium / ↓ Effect of anticoagulant due to ↑ breakdown by liver

EMS CONSIDERATIONS

See also *Anticonvulsants.*

Carbenicillin indanyl sodium
(kar-ben-ih-SILL-in)
Pregnancy Class: B
Geocillin **(Rx)**
Classification: Antibiotic, penicillin

Mechanism of Action: Acid stable drug.
Uses: Upper and lower UTIs or bacteriuria due to *Escherichia coli, Proteus vulgaris and P. mirabilis, Morganella morganii, Providencia rettgeri, Enterobacter, Pseudomonas,* and enterococci. Prostatitis due to *E. coli,*

Streptococcus faecalis (enterococci), *P. mirabilis,* and *Enterobacter* species.
Contraindications: Pregnancy.
Precautions: Safe use in children not established. Use with caution in patients with impaired renal function.

Route/Dosage
• **Tablets**
   UTIs due to E. coli, Proteus, Enterobacter.
382–764 mg carbenicillin q.i.d.
   UTIs due to Pseudomonas and enterococci.
764 mg carbenicillin q.i.d.
   Prostatitis due to E. coli, P. mirabilis, Enterobacter, and enterococci.
764 mg carbenicillin q.i.d.
How Supplied: *Tablet:* 382 mg
Drug Interactions: Blood levels of carbenicillin may be ↑ with administration of probenecid.**Additional:** When used in combination with gentamicin or tobramycin for *Pseudomonas* infections, effect of carbenicillin may be enhanced.

EMS CONSIDERATIONS

See also *Anti-Infectives* and *Penicillins.*

Carbidopa
Carbidopa/Levodopa
(KAR-bih-doh-pah)(KAR-bih-doh-pah/LEE-voh-doh-pah)
Carbidopa (Lodosyn **(Rx)**) Carbidopa/Levodopa (Sinemet-10/100, -25/100, or -25/250, Sinemet CR)
Classification: Antiparkinson agent

Mechanism of Action: Carbidopa inhibits peripheral decarboxylation of levodopa but not central decarboxylation because it does not cross the blood-brain barrier. Since peripheral decarboxylation is inhibited, this allows more levodopa to be available for transport to the brain, where it will be converted to dopamine, thus relieving the symptoms of parkinsonism. Carbidopa and levodopa are to be given together (e.g., Sinemet). However, *the dosage of levodopa must be reduced by up to 80% when combined with carbidopa.* This decreases the incidence of levodopa-induced side effects. *NOTE:* Pyridoxine will not reverse the action of carbidopa/levodopa.
Uses: All types of parkinsonism (idiopathic, postencephalitic, following injury to the nervous system due to carbon monoxide and manganese intoxication). Carbidopa alone is used in patients who require individual titration of carbidopa and levodopa. *Investigational:* Postanoxic intention myoclonus. **Warning:** Levodopa must be discontinued at least 8 hr before carbidopa/levodopa therapy is initiated. Also, patients taking carbidopa/levodopa must not take levodopa concomitantly, because the former is a combination of carbidopa and levodopa.
Contraindications: History of melanoma. MAO inhibitors should be stopped 2 weeks before therapy. Lactation.
Precautions: Use during pregnancy only if benefits outweigh risks. Safety and efficacy in children less than 18 years of age have not been determined. Lower doses may be necessary in geriatric patients due to aged-related decreases in peripheral dopa decarboxylase.

Route/Dosage
• **Tablets**
   Parkinsonism, patients not receiving levodopa.
Initial: 1 tablet of 10 mg carbidopa/100 mg levodopa t.i.d.–q.i.d. or 25 mg carbidopa/100 mg levodopa t.i.d.; **then,** increase by 1 tablet q 1–2 days until a total of 8 tablets/day is taken. If additional levodopa is required, substitute 1 tablet of 25 mg carbidopa/250 mg levodopa t.i.d.–q.i.d.
   Parkinsonism, patients receiving levodopa.
Initial: Carbidopa/levodopa dosage should be about 25% of prior levodopa dosage (levodopa dosage is discontinued 8 hr before carbidopa/levodopa is initiated); **then,** adjust

dosage as required. Suggested starting dose is 1 tablet of 25 mg carbidopa/250 mg levodopa t.i.d.–q.i.d. for patients taking more than 1500 mg levodopa or 25 mg carbidopa/100 mg levodopa for patients taking less than 1500 mg levodopa.

- **Sustained-Release Tablets**

Parkinsonism, patients not receiving levodopa.

1 tablet b.i.d. at intervals of not less than 6 hr. Depending on the response, dosage may be increased or decreased. Usual dose is 2–8 tablets/day in divided doses at intervals of 4–8 hr during waking hours (if divided doses are not equal, the smaller dose should be given at the end of the day).

Parkinsonism, patients receiving levodopa.

1 tablet b.i.d. Carbidopa is available alone for patients requiring additional carbidopa (i.e., inadequate reduction in N&V); in such patients, carbidopa may be given at a dose of 25 mg with the first daily dose of carbidopa/levodopa. If necessary, additional carbidopa, at doses of 12.5 or 25 mg, may be given with each dose of carbidopa/levodopa.

Patients receiving carbidopa/levodopa who require additional carbidopa.

In patients taking 10 mg carbidopa/100 mg levodopa, 25 mg carbidopa may be given with the first dose each day. Additional doses of 12.5 or 25 mg may be given during the day with each dose. If the patient is taking 25 mg carbidopa/250 mg levodopa, a dose of 25 mg carbidopa may be given with any dose, as needed. The maximum daily dose of carbidopa is 200 mg.

How Supplied: Carbidopa/Levodopa: Each 10/100 tablet contains: carbidopa, 10 mg, and levodopa, 100 mg. Each 25/100 tablets contains: carbidopa, 25 mg, and levodopa, 100 mg. Each 25/250 tablet contains: carbidopa, 25 mg, and levodopa, 250 mg. Each sustained-release tablet contains: carbidopa, 50 mg, and levodopa, 200 mg. Carbodopa:

Tablet: 25 mg. Carbidopa/Levodopa: See Content

Side Effects: Because more levodopa reaches the brain, dyskinesias may occur at lower doses with carbidopa/levodopa than with levodopa alone. Patients abruptly withdrawn from levodopa may experience neuroleptic malignant-like syndrome including symptoms of muscular rigidity, hyperthermia, increased serum phosphokinase, and changes in mental status. ·

Drug Interactions: Use with tricyclic antidepressants may cause hypertension and dyskinesia.

EMS CONSIDERATIONS

See also *Levodopa*.

Carisoprodol

(kar-eye-so-PROH-dohl)
Pregnancy Class: C
Soma **(Rx)**
Classification: Skeletal muscle relaxant, centrally acting

Mechanism of Action: Does not directly relax skeletal muscles. Sedative effects may be responsible for muscle relaxation.

Onset of Action: 30 min.

Duration of Action: 4-6 hr.

Uses: As an adjunct to rest, physical therapy, and other measures to treat skeletal muscle disorders including bursitis, low back disorders, contusions, fibrositis, spondylitis, sprains, muscle strains, and cerebral palsy.

Contraindications: Acute intermittent porphyria. Hypersensitivity to carisoprodol or meprobamate. Children under 12 years of age.

Precautions: Use with caution during lactation and in impaired liver kidney function. May cause GI upset and sedation in infants.

Route/Dosage

- **Tablets**

Skeletal muscle disorders.

Adults: 350 mg q.i.d. (take last dose at bedtime).

How Supplied: *Tablet:* 350 mg

Side Effects: *CNS:* Ataxia, dizziness, drowsiness, excitement, tremor, syncope, vertigo, insomnia, irritability, headache, depressive reactions. *GI:* N&V, gastric upset, hiccoughs. *CV:* Flushing of face, postural hypotension, tachycardia. *Allergic reactions:* Pruritus, skin rashes, erythema multiforme, eosinophilia, fever, dizziness, angioneurotic edema, asthmatic symptoms, "smarting" of the eyes, weakness, hypotension, *anaphylaxis.* **OD** **Overdose Management:** *Symptoms:* Stupor, coma, shock, respiratory depression, and rarely death. *Treatment:* Supportive measures. Diuresis, osmotic diuresis, peritoneal dialysis, hemodialysis. Monitor urinary output to avoid overhydration. Observe patient for possible relapse due to incomplete gastric emptying and delayed absorption.

Drug Interactions
Alcohol / Additive CNS depressant effects
Antidepressants, tricyclic / ↑ Effect of carisoprodol
Barbiturates / Possible ↑ effect of carisoprodol, followed by inhibition of carisoprodol
Chlorcyclizine / ↓ Effect of carisoprodol
CNS depressants / Additive CNS depression
MAO inhibitors / ↑ Effect of carisoprodol by ↓ breakdown by liver
Phenobarbital / ↓ Effect of carisoprodol by ↑ breakdown by liver
Phenothiazines / Additive depressant effects

EMS CONSIDERATIONS

See also *Skeletal Muscle Relaxants, Centrally Acting.*

Carteolol hydrochloride
(kar-TEE-oh-lohl)
Pregnancy Class: C
Cartrol, Ocupress **(Rx)**
Classification: Beta-adrenergic blocking agent

Mechanism of Action: Has both beta-1 and beta-2 receptor blocking activity. It has no membrane-stabilizing activity but does have moderate intrinsic sympathomimetic effects.

Uses: PO. Hypertension. *Investigational:* Reduce frequency of anginal attacks. **Ophthalmic.** Chronic open-angle glaucoma and intraocular hypertension alone or in combination with other drugs.

Contraindications: Severe, persistent bradycardia. Bronchial asthma or bronchospasm, including severe COPD.

Precautions: Dosage not established in children.

Route/Dosage
• **Tablets**
Hypertension.
Initial: 2.5 mg once daily either alone or with a diuretic. If response is inadequate, the dose may be increased gradually to 5 mg and then 10 mg/day as a single dose. **Maintenance:** 2.5–5 mg once daily. Doses greater than 10 mg/day are not likely to increase the beneficial effect and may decrease the response. Increase the dosage interval in patients with renal impairment.
Reduce frequency of anginal attacks.
10 mg/day.
• **Ophthalmic Solution**
Usual: 1 gtt in affected eye b.i.d. If the response is unsatisfactory, concomitant therapy may be initiated.
How Supplied: *Ophthalmic solution:* 1%; *Tablet:* 2.5 mg, 5 mg
Side Effects: Ophthalmic use: Transient irritation, burning, tearing, conjunctival hyperemia, edema, blurred or cloudy vision, photophobia, decreased night vision, ptosis, blepharoconjunctivitis, abnormal corneal staining, corneal sensitivity.

EMS CONSIDERATIONS

See also *Beta-Adrenergic Blocking Agents.*

Carvedilol
(kar-VAY-dih-lol)
Pregnancy Class: C

Coreg **(Rx)**
Classification: Alpha/beta-adrenergic blocking agent

C

Mechanism of Action: Has both alpha- and beta-adrenergic blocking activity. Decreases cardiac output, reduces exercise- or isoproterenol-induced tachycardia, reduces reflex orthostatic hypotension, causes vasodilation, and reduces peripheral vascular resistance. Significant beta-blocking activity occurs within 60 min while alpha-blocking action is observed within 30 min. BP is lowered more in the standing than in the supine position. Significantly lowers plasma renin activity when given for at least 4 weeks.

Uses: Essential hypertension used either alone or in combination with other antihypertensive drugs, especially thiazide diuretics. Used with digitalis, diuretics, and ACE inhibitors to reduce the progression of mild to moderate CHF of ischemic or cardiomyopathic origin. *Investigational:* Angina pectoris, idiopathic cardiomyopathy.

Contraindications: Patients with New York Heart Association Class IV decompensated cardiac failure, bronchial asthma, or related bronchospastic conditions, second- or third-degree AV block, sick sinus syndrome (unless a permanent pacemaker is in place), cardiogenic shock, severe bradycardia, drug hypersensitivity. Hepatic impairment. Lactation.

Precautions: Use with caution in hypertensive patients with CHF controlled with digitalis, diuretics, or an ACE inhibitor. Use with caution in peripheral vascular disease, in surgical procedures using anesthetic agents that depress myocardial function, in diabetics receiving insulin or oral hypoglycemic drugs, in those subject to spontaneous hypoglycemia, or in thyrotoxicosis. Patients with a history of severe anaphylactic reaction to a variety of allergen may be more reactive to repeated challenge while taking beta blocker. Safety and efficacy have not been established in children less than 18 years of age.

Route/Dosage
• **Tablets**
Essential hypertension.
Initial: 6.25 mg b.i.d. If this is tolerated, using standing systolic pressure measured about 1 hr after dosing, maintain the dose for 7–14 days. **Then,** increase to 12.5 mg b.i.d., if necessary, based on trough BP, using standing systolic pressure 2 hr after dosing. This dose should be maintained for 7–14 days and can then be adjusted upward to 25 mg b.i.d. if necessary and tolerated. The total daily dose should not exceed 50 mg.
Congestive heart failure.
Initial: 3.125 mg b.i.d. for 2 weeks. If this is tolerated, increase to 6.25 mg b.i.d. Dosing is doubled every 2 weeks to the highest tolerated level, up to a maximum of 25 mg b.i.d. in those weighing less than 85 kg and 50 mg b.i.d. in those weighing over 85 kg.
Angina pectoris.
25–50 mg b.i.d.
Idiopathic cardiomyopathy.
6.25–25 mg b.i.d.

How Supplied: *Tablet:* 3.125 mg, 6.25 mg, 12.5 mg, 25 mg

Side Effects: *CV:* Bradycardia, postural hypotension, dependent or peripheral edema, AV block, extrasystoles, hypertension, hypotension, palpitations, peripheral ischemia, syncope, angina, *cardiac failure,* myocardial ischemia, tachycardia, CV disorder. *CNS:* Dizziness, headache, somnolence, insomnia, ataxia, hypesthesia, paresthesia, vertigo, depression, nervousness, migraine, neuralgia, paresis, amnesia, confusion, sleep disorder, impaired concentration, abnormal thinking, paranoia, emotional lability. *Body as a whole:* Fatigue, viral infection, rash, allergy, asthenia, malaise, pain, injury, fever, infection, somnolence, sweating, *sudden death.* *GI:* Diarrhea, abdominal pain, bilirubinemia, N&V, flatulence, dry mouth, anorexia, dyspepsia, melena, periodontitis, increased hepatic enzymes, *GI hemorrhage. Respiratory:* Rhinitis, pharyngitis, sinusitis, bronchitis, dyspnea, **asthma, broncho-spasm,** pulmonary edema, respiratory alkalosis, dyspnea, respiratory disorder, URTI, coughing. *GU:* UTI, albuminuria, hematuria, frequency of micturition, abnormal renal function, impotence. *Dermatologic:* Pruritus; erythematous, maculopapular, and psoriaform rashes, photosensitivity reaction, exfoliative dermatitis. *Metabolic:* Hypertriglyceridemia, hypercholesterolemia, hyperglycemia, hypovolemia, hyperuricemia, increased weight, gout, dehydration, hypervolemia, glycosuria, hyponatremia, hypokalemia, hyperkalemia, diabetes mellitus. *Hematologic:* Thrombocytopenia, anemia, leukopenia, pancytopenia, purpura, atypical lymphocytes. *Musculoskeletal:* Back pain, arthralgia, myalgia, arthritis. *Otic:* Decreased hearing, tinnitus. *Miscellaneous:* Hot flushes, leg cramps, abnormal vision, **anaphylactoid reaction.**

OD **Overdose Management:** *Symptoms:* Severe hypotension, bradycardia, cardiac insufficiency, **cardiogenic shock, cardiac arrest, generalized seizures,** respiratory problems, bronchospasms, vomiting, lapse of consciousness. *Treatment:* Place the patient in a supine position and monitor carefully and treat under intensive care conditions. Treatment should continue for a long enough period of time consistent with the 7- to 10-hr half-life of the drug.

• Gastric lavage or induced emesis shortly after ingestion
• For excessive bradycardia, atropine, 2 mg IV. If the bradycardia is resistant to therapy, perform pacemaker therapy.
• To support cardiovascular function, give glucagon, 5–10 mg IV rapidly over 30 sec, followed by a continuous infusion of 5 mg/hr. Sympathomimetics (dobutamine, isoproterenol, epinephrine) may be given.
• For peripheral vasodilation, give epinephrine or norepinephrine with continuous monitoring of circulatory conditions.

• For bronchospasm, give beta sympathomimetics as aerosol or IV or give aminophylline IV.
• In the event of seizures, give a slow IV injection of diazepam or clonazepam.

Drug Interactions
Antidiabetic agents / The beta-blocking effect may ↑ the hypoglycemic effect of insulin and oral hypoglycemics
Calcium channel blocking agents / ↑ Risk of conduction disturbances
Clonidine / Potentiation of BP and heart rate lowering effects
Digoxin / ↑ Digoxin levels
Rifampin / ↓ Plasma levels of carvedilol

EMS CONSIDERATIONS
See also *Adrenergic Blocking Agents.*

Cefaclor
(SEF-ah-klor)
Pregnancy Class: B
Ceclor, Ceclor CD **(Rx)**
Classification: Cephalosporin, second-generation

Uses: Otitis media due to *Streptococcus pneumoniae, Hemophilus influenzae, Streptococcus pyogenes,* and staphylococci. Upper respiratory tract infections (including pharyngitis and tonsillitis) caused by *S. pyogenes.* Lower respiratory tract infections (including pneumonia) due to *S. pneumoniae, H. influenzae,* and *S. pyogenes.* Skin and skin structure infections due to *Staphylococcus aureus* and *S. pyogenes.* UTIs (including pyelonephritis and cystitis) caused by *Escherichia coli, Proteus mirabilis, Klebsiella,* and coagulase-negative staphylococci.

Extended-release tablets: Acute bacterial exacerbations of chronic bronchitis due to non-β-lactamase-producing strains of *H. influenzae, Moraxella catarrhalis* (including β-lactamase-producing strains)*,* or *S. pneumoniae.* Secondary bacterial infections of acute bronchitis due to *H. influenzae* (non-β-lactamase-producing strains only), *M. catarrhalis* (including β-lactamase-producing strains), or *S. pneumoniae*. Pharyngitis or tonsillitis due to *S. pyogenes*. Uncomplicated skin and skin structure infections due to *S. aureus* (methicillin-susceptible). *Investigational:* Acute uncomplicated UTIs in select populations using a single dose of 2 g. **Precautions:** Safety for use in infants less than 1 month of age has not been established.

Route/Dosage
• **Capsules, Oral Suspension**
   All uses.
Adults: 250 mg q 8 hr. Dose may be doubled in more severe infections or those caused by less susceptible organisms. Total daily dose should not exceed 4 g. **Children:** 20 mg/kg/day in divided doses q 8 hr. Dose may be doubled in more serious infections, otitis media, or for infections caused by less susceptible organisms. For otitis media and pharyngitis, the total daily dose may be divided and given q 12 hr. Total daily dose should not exceed 2 g.
• **Tablets, Extended Release**
   Acute bacterial exacerbations, chronic bronchitis, secondary bacterial infections of acute bronchitis.
500 mg q 12 hr for 7 days.
   Pharyngitis, tonsillitis.
375 mg q 12 hr for 10 days.
   Uncomplicated skin and skin structure infections.
375 mg q 12 hr for 7–10 days.
How Supplied: *Capsule:* 250 mg, 500 mg; *Powder for Reconstitution:* 125 mg/5 mL, 187 mg/5 mL, 250 mg/5 mL, 375 mg/5 mL; *Tablet, Extended Release:* 375 mg, 500 mg
Side Effects: Additional: Cholestatic jaundice, lymphocytosis.

EMS CONSIDERATIONS

See also *Anti-Infectives* and *Cephalosporins*.

Cefadroxil monohydrate
(sef-ah-DROX-ill)
Pregnancy Class: B

Duricef **(Rx)**
Classification: Cephalosporin, first-generation

Uses: UTIs caused by *Escherichia coli, Proteus mirabilis,* and *Klebsiella.* Skin and skin structure infections due to staphylococci or streptococci. Pharyngitis and tonsillitis due to group A beta-hemolytic streptococci. **Precautions:** Safe use in children not established.

Route/Dosage
• **Capsules, Oral Suspension, Tablets**
   Pharyngitis, tonsillitis.
Adults: 1 g/day in single or two divided doses for 10 days. **Children:** 30 mg/kg/day in single or two divided doses (for beta-hemolytic streptococcoal infection, dose should be given for 10 or more days).
   Skin and skin structure infections.
Adults: 1 g/day in single or two divided doses. **Children:** 30 mg/kg/day in divided doses q 12 hr.
   UTIs.
Adults: 1–2 g/day in single or two divided doses for uncomplicated lower UTI (e.g., cystitis). For all other UTIs, the usual dose is 2 g/day in two divided doses. **Children:** 30 mg/kg/day in divided doses q 12 hr.
   For patients with C_{CR} rates below 50 mL/min.
Initial: 1 g; **maintenance,** 500 mg at following dosage intervals: q 36 hr for C_{CR} rates of 0–10 mL/min; q 24 hr for C_{CR} rates of 10–25 mL/min; q 12 hr for C_{CR} rates of 25–50 mL/min.
How Supplied: *Capsule:* 500 mg; *Powder for Reconstitution:* 125 mg/5 mL, 250 mg/5 mL, 500 mg/5 mL; *Tablet:* 1 g

---

EMS CONSIDERATIONS

See also *Anti-Infectives* and *Cephalosporins*.

Cefazolin sodium
(sef-AYZ-oh-lin)
Pregnancy Class: B
Ancef, Kefzol, Zolicef **(Rx)**
Classification: Cephalosporin, first-generation

Uses: Respiratory tract infections due to *Streptococcus pneumoniae, Klebsiella, Haemophilus influenzae, Staphylococcus aureus,* and group A β–hemolytic streptococci. GU infections (prostatitis, epididymitis) due to *Escherichia coli, Proteus mirabilis, Klebsiella,* and some strains of *Enterobacter* and enterococci. Skin and skin structure infections due to *S. aureus,* group A β–hemolytic streptococci, and other strains of streptococci. Biliary tract infections due to *E. coli,* various strains of streptococci, *P. mirabilis, Klebsiella,* and *S. aureus.* Bone and joint infections due to *S. aureus.* Septicemia due to *S. pneumoniae, S. aureus, P. mirabilis, E. coli,* and *Klebsiella.* Endocarditis due to *S. aureus* and group A β–hemolytic streptococci. Perioperative prophylaxis may reduce the incidence of certain postoperative infections in those having contaminated or potentially contaminated surgical procedures (e.g., vaginal hysterectomy or cholecystectomy).

Precautions: Safety in infants under 1 month of age has not been determined.

Route/Dosage —————————
• **IM, IV Only**
   Mild infections due to gram-positive cocci.
Adults: 250–500 mg q 8 hr.
   Mild to moderate infections.
Children over 1 month: 25–50 mg/kg/day in three to four doses.
   Moderate to severe infections.
Adults: 0.5–1 g q 6–8 hr.
   Acute, uncomplicated UTIs.
Adults: 1 g q 12 hr. For severe infections, up to 100 mg/kg/day may be used.
   Endocarditis, septicemia.
Adults: 1–1.5 g q 6 hr (rarely, up to 12 g/day).
   Pneumococcal pneumonia.
Adults: 0.5 g q 12 hr.
   Preoperative prophylaxis.
Adults: 1 g 30–60 min prior to surgery.

   During surgery of 2 or more hours.
Adults: 0.5–1 g.
   Postoperative prophylaxis.
Adults: 0.5–1 g q 6–8 hr for 24 hr (may be given for 3–5 days, especially in open heart surgery or prosthetic arthroplasty).
   Impaired renal function.
Initial: 0.5 g; **then,** maintenance doses are given, depending on C_{CR}, according to schedule provided by manufacturer.
How Supplied: *Injection:* 1 g/50 mL, 500 mg/50 mL; *Powder for injection:* 500 mg, 1 g, 10 g, 20 g
Side Effects: Additional: When high doses are used in renal failure patients: extreme confusion, *tonic-clonic seizures,* mild hemiparesis.

EMS CONSIDERATIONS

See also *Anti-Infectives* and *Cephalosporins.*

Cefdinir
(SEF-dih-near)
Pregnancy Class: B
Omnicef **(Rx)**
Classification: Cephalosporin, third generation

Uses: Adults: (1) Community-acquired pneumonia or acute exacerbations of chronic bronchitis due to *Haemophilus influenzae* (including β-lactamase producing strains), *Haemophilus parainfluenzae* (including β-lactamase producing strains), *Streptococcus pneumoniae* (penicillin-susceptible strains only), and *Moraxella catarrhalis* (including β-lactamase producing strains). (2) Acute maxillary sinusitis due to *Haemophilus influenzae* (including β-lactamase producing strains), *Streptococcius pneumoniae* (penicillin-susceptible strains only), and *Moraxella catarrhalis* (including β-lactamase producing strains). (3) Uncomplicated skin and skin structure infections due to *Staphylococcus aureus* (including β-lactamase producing strains and *Streptococcus pyogenes.)*

---
bold italic = life threatening side effect

Children: (1) Acute bacterial otitis media due to *H. influenzae* (including β-lactamase producing strains), *S. pneumoniae* (penicillin-susceptible strains only), and *M. catarrhalis* (including β-lactamase producing strains). (2) Pharyngitis/tonsillitis due to *S. pyogenes.* (3) Uncomplicated skin and skin structure infections due to *S. aureus* (including β-lactamase producing strains) and *S. pyogenes.*

Contraindications: Allergy to cephalosporins.

Precautions: Safety and efficacy have not been determined in infants less than 6 months of age.

Route/Dosage ─────────────
• **Capsules**
Community-acquired pneumonia, uncomplicated skin and skin structure infections.
Adults and adolescents age 13 and older: 300 mg q 12 hr for 10 days.
Acute exacerbations of chronic bronchitis, acute maxillary sinusitis, or pharyngitis/tonsillitis.
Adults and adolescents age 13 and older: 300 mg q 12 hr or 600 mg q 24 hr for 10 days (5–10 days for pharyngitis/tonsillitis).
• **Oral Suspension**
Acute bacterial otitis media, acute maxillary sinusitis, pharyngitis/tonsillitis.
Children, 6 months through 12 years: 7 mg/kg q 12 hr or 14 mg/kg q 24 hr for 10 days (5–10 days for pharyngitis/tonsillitis).
Uncomplicated skin and skin structure infections.
Children, 6 months through 12 years: 7 mg/kg q 12 hr for 10 days.
How Supplied: *Capsules:* 300 mg; *Oral Suspension:* 125 mg/5mL
Side Effects: See Cephalosporins.
Drug Interactions
Antacids, aluminum– or magnesium–containing / ↓ Absorption of cefdinir
Probenecid / ↑ Plasma levels of cefdinir → enhanced effect

EMS CONSIDERATIONS

See also *Cephalosporins.*

Cefepime hydrochloride
(SEF-eh-pim)
Pregnancy Class: B
Maxipime **(Rx)**
Classification: Cephalosporin, third-generation

Mechanism of Action: Antibacterial activity against both gram-negative and gram-positive pathogens, including those resistant to other β-lactam antibiotics. High affinity for the multiple penicillin-binding proteins that are essential for cell wall synthesis.

Uses: Uncomplicated and complicated UTIs (including pyelonephritis) caused by *Escherichia coli* or *Klebsiella pneumoniae;* when the infection is severe or caused by *E. coli, K. pneumoniae,* or *Proteus mirabilis;* when the infection is mild to moderate, including infections associated with concurrent bacteremia with these microorganisms. Uncomplicated skin and skin structure infections caused by *Staphylococcus aureus* (methicillin-susceptible strains only) or *Streptococcus pyogenes.* Moderate to severe pneumonia due to *Streptococcus pneumoniae,* including cases associated with concurrent bacteremia, *Pseudomonas aeruginosa, K. pneumoniae,* or *Enterobacter* species. Monotherapy for empiric treatment of febrile neutropenia.

Contraindications: Use in those who have had an immediate hypersensitivity reaction to cefepime, cephalosporins, pencillins, or any other β-lactam antibiotics.

Precautions: Use with caution during lactation. Safety and efficacy have not been determined in children less than 12 years of age.

Route/Dosage ─────────────
• **IM, IV**
Mild to moderate uncomplicated or complicated UTIs, including pyelonephritis, due to E. coli, K. pneumoniae, *or* P. mirabilis.
Adults and children over 12 years: 0.5–1 g IV or IM (for *E. coli* infections) q 12 hr for 7–10 days.

Severe uncomplicated or complicated UTIs, including pyelonephritis, due to E. coli *or* K. pneumoniae.
Adults and children over 12 years: 2 g IV q 12 hr for 10 days.

Moderate to severe pneumonia due to S. pneumoniae, P. aeruginosa, K. pneumoniae, *or* Enterobacter *species.*
Adults and children over 12 years: 1–2 g IV q 12 hr for 10 days.

Moderate to severe uncomplicated skin and skin structure infections due to S. aureus *or* S. pyogenes.
Adults and children over 12 years: 2 g IV q 12 hr for 10 days.

Febrile neutropenia.
2 g IV q 8 hr for 7 days, or until resolution of neutropenia.
How Supplied: *Powder for injection:* 500 mg, 1 g, 2 g
Side Effects: See *Cephalosporins.* The most common side effects include rash, phlebitis, pain, and/or inflammation.
Drug Interactions
Aminoglycosides / ↑ Risk of nephrotoxicity and ototoxicity
Furosemide / ↑ Risk of nephrotoxicity

EMS CONSIDERATIONS

See also *Cephalosporins.*

Cefixime oral
(seh-FIX-eem)
Pregnancy Class: B
Suprax **(Rx)**
Classification: Cephalosporin, third-generation

Uses: Uncomplicated UTIs caused by *E. coli* and *P. mirabilis.* Otitis media due to *H. influenzae* (beta-lactamase positive and negative strains), *Moraxella catarrhalis,* and *S. pyogenes.* Pharyngitis and tonsillitis caused by *S. pyogenes.* Acute bronchitis and acute exacerbations of chronic bronchitis caused by *S. pneumoniae* and *H. influenzae* (beta-lactamase positive and negative strains). Uncomplicated cervical or urethral gonorrhea due to *N. gonor-*

rhoeae (both penicillinase- and non-penicillinase-producing strains).
Precautions: Safe use in infants less than 6 months old has not been established.

Route/Dosage
• **Oral Suspension, Tablets**
Adults: Either 400 mg once daily or 200 mg q 12 hr. **Children:** Either 8 mg/kg once daily or 4 mg/kg q 12 hr. Patients on renal dialysis or in whom C_{CR} is 21–60 mL/min, the dose should be 75% of the standard dose (i.e., 300 mg/day). If the C_{CR} is less than 20 mL/min, the dose should be 50% of the standard dose (i.e., 200 mg/day).

Uncomplicated gonorrhea.
One 400-mg tablet daily.
How Supplied: *Powder for Reconstitution:* 100 mg/5 mL; *Tablet:* 200 mg, 400 mg
Side Effects: Additional: *GI:* Flatulence. *Hepatic:* Elevated alkaline phosphatase levels. *Renal:* Transient increases in BUN or creatinine.

EMS CONSIDERATIONS

See also *Anti-Infectives* and *Cephalosporins.*

Cefoperazone sodium
(sef-oh-PER-ah-zohn)
Pregnancy Class: B
Cefobid **(Rx)**
Classification: Cephalosporin, third-generation

Uses: Respiratory tract infections due to *Streptococcus pneumoniae, Haemophilus influenzae, Staphylococcus aureus* (penicillinase/non-penicillinase producing), *S. pyogenes* (group A β–hemolytic streptococci), *Pseudomonas aeruginosa, Klebsiella pneumoniae, Escherichia coli, Proteus mirabilis,* and *Enterococcus* species. Peritonitis and other intra–abdominal infections due to *E. coli, P. aeruginosa,* enterococci, anaerobic gram–negative bacilli (including *Bacteroides fragilis).* Bacterial septicemia due to *S. pneumoniae, S. agalactiae, S. aureus,*

---

bold italic = life threatening side effect

enterococci, *P. aeruginosa, E. coli, Klebsiella* species, *Proteus* species, *Clostridium* species, and anaerobic gram–positive cocci. Skin and skin structure infections due to *S. aureus, S. pyogenes, P. aeruginosa,* and enterococci. Pelvic inflammatory disease, endometritis, and other female genital tract infections due to *N. gonorrhoeae, S. epidermidis, S. agalactiae, E. coli, Clostridium* species, enterococci, *Bacteroides* species, anaerobic gram–positive cocci. Urinary tract infections due to enterococci, *E. coli,* and *P. aeruginosa.*

Precautions: Use with caution in hepatic disease or biliary obstruction. Safety and effectiveness have not been determined in children.

Route/Dosage
• **IM, IV**
Adults, usual: 2–4 g/day in equally divided doses q 12 hr (up to 12–16 g/day has been used in severe infections or for less sensitive organisms).

NOTE: This drug is significantly excreted in the bile; thus, the daily dose should not exceed 4 g in hepatic disease or biliary obstruction.

How Supplied: *Powder for injection:* 1 g, 2 g, 10 g

Side Effects: Additional: Hypoprothrombinemia resulting from bleeding and/or bruising.

Drug Interactions: Additional: Concomitant use with ethanol may cause and Antabuse-like reaction.

EMS CONSIDERATIONS

See also *Anti-Infectives* and *Cephalosporins.*

Cefotaxime sodium
(sef-oh-TAX-eem)
Pregnancy Class: B
Claforan **(Rx)**
Classification: Cephalosporin, third-generation

Uses: Infections of the GU tract, lower respiratory tract (including pneumonia), skin, skin structures, bones, joints, and CNS (including ventriculitis and meningitis). Intra-abdominal infections (including peritonitis), gynecologic infections (including endometritis, pelvic cellulitis, pelvic inflammatory disease), septicemia, bacteremia, and prophylaxis in surgery. Used with aminoglycosides for gram-positive or gram-negative sepsis where the causative agent has not been identified.

The IV route is preferable for patients with severe or life-threatening infections; for patients after surgery; or for those manifesting malnutrition, trauma, malignancy, heart failure, or diabetes, especially if shock is present or possible.

Route/Dosage
• **IV, IM**
Uncomplicated infections.
Adults: 1 g q 12 hr.
Moderate to severe infections.
Adults: 1–2 g q 8 hr.
Septicemia.
Adults, IV: 2 g q 6–8 hr, not to exceed 12 g/day.
Life-threatening infections.
Adults, IV: 2 g q 4 hr, not to exceed 12 g/day.
Gonorrhea.
Adults, IM: Single dose of 1 g for rectal gonorrhea in males. **IM:** Single dose of 0.5 g for rectal gonorrhea in females or gonococcoal urethritis/cervicitis in males and females.
Preoperative prophylaxis.
Adults: 1 g 30–90 min prior to surgery.
Cesarean section.
IV: 1 g when the umbilical cord is clamped; **then,** give 1 g 6 and 12 hr after the first dose.
Use in children.
Pediatric, 1 month to 12 years, IM, IV: 50–180 mg/kg/day in four to six divided doses; **1–4 weeks, IV:** 50 mg/kg q 8 hr; **0–1 week, IV:** 50 mg/kg q 12 hr. *NOTE:* Use adult dose in children 50 kg or over.
Use in impaired renal function.
If C_{CR} is less than 20 mL/min/1.73m², reduce the dose by 50%. If only serum creatinine is available, use the following formulas to calculate C_{CR}:
Males: Weight (kg) x (140-age) / 72 x serum creatinine (mg/dL).

Females: 0.85 x above value.
How Supplied: *Injection:* 1 g/50 mL, 2 g/50 mL; *Powder for injection:* 500 mg, 1 g, 2 g, 10 g

EMS CONSIDERATIONS

See also *Anti-Infectives* and *Cephalosporins.*

Cefotetan disodium

(sef-oh-TEE-tan)
Pregnancy Class: B
Cefotan **(Rx)**
Classification: Cephalosporin, second-generation

Uses: Urinary tract infections due to *Escherichia coli, Klebsiella* species, *Proteus vulgaris, Providencia rettgeri,* and *Morganella morganii.* Lower respiratory tract infections due to *Streptococcus pneumoniae, Staphylococcus aureus, H. influenzae* (including ampicillin–resistant strains), *Klebsiella* species, *Proteus mirabilis, Serratia marcescens,* and *E. coli.* Skin and skin structure infections due to *S. aureus, S. epidermidis, S. pyogenes, Streptococcus* species (excluding enterococci), *Klebsiella* pneumonia, *Peptococcus niger, Peptostreptococcus* species, and *E. coli.* Gynecologic infections due to *S. aureus, S. epidermidis, Streptococcus* species (excluding enterococcus), *S. agalactiae, E. coli, P. mirabilis, N. gonorrhoeae, Bacteroides* species (excluding *B. distasonis, B. ovatus, B. thetaiotaomicron), Fusobacterium* species and gram–positive anaeroabic cocci (including *Peptococcus* and *Peptostreptococcus* species). Intra–abdominal infections due to *E. coli, Klebsiella* species (including *K. pneumoniae), Streptococcus* species (excluding enterococci), *Bacteroides* species (excluding *B. distasonis, B. ovatus, B. thetaiotaomicron),* and *Clostridium* species. Bone and joint infections due to *S. aureus.* Perioperatively to prevent infections in those underoing cesarian section, abdominal or vaginal hysterectomy, trans-

urethral surgery, or GI and biliary tract surgery.

The IV route is preferred with bacterial septicemia, bacteremia, or other severe or life-threatening infections. It's also preferred for poor-risk patients as the result of malnutrition, surgery, diabetes, trauma, heart failure, malignancy, or if shock is present or impending.
Precautions: Safety and effectiveness have not been determined in children.

Route/Dosage ————————
• **IV or IM**
Mild to moderate skin/skin structure infections.
Adults: 2 g q 24 hr IV or 1 g q 12 hr IV or IM. *Klebseilla pneumoniae* skin/skin structure infections: 1 or 2 g q 12 hr IV or IM.
Severe skin/skin structure infections.
Adults, IV: 2 g q 12 hr.
UTIs.
Adults: Either 0.5 g q 12 hr IV or IM, 1 or 2 g q 24 hr IV or IM, or 1 or 2 g q 12 hr IV or IM.
Infections of other sites.
Adults: 1 or 2 g q 12 hr IV or IM.
Severe infections.
Adults, IV: 2 g q 12 hr.
Life-threatening infections.
Adults, IV: 3 g q 12 hr.
Prophylaxis of postoperative infection.
Adults, IV: 1–2 g 30–60 min prior to surgery.
Use in impaired renal function.
May maintain q 12 hr dosing but reduce dose by ½ if the C_{CR} is 10–30 mL/min and reduce the dose by ¼ if the C_{CR} is less than 10 mL/min.
How Supplied: *Injection:* 1 g/50 mL, 2 g/50 mL; *Powder for injection:* 1 g, 2 g, 10 g
Side Effects: Additional: Concomitant use with ethanol produces a disulfiram-type reaction and hypotension.

EMS CONSIDERATIONS

See also *Anti-Infectives* and *Cephalosporins.*

---

bold italic = life threatening side effect

Cefoxitin sodium

(seh-FOX-ih-tin)
Pregnancy Class: B
Mefoxin **(Rx)**
Classification: Cephalosporin, second-generation

Mechanism of Action: Broad-spectrum cephalosporin that is penicillinase- and cephalosporinase-resistant and is stable in the presence of beta-lactamases.

Uses: Lower respiratory tract infections (pneumonia and abcess) due to *Streptococcus pneumoniae,* other streptococci (excluding enterococci such as *S. faecalis), Staphylococcus aureus, Escherichia coli, Klebsiella* species, *Haemophilus influenzae,* and *Bacteroides* species. UTIs due to *E. coli, Klebsiella* species, *Proteus mirabilis, Morganella morganii, Proteus vulgaris,* and *Providencia* species (including *P. rettgeri).* Uncomplicated gonorrhea due to *Neisseria gonorrhoeae* (penicillinase/non–penicillinase producing). Intra–abdominal infections (peritonitis and intra–abdominal abscess) due to *E. coli, Klebsiella* species, *Bacteroides* species (including *B. fragilis),* and *Clostridium* species. Gynecological infections (endometritis, pelvic cellulitis, pelvic inflammatory disease) due to *E. coli, N. gonorrhoeae, Bacteroides* species (including *B. fragilis* group), *Clostridium* species, *Peptococcus* species, *Peptostreptococcus* species, and group B streptococci. Septicemia due to *S. pneumoniae, S. aureus, E. coli, Klebsiella* species, and *Bacteroides* species (including *B. fragilis).* Bone and joint infections due to *S. aureus.* Skin and skin structure infections due to *S. aureus, S. epidermidis,* streptococci (excluding enterococci, especially *S. faecalis), E. coli, P. mirabilis, Klebsiella* species, *Bacteroides* species (including the *B. fragilis* group), *Clostridium* species, *Peptococcus* species, and *Peptostreptococcus* species. Perioperative prophylaxis, including vaginal hysterectomy, GI surgery, transurethral prostatectomy, prosthetic arthroplasty, and cesarean section.

NOTE: Many gram-negative infections resistant to certain cephalosporins and penicillins respond to cefoxitin.

Route/Dosage ─────────

• **IM, IV**
Uncomplicated infections (cutaneous, pneumonia, urinary tract).
Adults: 1 g q 6–8 hr IV.
Moderately severe or severe infections.
Adults: 1 g q 4 hr or 2 g q 6–8 hr IV.
Infections requiring higher dosage (e.g., gas gangrene).
Adults: 2 g q 4 hr or 3 g q 6 hr IV.
Gonorrhea.
Adults: 2 g IM with 1 g probenecid PO.
Prophylaxis in surgery.
Adults: 2 g IV 30–60 min before surgery followed by 2 g q 6 hr after first dose for 24 hr only (72 hr for prosthetic arthroplasty).
Cesarean section, prophylaxis.
2 g **IV** when cord is clamped; **then,** give two additional doses IV 4 and 8 hr later.
TURP, prophylaxis.
1 g before surgery; **then,** 1 g q 8 hr for up to 5 days.
Impaired renal function.
Initial: 1–2 g; **then,** follow maintenance schedule provided by manufacturer. When only creatinine level is available, use the following formulas to obtain C_{CR}:
Males: Weight (kg) x (140 - age) / 72 x serum creatinine (mg/dL).
Females: 0.85 x above value.
Use in children for infections.
Children over 3 months: 80–160 mg/kg/day in four to six divided doses. Total daily dosage should not exceed 12 g.
Use in children for prophylaxis.
Children over 3 months: 30–40 mg/kg q 6 hr.
How Supplied: *Injection:* 1 g/50 mL, 2 g/50 mL; *Powder for injection:* 1 g, 2 g, 10 g

EMS CONSIDERATIONS

See also *Anti-Infectives* and *Cephalosporins.*

Cefpodoxime proxetil

(sef-poh-DOX-eem)
Pregnancy Class: B
Vantin **(Rx)**
Classification: Cephalosporin, third-generation

Uses: Acute, community-acquired pneumonia due to *Streptococcus pneumoniae* or *Hemophilus influenzae* (non-β-lactamase-producing strains only). Acute bacterial exacerbation of chronic bronchitis caused by *S. pneumoniae*, non-beta-lactamase-producing *H. influenzae*, or M. catarrhalis. Acute otitis media caused by *S. pneumoniae*, *H. influenzae* (including beta-lactamase-producing strains), and *Moraxella catarrhalis*. Pharyngitis or tonsillitis due to *Streptococcus pyogenes*. Acute, uncomplicated urethral and cervical gonorrhea caused by *Neisseria gonorrhoeae* (including penicillinase-producing strains). Acute, uncomplicated anorectal infections in women due to *N. gonorrhoeae* (including penicillinase-producing strains). Uncomplicated skin and skin structure infections due to *Staphylococcus aureus* (including penicillinase-producing strains) or *S. pyogenes*. Uncomplicated UTIs (cystitis) due to *Escherichia coli*, *Klebsiella pneumoniae*, *Proteus mirabilis*, or *Staphyloccus saprophyticus*.

Route/Dosage
• **Tablets, Suspension**
Acute community-acquired pneumonia.
Adults and children over 13 years: 200 mg q 12 hr for 14 days.
Acute bacterial exacerbations of chronic bronchitis.
Adults and children over 13 years: 200 mg q 12 hr for 10 days. Use the tablets.
Uncomplicated gonorrhea (men and women) and rectal gonococcal infections (women).
Adults and children over 13 years: Single dose of 200 mg.
Skin and skin structure infections.
Adults and children over 13 years: 400 mg q 12 hr for 7–14 days.

Pharyngitis, tonsillitis.
Adults and children over 13 years: 100 mg q 12 hr for 5–10 days.
Children, 5 months–12 years: 5 mg/kg (maximum of 100 mg/dose) q 12 hr (maximum daily dose: 200 mg) for 5–10 days.
Uncomplicated UTIs.
Adults and children over 13 years: 100 mg q 12 hr for 7 days.
Acute otitis media.
Children, 5 months–12 years: 5 mg/kg (maximum of 200 mg/dose) q 12 hr or 10 mg/kg (maximum of 400 mg/dose) q 24 hr for 10 days.
How Supplied: *Granule for Reconstitution:* 50 mg/5 mL, 100 mg/5 mL; *Tablet:* 100 mg, 200 mg

EMS CONSIDERATIONS

See also *Anti-Infectives* and *Cephalosporins*.

Cefprozil

(SEF-proh-zill)
Pregnancy Class: B
Cefzil **(Rx)**
Classification: Cephalosporin, second-generation

Uses: Pharyngitis and tonsillitis due to *Streptococcus pyogenes*. Acute bacterial sinusitis due to *Streptococcus pneumoniae*, *Staphylococcus aureus*, *Haemophilus influenzae* (including β-lactamase producing strains), and *Morazella catarrhalis* (including β-lactamase producing strains). Otitis media caused by *S. pneumoniae*, *H. influenzae*, and *M. catarrhalis*. Uncomplicated skin and skin structure infections due to *S. aureus* (including penicillinase-producing strains) and *S. pyogenes*. Secondary bacterial infection of acute bronchitis and acute bacterial exacerbation of chronic bronchitis due to *S. pneumoniae*, *H. influenzae* (beta-lactamase positive and negative strains), and *M. catarrhalis*.

Route/Dosage
• **Suspension, Tablets**
Pharyngitis, tonsillitis.

---

bold italic = life threatening side effect

Adults and children over 13 years of age: 500 mg q 24 hr for at least 10 days (for *S. pyogenes* infections, give 10 or more days). **Children, 2–12 years of age:** 7.5 mg/kg q 12 hr for at least 10 days (for *S. pyogenes* infections,give 10 or more days).

Acute sinusitis.

Adults and children over 13 years of age: 250 mg q 12 hr or 500 mg q 12 hr for 10 days. Use the higher dose for moderate to severe infections. **Children, 6 months–12 years of age:** 7.5 mg/kg q 12 hr or 15 mg/kg q 12 hr for 10 days. Use the higher dose for moderate to severe infections.

Secondary bacterial infections of acute bronchitis and acute bacterial exacerbation of chronic bronchitis.

Adults and children over 13 years of age: 500 mg q 12 hr for 10 days.

Uncomplicated skin and skin structure infections.

Adults and children over 13 years of age: Either 250 mg q 12 hr, 500 mg q 24 hr, or 500 mg q 12 hr (all for a duration of 10 days). **Children, 2–12 years of age:** 20 mg/kg q 24 hr for 10 days.

Otitis media.

Infants and children 6 months–12 years: 15 mg/kg q 12 hr for 10 days.

How Supplied: *Powder for Reconstitution:* 125 mg/5 mL, 250 mg/5 mL; *Tablet:* 250 mg, 500 mg

EMS CONSIDERATIONS

See also *Anti-Infectives* and *Cephalosporins.*

Ceftazidime
(sef-TAY-zih-deem)
Pregnancy Class: B
Ceptaz, Fortaz, Tazicef, Tazidime **(Rx)**
Classification: Cephalosporin, third-generation

Uses: Lower respiratory tract infections (including pneumonia) due to *Pseudomonas aeruginosa* and other *Pseudomonas* species, *Haemophilus influenzae* (including ampicillin-resistant strains), *Klebsiella* species, *Enterobacter* species, *Proteus mirabilis, Escerichia coli, Serratia* species, *Citrobacter* species, *Streptococcus pneumoniae, Staphylococcus aureus* (methicillin-susceptible strains). Skin and skin structure infections due to *P. aeruginosa, Klebsiella* species, *E. coli, Proteus* species (including *P. mirabilis* and indole-positive *Proteus*), *Enterobacter* species, *Serratia* species, *S. aureus* (methicillin-susceptible strains), *S. pyogenes* (group A β-hemolytic streptococci). UTIs, both complicated and uncomplicated, due to *P. aeruginosa, Enterobacter* species, *Proteus* species (including *P. mirabilis* and indole-positive *Proteus*), *Klebsiella* species, and *E. coli.* Bacterial septicemia due to *P. aeruginosa, Klebsiella* species, *H. influenzae, E. coli, Serratia* species, *S. pneumoniae, S. aureus* (methicillin-susceptible strains). Bone and joint infections due to *P. aeruginosa, Klebsiella* species, *Enterobacter* species, *S. aureus* (methicillin-susceptible strains). GYN infections, including endometritis, pelvic cellulitis, and other infections of the female genital tract, due to *E. coli.* Intra-abdominal infections, including peritonitis, due to *E. coli, Klebsiella* species, *S. aureus* (methicillin-susceptible strains); polymicrobial infections due to aerobic and anaeraobic organisms and *Bacteroides* species (many strains of *B. fragilis* are resistant). CNS infections, including meningitis, due to *H. influenzae* and *Neisseria meningitidis* (limited effect against *P. aeruginosa* and *S. pneumoniae*). *Note:* May be used with aminoglycosides, vancomycin, and clindamycin in severe and life-threatening infections and in the immunocompromised patient.

Route/Dosage ———————
• **IM, IV**
Usual infections.
Adults,IM, IV: 1 g q 8–12 hr.
UTIs, uncomplicated.
Adults, IM, IV: 0.25 g q 12 hr.
UTIs, complicated.
Adults, IM, IV: 0.5 g q 8–12 hr.
Uncomplicated pneumonia, mild skin and skin structure infections.

Adults, IM, IV: 0.5–1 g q 8 hr.
Bone and joint infections.
Adults, IV: 2 g q 12 hr.
Serious gynecologic or intra-abdominal infections, meningitis, severe or life-threatening infections (especially in immunocompromised patients).
Adults, IV: 2 g q 8 hr.
Pseudomonal lung infections in cystic fibrosis patients with normal renal function.
IV: 30–50 mg/kg q 8 hr, not to exceed 6 g/day.
Use in neonates, infants, and children.
Neonates, 0–4 weeks, IV: 30 mg/kg q 12 hr, not to exceed the adult dose. **Infants and children, 1 month–12 years, IV:** 30–50 mg/kg q 8 hr not to exceed 6 g/day.
How Supplied: *Powder for injection:* 500 mg, 1 g, 2 g, 6 g, 10 g

EMS CONSIDERATIONS

See also *Anti-Infectives* and *Cephalosporins.*

Ceftibuten

(sef-TYE-byou-ten)
Pregnancy Class: B
Cedax **(Rx)**
Classification: Cephalosporin, third-generation

Uses: Acute bacterial exacerbations of chronic bronchitis due to *Haemophilus influenzae* (including β-lactamase-producing strains), *Moraxella catarrhalis* (including β-lactamase-producing strains), and penicillin-susceptible strains of *Streptococcus pneumoniae.* Acute bacterial otitis media due to *H. influenzae* (including β-lactamase-producing strains), *M. catarrhalis* (including β-lactamase-producing strains), and *Staphylococcus pyogenes.* Pharyngitis and tonsillitis due to *S. pyogenes.*

Route/Dosage
• **Capsules, Oral Suspension**
All uses.
Adults and children over 12 years of age: 400 mg once daily for 10

days. The maximum daily dose is 400 mg. Adjust the dose in patients with a creatinine clearance (C_{CR}) less than 50 mL/min as follows. If the C_{CR} is between 30 and 49 mL/min, the recommended dose is 4.5 mg/kg or 200 mg once daily. If the C_{CR} is between 5 and 29 mL/min, the recommended dose is 2.25 mg/kg or 100 mg once daily. In patients undergoing hemodialysis 2 or 3 times/week, a single 400-mg dose of ceftibuten capsules or a single dose of 9 mg/kg (maximum of 400 mg) of PO suspension can be given at the end of each hemodialysis session.
Children: pharyngitis, tonsillitis, acute bacterial otitis media.
9 mg/kg, up to a maximum of 400 mg daily, for a total of 10 days. Give children over 45 kg the maximum daily dose of 400 mg.
How Supplied: *Capsules:* 400 mg; *Oral Suspension:* 90 mg/5mL, 180 mg/5 mL.
Side Effects: See *Cephalosporins.* Ceftibuten is usually well tolerated. The most common side effect is diarrhea.

EMS CONSIDERATIONS

See also *Cephalosporins.*

Ceftizoxime sodium

(sef-tih-ZOX-eem)
Pregnancy Class: B
Cefizox **(Rx)**
Classification: Cephalosporin, third-generation

Uses: Lower respiratory tract infections due to *Streptococcus* species (including *S. pneumoniae,* but excluding enterococci), *Klebsiella* species, *Proteus mirabilis, Escherichia coli, Haemophilus influenzae* (including ampicillin-resistant strains), *Staphylococcus aureus* (penicillinase/nonpenicillinase-producing), *Serratia* species, *Enterobacter* species, and *Bacteroides* species. UTIs due to *S. aureus, E. coli, Pseudomonas* species (including *P. aeruginosa*), *P. mirabilis, P. vulgaris, Providencia* *rettgeri, Morganella morganii, Klebsiella* species, *Serratia* species (including *S. marcescens*), and *Enterobacter* species. Uncomplicated cervical and urethral gonorrhea due to *N. gonorrhoeae.* PID due to *N. gonorrhoeae, E. coli,* or *S. agalactiae.* Intra-abdominal infections due to *E. coli, S. epidermidis, Streptococcus* species (excluding enterococci), *Enterobacter* species, *Klebsiella* species, *Bacteroides* species (including *B. fragilis*) and anaerobic cocci (including *Peptococcus* and *Peptostreptococcus* species). Septicemia due to *Streptococcus* species (including *S. pneumoniae,* but excluding enterococci), *S. aureus, E. coli, Bacteroides* species (including *B. fragilis*), *Klebsiella* species, and *Serratia* species. Skin and skin structure infections due to *S. aureus, S. epidermidis, E. coli, Klebsiella* species, *Streptococcus* species (including *S. pyogenes,* but excluding enterococci), *P. mirabilis, Serratia* species, *Enterobacter* species, *Bacteroides* species (including *B. fragilis*) and anaerobic cocci (including *Peptococcus* and *Peptostreptococcus* species). Bone and joint infections due to *S. aureus, Streptococcus* species (excluding enterococci), *P. mirabilis, Bacteroides* species (including B. fragilis) and anaerobic cocci (including *Peptococcus* and *Peptostreptococcus* species). Meningitis due to *H. influenzae* and limited use for *S. pyogenes.*

Route/Dosage

- **IM, IV**
    Uncomplicated urinary tract infections.
Adults: 0.5 g q 12 hr IM or IV.
    Severe or resistant infections.
Adults: 1 g q 8 hr or 2 g q 8–12 hr IM or IV.
    Life-threatening infections.
Adults: Up to 3–4 g q 8 hr IV.
    Pelvic inflammatory disease.
2 g q 8 hr IV (doses up to 2 g q 4 hr have been used).
    Infections at other sites.
Adults: 1 g q 8–12 hr IM or IV.
- **IV**
    Uncomplicated gonorrhea.
Adults: 1 g as a single dose **IM.**

Use in children.
Pediatric, over 6 months: 50 mg/kg q 6–8 hr up to 200 mg/kg/day (not to exceed the maximum adult dose).
Impaired renal function.
Initial, IM, IV: 0.5–1 g; **then,** use maintenance schedule in package insert.
How Supplied: *Injection:* 1 g/50 mL, 2 g/50 mL; *Powder for injection:* 500 mg, 1 g, 2 g, 10 g

EMS CONSIDERATIONS

See also *Anti-Infectives* and *Cephalosporins.*

Ceftriaxone sodium

(sef-try-AX-ohn)
Pregnancy Class: B
Rocephin **(Rx)**
Classification: Cephalosporin, third-generation

Uses: Lower respiratory tract infections due to *Streptococcus pneumoniae, Staphylococcus aureus, Haemophilus influenzae, H. parainfluenzae, Klebsiella pneumonia, Serratia marcescens, Escherichia coli, E. aerogenes,* and *Proteus mirabilis.* Skin and skin structure infections due to *S. aureus, S. epidermidis, S. pyogenes,* Viridins group streptococci, *E. coli, Enterobacter cloacae, K. oxytoca, K. pneumoniae, P. mirabilis, Pseudomonas aeruginosa, Morganella morganii, S. marcescens. Acinetobacter calcoaceticus, Bacgeroides fragilis, Peptostreptococcus* species. UTIs (complicated and uncomplicted) due to *E. coli, P. mirabilis, P. vulgaris, M. morganii,* and *K. pneumoniae.* Uncomplicated cervical/urethral and rectal gonorrhea due to *Neisseria gonorrhoeae,* including penicillinase/non-penicillinase producing strains. Pharyngeal gonorrhea due to non-penicillinase producing strains of *N. gonorrhoeae.* PID due to *N. gonorrhoeae.* Bacterial septicemia due to *S. aureus, S. pneumoniae, E. coli, H. influenzae,* and *K. pneumoniae.* Bone and joint infections due to *S. aureus, S. pneumoniae, E. coli, P. mirabilis, K. pneumoniae,* and *Enterobacter* species. Intra-abdominal infections due to *E. coli, K. pneumoniae, B. fragilis, Clostridium* species (most strains of *C. difficle* are resistant), *Peptostreptococcus* species. Meningitis due to *H. influenzae, N. meningitidis,* and *S. pneumoniae.* Single preoperative doses may decrease the incidence of postoperative infections following vaginal or abdominal hysterectomy or in coronary artery bypass surgery. Pediatric otitis media. *Investigational:* Neurologic complications, arthritis, and carditis associated with Lyme disease in patients refractory to penicillin G.

Route/Dosage
• **IV, IM**
  General infections.
Adults, usual: 1–2 g/day in single or divided doses q 12 hr, not to exceed 4 g/day. Maintain therapy for 4–14 days, depending on the infection. **Pediatric:** *Other than meningitis:* 50–75 mg/kg/day not to exceed total daily dose of 2 g given in divided doses q 12 hr.
  Meningitis.
Pediatric: 100 mg/kg/day, not to exceed total daily dose of 4 g given once daily or in equally divided doses q 12 hr for 7–14 days.
  Skin and skin structure infections.
Pediatric: 50–75 mg/kg once daily or in equally divided doses q 12 hr. Do no exceed a daily dose of 2 g.
  Preoperative for prophylaxis of infection in surgery.
1 g 30–120 min prior to surgery.
  Uncomplicated gonorrhea.
Adults, IM: 125 mg as a single dose plus doxycycline, 100 mg b.i.d. for 7 days or azithromycin, 1 g, as a single PO dose. Or, a single dose of 250 mg IM.
  Disseminated gonococcal infection.
Adults: 1 g IM or IV q 24 hr.
  Gonococcal meningitis or endocarditis.
Adults: 1–2 g IV q 12 hr for 10–14 days (meningitis) or 4 weeks (endocarditis).
  Gonococcal conjunctivitis.

Adults and children over 20 kg: 1 g given as a single IM dose.
  Haemophilus ducreyi infection.
250 mg IM as a single dose.
  Acute pelvic inflammatory disease.
250 mg IM plus doxycycline or tetracycline.
  Lyme disease in those refractory to Pencillin G.
IV: 2 g/day for 14–28 days.
Note: Dosage adjustment is not required for renal or hepatic impairment; however, monitor blood levels.
  Acute bacterial otitis media.
IM: Single dose of 50 mg/kg, not to exceed 1 g.
How Supplied: *Injection:* 1 g/50 mL, 2 g/50 mL; *Kit:* 1 Gm-1%, 500 mg-1%; *Powder for injection:* 250 mg, 500 mg, 1 g, 2 g, 10 g

EMS CONSIDERATIONS

See also *Anti-Infectives* and *Cephalosporins.*

Cefuroxime axetil
Cefuroxime sodium
(sef-your-OX-eem)
Pregnancy Class: B
Cefuroxime axetil (Ceftin **(Rx)**) Cefuroxime sodium (Kefurox, Zinacef **(Rx)**)
Classification: Cephalosporin, second-generation

Mechanism of Action: Cefuroxime axetil is used PO, whereas cefuroxime sodium is used either IM or IV.
Uses: PO (axetil). Pharyngitis, tonsillitis, otitis media, acute bacterial maxillary sinusitis, acute bacterial exacerbations of chronic bronchitis and secondary bacterial infections of acute bronchitis, uncomplicated UTIs, uncomplicated skin and skin structure infections, uncomplicated gonorrhea (urethral and endocervical) caused by non-penicillinase-producing strains of *Neisseria gonorrhoeae.* Early Lyme disease due to *Borrelia burgdorferi.* The suspension is indicated for children from 3 months to 12 years to treat pharyngitis,

tonsillitis, acute bacterial otitis media, and impetigo.

IM, IV (sodium). Infections of the urinary tract, lower respiratory tract (including pneumonia), skin and skin structures, bones, and joints. Septicemia, meningitis, uncomplicated and disseminated gonococcal infections due to penicillinase- or non-penicillinase-producing strains of *N. gonorrhoeae* in men and women. Mixed infections in which several organisms have been identified. Prophylaxis of postoperative infections in surgical procedures such as vaginal hysterectomy.

Route/Dosage
CEFUROXIME AXETIL
• **Tablets (Cefuroxime Axetil)**
Pharyngitis, tonsillitis.
Adults and children over 13 years: 250 mg q 12 hr for 10 days. **Children:** 125 mg q 12 hr for 10 days.
Acute bacterial exacerbations of chronic bronchitis and secondary bacterial infections of acute bronchitis, uncomplicated skin and skin structure infections.
Adults and children over 13 years: 250 or 500 mg q 12 hr for 10 days (5 days for secondary bacterial infections of acute bronchitis).
Uncomplicated UTIs.
Adults and children over 13 years: 125 or 250 mg q 12 hr for 7–10 days. **Infants and children less than 12 years:** 125 mg b.i.d.
Acute otitis media.
Children: 250 mg b.i.d. for 10 days.
Uncomplicated gonorrhea.
Adults and children over 13 years: 1,000 mg as a single dose.
Early Lyme disease.
500 mg/day for 20 days.
• **Suspension**
Pharyngitis, tonsillitis.
Children, 3 months to 12 years: 20 mg/kg/day in 2 divided doses, not to exceed 500 mg total dose/day, for 10 days.
Acute otitis media, impetigo.
Children, 3 months to 12 years: 30 mg/kg/day in 2 divided doses,

not to exceed 1,000 mg total dose/day, for 10 days.
CEFUROXIME SODIUM
• **IM, IV**
Uncomplicated infections, including urinary tract, uncomplicated pneumonia, disseminated gonococcal, skin and skin structure.
Adults: 750 mg q 8 hr. **Pediatric, over 3 months:** 50–100 mg/kg/day in divided doses q 6–8 hr (not to exceed adult dose for severe infections).
Severe or complicated infections; bone and joint infections.
Adults: 1.5 g q 8 hr. **Pediatric, over 3 months:** bone and joint infections, **IV:** 150 mg/kg/day in divided doses q 8 hr (not to exceed adult dose).
Life-threatening infections or those due to less susceptible organisms.
Adults: 1.5 g q 6 hr.
Bacterial meningitis.
Adults: Up to 3 g q 8 hr. **Pediatric, over 3 months, initial, IV:** 200–240 mg/kg/day in divided doses q 6–8 hr; **then,** after clinical improvement, 100 mg/kg/day.
Gonorrhea (uncomplicated).
1.5 g as a single IM dose given at two different sites together with 1 g PO probenecid.
Prophylaxis in surgery.
Adults, IV: 1.5 g 30–60 min before surgery; if procedure is of long duration, **IM, IV,** 0.75 g q 8 hr.
Open heart surgery, prophylaxis.
IV: 1.5 g when anesthesia is initiated; **then,** 1.5 g q 12 hr for a total of 6 g.*Note:* Reduce the dose in impaired renal function as follows: C_{CR} over 20 mL/min: 0.75–1.5 g q 8 hr; C_{CR}, 10–20 mL/min: 0.75 g q 12 hr; C_{CR}, less than 10 mL/min: 0.75 g q 24 hr.
How Supplied: Cefuroxime axetil: *Powder for Reconstitution:* 125 mg/5 mL, 250 mg/5 mL; *Tablet:* 125 mg, 250 mg, 500 mg Cefuroxime sodium: *Injection:* 750 mg/50 mL, 1.5 g/50 mL; *Powder for injection:* 750 mg, 1.5 g, 7.5 g

EMS CONSIDERATIONS

See also *Anti-Infectives* and *Cephalosporins*.

Celecoxib

(sell-ah-KOX-ihb)
Pregnancy Class: C
Celebrex **(Rx)**
Classification: Nonsteroidal anti-inflammatory drug, COX-2 inhibitor

Mechanism of Action: Inhibits prostaglandin synthesis, primarily by inhibiting cyclooxygenase-2 (COX-2); it does not inhibit the cyclooxygenase-1 (COX-1) isoenzyme.

Uses: Relief of signs and symptoms of rheumatoid arthritis in adults and of osteoarthritis.

Contraindications: Use in severe hepatic impairment, in those who have shown an allergic reaction to sulfonamides, or in those who have experienced asthma, urticaria, or allergic-type reactions after taking aspirin or other NSAIDs. Use in late pregnancy (may cause premature closure of ductus arteriosus). Lactation.

Precautions: Use with caution in pre-existing asthma, with drugs that are known to inhibit P4502C9 in the liver, or when initiating the drug in significant dehydration. Use with extreme caution in those with a prior history of ulcer disease of GI bleeding. Safety and efficacy have not been determined in patients less than 18 years of age.

Route/Dosage

• **Capsules**
Osteoarthritis.
Adults: 100 mg b.i.d. or 200 mg as a single dose.
Rheumatoid arthritis.
Adults: 100–200 mg b.i.d.
How Supplied: *Capsules:* 100 mg, 200 mg

Side Effects: Listed are side effects with a frequency of 0.1% or greater. *GI:* Dyspepsia, diarrhea, abdominal pain, N&V, dry mouth, flatulence, constipation, GI bleeding, diverticulitis, dysphagia, eructation, esophagitis, gastritis, gastroenteritis, gastroesophageal reflux, hemorrhoids, hiatal hernia, melena, stomatitis, tooth disorder, abnormal hepatic function. *CNS:* Headache, dizziness, insomnia, anorexia, anxiety, depression, nervousness, somnolence, hypertonia, hypoesthesia, migraine, neuropathy, paresthesia, vertigo, increased appetite. *CV:* Aggravated hypertension, angina pectoris, coronary artery disorder, *MI,* palpitation, tachycardia, thrombocythemia. *Respiratory:* URI, sinusitis, pharyngitis, rhinitis, bronchitis, bronchospasm, coughing, dyspnea, laryngitis, pneumonia. *Dermatologic:* Rash, ecchymosis, alopecia, dermatitis, nail disorder, photosensitivity, pruritus, erythematous rash, maculopapular rash, skin disorder, dry skin, increased sweating, urticara. *Body as a whole:* Accidental injury, back pain, peripheral edema, aggravated allergy, allergic reaction, asthenia, chest pain, fluid retention, generalized edema, fatigue, fever, hot flushes, flu-like symptoms, pain, peripheral pain, weight increase. *Musculoskeletal:* Arthralgia, arthrosis, bone disorder, accidental fracture, myalgia, stiff neck, synovitis, tendinitis. *Infections:* Bacterial, fungal, or viral infection; herpes simplex, herpes zoster, soft tissue infection, moniliasis, genital moniliasis, otitis media. *GU:* Cystitis, dysuria, frequent urination, renal calculus, urinary incontinence, UTI, breast fibroadenosis, breast neoplasm, breast pain, dysmenorrhea, menstrual disorder, vaginal hemorrhage, vaginitis, prostatic disorder. *Ophthalmic:* Glaucoma, blurred vision, cataract, conjunctivitis, eye pain. *Otic:* Deafness, ear abnormality, earache, tinnitus. *Miscellaneous:* Tenesmus, facial edema, leg cramps, diabetes mellitus, epistaxis, anemia, taste perversion.

Drug Interactions
ACE Inhibitors / ↓ Antihypertensive effect
Antacids, aluminum- and magnesium-containing / ↓ Absorption of celecoxib
Aspirin / ↑ Risk of GI ulceration
Fluconazole / ↑ Plasma levels of celecoxib

---

bold italic = life threatening side effect

C

Furosemide / ↓ Natriuretic effect of furosemide
Lithium / ↑ Plasma levels of lithium
Thiazide diuretics / ↓ Natriuretic effect of thiazides

EMS CONSIDERATIONS

See also *Nonsteroidal Anti-Inflammatory Drugs.*

Cellulose sodium phosphate

(SELL-you-lohs)
Pregnancy Class: C
Calcibind **(Rx)**
Classification: Calcium-binding agent

Mechanism of Action: A synthetic, nonabsorbable compound insoluble in water. The sodium ion exchanges for calcium; the cellulose phospate-bound calcium (from both dietary and endogenous sources) is then excreted in the feces. Urinary calcium is decreased while urinary phosphorus and oxalate are increased.
Uses: Decrease incidence of new renal stone formation in absorptive hypercalciuria Type I. Diagnostic test for causes of hypercalciuria other than hyperabsorption.
Contraindications: Primary or secondary hyperparathyroidism, hypocalcemia, hypomagnesemia, enteric hyperoxaluria, osteoporosis, osteomalacia, osteitis, low intestinal absorption or renal excretion of calcium, when hypercalciuria is due to mobilization from bones. Children under age 16.
Precautions: Use with caution in CHF and ascites.

Route/Dosage ⸺
• **Powder**
   Urinary calcium greater than 300 mg/day.
5 g with each meal.
   Urinary calcium less than 150 mg/day.
2.5 g with breakfast and lunch and 5 g with dinner.
How Supplied: *Powder*

Side Effects: *GI:* Diarrhea, dyspepsia, loose bowel movements. *Other:* Hyperparathyroid bone disease, hyperoxaluria, hypomagnesiuria, loss of copper, zinc, iron. Long-term use may cause hyperoxaluria and hypomagnesiuria.

EMS CONSIDERATIONS

None.

Cephalexin hydrochloride monohydrate
Cephalexin monohydrate

(sef-ah-LEX-in)
Pregnancy Class: B
Cephalexin hydrochloride monohydrate (Keftab **(Rx)**) Cephalexin monohydrate (Keflex **(Rx)**)
Classification: Cephalosporin, first-generation

Uses: Respiratory tract infections caused by *Streptococcus pneumoniae* and group A β-hemolytic streptococci. Otitis media due to *S. pneumoniae, Hemophilus influenzae, Moraxella catarrhalis* (use monohydrate only), staphylococci, streptococci, and *N. catarrhalis*. GU infections (including acute prostatitis) due to *Escherichia coli, Proteus mirabilis,* or *Klebsiella* species. Bone infections caused by *P. mirabilis* or staphylococci. Skin and skin structure infections due to staphylococci and streptococci.
Precautions: Safety and effectiveness of the HCl monohydrate have not been determined in children.

Route/Dosage ⸺
• **Capsules, Oral Suspension, Tablets**
   General infections.
Adults, usual: 250 mg q 6 hr up to 4 g/day. **Pediatric:** *Monohydrate,* 25–50 mg/kg/day in four equally divided doses.
   Infections of skin and skin structures, streptococcal pharyngitis, uncomplicated cystitis, over 15 years.
Adults: 500 mg q 12 hr. Large doses may be needed for severe infections or for less susceptible organisms.

For streptococcal pharyngitis in children over 1 year and for skin and skin structure infections, the total daily dose should be divided and given q 12 hr. In severe infections, the dose should be doubled.

Otitis media.
Pediatric: 75–100 mg/kg/day in four divided doses.

How Supplied: Cephalexin hydrochloride monohydrate: *Tablet:* 500 mg. Cephalexin monohydrate: *Capsule:* 250 mg, 500 mg; *Powder for Reconstitution:* 125 mg/5 mL, 250 mg/5 mL; *Tablet:* 250 mg, 500 mg

Side Effects: Additional: Nephrotoxicity, cholestatic jaundice.

EMS CONSIDERATIONS

See also *Anti-Infectives* and *Cephalosporins.*

Cephapirin sodium
(sef-ah-PIE-rin)
Pregnancy Class: B
Cefadyl **(Rx)**
Classification: Cephalosporin, first-generation

Uses: Respiratory tract infections due to *Streptococcus pneumoniae, Staphylococcus aureus* (penicillinase/nonpenicillinase producing), *Klebsiella* species, *Haemophilus influenzae,* and group A β-hemolytic streptococci. Skin and skin structure infections due to *S. aureus, S. epidermidis* (methicillin-susceptible strains), *Escherichia coli, Proteus mirabilis, Klebsiella* species, and group A β-hemolytic streptococci. UTIs due to *S. aureus, E. coli, P. mirabilis,* and *Klebsiella* species. Septicemia due to *S. aureus, S. viridans, E. coli, Klebsiella* species, and group A β-hemolytic streptococci. Endocarditis due to *S. aureus* and *S. viridans.* Osteomyelitis due to *S. aureus, Klebsiella* species, *P. mirabilis,* and group A β-hemolytic streptococci. Preoperatively and postoperatively to reduce chance of infection during vaginal hysterectomy, open heart surgery, and prosthetic arthroplasty.

Precautions: Assess benefits vesus risks before use in children less than 3 months.

Route/Dosage
• **IM, IV only**
General infections.
Adults: 0.5–1 g q 4–6 hr up to 12 g/day for serious or life-threatening infections. **Pediatric, over 3 months:** 40–80 mg/kg/day in four equally divided doses, not to exceed adult doses.
Preoperatively.
Adults: 1–2 g 30–60 min before surgery.
During surgery.
Adults: 1–2 g.
Postoperatively.
Adults: 1–2 g q 6 hr for 24 hr.
In patients with impaired renal function, a dose of 7.5–15 mg/kg q 12 hr may be adequate.

How Supplied: *Powder for injection:* 1 g

EMS CONSIDERATIONS

See also *Anti-Infectives* and *Cephalosporins.*

Cephradine
(SEF-rah-deen)
Pregnancy Class: B
Velosef **(Rx)**
Classification: Cephalosporin, first-generation

Uses: Oral. Respiratory tract infections (tonsillitis, pharyngitis, lobar pneumonia) due to *Streptococcus pneumoniae* and group A β–hemolytic streptococci. Otitis media due to group A β–hemolytic streptococci, *S. pneumoniae, Haemophilus influenzae,* and staphylococci. Skin and skin structure infections due to staphylococci (penicillinase/nonpencilliase–producing) and β– streptococci. UTIs (including prostatitis) due to *Escherichia coli, Proteus mirabilis,* and *Klebsiella* species.

Parenteral. Respiratory tract infections due to *S. pneumoniae, Klebsiella* species, *H. influenzae, S. aure-*

---

bold italic = life threatening side effect

us (penicillinase/non–penicillinase–producing), and group A β–hemolytic streptococci. UTIs due to *E. coli, P. mirabilis,* and *Klebsiella* species. Skin and skin structure infections due to *S. aureus* and group A β–hemolytic streptococci. Bone infections due to *S. aureus.* Septicemia due to *S. pneumoniae, S. aureus, P. mirabilis,* and *E. coli.* To prevent infections before, during, and after surgery for vaginal hysterectomy and other surgical procedures.

Precautions: Safe use during pregnancy, of the parenteral form in infants under 1 month of age, and of the PO form in children less than 9 months of age have not been established.

Route/Dosage ⎯⎯⎯⎯⎯⎯⎯⎯⎯⎯
• **Capsules, Oral Suspension**
Skin and skin structures, respiratory tract infections (other than lobar pneumonia).
Adults, usual: 250 mg q 6 hr or 500 mg q 12 hr.
Lobar pneumonia.
Adults: 500 mg q 6 hr or 1 g q 12 hr.
Uncomplicated UTIs.
Adults, usual: 500 mg q 12 hr.
More serious UTIs and prostatitis.
500 mg q 6 hr or 1 g q 12 hr (severe, chronic infections may require up to 1 g q 6 hr).
Use in children.
Pediatric, over 9 months: 25–50 mg/kg/day in equally divided doses q 6–12 hr (75–100 mg/kg/day for otitis media). Do not exceed 4 g/day.
• **Deep IM, IV**
General infections.
Adults: 2–4 g/day in equally divided doses q.i.d.
Surgical prophylaxis.
Adults: 1 g 30–90 min before surgery; **then,** 1 g q 4–6 hr for one to two doses (or up to 24 hr postoperatively).
Cesarean section, prophylaxis.
IV: 1 g when the umbilical cord is clamped; **then,** give two additional 1-g doses **IV or IM** 6 and 12 hr after the initial dose.

Use in children.
Pediatric, over 1 year: 50–100 mg/kg/day in equally divided doses q.i.d. Do not exceed adult dose.*Note:* For patients not on dialysis, use the following dosage in renal impairment: C$_{CR}$, over 20 mL/min: 500 mg q 6 hr; C$_{CR}$, 5–20 mL/min: 250 mg q 6 hr; C$_{CR}$, less than 5 mL/min: 250 mg q 12 hr. For those on chronic, intermittent hemodialysis, give 250 mg initially; repeat at 12 hr and after 36–48 hr.

How Supplied: *Capsule:* 250 mg, 500 mg; *Powder for Reconstitution:* 125 mg/5 mL, 250 mg/5 mL

EMS CONSIDERATIONS

See also *Anti-Infectives* and *Cephalosporins.*

Cerivastatin sodium
(seh-RIHV-ah-stat-in)
Pregnancy Class: X
Baycol **(Rx)**
Classification: Antihyperlipidemic, HMG-CoA reductase inhibitor

Mechanism of Action: Competitive inhibitor of HMG-CoA reductase leading to inhibition of cholesterol synthesis and decrease in plasma cholesterol levels.

Uses: Adjunct to diet to reduce elevated total and LDL cholesterol in patients with primary hypercholesterolemia and mixed dyslipidemia (Types IIA and IIb) when response to diet or other non-pharmacologic approaches have not been adequate.

Contraindications: Use in active liver disease or unexplained elevation of serum transaminases. Pregnancy, lactation.

Precautions: Use in women of child-bearing age only when pregnancy is unlikely and they have been informed of potential risks. Drug has not been evaluated in rare homozygous familial hypercholesterolemia. Due to interference with cholesterol synthesis and lower cholesterol levels, may be blunting or adrenal or gonadal steroid hormone production. Use with caution in renal or hepatic insufficiency. Safety and efficacy have not been determined in children.

Route/Dosage
• **Tablets**
  Hypercholesterolemia.
Adults: 0.3 mg once daily in evening. Recommended starting dose in those with significant renal impairment (C_{CR} less than 60 mL/min/1.73 m²) is 0.2 mg once daily in evening.
How Supplied: *Tablets:* 0.2 mg, 0.3 mg
Side Effects: See also *HMG-CoA Reductase Inhibitors. Musculoskeletal:* Rarely, rhabdomyolysis with acute renal failure secondary to myoglobinemia.
Drug Interactions: ↑ Risk of myopathy when used with azole antifungals, cyclosporine, erythromycin, fibric acid derivatives, and lipid-lowering doses of niacin.

EMS CONSIDERATIONS

None.

Cetirizine hydrochloride
(seh-TIH-rah-zeen)
Pregnancy Class: B
Zyrtec **(Rx)**
Classification: Antihistamine

Mechanism of Action: A potent H_1-receptor antagonist. A mild bronchodilator that protects against histmine-induced bronchospasm; negligible anticholinergic and sedative activity.
Uses: Relief of symptoms associated with seasonal allergic rhinitis due to ragweed, grass, and tree pollens; perennial allergic rhinitis due to allergens such as dust mites, animal dander, and molds. Chronic idiopathic urticaria.
Contraindications: Lactation. In those hypersensitive to hydroxyzine.
Precautions: Due to the possibility of sedation, use with caution in situations requiring mental altetness. Safety and efficacy have not been deter-

mined in children less than 12 years of age.

Route/Dosage
• **Tablets**
  Seasonal or perennial allergic rhinitis, chronic urticaria.
Adults and children over 6 years of age, initial: Depending on the severity of the symptoms, 5 or 10 mg (most common initial dose) once daily. In patients with decreased renal function (C_{CR}: 11–31 mL/min), in hemodialysis patients (C_{CR} less than 7 mL/min), and in those with impaired hepatic function, the dose is 5 mg once daily. **Children, 2 to 5 years, initial:** 2.5 mg once daily.
How Supplied: *Syrup:* 1 mg/mL; *Tablets:* 5 mg, 10 mg.
Side Effects: See *Antihistamines.* The most common side effects are somnolence, dry mouth, fatigue, pharyngitis, and dizziness.
OD Overdose Management: *Symptoms:* Somnolence. *Treatment:* Symptomatic and supportive. Dialysis is not effective in removing the drug from the body.

EMS CONSIDERATIONS

See also *Antihistamines.*

Chenodiol (Chenodeoxycholic acid)
(kee-noh-DYE-ohl)
Pregnancy Class: X
Chenix **(Rx)**
Classification: Naturally occurring human bile acid

Mechanism of Action: By reducing hepatic synthesis of cholesterol and cholic acid, replaces both cholic and deoxycholic acids in the bile acid pool. This helps desaturation of biliary cholesterol and leads to dissolution of radiolucent cholesterol gallstones. Is ineffective on calcified gallstones or on radiolucent bile pigment stones. Fifty percent of patients have stone recurrence within 5 years. Also increases LDLs and inhibits absorption of fluid from the colon.

Uses: In radiolucent cholesterol gallstones where surgery is a risk due to age or systemic disease. Ineffective in some. Best results in thin females with a serum cholesterol not higher than 227 mg/dL and who have a small number of radiolucent cholesterol gallstones.

Contraindications: Known hepatic dysfunction or bile ductal abnormalities. Colon cancer. Pregnancy or in those who may become pregnant.

Precautions: Safety and efficacy in lactation and in children have not been established.

Route/Dosage ————————————
• **Tablets**
  Radiolucent cholesterol gallstones.
Adults, initial: 250 mg b.i.d. for 2 weeks; **then,** increase by 250 mg/week until maximum tolerated or recommended dose is reached (13–16 mg/kg/day in two divided doses morning and night with milk or food). *NOTE:* Doses less than 10 mg/kg are usually ineffective and may result in increased risk of cholecystectomy.

How Supplied: *Tablet:* 250 mg

Side Effects: Hepatotoxicity including increased ALT in one-third of patients, intrahepatic cholestasis. *GI:* Diarrhea (common), anorexia, constipation, dyspepsia, flatulence, heartburn, cramps, epigastric distress, N&V, abdominal pain. *Hematologic:* Decreased white cell count. ***Chenodiol may contribute to colon cancer in susceptible patients.***

Drug Interactions
Antacids, aluminum / ↓ Effect of chenodiol due to ↓ absorption from GI tract
Cholestyramine / See *Antacids*
Clofibrate / ↓ Effect of chenodiol due to ↑ biliary cholesterol secretion
Colestipol / See *Antacids*
Estrogens, oral contraceptives / ↓ Effect of chenodiol due to ↑ biliary cholesterol secretion

EMS CONSIDERATIONS
None.

Chloral hydrate
(KLOH-ral HY-drayt)
Pregnancy Class: C
Classification: Nonbenzodiazepine, nonbarbiturate sedative-hypnotic

Mechanism of Action: Metabolized to trichloroethanol, which is the active metabolite causing CNS depression. Produces only slight hangover effects and is said not to affect REM sleep. High doses lead to severe CNS depression, as well as depression of respiratory and vasomotor centers (hypotension). Both psychologic and physical dependence develop.

Onset of Action: Within 30 min.
Duration of Action: 4–8 hr.
Uses: Short-term hypnotic. Daytime sedative and sedation prior to EEG procedures. Preoperative sedative and postoperative as adjunct to analgesics. Prevent or reduce symptoms of alcohol withdrawal.

Contraindications: Marked hepatic or renal impairment, severe cardiac disease, lactation. PO use in patients with esophagitis, gastritis, or gastric or duodenal ulcer.

Precautions: Use by nursing mothers may cause sedation in the infant. Dose decrease may be necessary in geriatric patients due to age-related decrease in both hepatic and renal function.

Route/Dosage ————————————
• **Capsules, Syrup**
  Daytime sedative.
Adults: 250 mg t.i.d. after meals.
  Preoperative sedative.
Adults: 0.5–1.0 g 30 min before surgery.
  Hypnotic.
Adults: 0.5–1 g 15–30 min before bedtime. **Pediatric:** 50 mg/kg (1.5 g/m²) at bedtime (up to 1 g may be given as a single dose).
  Daytime sedative.
Pediatric: 8.3 mg/kg (250 mg/m²) up to a maximum of 500 mg t.i.d. after meals.
  Premedication prior to EEG procedures.
Pediatric: 20–25 mg/kg.
• **Suppositories, Rectal**

Daytime sedative.
Adults: 325 mg t.i.d. **Pediatric:** 8.3 mg/kg (250 mg/m^2) t.i.d.
Hypnotic.
Adults: 0.5–1 g at bedtime. **Pediatric:** 50 mg/kg (1.5 g/m^2) at bedtime (up to 1 g as a single dose).
How Supplied: *Capsule:* 500 mg; *Suppository:* 325 mg, 500 mg, 650 mg; *Syrup:* 500 mg/5 mL
Side Effects: *CNS:* Paradoxical paranoid reactions. Sudden withdrawal in dependent patients may result in "chloral delirium." *Sudden intolerance to the drug following prolonged use may result in respiratory depression, hypotension, cardiac effects, and possibly death. GI:* N&V, diarrhea, bad taste in mouth, gastritis, increased peristalsis. *GU:* Renal damage, decreased urine flow and uric acid excretion. *Miscellaneous:* Skin reactions, hepatic damage, allergic reactions, leukopenia, eosinophilia.

Chronic toxicity is treated by gradual withdrawal and rehabilitative measures such as those used in treatment of the chronic alcoholic. Poisoning by chloral hydrate resembles acute barbiturate intoxication; the same supportive treatment is indicated (see *Barbiturates*).
Drug Interactions
Anticoagulants, oral / ↑ Effect of anticoagulants by ↓ plasma protein binding
CNS depressants / Additive CNS depression; concomitant use may lead to drowsiness, lethargy, stupor, respiratory collapse, coma, or death
Furosemide (IV) / Concomitant use results in diaphoresis, tachycardia, hypertension, flushing

EMS CONSIDERATIONS
See also *Pentobarbital Sodium.*

Chlorambucil
(klor-AM-byou-sill)
Pregnancy Class: D
Leukeran (CHL) **(Rx)**
Classification: Antineoplastic, alkylating agent

Mechanism of Action: Cell-cycle nonspecific; cytotoxic to nonproliferating cells and has immunosuppressant activity. Forms an unstable ethylenimmonium ion which binds (alkylates) with intracellular substances such as nucleic acids. The cytotoxic effect is due to cross-linking of strands of DNA and RNA and inhibition of protein synthesis.
Uses: Palliation in chronic lymphocytic leukemia, malignant lymphomas (including lymphosarcoma), giant follicular lymphomas, and Hodgkin's disease. *Investigational:* Uveitis and meningoencephalitis associated with Behcet's disease. With a corticosteroid for idiopathic membranous nephropathy. Rheumatoid arthritis. Possible alternative to MOPP in combination with vinblastine, procarbazine, and prednisone.
Precautions: Use during lactation only if benefits outweigh risks. Safety and efficacy have not been established in children. The drug is carcinogenic in humans and may be both mutagenis and teratogenic in humans. It also affects fertility. May be cross-hypersensitivity with other alkylating agents.

Route/Dosage ——————
• **Tablets**
Leukemia, lymphomas.
Individualized according to response of patient. **Adults, children, initial dose:** 0.1–0.2 mg/kg (or 4–10 mg) daily in single or divided doses for 3–6 weeks; **maintenance:** 0.03–0.1 mg/kg/day depending on blood counts.
Alternative for chronic lymphocytic leukemia.
Initial: 0.4 mg/kg; **then,** repeat this dose every 2 weeks increasing by 0.1 mg/kg until either toxicity or control of condition is observed.
Nephrotic syndrome, immunosuppressant.
Adults, children: 0.1–0.2 mg/kg body weight daily for 8–12 weeks.
Uveitis and meningoencephalitis associated with Behcet's disease.
0.1 mg/kg/day.

---

bold italic = life threatening side effect

C

Idiopathic membranous nephropathy.
0.1–0.2 mg/kg/day every other month, alternating with a corticosteroid for 6 months duration.
Rheumatoid arthritis.
0.1–0.3 mg/kg/day.
How Supplied: *Tablet:* 2 mg
OD **Overdose Management:**
Symptoms: Pancytopenia (reversible), ataxia, agitated behavior, *clonic-tonic seizures.* *Treatment:* General supportive measures. Monitor blood profiles carefully; blood transfusions may be required.

EMS CONSIDERATIONS

None.

Chloramphenicol
Chloramphenicol ophthalmic
Chloramphenicol sodium succinate

(klor-am-FEN-ih-kohl)
Chloramphenicol (Chloromycetin (Cream and Otic), Mychel **(Rx)**)
Chloramphenicol ophthalmic (AK Chlor, Chloromycetin Ophthalmic, Chloroptic Ophthalmic, Chloroptic S.O.P. Ophthalamic **(Rx)**) Chloramphenicol sodium succinate (Chloromycetin Sodium Succinate **(Rx)**)
Classification: Anti-infective

Mechanism of Action: Interferes with or inhibits protein synthesis in bacteria by binding to 50S ribosomal subunits.

Uses: *Not to be used for trivial infections, prophylaxis of bacterial infections, or to treat colds, flu, or throat infections.* **Systemic Use.** Treatment of choice for typhoid fever but not for typhoid carrier state. Serious infections caused by *Salmonella, Rickettsia, Chlamydia,* and lymphogranuloma-psittacosis group. Meningitis due to *Haemophilus influenzae.* Brain abscesses due to *Bacteroides fragilis.* Cystic fibrosis anti-infective. Meningococcal or pneumococcal meningitis. **Topical Use.** Otitis externa. Prophylaxis of infection in minor cuts, wounds, skin abrasions, burns; promote healing in superficial infections of the skin. **Ophthalmic Use.** Superficial ocular infections due to *Staphylococcus aureus; Streptococcus* species, including *S. pneumoniae; Escherichia coli, H. influenzae, H. aegyptius, H. ducreyi, Klebsiella* species, *Neisseria* species, *Enterobacter* species, *Moraxella* species, and *Vibrio* species. Use only for serious ocular infections for which less dangerous drugs are either contraindicated or ineffective.

Contraindications: Hypersensitivity to chloramphenicol; pregnancy, especially near term and during labor; lactation. Avoid simultaneous administration of other drugs that may depress bone marrow. Ophthalmically in the presence of dendritic keratitis, vaccinia, varicella, mycobacterial or fungal eye infections, or following removal of a corneal foreign body. Topical products should not be used near or in the eye.

Precautions: Use with caution in patients with intermittent porphyria or G6PD deficiency. To avoid gray syndrom, use with caution and in reduced doses in premature and full-term infants. Ophthalmic ointments may retard corneal epithelial healing.

Route/Dosage ────────
• **IV: Chloramphenicol**
Adults: 50 mg/kg/day in four equally divided doses q 6 hr. Can be increased to 100 mg/kg/day in severe infections, but dosage should be reduced as soon as possible. **Neonates and children with immature metabolic function:** 25 mg/kg once daily in divided doses q 12 hr. **Neonates, less than 2 kg:** 25 mg/kg once daily. **Neonates, over 2 kg, over 7 days of age:** 50 mg/kg/day q 12 hr in divided doses. **Neonates, over 2 kg, from birth to 7 days of age:** 50 mg/kg once daily. **Children:** 50–75 mg/kg/day in divided doses q 6 hr (50–100 mg/kg/day in divided doses q 6 hr for meningitis). *NOTE:* Carefully follow dosage for premature and newborn

infants less than 2 weeks of age because blood levels differ significantly from those of other age groups.

• **Chloramphenicol Sodium Succinate—IV Only**

Same dosage as chloramphenicol (see the preceding). Switch to **PO** as soon as possible.

• **Chloramphenicol Ophthalmic Ointment 1%**

0.5-in. ribbon placed in lower conjunctival sac q 3–4 hr for acute infections and b.i.d.–t.i.d. for mild to moderate infections.

• **Chloramphenicol Ophthalmic Solution 0.5%**

1–2 gtt in lower conjunctival sac 2–6 times/day (or more for acute infections).

• **Chloramphenicol Otic Solution 0.5%**

2–3 gtt in ear t.i.d.

• **Chloramphenicol Topical Cream 1%**

Apply 1–4 times/day.

How Supplied: Chloramphenicol ophthalmic: *Ointment:* 1%; *Powder for reconstitution:* 25 mg; *Solution:* 0.5% Chloramphenicol sodium succinate: *Powder for injection:* 1 g

Side Effects: *Hematologic* (most serious): ***Aplastic anemia, hypoplastic anemia,*** thrombocytopenia, granulocytopenia, ***hemolytic anemia,*** pancytopenia, hemoglobinuria (paroxysmal nocturnal). *Hematologic studies should be undertaken before and every 2 days during therapy. GI:* N&V, diarrhea, glossitis, stomatitis, unpleasant taste, enterocolitis, pruritus ani. *Allergic:* Fever, angioedema, macular and vesicular rashes, urticaria, hemorrhages of the skin, intestine, bladder, mouth. ***Anaphylaxis.*** *CNS:* Headache, delirium, confusion, mental depression. *Neurologic:* Optic neuritis, peripheral neuritis. *Following topical use:* Burning, itching, irritation, redness of skin. Hypersensitive patients may exhibit ***angioneurotic edema,*** urticaria, vesicular and maculopapular dermatoses. *Miscellaneous:* Superinfection. Jaundice (rare). Herxheimer-like reactions when

used for typhoid fever (may be due to release of bacterial endotoxins). ***Gray syndrome in infants:*** Rapid respiration, ashen gray color, failure to feed, abdominal distention with or without vomiting, progressive pallid cyanosis, vasomotor collapse, death. Can be reversed when drug is discontinued. *NOTE: Neonates should be observed closely, since the drug accumulates in the bloodstream and the infant is thus subject to greater hazards of toxicity.*

After ophthalmic use: Temporary blurring of vision, stinging, itching, burning, redness, irritation, swelling, decreased vision, persistent or worse pain.

Drug Interactions

Acetaminophen / ↑ Effect of chloramphenicol due to ↑ serum levels
Anticoagulants, oral / ↑ Effect of anticoagulants due to ↓ breakdown by liver
Antidiabetics, oral / ↑ Effect of antidiabetics due to ↓ breakdown by liver
Barbiturates / ↑ Effect of barbiturates due to ↓ breakdown by liver; also, ↓ serum levels of chloramphenicol
Chymotrypsin / Chloramphenicol will inhibit chymotrypsin
Cyclophosphamide / Delayed or ↓ activation of cyclophosphamide
Iron preparations / ↑ Serum iron levels
Penicillins / Either ↑ or ↓ effect when combined to treat certain microorganisms
Phenytoin / ↑ Effect of phenytoin due to ↓ breakdown by liver; also, chloramphenicol levels may be ↑ or ↓
Rifampin / ↓ Effect of chloramphenicol due to ↑ breakdown by liver
Vitamin B_{12} / ↓ Response to vitamin B_{12} when treating pernicious anemia

---

EMS CONSIDERATIONS

See also *Anti-Infectives.*

---

bold italic = life threatening side effect

Chlordiazepoxide

(klor-dye-AYZ-eh-POX-eyed)
Pregnancy Class: D
Libritabs, Librium **(Rx)**
Classification: Antianxiety agent,
benzodiazepine

Mechanism of Action: Has less anticonvulsant activity and is less potent than diazepam.
Onset of Action: PO:30-60 min; **IM:**15-30 min (absorption may be slow and erratic); **IV:** 3-30 min.
Duration of Action: t½: 5-30 hr.
Uses: Anxiety, acute withdrawal symptoms in chronic alcoholics. Sedative-hypnotic. Preoperatively to reduce anxiety and tension. Tension headache. Antitremor agent (PO). Antipanic (parenteral).

Route/Dosage
• **Capsules, Tablets**
Anxiety and tension.
Adults: 5–10 mg t.i.d.–q.i.d. (up to 20–25 mg t.i.d.–q.i.d. in severe cases). Reduce dose to 5 mg b.i.d.–q.i.d. in geriatric or debilitated patients. **Pediatric, over 6 years, initial,** 5 mg b.i.d.–q.i.d. May be increased to 10 mg b.i.d.–q.i.d.
Preoperatively.
Adults: 5–10 mg t.i.d.–q.i.d. on day before surgery.
Alcohol withdrawal/sedative-hypnotic.
Adults: 50–100 mg; may be increased to 300 mg/day; **then,** reduce to maintenance levels.
• **IM, IV (not recommended for children under 12 years)**
Acute/severe agitation, anxiety.
Initial: 50–100 mg; **then,** 25–50 mg t.i.d.–q.i.d.
Preoperatively.
Adults: 50–100 mg IM 1 hr before surgery.
Alcohol withdrawal.
Adults: 50–100 mg IM or IV; repeat in 2–4 hr if necessary. Dosage should not exceed 300 mg/day.
Antipanic.
Adults, initial: 50–100 mg; dose may be repeated in 4–6 hr if needed.
How Supplied: *Capsule:* 5 mg, 10 mg, 25 mg; *Powder for injection:* 100 mg

Side Effects: Additional: Jaundice, acute hepatic necrosis, hepatic dysfunction.

EMS CONSIDERATIONS

See also *Tranquilizers* and *Hypnotics.*

Chloroquine hydrochloride
Chloroquine phosphate

(KLOR-oh-kwin)
Chloroquine hydrochloride (Aralen HCl **(Rx)**) Chloroquine phosphate (Aralen Phosphate **(Rx)**)
Classification: 4-Aminoquinoline, antimalarial, amebicide

Precautions: Use during pregnancy only if benefits outweigh risks.

Route/Dosage
CHLOROQUINE HYDROHLORIDE
• **IM**
Acute malarial attack.
Adults, initial: 200–250 mg (160–200 mg base); repeat dosage in 6 hr if necessary. Total daily dose in first 24 hr should not exceed 1 g (800 mg base). Begin PO therapy as soon as possible. **IM, SC. Children and infants:** 6.25 mg/kg (5 mg base/kg) repeated in 6 hr; dose should not exceed 12.5 mg/kg/day (10 mg base/kg/day).
Extraintestinal amebiasis.
Adults: 200–250 mg/day (160–200 mg of the base) for 10–12 days. Begin PO therapy as soon as possible. **Children:** 7.5 mg/kg/day for 10–12 days.
• **IV Infusion**
Acute malarial attack.
Adults, initial: 16.6 mg/kg over 8 hr; **then,** 8.3 mg/kg q 6–8 hr by continuous infusion.
CHLOROQUINE PHOSPHATE
• **Tablets**
Acute malarial attack.
Adults, Day 1: 1 g (600 mg base); **then,** 500 mg (300 mg base) 6 hr later. **Days 2 and 3:** 500 mg/day (300 mg base/day). **Children, Day 1:** 10 mg base/kg; **then,** 5 mg base/kg 6 hr later. **Days 2 and 3:** 5 mg base/kg/day.

Suppression (prophylaxis) of malaria.
Adults: 500 mg/week (300 mg base/week) on same day each week. If therapy has not been initiated 14 days before exposure, an initial loading dose of 1 g (600 mg base) may be given in 500-mg doses 6 hr apart. **Children:** 5 mg base/kg/week, not to exceed the adult dose of 300 mg of the base, given on same day each week. If therapy has not been initiated 14 days before exposure, an initial loading dose of 10 mg/kg of the base may be given in two divided doses 6 hr apart.
Extraintestinal amebiasis.
Adults: 1 g (600 mg base) given as 250 mg q.i.d. for 2 days; **then,** 500 mg (300 mg base) given as 250 mg b.i.d. for 2–3 weeks (combine with an intestinal amebicide). **Children:** 10 mg/kg (not to exceed 500 mg) daily for 3 weeks.
How Supplied: Chloroquine hydrochloride: *Injection:* 50 mg/mL Chloroquine phosphate: *Tablet:* 250 mg, 500 mg
Side Effects: Additional: Chloroquine may exacerbate psoriasis and precipitate an acute attack.
Drug Interactions
Cimetidine / ↓ Oral clearance rate and metabolism of chloroquine
Kaolin / ↓ Effect of chloroquine due to ↓ absorption from GI tract
Magnesium trisilicate / ↓ Effect of chloroquine due to ↓ absorption from GI tract

EMS CONSIDERATIONS
None.

Chlorothiazide
Chlorothiazide sodium
(klor-oh-THIGH-ah-zyd)
Pregnancy Class: C
Chlorothiazide (Diuril **(Rx)**) Chlorothiazide sodium (Sodium Diuril **(Rx)**)
Classification: Diuretic, thiazide type

Mechanism of Action: Produces a greater diuretic effect if given in divided doses.

Onset of Action: PO: 2 hr; **IV:** 15 min; **Peak effect:** 4 hr for PO, 30 min for IV.
Duration of Action: 6-12 hr. **t½:** 45-120 min.

Route/Dosage
• **Oral Suspension, Tablets, IV**
Diuretic.
Adults: 0.5–2 g 1–2 times/day either PO or IV (reserved for patients unable to take PO medication or in emergencies). Some patients may respond to the drug given 3–5 days each week.
Antihypertensive.
Adults, IV, PO: 0.5–1 g/day in one or more divided doses. **Pediatric, 6 months and older, PO:** 22 mg/kg/day (10 mg/lb/day) in two divided doses; **6 months and younger, PO:** 33 mg/kg/day (15 mg/lb/day) in two divided doses. Thus, children up to 2 years of age may be given 125–375 mg/day in two doses while children 2–12 years of age may be given 375 mg–1 g/day in two doses. IV use in children is not recommended.
How Supplied: Chlorothiazide: *Suspension:* 250 mg/5 mL; *Tablet:* 250 mg, 500 mg. Chlorothiazide sodium: *Powder for injection:* 0.5 g
Side Effects: Additional: Hypotension, renal failure, renal dysfunction, interstitial nephritis. Following IV use: Alopecia, hematuria, exfoliative dermatitis, toxic epidermal necrolysis, erythema multiforme, **Stevens-Johnson syndrome.**

EMS CONSIDERATIONS
See also *Diuretics, Thiazides.*

Chlorpheniramine maleate
(klor-fen-EAR-ah-meen)
Pregnancy Class: B
Syrup, Tablets, Chewable Tablets: Aller-Chlor, Allergy, Chlo-Amine, Chlor-Trimeton Allergy 4 Hour **(OTC)**, **Extended-release Tablets:** Chlor-Trimeton 8 Hour and 12 Hour **(OTC)**, **Injectable:** Chlorpheniramine maleate **(Rx)**
Classification: Antihistamine, alkylamine type

Mechanism of Action: Moderate anticholinergic and low sedative activity.

Onset of Action: 15-30 min, **Time to peak effect:** 6 hr.

Duration of Action: 3-6 hr.

Uses: PO: Allergic rhinitis. **IM, SC:** Allergic reactions to blood and plasma and adjunct to anaphylaxis therapy.

Contraindications: IV or intradermal use. Parenteral route for neonates. Use for children under 6 years of age.

Precautions: Geritaric patients may be more sensitive to the adult dose.

Route/Dosage ⎯⎯⎯⎯⎯⎯⎯
• **Syrup, Tablets, Chewable Tablets**
Adults and children over 12 years: 4 mg q 6 hr, not to exceed 24 mg in 24 hr. **Pediatric, 6–12 years:** 2 mg (break 4-mg tablets in half) q 4–6 hr, not to exceed 12 mg in 24 hr. **2–6 years:** 1 mg (¼ of a 4-mg tablet) q 4–6 hr.

• **Extended-Release Tablets**
Adults and children over 12 years: 8 mg q 8–12 hr or 12 mg q 12 hr, not to exceed 24 mg in 24 hr.

• **IM, SC**
Adults and children over 12 years: 5–40 mg for uncomplicated allergic reactions; 10–20 mg for amelioration of allergic reactions to blood or plasma or to treat anaphylaxis. Maximum dose per 24 hr: 40 mg.

How Supplied: *Capsule, Extended Release:* 8 mg, 12 mg; *Injection:* 10 mg/mL; *Syrup:* 2 mg/5 mL; *Tablet:* 4 mg; *Tablet, Extended Release:* 8 mg, 12 mg, 16 mg

⎯⎯⎯⎯⎯⎯⎯⎯⎯⎯⎯⎯⎯⎯⎯⎯⎯

EMS CONSIDERATIONS

See also *Antihistamines*.

⎯⎯⎯⎯⎯⎯⎯⎯⎯⎯⎯⎯⎯⎯⎯⎯⎯

Chlorpromazine hydrochloride

(klor-PROH-mah-zeen)
Pregnancy Class: C
Thorazine **(Rx)**
Classification: Antipsychotic, dimethylamino-type phenothiazine

Mechanism of Action: Has significant antiemetic, hypotensive, and sedative effects; moderate anticholinergic and extrapyramidal effects.

Uses: Acute and chronic psychoses, including schizophrenia; manic phase of manic-depressive illness. Acute intermittent porphyria. Preanesthetic, adjunct to treat tetanus, intractable hiccoughs, severe behavioral problems in children, and N&V. *Investigational:* Treatment of phencyclidine psychosis. IM or IV to treat migraine headaches.

Precautions: Use during pregnancy only if benefits outweigh risks. Safety for use during lactation has not been established, PO dosage for psychoses and N&V has not been established in children less than 6 months of age.

Route/Dosage ⎯⎯⎯⎯⎯⎯⎯
• **Tablets, Extended-Release Capsules, Oral Concentrate, Syrup**
  Outpatients, general uses.
Adults: 10 mg t.i.d. or q.i.d. or 25 mg b.i.d.–t.i.d. For more serious cases, 25 mg t.i.d. After 1 or 2 days, increase daily dose by 20 to 50 mg semiweekly, until patient becomes calm and cooperative. Maximum improvement may not be seen for weeks or months. Continue optimum dosage for 2 weeks; then, reduce gradually to maintenance levels (200 mg/day is usual). Up to 800 mg/day may be needed in discharged mental patients.
  Psychotic disorders, less acutely disturbed.
Adults and adolescents: 25 mg t.i.d.; dosage may be increased by 20–50 mg/day q 3–4 days as needed, up to 400 mg/day.
  Behavioral disorders in children.
Outpatients: 0.5 mg/kg (0.25 mg/lb) q 4–6 hr, as needed. **Hospitalized:** Start with low doses and increase gradually. For severe conditions: 50–100 mg/day. In older children, 200 mg or more/day may be needed.
  N&V.
Adults and adolescents: 10–25 mg (of the base) q 4 hr; dosage may be increased as needed. **Pediatric:** 0.55 mg/kg (15 mg/m^2) q 4–6 hr.

Preoperative sedation.
Adults and adolescents: 25–50 mg 2–3 hr before surgery. **Pediatric:** 0.5 mg/kg (15 mg/m²) 2–3 hr before surgery.
Hiccoughs or porphyria.
Adults and adolescents: 25–50 mg t.i.d.–q.i.d.

• **IM**
Psychotic disorders, acutely manic or disturbed.
Adults, initial: 25 mg. If necessary, give an additional 25–50 mg in 1 hr. Increase gradually over several days; up to 400 mg q 4–6 hr may be needed in severe cases. Patient usually becomes quiet and cooperative within 24–48 hr. Substitute PO dosage and increase until patient is calm (usually 500 mg/day). **Pediatric, over 6 months:** 0.5 mg/kg (0.25 mg/lb) q 6–8 hr as needed. Do not exceed 75 mg/day in children 5 to 12 years of age or 40 mg/day in children up to 5 years of age.
Intraoperative to control N&V.
Adults: 12.5 mg; repeat in 30 min if necessary and if no hypotension occurs. **Pediatric:** 0.25 mg/kg (0.125 mg/lb); repeat in 30 min if necessary and if no hypotension occurs.
Preoperative sedative.
Adults: 12.5–25 mg 1–2 hr before surgery. **Pediatric:** 0.5 mg/kg (0.25 mg/lb) 1–2 hr before surgery.
Hiccoughs.
Adults: 25–50 mg (base) t.i.d.–q.i.d.
Acute intermittent porphyria.
Adults: 25 mg q 6–8 hr until patient can take PO therapy.
Tetanus.
Adults: 25–50 mg t.i.d.–q.i.d., usually with barbiturates.

• **IV**
Intraoperative to control N&V.
Adults: 2 mg/fractional injection at 2–min intervals, not to exceed 25 mg (dilute with 1 mg/mL saline). **Pediatric:** 1 mg/fractional injection at 2–min intervals, not to exceed IM dosage (always dilute to 1 mg/mL saline).
Tetanus.

Adults: 25–50 mg diluted to 1 mg/mL with 0.9% NaCl injection and given at a rate of 1 mg/min. **Pediatric:** 0.5 mg/kg diluted to 1 mg/mL with 0.9% NaCl injection and given at a rate of 1 mg/2 min. Do not exceed 40 mg/day in children who weigh up to 23 kg (50 lb) or 75 mg/day in children who weigh 23–45 kg (50–100 lb).

• **Suppositories**
Behavioral disorders in children.
1 mg/kg (0.5 mg/lb) q 6–8 hr, as needed.
How Supplied: Chlorpromazine hydrochloride: *Capsule, Extended Release:* 30 mg, 75 mg, 150 mg; *Concentrate:* 30 mg/mL, 100 mg/mL; *Injection:* 25 mg/mL; *Rectal Suppository:* 25 mg, 100 mg; *Syrup:* 10 mg/5 mL; *Tablet:* 10 mg, 25 mg, 50 mg, 100 mg, 200 mg
Drug Interactions: Additional: *Epinephrine*/Chlorpromazine ↓ peripheral vasoconstriction and may reverse action of epinephrine *Norepinephrine*/Chlorpromazine ↓ pressor effect and eliminates bradycardia due to norepinephrine *Valproic acid*/↑ Effect of valproic acid due to ↓ clearance.

EMS CONSIDERATIONS

See also *Antipsychotic Agents.*

Chlorpropamide
(klor-PROH-pah-myd)
Pregnancy Class: C
Diabinese **(Rx)**
Classification: Sulfonylurea, first-generation

Mechanism of Action: May be effective in patients who do not respond well to other antidiabetic agents.
Onset of Action: 1 hr.
Duration of Action: Up to 60 hr (due to slow excretion).
Uses: Additional: *Investigational:* Neurogenic diabetes insipidus.
Precautions: Monitor frequently in those susceptible to fluid retention or impaired cardiac function.

---

bold italic = life threatening side effect

Route/Dosage ───────────
• **Tablets**
Diabetes.
Adults, middle-aged patients, mild to moderate diabetes, initial: 250 mg/day as a single or divided dose; **geriatric, initial:** 100–125 mg/day. **All patients, maintenance:** 100–250 mg/day as single or divided doses. Severe diabetics may require 500 mg/day; doses greater than 750 mg/day are not recommended.
Neurogenic diabetes insipidus.
Adults: 200–500 mg/day.
How Supplied: *Tablet:* 100 mg, 250 mg

Side Effects: Additional: Side effects are frequent. Severe diarrhea, occasionally accompanied by bleeding in the lower bowel. Relieve severe GI distress by dividing total daily dose in half. In older patients, hypoglycemia may be severe. Inappropriate ADH secretion, leading to hyponatremia, water retention, low serum osmolality, and high urine osmolality.

Drug Interactions: Additional:*Ammonium chloride/* ↑ Effect of chlorpropamide due to ↑ excretion by kidney */dusykfuran/* More likely to interact with chlorpropamide than other oral antidiabetics *Probenecid/* ↑ Effect of chlorpropamide *Sodium bicarbonate/* ↓ Effect of chlorpropamide due to ↑ excretion by kidney.

EMS CONSIDERATIONS

See also *Antidiabetic Agents: Hypoglycemic Agents and Insulin.*

Chlorthalidone
(klor-THAL-ih-dohn)
Pregnancy Class: B
Hygroton **(Rx)**
Classification: Diuretic, thiazide

Onset of Action: 2-3 hr; **Peak effect:** 2-6 hr.
Duration of Action: 24-72 hr.
Uses: Additional: To potentiate and reduce dosage of other antihypertensive agents.

Precautions: Geriatric patients may be more sensitive to the usual adult dose.

Route/Dosage ───────────
• **Tablets**
Edema.
Adults, initial: 50–100 mg/day (30–60 mg Thalitone) or 100–200 mg (60 mg Thalitone) on alternate days. Some patients require 150 or 200 mg (90–120 mg Thalitone). **Maximum daily dose:** 200 mg (120 mg Thalitone). **Pediatric:** All uses, 2 mg/kg (60 mg/m²) 3 times/week.
Hypertension.
Adults, initial: Single dose of 25 mg (15 mg Thalitone); if response is not sufficient, dose may be increased to 50 mg (30 mg Thalitone). For additional control, increase the dose to 100 mg/day (except Thalitone) or a second antihypertensive drug may be added to the regimen. **Maintenance:** Determined by patient response. *NOTE:* Doses greater than 25 mg/day are likely to increase potassium excretion but not cause further benefit in sodium excretion or BP reduction.
How Supplied: *Tablet:* 15 mg, 25 mg, 50 mg, 100 mg

Side Effects: Additional: Exfoliative dermatitis, toxic epidermal necrolysis.

EMS CONSIDERATIONS

See also *Diuretics, Thiazides.*

Chlorzoxazone
(klor-ZOX-ah-zohn)
Parafon Forte DSC, Remular-S **(Rx)**
Classification: Muscle relaxant, centrally acting

Mechanism of Action: Inhibits polysynaptic reflexes at both the spinal cord and subcortical areas of the brain. Effects may also be due to sedation.
Onset of Action: 1 hr.
Duration of Action: 3-4 hr.
Uses: As adjunct to rest, physical therapy, and other approaches for treatment of acute, painful muscu-

loskeletal conditions (e.g., muscle spasms, sprains, muscle strain).

Precautions: Use during pregnancy only if benefits clearly outweigh risks. Use with caution in patients with known allergies or a history of allergic reactions to drugs.

Route/Dosage
• **Tablets**
  Skeletal muscle disorders.
  Adults: 250–750 mg t.i.d.–q.i.d. with meals and at bedtime; **pediatric:** 125–500 mg t.i.d.–q.i.d. (or 20 mg/kg in three to four divided doses daily).

How Supplied: *Tablet:* 250 mg, 500 mg

Side Effects: *CNS:* Dizziness, drowsiness, lightheadedness, overstimulation, malaise. *Dermatologic:* Allergic-type skin rashes, petechiae, ecchymoses (rare). *GI:* GI upset, GI bleeding (rare). *Allergic Reactions:* **Angioneurotic edema, anaphylaxis** (rare). *Miscellaneous:* Discoloration of urine, liver damage.

OD Overdose Management: *Symptoms:* N&V, diarrhea, drowsiness, dizziness, lightheadedness, headache, malaise, sluggishness. May be followed by marked loss of muscle tone (voluntary movement may be impossible), decreased or absent deep tendon reflexes, respiratory depression, decreased BP. *Treatment:* Supportive.

EMS CONSIDERATIONS

See also *Skeletal Muscle Relaxants, Centrally Acting.*

Cholestyramine resin
(koh-less-TEER-ah-meen)
Prevalite, Questran, Questran Light **(Rx)**
Classification: Hypocholesterolemic agent, bile acid sequestrant

Mechanism of Action: Binds sodium cholate (bile salts) in the intestine; thus, the principal precursor of cholesterol is not absorbed due to formation of an insoluble complex, which is excreted in the feces. Decreases cholesterol and LDL and either has no effect or increases triglycerides, VLDL, and HDL. Also, itching is relieved as a result of removing irritating bile salts. The antidiarrheal effect results from the binding and removal of bile acids.

Onset of Action: To reduce plasma cholesterol: Within 24–48 hr, but levels may continue to fall for 1 yr; **to relieve pruritus:** 1–3 weeks; **relief of diarrhea associated with bile acids:** 24 hr.

Uses: Adjunct to reduce elevated serum cholesterol in primary hypercholesterolemia in those who do not respond adequately to diet. Pruritus associated with partial biliary obstruction. Diarrhea due to bile acids. *Investigational:* Antibiotic-induced pseudomembranous colitis (i.e., due to toxin produced by *Clostridium difficile*), digitalis toxicity, treatment of chlordecone (Kepone) poisoning, treatment of thyroid hormone overdose.

Contraindications: Complete obstruction or atresia of bile duct.

Precautions: Use during pregnancy only if benefits outweigh risks. Use with caution during lactation and in children. Long-term effects and efficacy in decreasing cholesterol levels in pediatric patients are not known. Geriatric patients may be more likely to manifest GI side effects as well as adverse nutritional effects. Exercise caution in phenylketonurics as Prevalilte contains 14.1 mg phenylalanine per 5.5-g dose.

Route/Dosage
• **Powder**
  Adults, initial: 1 g 1–2 times/day. Dose is individualized. For Prevalite, give 1 packet or 1 level scoopful (5.5 g Prevalite: 4 g anhydrous cholestyramine). **Maintenance:** 2–4 packets or scoopfuls/day (8–16 g anhydrous cholestyramine resin) mixed with 60–180 mL water or noncarbonated beverage. The recommended dosing schedule is b.i.d. but it can be given in one to six doses/day. Maximum

daily dose: 6 packets or scoopsful (equivalent to 24 g cholestyramine).

How Supplied: *Powder for Reconstitution:* 4 g/5 g, 4 g/5.5 g, 4 g/5.7 g, 4 g/9 g

Side Effects: *GI:* Constipation (may be severe), N&V, diarrhea, heartburn, GI bleeding, anorexia, flatulence, belching, abdominal distention, abdominal pain or cramping, loose stools, indigestion, aggravation of hemorrhoids, rectal bleeding or pain, black stools, bleeding duodenal ulcer, peptic ulceration, GI irritation, dysphagia, dental bleeding, hiccoughs, sour taste, pancreatitis, diverticulitis, cholescystitis, cholelithiasis. Fecal impaction in elderly patients. Large doses may cause steatorrhea. *CNS:* Migraine or sinus headaches, dizziness, anxiety, vertigo, insomnia, fatigue, lightheadedness, syncope, drowsiness, femoral nerve pain, paresthesia. *Hypersensitivity:* Urticaria, dermatitis, asthma, wheezing, rash. *Hematologic:* Increased PT, ecchymosis, anemia. *Musculoskeletal:* Muscle or joint pain, backache, arthritis, osteoporosis. *GU:* Hematuria, dysuria, burnt odor to urine, diuresis. *Other:* Bleeding tendencies (due to hypoprothrombinemia). Deficiencies of vitamins A and D. Uveitis, weight loss or gain, osteoporosis, swollen glands, increased libido, weakness, SOB, edema, swelling of hands/feet; hyperchloremic acidosis in children, rash and irritation of the skin, tongue, and perianal area.

OD **Overdose Management:** *Symptoms:* GI tract obstruction.

Drug Interactions
Anticoagulants, PO / ↓ Anticoagulant effect due to ↓ absorption from GI tract
Aspirin / ↓ Absorption of aspirin from GI tract
Clindamycin / ↓ Absorption of clindamycin from GI tract
Clofibrate / ↓ Absorption of clofibrate from GI tract
Digitalis glycosides / ↓ Effect of digitalis due to ↓ absorption from the GI tract
Furosemide / ↓ Absorption of furosemide from GI tract

Gemfibrozil / ↓ Bioavailability of gemfibrozil
Glipizide / ↓ Serum glipizide levels
Hydrocortisone / ↓ Effect of hydrocortisone due to ↓ absorption from GI tract
Imipramine / ↓ Absorption of imipramine from GI tract
Iopanoic acid / Results in abnormal cholecystography
Lovastatin / Effects may be additive
Methyldopa / ↓ Absorption of methyldopa from GI tract
Nicotinic acid / ↓ Absorption of nicotinic acid from GI tract
Penicillin G / ↓ Effect of penicillin G due to ↓ absorption from GI tract
Phenytoin / ↓ Absorption of phenytoin from GI tract
Phosphate supplements / ↓ Absorption of phosphate supplements from GI tract
Piroxicam / ↑ Elimination
Propranolol / ↓ Effect of propranolol due to ↓ absorption from GI tract
Tetracyclines / ↓ Effect of tetracyclines due to ↓ absorption from GI tract
Thiazide diuretics / ↓ Effect of thiazides due to ↓ absorption from GI tract
Thyroid hormones / ↓ Effect of thyroid hormones due to ↓ absorption from GI tract
Tolbutamide / ↓ Absorption of tolbutamide from GI tract
Troglitazone / ↓ Absorption of troglitazone from GI tract
Ursodiol / ↓ Effect of ursodiol due to ↓ absorption from GI tract
Vitamins A, D, E, K / Malabsorption of fat-soluble vitamins

NOTE: These drug interactions may also be observed with colestipol.

EMS CONSIDERATIONS

None.

Chorionic gonadotropin (HCG)

(kor-ee-ON-ik go-NAD-troh-pin)
Pregnancy Class: X

A.P.L., Chorex-5 and -10, Choran 10, Gonic, Pregnyl, Profasi **(Rx)**
Classification: Gonadotropic hormone

Mechanism of Action: The actions of HCG, produced by the trophoblasts of the fertilized ovum and then by the placenta, resemble those of LH. In males, HCG stimulates androgen production by the testes, the development of secondary sex characteristics, and testicular descent when no anatomic impediment is present. In women, HCG stimulates progesterone production by the corpus luteum and completes expulsion of the ovum from a mature follicle. No significant evidence that HCG causes a more attractive or "normal" distribution of fat or that it decreases hunger and discomfort due to calorie-restricted diets.
Uses: Males: Prepubertal cryptorchidism, hypogonadism due to pituitary insufficiency. **Females:** Infertility not due to primary ovarian failure (used with menotropins).
Contraindications: Precocious puberty, prostatic cancer or other androgen-dependent neoplasm, hypersensitivity to drug. Development of precocious puberty is cause for discontinuation of therapy. Pregnancy.
Precautions: Since HCG increases androgen production, drug should be used with caution in patients in whom androgen-induced edema may be harmful (epilepsy, migraines, asthma, cardiac or renal diseases). Use with caution during lactation. Safety and efficacy have not been shown in children less than 4 years of age.

Route/Dosage ───────────
• **IM Only**
   Prepubertal cryptorchidism, not due to anatomic obstruction.
Various regimens including (1) 4,000 USP units 3 times/week for 3 weeks; (2) 5,000 USP units every other day for 4 injections; (3) 15 injections over a period of 6 weeks of 500–1,000 USP units/injection; (4) 500 USP units 3

times/week for 4–6 weeks; may be repeated after 1 month using 1,000 USP units.
   Hypogonadotropic hypogonadism in males.
The following regimens may be used: (1) 500–1,000 USP units 3 times/week for 3 weeks; **then,** same dose twice weekly for 3 weeks; (2) 4,000 USP units 3 times/week for 6–9 months; then, 2,000 USP units 3 times/week for 3 more months; (3) 1,000–2,000 USP units 3 times/week.
How Supplied: *Powder for injection:* 5,000 U, 10,000 U, 20,000 U
Side Effects: *CNS:* Headache, irritability, restlessness, depression, fatigue, aggressive behavior. *GU:* Precocious puberty, ovarian hyperstimulation syndrome, ovarian malignancy (rare), ***enlargement of preexisting ovarian cysts with possible rupture.*** *Miscellaneous:* Edema, gynecomastia, pain at injection site, fluid retention, arterial thromboembolism.

EMS CONSIDERATIONS
None.

Ciclopirox olamine
(sye-kloh-PEER-ox)
Pregnancy Class: B
Loprox **(Rx)**
Classification: Broad-spectrum topical antifungal

Mechanism of Action: At lower concentrations the drug blocks the transport of amino acids into the cell, whereas at higher concentrations the cell membrane of the fungus is altered so that intracellular material leaks out. May also inhibit synthesis of RNA, DNA, and protein in growing fungal cells. A small amount of drug is absorbed through the skin; it also penetrates to the sebaceous glands and dermis as well as into the hair.
Uses: Effective against dermatophytes, yeast, *Malassezia furfur, Trichophyton rubrum, T. mentagrophytes, Epidermophyton floccosum, Microsporum canis,* and *Candida albicans* that

---

bold italic = life threatening side effect

cause tinea pedis, tinea corporis, tinea cruris, tinea versicolor, candidiasis. **Contraindications:** Use in or around the eyes.

Precautions: Safety and efficacy in lactation and in children under 10 years of age not established.

Route/Dosage
• **Lotion (1%), Topical Cream (1%)**
Massage gently into the affected area and surrounding skin morning and evening. If there is no improvement after 4 weeks, reevaluate diagnosis.
How Supplied: *Cream:* 1%; *Gel; Lotion:* 0.77%, 1%
Side Effects: *Dermatologic:* Irritation, redness, burning, pain, skin sensitivity, pruritus at application site.

EMS CONSIDERATIONS

None.

Cilostazol
(sih-LESS-tah-zohl)
Pregnancy Class: C
Pletal
Classification: Antiplatelet drug

Mechanism of Action: Inhibits cellular phosphodiesterase (PDE), especially PDE III. Cilostazol and several metabolites inhibit cyclic AMP PDE III. Suppression of this isoenzyme causes increased levels of cyclic AMP resulting in vasodilation and inhibition of platelet aggregation. Inhibits platelet aggregation caused by thrombin, ADP, collagen, arachidonic acid, epinephrine, and shear stress.
Uses: Reduce symptoms of intermittent claudication.
Contraindications: CHF of any severity (may cause a decreased survival rate in patients with class III-IV CHF). Concurrent use of grapefruit juice. Lactation.
Precautions: Safety and efficacy have not been determined in children.

Route/Dosage
• **Tablets**

Intermittent claudication.
100 mg b.i.d. taken 30 min or more before or 2 hr after breakfast and dinner. Consider a dose of 50 mg b.i.d. during coadministration of diltiazem, erythromycin, itraconazole, or ketoconazole.
How Supplied: *Tablets:* 50 mg, 100 mg
Side Effects: *GI:* Abnormal stool, diarrhea, dyspepsia, flatulence, N&V, abdominal pain, anorexia, cholelithiasis, colitis, duodenal ulcer, duodenitis, esophageal hemorrhage, esophagitis, gastritis, gastroenteritis, gum hemorrhage, hematemesis, melena, gastric ulcer, periodontal abscess, rectal hemorrhage, stomach ulcer, tongue edema. *CNS:* Headache, dizziness, vertigo, anxiety, insomnia, neuralgia. *CV:* Palpitation, tachycardia, hypertension, angina pectoris, atrial fibrillation/flutter, cerebral infarct, cerebral ischemia, CHF, **heart arrest, hemorrhage,** hypotension, MI, myocardial ischemia, nodal arrhythmia, postural hypotension, supraventricular tachycardia, syncope, varicose veins, vasodilation, ventricular extrasystole or **V.tach.** *Respiratory:* Rhinitis, pharyngitis, increased cough, dyspnea, bronchitis, asthma, epistaxis, hemoptysis, pneumonia, sinusitis. *Musculoskeletal:* Back pain, myalgia, asthenia, leg cramps, arthritis, arthralgia, bone pain, bursitis. *Dermatologic:* Rash, dry skin, furunculosis, skin hypertrophy, urticaria. *GU:* Hematuria, UTI, cystitis, urinary frequency, vaginal hemorrhage, vaginitis. *Hematologic:* Anemia, ecchymosis, iron deficiency anemia, polycythemia, purpura. *Ophthalmic:* Amblyopia, blindness, conjunctivitis, diplopia, eye hemorrhage, retinal hemorrhage. *Miscellaneous:* Infection, peripheral edema, hyperesthesia, paresthesia, flu syndrome, ear pain, tinnitus, chills, facial edema, fever, generalized edema, malaise, neck rigidity, pelvic pain, **retroperitoneal hemorrhage,** diabetes mellitus.
OD **Overdose Management:** *Symptoms:* Severe headache, diarrhea, hypotension, tachycardia, possible cardiac arrhythmias. *Treatment:* Observe

patient carefully and provide symptomatic treatment.

Drug Interactions

Diltiazem / ↑ Plasma levels of cilostazol; start therapy at ½ dose

Macrolide antibiotics / ↑ Plasma levels of cilostazol

Omeprazole / ↑ Plasma levels of one of the active metabolites of cilostazol

EMS CONSIDERATIONS

None.

Cimetidine

(sye-MET-ih-deen)
Pregnancy Class: B
Tagamet **(Rx)** Tagamet HB **(OTC)**
Classification: Histamine H$_2$ receptor blocking agent

Mechanism of Action: Reduces postprandial daytime and nighttime gastric acid secretion by about 50%–80%. May increase gastromucosal defense and healing in acid-related disorders (e.g., stress-induced ulcers) by increasing production of gastric mucus, increasing mucosal secretion of bicarbonate and gastric mucosal blood flow as well as increasing endogenous mucosal synthesis of prostaglandins. It also inhibits cytochrome P-450 and P-448, which will affect metabolism of drugs. Also possesses antiandrogenic activity and will increase prolactin levels following an IV bolus injection.

Uses: Rx. Treatment and maintenance of active duodenal ulcers. Short-term (6 weeks) treatment of benign gastric ulcers (in rare cases, healing has occurred). As part of multidrug regimen to eradicate *Helicobacter pylori.* Management of gastric acid hypersecretory states (Zollinger-Ellison syndrome, systemic mastocytosis). GERD, including erosive esophagitis. Prophylaxis of UGI bleeding in critically ill hospitalized patients. *Investigational:* Prior to surgery to prevent aspiration pneumonia, secondary hyperparathyroidism in chronic hemodialysis patients, prophylaxis of stress-induced ulcers, hyperparathyroidism, dyspepsia, herpes virus infections, tinea capitis, hirsute women, chronic idiopathic urticaria, dermatologic anaphylaxis, acetaminophen overdosage, warts, colorectal cancer.

OTC. Relief of symptoms of heartburn, acid indigestion, and sour stomach.

Contraindications: Children under 16, lactation. Cirrhosis, impaired liver and renal function.

Precautions: In geriatric patients with impaired renal or hepatic function, confusion is more likely to occur. Not recommended for children less than 16 years of age.

Route/Dosage —————————

• **Tablets, Oral Solution**

Duodenal ulcers, short-term.

Adults: 800 mg at bedtime. Alternate dosage: 300 mg q.i.d. with meals and at bedtime for 4–6 weeks (administer with antacids, staggering the dose of antacids) or 400 mg b.i.d. (in the morning and evening). **Maintenance:** 400 mg at bedtime.

Active benign gastric ulcers.

Adults: 800 mg at bedtime (preferred regimen) or 300 mg q.i.d. with meals and at bedtime for no more than 8 weeks.

Pathologic hypersecretory conditions.

Adults: 300 mg q.i.d. with meals and at bedtime up to a maximum of 2,400 mg/day for as long as needed.

Erosive gastroesophageal reflux disease.

Adults: 800 mg b.i.d. or 400 mg q.i.d. for 12 weeks. Use beyond 12 weeks has not been determined.

Heartburn, acid indigestion, sour stomach (OTC only).

200 mg with water as symptoms present up to b.i.d.

Dyspepsia.

Adults: 400 mg b.i.d.

Prophylaxis of aspiration pneumonitis.

Adults: 400–600 mg 60–90 min before anesthesia.

---

bold italic = life threatening side effect

Primary hyperparathyroidism, secondary hyperparathyroidism in chronic hemodialysis patients.
Up to 1 g/day.

- **IM, IV, IV Infusion**

Hospitalized patients with pathologic hypersecretory conditions or intractable ulcers or those unable to take PO medication.
Adults: 300 mg IM or IV q 6–8 hr. If an increased dose is necessary, administer 300 mg more frequently than q 6–8 hr, not to exceed 2,400 mg/day.

Prophylaxis of upper GI bleeding.
Adults: 50 mg/hr by continuous IV infusion. If C_{CR} is less than 30 mL/min, use one-half the recommended dose. Treatment beyond 7 days has not been studied.

Prophylaxis of aspiration pneumonitis.
Adults: 300 mg IV 60–90 min before induction of anesthetic.

How Supplied: *Injection:* 150 mg/mL, 300 mg/50 mL; *Solution:* 300 mg/5 mL; *Tablet:* 100 mg, 200 mg, 300 mg, 400 mg, 800 mg

Side Effects: *GI:* Diarrhea, pancreatitis (rare), hepatitis, hepatic fibrosis. *CNS:* Dizziness, sleepiness, headache, confusion, delirium, hallucinations, double vision, dysarthria, ataxia. Severely ill patients may manifest agitation, anxiety, depression, disorientation, hallucinations, mental confusion, and psychosis. *CV:* Hypotension and arrhythmias following rapid IV administration. *Hematologic:* Agranulocytosis, thrombocytopenia, **hemolytic or aplastic anemia,** granulocytopenia. *GU:* Impotence (high doses for prolonged periods of time), gynecomastia (long-term treatment). *Dermatologic:* Exfoliative dermatitis, erythroderma, erythema multiforme. *Musculoskeletal:* Arthralgia, reversible worsening of joint symptoms with preexisting arthritis (including gouty arthritis). *Other:* Hypersensitivity reactions, pain at injection site, myalgia, rash, cutaneous vasculitis, peripheral neuropathy, galactorrhea, alopecia, bronchoconstriction.

Drug Interactions
Antacids / ↓ Effect of cimetidine due to ↓ absorption from GI tract

Anticholinergics / ↓ Effect of cimetidine due to ↓ absorption from GI tract

Benzodiazepines / ↑ Effect of benzodiazepines due to ↓ breakdown by liver

Beta-adrenergic blocking drugs / ↑ Effect of beta blockers due to ↓ breakdown by liver

Caffeine / ↑ Effect of caffeine due to ↓ breakdown by liver

Calcium channel blockers / ↑ Effect of calcium channel blockers due to ↓ breakdown by liver

Carbamazepine / ↑ Effect of carbamazepine due to ↓ breakdown by liver

Carmustine / Additive bone marrow depression

Chloroquine / ↑ Effect of chloroquine due to ↓ breakdown by liver

Chlorpromazine / ↓ Effect of chlorpromazine due to ↓ absorption from GI tract

Digoxin / ↓ Serum levels of digoxin

Flecainide / ↑ Effect of flecainide

Fluconazole / ↓ Effect of fluconazole due to ↓ absorption from GI tract

Fluorouracil / ↑ Serum levels of fluorouracil following chronic cimetidine use

Indomethacin / ↓ Effect of indomethacin due to ↓ absorption from GI tract

Iron salts / ↓ Effect of iron due to ↓ absorption from GI tract

Ketoconazole / ↓ Effect of ketoconazole due to ↓ absorption from GI tract

Labetalol / ↑ Effect of labetalol due to ↓ breakdown by liver

Lidocaine / ↑ Effect of lidocaine due to ↓ breakdown by liver

Metoclopramide / ↓ Effect of cimetidine due to ↓ absorption from GI tract

Metoprolol / ↑ Effect of metoprolol due to ↓ breakdown by liver

Metronidazole / ↑ Effect of metronidazole due to ↓ breakdown by liver

Moricizine / ↑ Effect of moricizine due to ↓ breakdown by liver

Narcotics / Possible ↑ toxic effects (respiratory depression) of narcotics

Pentoxifylline / ↑ Effect of pentoxifylline due to ↓ breakdown by liver

Phenytoin / ↑ Effect of phenytoin due to ↓ breakdown by liver

Procainamide / ↑ Effect of procainamide due to ↓ excretion by kidney

Propafenone / ↑ Effect of propafenone due to ↓ breakdown by liver

Propranolol / ↑ Effect of propranolol due to ↓ breakdown by liver

Quinidine / ↑ Effect of quinidine due to ↓ breakdown by liver

Quinine / ↑ Effect of quinine due to ↓ breakdown by liver

Sildenafil / ↑ Effect of sildenafil due to ↓ breakdown by liver

Succinylcholine / ↑ Neuromuscular blockade → respiratory depression and extended apnea

Sulfonylureas / ↑ Effect of sulfonylureas due to ↓ breakdown by liver

Tacrine / ↑ Effect of tacrine due to ↓ breakdown by liver

Tetracyclines / ↓ Effect of tetracyclines due to ↓ absorption from GI tract

Theophyllines / ↑ Effect of theophyllines due to ↓ breakdown by liver

Tocainide / ↓ Effect of tocainide

Triamterene / ↑ Effect of triamterene due to ↓ breakdown by liver

Tricyclic antidepressants / ↑ Effect of tricyclic antidepressants due to ↓ breakdown by liver

Valproic acid / ↑ Effect of valproic acid due to ↓ breakdown by liver

Warfarin / ↑ Effect of anticoagulant due to ↓ breakdown by liver

EMS CONSIDERATIONS

See also *Histamine H₂* Antagonists.

Cinoxacin
(sin-OX-ah-sin)
Pregnancy Class: B
Cinobac Pulvules **(Rx)**
Classification: Urinary anti-infective

Mechanism of Action: Related chemically to nalidixic acid. Acts by inhibiting DNA replication, resulting in a bactericidal action.

Uses: Initial and recurrent UTIs caused by *Escherichia coli, Proteus mirabilis, P. vulgaris, Klebsiella,* and *Enterobacter* species. Prevents UTIs for up to 5 months in women with a history of UTIs. *NOTE:* Cinoxacin is ineffective against *Pseudomonas,* staphylococci, and enterococci infections. Prophylaxis of UTIs.

Contraindications: Hypersensitivity to cinoxacin or other quinolones. Infants and prepubertal children. Anuric patients. Lactation.

Precautions: Use with caution in patients with hepatic or kidney disease. Safety and efficacy in children less than 18 years of age have not been determined.

Route/Dosage
- **Capsules**
  UTIs.

Adults: 1 g/day in two to four divided doses for 7–14 days. *In patients with impaired renal function:* **Initial,** 500 mg; **then,** dosage schedule based on creatinine clearance (see package insert).

Prophylaxis of UTIs in women.
250 mg at bedtime for up to 5 months.

How Supplied: *Capsule:* 250 mg, 500 mg

Side Effects: *GI:* N&V, anorexia, abdominal cramps and pain, diarrhea, altered sensation of taste. *CNS:* Headache, dizziness, insomnia, drowsiness, confusion, nervousness. *Hypersensitivity:* Rash, pruritus, urticaria, edema, angioedema, eosinophilia, ***anaphylaxis (rare),*** toxic epidermal necrolysis (rare), erythema multiforme, ***Stevens-Johnson syndrome.*** *Other:* Tingling sensation, photophobia, perineal burning, tinnitus, thrombocytopenia.

OD Overdose Management: *Symptoms:* Anorexia, N&V, epigastric distress, diarrhea, headache, dizziness, insomnia, photophobia, tinnitus, and a tingling sensation. *Treatment:* Well hydrate the patient to prevent crystalluria. Maintain an airway and support ventilation and perfusion. Carefully

---

bold italic = life threatening side effect

monitor VS, blood gases, and serum electrolytes. Give activated charcoal to decrease absorption.

Drug Interactions: Probenecid ↓ excretion of cinoxacin → ↓ concentration in the urine.

EMS CONSIDERATIONS

See also *Anti-Infectives.*

Ciprofloxacin hydrochloride

(sip-row-FLOX-ah-sin)

Pregnancy Class: C

Ciloxan Ophthalmic, Cipro, Cipro Cystitis Pack, Cipro I.V. **(Rx)**

Classification: Fluoroquinolone antiinfective

Mechanism of Action: Effective against both gram-positive and gram-negative organisms.

Uses: Systemic. UTIs caused by *Escherichia coli, Enterobacter cloacae, Citrobacter diversus, Citrobacter freundii, Klebsiella pneumoniae, Proteus mirabilis, Providencia rettgeri, Pseudomonas aeruginosa, Morganella morganii, Serratia marcescens, Serratia epidermidis,* and *Streptococcus faecalis.* Uncomplicated cervical and urethral gonorrhea due to *Neisseria gonorrhoeae.* Chancroid due to *Haemophilus ducreyi;* uncomplicated or disseminated gonococcal infections.

Mild to moderate chronic bacterial prostatitis due to *E. coli* or *P. mirabilis.*

Mild to moderate sinusitis due to *S. pneumoniae, H. influenzae,* or *M. catarrhalis.*

Lower respiratory tract infections caused by *E. coli, E. cloacae, K. pneumoniae, P. mirabilis, P. aeruginosa, Haemophilus influenzae, H. parainfluenzae,* and *Streptococcus pneumoniae.*

Bone and joint infections due to *E. cloacae, P. aeruginosa,* and *S. marcescens.*

Skin and skin structure infections caused by *E. coli, E. cloacae, Citrobacter freundii, M. morganii, K. pneumoniae, P. aeruginosa, P. mi-*

rabilis, Proteus vulgaris, Providencia stuartii, Staphylococcus pyogenes, Staphylococcus epidermidis, and penicillinase- and non-penicillinase-producing strains of *Staphylococcus aureus.*

Infectious diarrhea caused by enterotoxigenic strains of *E. coli.* Also, *Campylobacter jejuni, Shigella flexneri,* and *Shigella sonnei.*

Typhoid fever (enteric fever) due to *Salmonella typhi.* Efficacy in eradicating the chronic typhoid carrier state has not been shown.

IV as empirical therapy in febrile neutropenia.

Investigational: Patients, over 14 years of age, with cystic fibrosis who have pulmonary exacerbations due to susceptible microorganisms. Malignant external otitis. In combination with rifampin and other tuberculostatics for tuberculosis.

Ophthalmic. Superficial ocular infections due to *Staphylococcus* species (including *S. aureus*), *Streptococcus* species (including *S. pneumoniae, S. pyogenes*), *E. coli, H. ducreyi, H. influenzae, H. parainfluenzae, K. pneumoniae, N. gonorrhoeae, Proteus* species, *Klebsiella* species, *Acinetobacter calcoaceticus, Enterobacter aerogenes, P. aeruginosa, S. marcescens, Chlamydia trachomatis, Vibrio* species, and *Providencia* species.

Contraindications: Hypersensitivity to quinolones. Use in children. Lactation. Ophthalmic use in the presence of dendritic keratitis, varicella, vaccinia, and mycobacterial and fungal eye infections and after removal of foreign bodies from the cornea.

Precautions: Safety and effectiveness of ophthalmic, PO, or IV use have not been determined in children.

Route/Dosage

• **Tablets**

UTIs.

250 mg (mild to moderate) to 500 mg (severe/complicated) q 12 hr for 7–14 days.

Mild to moderate chronic bacterial prostatitis.
Adults: 500 mg b.i.d. for 28 days.
Mild to moderate sinusitis.
Adults: 500 mg b.i.d. for 10 days.
Urethral or cervical gonococcal infections, uncomplicated.
250 mg in a single dose.
Infectious diarrhea.
500 mg q 12 hr for 5–7 days.
Skin, skin structures, lower respiratory tract, bone and joint infections.
500 mg (mild to moderate) to 750 mg (severe or complicated) q 12 hr for 7–14 days. Treatment may be required for 4–6 weeks in bone and joint infections.
Typhoid fever.
500 mg (mild to moderate) q 12 hr for 10 days.
*Chancroid (*H. ducreyi infection).
500 mg b.i.d. for 3 days.
Disseminated gonococcal infections.
500 mg b.i.d. to complete a full week of therapy after initial treatment with ceftriaxone, 1 g IM or IV q 24 hr for 24–48 hr after improvement begins.
Uncomplicated gonococcal infections.
500 mg in a single dose plus doxycycline.
NOTE: Dose must be reduced with a C_{CR} less than 50 mL/min. The PO dose should be 250–500 mg q 12 hr if the C_{CR} is 30–50 mL/min and 250–500 mg q 18 hr (IV: 200–400 mg q 18–24 hr) if the C_{CR} is 5–29 mL/min. If the patient is on hemodialysis or peritoneal dialysis, the PO dose should be 250–500 mg q 24 hr after dialysis.
• **Cipro Cystitis Pack**
Uncomplicated UTI infections.
100 mg b.i.d. for 3 days. The pack contains six 100-mg tablets of ciprofloxacin and is intended to increase compliance.
• **IV Infusion**
UTIs.

200 mg (mild to moderate) to 400 mg (severe or complicated) q 12 hr for 7–14 days.
Skin, skin structures, respiratory tract, bone and joint infections.
400 mg (for mild to moderate infections) q 12 hr for 7–14 days.
• **Ophthalmic Solution**
Acute infections.
Initial, 1–2 gtt q 15–30 min; **then,** reduce dosage as infection improves.
Moderate infections.
1–2 gtt 4–6 (or more) times/day.
How Supplied: *Injection:* 10 mg/mL, 200 mg/100 mL, 400 mg/200 mL; *Ophthalmic solution:* 0.3%; *Ophthalmic ointment:* 0.3%; *Powder for Reconstitution:* 250 mg/5 mL, 500 mg/5 mL; *Tablet:* 100 mg, 250 mg, 500 mg, 750 mg

EMS CONSIDERATIONS

See also *Anti-Infectives.*
Administration/Storage
IV 1. Due to slower times of onset in geriatric patients and those with impaired renal function, extend the interval between administration of the drug and intubation.
2. Spontaneous recovery following infusion will proceed at a rate comparable to that following administration of a bolus dose.
3. Cisatracurium is acidic; thus, it may not be compatible with alkaline solutions with a pH greater than 8.5 (e.g., barbiturate solutions).
4. Cisatracurium is compatible with 5% dextrose injection, 0.9% NaCl injection, D5/0.9% NaCl injection, sufentanil, alfentanil hydrochloride, fentanyl, midazolam hydrochloride, and droperidol. Drug is not compatible with propofol or ketorolac for Y-site administration.
5. Refrigerate vials at 2°C–8°C (36°F–46°F) and protect from light. Once removed from the refrigerator, use vials within 21 days, even if rerefrigerated.
6. Cisatracurium diluted in 5% dextrose injection, 0.9% NaCl injection, or D5/0.9% NaCl injection may be refrig-

erated or stored at room temperature for 24 hr without significant loss of potency. Dilutions to 0.1 or 0.2 mg/mL in D5%/RL injection may be refrigerated for 24 hr. Due to chemical instability, do not dilute in RL injection.

Assessment
1. Document indications for therapy, other agents trialed, and anticipated duration of therapy.
2. Note any hypersensitivity to benzyl alcohol.
3. Obtain baseline neurologic assessment and note findings.

Interventions
1. To be administered only by those trained in administration of neuromuscular blocking agents.
2. Patient requires constant monitoring and respiratory support.
3. Medicate with analgesics for pain and agents for anxiety based on assessed need.
4. Utilize a peripheral nerve stimulator to evaluate response to therapy and to ensure partial recovery between doses.

Citalopram hydrobromide
(sigh-TAL-oh-pram)
Pregnancy Class: Pregnancy Class: C
Celexa **(Rx)**
Classification: Antidepressant, selective serotonin-reuptake inhibitor

Mechanism of Action: Acts to inhibit reuptake of serotonin into CNS neurons resulting in increased levels of serotonin in synapses. Has minimal effects on reuptake of norepinephrine and dopamine.
Uses: Treatment of depression in those with DSM-III or DSM-III-R category of major depressive disorder.
Contraindications: Use with MAO inhibitors or with alcohol. Lactation.
Precautions: Use with caution in severe renal impairment, a history of seizure disorders, or in diseases or conditions that produce altered metabolism or hemodynamic responses. Safety and efficacy have not been determined in children.

Route/Dosage
• **Tablets**
Depression.
Adults, initial: 20 mg once daily in the a.m. or p.m. with or without food. Increase the dose in increments of 20 mg at intervals of no less than 1 week. Doses greater than 40 mg/day are not recommended. For the elderly or those with hepatic impairment, 20 mg/day is recommended; titrate to 40 mg/day only for nonresponders. Initial treatment is continued for 6 or 8 weeks. **Maintenance:** Up to 24 weeks.
How Supplied: *Tablets:* 20 mg, 40 mg
Side Effects: *CNS:* Activation of mania/hypomania, dizziness, insomnia, agitation, somnolence, insomnia, anorexia, paresthesia, migraine, hyperkinesia, vertigo, hypertonia, extrapyramidal disorder, neuralgia, dystonia, abnormal gait, hypesthesia, ataxia, aggravated depression, suicide attempt, confusion, aggressive reaction, drug dependence, depersonalization, hallucinations, euphoria, psychotic depression, delusions, paranoid reaction, emotional lability, panic reaction, psychosis. *GI:* N&V, dry mouth, diarrhea, dyspepsia, abdominal pain, increased salivation, flatulence, gastritis, gastroenteritis, stomatitis, eructation, hemorrhoids, dysphagia, teeth grinding, gingivitis, esophagitis. *CV:* Tachycardia, postural hypotension, hypertension, bradycardia, edema of extremities, angina pectoris, extrasystoles, *cardiac failure, MI, CVA,* flushing, myocardial ischemia. *Musculoskeletal:* Arthralgia, myalgia, arthritis, muscle weakness, skeletal pain, leg cramps, involuntary muscle contraction. *Hematologic:* Purpura, anemia, leukocytosis, lymphadenopathy. *Metabolic/nutritional:* Decreased or increased weight, thirst. *GU:* Ejaculation disorder, impotence, dysmenorrhea, decreased or increased libido, amenorrhea, galactorrhea, breast pain, breast enlargement, vaginal hemorrhage, polyuria, frequent micturition, urinary incontinence, urinary retention, dysuria. *Respiratory:* Coughing, epistaxis, bronchitis, dyspnea, pneumonia.

Dermatologic: Rash, pruritus, photosensitivity reaction, urticaria, acne, skin discoloration, eczema, dermatitis, dry skin, psoriasis. *Ophthalmic:* Abnormal accommodation, conjunctivitis, eye pain. *Body as a whole:* Asthenia, fatigue, fever. *Miscellaneous:* Hyponatremia, increased sweating, yawning, hot flushes, rigors, alcohol intolerance, syncope, flu-like symptoms, taste perversion, tinnitus.

OD **Overdose Management:** *Symptoms:* Dizziness, sweating, N&V, tremor, somnolence, sinus tachycardia. Rarely, amnesia, confusion, coma, convulsions, hyperventilation, cyanosis, rhabdomyolysis, ECG changes (including QTc prolongation, nodal rhythm, ventricular arrhythmias). *Treatment:* Establish and maintain an airway. Gastric lavage with use of activated charcoal. Monitor cardiac and vital signs. General symptomatic and supportive care.

Drug Interactions
Azole antifungals / ↑ Citalopram plasma levels
Carbamazepine / ↓ Citalopram plasma levels
Imipramine / ↑ Imipramine metabolite (desimipramine) by 50%
Lithium / Possible ↑ serotonergic effects of citalopram
Macrolide antibiotics / ↑ Citalopram plasma levels
MAO inhibitors / Possible serious and sometimes fatal reactions, including hyperthermia, rigidity, myoclonus, autonomic instability, mental status changes (extreme agitation, delirium, coma)

EMS CONSIDERATIONS
Administration/Storage: Allow at least 14 days to elapse between discontinuation of a monoamine oxidase inhibitor and initiation of citalopram or vice versa.
Assessment
1. Note indications for therapy, onset and characteristics of symptoms.
2. Note other drugs prescribed to ensure none interact. Avoid use with

MAOs or within 14 days before or after MAO use.
3. Determine any liver or renal dysfunction or seizure disorder.
4. Assess for altered metabolic/hemodynamics; reduce dose with liver or renal dysfunction.

Clarithromycin
(klah-rith-roh-MY-sin)
Pregnancy Class: C
Biaxin (Rx)
Classification: Antibiotic, macrolide

Mechanism of Action: Macrolide antibiotic that acts by binding to the 50S ribosomal subunit of susceptible organisms, thus interfering with or inhibiting microbial protein synthesis.

Uses: Mild to moderate infections caused by susceptible strains of the following. **Adults.** Pharyngitis/tonsillitis due to *Streptococcus pyogenes.* Acute maxillary sinusitis or acute bacterial exacerbaton of chronic bronchitis due to *Sreptococcus pneumoniae, Haemophilus influenzae,* and *Moraxella catarrhalis.* The active metabolite, 14-OH clarithromycin, has significant activity (twice the parent compound) against *H. influenzae.* Pneumonia due to *Mycoplasma pneumoniae, S. pneumoniae,* or *Chlamydia pneumoniae.* Uncomplicated skin and skin structure infections due to *Staphylococcus aureus* or *S. pyogenes.* Treatment of disseminated mycobacterial infections due to *Mycobacterium avium* (commonly seen in AIDS patients) and *M. intracellulare.* Prevention of disseminated *M. avium* complex in individuals with advanced HIV.

Used with omeprazole or ranitidine bismuth citrate (Tritec) for the eradication of *Helicobacter pylori* infection in patients with active duodenal ulcers associated with *H. pylori* infection. Also with amoxicillin and lansoprazole for the same purpose.

Children. Pharyngitis or tonsillitis due to *S. pyogenes.* Acute maxillary sinusitis or acute otitis media due to *S.*

pneumoniae, H. influenzae, and *M. catarrhalis.* Uncomplicated skin and skin structure infections due to *S. aureus* or *S. pyogenes.* Disseminated mycobacterial infections due to *M. avium* or *M. intracellulare.* Prevention of disseminated *M. avium* complex disease in patients with advanced HIV infection. Community-acquired pneumonia caused by *M. pneumoniae, Chlamydia pneumoniae,* and *S. pneumoniae.*

Contraindications: Hypersensitivity to clarithromycin, other macrolide antibiotics, or erythromycin. Patients taking astemizole, terfenadine, cisapride, or pimozide. Use with ranitidine bismuth citrate in those with a history of acute porphyria.

Precautions: Use with caution in severe renal impairment with or without concomitant hepataic impairment and during lactation. Safety and effectiveness in children less than 6 months of age have not been determined. Safety has not been determined. Safety has not been determined in MAC patients less than 20 months of age.

Route/Dosage ———————
• **Tablets, Oral Suspension**
Pharyngitis, tonsillitis.
Adults: 250 mg q 12 hr for 10 days.
Acute exacerbation of chronic bronchitis due to S. pneumoniae or M. catarrhalis; pneumonia due to S. pneumoniae or M. pneumoniae; uncomplicated skin and skin structure infections.
Adults: 250 mg q 12 hr for 7–14 days.
Acute maxillary sinusitis, acute exacerbation of chronic bronchitis due to H. influenzae.
Adults: 500 mg q 12 hr for 7–14 days.
Disseminated M. avium complex or prophylaxis of M. avium complex.
Adults: 500 mg b.i.d.; **children:** 7.5 mg/kg b.i.d. up to 500 mg b.i.d.
NOTE: The usual daily dose for children is 15 mg/kg q 12 hr for 10 days.
Community-acquired pneumonia in children.

15 mg/kg/day of the suspension, divided and given q 12 hr for 10 days.
Active duodenal ulcers associated with H. pylori *infection.*
Clarithromycin, 500 mg t.i.d., with omeprazole, 40 mg, each morning for 2 weeks. **Then,** omeprazole is given alone at a dose of 20 mg/day for 2 more weeks. Or, clarithromycin, 500 mg t.i.d., with ranitidine bismuth citrate, 400 mg b.i.d., for 2 weeks. **Then,** ranitidine bismuth citrate is given alone at a dose of 400 mg b.i.d. for 2 more weeks. Or, clarithromycin 500 mg, plus lansoprazole, 30 mg, and amoxicillin, 1 g b.i.d. for 10 days.

How Supplied: *Granules for Oral Suspension after Reconstitution:* 125 mg/5 mL, 250 mg/5 mL; *Tablet:* 250 mg, 500 mg

Side Effects: *GI:* Diarrhea, nausea, abnormal taste, dyspepsia, abdominal discomfort or pain, pseudomembranous colitis, glossitis, stomatitis, oral moniliasis, vomiting. *CNS:* Headache, dizziness, behavioral changes, confusion, depersonalization, disorientation, hallucinations, insomnia, nightmares, vertigo. *Allergic:* Urticaria, mild skin eruptions and, rarely, ***anaphylaxis and Stevens-Johnson syndrome.*** *Hepatic:* Hepatocellular cholestatic hepatitis with or without jaundice, increased liver enzymes, ***hepatic failure.*** *Miscellaneous:* Hearing loss (usually reversible), alteration of sense of smell (usually with taste perversion).

In children, the most common side effects are diarrhea, vomiting, abdominal pain, rash, and headache.

Drug Interactions
See also Drug Interactions for Erythromycins.
Anticoagulants / ↑ Anticoagulant effects
Astemizole / ↑ Astemizole levels; side effects, including ventricular arrhythmias, torsades de pointes, cardiac arrest, and death
Benzodiazepines / ↑ Plasma levels of certain benzodizepines → ↑ and prolonged CNS effects

Buspirone / ↑ Plasma levels of buspirone → ↑ risk of side effects

Carbamazepine / ↑ Blood levels of carbamazepine

Cisapride / Possibility of serious cardiac arrhythmias, including ventricular tachycardia, ventricular fibrillation, torsade de pointes, and QT prolongation

Cyclosporine ↑ Levels of cyclosporine → ↑ risk of nephrotoxicity and neurotoxicity

Digoxin / ↑ Plasma levels of digoxin due to ↓ metabolism of digoxin by the gut flora

Disopyramide / ↑ Plasma levels → arrhythmias and ↑ QTc intervals

Ergot alkaloids / Acute ergot toxicity, including severe peripheral vasospasm and dysesthesia

Fluconazole / ↑ Blood levels of clarithromycin

HMG–CoA Reductase Inhibitors / ↑ Risk of severe myopathy or rhabdomyolysis

Omeprazole / ↑ Plasma levels of omeprazole, clarithromycin, and 14-OH-clarithromycin

Pimozide / ↑ Risk of sudden death; do not use together

Ranitidine bismuth citrate / ↑ Levels of ranitidine, bismuth citrate, and 14–OH clarithromycin

Rifabutin, Rifampin / ↓ Effect of clarithromycin and ↑ GI side effects

Tacrolimus / ↑ Plasma tacrolimus levels → ↑ risk of toxicity (e.g., nephrotoxicity)

Terfenadine / ↑ Plasma levels of the active acid metabolite of terfenadine; ↑ risk of cardiac arrhythmias, including QT interval prolongation

Theophylline / ↑ Serum levels of theophylline

Triazolam / ↑ Risk of somnolence and confusion

AZT / ↓ Steady-state AZT levels in HIV-infected patients; however, peak serum AZT levels may be ↑ or ↓

EMS CONSIDERATIONS

See also *Anti-Infectives*.

Clemastine fumarate

(kleh-MAS-teen)
Pregnancy Class: B
Antihist-1 **(OTC)**, Tavist **(Rx)**
Classification: Antihistamine

Mechanism of Action: Moderate sedative effects, high anticholinergic activity, and moderate to high antiemetic effects.

Onset of Action: Peak effects: 5-7 hr.

Duration of Action: 10-12 hr (up to 24 hr in some patients).

Uses: Allergic rhinitis. Urticaria and angioedema.

Contraindications: Use in newborns or premature infants. Lactation. Treatment of lower respiratory tract symptoms, including asthma. Use with monoamine oxidase (MAO) inhibitors.

Precautions: Use with caution in patients with narrow angle glaucome, stenosing peptic ulcer, pyloroduodenal obstruction, symptomatic prostatic hypertrophy, and bladder nect obstruction. Use with caution in patients 60 years of age and older and in those with a history of bronchial asthma, increased intraocular pressure, hyperthyroidism, CV disease, and hypertension. Safety and efficacy have not been determined in children less than 12 years of age.

Route/Dosage

• **Syrup, Tablets**
Allergic rhinitis.
Adults and children over 12 years of age, initial: 1.34 mg (1 mg clemastine) b.i.d., up to a maximum dose of 8.04 mg (60 mL of syrup or 6 tablets) daily. **Children, aged 6 to 12 years of age, initial:** 0.67 mg (0.5 mg clemastine) b.i.d., up to a maximum of 4.02 mg (3 mg) daily. Use only the syrup in children.
Urticaria and angioedema.
Adults and children over 12 years of age, initial: 2.68 mg (use tablet) 1–3 times/day, not to exceed 8.04 mg (6 tablets) daily. **Children, aged**

---

bold italic = life threatening side effect

6 to 12 years, initial: 1.34 mg (use syrup only) b.i.d., not to exceed 4.02 mg daily.

How Supplied: *Syrup:* 0.5 mg/5 mL; *Tablets:* 1.34 mg, 2.68 mg.

Side Effects: *CNS:* Drowsiness (common), sedation, sleepiness, dizziness, incoordination, fatigue, confusion, restlessness, excitation, nervousness, tremor, irritability, insomnia, euphoria, paresthesia, blurred vision, diplopia, vertigo, tinnitus, acute labyrinthitis, hysteria, neuritis, **convulsions.** *GI:* Epigastric distress, anorexia, N&V, diarrhea, constipation. *CV:* Hypotension, headache, palpitations, tachycardia, extrasystoles. *Respiratory:* Thickening of bronchial secretions, tightness of chest, wheezing, nasal stuffiness. *Hematologic:* Hemolytic anemia, thrombocytopenia, agranulocytosis. *GU:* Urinary frequency, difficulty in urination, urinary retention, early menses.

EMS CONSIDERATIONS

See also *Antihistamines.*

Clindamycin hydrochloride
Clindamycin palmitate hydrochloride
Clindamycin phosphate
(klin-dah-MY-sin)

Pregnancy Class: B
Clindamycin hydrochloride (Cleocin **(Rx)**) Clindamycin palmitate hydrochloride (Cleocin Pediatric **(Rx)**) Clindamycin phosphate (Cleocin Vaginal Cream, Cleocin Phosphate, Cleocin T, Clinda-Derm, C/T/S **(Rx)**)
Classification: Antibiotic, clindamycin and lincomycin

Mechanism of Action: A semisynthetic antibiotic that suppresses protein synthesis by microorganism by binding to ribosomes (50S subunit) and preventing peptide bond formation. Is both bacteriostatic and bactericidal.

Uses: Should not be used for trivial infections. **Systemic.** *Anaerobes:* Serious respiratory tract infections (e.g., empyema, lung abscess, anaerobic pneumonitis). Serious skin and soft tissue infections, septicemia, intra-abdominal infections (e.g., peritonitis, intra–abdominal abscess), infections of the female pelvis and genital tract (e.g., PID, endometritis, nongonococcal tubo–ovarian abscess, pelvic cellulitis, postsurgical vaginal cuff infection). *Streptococci/staphylococci:* Serious respiratory tract infections, serious skin and soft tissue infections, septicemia (parenteral use), acute staphylococcal hematogenous osteomyelitis (parenteral use). *Pneumonococcus:* Serious respiratory tract infections. Adjunct to surgery for chronic bone/joint infections. *Investigational:* Alternative to sulfonamides in combination with pyrimethamine in the acute treatment of CNS toxoplasmosis in AIDS patients. In combination with primaquine to treat *Pneumocystis carinii* pneumonia. Chlamydial infections in women. Bacterial vaginosis due to *Gardnerella vaginalis.* **Topical Use.** Used topically for inflammatory acne vulgaris. Vaginally to treat bacterial vaginosis. *Investigational:* Treatment of rosacea (lotion used).

Contraindications: Hypersensitivity to either clindamycin or lincomycin. Use in treating viral and minor bacterial infections or in patients with a history of regional enteritis, nonbacterial infections (e.g., most URIs), ulcerative colitis, meningitis, or antibiotic-associated colitis. Lactation.

Precautions: Use with caution in infants up to 1 month of age, in patients with GI disease, liver or renal disease, or a history of allergy or asthma. Safety and efficacy of topical products have not been established in children less than 12 years of age.

Route/Dosage

• **Capsules, Oral Solution**
  Serious infections.
Adults: 150–300 mg q 6 hr. **Pediatric, Clindamycin hydrochloride:** 8–16 mg/kg/day divided into three or four equal doses. **Pediatric, clindamycin palmitate hydrochloride:** 8–12 mg/kg/day divided into three or four equal doses.

More severe infections.
Adults: 300–450 mg q 6 hr. **Pediatric, Clindamycin hydrochloride:** 16–20 mg/kg/day divided into three or four equal doses. **Pediatric, clindamycin palmitate hydrochloride:** 13–25 mg/kg/day divided into three or four equal doses. **Children less than 10 kg:** Minimum recommended dose is 37.5 mg t.i.d.

• **IM, IV**
Serious infections due to aerobic gram–positive cocci.
Adults: 600–1,200 mg/day in two to four equal doses. **Pediatric, over 1 month to 16 years:** 350 mg/m²/day.

More severe infections due to B. fragilis, Peptococcus, or Clostridium (other than C.perfringens).
Adults: 1,200–2,700 mg/day in two to four equal doses. May have to be increased in more serious infections. **Pediatric, over 1 month to16 years:** 450 mg/m²/day.

Life-threatening infections.
Adults: 4.8 g IV. **Pediatric, 1 month to 16 years:** 20–40 mg/kg/day in three to four equal doses depending on severity of infections. **Pediatric, less than 1 month of age:** 15–20 mg/kg/day in three or four equal doses.

Acute pelvic inflammatory disease.
IV: 900 mg q 8 hr plus gentamicin loading dose of 2 mg/kg IV or IM; **then,** gentamicin, 1.5 mg/kg q 8 hr IV or IM. Therapy may be discontinued 24 hr after patient improves. After discharge from the hospital, continue with doxycycline PO, 100 mg b.i.d. for 10–14 days. Alternatively, give clindamycin, PO, 450 mg q.i.d. for 14 days.

• **Topical Gel, Lotion, or Solution**
Apply thin film b.i.d. to affected areas. One or more pledgets may also be used.

• **Vaginal Cream (2%)**
Bacterial vaginosis
One applicatorful (containing about 100 mg clindamycin phosphate),

preferably at bedtime, for 3 or 7 consecutive days.

How Supplied: Clindamycin hydrochloride: *Capsule:* 75 mg, 150 mg, 300 mg Clindamycin palmitate: *Granule for oral solution: 75 mg/5 mL* Clindamycin phosphate: *Vaginal cream:* 2%; *Gel:* 1%; *Injection:* 150 mg/mL, 300 mg/50 mL, 600 mg/50 mL, 900 mg/50 mL; *Lotion:* 1%; *Solution:* 1%; *Swab:* 1%

Side Effects: *GI:* N&V, diarrhea, ***pseudomembranous colitis*** (more frequent after PO use), abdominal pain, esophagitis, unpleasant or metallic taste (after high IV doses), glossitis, stomatitis. *CV:* Hypotension, ***rarely, cardiopulmonary arrest after too rapid IV use.*** *Allergic:* Morbilliform rash (most common), skin rashes, urticaria, erythema multiforme, ***anaphylaxis, Stevens-Johnson-like syndrome,*** maculopapular rash, angioneurotic edema. *Hematologic:* Leukopenia, neutropenia, thrombocytopenia, transient eosinophilia, ***agranulocytosis, aplastic anemia.*** *Hepatic:* Jaundice, abnormal LFT's. *GU:* Renal dysfunction (azotemia, oliguria, proteinuria), vaginitis. *Miscellaneous:* Superinfection, tinnitus, polyarthritis. Also sore throat, fatigue, urinary frequency, headache.

Following IV use: Thrombophlebitis, erythema, pain, swelling. *Following IM use:* Pain, induration, sterile abscesses.

Following topical use: Erythema, irritation, dryness, peeling, itching, burning, oiliness of skin.

Following vaginal use: Cervicitis, vaginitis, vulvar irritation, urticaria, rash.

NOTE: The injection contains benzyl alcohol, which has been associated with ***a fatal "gasping syndrome"*** in infants.

Drug Interactions
Antiperistaltic antidiarrheals (opiates, Lomotil) / ↑ Diarrhea due to ↓ removal of toxins from colon
Ciprofloxacin HCl / Additive antibacterial activity

---

bold italic = life threatening side effect

Erythromycin / Cross-interference → ↓ effect of both drugs
Kaolin/Pectin (e.g., Kaopectate) / ↓ Effect due to ↓ absorption from GI tract
Neuromuscular blocking agents / ↑ Effect of blocking agents

EMS CONSIDERATIONS

See also *Anti-Infectives*.

Clobetasol propionate
(kloh-BAY-tah-sohl)
Pregnancy Class: C
Temovate **(Rx)**
Classification: Corticosteroid, topical

Mechanism of Action: Has anti-inflammatory, antipruritic, and vasoconstrictive effects.
Uses: Relief of inflammatory and pruritic dermatoses.
Contraindications: Use in children less than 12 years old, use for more than 2 weeks, to treat rosacea or perioral dermatitis, and use on face, groin, axillae.
Precautions: May suppress hypothalamic-pituitary-adrenal (HPA) axis at doses as low as 2 g/day. Use with caution during lactation.

Route/Dosage
• **Topical gel**
Dermatoses.
Apply thin layer to affected skin b.i.d. once in the morning and once in the evening. Rub in gently and completely. Use no more than 50 g/week.
How Supplied: *Cream:* 0.05%; *Gel:* 0.05%

Side Effects: *Dermatologic:* Burning sensation, itching, stinging, irritation, dryness, pruritus, erythema, folliculitis, hypertrichosis, acneform eruptions, hypopigmentation, perioral dermatitis, allergic contact dermatitis, skin maceration, secondary infection, striae, millaria, cracking and fissuring of the skin, skin atrophy, numbness of fingers, telangiectasia. *Miscellaneous:* Cushing's syndrome.

EMS CONSIDERATIONS

See also *Corticosteroids*.

Clofazimine
(kloh-FAYZ-ih-meen)
Pregnancy Class: C
Lamprene **(Rx)**
Classification: Leprostatic

Mechanism of Action: Inhibits mycobacterial growth (is bactericidal) and binding to mycobacterial DNA in *Mycobacterium leprae.* Is also an anti-inflammatory by controlling erythema nodosum leprosum reactions. Cross-resistance with rifampin or dapsone is not observed.
Uses: Lepromatous leprosy (including dapsone-resistant leprosy and leprosy complicated by erythema nodosum leprosum). In combination with other drugs to prevent resistance in multibacillary leprosy.
Precautions: Use with caution in patients with abdominal pain or diarrhea. Use during lactation only if benefits outweigh risks. Safety and efficacy have not been determined in children.

Route/Dosage
• **Capsules**
Leprosy resistant to dapsone.
100 mg/day together with one or more other leprostatic drugs for a period of 3 years; **maintenance:** clofazimine alone, 100 mg/day.
Erythema nodosum leprosum.
Dosage depends on severity of symptoms, but doses greater than 200 mg/day are not recommended. Goal is 100 mg/day.
How Supplied: *Capsule:* 50 mg
Side Effects: *GI:* N&V, diarrhea, abdominal or epigastric pain, GI intolerance, GI bleeding, intestinal obstruction, anorexia, constipation, liver enlargement, eosinophilic enteritis, taste disorder. *Dermatologic:* Pink to brownish black pigmentation of skin in nearly all patients, ichthyosis, dryness of skin, pruritus, rash, erythroderma, acneiform eruptions, monilial cheilosis. *Ophthalmologic:* Pigmentation of conjunctiva and cornea (due to clofazimine crystals), phototoxicity, decreased vision, eye irritation, burning, itching, or dryness. *CNS:* Headache, dizziness,

drowsiness, neuralgia, fatigue, depression, giddiness. Depression due to skin discoloration. *Miscellaneous:* Jaundice, weight loss, hepatitis, anemia, ***thromboembolism,*** bone pain, edema, cystitis, fever, vascular pain, lymphadenopathy, eosinophilia, hypokalemia. Discoloration of urine, feces, sweat, or sputum.

OD Overdose Management: *Treatment:* Gastric lavage or induction of vomiting. General supportive measures.

EMS CONSIDERATIONS

None.

Clofibrate
(kloh-FYE-brayt)
Pregnancy Class: C
Atromid-S **(Rx)**
Classification: Antihyperlipidemic agent

Mechanism of Action: Decreases triglycerides and VLDL; cholesterol and LDL are decreased less predictably and less effectively. Mechanism may be due to increased catabolism of VLDL to LDL and decreased synthesis of VLDL by the liver. Cholesterol formation is inhibited early in the biosynthetic chain; excretion of neutral streoids is increased.

Onset of Action: 2-5 days; **maximum effect:** 3 weeks. Triglycerides return to pretreatment levels 2-3 weeks after therapy is terminated.

Uses: Dysbetalipoproteinemia (type III hyperlipidemia) not responding to diet. Hyperlipidemia (types IV and V) with a risk of abdominal pain and pancreatitis not responding to diet.

Contraindications: Impaired hepatic or renal function, primary biliary cirrhosis, lactation, pregnancy, children.

Precautions: Use with caution in patients with gout and peptic ulcer. Reduced dosage may be required in geriatric patients due to age-related decreases in renal function.

Route/Dosage
• **Capsules**
  Antihyperlipidemic.
Adults: 500 mg q.i.d. Therapeutic response may take several weeks to become apparent. Drug must be administered on a continuous basis because lowered levels of cholesterol and other lipids will return to elevated state within several weeks after administration is stopped. Discontinue after 3 months if response is poor.

How Supplied: *Capsule:* 500 mg
Side Effects: *GI:* Nausea, dyspepsia, weight gain, gastritis, vomiting, bloating, flatulence, abdominal distress, stomatitis, loose stools, diarrhea, hepatomegaly, cholelithiasis, gallstones. *CNS:* Headaches, dizziness, fatigue, weakness, drowsiness. *CV:* Changes in blood-clotting time, arrhythmias, increased or decreased angina, intermittent claudication, thromboembolic events, thrombophlebitis, swelling and phlebitis at xanthoma site, pulmonary embolism. *Skeletal muscle:* Asthenia, arthralgia, myalgia, weakness, muscle cramps, aches. *GU:* Impotence, dysuria, hematuria, decreased urine output, decreased libido, proteinuria. *Hematologic:* Anemia, leukopenia, eosinophilia. *Dermatologic:* Allergic reactions, including urticaria, skin rash, dry skin, pruritus, dry brittle hair, alopecia. *Other:* Dyspnea, polyphagia, flu-like symptoms, ***noncardiovascular death.***

Drug Interactions
Anticoagulants / Clofibrate ↑ anticoagulant effect by ↓ plasma protein binding
Antidiabetics (sulfonylureas) / Clofibrate ↑ effect of antidiabetics
Furosemide / Exaggerated diuretic response
Insulin / Clofibrate ↑ effect of insulin
Probenecid / ↑ Therapeutic and toxic effects of clofibrate due to ↓ breakdown by liver and ↓ kidney excretion

---

bold italic = life threatening side effect

Ursodiol / ↑ Risk of gallstone formation

EMS CONSIDERATIONS
None.

Clomiphene citrate
(KLOH-mih-feen)
Clomid, Serophene **(Rx)**
Classification: Ovarian stimulant

Mechanism of Action: Combines with estrogen receptors, thus decreasing the number of available receptor sites. Through negative feedback, the hypothalamus and pituitary are thus stimulated to increase secretion of LH and FSH. Under the influence of increased levels of these hormones, an ovarian follicle develops, followed by ovulation and corpus luteum development. Most women ovulate after the first course of therapy. Further treatment may be inadvisable if pregnancy fails to occur after ovulatory responses.
Onset of Action: Time to peak effect: 4-10 days after the last day of treatment for ovulation.
Uses: To treat ovulatory failure in women desiring pregnancy and whose partners are fertile and potent. Normal liver function and normal levels of endogenous estrogen are necessary criteria to clomiphene use. Therapy is ineffective in patients with ovarian or pituitary failure. *Investigational:* Male infertility (controversial).
Contraindications: Pregnancy, liver disease or history thereof, abnormal bleeding of undetermined origin. Ovarian cysts or enlargement not due to polycystic ovarian syndrome. Uncontrolled thyroid or adrenal dysfunction, organic intracranial lesion (e.g., pituitary tumor). The absence of neoplastic disease should be established before treatment is initiated.
Precautions: Multiple births are possible.

Route/Dosage ────────────
• **Tablets**
First course.

50 mg/day for 5 days. Therapy may be initiated at any time in patients who have had no recent uterine bleeding.
Second course.
Same dosage if ovulation has occurred. In absence of ovulation, dose may be increased to 100 mg/day for 5 days. This course may be started as early as 30 days after the previous one.
Third course.
Most patients who are going to respond will do so during the first course of therapy. Three courses are an adequate therapeutic trial. If ovulatory menses has not occurred, re-evaluate diagnosis.
How Supplied: *Tablet:* 50 mg
Side Effects: *Ovarian:* Ovarian overstimulation and/or enlargement and subsequent symptoms resembling those of PMS. *Ophthalmologic:* Blurred vision, spots, or flashes, probably due to intensification of after images. Although cause and effect have not been established, the following have been noted in users of clomiphene: posterior capsular cataract, detachment of the posterior vitreous, spasm of retinal arteriole, and thrombosis of temporal arteries of retina. *GI:* Abdominal distention, pain, bloating, or soreness; N&V. *GU:* Abnormal uterine bleeding, breast tenderness, increased urination. *CNS:* Insomnia, nervousness, headache, depression, fatigue, lightheadedness, dizziness. *Other:* Hot flashes, allergic dermatitis, urticaria, weight gain, alopecia (reversible).

EMS CONSIDERATIONS
None.

Clomipramine hydrochloride
(kloh-MIP-rah-meen)
Pregnancy Class: C
Anafranil **(Rx)**
Classification: Antidepressant, tricyclic

Mechanism of Action: Significant anticholinergic and sedative effects as well as moderate orthostatic hypotension. Significant serotonin uptake blocking activity and moderate blocking activity for norepinephrine.

Uses: Obsessive-compulsive disorder in which the obsessions or compulsions cause marked distress, significantly interfere with social or occupational activities, or are time-consuming. Panic attacks and cataplexy associated with narcolepsy.

Contraindications: To relieve symptoms of depression.

Precautions: Safety has not been established for use during lactation or in children less than 10 years of age.

Route/Dosage
• **Capsules**
Adult, initial: 25 mg/day; **then,** increase gradually to approximately 100 mg during the first 2 weeks (depending on patient tolerance). The dose may then be increased slowly to a maximum of 250 mg/day over the next several weeks. **Adolescents, children, initial:** 25 mg/day; **then,** increase gradually during the first 2 weeks to a maximum of 100 mg or 3 mg/kg, whichever is less. The dose may then be increased to a maximum daily dose of 3 mg/kg or 200 mg, whichever is less. **Maintenance, adults and children:** Adjust the dose to the lowest effective dose with periodic reassessment to determine need for continued therapy.

How Supplied: *Capsule:* 25 mg, 50 mg, 75 mg

Side Effects: Additional: Hyperthermia, especially when used with other drugs. Increased risk of **seizures.** Agressive reactions, asthenia, anemia, eructation, failure to ejaculate, laryngitis, vestibular disorders, muscle weakness.

EMS CONSIDERATIONS

See also *Antidepressants, Tricyclic.*

Clonazepam
(kloh-NAY-zeh-pam)

Klonopin **(Rx)**
Classification: Anticonvulsant, miscellaneous

Mechanism of Action: Benzodiazepine derivative which increases presynaptic inhibition and suppresses the spread of seizure activity.

Even though a benzodiazepine, clonazepam, is used only as an anticonvulsant. However, contraindications, side effects, and so forth are similar to those for diazepam.

Uses: Absence seizures (petit mal) including Lennox-Gastaut syndrome, akinetic and myoclonic seizures. Some effectiveness in patients resistant to succinimide therapy. *Investigational:* Parkinsonian dysarthria, acute manic episodes of bipolar affective disorder, leg movements (periodic) during sleep, adjunct in treating schizophrenia, neuralgias, multifocal tic disorders.

Contraindications: Sensitivity to benzodiazepines. Severe liver disease, acute narrow-angle glaucoma. Pregnancy.

Precautions: Effects on lactation not known.

Route/Dosage
• **Tablets**
Seizure disorders.
Adults, initial: 0.5 mg t.i.d. Increase by 0.5–1 mg/day q 3 days until seizures are under control or side effects become excessive; **maximum:** 20 mg/day. **Pediatric up to 10 years or 30 kg:** 0.01–0.03 mg/kg/day in two to three divided doses up to a maximum of 0.05 mg/kg/day. Increase by increments of 0.25–0.5 mg q 3 days until seizures are under control or maintenance of 0.1–0.2 mg/kg is attained.
Parkinsonian dysarthria.
Adults: 0.25–0.5 mg/day.
Acute manic episodes of bipolar affective disorder.
Adults: 0.75–16 mg/day.
Periodic leg movements during sleep.
Adults: 0.5–2 mg nightly.
Adjunct to treat schizophrenia.

Adults: 0.5–2 mg/day.
Neuralgias.
Adults: 2–4 mg/day.
Multifocal tic disorders.
Adults: 1.5–12 mg/day.
How Supplied: *Tablet:* 0.5 mg, 1 mg, 2 mg

Side Effects: Additional: In patients in whom different types of seizure disorders exist, clonazepam may elicit or precipitate **grand mal seizures.**

Drug Interactions
CNS depressants / Potentiation of CNS depressant effect of clonazepam
Phenobarbital / ↓ Effect of clonazepam due to ↑ breakdown by liver
Phenytoin / ↓ Effect of clonazepam due to ↑ breakdown by liver
Valproic acid / ↑ Chance of absence seizures

EMS CONSIDERATIONS

See also *Anticonvulsants.*

Clonidine hydrochloride
(KLOH-nih-deen)
Pregnancy Class: C
Catapres; Catapres-TTS-1, -2, and -3
Classification: Antihypertensive, centrally acting antiadrenergic

Mechanism of Action: Stimulates alpha-adrenergic receptors of the CNS, which results in inhibition of the sympathetic vasomotor centers and decreased nerve impulses. Thus, bradycardia and a fall in both SBP and DBP occur. Plasma renin levels are decreased, while peripheral venous pressure remains unchanged. Few orthostatic effects. Although NaCl excretion is markedly decreased, potassium excretion remains unchanged. To relieve spasticity, it decreases excitatory amino acids by central presynaptic α–receptor agonism. Tolerance to the drug may develop.

The transdermal dosage form contains the following levels of drug: Catapres-TTS-1 contains 2.5 mg clonidine (surface area 3.5 cm²), with 0.1 mg released daily; Catapres-TTS-2 contains 5 mg clonidine (surface area 7 cm²), with 0.2 mg released daily; and Catapres-TTS-3 contains 7.5 mg clonidine (surface area 10.5 cm²), with 0.3 mg released daily.

Epidural use causes analgesia at presynaptic and postjunctional alpha-2-adrenergic receptors in the spinal cord due to prevention of pain signal transmission to the brain.
Onset of Action: PO: 30-60 min; **transdermal:** 2-3 days. **Maximum effect, PO:** 2-4 hr.
Duration of Action: PO: 12-24 hr; **transdermal:** 7 days (with system in place).

Uses: Oral, Transdermal: Mild to moderate hypertension. A diuretic or other antihypertensive drugs, or both, are often used concomitantly. Treat spasticity. *Investigational:* Alcohol withdrawal, atrial fibrillation, attention deficit hyperactivity disorder, constitutional growth delay in children, cyclosporine-associated nephrotoxicity, diabetic diarrhea, Gilles de la Tourette's syndrome, hyperhidrosis, hypertensive emergencies, mania, menopausal flushing, opiate detoxification, diagnosis of pheochromocytoma, postherpetic neuralgia, psychosis in schizophrenia, reduce allergen-induced inflammatory reactions in extrinsic asthma, restless leg syndrome, facilitate smoking cessation, ulcerative colitis.

Epidural: With opiates for severe pain in cancer patients not relieved by opiate analgesics alone. Most effective for neuropathic pain.
Contraindications: Epidurally: Presence of an injection site infection, patients on anticoagulant therapy, in bleeding diathesis, administration above the C4 dermatome. For obstetric, postpartum, or perioperative pain.
Precautions: Use with caution during lactation and in the presence of severe coronary insufficiency, recent MI, cerebrovascular disease, or chronic renal failure. Safe use in children not established. Geriatric patients may be more sensitive to the hypotensive effects; a decreased dosage may also be necessary in these patients due to

age-related decreases in renal function. For children, restrict epidural use to severe intractable pain from malignancy that is not responsive to epidural or spinal opiates or other analgesic approaches.

Route/Dosage

• **Tablets**

Hypertension.

Initial: 100 mcg b.i.d.; **then,** increase by 100–200 mcg/day until desired response is attained; **maintenance:** 200–600 mcg/day in divided doses (maximum: 2400 mcg/day). Tolerance necessitates increased dosage or concomitant administration of a diuretic. Gradual increase of dosage after initiation minimizes side effects. **Pediatric:** 50–400 mcg b.i.d.

NOTE: In hypertensive patients unable to take PO medication, clonidine may be administered sublingually at doses of 200–400 mcg/day.

Treat spasticity.

Adults and children: 0.1–0.3 mg/day, given in divided doses.

Alcohol withdrawal.

300–600 mcg q 6 hr.

Atrial fibrillation.

75 mcg 1–2 times/day with or without digoxin.

Attention deficit hyperactivity disorder.

5 mcg/kg/day for 8 weeks.

Constitutional growth delay in children.

37.5–150 mcg/m²/day.

Diabetic diarrhea.

100–600 mcg q 12 hr.

Gilles de la Tourette syndrome.

150–200 mcg/day.

Hyperhidrosis.

250 mcg 3–5 times/day.

Hypertensive urgency (diastolic > 120 mm Hg).

Initial: 100–200 mcg; **then,** 50– 100 mcg q hr to a maximum of 800 mcg.

Menopausal flushing.

100–400 mcg/day.

Withdrawal from opiate dependence.

15–16 mcg/kg/day.

Diagnosis of pheochromocytoma.

300 mcg.

Postherpetic neuralgia.

200 mcg/day.

Psychosis in schizophrenia.

Less than 900 mcg/day.

Reduce allergen-induced inflammation in extrinsic asthma.

150 mcg for 3 days or 75 mcg/1.5 mL saline by inhalation.

Restless leg syndrome.

100–300 mcg/day, up to 900 mcg/ day.

Facilitate cessation of smoking.

150–400 mcg/day.

Ulcerative colitis.

300 mcg t.i.d.

• **Transdermal**

Hypertension.

Initial: Use 0.1-mg system; **then,** if after 1–2 weeks adequate control has not been achieved, can use another 0.1-mg system or a larger system. The antihypertensive effect may not be seen for 2–3 days. The system should be changed q 7 days.

Treat spasticity.

Adults and children: 0.1–0.3 mg; apply patch q 7 days.

Cyclosporine-associated nephrotoxicity.

100–200 mcg/day.

Diabetic diarrhea.

0.3 mg/24 hr patch (1 or 2 patches/week).

Menopausal flushing.

100 mcg/24-hr patch.

Facilitate cessation of smoking.

200 mcg/24-hr patch.

• **Epidural infusion**

Analgesia.

Initial: 30 mcg/hr. Dose may then be titrated up or down, depending on pain relief and side effects.

How Supplied: *Film, Extended Release:* 0.1 mg/24 hrs, 0.2 mg/24 hrs, 0.3 mg/24 hrs; *Injection:* 0.1 mg/mL; *Tablet:* 0.1 mg, 0.2 mg, 0.3 mg

Side Effects: *CNS:* Drowsiness (common), sedation, confusion, dizziness, headache, fatigue, malaise, nightmares, nervousness, restlessness, anxiety, mental depression, increased dreaming, insomnia, hallucinations, delirium, agitation. *GI:* Dry

---

bold italic = life threatening side effect

mouth (common), constipation, anorexia, N&V, parotid pain, weight gain, hepatitis, parotitis, ileus, pseudo-obstruction, abdominal pain. *CV:* CHF, severe hypotension, Raynaud's phenomenon, abnormalities in ECG, palpitations, tachycardia and bradycardia, postural hypotension, conduction disturbances, sinus bradycardia, *CVA*. *Dermatologic:* Urticaria, skin rashes, sweating, **angioneurotic edema,** pruritus, thinning of hair, alopecia, skin ulcer. *GU:* Impotence, urinary retention, decreased sexual activity, loss of libido, nocturia, difficulty in urination, UTI. *Respiratory:* Hypoventilation, dyspnea. *Musculoskeletal:* Muscle or joint pain, leg cramps, weakness. *Other:* Gynecomastia, increase in blood glucose (transient), increased sensitivity to alcohol, chest pain, tinnitus, hyperaesthesia, pain, infection, thrombocytopenia, syncope, blurred vision, withdrawal syndrome, dryness of mucous membranes of nose; itching, burning, dryness of eyes; skin pallor, fever.

Transdermal products: Localized skin reactions, pruritus, erythema, allergic contact sensitization and contact dermatitis, localized vesiculation, hyperpigmentation, edema, excoriation, burning, papules, throbbing, blanching, generalized macular rash.

NOTE: Rebound hypertension may be manifested if clonidine is withdrawn abruptly.

OD **Overdose Management:** *Symptoms:* Hypotension, bradycardia, respiratory and CNS depression, hypoventilation, hypothermia, apnea, miosis, agitation, irritability, lethargy, **seizures, cardiac conduction defects, arrhythmias,** transient hypertension, diarrhea, vomiting. *Treatment:* Maintain respiration; perform gastric lavage followed by activated charcoal. Magnesium sulfate may be used to hasten the rate of transport through the GI tract. IV atropine sulfate (0.6 mg for adults; 0.01 mg/kg for children), epinephrine, tolazoline, or dopamine to treat persistent bradycardia. IV fluids and elevation of the legs are used to reverse hypotension; if unresponsive to these measures, dopamine (2–20 mcg/kg/min) or tolazoline (1 mg/kg IV, up to a maximum of 10 mg/dose) may be used. To treat hypertension, diazoxide, IV furosemide, or an alpha-adrenergic blocking drug may be used.

Drug Interactions
Alcohol / ↑ Depressant effects
Beta-adrenergic blocking agents / Paradoxical hypertension; also, ↑ severity of rebound hypertension following clonidine withdrawal
CNS depressants / ↑ Depressant effect
Levodopa / ↓ Effect of levodopa
Local anesthetics / Epidural clonidine → prolonged duration of epidural local anesthetics
Prazosin / ↓ Antihypertensive effect of clonidine
Narcotic analgesics / Potentiation of hypotensive effect of clonidine
Tolazoline / Blocks antihypertensive effect
Tricyclic antidepressants / Blocks antihypertensive effect
Verapamil / ↑ Risk of AV block and severe hypotension

EMS CONSIDERATIONS

See also *Antihypertensive Agents.*

Clopidogrel bisulfate
(kloh-PID-oh-grel)
Pregnancy Class: B
Plavix **(Rx)**
Classification: Antiplatelet drug

Mechanism of Action: Inhibits platelet aggregation by inhibiting binding of adenosine diphosphate (ADP) to its platelet receptor and subsequent ADP-mediative activation of glycoprotein GPIIb/IIIa complex. Modifies receptor irreversibly; thus, platelets are affected for remainder of their lifespan. Also inhibits platelet aggregation caused by agonists other than ADP by blocking amplification of platelet activation by released ADP.

Uses: Reduction of MI, stroke, and vascular death in patients with atherosclerosis documented by recent stroke, MI, or established peripheral arterial disease.

Contraindications: Lactation. Active pathological bleeding such as peptic ulcer or intracranial hemorrhage.
Precautions: Use with caution in those at risk of increased bleeding from trauma, surgery, or other pathological conditions. Safety and efficacy have not been determined in children.

Route/Dosage
• **Tablets**
Reduction of atherosclerotic events.
Adults: 75 mg once daily with or without food.
How Supplied: *Tablets:* 75 mg
Side Effects: *CV:* Edema, hypertension, *intracranial hemorrhage. GI:* Abdominal pain, dyspepsia, diarrhea, nausea, hemorrhage, ulcers (peptic, gastric, duodenal). *CNS:* Headache, dizziness, depression. *Body as a whole:* Chest pain, accidental injury, flu-like symptoms, pain, fatigue. *Respiratory:* URTI, dyspnea, rhinitis, bronchitis, coughing. *Hematologic:* Purpura, epistaxis. *Musculoskeletal:* Arthralgia, back pain. *Dermatologic:* Disorders of skin/appendages, rash, pruritus. *Miscellaneous:* UTI.
Drug Interactions
NSAIDs / ↑ Risk of occult blood loss
Warfarin / Clopidogrel prolongs bleeding time; safety of use with warfarin not established

EMS CONSIDERATIONS
None.

Clorazepate dipotassium
(klor-AYZ-eh-payt)
Pregnancy Class: D
Tranxene-SD, Tranxene-T **(C-IV) (Rx)**
Classification: Antianxiety agent, benzodiazepine type; anticonvulsant

Uses: Anxiety, tension. Acute alcohol withdrawal, as adjunct in treatment of seizures. Adjunct for treating partial seizures.
Contraindications: Additional: Depressed patients, nursing mothers.
Precautions: Use with caution with impaired renal or hepatic function.

Route/Dosage
• **Extended-Release Tablets, Tablets**
Anxiety.
Initial: 7.5–15 mg b.i.d.–q.i.d.; **maintenance:** 15–60 mg/day in divided doses. **Elderly or debilitated patients, initial:** 7.5–15 mg/day. **Alternative.** Single daily dosage: **Adult, initial:** 15 mg; **then,** 11.25–22.5 mg once daily.
Acute alcohol withdrawal.
Day 1, initial: 30 mg; **then,** 15 mg b.i.d.–q.i.d. the first day; **day 2:** 45–90 mg in divided doses; **day 3:** 22.5–45 mg in divided doses; **day 4:** 15–30 mg in divided doses. Thereafter, reduce to 7.5/day and discontinue as soon as possible. Maximum daily dose: 90 mg.
Partial seizures.
Adults and children over 12 years, initial: 7.5 mg t.i.d.; increase no more than 7.5 mg/week to maximum of 90 mg/day. **Children (9–12 years), initial:** 7.5 mg b.i.d.; increase by no more than 7.5 mg/week to maximum of 60 mg/day. Not recommended for children under 9 years of age.
How Supplied: *Tablet:* 3.75 mg, 7.5 mg, 15 mg; *Tablet, Extended Release:* 11.25 mg, 22.5 mg

EMS CONSIDERATIONS
See also *Tranquilizers.*

Clotrimazole
(kloh-TRY-mah-zohl)
Pregnancy Class: C (systemic use); B (topical/vaginal use)
FemCare, Gyne-Lotrimin, Lotrimin, Lotrimin AF, Mycelex, Mycelex-7, Mycelex-G, Mycelex OTC, Neo-Zol **(OTC) (Rx)**
Classification: Antifungal

Mechanism of Action: Depending on concentration, may be fungistatic or fungicidal. Acts by inhibiting the biosynthesis of sterols, resulting in damage to the cell wall and subsequent loss of essential intracellular elements due to altered permeabil-

bold italic = life threatening side effect

ity. May also inhibit oxidative and peroxidative enzyme activity and inhibit the biosynthesis of triglycerides and phospholipids by fungi. When used for *Candida albicans,* the drug inhibits transformation of blastophores into the invasive mycelial form.

Uses: Broad-spectrum antifungal effective against *Malassezia furfur, Trichophyton rubrum, Trichophyton mentagrophytes, Epidermophyton floccosum, Microsporum canis, C. albicans. Oral troche:* Oropharyngeal candidiasis. Reduce incidence of oropharyngeal candidiasis in patients who are immunocompromised due to chemotherapy, radiotherapy, or steroid therapy used for leukemia, solid tumors, or kidney transplant. *Topical OTC products:* Topically to treat tinea pedis, tinea cruris, and tinea corporis. *Topical prescription products:* Same as OTC plus candidiasis and tinea versicolor. *Vaginal products:* Vulvovaginal candidiasis.

Contraindications: Hypersensitivity. First trimester of pregnancy.

Precautions: Use with caution during lactation. Safety and effectiveness for PO use in children less than 3 years of age has not been determined.

Route/Dosage —————————
• **Troche**
Treatment of oropharyngeal candidiasis.
One troche (10 mg) 5 times/day for 14 consecutive days.
Prophylaxis of oropharyngeal candidiasis.
One troche t.i.d. for duration of chemotherapy or until maintenance doses of steroids are instituted.
• **Topical Cream, Lotion, Solution (each 1%)**
Massage into affected skin and surrounding areas b.i.d. in morning and evening for 7 consecutive days. Diagnosis should be reevaluated if no improvement occurs in 4 weeks.
• **Vaginal Tablets**
One 100-mg tablet/day at bedtime for 7 days. One 500-mg tablet can be inserted once at bedtime.

• **Vaginal Cream (1%)**
5 g (one full applicator)/day at bedtime for 7 consecutive days.
• **Vaginal Inserts and Clotrimazole, 1%**
Vaginal yeast infections.
Insert daily for 3 consecutive days.
How Supplied: *Kit; Lotion:* 1%; *Lozenge/Troche:* 10 mg; *Solution:* 1%; *Topical cream:* 1%; *Vaginal cream:* 1%; *Vaginal tablet:* 100 mg, 500 mg
Side Effects: *Skin:* Irritation including rash, stinging, pruritus, urticaria, erythema, peeling, blistering, edema. *Vaginal:* Lower abdominal cramps; urinary frequency; bloating; vaginal irritation, itching or burning; dyspareunia. *Hepatic:* Abnormal liver function tests. *GI:* N&V following use of troche.

EMS CONSIDERATIONS

See slso *Anti-Infectives.*

Cloxacillin sodium
(klox-ah-SILL-in)
Pregnancy Class: B
Classification: Antibiotic, penicillin

Uses: Infections caused by penicillinase-producing staphylococci, including pneumococci, group A beta-hemolytic streptococci, and penicillin G-sensitive and penicillin G-resistant staphylococci.

Route/Dosage —————————
• **Capsules, Oral Solution**
Skin and soft tissue infections, mild to moderate URTIs.
Adults and children over 20 kg: 250 mg q 6 hr; **pediatric, less than 20 kg:** 50 mg/kg/day in divided doses q 6 hr.
Lower respiratory tract infections or disseminated infections.
Adults and children over 20 kg: 500 mg q 6 hr; **pediatric, less than 20 kg:** 100 mg/kg/day in divided doses q 6 hr. Alternatively, a dose of 50–100 mg/kg/day (up to a maximum of 4 g/day) divided q 6 hr may be used for infants and children.
How Supplied: *Capsule:* 250 mg, 500 mg; *Powder for Reconstitution:* 125 mg/5 mL when reconstituted

EMS CONSIDERATIONS

See also *Anti-Infectives* and *Penicillins.*

Clozapine

(KLOH-zah-peen)
Pregnancy Class: B
Clozaril **(Rx)**
Classification: Antipsychotic

Mechanism of Action: Interferes with the binding of dopamine to both D-1 and D-2 receptors; more active at limbic than at striatal dopamine receptors. Thus, is relatively free from extrapyramidal side effects and does not induce catalepsy. Also acts as an antagonist at adrenergic, cholinergic, histaminergic, and serotonergic receptors. Increases the amount of time spent in REM sleep.

Uses: Severely ill schizophrenic patients who do not respond adequately to conventional antipsychotic therapy, either because of ineffectiveness or intolerable side effects from other drugs. Due to the possibility of development of agranulocytosis and seizures, avoid continued use in patients failing to respond.

Contraindications: Myeloproliferative disorders. Use in those with a history of clozapine–induced agranulocytosis or severe granulocytopenia; use with other agents known to suppress bone marrow function . Severe CNS depression or coma due to any cause. Lactation.

Precautions: Use with caution in patients with known CV disease, prostatic hypertrophy, narrow angle glaucoma, hepatic or renal disease.

Route/Dosage ———————
• **Tablets**
  Schizophrenia.
Adults, initial: 25 mg 1–2 times/day; **then,** if drug is tolerated, the dose can be increased by 25–50 mg/day to a dose of 300–450 mg/day at the end of 2 weeks. Subsequent dosage increments should occur no more often than once or twice a week in increments not to exceed

100 mg. **Usual maintenance dose:** 300–600 mg/day (although doses up to 900 mg/day may be required in some patients). Total daily dose should not exceed 900 mg.

How Supplied: *Tablet:* 25 mg, 100 mg

Side Effects: *Hematologic:* **Agranulocytosis,** leukopenia, neutropenia, eosinophilia. *CNS:* **Seizures** (appear to be dose dependent), drowsiness or sedation, dizziness, vertigo, headache, tremor, restlessness, nightmares, hypokinesia, akinesia, agitation, akathisia, confusion, rigidity, fatigue, insomnia, hyperkinesia, weakness, lethargy, slurred speech, ataxia, depression, anxiety, epileptiform movements. *CV:* Orthostatic hypotension (especially initially), tachycardia, syncope, hypertension, angina, chest pain, **cardiac abnormalities,** changes in ECG. *Neuroleptic malignant syndrome:* **Hyperpyrexia,** muscle rigidity, altered mental status, irregular pulse or BP, tachycardia, diaphoresis, cardiac dysrhythmias. *GI:* Constipation, nausea, heartburn, abdominal discomfort, vomiting, diarrhea, anorexia. *GU:* Urinary abnormalities, incontinence, abnormal ejaculation, urinary frequency or urgency, urinary retention. *Musculoskeletal:* Muscle weakness, pain (back, legs, neck), muscle spasm, muscle ache. *Respiratory:* Dyspnea, SOB, throat discomfort, nasal congestion. *Miscellaneous:* Salivation, sweating, visual disturbances, fever (transient), dry mouth, rash, weight gain, numb or sore tongue.

OD Overdose Management: *Symptoms:* Drowsiness, delirium, tachycardia, **respiratory depression,** hypotension, hypersalivation, **seizures, coma.** *Treatment:* Establish an airway and maintain with adequate oxygenation and ventilation. Give activated charcoal and sorbitol. Monitor cardiac status and VS. General supportive measures.

Drug Interactions
Anticholinergic drugs / Additive anticholinergic effects
Antihypertensive drugs / Additive hypotensive effects

---

bold italic = life threatening side effect

Benzodiazepines / Possible respiratory depression and collapse

Digoxin / ↑ Effect of digoxin due to ↓ binding to plasma protein

Epinephrine / Clozapine may reverse effects if epinephrine is given for hypotension

Warfarin / ↑ Effect of warfarin due to ↓ binding to plasma protein

EMS CONSIDERATIONS

None.

Codeine phosphate
Codeine sulfate

(KOH-deen)
Pregnancy Class: C
(C-II) (Rx)
Classification: Narcotic analgesic, morphine type

Mechanism of Action: Produces less respiratory depression and N&V than morphine. Moderately habit-forming and constipating. Dosages over 60 mg often cause restlessness and excitement and irritate the cough center. In lower doses it is a potent antitussive and is an ingredient in many cough syrups. **Onset of Action:** 10-30 min. **Peak effect:** 30-60 min.

Duration of Action: 4-6 hr. Codeine is two-thirds as effective PO as parenterally.

Uses: Relief of mild to moderate pain. Antitussive to relieve chemical or mechanical respiratory tract irritation. In combination with aspirin or acetaminophen to enhance analgesia.

Contraindications: Premature infants or during labor when delivery of a premature infant is expected.

Precautions: May increase the duration of labor. Use with caution and reduce the initial dose in patients with seizure disorders, acute abdominal conditions, renal or hepatic disease, fever, Addison's disease, hypothyroidism, prostatic hypertrophy, ulcerative colitis, urethral stricture, following recent GI or GU tract surgery, and in the young, geriatric, or debilitataed patients.

Route/Dosage
• **Solution, Tablets, IM, IV, SC**
   Analgesia.
Adults: 15–60 mg q 4–6 hr, not to exceed 360 mg/day. **Pediatric, over 1 year:** 0.5 mg/kg q 4–6 hr. IV should not be used in children.
   Antitussive.
Adults: 10–20 mg q 4–6 hr, up to maximum of 120 mg/day. **Pediatric, 2–6 years:** 2.5–5 mg PO q 4–6 hr, not to exceed 30 mg/day; **6–12 years:** 5–10 mg q 4–6 hr, not to exceed 60 mg/day.

How Supplied: Codeine Phosphate: *Injection:* 15 mg/mL, 30 mg/mL, 60 mg/mL; *Solution:* 15 mg/5 mL; *Tablet:* 30 mg, 60 mg Codeine Sulfate: *Tablet:* 15 mg, 30 mg, 60 mg

Drug Interactions: Additional: Combination with chlordiazepoxide may induce coma.

EMS CONSIDERATIONS

See also *Narcotic Analgestics*.

———COMBINATION DRUG———
Codeine phosphate and guaifenesin

(KOH-deen FOS-fayt, gwye-FEN-eh-sin)
Pregnancy Class: C
Brontex **(C-III) (Rx)**
Classification: Antitussive/expectorant

Uses: Relief of cough due to a cold or inhaled irritants. To loosen mucus and thin bronchial secretions.

Contraindications: Asthma, during labor and delivery. Use of tablets in children less than 12 years of age and use of the liquid in children less than 6 years of age.

Precautions: Use with caution in patients with severe CNS depression, respiratory depression, acute alcoholism, chronic pulmonary disease, acute abdominal conditions, seizure disorders, fever, hypothyroidism, Addison's disease, ulcerative colitis, prostatic hypertrophy, following recent GI or urinary tract surgery, and in significant renal or hepatic dysfunction, in the very young and eldery, and during lactation.

Route/Dosage
- **Oral Solution, Tablets**
  Cough/colds, bronchial congestion.

Adults and children over 12 years of age: One tablet q 4 hr or 20 mL (4 teaspoonfuls) q 4 hr. **Children, 6–12 years of age:** 10 mL (2 teaspoonfuls) q 4 hr.

How Supplied: *Antitussive:* Codeine phosphate, 10 mg/tablet or 20 mL. *Expectorant:* Guaifenesin, 300 mg/tablet or 20 mL.

Side Effects: *CNS:* CNS depression, lightheadedness, dizziness, sedation, headache, euphoria or dysphoria, transient hallucinations, disorientation, visual disturbances, **seizures.** *CV:* Tachycardia, bradycardia, palpitations, syncope, faintness, orthostatic hypotension, circulatory depression. *GI:* N&V, stomach pain, constipation, biliary tract spasm, increased colonic motility in those with ulcerative colitis. *GU:* Oliguria, urinary retention. *Allergic:* Pruritus, urticaria, **angioneurotic edema, laryngeal edema, anaphylaxis.** *Miscellaneous:* Flushing of the face, sweating, weakness.

Drug Interactions: Additive CNS depression if used with alcohol, sedatives, antianxiety agents, and MAO inhibitors

EMS CONSIDERATIONS
See also *Narcotic analgestics.*

Colchicine
(KOHL-chih-seen)
Pregnancy Class: C (oral use): D (parenteral use)
(Rx)
Classification: Antigout agent

Mechanism of Action: Colchicine is not uricosuric. It may reduce the crystal-induced inflammation by reducing lactic acid production by leukocytes (resulting in a decreased deposition of sodium urate), by inhibiting leukocyte migration, and by reducing phagocytosis. May also inhibit the synthesis of kinins and leukotrienes.

Onset of Action: IV:6-12 hr; **PO:** 12 hr.

Uses: Prophylaxis and treatment of acute attacks of gout. *Investigational:* To slow progression of chronic progressive multiple sclerosis, to decrease frequency and severity of fever and to prevent amyloidosis in familiar Mediterranean fever, primary biliary cirrhosis, hepatic cirrhosis, adjunct in the treatment of primary amyloidosis, Behcet's disease, pseudogout due to chondrocalcinosis, refractory idiopathic thrombocytopenic purpura, progressive systemic sclerosis, dermatologic disorders including dermatitis herpetiformis, psoriasis, palmoplantar pustulosis, and pyoderma associated with Crohn's disease.

Contraindications: Blood dyscrasias. Serious GI, hepatic, cardiac, or renal disorders.

Precautions: Use with caution during lactation. Dosage has not been established for children. Geriatric patients may be at grreater risk of developing cumulative toxicity. Use with extreme caution for elderly, debilitated patients, expecially in the presence of chronic renal, hepatic, GI, or CV disease. May impair fertility.

Route/Dosage
- **Tablets**
  Acute attack of gout.

Adults, initial: 1–1.2 mg followed by 0.5–1.2 mg q 1–2 hr until pain is relieved or nausea, vomiting, or diarrhea occurs. **Total amount required:** 4–8 mg.
  Prophylaxis for gout.

Adults: 0.5–0.65 mg/day for 3–4 days a week if the patient has less than one attack per year or 0.5–0.65 mg/day if the patient has more than one attack per year.
  Prophylaxis for surgical patients.

Adults: 0.5–0.65 mg t.i.d. for 3 days before and 3 days after surgery.
- **IV Only**
  Acute attack of gout.

Adults, initial: 2 mg; **then,** 0.5 mg q 6 hr until pain is relieved; give no more than 4 mg in a 24-hr period. Some physicians recommend a single IV dose of 3 mg while others recommend no more than 1 mg for the initial dose, followed by 0.5 mg once or twice daily, if needed. If pain recurs, 1–2 mg/day may be given for several days; however, colchicine should not be given by any route for at least 7 days after a full course of IV therapy (i.e., 4 mg).

Prophylaxis or maintenance of recurrent or chronic gouty arthritis.
0.5–1 mg 1–2 times/day. However, PO colchicine is preferred (usually with a uricosuric drug).

How Supplied: *Injection:* 0.5 mg/ml; *Tablet:* 0.5 mg, 0.6 mg

Side Effects: The drug is toxic; thus patients must be carefully monitored. *GI:* N&V, diarrhea, abdominal cramping. *Hematologic: **Aplastic anemia, agranulocytosis,*** or thrombocytopenia following long-term therapy. *Miscellaneous:* Peripheral neuritis, purpura, myopathy, neuropathy, alopecia, reversible azoospermia, dermatoses, hypersensitivity, thrombophlebitis at injection site (rare), liver dysfunction. If such symptoms appear, discontinue drug at once and wait at least 48 hr before reinstating drug therapy.

OD Overdose Management: *Symptoms (Acute Intoxication):* Characterized at first by violent GI tract symptoms such as N&V, abdominal pain, and diarrhea. The latter may be profuse, watery, bloody, and associated with severe fluid and electrolyte loss. Also, burning of throat and skin, hematuria and oliguria, rapid and weak pulse, general exhaustion, muscular depression, and CNS involvement. ***Death is usually caused by respiratory paralysis.*** *Treatment (Acute Poisoning):* Gastric lavage, symptomatic support, including atropine and morphine, artificial respiration, hemodialysis, peritoneal dialysis, and treatment of shock.

Drug Interactions
Acidifying agents / Inhibit the action of colchicine

Alkalinizing agents / Potentiate the action of colchicine
CNS depressants / Patients on colchicine may be more sensitive to CNS depressant effect of these drugs
Sympathomimetic agents / Enhanced by colchicine
Vitamin B_{12} / Colchicine may interfere with absorption from the gut

EMS CONSIDERATIONS

None.

Colestipol hydrochloride
(koh-LESS-tih-poll)
Colestid **(Rx)**
Classification: Hypocholesterolemic, bile acid sequestrant

Mechanism of Action: An anion exchange resin that binds bile acids in the intestine, forming an insoluble complex excreted in the feces. The loss of bile acids results in increased oxidation of cholesterol to bile acids and a decrease in LDL and serum cholesterol. Does not affect (or may increase) triglycerides or HDL and may increase VLDL.

Onset of Action: 1-2 days; **maximum effect:** 1 month. Return to pretreatment cholesterol levels after discontinuance of therapy: 1 month.

Uses: As adjunctive therapy in hyperlipoproteinemia (types IIA and IIB) to reduce serum cholesterol in patients who do not respond adequately to diet. *Investigational:* Digitalis toxicity.

Contraindications: Complete obstruction or atresia of bile duct.

Precautions: Use during pregnancy only if benefits outweigh risks. Use with caution during lactation and in children. Children may be more likely to develop hyperchloremic acidosis although dosage has not been established. Patients over 60 years of age may be at greater risk of GI side effects and adverse nutritional effects.

Route/Dosage

• **Oral Granules**
  Antihyperlipidemic.

Adults, initial: 5 g 1–2 times/day; **then,** can increase 5 g/day at 1–2-month intervals. **Total dose:** 5–30 g/day given once or in two to three divided doses.

• **Tablets**

Adults, initial: 2 g 1–2 times/day. Dose can be increased by 2 g, once or twice daily, at 1–2-month intervals. **Total dose:** 2–16 g/day given once or in divided doses.

Digitalis toxicity.

10 g followed by 5 g q 6–8 hr.

How Supplied: *Granule for Reconstitution:* 5 g/7.5 g, 5 g/packet, 5 g/scoopful; *Tablet:* 1 g

Side Effects: *GI:* Constipation (may be severe and accompanied by fecal impaction), N&V, diarrhea, heartburn, GI bleeding, anorexia, flatulence, steatorrhea, abdominal distention/cramping, bloating, loose stools, indigestion, rectal bleeding/pain, black stools, hemorrhoidal bleeding, ***bleeding duodenal ulcer, peptic ulceration,*** ulcer attack, GI irritation, dysphagia, dental bleeding/caries, hiccoughs, sour taste, pancreatitis, diverticulitis, cholecystitis, cholelithiasis. *CV:* Chest pain, angina, tachycardia (rare). *CNS:* Migraine or sinus headache, anxiety, vertigo, dizziness, lightheadedness, insomnia, fatigue, tinnitus, syncope, drowsiness, femoral nerve pain, paresthesia. *Hematologic:* Ecchymosis, anemia, beeding tendencies due to hypoprothrombinemia. *Allergic:* Urticaria, dermatitis, asthma, wheezing, rash. *Musculoskeletal:* Backache, muscle/joint pain, arthritis. *Renal:* Hematuria, burnt odor to urine, dysuria, diuresis. *Miscellaneous:* Uveitis, fatigue, weight loss or gain, increased libido, swollen glands, SOB, edema, weakness, swelling of hands/feet, osteoporosis, calcified material in biliary tree and gall bladder, hyperchloremic acidosis in children.

Drug Interactions: See *Cholestyramine.*

EMS CONSIDERATIONS

None.

Collagenase
(koh-LAJ-eh-nace)
Biozyme-C, Santyl **(Rx)**
Classification: Topical enzyme

Mechanism of Action: Digests collagen, thus, effectively removing tissue debris. Assists in the formation of granulation tissue and subsequent epithelialization of dermal ulcers and severely burned areas. May also reduce the incidence of hypertrophic scarring. Collagen in healthy tissue or newly formed granulation is not affected.

Uses: Reduces pus, odor, necrosis, and inflammation in chronic dermal ulcers and severely burned areas.

Contraindications: Local or systemic hypersensitivity to collagenase.

Route/Dosage

• **Ointment**

Chronic dermal ulcers, burns.

Apply once daily (more frequently if the dressing becomes soiled).

How Supplied: *Ointment:* 250 U/g

Side Effects: No allergic sensitivity or toxic reactions have been noted.

Drug Interactions: Detergents, benzalkonium chloride, hexachlorophene, nitrofurazone, tincture of iodine, and certain heavy metal ions used in some antiseptics (e.g., mercury, silver) inhibit the activity of collagenase.

EMS CONSIDERATIONS

None.

Conjugated estrogens and Medroxyprogesterone acetate
(KON-jyou-gay-ted ES-troh-jens meh-drox-see-proh-JESS-ter-ohn)
Pregnancy Class: X
PremPro **(Rx)**
Classification: Hormones

Uses: Moderate to severe vasomotor symptoms associated with menopause in women with an intact uterus. Vulvular and vaginal atrophy. Prevention of osteoporosis.

Contraindications: Known or suspected pregnancy, including use for missed abortion or as a diagnostic test for pregnancy. Known or suspected cancer of the breast or estrogen-dependent neoplasia. Undiagnosed abnormal genital bleeding. Active or past history of thrombophlebitis, thromboembolic disease, or stroke. Liver dysfunction or disease. Lactation.

Precautions: Estrogens reportedly increase the risk of endometrial carcinoma in postmenopausal women. Use with caution in conditions aggravated by fluid retention, including asthma, epilepsy, migraine, and cardiac or renal dysfunction. Estrogens may cause significant increases in plasma triglycerides that may cause pancreatitis and other complications in patients with familial defects of lipoprotein metabolism.

Route/Dosage
- **Tablets**

Vasomotor symptoms due to menopause, vulvar and vaginal atrophy, prevention of osteoporosis.

Initial: 0.625 mg/2.5 mg estrogen/medroxyprogesterone per day; **then,** increase to 0.625/5 mg estrogen/medroxyprogestrone per day.

How Supplied: Each tablet contains: conjugated estrogens, 0.625 mg, and medroxyprogesterone acetate, 2.5 mg or 5 mg.

Side Effects: See individual drug entries.

Drug Interactions: See individual drug entries.

EMS CONSIDERATIONS

None.

Corticotropin injection (ACTH, Adrenocorticotropic hormone)

Corticotropin repository injection (ACTH gel, Corticotropin gel)

(kor-tih-koh-TROH-pin)

Pregnancy Class: C

Corticotropin injection (ACTH, Adrenocorticotropic hormone) (ACTH, Acthar **(Rx)**) Corticotropin repository injection (ACTH gel, Corticotropin gel) (ACTH-80, H.P. Acthar Gel **(Rx)**)

Classification: Anterior pituitary hormone

Mechanism of Action: The hormone stimulates the functional adrenal cortex to secrete its entire spectrum of hormones, including the corticosteroids. Thus, the overall physiologic effects of corticotropin are similar to those of cortisone. Since the latter is more easily obtainable, is more predictable, and has more prolonged activity, it is usually used for therapeutic purposes. Is useful for the diagnosis of Addison's disease and other conditions in which the functionality of the adrenal cortex is to be determined. *Corticotropin cannot elicit a hormonal response from a nonfunctioning adrenal gland.*

Uses: Diagnosis of adrenal insufficiency syndromes, nonsuppurative thyroiditis, hypercalcemia associated with cancer, tuberculous meningitis with subarachnoid block or impending block (with tuberculostatic drugs). *Investigational:* Infant spasm, multiple sclerosis. For same diseases as glucocorticosteroids.

Contraindications: Additional: Cushing's syndrome, psychotic or psychopathic patients, active tuberculosis, active peptic ulcers. Lactation.

Precautions: Use with caution in patients who have diabetes and hypotension.

Route/Dosage
- **Injection: SC, IM, or Slow IV Drip**

Most uses.

Highly individualized. Usual, using aqueous solution IM or SC: 20 units q.i.d. **IV:** 10–25 units of aqueous solution in 500 mL 5% dextrose injection over period of 8 hr. Infants and young children require larger dose per body weight than do older children or adults.

Acute exacerbation of multiple sclerosis.
IM: 80–120 units/day for 2–3 weeks.

Infantile spasms.
IM: 20–40 units/day or 80 units every other day for 3 months (or 1 month after cessations of seizures).
• **Repository Gel: IM, SC**
40–80 units q 24–72 hr. A dose of 12.5 units q.i.d. causes little metabolic disturbance; 25 units q.i.d. causes definite metabolic alterations.

As a general rule, patients are started on 10–12.5 units q.i.d. If no clinical effect is noted in 72–96 hr, dosage is increased by 5 units every few days to a final maximum of 25 units q.i.d.
How Supplied: Corticotropin injection: *Powder for injection:* 25 U. Corticotropin repository injection: *Injection:* 80 U/mL.

EMS CONSIDERATIONS

None.

Cortisone acetate (Compound E)
(KOR-tih-zohn)
Cortone Acetate, Cortone Acetate Sterile Suspension **(Rx)**
Classification: Corticosteroid, glucocorticoid-type

Mechanism of Action: Possesses both glucocorticoid and mineralocorticoid activity. Short-acting.
Uses: Replacement therapy in chronic cortical insufficiency. Short-term (due to strong mineralocorticoid effect) for inflammatory or allergic disorders. Sterile suspension: Congenital adrenal hyperplasia in children.
Precautions: Use during pregnancy only if benefits outweigh risks.

Route/Dosage
• **Tablets, Injection**
Initial or during crisis.

25–300 mg/day. Decrease gradually to lowest effective dose.
Anti-inflammatory.
25–150 mg/day, depending on severity of the disease.
Acute rheumatic fever.
200 mg b.i.d. day 1, thereafter, 200 mg/day.
Addison's disease.
Maintenance: 0.5–0.75 mg/kg/day.
How Supplied: *Injection:* 50 mg/mL; *Tablet:* 5 mg, 10 mg, 25 mg

EMS CONSIDERATIONS

See also *Corticosteroids.*

Cromolyn sodium (Sodium cromoglycate)
(CROH-moh-lin)
Pregnancy Class: B
Intal, Nasalcrom **(OTC) (Rx)**
Classification: Antiasthmatic, antiallergic drug

Mechanism of Action: Acts locally to inhibit the degranulation of sensitized mast cells that occurs after exposure to certain antigens. Prevents the release of histamine, slow-reacting substance of anaphylaxis, and other endogenous substances causing hypersensitivity reactions. When effective, reduces the number and intensity of asthmatic attacks as well as decreasing allergic reactions in the eye. No antihistaminic, anti-inflammatory, or bronchodilator effects and has no role in terminating an acute attack of asthma. After inhalation, some drug is absorbed systemically.
Onset of Action: Ophthalmic: several days; **nasal:** less than 1 week, **Time to peak effect, nasal:** up to 4 weeks.
Uses: Inhalation: Prophylactic and adjunct in the management of severe bronchial asthma in selected patients. Prophylaxis of exercise-induced bronchospasms and bronchospasms due to allergens, cold dry air, or environmental pollutants.
Ophthalmologic: Conjunctivitis, including vernal keratoconjunctivitis,

C

---

bold italic = life threatening side effect

vernal conjunctivitis, and vernal keratitis. **Nasal, OTC:** Prophylaxis and treatment of allergic rhinitis. **PO:** Mastocytosis (improves symptoms including diarrhea, flushing, headaches, vomiting, urticaria, nausea, abdominal pain, and itching). *Investigational:* PO to treat food allergies. **Contraindications:** Hypersensitivity. Acute attacks and status asthmaticus. Due to the presence of benzalkonium chloride in the product, soft contact lenses should not be worn if the drug is used in the eye. For mastocytosis in premature infants.

Precautions: Dosage of the ophthalmic product has not been established in children less than 4 years of age; dosage of the nasal product has not been established in children less than 6 years of age. Use with caution for long periods of time, in the presence of renal of hepatic disease, and during lactation.

Route/Dosage

• **Capsules or Metered Dose Inhaler**
Prophylaxis of bronchial asthma.
Adults: 20 mg q.i.d. at regular intervals. Adjust dosage as required.
Prophylaxis of bronchospasm.
Adults: 20 mg as a single dose just prior to exposure to the precipitating factor. If used chronically, 20 mg q.i.d, up to a maximum of 160 mg/day.

• **Ophthalmic Solution**
Allergic ocular disorders.
Adults and children over 4 years: 1–2 gtt of the 4% solution in each eye 4–6 times/day at regular intervals.

• **Nasal Spray (OTC)**
Allergic rhinitis.
Adults and children over 6 years: 5.2 mg in each nostril 3–4 times/day at regular intervals (e.g., q 4–6 hr). May be used up to 6 times/day.

• **Oral Capsules**
Mastocytosis.
Adults: 200 mg q.i.d. 30 min before meals and at bedtime. **Pediatric, term to 2 years:** 20 mg/kg/day in four divided doses; should be used in this age group only in severe incapac-

itating disease where benefits outweigh risks. **Pediatric, 2–12 years:** 100 mg q.i.d. 30 min before meals and at bedtime. If relief is not seen within 2–3 weeks, dose may be increased, but should not exceed 40 mg/kg/day for adults and children over 2 years of age and 30 mg/kg/day for children 6 months–2 years.

How Supplied: *Concentrate:* 100 mg/5 mL; *Metered dose inhaler:* 0.8 mg/inh; *Ophthalmic solution:* 4%; *Solution:* 10 mg/mL; *Nasal spray:* 5.2 mg/inh

Side Effects: *Respiratory:* **Bronchospasm, laryngeal edema (rare),** cough, eosinophilic pneumonia. *CNS:* Dizziness, drowsiness, headache. *Allergic:* Urticaria, rash, angioedema, serum sickness, **anaphylaxis.** *Other:* Nausea, urinary frequency, dysuria, joint swelling and pain, lacrimation, swollen parotid gland.

Following nebulization: Sneezing, wheezing, itching, nose bleeds, burning, nasal congestion. **Following nasal solution:** Burning, stinging, irritation of nose; sneezing, nose bleeds, headache, bad taste in mouth, postnasal drip. **Following ophthalmic use:** Stinging and burning after use. Also, conjunctival injection, watery or itchy eyes, dryness around the eye, puffy eyes, eye irritation, styes.

Following PO use: *GI:* Diarrhea, taste perversion, spasm of esophagus, flatulence, dysphagia, burning of mouth and throat. *CNS:* Headache, dizziness, fatigue, migraine, paresthesia, anxiety, depression, psychosis, behavior changes, insomnia, hallucinations, lethargy, lightheadedness after eating. *Dermatologic:* Flushing, angioedema, urticaria, skin burning, skin erythema. *Musculoskeletal:* Arthralgia, stiffness and weakness in legs. *Miscellaneous:* Altered liver function test, dyspnea, dysuria, polycythemia, neutropenia.

EMS CONSIDERATIONS

None.

Cyanocobalamin (Vitamin B₁₂)
Cyanocobalamin crystalline

(sye-an-oh-koh-BAL-ah-min)
Pregnancy Class: C
Cyanocobalamin (Vitamin B₁₂) (**Nasal gel:** Ener-B, Nascobal **(OTC) Parenteral:** Berubigen, Kaybovite-1000 **(OTC) (Rx)**) Cyanocobalamin crystalline (Crystamine, Crysti 1000, Cyanoject, Cyomin, rubesol-1000, Vitamin B₁₂)
Classification: Vitamin ₆12

Mechanism of Action: Cyanocobalamin (vitamin B₁₂), a cobalt-containing vitamin, can be isolated from liver and is identical to that of the antianemic factor of liver. Required for hematopoiesis, cell reproduction, nucleoprotein and myelin synthesis.

Intrinsic factor is required for adequate absorption of PO vitamin B₁₂, and in pernicious anemia and malabsorption diseases intrinsic factor is administered simultaneously. Rapidly absorbed following IM or SC administration. Following absorption, vitamin B₁₂ is carried by plasma proteins to the liver where it is stored until required for various metabolic functions.

Products containing less than 500 mcg vitamin B₁₂ are nutritional supplements and are not to be used for the treatment of pernicious anemia.
Uses: Nutritional vitamin B₁₂ deficiency, including cancer of the bowel or pancreas, sprue, total or partial gastrectomy, accompanying folic acid deficiency, GI surgery or pathology, gluten enteropathy, fish tapeworm infestation, bacterial overgrowth of the small intestine. Do not use PO products to treat pernicious anemia. Also, in conditions with an increased need for vitamin B₁₂ such as thyrotoxicosis, hemorrhage, malignancy, pregnancy, and in liver and kidney disease. Vitamin B₁₂ is particularly suitable for the treatment of patients allergic to liver extract.

Investigational: Diagnosis of vitamin B₁₂ deficiency.
NOTE: Folic acid is not a substitute for vitamin B₁₂ although concurrent folic acid therapy may be required.
Contraindications: Hypersensitivity to cobalt, Leber's disease.
Precautions: Use with caution in patients with gout.

Route/Dosage
CYANOCOBALAMIN
• **Tablets, Extended-Release Tablets**
Nutritional supplement.
Adults: 1 mcg/day (up to 25 mcg for increased requirements). The RDA is 2 mcg/day. **Pediatric, up to 1 year:** 0.3 mcg/day; **over 1 year:** 1 mcg/day.
Nutritional deficiency.
25–250 mcg/day.
• **Nasal gel**
Nutritional deficiency.
500 mcg/0.1 mL weekly given intranasally.
CYANOCOBALAMIN CRYSTALLINE
• **IM, Deep SC**
Addisonian pernicious anemia.
Adults: 100 mcg/day for 6–7 days; **then,** 100 mcg every other day for seven doses. If improvement is noted along with a reticulocyte response, 100 mcg q 3–4 days for 2–3 weeks; **maintenance, IM:** 100 mcg once a month for life. Give folic acid if necessary.
Vitamin B₁₂ deficiency.
Adults: 30 mcg daily for 5–10 days; **then,** 100–200 mcg/month. Doses up to 1,000 mcg have been recommended. **Pediatric, for hematologic signs:** 10–50 mcg/day for 5–10 days followed by 100–250 mcg/dose q 2–4 weeks. **Pediatric, for neurologic signs:** 100 mcg/day for 10–15 days; **then,** 1–2 times/week for several months (can possibly be tapered to 250–1,000 mcg/month by 1 year).
Diagnosis of vitamin B₁₂ deficiency.
Adults: 1 mcg/day IM for 10 days plus low dietary folic acid and vitamin

B_{12}. Loading dose for the Schilling test is 1,000 mcg given IM.

How Supplied: Cyanocobalamin: *Lozenge:* 100 mcg, 250 mcg, 300 mcg; *Tablet:* 50 mcg, 100 mcg, 250 mcg, 500 mcg, 1,000 mcg, 2,000 mcg 2,500 mcg, 5,000 mcg; *Tablet, Extended Release:* 1,000 mcg, 1,500 mcg Cyanocobalamin crystalline: *Injection:* 2 mcg/mL, 100 mcg/mL, 1,000 mcg/mL

Side Effects: Following parenteral use. *Allergic:* Urticaria, itching, transitory exanthema, ***anaphylaxis, shock, death.*** *CV: **Peripheral vascular thrombosis,*** CHF, ***pulmonary edema.*** *Other:* Polycythemia vera, optic nerve atrophy in patients with hereditary optic nerve atrophy, diarrhea, hypokalemia, body feels swollen.

Following intranasal use. *GI:* Glossitis, N&V. *Miscellaneous:* Asthenia, headache, infection (sore throat, common cold), paresthesia, rhinitis.

NOTE: Benzyl alcohol, which is present in certain products, may cause ***a fatal "gasping syndrome"*** in premature infants.

Drug Interactions
Alcohol / ↓ Vitamin B_{12} absorption
Chloramphenicol / ↓ Response to vitamin B_{12} therapy
Cholestyramine / ↓ Vitamin B_{12} absorption
Cimetidine / ↓ Digestion and release of vitamin B_{12}
Colchicine / ↓ Vitamin B_{12} absorption
Neomycin / ↓ Vitamin B_{12} absorption
PAS / ↓ Vitamin B_{12} absorption
Potassium, timed-release / ↓ Vitamin B_{12} absorption

EMS CONSIDERATIONS

None.

Cyclobenzaprine hydrochloride

(sye-kloh-BENZ-ah-preen)
Pregnancy Class: B
Flexeril **(Rx)**
Classification: Skeletal muscle relaxant, centrally acting

Mechanism of Action: Related to the tricyclic antidepressants; possesses both sedative and anticholinergic properties. Thought to inhibit reflexes by reducing tonic somatic motor activity.

Onset of Action: 1 hr.

Duration of Action: 12–24 hr.

Uses: Adjunct to rest and physical therapy for relief of muscle spasms associated with acute and/or painful musculoskeletal conditions. Not indicated for the treatment of spastic diseases or for cerebral palsy. *Investigational:* Adjunct in the treatment of fibrositis syndrome.

Contraindications: Hypersensitivity. Arrhythmias, heart block or conduction disturbances, CHF, or during acute recovery phase of MI. Hyperthyroidism. Concomitant use of MAO inhibitors or within 14 days of their discontinuation.

Precautions: Safe use during lactation and in children under age 15 has not been established. Due to atropine-like effects, use with caution in situations where cholinegic blockade is not desired (e.g., history of urinary retention, angle-closure glaucoma, recreased intraocular pressure). Geriatric patients may be more sensitive to cholinergic blockade.

Route/Dosage ─────────
• **Tablets**
  Skeletal muscle disorders.

Adults: 20–40 mg/day in three to four divided doses (usual: 10 mg t.i.d.), up to a maximum of 60 mg/day in divided doses.

How Supplied: *Tablet:* 10 mg

Side Effects: Since cyclobenzaprine resembles tricyclic antidepressants, side effects to these drugs should also be noted. *GI:* Dry mouth, N&V, constipation, dyspepsia, unpleasant taste, anorexia, diarrhea, GI pain, gastritis, thirst, flatulence, ageusia, paralytic ileus, discoloration of tongue, stomatitis, parotid swelling. *CNS:* Drowsiness, dizziness, fatigue, asthenia, blurred vision, nervousness, headache, ***convulsions,*** ataxia, vertigo, dysarthria, paresthesia, hypertonia, tremors, malaise, abnormal gait, delusions, Bell's palsy, alteration in EEG patterns, extrapyramidal symptoms. Psychiatric symptoms include: confusion, insomnia, disorientation, depressed mood, abnormal sensations, anxiety, agitation, abnormal thinking or dreaming, excitement, hallucinations. *CV:* Tachycardia, syncope, **arrhythmias,** vasodilation, palpitations, hypotension, edema, chest pain, hypertension, MI, heart block, stroke. *GU:* Urinary frequency or retention, impaired urination, dilation of urinary tract, impotence, decreased or increased libido, testicular swelling, gynecomastia, breast enlargement, galactorrhea. *Dermatologic:* Sweating, skin rashes, urticaria, pruritus, photosensitivity, alopecia. *Musculoskeletal:* Muscle twitching, weakness, myalgia. *Hematologic:* Purpura, bone marrow depression, leukopenia, eosinophilia, thrombocytopenia. *Hepatic:* Abnormal liver function, hepatitis, jaundice, cholestasis. *Miscellaneous:* Tinnitus, diplopia, peripheral neuropathy, increase and decrease of blood sugar, weight gain or loss, **edema of the face and tongue,** inappropriate ADH syndrome, dyspnea.

OD **Overdose Management:** *Symptoms:* Temporary confusion, disturbed concentration, transient visual hallucinations, agitation, hyperactive reflexes, muscle rigidity, vomiting, **hyperpyrexia.** Also, drowsiness, hypothermia, tachycardia, **cardiac arrhythmias such as bundle branch block, ECG evidence of impaired conduction,** CHF, dilated pupils, **seizures, severe hypotension,** stupor, **coma,** paradoxical diaphoresis. *Treatment:* In addition to the treatment outlined in , for physostigmine salicylate, 1–3 mg IV may be used to reverse symptoms of severe cholinergic blockade.

Drug Interactions: *NOTE:* Because of the similarity of cyclobenzaprine to tricyclic antidepressants, the drug interactions for tricyclics should also be consulted.

Anticholinergics / Additive anticholinergic side effects

CNS depressants / Additive depressant effects

Guanethidine / Cyclobenzaprine may block effect

MAO inhibitors / Hypertensive crisis, severe convulsions

Tricyclic antidepressants / Additive side effects

EMS CONSIDERATIONS

See also *Skeletal Muscle Relaxants.*

Cyclophosphamide
(sye-kloh-FOS-fah-myd)
Pregnancy Class: D
Cytoxan, Cytoxan Lyophilized, Neosar, (Abbreviation: CYC) **(Rx)**
Classification: Antineoplastic, alkylating agent

Mechanism of Action: Metabolized in the liver to both active antineoplastic alkylating agents and inactive metabolites. The active metabolites alkylate nucleic acids, thus interfering with the growth of neoplastic and normal tissues. The cytotoxic action is due to cross-linking of strands of DNA and RNA and inhibition of protein synthesis. Also possesses immunosuppressive activity.

Uses: Often used in combination with other antineoplastic drugs. *Malignancies:* Malignant lymphomas (Stages III and IV, Ann Arbor Staging System), Hodgkin's disease, lymphocytic lymphoma (nodular or diffuse), mixed-cell-type lymphoma, histiocytic lymphoma, Burkitt's lymphoma, multiple myeloma, neuroblastoma (disseminated), adenocarcinoma of the ovary, retinoblastoma, carcinoma of the breast. *Leukemias:* Chronic lymphocytic and granulocytic leukemia, acute myelogenous and monocytic leukemia, acute lymphoblastic leukemia in children. *Other:* Mycosis fungoides, nephrotic syndrome in children. *Investigational:* Rheumatic diseases including rheumatoid arthritis and lupus erythematosus, Wegemer's granulomatosis, multiple sclerosis, polyarteritis nodosa, polymyositis (use with corticosteroids), severe neuropsychiatric lupus erythematosus.

Contraindications: Lactation. Severe bone marrow depression.

Precautions: Use with caution in patients with thrombocytopenia, leukopenia, previous radiation therapy, bone marrow infiltration of tumor cells, previous therapy causing cytotoxicity, and impaired liver and kidney function. May interfere with wound healing.

Route/Dosage ─────────
• **IV**
Malignancies.
Initial, with no hematologic deficiency: 40–50 mg/kg in divided doses over 2–5 days. *Alternative therapy:* 10–15 mg/kg q 7–10 days or 3–5 mg/kg twice weekly.
• **Tablets**
Malignancies.
Initial and maintenance: 1–5 mg/kg depending on patient tolerance. Attempt to maintain leukocyte count at 3,000–4,000/mm³. Adjust dosage for kidney or liver disease.
Nephrotic syndrome in children.
2.5–3 mg/kg/day for 60–90 days.
How Supplied: *Powder for injection:* 100 mg, 200 mg, 500 mg, 1 g, 2 g; *Tablet:* 25 mg, 50 mg
Side Effects: Additional: Acute hemorrhagic cystitis. **Bone marrow depression** appears frequently during days 9-14 of therapy. Alopecia occurs more frequently than with other drugs. **Secondary neoplasia (especially of urinary bladder), pulmonary fibrosis, cardiotoxicity,** darkening of skin or fingernails. Interference with oogenesis and spermatogenesis.
OD **Overdose Management:** *Treatment:* General supportive measures. Dialysis.
Drug Interactions
Allopurinol / ↑ Chance of bone marrow toxicity
Anticoagulants / ↑ Effect of anticoagulants
Chloramphenicol / ↓ Metabolism of cyclophosphamide to active metabolites → ↓ pharmacologic effect

Digoxin / ↓ Serum digoxin levels
Doxorubicin / ↑ Cardiotoxicity due to doxorubicin
Insulin / ↑ Hypoglycemia
Phenobarbital / ↑ Rate of metabolism of cyclophosphamide in liver
Quinolone antibiotics / ↓ Antimicrobial effect of quinolones
Succinylcholine / ↑ Neuromuscular blockade due to ↓ cholinesterase activity
Thiazide diuretics / ↑ Chance of leukopenia

EMS CONSIDERATIONS
None.

Cycloserine
(sye-kloh-SEE-reen)
Pregnancy Class: C
Seromycin **(Rx)**
Classification: Antitubercular agent for retreatment regimens

Mechanism of Action: Produced by a strain of *Streptomyces orchidaceus* or *Garyphalus lavendulae.* Acts by inhibiting cell wall synthesis by interfering with the incorporation of the amino acid alanine.

Uses: With other drugs to treat active pulmonary and extrapulmonary tuberculosis only when primary therapy cannot be used. To treat UTIs when other therapy has failed or if the organism has demonstrated sensitivity.

Contraindications: Hypersensitivity to cycloserine, epilepsy, depression, severe anxiety, psychosis, severe renal insufficiency, and alcoholism. Lactation.

Precautions: Safe use during pregnancy and in children has not been established.

Route/Dosage ─────────
• **Capsules**
Adults, initially: 250 mg q 12 hr for first 2 weeks; **then,** 0.5–1 g/day in divided doses based on blood levels. Dosage should not exceed 1 g/day.
Pediatric: 10–20 mg/kg/day, not to exceed 0.75–1 g/day. *NOTE:* Pyridoxine, 200–300 mg/day may prevent neurotoxic effects.

How Supplied: *Capsule:* 25 mg

Side Effects: *CNS:* Drowsiness, headache, mental confusion, tremors, vertigo, loss of memory, psychoses (possibly with *suicidal tendencies),* character changes, hyperirritability, aggression, increased reflexes, *seizures,* paresthesias, paresis, coma. Neurotoxic effects depend on blood levels of cycloserine. Hence, frequent determinations of cycloserine blood levels are indicated, especially during the initial period of therapy. *Other:* Sudden development of CHF, skin rashes, increased transaminase.

OD **Overdose Management:** *Symptoms:* CNS depression, including drowsiness, mental confusion, headache, vertigo, paresthesias, dysarthrias, hyperirritability, psychosis, paresis, *seizures,* and *coma.* *Treatment:* Supportive therapy. Charcoal may be more effective than emesis or gastric lavage. Hemodialysis may be used for life-threatening toxicity. Pyridoxine may treat neurotoxic effects.

Drug Interactions

Ethanol / ↑ Risk of epileptic episodes

Isoniazid / ↑ Risk of cycloserine CNS side effects (especially dizziness)

EMS CONSIDERATIONS

See also *Anti-Infectives.*

Cyclosporine

(sye-kloh-SPOR-een)

Pregnancy Class: C

Neoral, Sandimmune **(Rx)**

Classification: Immunosuppressant

Mechanism of Action: Thought to act by inhibiting the immunocompetent lymphocytes in the G_0 or G_1 phase of the cell cycle. T-lymphocytes are specifically inhibited; both the T-helper cell and the T-suppressor cell may be affected. Also inhibits interleukin 2 or T-cell growth factor production and release. Children often require larger PO doses than

adults, which may be due to the smaller absorptive surface area of their intestines.

Uses: Prophylaxis of rejection in kidney, liver, and heart allogeneic transplants. Sandimmune is always to be taken with adrenal corticosteroids while Neoral has been used in combination with azathioprine and corticosteroids. Neoral microemulsion: Alone or in combination with methotrexate for severe, active rheumatoid arthritis which has not responded to methotrexate alone. Neoral microemulsion: Severe recalcitrant plaque psoriasis. Sandimmune: Treatment of chronic rejection in patients previously treated with other immunosuppressants. Sandimmune has been used in children as young as 6 months with no unusual side effects. *Investigational:* Aplastic anemia, myasthenia gravis, atopic dermatitis, Crohn's disease, Graves ophthalmology, severe psoriasis, multiple sclerosis, polymyositis, Behcet's disease, biliary cirrhosis, corneal transplantation (or other diseases of the eye which have an autoimmune component), dermatomyositis, insulin-dependent diabetes mellitus, lichen planus, lupus nephritis, nephrotic syndrome, pemphigus and pemphigoid, psoriatic arthritis, pulmonary sarcoidosis, pyoderma gangrenosum, alopecia areata, ulcerative colitis, uveitis.

Contraindications: Hypersensitivity to cyclosporine or polyoxyethylated castor oil. Lactation. Use of potassium-sparing diuretics. Neoral in psoriasis or rheumatoid arthritis with abnormal renal function, uncontrolled hypertension, or malignancies. Neoral together with PUVA or UVB in psoriasis.

Precautions: Use with caution in patients with impaired renal or hepatic function. Safety and efficacy have not been established in children. Patients with malabsorption may not achieve therappeutic levels following PO use.

C

C

Route/Dosage

• Capsules, Oral Solution

Allogenic transplants.

Adults and children, initial: A single 15 mg/kg dose given 4–12 hr before transplantation; there is a trend to use lower initial doses of 10–14 mg/kg/day. The dose should be continued postoperatively for 1–2 weeks followed by 5% decrease in dose per week to maintenance dose of 5–10 mg/kg/day (some have used a dose of 3 mg/kg/day successfully). Compared with Sandimmune, lower maintenance doses of Neoral may be sufficient.

If converting from Sandimmune to Neoral, start with a 1:1 conversion. Then, adjust the Neoral dose to reach the pre-conversion cyclosporine blood trough levels. Until this level is reached, monitor the cyclosporine trough level q 4–7 days.

Rheumatoid arthritis (Neoral only).

Initial: 1.25 mg/kg b.i.d. PO. Salicylates, NSAIDs, and PO corticosteroids may be continued. If sufficient beneficial effect is not seen and the patient is tolerating the medication, the dose may be increased by 0.5–0.75 mg/kg/day after 8 weeks and again after 12 weeks to a maximum dose of 4 mg/kg/day. If no benefit is seen after 16 weeks, discontinue therapy. If Neoral is combined with methotrexate, the same initial dose and dose range of Neoral can be used.

Psoriasis (Neoral only).

Initial: 1.25 mg/kg b.i.d. PO. Maintain this dose for 4 weeks if tolerated. If significant improvement is not seen, increase the dose at 2-week intervals. Based on patient response, make dose increases of about 0.5 mg/kg/day to a maximum of 4 mg/kg/day. Discontinue treatment if beneficial effects can not be achieved after 6 weeks at 4 mg/kg/day. Once beneficial effects are seen, decrease the dose (doses less than 2.5 mg/kg/day may be effective). To control side effects, make dose decreases by 25% to 50% at any time.

• IV (only in patients unable to take PO medication)

Allogenic transplants.

Adults: 5–6 mg/kg/day 4–12 hr prior to transplantation and postoperatively until patient can be switched to PO dosage. *NOTE:* Steroid therapy must be used concomitantly.

Investigational uses.

Oral doses ranging from 1 to 10 mg/kg/day.

How Supplied: *Capsule:* 25 mg, 100 mg, 250 mg; *Injection:* 50 mg/mL; *Solution:* 100 mg/mL

Side Effects: *GI:* N&V, diarrhea, gum hyperplasia, anorexia, gastritis, hiccoughs, peptic ulcer, abdominal discomfort, upper GI bleeding, pancreatitis, constipation, mouth sores, difficulty in swallowing. *Hematologic:* Leukopenia, lymphoma, thrombocytopenia, anemia, microangiopathic hemolytic anemia syndrome. *Allergic:* **Anaphylaxis (rare).** *CV:* Hypertension, edema, chest pain, cramps, **MI** (rare). *CNS:* Headache, tremor, confusion, fever, **seizures,** anxiety, depression, weakness, lethargy, ataxia. *GU:* Renal dysfunction, glomerular capillary thrombosis, nephrotoxicity. *Dermatologic:* Acne, hirsutism, brittle finger nails, hair breaking, pruritus. *Miscellaneous:* Hepatotoxicity, flushing, paresthesia, sinusitis, gynecomastia, conjunctivitis, hearing loss, tinnitus, muscle pain, infections (including fungal, viral), *Pneumocystis carinii* pneumonia, hematuria, blurred vision, weight loss, joint pain, night sweats, tingling, hypomagnesemia in some patients with seizures, infectious complications, increased risk of cancer.

OD **Overdose Management:** *Symptoms:* Transient hepatotoxicity and nephrotoxicity. *Treatment:* Induction of vomiting (up to 2 hr after ingestion). General supportive measures.

Drug Interactions

Aminoglycosides / ↑ Risk of nephrotoxicity

Amiodarone / ↑ Blood levels of cyclosporine → ↑ risk of nephrotoxicity

Amphotericin B / ↑ Risk of nephrotoxicity

Azathioprine / ↑ Immunosuppression due to suppression of lymphocytes → possible infection and malignancy

Bromocriptine / ↑ Plasma level of cyclosporine due to ↓ breakdown by liver

Calcium channel blockers / / ↑ Plasma levels of cyclosporine due to ↓ breakdown by liver; ↑ risk of toxicity

Carbamazepine / ↓ Plasma level of cyclosporine due to ↑ breakdown by liver

Cimetidine / ↑ Risk of nephrotoxicity

Clarithromycin / ↑ Plasma levels of cyclosporine due to ↓ breakdown by liver; ↑ risk of nephrotoxicity, neurotoxicity

Colchicine / Severe side effects, including GI, hepatic, renal, and neuromuscular toxicity

Corticosteroids / ↑ Immunosuppression due to suppression of lymphocytes → possible infection and malignancy

Cyclophosphamide / ↑ Immunosuppression due to suppression of lymphocytes → possible infection and malignancy

Danazol / ↑ Plasma level of cyclosporine due to ↓ breakdown by liver

Diclofenac / ↑ Risk of nephrotoxicity

Digoxin / ↑ Digoxin levels due to ↓ clearance; also, ↓ volume of distribution of digoxin → toxicity

Diltiazem / ↑ Plasma level of cyclosporine due to ↓ breakdown by liver → possible nephrotoxicity

Erythromycin / ↑ Plasma level of cyclosporine due to ↓ breakdown by liver and ↓ biliary excretion → possible nephrotoxicity

Etoposide / ↓ Etoposide renal clearance → increased toxicity

Fluconazole / ↑ Plasma level of cyclosporine due to ↓ gut and liver metabolism → possible nephrotoxicity

Foscarnet ↑ Risk of renal failure

HIV Protease Inhibitors / ↑ Plasma levels of cyclosporine due to ↓ breakdown by liver → toxicity

Imipenem-cilastatin / ↑ Blood levels of cyclosporine → CNS toxicity

Isoniazid / ↓ Plasma level of cyclosporine due to ↑ breakdown by liver

Itraconazole / ↑ Plasma level of cyclosporine due to ↓ breakdown by liver

Ketoconazole / ↑ Plasma level of cyclosporine due to ↓ breakdown by gut and liver metabolism → possible nephrotoxicity

Lovastatin / ↑ Risk of myopathy and rhabdomyolysis

Melphalan / ↑ Risk of nephrotoxicity

Methylprednisolone / ↑ Blood levels of cyclosporine due to ↓ breakdown by liver → toxicity

Metoclopramide / ↑ Plasma level of cyclosporine due to ↓ breakdown by liver → toxicity

Naproxen / ↑ Risk of nephrotoxicity

Nephrotoxic drugs / Additive nephrotoxicity

Nicardipine / ↑ Plasma level of cyclosporine due to ↓ breakdown by liver → possible nephrotoxicity

Nifedipine / ↑ Risk of gingival hyperplasia

Octreotide / ↓ Plasma level of cyclosporine due to ↑ breakdown by liver

Oral contraceptives / ↑ Plasma level of cyclosporine due to ↓ breakdown by liver; possible severe hepatotoxicity

Phenobarbital / ↓ Plasma level of cyclosporine due to ↑ breakdown by liver

Phenytoin / ↓ Plasma level of cyclosporine due to ↑ breakdown by liver

Probucol / ↓ Bioavailability of cyclosporine → ↓ clinical effect

Ranitidine / ↑ Risk of nephrotoxicity

Rifabutin/Rifampin / ↓ Plasma level of cyclosporine due to ↑ breakdown by liver

---

bold italic = life threatening side effect

C

Sulfamethoxazole and/or trimethoprim / ↑ Risk of nephrotoxicity; also, ↓ serum levels of cyclosporine → possible rejection

Sulindac / ↑ Risk of nephrotoxicity

Tacrolimus / ↑ Risk of nephrotoxicity

Terbenafine / ↓ Serum levels of cyclosporine due to ↑ breakdown by liver

Vancomycin / ↑ Risk of nephrotoxicity

Verapamil / ↑ Immunosuppression

EMS CONSIDERATIONS

None.

Cyproheptadine hydrochloride

(sye-proh-HEP-tah-deen)
Pregnancy Class: B
Periactin **(Rx)**
Classification: Antihistamine, piperidine-type

Mechanism of Action: Moderate anticholinergic activity and low sedative effects.

Onset of Action: 15-30 min.

Duration of Action: 3-6 hr.

Uses: Hypersensitivity reactions: Perennial and seasonal allergic rhinitis, vasomotor rhinitis, allergic conjunctivitis, uncomplicated allergic skin reactions of urticaria and angioedema, allergic reactions to blood or plasma, cold urticaria, adjunct to treat anaphylaxis, dermographism. *Investigational:* Stimulate appetite in anorexia nervosa and for cachexia associated with cancer. Vascular cluster headaches.

Contraindications: **Additional:** Glaucoma, urinary retention.

Precautions: Geriatric patients may be more sensitive to the usual adult dose.

Route/Dosage ————

• **Syrup, Tablets**
Hypersensitivity reactions.

Adults, initial: 4 mg q 8 hr; **then,** 4–20 mg/day, not to exceed 0.5 mg/kg/day. **Pediatric, 2–6 years:** 2 mg q 8–12 hr, not to exceed 12 mg/day; **6–14 years:** 4 mg q 8–12 hr, not to exceed 16 mg/day.

Appetite stimulant.

Adults: 4 mg t.i.d. with meals. **Pediatric, 6–14 years, initial:** 2 mg t.i.d.–q.i.d. with meals; **then,** reduce dose to 4 mg t.i.d. **Pediatric, 2–6 years, initial:** 2 mg t.i.d. with meals; **then,** dose may be increased to a total of 8 mg/day.

How Supplied: *Syrup:* 2 mg/5 mL; *Tablet:* 4 mg

Side Effects: **Additional:** Increased appetite.

EMS CONSIDERATIONS

See also *Antihistamines.*

Cysteamine bitartrate

(SIS-tee-ah-meen)
Pregnancy Class: C
Cystagon **(Rx)**
Classification: Urinary tract product

Mechanism of Action: Lowers cystine levels of cells in cystinosis, which is an inherited defect of lysosomal transport. In those with cystinosis, cystine transport out of lysosomes is abnormal, resulting in the formation of crystals which damage the kidney. Other tissues are damaged as well, including the retina, muscles, and CNS. Acts within the cell to convert cystine into both cysteine and cysteine-cysteamine mixed disulfide, which can leave the lysosome in those with cystinosis.

Uses: Management of nephropathic cystinosis in adults and children.

Contraindications: Hypersensitivity to cysteamine or penicillamine. Use during lactation.

Route/Dosage ————

• **Capsules**
Nephropathic cystinosis.

Initial: New patients should be started on one-fourth to one-sixth of the maintenance dose. The dose is then raised gradually over 4–6 weeks to avoid intolerance. **Maintenance, children up to age 12 years:** 1.3 g/m^2/day (of the free base) given in four divided doses. **Maintenance, children over 12**

years and over 110 lb: 2 g/day in four divided doses.

How Supplied: *Capsule:* 50 mg, 150 mg

Side Effects: *CNS:*Lethargy, somnolence, depression, encephalopathy, *seizures,* headache, ataxia, confusion, tremor, hyperkinesia, dizziness, jitteriness, nervousness, abnormal thinking, emotional lability, hallucinations, nightmares. *GI:* N&V, anorexia, abdominal pain (may be severe), diarrhea, bad breath, dyspepsia, constipation, gastroenteritis, duodenitis, duodenal ulceration. *He-* *matologic:* Reversible leukopenia, anemia. *Miscellaneous;* Decreased hearing, fever, rash, dehydration, hypertension, urticaria.

OD **Overdose Management:** *Symptoms:* Extension of side effects, respiratory symptoms. *Treatment:* Support the cardiovascular and respiratory systems. Hemodialysis may be effective in removing the drug from the body.

EMS CONSIDERATIONS

None.

Dalteparin sodium injection

(DAL-tih-pair-in)

Pregnancy Class: B

Fragmin **(Rx)**

Classification: Anticoagulant

Mechanism of Action: A low molecular weight heparin prepared through depolymerization of sodium heparin from porcine intestinal mucosa. Acts by increasing the inhibition of factor Xa and thrombin by antithrombin. Causes a significant change in platelet aggregation, fibrinolysis, or global clotting tests (e.g., PT, APTT, or thrombin time).

Uses: To prevent deep vein thrombosis (DVT) in patients undergoing abdominal surgery who are at risk for thromboembolic complications (i.e., pulmonary embolism). High risk includes obesity, general anesthesia more than 30 min, malignancy, history of DVT or pulmonary embolism, age 40 and over. *Investigational:* Systemic anticoagulation in venous and arterial thromboembolic complications.

Contraindications: Active major bleeding or thrombocytopenia. Known hypersensitivity to heparin or pork products. IM use.

Precautions: Cannot be used interchangeably with unfractionated heparin or other low molecular weight heparins. Use with extreme caution in those with a history of heparin-induced thrombocytopenia. Use with caution in patients with an increased risk of ehmorrhage, icluding those with severe uncontrolled hypertension, bacterial endocarditis, congenital or acquired bleeding disorders, active ulceration and angiodysplastic GI disease, or hemorrhagic stroke or shortly after brain, spinal, or opthalmologic surgery. Also, use with caution in patients with bleeding diathesis, severe liver or kidney disease, hypertensive or diabetic retinopathy, and recent GI bleeding. Use with caution during lactation. Safety and efficacy have not been determined in children.

Route/Dosage

• **SC Only**
  Prevention of DVT in abdominal surgery.

Adults: 2,500 IU each day starting 1–2 hr prior to surgery and repeated once daily for 5–10 days postoperatively. High-risk patients: 5,000 IU the night before surgery and repeated once daily for 5–10 days. In malignancy: 2,500 IU 1–2 hr before surgery followed by 2,500 IU 12 hr later and 5,000 IU once daily for 5–10 days.

Systemic anticoagulation.
200 IU/kg SC daily or 100 IU/day b.i.d.

How Supplied: *Injection:* 2,500 IU/0.2 mL, 5,000 IU/0.2 mL, 10,000 IU/mL

Side Effects: *CV: Hemorrhage,* hematoma at injection site, wound hematoma, reoperation due to bleeding, postoperational transfusions. *Hematologic:* Thrombocytopenia. *Hypersensitivity:* Allergic reactions, including pruritus, rash, fever, injection site reaction, bulleous eruption, skin necrosis (rare), *anaphylaxis.* *Miscellaneous:* Pain at injection site.

OD Overdose Management: *Symptoms:* Hemorrhagic complications. *Treatment:* Slow IV protamine sulfate (1%) at a dose of 1 mg protamine sulfate for every 100 anti-Xa IU of fragmin given. A second infusion protamine sulfate, 0.5 mg for every 100 anti-Xa IU of fragmin, may be given if the APTT measured 2–4 hr after the first infusion of protamine sulfate remains prolonged. Care should be taken not to give an overdose of protamine sulfate.

Drug Interactions: Increased anticoagulant effect, and therefore increased risk of bleeding or hemorrhage, when used with oral anticoagulants or other platelet inhibitors.

EMS CONSIDERATIONS

None.

Danaparoid sodium
(dah-NAP-ah-royd)
Pregnancy Class: B
Orgaran **(Rx)**
Classification: Anticoagulant, glycosaminoglycan

Mechanism of Action: A low molecular weight sulfated glycosaminoglycans obtained from porcine mucosa. Prevents fibrin formation in the coagulation pathway via thrombin generation inhibition by anti-Xa and anti-IIa effects. Minimal effect on clotting assays, fibrinolytic activity, or bleeding time.

Uses: Prophylaxis of postoperative deep vein thrombosis (DVT) in patients undergoing elective hip replacement surgery. *Investigational:* Thromboembolism, anticoagulation during hemodialysis, hemofiltration during CV operation, and increased risk of thrombosis during pregnancy.

Contraindications: Use in hemophilia, idiopathic thrombocytopenic purpura, active major bleeding state (including hemorrhagic stroke in the acute phase), and type II thrombocytopenia associated with a positive in vitro test for antiplatelet antibody in the presence of danaparoid. Hypersensitivity to pork products. IM use.

Precautions: Cannot be dosed interchangeably (unit for unit) with either heparin or low molecular weight heparins. Use with extreme caution in disease states where there is an increased risk of hemorrhage, including severe uncontrolled hypertension, acute bacterial endocarditis, congenital or acquired bleeding disorders, active ulcerative and angiodysplastic GI disease, nonhemorrhagic stroke, postoperative indwelling epidural catheter use, and shortly after brain, spinal, or ophthalmologic surgery. Use with caution during lactation and in those with severely impaired renal function. Use with caution in patients receiving oral anticoagulants or platelet inhibitors. Safety and efficacy have not been determined in children.

Route/Dosage —————
• **SC only**
  Prophylaxis of DVT in hip replacement surgery.
Adults: 750 anti-Xa units b.i.d. SC, beginning 1 to 4 hr preoperatively and then not sooner than 2 hr postoperatively. Continue treatment throughout the postoperative period until the risk of deep vein thrombosis has decreased. Average duration of treatment is 7 to 10 days, up to 14 days.

How Supplied: *Injection:* 750 anti-Xa units/0.6 mL.

Side Effects: *CV:* Intraoperative blood loss, postoperative blood loss. *GI:* N&V, constipation. *CNS:* Insomnia, headache, dizziness. *Dermatologic:* Rash, pruritus. *GU:* UTI, urinary retention. *Miscellaneous:* Fever, pain at injection site, peripheral edema, joint disorder, edema, asthenia, anemia, pain, infection.

OD Overdose Management: *Symptoms:* Bleeding disorders, including hemorrhage. *Treatment:* Protamine sulfate partially neutralizes the anti-Xa activity of the drug; however, there is no evidence that protamine sulfate will reduce severe non-surgical bleeding. For serious bleeding, discontinue danaparoid and give blood or blood product transfusions as needed.

EMS CONSIDERATIONS

See also *Anticoagulants.*

Danazol
(DAN-ah-zohl)
Danocrine **(Rx)**
Classification: Synthetic androgen (gonadotropin inhibitor)

Mechanism of Action: Inhibits the release of gonadotropins (FSH and LH) by the anterior pituitary; thus, inhibits synthesis of sex steroids and competitively inhibits binding of steroids to their cytoplasmic receptors in target tissues. In women this action arrests ovarian function, induces amenorrhea, and causes atrophy of normal and ectopic endometrial tissue. Has weak androgenic effects.

Onset of Action: Fibrocystic disease: 4 weeks; **time to peak effect, amenorrhea and anovulation:** 6-8 weeks; **fibrocystic disease:** 2-3 months to eliminate breast pain and tenderness and 4-6 months for elimination of nodules.

Uses: Endometriosis amenable to hormonal management in patients who cannot tolerate or who have not responded to other drug therapy. Fibrocystic breast disease. Hereditary angioedema in males and females. *Investigational:* Gynecomas-

tia, menorrhagia, precocious puberty, idiopathic immune thrombocytopenia, lupus-associated thrombocytopenia, and autoimmune hemolytic anemia.

Contraindications: Undiagnosed genital bleeding; markedly impaired hepatic, renal, and cardiac function; pregnancy and lactation.

Precautions: Use with caution in children treated for hereditary angioedema due to the possibility of virilization in females and precocious sexual development in males. Use with caution in conditions aggravated by fluid retention (e.g., epilepsy, migraine, cardiac, or renal dysfunction). Geriatric patients may have an increased risk of prostatic hypertrophy or prostatic carcinoma.

Route/Dosage
• **Capsules**
Endometriosis.
400 mg b.i.d. (moderate to severe) or 100–200 mg b.i.d. (mild) for 3–6 months (up to 9 months may be required in some patients). Begin therapy during menses, if possible, to be sure that patient is not pregnant.
Fibrocystic breast disease.
50–200 mg b.i.d. beginning on day 2 of menses. Begin therapy during menses to assure patient is not pregnant.
Hereditary angioedema.
Initial: 200 mg b.i.d.–t.i.d.; after desired response, decrease dosage by 50% (or less) at 1–3-month intervals. Treat subsequent attacks by giving up to 200 mg/day. No more than 800 mg/day should be given to adults.

How Supplied: *Capsule:* 50 mg, 100 mg, 200 mg

Side Effects: *Androgenic:* Acne, decrease in breast size, oily hair and skin, weight gain, deepening of voice and hair growth, clitoral hypertrophy, testicular atrophy. *Estrogen deficiency:* Flushing, sweating, vaginitis, nervousness, changes in emotions. *GI:* N&V, constipation, gastroenteritis. *Hepatic:* Jaundice, dys-

D

function. *CNS:* Fatigue, tremor, headache, dizziness, sleep problems, paresthesia of extremities, anxiety, depression, appetite changes. *Musculoskeletal:* Muscle cramps or spasms, joint swelling or lock-up, pain in back, legs, or neck. *Miscellaneous:* Allergic reactions (skin rashes and rarely nasal congestion), hematuria, increased BP, chills, pelvic pain, carpal tunnel syndrome, hair loss, change in libido.

Drug Interactions

Insulin / Danazol ↑ insulin requirements

Warfarin / Danazol ↑ PT in warfarin-stabilized patients

EMS CONSIDERATIONS

None.

Dantrolene sodium

(DAN-troh-leen)
Pregnancy Class: C (parenteral use)
Dantrium, Dantrium IV **(Rx)**
Classification: Muscle relaxant, centrally acting

Mechanism of Action: Not related to other skeletal muscle relaxants. Acts directly on skeletal muscle, probably by dissociating the excitation-contraction coupling mechanism as a result of interference of release of calcium from the sarcoplasmic reticulum. This results in a decreased force of reflex muscle contraction and a reduction of hyperreflexia, spasticity, involuntary movements, and clonus. Effectiveness in malignant hyperthermia is due to an inhibition of release of calcium from the sarcoplasmic reticulum. This results in prevention or reduction of the increased myoplasmic calcium ion concentration that activates the acute catabolic processes associated with malignant hyperthermia.

Uses: PO: Muscle spasticity associated with severe chronic disorders, such as multiple sclerosis, cerebral palsy, spinal cord injury, and stroke. Preoperatively to prevent or reduce the development of signs of malignant hyperthermia. To prevent recurrence following a malignant hyper-

thermia crisis. **IV:** Malignant hyperthermia due to hypermetabolism of skeletal muscle. Preoperatively or postoperatively to prevent or reduce the development of signs of malignant hyperthermia in susceptible patients. *Investigational:*   Exercise-induced muscle pain, heat stroke, and neuroleptic malignant syndrome.

Contraindications: Orally in active hepatitis or cirrhosis, where spasticity is used to sustain upright posture and balance in locomotion or to obtain or maintain increased function, and to treat skeletal muscle spasm due to rheumatic disease. Pregnancy, lactation, or children under 5 years of age.

Precautions: Use with caution in patients with impaired pulmonary function, especially those with obstructive pulmonary disease; severely imparied cadiac function due to myocardial disease; and a history of previous liver disease of dysfunction.

Route/Dosage ────────
• **Capsules**
Spastic conditions.
Adults, initial: 25 mg once daily; **then,** increase to 25 mg b.i.d.–q.i.d.; dose may then be increased by 25-mg increments up to 100 mg b.i.d.–q.i.d. (doses in excess of 400 mg/day not recommended). **Pediatric: initial,** 0.5 mg/kg b.i.d.; **then,** increase to 0.5 mg/kg t.i.d.–q.i.d.; dose may then be increased by increments of 0.5 mg/kg to 3 mg/kg b.i.d.–q.i.d. (doses should not exceed 400 mg/day).
Malignant hyperthermia, preoperatively.
Adults and children: 4–8 mg/kg/day in three to four divided doses 1–2 days before surgery with the last dose given 3 to 4 hr before surgery.
Postmalignant hyperthermic crisis.
Adults and children: 4–8 mg/kg/day in four divided doses for 1–3 days.
• **IV Infusion**
Malignant hyperthermia, crisis treatment.

Adults and children, initial: 2.5 mg/kg 60 min prior to surgery and infused over 1 hr. Additional IV dantrolene may be given during anesthesia and surgery, depending on symptoms.

- **IV Push**
  Malignant hyperthermia, crisis treatment.

Initial: At least 1 mg/kg; continue administration until symptoms decrease or a cumulative dose of 10 mg/kg has been administered.

How Supplied: *Capsule:* 25 mg, 50 mg, 100 mg; *Powder for injection:* 20 mg

Side Effects: Following PO use: Side effects are dose-related and decrease with usage. *Fatal* and nonfatal *hepatotoxicity. CNS:* Drowsiness, dizziness, weakness, malaise, lightheadedness, headaches, insomnia, seizures, speech disturbances, fatigue, confusion, depression, nervousness. *GI:* Diarrhea (common), anorexia, constipation, GI bleeding, dysphagia, gastric irritation, abdominal cramps. *Musculoskeletal:* Backache, myalgia. *Dermatologic:* Rash (acne-like), photosensitivity, pruritus, urticaria, hair growth, sweating, eczematoid eruption. *CV:* BP changes, phlebitis, tachycardia. *GU:* Urinary retention, increased urinary frequency, urinary incontinence, hematuria, crystalluria, nocturia, impotence. *Ophthalmic:* Visual disturbances, diplopia. *Miscellaneous:* Chills, fever, tearing, feeling of suffocation, alteration of taste, ***pleural effusion with pericarditis.***

Following IV use: Pulmonary edema, ***thrombophlebitis,*** urticaria, erythema.

OD Overdose Management: *Symptoms:* Extension of side effects. *Treatment:* Immediate gastric lavage. Maintain airway and have artificial resuscitation equipment available. Large quantities of IV fluids to prevent crystalluria. Monitor ECG.

Drug Interactions:
Clofibrate / ↓ Plasma protein binding of dantrolene

CNS depressants / ↑ CNS depression
Estrogens / ↑ Risk of hepatotoxicity
Warfarin / ↓ Plasma protein binding of dantrolene

EMS CONSIDERATIONS

See also *Skeletal Muscle Relaxants, Centrally Acting.*

Dapiprazole hydrochloride
(dah-PIP-rah-zol)
Pregnancy Class: B
RevEyes **(Rx)**
Classification: Ophthalmic alpha-adrenergic blocking agent

Mechanism of Action: Produces miosis by blocking the alpha-adrenergic receptors on the dilator muscle of the iris. No significant action on ciliary muscle contraction; thus, there are no changes in the depth of the anterior chamber of the thickness of the lens. Does not alter the IOP either in normal eyes or in eyes with elevated IOP. The rate of pupillary constriction may be slightly slower in patients with brown irides than in patients with blue or green irides.

Uses: To reverse diagnostic mydriasis induced by adrenergic (e.g., phenylephrine) or parasympatholytic (e.g., tropicamide) agents.

Contraindications: Acute iritis or other conditions where miosis is not desirable. To reduce intraocular pressure or to treat open-angle glaucoma.

Precautions: Use with caution during lactation. Safety and effectiveness have not been determined in children. The drug may cause difficulty in adaptation to dark and may reduce the field of vision.

Route/Dosage
- **Ophthalmic Solution**
  Reverse mydriasis.
2 gtt followed in 5 min by 2 more gtt applied to the conjunctiva of the eye after ophthalmic examination.

How Supplied: *Ophthalmic Powder for Reconstitution:* 0.5%

---

bold italic = life threatening side effect

Side Effects: *Ophthalmic:* Conjunctival injection lasting 20 min, burning on instillation, ptosis, lid erythema, itching, lid edema, chemosis, corneal edema, punctate keratitis, photophobia, tearing and blurring of vision, dryness of eyes. *Miscellaneous:* Headaches, browache.

EMS CONSIDERATIONS

None.

Dapsone (DDS, Diphenylsulfone)

(DAP-sohn)
Pregnancy Class: C
Classification: Sulfone, leprostatic

Mechanism of Action: Has both bacteriostatic and bactericidal activity, especially against *Mycobacterium leprae* (Hansen's bacillus). Thought to interfere with the metabolism of the infectious organism.

Uses: Lepromatous and tuberculoid types of leprosy, dermatitis herpetiformis. *Investigational:* Relapsing polychondritis, prophylaxis of malaria, inflammatory bowel disease, leishmaniasis, *Pneumocystis carinii* pneumonia, rheumatoid arthritis, lupus erythematosus, bites of the brown recluse spider.

Contraindications: Advanced amyloidosis of kidneys. Lactation.

Route/Dosage

• **Tablets**

Leprosy.

Adults: 50–100 mg/day. Initiate and continue the full dose without interruption.

Leprosy, bacteriologically negative tuberculoid and indeterminate type.

Adults: 100 mg/day with rifampin, 600 mg/day for 6 months; **then,** continue for a minimum of 3 years.

Leprosy, lepromatous and borderline patients.

100 mg/day for at least 2 years with rifampin, 600 mg/day. A third antileprosy drug may be added such as clofazimine, 50–100 mg/day or ethionamide, 250–500 mg/day. Dapsone is continued for up to 10 years until skin scrapings and biopsies are negative for 1 year.

Dermatitis herpetiformis.

Adults, initial: 50 mg/day; dosage may be increased to 300 mg/day or higher, if necessary. **Maintenance:** Reduce dosage to minimum maintenance dose as soon as possible; maintenance dosage may be reduced or eliminated in patients on a gluten-free diet. Dosage is correspondingly less in children.

How Supplied: *Tablet:* 25 mg, 100 mg

Side Effects: *Hematologic:* **Hemolytic anemia, agranulocytosis,** methemoglobinemia. *GI:* N&V, anorexia, abdominal discomfort. *CNS:* Headache, insomnia, vertigo, paresthesia, psychoses, peripheral neuropathy. *Dermatologic:* Photosensitivity, lupus-like syndrome. *Hypersensitivity:* Severe skin reactions including exfoliative dermatitis, erythema multiforme, toxic erythema, urticaria, erythema nodosum, toxic erythema, toxic epidermal necrolysis, morbilliform and scarlatiniform reactions. *Sulfone syndrome:* **Potentially fatal hypersensitivity reaction**, including symptoms of fever, malaise, jaundice with **hepatic necrosis,** exfoliative dermatitis, lymphadenopathy, methemoglobinemia, and **hemolytic anemia.** *Renal:* Nephrotic syndrome, renal papillary necrosis, albuminuria. *Miscellaneous:* Muscle weakness, blurred vision, tinnitus, male infertility, fever, tachycardia, mononucleosis-type syndrome, pulmonary eosinophilia, pancreatitis.

A leprosy-reactional state may occur in large numbers of patients during therapy with dapsone. Type 1 occurs soon after therapy is initiated. Patients manifest an enhanced delayed hypersensitivity syndrome, leading to swelling of existing nerve and skin lesions with possible neuritis. However, this is not an indication to discontinue therapy. Steroids, analgesics, and surgical decompression of swollen nerve trunks may be used to reduce symptoms. Type 2 occurs in nearly 50% of patients during the first year of therapy. Symptoms include fever, erythematous skin nodules, joint swelling, neuritis, orchitis, malaise, depression, iritis, or epistaxis. Usually therapy is continued with the use of analgesics, steroids, or clofazimine to suppress the reaction.

OD **Overdose Management:** *Symptoms:* N&V, hyperexcitability (up to 24 hr after ingestion of an overdose). Methemoglobin-induced depression, *seizures,* severe cyanosis, headache, hemolysis. *Treatment:* Gastric lavage. In normal and methemoglobin-reductase deficient patients, give methylene blue, 1–2 mg/kg by slow IV (may need to be repeated if methemoglobin reaccumulates). In nonemergencies, methylene blue may be given PO, 3–5 mg/kg/4–6 hr.

Drug Interactions
Charcoal, activated / ↓ Absorption of dapsone from GI tract
Didanosine / Possible therapeutic failure of dapsone → increased infection
Para-aminobenzoic acid / ↓ Effect of dapsone
Probenecid / ↑ Effect of dapsone due to inhibition of renal excretion
Pyrimethamine / ↑ Risk of hematologic reactions
Rifampin / ↓ Effect of dapsone due to ↑ plasma clearance
Trimethoprim / ↑ Serum levels of both drugs → pharmacologic and toxic effects of both

EMS CONSIDERATIONS
None.

Darvocet-N 50 and Darvocet-N 100
(DAR-voh-set)
(Rx)
Classification: Analgesic

Uses: Mild to moderate pain (may be used if fever is present).
Precautions: Use during pregnancy only if benefits outweigh risks. Safety and a suitable dosage regimen have not been established in children. Increased dosing intervals should be considered in geriatric patients.

Route/Dosage
• **Tablets**
  Analgesia.
Two Darvocet-N 50 tablets or 1 Darvocet-N 100 tablet q 4 hr, not to exceed 600 mg/day of propoxyhene napsylate. Reduce total daily dose in impaired hepatic or renal function.
How Supplied: *Nonnarcotic analgesic:* Acetaminophen, 325 (Darvocet-N 50) or 650 mg (Darvocet-N 100). *Analgesic:* Propoxyphene napsylate, 50 or 100 mg.

EMS CONSIDERATIONS
See also *Acetaminophen.*

Darvon Compound 65
(DAR-von)
(Rx)
Classification: Analgesic

Uses: Mild to moderate pain, with or without accompanying fever.
Precautions: Use during pregnancy only if benefits outweigh risks.

Route/Dosage
• **Capsules**
  Analgesia.
One capsule q 4 hr. Total daily dose of propoxyphene HCl should not exceed 390 mg. Decrease total daily dosage in hepatic or renal impairment.
How Supplied: Darvon Compound 65: *Analgesic:*Propoxyphene HCl, 65 mg. *Nonnarcotic analgesic:* Aspirin, 389 mg. *CNS stimulant:* Caffeine, 32.4 mg.

EMS CONSIDERATIONS
See also *Acetylsalicylic acid.*

Deferoxamine mesylate
(deh-fer-OX-ah-meen)
Pregnancy Class: C
Desferal **(Rx)**
Classification: Heavy metal antagonist (iron chelator)

---

bold italic = life threatening side effect

Mechanism of Action: Binds to free iron, iron of ferritin, and hemosiderin forming ferrioxamine, which is a water-soluble chelate excreted by the kidneys (urine is a reddish color) as well as in the feces via the bile. Iron is not removed from hemoglobin, myoglobin, or cytochromes. Must be given parenterally for systemic activity.

Uses: Adjunct in treatment of acute iron intoxication. Chronic iron overload including thalassemia. *Investigational:* Accumulation of aluminum in bone in renal failure and in encephalopathy due to aluminum. May be helpful in Alzheimer's disease and some cancers.

Contraindications: Severe renal disease, anuria. Treatment of primary hemochromatosis.

Precautions: Use in pregnancy only if clearly necessary. Use with caution for patients with pyelonephritis. Should not be used in children under the age of 3 years unless mobilization of 1 mg iron/day or more can be shown. Use deferoxamine and ascorbic acid with caution in geriatric patients due to greater risk of cardiac decompensation.

Route/Dosage ——————————
• **IM, IV, SC**
Acute iron intoxication.
Adults and children over 3 years of age, IM (preferred), initial: 1 g; **then,** 0.5 g q 4 hr for two doses; if necessary, then give 0.5 g q 4–12 hr, not to exceed 6 g/day. **IV infusion** (*only in emergencies such as CV collapse:*) Same as IM at a rate not to exceed 15 mg/kg/hr. Begin IM therapy as soon as possible.
Chronic iron overload.
IM: 0.5–1.0 g/day; **SC:** 1–2 g (20–40 mg/kg/day) given by mini-infusion pump over an 8–24-hr period; **IV:** 2 g (given separately but at same time as each unit of blood and in addition to IM administration); IV rate not to exceed 15 mg/kg/hr.

How Supplied: *Powder for injection:* 500 mg

Side Effects: Following long-term therapy. *Allergic:* Rash, itching, wheal formation, *anaphylaxis.* *GI:* Ab-

dominal discomfort, diarrhea. *Ophthalmologic:* Blurred vision. Rarely, impaired peripheral, night, or color vision; cataracts, decreased visual acuity, retinal pigmentation abnormalities. *Other:* Dysuria, leg cramps, fever, tachycardia, high-frequency hearing loss. **Following rapid IV use.** Hypotension, urticaria, erythema. **Following SC use.** Local pain, erythema, swelling, pruritus, skin irritation.

EMS CONSIDERATIONS

None.

Delavirdine mesylate
(deh-lah-VIR-deen)
Pregnancy Class: C
Rescriptor **(Rx)**
Classification: Antiviral drug, reverse transcriptase inhibitor

Mechanism of Action: Non-nucleoside reverse transcriptase inhibitor that binds directly to reverse transcriptase and blocks RNA-dependent and DNA-dependent DNA polymerase activities. Effect is additive if used with other antiviral drugs. Delavirdine may confer cross-resistance to other non-nucleoside reverse transcriptase inhibitors when used alone or in combination.

Uses: Treatment of HIV-1 infections in combination with appropriate antiretroviral agents.

Precautions: Use with caution in impaired hepatic function. Safety and efficacy in combination with other antiretroviral drugs have not been determined in HIV-1-infected patients less than 16 years of age.

Route/Dosage ——————————
• **Tablets**
HIV-1 infection.
400 mg (4-100 mg tablets) t.i.d. in combination with other antiretroviral therapy.

How Supplied: *Tablets:* 100 mg

Side Effects: *Body as a whole:* Headache, fatigue, asthenia, allergic reaction, chest pain, chills, general or local edema, fever, flu syndrome, lethargy, malaise, neck rigidity, general or local pain, trauma. *CV:* Bradycardia, migraine, pallor, palpitation, postural hypotension, syncope, tachycardia, vasodilation. *CNS:* Abnormal coordination, agitation, amnesia, anxiety, change in dreams, cognitive impairment, confusion, decreased libido, depression, disorientation, dizziness, emotional lability, hallucinations, hyperesthesia, hyperreflexia, hypesthesia, impaired coordination, insomnia, mania, nervousness, neuropathy, nightmares, paralysis, paranoia, paresthesia, restlessness, somnolence, tingling, tremor, vertigo, weakness. *GI:* N&V, diarrhea, anorexia, aphthous stomatitis, bloody stool, colitis, constipation, appetite decreased or increased, diarrhea, duodenitis, dry mouth, diverticulitis, dyspepsia, dysphagia, fecal incontinence, flatulence, enteritis, esophagitis, gastritis, gagging, gastroesophageal reflux, GI bleeding or disorder, gingivitis, gum hemorrhage, increased saliva, increased thirst, mouth ulcer, abdominal cramps/distention/pain, lip edema, hepatitis (nonspecified), pancreatitis, rectal disorder, sialadenitis, stomatitis, tongue edema, ulceration. *Dermatologic:* Skin rashes, maculopapular rash, pruritus, angioedema, dermal leukocytoblastic vasculitis, dermatitis, desquamation, diaphoresis, dry skin, erythema, erythema multiforme, folliculitis, fungal dermatitis, alopecia, nail disorder, petechial rash, seborrhea, skin disorder, skin nodule, ***Stevens-Johnson syndrome,*** vesiculobullous rash, sebaceous cyst. *GU:* Breast enlargement, kidney calculi, epididymitis, hematuria, hemospermia, impotence, kidney pain, metrorrhagia, nocturia, polyuria, proteinuria, vaginal moniliasis. *Musculoskeletal:* Back pain, neck rigidity, arthritis or arthralgia of single or multiple joints, bone disorder or pain, leg cramps, muscle weakness, myalgia, tendon disorder, tenosynovitis, tetany, muscle cramps. *Respiratory:* Upper respiratory infection, bronchitis, chest congestion, cough,

dyspnea, epistaxis, laryngismus, pharyngitis, rhinitis, sinusitis. *Hematologic:* Anemia, bruises, ecchymosis, eosinophilia, granulocytosis, neutropenia, pancytopenia, petechiae, purpura, spleen disorder, thrombocytopenia. *Ophthalmic:* Nystagmus, blepharitis, conjunctivitis, diplopia, dry eyes, photophobia. *Miscellaneous:* Alcohol intolerance, peripheral edema, weight increase or decrease, taste perversion, tinnitus, ear pain.

Drug Interactions

Antacids / ↓ Absorption of delavirdine; separate doses by 1 hr

Anticonvulsants / ↓ Plasma levels of delavirdine due to ↑ hepatic metabolism

Astemizole / Possible serious or life-threatening side effects of astemizole due to ↓ metabolism

Benzodiazpines / Possible serious or life-threatening side effects of benzodiazepines due to ↓ metabolism

Calcium channel blockers, dihydropyridine-type / Possible serious or life-threatening side effects of calcium channel blocker due to ↓ metabolism

Cisapride / Possible serious or life-threatening side effects of cisapride due to ↓ metabolism

Clarithromycin / Significant ↑ in amount absorbed of both drugs; possible serious side effects

Dapsone / Possible serious or life-threatening side effects of dapsone due to ↓ metabolism

Didanosine / ↓ Absorption of both drugs; separate administration by at least 1 hr

Ergot derivatives / Possible serious or life-threatening side effects of ergot due to ↓ metabolism

Fluoxetine / ↑ Trough levels of delavirdine by 50%

Indinavir / ↑ Levels of indinavir due to ↓ metabolism; possible serious side effects

Quinidine / Possible serious or life-threatening side effects of quinidine due to ↓ metabolism

---

bold italic = life threatening side effect

Rifabutin, Rifampin / ↓ Plasma levels of delavirdine due to ↑ hepatic metabolism

Saquinavir / ↑ Levels of saquinavir due to ↓ metabolism; possible serious side effects

Terfenadine / Possible serious or life-threatening side effects of terfenadine due to ↓ metabolism

Warfarin / Possible serious or life-threatening side effects of warfarin due to ↓ metabolism

EMS CONSIDERATIONS

See also *Antiviral Drugs.*

Desipramine hydrochloride
(dess-IP-rah-meen)
Desipramine **(Rx)**
Classification: Antidepressant, tricyclic

Mechanism of Action: Slight anticholinergic, sedative, and orthostatic hypotensive effects.
Onset of Action: Response usually seen within the first week.
Uses: Symptoms of depression. Bulimia nervosa. To decrease craving and depression during cocaine withdrawal. To treat severe neurogenic pain. Cataplexy associated with narcolepsy. Attention deficit disorders with or without hyperactivity in children over 6 years of age.
Contraindications: Use in children less than 12 years of age.
Precautions: Safe use during pregnancy has not been established. Safety and efficacy have not been established in children.

Route/Dosage
• **Tablets**
  Antidepressant.
Initial: 100–200 mg/day in single or divided doses. **Maximum daily dose:** 300 mg in severely ill patients. **Maintenance:** 50–100 mg/day. **Geriatric patients:** 25–50 mg/day in divided doses up to a maximum of 150 mg/day. **Adolescents and geriatric patients:** 25–50 mg/day in divided doses up to a maximum of 150 mg.

  Cocaine withdrawal.
50–200 mg/day.
How Supplied: *Tablet:* 10 mg, 25 mg, 50 mg, 75 mg, 100 mg, 150 mg
Side Effects: Additional: Bad taste in mouth, hypertension during surgery.

EMS CONSIDERATIONS

See also *Antidepressants.*

Desmopressin acetate
(des-moh-PRESS-in)
Pregnancy Class: B
DDAVP, DDAVP Nasal Solution **(Rx)**
Classification: Antidiuretic hormone, synthetic

Mechanism of Action: A synthetic analog of arginine vasopressin which possesses antidiuretic activity but is devoid of vasopressor and oxytocic effects. Acts to increase absorption of water in the kidney by increasing permeability of cells in the collecting ducts.
Onset of Action: 1 hr. **Peak, intranasal:** 1-5 hr; **peak, PO:** 4-7 hr.
Duration of Action: 8-20 hr.
Uses: DDAVP: Primary noctural enuresis (intranasal, tablet), central cranial DI (intranasal, oral, parenteral), hemophilia A with factor VIII levels greater than 5% (intranasal, parenteral), von Willebrand's disease (type I) with factor VIII levels greater than 5% (intranasal, parenteral). **Stimate:** Hemophilia A with factor VIII levels greater than 5%, von Willebrand's disease with factor VIII levels greater than 5%.
Investigational: Chronic autonomic failure (nocturnal polyuria, overnight weight loss, morning postural hypotension).
Contraindications: Hypersensitivity to drug. Use for treatment of hemophilia A with factor VIII levels less than or equal to 5%, treatment of hemophilia B or in patients who have factor VIII antibodies. Treatment of severe classic von Willebrand's disease (type I) and when an abnormal molecular form of factor VIII antigen is present. Use for type IIB von Willebrand's disease. Paren-

teral administration for DI in infants under 3 months and intranasal administration in infants less than 11 months. Nephrogenic DI, polyuria due to psychogenic DI, renal disease, hypercalcemia, hyperkalemia, or administration of demeclocycline or lithium.

Precautions: Safety for use during lactation not established. Use with caution and with restricted fluid intake in infants due to an increased risk of hyponatremia and water intoxication. Geriatric patients may have a greater risk of developing hyponatremia and water intoxication. Use with caution in patients with coronary artery insufficiency and/or hypertensive CV disease. Use cautiously with other pressor agents. Safety and efficacy have not been determined in children less than 12 years of age (parenteral) or less than 2 months of age (intranasal) with DI.

Route/Dosage ⎯⎯⎯⎯⎯⎯⎯⎯
- **SC, Direct IV**
  Neurogenic DI.
  Adults: 0.5–1 mL/day in two divided doses, adjusted separately for an adequate diurnal rhythm of water turnover. If switching from intranasal to IV, the comparable IV antidiuretic dose is about ¹⁄₁₀ the intranasal dose.
  Hemophilia A, von Willebrand's disease (type I).
  Adults: 0.0003 mg/kg diluted in 50 mL 0.9% NaCl injection infused IV over 15–30 min; dose may be repeated, if necessary. **Pediatric, 3 months or older, weighing 10 kg or less, IV:** 0.0003 mg/kg diluted in 10 mL of 0.9% NaCl injection and given over 15–30 min; repeat if necessary. **Pediatric, 3 months or older, weighing 10 kg or more, IV:** 0.0003 mg/kg diluted in 50 mL of 0.9% NaCl injection and given over 15–30 min; repeat if necessary.
- **Intranasal**
  Neurogenic DI.
  Adults: 0.1–0.4 mL/day, either as a single dose or divided into two to three doses (usual: 0.2 mL/day in

two divided doses). Adjust morning and evening doses separately for an adequate diurnal rhythm of water turnover. **Children, 3 months to 12 years:** 0.05–0.3 mL/day, either as a single dose or two divided doses.
  Nocturnal enuresis.
  Age 6 years and older, initial: 0.02 mg (0.2 mL) at bedtime with one-half the dose in each nostril; if no response, the dose may be increased to 0.04 mg.
  Hemophilia A and type I von Willenbrand's disease.
  In patients weighing 50 kg or more: One spray per nostril (total dose of 300 mcg). **In patients weighing less than 50 kg:** Given as a single spray of 150 mcg. The drug may be given 2 hr prior to minor surgery in the same doses as described above.
  Renal concentration capacity test.
  Adults: 0.040 mg (0.020 mg in each nostril) given any time during the day. **Children, 3–12 years:** 0.020 mg given in the morning.
- **Tablets**
  Central cranial DI.
  Adults, initial: 0.05 mg b.i.d.; adjust individually to optimum therapeutic dose and adjust each dose for an adequate diurnal rhythm of water turnover. Total daily dose should be increased or decreased (range 0.1–1.2 mg divided b.i.d.–t.i.d.) as needed to obtain adequate antidiuresis. **Children, initial:** 0.05 mg. Careful restriction of fluid intake in children is required to prevent hyponatremia and water intoxication.
  Primary nocturnal enuresis.
  Age 6 years and older, initial: 0.2 mg at bedtime. May be increased to 0.6 mg, depending on patient response.
  How Supplied: *Injection:* 4 mcg/mL, 15 mcg/mL; *Solution:* 0.01%; *Spray:* 0.01 mg/inh, 0.15 mg/inh; *Tablet:* 0.1 mg, 0.2 mg
  Side Effects: DDAVP: *Intranasal:* Transient headaches, nausea, nasal congestion, rhinitis, facial flushing, asthenia, chills, conjunctivitis,

cough, dizziness, epistaxis, eye edema, GI disorder, lacrimation, nosebleed, nostril pain, sore throat, URIs. *Parenteral:* Mild abdominal pain, facial flushing, transient headache, nausea, vulval pain, BP changes, burning pain, edema, local erythema, *anaphylaxis (rare).*

Stimate: I*ntranasal:* Agitation, balanitis, chest pain, chills, dizziness, dyspepsia, edema, insomnia, itch or light-sensitive eyes, pain, palpitations, somnolence, tachycardia, vomiting, warm feeling.

OD Overdose Management: *Symptoms:* Headache, abdominal cramps, facial flushing, dyspnea, fluid retention, mucous membrane irritation. *Treatment:* Reduce dose, decrease frequency of administration, or withdraw the drug depending on the severity of the condition.

Drug Interactions: Chlorpropamide, clofibrate, and carbamazepine may potentiate the effects of desmopressin.

EMS CONSIDERATIONS

None.

Dexamethasone
(dex-ah-METH-ah-zohn)

Oral: Decadron, Dexone, Hexadrol **(Rx), Topical:** Aeroseb-Dex, Decaderm **(Rx), Ophthalmic:** Maxidex Ophthalmic **(Rx)**
Classification: Glucocorticoid, synthetic

Mechanism of Action: Long-acting. Low degree of sodium and water retention. Diuresis may ensue when transferred from other corticosteroids to dexamethasone.

Uses: Additional: In acute allergic disorder, PO dexamethasone may be combined with dexamethasone sodium phosphate injection and used for 6 days. To test for adrenal cortical hyperfunction. Cerebral edema due to brain tumor, craniotomy, or head injury. *Investigational:* Diagnosis of depression. Antiemetic in cisplatin-induced vomiting. Prophylaxis or treatment of acute mountain sickness. Decrease hearing loss in bacterial meningitis. Bronchopulmonary dysplasia in preterm infants. Hirsutism.

Contraindications: Use for replacement therapy in adrenal cortical insufficiency.

Precautions: Use during pregnancy only if benefits outweigh risks.

Route/Dosage

• **Oral Concentrate Tablets, Elixir**
   Most uses.
Initial: 0.75–9 mg/day; **maintenance:** gradually reduce to minimum effective dose (0.5–3 mg/day).
   Suppression test for Cushing's syndrome.
0.5 mg q 6 hr for 2 days for 24-hr urine collection (or 1 mg at 11 p.m. with blood withdrawn at 8 a.m. for blood cortisol determination).
   Suppression test to determine cause of pituitary ACTH excess.
2 mg q 6 hr for 2 days (for 24-hr urine collection).
   Acute allergic disorders or acute worsening of chronic allergic disorders.
Day 1: Dexamethasone sodium phosphate injection, 4–8 mg IM. **Days 2 and 3:** Two 0.75-mg dexamethasone tablets b.i.d. **Day 4:** One 0.75-mg dexamethasone tablet b.i.d. **Days 5 and 6:** One 0.75-mg dexamethasone tablet. **Day 7:** No treatment. **Day 8:** Follow-up visit to physician.

• **Topical Aerosol, Cream**
Apply sparingly as a light film to affected area b.i.d.–t.i.d.

• **Ophthalmic Suspension**
1–2 gtt in the conjunctival sac q hr during day and q 2 hr during night until a satisfactory response obtained; **then,** 1 gtt q 4 hr and finally 1 gtt q 6–8 hr.

How Supplied: *Concentrate:* 1 mg/mL; *Elixir:* 0.5 mg/5 mL; *Ophthalmic suspension:* 0.1%; *Tablet:* 0.25 mg, 0.5 mg, 0.75 mg, 1 mg, 1.5 mg, 2 mg, 4 mg, 6 mg

EMS CONSIDERATIONS

See also *Corticosteroids.*

Dexamethasone acetate

(dex-ah-METH-ah-zohn)
Dalalone D.P., Dalalone L.A., Decadron-LA, Decaject-L.A., Dexasone L.A., Dexone LA, Solurex LA **(Rx)**
Classification: Glucocorticoid, synthetic

Precautions: Use during pregnancy only if benefits outweigh risks.

Route/Dosage

- **Repository Injection, IM**
8–16 mg q 1–3 weeks, if necessary.
- **Intralesional**
0.8–1.6 mg.
- **Soft Tissue and Intra-articular**
4–16 mg repeated at 1–3-week intervals.

How Supplied: *Injection:* 8 mg/mL, 16 mg/mL

EMS CONSIDERATIONS

See also *Corticosteroids.*

Dexamethasone sodium phosphate

(dex-ah-METH-ah-zohn)
Systemic: Decadron Phasphate, Solurex **(Rx)**, **Inhaler:** Decadron Phosphate Respihaler **(Rx)**, **Nasal:** Decadron Phosphate Turbinaire **(Rx)**, **Ophthalmic:** AK-Dex, Decadron Phosphate Ophthalmic **(Rx)**, **Otic:** AK-Dex, Decadron, I-Methasone **(Rx)**, **Topical:** Decadron Phosphate **(Rx)**
Classification: Glucocorticoid, synthetic

Mechanism of Action: Rapid onset and short duration of action.
Uses: Additional: For IV or IM use in emergency situation when dexamethasone cannot be given PO. Intranasally for nasal polyps, allergic or inflammatory nasal conditions.
Contraindications: Acute infections, persistent positive sputum cultures of *Candida albicans.* Lactation.
Precautions: Use during pregnancy only if benefits outweigh risks.

Route/Dosage

- **IM, IV**
Most uses.
Range: 0.5–9 mg/day (⅓–½ the PO dose q 12 hr).
Cerebral edema.
Adults, initial: 10 mg IV; **then,** 4 mg IM q 6 hr until maximum effect obtained (usually within 12–24 hr). Switch to PO therapy (1–3 mg t.i.d.) as soon as feasible and then slowly withdraw over 5–7 days.
Shock, unresponsive.
Initial: either 1–6 mg/kg IV or 40 mg IV; **then,** repeat IV dose q 2–6 hr as long as necessary.
- **Intralesional, Intra-articular, Soft Tissue Injections**
0.4–6 mg, depending on the site (e.g., small joints: 0.8–1 mg; large joints: 2–4 mg; soft tissue infiltration: 2–6 mg; ganglia: 1–2 mg; bursae: 2–3 mg; tendon sheaths: 0.4–1 mg.
- **Metered Dose Inhaler**
Bronchial asthma.
Adults, initial: 3 inhalations (84 mcg dexamethasone/inhalation) t.i.d.–q.i.d.; **maximum:** 3 inhalations/dose; 12 inhalations/day. **Pediatric: initial,** 2 inhalations t.i.d.–q.i.d.; **maximum:** 2 inhalations/dose; 8 inhalations/day.
- **Intranasal**
Allergies, nasal polyps.
Adults: 2 sprays (total of 168 mcg dexamethasone) in each nostril b.i.d.–t.i.d. (maximum: 12 sprays/day); **pediatric, 6–12 years:** 1–2 sprays (total of 84–168 mcg dexamethasone) in each nostril b.i.d. (maximum: 8 sprays/day).
- **Ophthalmic Ointment**
Instill a small amount of the ointment into the conjunctival sac t.i.d.–q.i.d. As response is obtained, reduce the number of applications.
- **Ophthalmic Solution**
Initial: Instill 1–2 gtt into the conjunctival sac q hr during the day and q 2 hr at night until response obtained. After a favorable response, reduce to 1 gtt q 4 hr and later 1 gtt t.i.d.–q.i.d.
- **Otic Solution**
3–4 gtt into the ear canal b.i.d.–t.i.d.
- **Topical Cream**

Apply sparingly to affected areas and rub in.

How Supplied: *Metered dose inhaler* 0.1 mg/inh; *Injection:* 4 mg/mL, 10 mg/mL, 24 mg/mL; *Ophthalmic ointment:* 0.05%; *Ophthalmic solution:* 0.1%

Side Effects: *Following inhalation:* Nasal and nasopharyngeal irritation, burning, dryness, stinging, headache.

EMS CONSIDERATIONS

See also *Corticosteroids*.

Administration/Storage: **IV** For IV administration may give undiluted over 1 min. Do not use preparation containing lidocaine IV.

Dexchlorpheniramine maleate

(dex-klor-fen-EAR-ah-meen)
Pregnancy Class: B
Polaramine **(Rx)**
Classification: Antihistamine, alkylamine type

Mechanism of Action: Minimal sedative and moderate anticholinergic effects. **Duration:** 8 hr.

Duration of Action: 8 hr.

Contraindications: Use of extended-release tablets in children.

Precautions: Geriatric patients may be more sensitive to the usual adult dose.

Route/Dosage ────────────
• **Syrup, Tablets**
Adults: 2 mg q 4–6 hr. **Pediatric, 5–12 years:** 1 mg q 4–6 hr; **2–5 years:** 0.5 mg q 4–6 hr.
• **Extended-Release Tablets**
Adults and children over 12 years: 4–6 mg at bedtime or q 8–10 hr. **Children, 6–12 years:** 4 mg/day, taken preferably at bedtime.

How Supplied: *Syrup:* 2 mg/5 mL; *Tablet:* 2 mg; *Tablet, Extended Release:* 4 mg, 6 mg

EMS CONSIDERATIONS

See also *Antihistamines*.

Dextroamphetamine sulfate

(dex-troh-am-FET-ah-meen)
Pregnancy Class: C
Dexedrine, Oxydess II, Spancap No. 1 **(C-II) (Rx)**
Classification: Central nervous system stimulant, amphetamine type

Mechanism of Action: Stronger CNS effects and weaker peripheral action than amphetamine; thus, dextroamphetamine manifests fewer undesirable CV effects.

Duration of Action: PO: 4–24 hr.

Uses: Attention deficit disorders in children, narcolepsy.

Contraindications: Additional: Lactation. Use for obesity.

Precautions: Use of extended-release capsulte for attention deficit disorders in children less than 6 years of age and the elixir or tablets for attention deficit disorders in children less than 3 years of age is not recommended. Dosgae for narcolepsy has not been determined in children less than 6 years of age.

Route/Dosage ────────────
• **Tablets**
Attention deficit disorders in children.
3–5 years, initial: 2.5 mg/day; increase by 2.5 mg/day at weekly intervals until optimum dose is achieved (usual range 0.1–0.5 mg/kg/dose each morning). **6 years and older, initial:** 5 mg 1–2 times/day; increase in increments of 5 mg/week until optimum dose is achieved (rarely over 40 mg/day).
Narcolepsy.
Adults: 5–60 mg in divided doses daily. **Children over 12 years, initial:** 10 mg/day; increase in increments of 10 mg/day at weekly intervals until optimum dose is reached. **Children, 6–12 years, initial:** 5 mg/day; increase in increments of 5 mg/week until optimum dose is reached (maximum is 60 mg/day).
• **Extended-Release Capsule**
Attention deficit disorders.
Children, 6 years and older: 5–15 mg/day.

Narcolepsy.
Adults: 5–30 mg/day. **Children, 6–12 years:** 5–15 mg/day; **12 years and older:** 10–15 mg/day.
How Supplied: *Capsule, Extended Release:* 5 mg, 10 mg, 15 mg; *Tablet:* 5 mg, 10 mg

EMS CONSIDERATIONS

See also *Amphetamines and Derivatives.*

Dextromethorphan hydrobromide

(dex-troh-meth-OR-fan)
Benylin DM, Benylin DM for Children, Children's Hold, Delsym, Drixoral Cough Liquid Caps, Pertussin CS, Pertussin ES, Robitussin Cough Calmers, Robitussin Pediatric, St. Joseph Cough Suppressant, Scot-Tussin DM Cough Chasers, Sucrets Cough Control, Suppress, Triaminic DM, Triaminic DM Long Lasting for Children, Trocal, Vick's Formula 44, Vick's Formula 44 Pediatric Formula **(OTC)**
Classification: Nonnarcotic antitussive

Mechanism of Action: Selectively depresses the cough center in the medulla. Dextromethorphan 15–30 mg is equal to 8–15 mg codeine as an antitussive. Does not produce physical dependence or respiratory depression.
Onset of Action: 15-30 min.
Duration of Action: 3-6 hr.
Uses: Symptomatic relief of nonproductive cough due to colds or inhaled irritants.
Contraindications: Persistent or chronic cough or when cough is accompanied by excessive secretions. Use during first trimester of pregnancy unless directed otherwise by physician. Use in children less than 2 years of age.
Precautions: Use with caution in patients with nausea, vomiting, high fever, rash, or persistent headache.

Route/Dosage ———————
• **Capsules, Liquid, Lozenges, Syrup, Concentrate, Tablets**

Antitussive.
Adults and children over 12 years: 10–30 mg q 4–8 hr, not to exceed 120 mg/day; **pediatric, 6–12 years:** either 5–10 mg q 4 hr or 15 mg q 6–8 hr, not to exceed 60 mg/day; **pediatric, 2–6 years:** either 2.5–7.5 mg q 4 hr or 7.5 mg q 6–8 hr of the syrup, not to exceed 30 mg/day.
• **Sustained-Release Suspension**
Antitussive.
Adults: 60 mg q 12 hr. **Pediatric, 6–12 years:** 30 mg q 12 hr, not to exceed 60 mg/day; **pediatric, 2–6 years:** 15 mg q 12 hr, not to exceed 30 mg/day.
How Supplied: *Concentrate:* 40 mg/5 mL; *Liquid:* 3.5 mg/5 mL, 5 mg/5 mL, 7.5 mg/5 mL, 15 mg/5 mL; *Lozenge/troche:* 2.5 mg, 5 mg, 15 mg; *Suspension, Extended Release:* 30 mg/5 mL; *Syrup:* 3.5 mg/5 mL, 5 mg/5 mL, 7.5 mg/5 mL, 10 mg/5 mL, 15 mg/5 mL, 20 mg/15 mL; *Tablet:* 15 mg

Side Effects: *CNS:* Dizziness, drowsiness. *GI:* N&V, stomach pain.
OD Overdose Management: *Symptoms:* **Adults:** Dysphoria, slurred speech, ataxia, altered sensory perception. **Children:** Ataxia, *convulsions, respiratory depression. Treatment:* Treat symptoms and provide support.
Drug Interactions: Use with MAO inhibitors may cause nausea, hypotension, hyperpyrexia, myoclonic leg jerks, and coma.

EMS CONSIDERATIONS

None.

Dextrose and electrolytes

(DEX-trohs)
Pedialyte, Rehydralyte, Resol **(Rx)**
Classification: Electrolyte replenisher

Mechanism of Action: PO products that contain varying amounts of sodium, potassium, chloride, citrate, and dextrose (Lytren and Resol contain 20 g/L whereas Pedialyte and Rehydralyte contain 25 g/L). In addition, Resol contains magnesium, calcium, and phosphate.

---

bold italic = life threatening side effect

Onset of Action: Time to peak effect: 8-12 hr.

Uses: Diarrhea. Prophylaxis and treatment of electrolyte depletion in diarrhea or in continuing fluid loss. Maintenance of hydration.

Contraindications: Anuria, oliguria. Severe dehydration including severe diarrhea (IV therapy is necessary for prompt replacement of fluids and electrolytes). Malabsorption of glucose. Severe and sustained vomiting when the patient is unable to drink. Intestinal obstruction, perforated bowel, paralytic ileus.

Precautions: Use with caution in premature infants.

Route/Dosage
• **Oral Solution**
   Mild dehydration.

Adults and children over 10 years, initial: 50 mL/kg over 4–6 hr; **maintenance:** 100–200 mL/kg over 24 hr until diarrhea stops.

Moderate dehydration.

Adults and children over 10 years, initial: 100 mL/kg over 6 hr; **maintenance:** 15 mL/kg q hr until diarrhea stops.

Moderate to severe dehydration.

Pediatric, 2–10 years, initial: 50 mL/kg over the first 4–6 hr followed by 100 mL/kg over the next 18–24 hr; **less than 2 years, initial:** 75 mL/kg during the first 8 hr and 75 mL/kg during the next 16 hr.

How Supplied: *Powder for Reconstitution; Solution; Tablet*

Side Effects: Overhydration indicated by puffy eyelids. Hypernatremia, vomiting (usually shortly after treatment has started).

EMS CONSIDERATIONS

None.

Dezocine
(DEZ-oh-seen)
Pregnancy Class: C
Dalgan (Rx)
Classification: Narcotic agonist-antagonist analgesic

Mechanism of Action: Parenteral narcotic analgesic possessing both agonist and antagonist activity. Similar to morphine with respect to analgesic potency and onset and duration of action. Less risk of abuse due to the mixed agonist-antagonist properties of the drug. The narcotic antagonist activity is greater than that of pentazocine.

Onset of Action: IM: approximately 30 min; **IV:** approximately 15 min.

Peak effect: 30-150 min.

Duration of Action: 2-4 hr.

Uses: Analgesic when use of a narcotic is desirable.

Contraindications: Lactation. Individuals dependent on narcotics. SC administration.

Precautions: Elderly patients are at an increased risk of altered respiratory patterns and mental changes.

Route/Dosage
• **IM**
   Analgesia.

Adults: 5–20 mg (usual is 10 mg) as a single dose; dose may be repeated q 3–6 hr with dosage adjusted, if necessary, depending on the status of the patient.
• **IV**
   Analgesia.

Adults: 2.5–10 mg (usual initial dose is 5 mg) repeated q 2–4 hr.

How Supplied: *Injection:* 5 mg/mL, 10 mg/mL, 15 mg/mL

Side Effects: *CNS:* Sedation (common), dizziness, vertigo, confusion, anxiety, crying, sleep disturbances, delusions, headache, depression, delirium. *Respiratory:* Respiratory depression, atelectasis. *CV:* Hypotension, irregular heart or pulse, hypertension, chest pain, pallor, thrombophlebitis. *GI:* N&V, dry mouth, constipation, abdominal pain, diarrhea. *Dermatologic:* Reactions at the injection site, pruritus, rash, erythema. *EENT:* Diplopia, blurred vision, congestion in ears, tinnitus. *GU:* Urinary frequency, retention, or hesitancy. *Miscellaneous:* Sweating, chills, edema, flushing, low hemoglobin, muscle cramps or aches, muscle pain, slurred speech.

OD **Overdose Management:** *Treatment:* Naloxone IV with appropriate supportive measures including oxygen, IV fluids, vasopressors, and artificial respiration.

Drug Interactions: Additive depressant effect when used with general anesthetics, sedatives, antianxiety drugs, hypnotics, alcohol, and other opiate analgesics.

EMS CONSIDERATIONS

See also *Narcotic Analgesics.*

Diazepam
(dye-AYZ-eh-pam)
Pregnancy Class: D
Valium **(C-IV) (Rx)**
Classification: Antianxiety agent, anticonvulsant, skeletal muscle relaxant

Mechanism of Action: The skeletal muscle relaxant effect of diazepam may be due to enhancement of GABA-mediated presynaptic inhibition at the spinal level as well as in the brain stem reticular formation.

Onset of Action: PO: 30-60 min; **IM:** 15-30 min; **IV:** more rapid.

Duration of Action: 3 hr.

Uses: Anxiety, tension (more effective than chlordiazepoxide), alcohol withdrawal, muscle relaxant, adjunct to treat seizure disorders, antipanic drug. Used prior to gastroscopy and esophagoscopy, preoperatively and prior to cardioversion. In dentistry to induce sedation. Treatment of status epilepticus. Relief of skeletal muscle spasm due to inflammation of muscles or joints or trauma; spasticity caused by upper motor neuron disorders such as cerebral palsy and paraplegia; athetosis; and stiff-man syndrome. Relieve spasms of facial muscles in occlusion and temporomandibular joint disorders. **IV:** Status epilepticus, severe recurrent seizures, and tetanus. Rectal gel: Treat epilepsy in those with stable regimens of anticonvulsant drugs who require intermittent diazepam to control increased seizure activity.

Contraindications: Additional: Narrow-angle glaucoma, children under 6 months, lactation, and parenterally in children under 12 years.

Precautions: When used as an adjunct for seizure disorders, diazepam may increase the frequency of severity of clonic-tonic seizures, for which an increase in the dose of anticonvulsant medication is necessary. Safety and efficacy of parenteral diazepam have not been determined in neonates less than 30 days of age. Prolonged CNS depression has been observed in neonates, probably due to inability to biotransform diazepam into inactive metabolites.

Route/Dosage

• **Tablets, Oral Solution**

Antianxiety, anticonvulsant, adjunct to skeletal muscle relaxants.

Adults: 2–10 mg b.i.d.–q.i.d. **Elderly, debilitated patients:** 2–2.5 mg 1–2 times/day. May be gradually increased to adult level. **Pediatric, over 6 months, initial:** 1–2.5 mg (0.04–0.2 mg/kg or 1.17–6 mg/m^2) b.i.d.–t.i.d.

Alcohol withdrawal.

Adults: 10 mg t.i.d.–q.i.d. during the first 24 hr; **then,** decrease to 5 mg t.i.d.–q.i.d. as required.

Anticonvulsant.

Adults: 15–30 mg once daily.

• **Rectal Gel**

Anticonvulsant.

Over 12 years: 0.2 mg/kg. **Children, 6–11 years:** 0.3 mg/kg; **2–5 years:** 0.5 mg/kg. If required, a second dose can be given 4 to 12 hr after the first dose. Do not treat more than five episodes per month or more than one episode every 5 days. Adjust dose downward in elderly or debilitated patients to reduce ataxia or oversedation.

• **IM, IV**

Preoperative or diagnostic use.

Adults: 10 mg IM 5–30 min before procedure.

Adjunct to treat skeletal muscle spasm.

Adults, initial: 5–10 mg IM or IV; **then,** repeat in 3–4 hr if needed (larger doses may be required for tetanus).

Moderate anxiety.
Adults: 2–5 mg IM or IV q 3–4 hr if necessary.

Severe anxiety, muscle spasm.
Adults: 5–10 mg IM or IV q 3–4 hr, if necessary.

Acute alcohol withdrawal.
Initial: 10 mg IM or IV; **then,** 5–10 mg q 3–4 hr.

Preoperatively.
Adults: 10 mg IM prior to surgery.

Endoscopy.
IV: 10 mg or less although doses up to 20 mg can be used; **IM:** 5–10 mg 30 min prior to procedure.

Cardioversion.
IV: 5–15 mg 5–10 min prior to procedure.

Tetanus in children.
IM, IV, over 1 month: 1–2 mg, repeated q 3–4 hr as necessary; **5 years and over:** 5–10 mg q 3–4 hr.

• **IV**

Status epilepticus.
Adults, initial: 5–10 mg; **then,** dose may be repeated at 10–15-min intervals up to a maximum dose of 30 mg. Dosage may be repeated after 2–4 hr. **Children, 1 month–5 years:** 0.2–0.5 mg q 2–5 min, up to maximum of 5 mg. Can be repeated in 2–4 hr. **5 years and older:** 1 mg q 2–5 min up to a maximum of 10 mg; dose can be repeated in 2–4 hr, if needed.

NOTE: Elderly or debilitated patients should not receive more than 5 mg parenterally at any one time.

How Supplied: *Concentrate:* 5 mg/mL; *Injection:* 5 mg/mL; *Rectal Gel:* 2.5 mg/0.5 mL, 5 mg/mL, 10 mg/2 mL, 15 mg/3 mL, 20 mg/4 mL; *Solution:* 5 mg/5 mL; *Tablet* 2 mg, 5 mg, 10 mg

Drug Interactions: Additional: Diazepam potentiates antihypertensive effects of thiazides and other diuretics. Diazepam potentiates muscle relaxant effects of *d*-tubocruaring and gallamine.*Fluoxetine/↑* half-life of diazepam.*Isoniazid/↑* half-life of diazepam.*Ranitidine/↓* GI absorption of diazepam.

EMS CONSIDERATIONS
See also *Tranquilizers.*
Administration/Storage
IV 1. The IV route is preferred in the convulsing patient.
2. Dizac, which is an emulsified injection, should only be given IV; it is not to be given IM or SC.
3. Parenteral administration may cause bradycardia, respiratory or cardiac arrest; have emergency equipment and drugs available.
4. To reduce reactions at the IV site, give diazepam slowly (5 mg/min); avoid small veins. For pediatric use, give the IV solution slowly over a 3-min period at a dose not exceeding 0.25 mg/kg. The initial dose can be repeated after 15–30 min.
Assessment: Elderly patients may experience adverse reactions more quickly than younger patients; use a lower dose in this group.

Diazoxide IV
(dye-az-OX-eyed)
Pregnancy Class: C
Hyperstat IV **(Rx)**
Classification: Antihypertensive, direct action on vascular smooth muscle

Mechanism of Action: Exerts a direct action on vascular smooth muscle to cause arteriolar vasodilation and decreased peripheral resistance.
Onset of Action: 1-5 min. **Time to peak effect:**2-5 min.
Duration of Action: Variable: usual, 3-12 hr.
Uses: May be the drug of choice for hypertensive crisis (malignant and nonmalignant hypertension) in hospitalized adults and children. Often given concomitantly with a diuretic. Especially suitable for patients with impaired renal function, hypertensive encephalopathy, hypertension complicated by LV failure, and eclampsia. Ineffective for hypertension due to pheochromocytoma.
Contraindications: Hypersensitivity to drug or thiazide diuretics. Treatment of compensatory hyper-

tension due to aortic coarctation or AV shunt. Dissecting aortic aneurysm.

Precautions: A decrease in dose may be necessary in geriatric patients due to age-related decreases in renal function. If given prior to delivery, fetal or neonatal hyperbilirubinemia, thrombocytopenia, or altered carbohydrate metabilism may result. Use with caution during lactation and in patients with impaired cerebral or cardiac circulation.

Route/Dosage
• **IV Push (30 sec or less)**
Hypertensive crisis.
Adults: 1–3 mg/kg up to a maximum of 150 mg; may be repeated at 5–15-min intervals until adequate BP response obtained. Drug may then be repeated at 4–24-hr intervals for 4–5 days or until oral antihypertensive therapy can be initiated. **Pediatric:** 1–3 mg/kg (30–90 mg/m^2) using the same dosing intervals as adults.

Repeated use can result in sodium and water retention; therefore, a diuretic may be needed to avoid CHF and for maximum reduction of BP.

How Supplied: *Injection:* 15 mg/mL

Side Effects: *CV:* Hypotension (may be severe enough to cause shock), sodium and water retention, especially in patients with impaired cardiac reserve, ***atrial or ventricular arrhythmias, cerebral or myocardial ischemia,*** marked ECG changes with possibility of ***MI,*** palpitations, bradycardia, SVT, chest discomfort or nonanginal chest tightness. *CNS:* Cerebral ischemia manifested by unconsciousness, ***seizures,*** paralysis, confusion, numbness of the hands. Headache, dizziness, weakness, drowsiness, lightheadedness, somnolence, lethargy, euphoria, weakness of short duration, apprehension, anxiety, malaise, blurred vision. *Respiratory:* Tightness in chest, cough, dyspnea, sensation of choking. *GI:* N&V, diarrhea, anorexia, parotid swelling, change in sense of taste, salivation, dry mouth, ileus, constipation, acute pancreatitis (rare). *Other:* Hyperglycemia (may be serious enough to require treatment), sweating, flushing, sensation of warmth, transient neurologic findings due to alteration in regional blood flow to the brain, hyperosmolar coma in infants, tinnitus, hearing loss, retention of nitrogenous wastes, acute pancreatitis, back pain, increased nocturia, lacrimation, hypersensitivity reactions, papilledema, hirsutism, decreased libido. Pain, cellulitis without sloughing, warmth or pain along injected vein, phlebitis at injection site, extravasation.

OD Overdose Management: *Symptoms:* Hypotension, excessive hyperglycemia. *Treatment:* Use the Trendelenburg maneuver to reverse hypotension.

Drug Interactions
Anticoagulants, oral / ↑ Effect of oral anticoagulants due to ↓ plasma protein binding
Nitrites / ↑ Hypotensive effect
Phenytoin / Diazoxide ↓ anticonvulsant effect of phenytoin
Reserpine / ↑ Hypotensive effect
Sulfonylureas / Destablization of the patient resulting in hyperglycemia
Thiazide diuretics / ↑ Hyperglycemic, hyperuricemic, and antihypertensive effect of diazoxide
Vasodilators, peripheral / ↑ Hypotensive effect

EMS CONSIDERATIONS

See also *Antihypertensive Agents and Diazoxide oral.*
Administration/Storage
IV 1. Do not administer IM or SC. Medication is highly alkaline.
2. Ensure patency and inject rapidly (30 sec) undiluted into a peripheral vein to maximize response.
3. Assess site for signs of irritation or extravasation. If extravasation occurs, apply ice packs.
4. Have a sympathomimetic drug, such as norepinephrine, to treat severe hypotension should it occur.

---

bold italic = life threatening side effect

Assessment
1. With diabetics, can cause serious elevations in blood sugar levels. Note complaints of sweating, flushing, or evidence of hyperglycemia.
2. Monitor BP frequently until stabilized. Keep recumbent during and for 30 min after injection to avoid orthostatic hypotension.

Diazoxide oral
(dye-az-OX-eyed)
Pregnancy Class: C
Proglycem **(Rx)**
Classification: Insulin antagonist, hypotensive agent

Mechanism of Action: Related to the thiazide diuretics. It inhibits the release of insulin from beta islet cells of the pancreas, leading to an increase in blood glucose levels. Effect is dose related. Causes sodium, potassium, uric acid, and water retention. Other effects include increased pulse rate, increased serum uric acid levels, increased serum free fatty acids, decreased para-aminohippuric acid clearance from the kidneys (little effect on GFR).
Onset of Action: 1 hr.
Duration of Action: 8 hr.
Uses: Management of hypoglycemia due to hyperinsulinism, including inoperable islet cell adenoma or carcinoma or extrapancreatic malignancies in adults. In children, for treatment of hyperinsulinemia due to leucine sensitivity, islet cell hyperplasia, nesidioblastosis, extrapancreatic malignancy, islet cell adenoma or adenomatosis. The drug is used parenterally as an antihypertensive agent (see *Diazoxide IV*).
Contraindications: Functional hypoglycemia, hypersensitivity to diazoxide or thiazides.
Precautions: Infants are particularly prone to development of edema. Use with extreme caution in patients with history of gout and in those in whom edema presents a risk (cardiac disease).

Route/Dosage
• **Capsules, Oral Suspension**

Diabetes.
Dosage is individualized on the basis of blood glucose level and response of patient. **Adults and children, usual, initial:** 1 mg/kg q 8 hr (adjust according to response); **maintenance:** 3–8 mg/kg/day divided into two or three equal doses q 8–12 hr. **Infants and newborns, initial:** 3.3 mg/kg q 8 hr (adjust according to response); **maintenance:** 8–15 mg/kg/day divided into two or three equal doses q 8–12 hr.
How Supplied: *Capsule:* 50 mg; *Suspension:* 50 mg/mL
Side Effects: *CV:* Sodium and fluid retention (common); precipitation of CHF in patients with compromised cardiac reserve, palpitations, increased HR, hypotension, transient hypertension, chest pain (rare). *Metabolic:* Hyperglycemia, glycosuria, *diabetic ketoacidosis, hyperosmolar nonketotic coma.* *GI:* N&V, diarrhea, transient taste loss, anorexia, ileus, abdominal pain. *CNS:* Weakness, headache, insomnia, extrapyramidal symptoms, dizziness, paresthesia, fever, malaise, anxiety, polyneuritis. *Hematologic:* Thrombocytopenia with or without purpura, eosinophilia, neutropenia, decreased hemoglobin/hematocrit, excessive bleeding, decreased IgG. *Dermatologic:* Skin rashes, hirsutism, herpes, loss of hair from scalp, monilial dermatitis, pruritus. *GU:* Hematuria, decrease in urine production, nephrotic syndrome (reversible), azotemia, albuminuria. *Ophthalmologic:* Blurred or double vision, lacrimation, transient cataracts, ring scotoma, subconjunctival hemorrhage. *Other:* Pancreatitis, *pancreatic necrosis,* galactorrhea, gout, premature aging of bone, polyneuritis, enlargement of lump in breast.
OD Overdose Management: *Symptoms:* Hypotension; excessive hyperglycemia. *Treatment:* Insulin to treat hyperglycemia; use Trendelenburg maneuver to reverse hypotension.
Drug Interactions
Alpha-adrenergic blocking agents /
↓ Effect of diazoxide

Anticoagulants, oral / ↑ Effect of anticoagulant due to ↓ plasma protein binding
Antihypertensives / Excessive ↓ BP due to additive effects
Phenothiazines / ↑ Effects of diazoxide, including hyperglycemia
Phenytoin / ↓ Effect of phenytoin due to ↑ breakdown by liver
Sulfonylureas / ↓ Effect of both drugs
Thiazide diuretics / ↑ Hyperglycemic and hyperuricemic effects; hypotension may occur.

EMS CONSIDERATIONS
None.

Diclofenac potassium
Diclofenac sodium
(dye-KLOH-fen-ack)
Pregnancy Class: B
Diclofenac potassium (Cataflam **(Rx)**) Diclofenac sodium (Voltaren, Voltaren Ophthalmic, Voltaren-XR **(Rx)**)
Classification: Nonsteroidal anti-inflammatory analgesic

Mechanism of Action: Available as both the potassium (immediate-release) and sodium (delayed-release) salts. *Immediate-release product.*
Onset of Action: 30 min. **Peak plasma levels:** 1 hr.
Duration of Action: 8 hr.
Uses: PO, Immediate-release: Analgesic, primary dysmenorrhea. **PO, Immediate- or Delayed-release:** Rheumatoid arthritis, osteoarthritis, ankylosing spondylitis. **PO, Delayed-release:** Osteoarthritis, rheumatoid arthritis. *Investigational:* Mild to moderate pain, juvenile rheumatoid arthritis, acute painful shoulder, sunburn. **Ophthalmic:** Postoperative inflammation following cataract or corneal refractive surgery.
Contraindications: Wearers of soft contact lenses.
Precautions: Use with caution during lactation. Saftey and effectiveness have not been determined in children. When used ophthalmically,

may cause increased bleeding of ocular tissues in conjunction with ocular surgery. Healing may be slowed or delayed.

Route/Dosage
• **Immediate-Release Tablets, Delayed-Release Tablets**
Analgesia, primary dysmenorrhea.
Adults: 50 mg t.i.d. of immediate-release tablets. In some, an initial dose of 100 mg followed by 50-mg doses may achieve better results. After the first day, the total daily dose should not exceed 150 mg.
Rheumatoid arthritis.
Adults: 100–200 mg/day in divided doses (e.g., 50 mg t.i.d. or q.i.d.; 75 mg b.i.d. of the sodium salt). For chronic therapy, use extended-release tablets, 100 mg once or twice daily, not to exceed 225 mg/day.
Osteoarthritis.
Adults: 100–150 mg/day in divided doses (e.g., 50 mg b.i.d. or t.i.d.; 75 mg b.i.d. of the sodium salt). For chronic therapy, use extended-release tablets, 100 mg/day. Doses greater than 200 mg/day have been evaluated.
Ankylosing spondylitis.
Adults: 25 mg q.i.d. with an extra 25-mg dose at bedtime, if necessary. Doses greater than 125 mg/day have not been evaluated.
• **Ophthalmic Solution, 0.1%**
Following cataract surgery.
1 gtt in the affected eye q.i.d. beginning 24 hr after cataract surgery and for 2 weeks thereafter.
Corneal refractive surgery.
1–2 gtt within 1 hr prior to surgery; then, apply 1–2 gtt within 15 min of surgery and continue q.i.d. for three days or less.
How Supplied: Diclofenac potassium: *Tablet:* 50 mg Diclofenac sodium: *Enteric Coated Tablet:* 25 mg, 50 mg, 75 mg; *Ophthalmic solution:* 0.1%; *Tablet, Extended Release:* 100 mg
Side Effects: *Following ophthalmic use:* Keratitis, increased intraocular

---

bold italic = life threatening side effect

pressure, ocular allergy, N&V, anterior chamber reaction, viral infections, transient burning and stinging on administration. When used with soft contact lenses, may cause ocular irritation, including redness and burning.

EMS CONSIDERATIONS

None.

————COMBINATION DRUG————
Diclofenac sodium and Misoprostol
(dye-KLOH-fen-ack/my-soh-PROST-ohl)
Pregnancy Class: X
Arthrotec 50, Arthrotec 75 **(Rx)**
Classification: Nonsteroidal Anti-Inflammatory

Mechanism of Action: Diclofenac is a NSAID with anti-inflammatory and analgesic effects. Misoprostol, a synthetic prostaglandin E1 analog, maintains gastroduodenal integrity and minimizes NSAID-induced gastric and duodenal ulcer formation. See individual drugs.

Uses: Treatment of osteoarthritis and rheumatoid arthritis in those at high risk of developing NSAID-induced gastric and duodenal ulcers.

Contraindications: Use in those with active GI bleeding, gastric and/or duodenal ulceration, porphyria. Pregnancy or in women planning pregnancy. Lactation. Known hypersensitivity to diclofenac, aspirin, other NSAIDs, misoprostol, or other prostaglandins.

Precautions: Use in premenopausal women only if effective contraception has been used and they have been advised of the risks or taking the drug if pregnant. Use with caution in renal, cardiac, or hepatic impairment. Safety and efficacy have not been determined in children.

Route/Dosage ————
• **Tablets**
    Osteoarthritis.
Adults: 1 Arthrotec 50 tablet with food t.i.d.
    Rheumatoid arthritis.

Adults: 1 Arthrotec 50 tablet with food t.i.d. or q.i.d.*Note:* For patients who experience intolerance, Arthrotec 75 b.i.d. or Arthrotec 50 b.i.d. can be used, but are less effective in preventing ulcers.

How Supplied: Arthrotec 50 contains: *NSAID:* Diclofenac sodium, 50 mg and *Prostaglandin:* Misoprostol, 200 mcg. Arthrotec 75 contains: Diclofenac sodium, 75 mg and Misoprostol, 200 mcg.

Side Effects: See individual drugs. *GI:* Abdominal pain, diarrhea, nausea, dyspepsia, flatulence, vomiting, gastritis, constipation, eructation, GI bleeding, GI perforation, gastroduodenal ulcerations or erosions. *CNS:* Headache, dizziness. *GU:* Menorrhagia, intermenstrual bleeding, vaginal bleeding, papillary necrosis, interstitial nephritis. *Hematologic:* Decreased platelet aggregation, prolonged bleeding time, anemia. *Miscellaneous:* Skin rashes, allergic reactions, **anaphylaxis,** fluid retention, edema.

Drug Interactions
Antacids, magnesium-containing / Worsening of diarrhea
Aspirin / ↓ Effect of diclofenac
Cyclosporine / ↑ Nephrotoxicity
Digoxin / ↑ Plasma digoxin levels
Diuretics / ↓ Effect of diuretics
Diuretics, potassium-sparing / ↑ Serum potassium levels
Lithium / ↑ Plasma lithium levels
Methotrexate / Possible enhanced methotrexate toxicity due to ↑ plasma levels
Warfarin / ↑ Risk of GI bleeding

EMS CONSIDERATIONS

None.

Dicloxacillin sodium
(dye-klox-ah-SILL-in)
Pregnancy Class: B
Dycill, Dynapen, Pathocil **(Rx)**
Classification: Antibiotic, penicillin

Uses: Infections due to penicillinase–producing staphylococci. To initiate therapy in any suspected

staphylococcal infection. Infections due to *Streptococcus pneumoniae.*
Contraindications: Treatment of meningitis. Use in newborns.

Route/Dosage
• **Capsules, Oral Suspension**
   Skin and soft tissue infections, mild to moderate URTIs.
Adults and children over 40 kg: 125 mg q 6 hr; **pediatric, less than 40 kg:** 12.5 mg/kg/day in four equal doses given q 6 hr.
   More severe lower respiratory tract infections or disseminated infections.
Adults and children over 40 kg: 250 mg q 6 hr, up to a maximum of 4 g/day; **pediatric, less than 40 kg:** 25 mg/kg/day in four equal doses given q 6 hr.
How Supplied: *Capsule:* 250 mg, 500 mg; *Powder for reconstitution:* 62.5 mg/5 mL

EMS CONSIDERATIONS

See also *Anti-Infectives* and *Penicillins.*

Dicyclomine hydrochloride
(dye-SYE-kloh-meen)
Pregnancy Class: C
Antispas, A-Spas, Bentyl, Byclomine, Dibent, Di-Cyclonex, Dilomine, Di-Spaz, Or-Tyl **(Rx)**
Classification: Cholinergic blocking agent

Uses: Hypermotility and spasms of GI tract associated with irritable colon and spastic colitis, mucous colitis.
Contraindications: Additional: Use for peptic ulcer.
Precautions: Lower doses may be needed in elderly patients due to confusion, agitation, excitement, or drowsiness.

Route/Dosage
• **Capsules, Syrup, Tablets**
   Hypermotility and spasms of GI tract.

Adults: 10–20 mg t.i.d.–q.i.d.; **then,** may increase to total daily dose of 160 mg if side effects do not limit this dosage. **Pediatric, 6 years and older, capsules or tablets:** 10 mg t.i.d.–q.i.d.; adjust dosage to need and incidence of side effects. **Pediatric, 6 months–2 years, syrup:** 5–10 mg t.i.d.–q.i.d.; **2 years and older:** 10 mg t.i.d.–q.i.d. The dose should be adjusted to need and incidence of side effects.
• **IM**
   Hypermotility and spasms of GI tract.
Adults: 20 mg q 4–6 hr. **Not for IV use.**
How Supplied: *Capsules:* 10 mg; *Injection:* 10 mg/mL; *Syrup:* 10 mg/1.5 mL; *Tablets:* 20 mg
Side Effects: Additional: Brief euphoria, slight dizziness, feeling of abdominal distention. **Use of the syrup in infants less than 3 months of age; Seizures,**syncope, respiratory symptoms, fluctuations in pulse rate, **asphyxia,**muscular hypotonia, **coma.**

EMS CONSIDERATIONS

See also *Cholinergic Blocking Agents.*

Didanosine (ddI, dideoxyinosine)
(die-DAN-oh-seen)
Pregnancy Class: B
Videx **(Rx)**
Classification: Antiviral

Mechanism of Action: A nucleoside analog of deoxyadenosine. After entering the cell, it is converted to the active dideoxyadenosine triphosphate (ddATP) by cellular enzymes. Due to the chemical structure of ddATP, its incorporation into viral DNA leads to chain termination and therefore inhibition of viral replication. ddATP also inhibits viral replication by interfering with the HIV–RNA-dependent DNA polymerase by competing with the natural nucleoside triphosphate for binding to the active site of the enzyme. Didanosine has shown in vitro antiviral activity in a variety of HIV-infected T cell and monocyte/macrophage cell cultures.

Uses: Advanced HIV infection in adult and pediatric (over 6 months of age) patients who are intolerant of AZT therapy or who have demonstrated decreased effectiveness of AZT therapy. Use in adults with HIV infection who have received prolonged AZT therapy. Treatment of HIV infection when antiretroviral therapy is indicated. AZT should be considered as initial therapy for the treatment of advanced HIV infection, unless contraindicated, since this drug prolongs survival and decreases the incidence of opportunistic infections. May be used as monotherapy for the treatment of AIDS.

Contraindications: Lactation.

Precautions: Use with caution in renal and hepatic impairment and in those on sodium-restricted diets. Opportunistic infections and other complications of HIV infection may continue to develop; thus, keep patients under close observation.

Route/Dosage ⸻

• **Chewable/Dispersible Buffered Tablets, Buffered Powder for Oral Solution, Powder for Pediatric Oral Solution**

Adults, initial, weight over 60 kg: 200 mg q 12 hr (with 250 mg buffered powder q 12 hr). **Weight less than 60 kg:** 125 mg q 12 hr (with 167 mg buffered powder q 12 hr). **Pediatric, BSA 1.1–1.4 m²:** Two 50-mg tablets q 12 hr or 125 mg of the pediatric powder q 12 hr; BSA 0.8–1.0 m²: **One 50- and one 25-mg tablet q 12 hr or 94 mg of the pediatric powder q 12 hr.** BSA 0.5–0.7 m²: **Two 25-mg tablets q 12 hr or 62 mg of the pediatric powder q 12 hr.** BSA less than 0.4 m²: **One 25-mg tablet q 12 hr or 31 mg of the pediatric powder q 12 hr.**

How Supplied: *Chew Tablet:* 25 mg, 50 mg, 100 mg, 150 mg; *Powder*

for reconstitution: 10 mg/mL, 100 mg, 167 mg, 250 mg

Side Effects: Commonly pancreatitis and peripheral neuropathy (manifested by distal numbness, tingling, or pain in the feet or hands). Neuropathy occurs more frequently in patients with a history of neuropathy or neurotoxic drug therapy.

In adults. *GI:* Diarrhea, abdominal pain, N&V, anorexia, dry mouth, ileus, colitis, constipation, eructation, flatulence, gastroenteritis, *GI hemorrhage,* oral moniliasis, stomatitis, mouth sores, sialadenitis, *stomach ulcer hemorrhage,* melena, oral thrush, liver abnormalities. *CNS:* Headache, *tonic-clonic seizures,* abnormal thinking, anxiety, nervousness, twitching, confusion, depression, acute brain syndrome, amnesia, aphasia, ataxia, dizziness, hyperesthesia, hypertonia, incoordination, *intracranial hemorrhage,* paralysis, paranoid reaction, psychosis, insomnia, sleep disorders, speech disorders, tremor. *Hematologic:* Leukopenia, granulocytopenia, thrombocytopenia, microcytic anemia, *hemorrhage,* ecchymosis, petechiae. *Dermatologic:* Rash, pruritus, herpes simplex, skin disorder, sweating, eczema, impetigo, excoriation, erythema. *Musculoskeletal:* Asthenia, myopathy, arthralgia, arthritis, myalgia, muscle atrophy, decreased strength, hemiparesis, neck rigidity, joint disorder, leg cramps. *CV:* Chest pain, hypertension, hypotension, migraine, palpitation, peripheral vascular disorder, syncope, vasodilation, arrhythmias. *Body as a whole:* Chills, fever, infection, allergic reaction, pain, abscess, cellulitis, cyst, dehydration, malaise, flu syndrome, numbness of hands and feet, weight loss, alopecia. *Respiratory:* Pneumonia, dyspnea, asthma, bronchitis, increased cough, rhinitis, rhinorrhea, epistaxis, laryngitis, decreased lung function, pharyngitis, hypoventilation, sinusitis, rhonchi, rales, congestion, interstitial pneumonia, respiratory disorders. *Ophthalmic:* Blurred vision, conjunctivitis, diplopia, dry eye, glaucoma, retinitis, photophobia, strabismus. *Otic:* Ear disorder, otitis (externa and media), ear pain. *GU:* Impotency, kidney calculus, kidney failure, abnormal kidney function, nocturia, urinary frequency, vaginal hemorrhage. *Miscellaneous:* Peripheral edema, sarcoma, hernia, hypokalemia, lymphoma-like reaction.

In children. *GI:* Diarrhea, N&V, liver abnormalities, abdominal pain, stomatitis, mouth sores, pancreatitis, anorexia, increase in appetite, constipation, oral thrush, melena, dry mouth. *CNS:* Headache, nervousness, insomnia, dizziness, poor coordination, lethargy, neurologic symptoms, *seizures.* *Hematologic:* Ecchymosis, *hemorrhage,* petechaie, leukopenia, granulocytopenia, thrombocytopenia, anemia. *Dermatologic:* Rash, pruritus, skin disorder, eczema, sweating, impetigo, excoriation, erythema. *Musculoskeletal:* Arthritis, myalgia, muscle atrophy, decreased strength. *Body as a whole:* Chills, fever, asthenia, pain, malaise, failure to thrive, weight loss, flu syndrome, alopecia, dehydration. *CV:* Vasodilation, arrhythmia. *Respiratory:* Cough, rhinitis, dyspnea, asthma, rhinorrhea, epistaxis, pharyngitis, hypoventilation, sinusitis, rhonchi, rales, congestion, pneumonia. *Ophthalmic:* Photophobia, strabismus, visual impairment. *Otic:* Ear pain, otitis. *Miscellaneous:* Urinary frequency, diabetes mellitus, diabetes insipidus, liver abnormalities.

OD Overdose Management: *Symptoms:* Pancreatitis, peripheral neuropathy, diarrhea, hyperuricemia, hepatic dysfunction. *Treatment:* There are no antidotes; treatment should be symptomatic.

Drug Interactions
Ketoconazole / ↓ Absorption of ketoconazole due to gastric pH change caused by buffering agents in didanosine
Pentamidine (IV) / ↑ Risk of pancreatitis
Quinolone antibiotics / ↓ Plasma levels of quinolone antibiotics
Ranitidine / ↓ Absorption of ranitidine due to gastric pH change

caused by buffering agents in didanosine
Tetracyclines / ↓ Absorption of tetracyclines from the stomach due to the buffering agents in didanosine

EMS CONSIDERATIONS
See also *Antiviral Agents.*

D

Diethylstilbestrol diphosphate
(dye-eth-ill-still-BESS-trohl)
Pregnancy Class: X
Stilphostrol (Abbreviation: DES) **(Rx)**
Classification: Estrogen, synthetic, nonsteroidal

Mechanism of Action: Synthetic estrogen, which competes with androgen receptors, thereby preventing androgen from inducing further growth of the neoplasm. Also binds to cytoplasmic receptor protein. The estrogen-receptor complex translocates to the nucleus, where metabolic alterations ensue.

Uses: Palliative treatment of inoperable, progressive prostatic cancer. Postcoital contraceptive (emergency use only).

Contraindications: Known or suspected breast cancer, estrogen-dependent neoplasia, active thrombophlebitis, thromboembolic disease, markedly impaired liver function. **Not to be used during pregnancy because of the possibility of vaginal cancer in female offspring.** The diphosphate is not to be used to treat any disorder in women.

Precautions: Use with caution in presence of hypercalcemia, elilepsy, migraine, asthma, cardiac and renal disease. Use with caution in childern in whom bone growth is incomplete.

Route/Dosage
• **Tablets**
   Palliative treatment of prostatic carcinoma.
   50 mg t.i.d. up to 200 mg t.i.d., not to exceed 1 g/day.

---

bold italic = life threatening side effect

- **IV**

  Palliative treatment of prostatic carcinoma.

  500 mg (in 250 mL 5% dextrose or saline) on day 1 followed by 1 g (in 250–500 mL 5% dextrose or saline) daily for 5 days. **Maintenance, IV:** 250–500 mg 1–2 times/week. Maintenance dose may also be given PO.

How Supplied: *Injection:* 250 mg/5 mL

Side Effects: *CV:* ***Thrombophlebitis, pulmonary embolism, cerebral thrombosis,*** neuro-ocular lesions. *GI:* N&V, anorexia. *CNS:* Headaches, malaise, irritability. *Skin:* Allergic rash, itching. *GU:* Gynecomastia, changes in libido. *Other:* Porphyria, backache, pain and sterile abscess at injection site, postinjection flare.

EMS CONSIDERATIONS

None.

Difenoxin hydrochloride with Atropine sulfate

(dye-fen-OX-in, AH-troh-peen)
Pregnancy Class: C
Motofen **(Rx)**
Classification: Antidiarrheal

Mechanism of Action: Related chemically to meperidine; thus, atropine sulfate is incorporated to prevent deliberate overdosage.

Uses: Management of acute nonspecific diarrhea and acute episodes of chronic functional diarrhea.

Contraindications: Diarrhea caused by *Escherichia coli, Salmonella,* or *Shigella;* pseudomembranous colitis caused by broad-spectrum antibiotics; jaundice; children less than 2 years of age.

Precautions: Use with caution in ulcerative colitis, liver and kidney disease, lactation, and in patients receiving dependence-producing drugs or in those who are addiction prone. Safety and effectiveness in children less than 12 years of age have not been determined.

Route/Dosage ——————
- **Tablets**

Adults, initial: 2 tablets (2 mg difenoxin); **then,** 1 tablet (1 mg difenoxin) after each loose stool or 1 tablet q 3–4 hr as needed. Total dose during a 24-hr period should not exceed 8 mg (i.e., 8 tablets).

How Supplied: Each tablet contains: *Antidiarrheal:* Difenoxin HCl, 1 mg. *Anticholinergic:* Atropine sulfate, 0.025 mg.

Side Effects: *GI:* N&V, dry mouth, epigastric distress, constipation. *CNS:* Lightheadedness, dizziness, drowsiness, headache, tiredness, nervousness, confusion, insomnia. *Ophthalmic:* Blurred vision, burning eyes.

OD Overdose Management: *Symptoms:* Initially include dry skin and mucous membranes, hyperthermia, flushing, and tachycardia. These are followed by hypotonic reflexes, nystagmus, miosis, lethargy, coma, and *respiratory depression* (may occur up to 30 hr after overdose taken). *Treatment:* Naloxone may be used to treat respiratory depression.

Drug Interactions

Antianxiety agents / Potentiation or addition of CNS depressant effects
Barbiturates / Potentiation or addition of CNS depressant effects
Ethanol / Potentiation or addition of CNS depressant effects
MAO inhibitors / Precipitation of hypertensive crisis
Narcotics / Potentiation or addition of CNS depressant effects

EMS CONSIDERATIONS

See also *Cholinergic Blocking Agents.*

Assessment

1. Assess for evidence of dehydration (weakness, weight loss, poor skin turgor, higher temperature, rapid weak pulse, or decreased urinary output) or electrolyte imbalance (weakness, irritability, anorexia, nausea, and dysrhythmias).

2. May precipitate hypertensive crisis with MAO inhibitors.

3. With overdose, hospitalize, since latent (12–30 hr later) respiratory depression may occur.

Diflunisal
(dye-FLEW-nih-sal)
Pregnancy Class: C
Dolobid **(Rx)**
Classification: Nonsteroidal analgesic, anti-inflammatory, antipyretic

Mechanism of Action: A salicylic acid derivative, although not metabolized to salicylic acid. Mechanism not known; may be an inhibitor of prostaglandin synthetase.
Onset of Action: 20 min (analgesic, antipyretic). **Peak effect:** 2-3 hr.
Duration of Action: 4-6 hr.
Uses: Analgesic, rheumatoid arthritis, osteoarthritis, ankylosing spondylitis, psoriatic arthritis, musculoskeletal pain. Prophylaxis and treatment of vascular headaches.
Contraindications: Hypersensitivity to diflunisal, aspirin, or other anti-inflammatory drugs. Acute asthmatic attacks, urticaria, or rhinitis precipitated by aspirin. During lactation and in children less than 12 years of age.
Precautions: Use with caution in presence of ulcers or in patients with a history thereof, in patients with hypertension, compromised cardiac function, or in conditions leading to fluid retention. Use with caution in only first two trimesters of pregnancy. Geriatric patients may be at greater risk of GI toxicity.

Route/Dosage
• **Tablets**
  Mild to moderate pain.
Adults, initial: 1,000 mg; **then,** 250–500 mg q 8–12 hr.
  Rheumatoid arthritis, osteoarthritis.
Adults: 250–500 mg b.i.d. Doses in excess of 1,500 mg/day are not recommended. For some, an initial dose of 500 mg followed by 250 mg q 8–12 hr may be effective. Reduce dosage with impaired renal function.
How Supplied: *Tablet:* 250 mg, 500 mg
Side Effects: *GI:* Nausea, dyspepsia, GI pain and bleeding, diarrhea, vomiting, constipation, flatulence, peptic ulcer, eructation, anorexia.

CNS: Headache, fatigue, fever, malaise, dizziness, somnolence, insomnia, nervousness, vertigo, depression, paresthesias. *Dermatologic:* Rashes, pruritus, sweating, ***Stevens-Johnson syndrome,*** dry mucous membranes, erythema multiforme. *CV:* Palpitations, syncope, edema. *Other:* Tinnitus, asthenia, chest pain, hypersensitivity reactions, ***anaphylaxis,*** dyspnea, dysuria, muscle cramps, thrombocytopenia.
OD **Overdose Management:** *Symptoms:* Drowsiness, N&V, diarrhea, tachycardia, hyperventilation, stupor, disorientation, diminished urine output, ***coma, cardiorespiratory arrest.*** *Treatment:* Supportive measures. To empty the stomach, induce vomiting, or perform gastric lavage. Hemodialysis may not be effective since the drug is significantly bound to plasma protein.
Drug Interactions
Acetaminophen / ↑ Plasma levels of acetaminophen
Antacids / ↓ Plasma levels of diflunisal
Anticoagulants / ↑ PT
Furosemide / ↓ Hyperuricemic effect of furosemide
Hydrochlorothiazide / ↑ Plasma levels and ↓ hyperuricemic effect of hydrochlorothiazide
Indomethacin / ↓ Renal clearance of indomethacin → ↑ plasma levels
Naproxen / ↓ Urinary excretion of naproxen and metabolite

EMS CONSIDERATIONS
None.

Digoxin
(dih-JOX-in)
Pregnancy Class: A
Lanoxicaps, Lanoxin, **(Rx)**
Classification: Cardiac glycoside

Onset of Action: PO: 0.5-2 hr; **time to peak effect:** 2-6 hr, **IV:** 5-30 min; **time to peak effect:** 1-4 hr.
Duration of Action: PO: Over 24 hr; **IV:** 6 days.

---
bold italic = life threatening side effect

Uses: May be drug of choice for CHF because of rapid onset, relatively short duration, and ability to be administered PO or IV.

Route/Dosage —————————
- **Capsules**
  Digitalization: Rapid.
  Adults: 0.4–0.6 mg initially followed by 0.1–0.3 mg q 6–8 hr until desired effect achieved.
  Digitalization: Slow.
  Adults: A total of 0.05–0.35 mg/day divided in two doses for a period of 7–22 days to reach steady-state serum levels. **Pediatric.** Digitalizing dosage is divided into three or more doses with the initial dose being about one-half the total dose; doses are given q 4–8 hr. **Children, 10 years and older:** 0.008–0.012 mg/kg. **5–10 years:** 0.015–0.03 mg/kg. **2–5 years:** 0.025–0.035 mg/kg. **1 month–2 years:** 0.03–0.05 mg/kg. **Neonates, full-term:** 0.02–0.03 mg/kg. **Neonates, premature:** 0.015–0.025 mg/kg.
  Maintenance.
  Adults: 0.05–0.35 mg once or twice daily. **Premature neonates:** 20%–30% of total digitalizing dose divided and given in two to three daily doses. **Neonates to 10 years:** 25%–35% of the total digitalizing dose divided and given in two to three daily doses.
- **Elixir, Tablets**
  Digitalization: Rapid.
  Adults: A total of 0.75–1.25 mg divided into two or more doses each given at 6–8-hr intervals.
  Digitalization: Slow.
  Adults: 0.125–0.5 mg/day for 7 days. **Pediatric.** (Digitalizing dose is divided into two or more doses and given at 6–8-hr intervals.) **Children, 10 years and older, rapid or slow:** Same as adult dose. **5–10 years:** 0.02–0.035 mg/kg. **2–5 years:** 0.03–0.05 mg/kg. **1 month–2 years:** 0.035–0.06 mg/kg. **Premature and newborn infants to 1 month:** 0.02–0.035 mg/kg.
  Maintenance.
  Adults: 0.125–0.5 mg/day. **Pediatric:** One-fifth to one-third the total

digitalizing dose daily. *NOTE:* An alternate regimen (referred to as the "small-dose" method) is 0.017 mg/kg/day. This dose causes less toxicity.
- **IV**
  Digitalization.
  Adults: Same as tablets. **Maintenance:** 0.125–0.5 mg/day in divided doses or as a single dose. **Pediatric:** Same as tablets.

How Supplied: *Capsule:* 0.05 mg, 0.1 mg, 0.2 mg; *Elixir:* 0.05 mg/mL; *Injection:* 0.1 mg/mL, 0.25 mg/mL; *Tablet:* 0.125 mg, 0.25 mg, 0.5 mg

OD Overdose Management: *Treatment:* See Digoxin immune Fab.

Drug Interactions: Additional: 1. The following drugs increase serum digoxin levels, leading to possible toxicity: Aminoglycosides, amiodarone, anticholinergics, benzodiazepines, captopril, diltiazem, erythromycin, esmolol, flecainide, hydroxychloroquine, ibuprofen, indomethacin, nifedipine, quinidine, quinine, tetracyclines, tolbutamide, verapamil. 2. Disopyramide may alter the pharmacologic effect of digoxin. 3. Pencillamine decreases serum digoxin levels.

EMS CONSIDERATIONS

See also *Cardiac Glycosides.*
Administration/Storage: IV Give IV injections over 5 min (or longer) either undiluted or diluted fourfold or greater with sterile water for injection, 0.9% NaCl injection, RL injection, or D5W.

Digoxin Immune Fab (Ovine)
(dih-JOX-in)
Pregnancy Class: C
Digibind **(Rx)**
Classification: Digoxin antidote

Mechanism of Action: Digoxin immune Fab are antibodies that bind to digoxin. In cases of digoxin toxicity, the antibodies bind to digoxin and the complex is excreted through the kidneys. As serum levels of digoxin decrease, digoxin bound to tissue is released into the serum to maintain equilibrium and this is then bound and excreted. The net result is a decrease in both tissue and serum digoxin.

Onset of Action: Less than 1 min. Improvement in signs of toxicity occurs within 30 min.

Uses: Life-threatening digoxin or digitoxin toxicity or overdosage. Symptoms of toxicity include severe sinus bradycardia, second- or third-degree heart block which does not respond to atropine, ventricular tachycardia, ventricular fibrillation.

NOTE: Cardiac arrest can be expected if a healthy adult ingests more than 10 mg digoxin or a healthy child ingests more than 4 mg. Also, steady-state serum concentrations of digoxin greater than 10 ng/mL or potassium concentrations greater than 5 mEq/L as a result of digoxin therapy require use of digoxin immune Fab.

Precautions: Use with caution during lactation. Use in infants only if benefits outweigh risks. Patients sensitive to products of sheep origin may also be sensitive to digoxin immune Fab. Skin testing may be appropriate for high-risk patients.

Route/Dosage —————————
• **IV**
Dosage depends on the serum digoxin concentration. A large dose has a faster onset but there is an increased risk of allergic or febrile reactions. The package insert should be carefully consulted. **Adults, usual:** Six vials (228 mg) is usuallly enough to reverse most cases of toxicity. **Children, less than 20 kg:** A single vial (38 mg) should be sufficient.

How Supplied: *Injection:* 10 mg/mL

Side Effects: *CV:* Worsening of CHF or low CO, atrial fibrillation (all due to withdrawal of the effects of digoxin). *Other:* Hypokalemia. Rarely, hypersensitivity reactions occur, including fever and *anaphylaxis.*

EMS CONSIDERATIONS

Administration/Storage
IV 1. Reconstitute the lyophilized material with 4 mL of sterile water for injection to give a concentration of 10 mg/mL. If small doses are required (e.g., in infants), can be further diluted with 36 mL sterile isotonic saline for a concentration of 1 mg/mL.
2. Administer over a 30-min period through a 0.22-μm membrane filter.
3. If acute digoxin ingestion results in severe symptoms and a serum concentration is not known, 800 mg (20 vials) of digoxin immune Fab may be given.

Assessment: Monitor VS and cardiac rhythm.

Dihydroergotamine mesylate
(dye-hy-droh-er-GOT-ah-meen)
Pregnancy Class: X
Migranal Nasal Spray **(Rx)**
Classification: Alpha-adrenergic blocking agent

Mechanism of Action: Manifests alpha-adrenergic receptor blocking activity as well as a direct stimulatory action on vascular smooth muscle of peripheral and cranial blood vessels, resulting in vasoconstriction, thus preventing the onset of a migraine attack. Manifests greater adrenergic blocking activity, less pronounced vasoconstriction, less N&V, and less oxytocic properties than does ergotamine. More effective when given early in the course of a migraine attack.

Onset of Action: IM: 15-30 min; **IV:** <5 min.

Duration of Action: IM: 3-4 hr.

Uses: IM, IV. To prevent or abort migraine, migraine variant, histaminic cephalalgia (cluster headaches). Especially useful when rapid effect is desired or when other routes of administration are not possible. **Nasal Spray.** Acute treatment of migraine headaches with or without aura.

Contraindications: Lactation. Pregnancy. Peripheral vascular disease, coronary heart disease, hypertension, impaired hepatic or renal function, sepsis, hypersensitivity, malnutrition, severe pruritus, presence of infection.

Precautions: Safety and efficacy have not been determined in children. Geriatric patients may be more affected by peripheral vasoconstriction that results in hypothermia. Prolonged administration may cause ergotism and gangrene.

Route/Dosage

• **IM**
Suppress vascular headache.
Adults, initial: 1 mg at first sign of headache; repeat q hr for a total of 3 mg (not to exceed 6 mg/week).

• **IV**
Suppress vascular headache.
Similar to IM but to a maximum of 2 mg/attack or 6 mg/week.

• **Nasal spray**
Acute migraine headaches.
Single treatment of 0.5 mg spray in each nostril followed in 15 min by a second 0.5 mg spray in each nostil (i.e., total of 2 mg).

How Supplied: *Injection:* 1 mg/mL; *Nasal Spray:* 0.5 mg/inh

Side Effects: *CV:* Precordial pain, transient tachycardia or bradycardia. Large doses may cause increased BP, vasoconstriction of coronary arteries, and bradycardia. *GI:* N&V, diarrhea. *Other:* Numbness and tingling of fingers and toes, muscle pain in extremities, weakness in legs, localized edema, and itching. *Prolonged use:* Gangrene, ergotism.

OD **Overdose Management:** *Symptoms:* N&V, pain in limb muscles, tachycardia or bradycardia, precordial pain, numbness and tingling of fingers and toes, weakness of the legs, hypertension or hypotension, localized edema, S&S of ischemia due to vasoconstriction of peripheral arteries and arterioles. Symptoms of ischemia include the feet and hands becoming cold, pale, and numb; muscle pain, gangrene. Occasionally confusion, depression, drowsiness, and *seizures. Treatment:* Maintain adequate circulation. IV nitroglycerin and nitroprusside to treat

vasospasm. IV heparin and low molecular weight dextran to minimize thrombosis.

Drug Interactions
Beta-adrenergic blockers / ↑ Peripheral ischemia resulting in cold extremities and possibly peripheral gangrene
Macrolide antibiotics / Acute ergotism resulting in peripheral ischemia
Nitrates / ↑ Bioavailability of hydroergotamine and ↓ anginal effects of nitrates

EMS CONSIDERATIONS
None.

Diltiazem hydrochloride
(dill-TIE-ah-zem)
Pregnancy Class: C
Cardizem, Cardizem CD, Cardizem Injectable, Cardizem Lyo-Ject, Cardizem-SR, Dilacor XR, Diltiazem HCl Extended Release, Tiamate, Tiazac **(Rx)**
Classification: Calcium channel blocking agent (antianginal, antihypertensive)

Mechanism of Action: Decreases SA and AV conduction and prolongs AV node effective and functional refractory periods. Also decreases myocardial contractility and peripheral vascular resistance.

Onset of Action: Tablets: 30-60 min; **Extended-Release Capsules:** 2-3 hr.

Duration of Action: Tablets: 4-8 hr; **Extended-Release Capsules:** 12 hr.

Uses: Tablets: Vasospastic angina (Prinzmetal's variant). Chronic stable angina (classic effort-associated angina), especially in patients who cannot use beta-adrenergic blockers or nitrates or who remain symptomatic after clinical doses of these agents. **Sustained-Release Capsules:** Essential hypertension, angina. **Parenteral:** Atrial fibrillation or flutter. Paroxysmal SVT. Cardizem Lyo-Ject is used on an emergency basis for atrial fibrillation or atrial flutter. Cardizem Monovial is used to maintain control of HR for up to 24 hr in atrial fibrillation or flutter. *Investigational:* Prophylaxis of reinfarction of nonQ wave MI; tardive dyskinesia, Raynaud's syndrome.

Contraindications: Hypotension. Second- or third-degree AV block and sick sinus syndrome except in presence of a functioning ventricular pacemaker. Acute MI, pulmonary congestion. Lactation.

Precautions: Safety and effectiveness in children have not been determined. The half-life may be increased in geriatric patients. Use with caution in hepatic disease and in CHF. Abrupt withdrawal may cause an increase in the frequency and duration of chest pain. Use with beta blockers or digitalis is usually well tolerated, although the effects of co-administration cannot be predicted (especially in patients with left ventricular dysfunction or cardiac conduction abnormalities).

Route/Dosage ————————————
• **Tablets**
Angina.

Adults, initial: 30 mg q.i.d. before meals and at bedtime; **then,** increase gradually to total daily dose of 180–360 mg (given in three to four divided doses). Increments may be made q 1–2 days until the optimum response is attained.

• **Capsules, Sustained-Release**
Angina.

Cardizem CD: Adults, initial: 120 or 180 mg once daily. Up to 480 mg/day may be required. Dosage adjustments should be carried out over a 7–14-day period.

Dilacor XR: Adults, initial: 120 mg once daily; **then,** dose may be titrated, depending on the needs of the patient, up to 480 mg once daily. Titration may be carried out over a 7–14-day period.

Hypertension.

Cardizem CD: Adults, initial: 180–240 mg once daily. Maximum antihypertensive effect usually reached within 14 days. Usual range is 240–360 mg once daily.

Cardizem SR: Adults, initial: 60–120 mg b.i.d.; **then,** when maximum antihypertensive effect is reached (approximately 14 days), adjust dosage to a range of 240–360 mg/day.

Dilacor XR: Adults, initial: 180–240 mg once daily. Usual range is 180–480 mg once daily. The dose may be increased to 540 mg/day with little or no increased risk of side effects.

Tiazac: Adults, initial: 120–240 mg once daily. Usual range is 120–360 mg once daily, although doses up to 540 mg once daily have been used.

• **IV Bolus**
Atrial fibrillation/flutter; paroxysmal SVT.

Adults, initial: 0.25 mg/kg (average 20 mg) given over 2 min; **then,** if response is inadequate, a second dose may be given after 15 min. The second bolus dose is 0.35 mg/kg (average 25 mg) given over 2 min. Subsequent doses should be individualized. Some patients may respond to an initial dose of 0.15 mg/kg (duration of action may be shorter).

• **IV Infusion**
Atrial fibrillation/flutter.

Adults: 10 mg/hr following IV bolus dose(s) of 0.25 mg/kg or 0.35 mg/kg. Some patients may require 5 mg/hr while others may require 15 mg/hr. Infusion may be maintained for 24 hr.

• **Cardizem Lyo-Ject**
Atrial fibrillation/atrial flutter.
Delivery system consists of a dual-chamber, prefilled, calibrated syringe containing 25 mg of diltiazem hydrochloride in one chamber and 5 mL of diluent in the other chamber.

How Supplied: *Capsule, Extended Release:* 60 mg, 90 mg, 120 mg, 180 mg, 240 mg, 300 mg, 360 mg; *Injection:* 5 mg/mL; *Monovial:* 100 mg freeze-dried diltiazem; *Powder for Injection:* 10 mg, 25 mg; *Tablet:* 30 mg, 60 mg, 90 mg, 120 mg; *Tablet, Extended Release:* 120 mg, 180 mg, 240 mg

Side Effects: *CV:* AV block, bradycardia, CHF, hypotension, syncope, palpitations, peripheral edema, *arrhythmias,* angina, tachycardia, *abnormal ECG, ventricular extrasystoles.* *GI:* N&V, diarrhea, constipation, anorexia, abdominal discomfort, cramps, dry mouth, dysgeusia. *CNS:* Weakness, nervousness, dizziness, lightheadedness, headache, depression, psychoses, hallucinations, disturbances in sleep, somnolence, insomnia, amnesia, abnormal dreams. *Dermatologic:* Rashes, dermatitis, pruritus, urticaria, erythema multiforme, *Stevens-Johnson syndrome. Other:* Photosensitivity, joint pain or stiffness, flushing, nasal or chest congestion, dyspnea, SOB, nocturia/polyuria, sexual difficulties, weight gain, paresthesia, tinnitus, tremor, asthenia, gynecomastia, gingival hyperplasia, petechiae, ecchymosis, purpura, bruising, hematoma, leukopenia, double vision, epistaxis, eye irritation, thirst, alopecia, *bundle branch block,* abnormal gait, hyperglycemia.

EMS CONSIDERATIONS

See also *Calcium Channel Blocking Agents.*

Dimenhydrinate
(dye-men-HY-drih-nayt)
Pregnancy Class: B
Oral Liquid, Syrup, Tablets, Chewable Tablets: Calm-X, Dimentabs, Dramamine, Travamine **(OTC). Injection:** Dinate, Dramanate, Dramillin, Dymenage, Hydrate, Marmine, Reidamine **(Rx)**
Classification: Antihistamine, antiemetic

Mechanism of Action: Contains both diphenhydramine and chlorotheophylline. Antiemetic mechanism not known, but it does depress labyrinthine and vestibular function. Possesses anticholinergic activity.
Duration of Action: 3-6 hr.
Uses: Motion sickness, especially to relieve nausea, vomiting, or dizziness. Treat vertigo.
Precautions: Use of the injectable form is not recommended in neonates. Geriatric patients may be more sensitive to the usual adult dose.

Route/Dosage
• **Elixir, Syrup, Tablets, Chewable Tablets**
Motion sickness.
Adults: 50–100 mg q 4 hr, not to exceed 400 mg/day. **Pediatric, 6–12 years:** 25–50 mg q 6–8 hr, not to exceed 150 mg/day; **2–6 years:** 12.5–25 mg q 6–8 hr, not to exceed 75 mg/day.
• **IM, IV**
Adults: 50 mg as required. **Pediatric, over 2 years:** 1.25 mg/kg (37.5 mg/m^2) q.i.d., not to exceed 300 mg/day.
• **IV**
Adults: 50 mg in 10 mL sodium chloride injection given over 2 min; may be repeated q 4 hr as needed. **Pediatric:** 1.25 mg/kg (37.5 mg/m^2) in 10 mL of 0.9% sodium chloride injection given slowly over 2 min; may be repeated q 6 hr, not to exceed 300 mg/day.

How Supplied: *Chew Tablet:* 50 mg; *Injection:* 50 mg/mL; *Liquid:* 12.5 mg/4 mL, 12.5 mg/5 mL; *Tablet:* 25 mg, 50 mg

EMS CONSIDERATIONS

See also *Antihistamines* and *Antiemetics.*

Dimercaprol
(dye-mer-KAP-rohl)
Pregnancy Class: C
BAL In Oil **(Rx)**
Classification: Chelating agent for heavy metals

Mechanism of Action: Forms a chelate by binding sulfhydryl groups with arsenic, mercury, lead, and gold, thus increasing both urinary and fecal excretion of the metals. Because the drug has a higher affinity for the metal than it does for sulfhydryl groups on protein in the body, BAL reverses enzyme inhibition by regenerating free sulfhydryl groups. To be fully effective, administer 1–2 hr after exposure.
Uses: Acute arsenic, mercury, and gold poisoning. With EDTA in acute

lead poisoning. Not effective for chronic mercury poisoning.

Contraindications: Iron, cadmium, silver, uranium, or selenium poisoning. Hepatic or renal insufficiency, except postarsenical jaundice.

Precautions: Use during pregnancy only if poisoning is life-threatening. Use with caution in patients with G6PD deficiency and during lactation. Of questionable value in bismuth or antimony poisoning.

Route/Dosage

• **Deep IM Only**

Mild arsenic and gold poisoning.
Adults: 2.5 mg/kg q.i.d. for 2 days; then, b.i.d. on the third day, and once daily thereafter for 10 days.

Severe arsenic or gold poisoning.
Adults: 3 mg/kg q 4 hr for days 1 and 2; q.i.d. on day 3; b.i.d. for 10 more days.

Mercury poisoning, mild.
Adults, initial: 5 mg/kg; **then,** 2.5 mg/kg 1 or 2 times/day for 10 days. Alternate dosing regimen: 2.5 mg/kg q 4 hr on day 1, q 6 hr on day 2, q 12 hr on day 3, and thereafter, once daily for the next 10 days or until recovery occurs.

Mercury poisoning, severe.
Adults: 5 mg/kg for the first dose followed by 2.5 mg/kg q 3 hr for the first 24 hr; **then,** 2 mg/kg q 4 hr on day 2; 3 mg/kg q 6 hr on day 3; and 3 mg/kg q 12 hr for the next 10 days or until recovery.

Mild lead encephalopathy.
Adults: 4 mg/kg alone initially; **then,** 3 mg/kg q 4 hr in combination with calcium EDTA administered in a separate site. Treatment should be continued for 2–7 days only if the blood level at the end of the first course of combined BAL-CaEDTA therapy exceeds 80–90 mcg/dL.

Severe lead encephalopathy.
Adults: 4 mg/kg alone initially; **then,** 4 mg/kg q 4 hr in combination with calcium EDTA administered in a separate site. Treatment should be continued for 2–7 days and repeated after an interval of 2 days for 5 additional days only if the blood lead level at the end of the first course of combined BAL-CaEDTA therapy exceeds 80–90 mcg/dL.

Lead toxicity in symptomatic children, acute encephalopathy.
75 mg/m² q 4 hr (up to 450 mg/m² in 24 hr). After the first dose, give calcium EDTA, 1,500 mg/m² over a 24-hr period in divided doses q 4 hr at a separate IM site; maintain treatment for 5 days and after an interval of 2 days, the treatment may be repeated for 5 additional days.

Lead toxicity in children, other symptoms.
50 mg/m² q 4 hr. After the first dose, give calcium EDTA, 1,000 mg/m² over a 24-hr period in divided doses q 4 hr at a separate IM site; maintain treatment for 5 days and after an interval of 2 days, the treatment may be repeated for 5 more days if the lead levels are still high.

How Supplied: *Injection:* 10%

Side Effects: *CV:* Most common including hypertension and tachycardia (dose dependent). *GI:* N&V, salivation, abdominal pain, burning feeling of the lips, mouth and throat. *CNS:* Anxiety, weakness, restlessness, headache. *Other:* Constriction and pain in the throat, chest, or hands; sweating of the hands and forehead, conjunctivitis, blepharal spasm, lacrimation, salivation, rhinorrhea, tingling of hands, burning feeling in the penis, sterile abscesses, local pain at injection site. Children may also develop fever. *At high doses dimercaprol may cause coma or convulsions* and metabolic acidosis.

OD Overdose Management: *Symptoms:* Doses exceeding 5 mg/kg usually result in vomiting, convulsions, and stupor. *Treatment:* Reduce dose; symptoms usually subside within 6 hr.

Drug Interactions: Dimercaprol may increase the toxicity of cadmium, iron, selenium, or uranium salts.

EMS CONSIDERATIONS

None.

---

bold italic = life threatening side effect

Diphenhydramine hydrochloride

(dye-fen-HY-drah-meen)

Pregnancy Class: B

AllerMax, AllerMax Allegy & Cough Formula, Banophen Caplets, Benadryl, Benadryl Allergy, Benadryl Allergy Ultratabs, Benadryl Dye-Free Allergy, Benadryl Dye-Free Allergy Liqui Gels, Diphen AF, Diphen Cough, Diphenhist, Genahist, Hyrexin-50, Scot-Tussin DM, Siladryl, Tusstat **(OTC and Rx)., Sleep-Aids:** Dormin, Miles Nervine, Nighttime Sleep Aid, Nytol, Sleepeze 3, Sleepwell 2-nite, Sominex **(OTC)**

Classification: Antihistamine, ethanolamine-type; antiemetic

Mechanism of Action: High sedative, anticholinergic, and antiemetic effects.

Uses: Hypersensitivity reactions, motion sickness (PO only), parkinsonism, nighttime sleep aid (PO only), antitussive (syrup only).

Contraindications: Topically to treat chickenpox, poison ivy, or sunburn. Topically on large areas of the body or on blistered or oozing skin.

Route/Dosage

• **Capsules, Chewable Tablets, Elixir, Liquid, Syrup, Tablets**

Antihistamine, antiemetic, anti-motion sickness, parkinsonism.

Adults: 25–50 mg t.i.d.–q.i.d.; **pediatric, over 10 kg:** 12.5–25 mg t.i.d.–q.i.d. (or 5 mg/kg/day not to exceed 300 mg/day or 150 mg/m²/day).

Sleep aid.

Adults and children over 12 years: 50 mg at bedtime.

Antitussive (Syrup only).

Adults: 25 mg q 4 hr, not to exceed 100 mg/day; **pediatric, 6–12 years:** 12.5–25 mg q 4 hr, not to exceed 50 mg/day; **pediatric, 2–6 years:** 6.25 mg q 4 hr, not to exceed 25 mg/day.

• **IV, Deep IM**

Parkinsonism.

Adults: 10–50 mg up to 100 mg if needed (not to exceed 400 mg/day); **pediatric:** 1.25 mg/kg (or 37.5 mg/m²) q.i.d., not to exceed a total of 300 mg/day.

How Supplied: *Balm:* 2%; *Capsule:* 25 mg, 50 mg; *Chew Tablet:* 12.5 mg; *Cream:* 2%; *Elixir:* 12.5 mg/5 mL; *Injection:* 10 mg/mL, 50 mg/mL; *Liquid:* 6.25 mg/5 mL, 12.5 mg/5 mL, 50 mg/15 mL; *Lotion:* 0.5%; *Spray:* 1%, 2%; *Syrup:* 12.5 mg/5 mL; *Tablet:* 25 mg, 50 mg

EMS CONSIDERATIONS

See also *Antihistamines* and *Antiemetics.*

Administration/Storage:

IV For IV, may give undiluted; each 25 mg over at least 1 min.

Diphenoxylate hydrochloride with Atropine sulfate

(dye-fen-OX-ih-layt, AH-troh-peen)

Pregnancy Class: C

Lofene, Logen, Lomanate, Lomodix, Lomotil, Lonox, Low-Quel **(C-V) (Rx)**

Classification: Antidiarrheal agent, systemic

Mechanism of Action: Chemically related to the narcotic analgesic drug meperidine but without the analgesic properties. Inhibits GI motility and has a constipating effect. May aggravate diarrhea due to organisms that penetrate the intestinal mucosa (e.g., *Escherichia coli, Salmonella, Shigella)* or in antibiotic-induced pseudomembranous colitis. High doses over prolonged periods may cause euphoria and physical dependence. The product also contains small amounts of atropine sulfate which will prevent abuse by deliberate overdosage.

Onset of Action: 45-60 min.

Duration of Action: 2-4 hr.

Uses: Symptomatic treatment of chronic and functional diarrhea. Also, diarrhea associated with gastroenteritis, irritable bowel, regional enteritis, malabsorption syndrome, ulcerative colitis, acute infections, food poisoning, postgastrectomy, and drug-induced diarrhea. Therapeutic results for control of acute diarrhea are inconsistent. Also used in the control of intestinal passage time in patients with ileostomies and colostomies.

Contraindications: Obstructive jaundice, liver disease, diarrhea associated with pseudomembranous enterocolitis after antibiotic therapy or enterotoxin-producing bacteria, children under the age of 2.

Precautions: Use with caution during lactation, when acticholinergics may be contgraindicated, and in advanced hepatic-renal disease or abnormal renal functions. Children (especially those with Down syndrome) are susceptible to atropine toxicity. Children and geriatric patients may be more sensitive to the respiratory depressant effects of diphenoxylate. Dehydration, especially in young children, may cause a delayed diphenoxylate toxicity.

Route/Dosage

• **Oral Solution, Tablets**

Adults, initial: 2.5–5 mg (of diphenoxylate) t.i.d.–q.i.d.; **maintenance:** 2.5 mg b.i.d.–t.i.d. **Pediatric, 2–12 years:** 0.3–0.4 mg/kg/day (of diphenoxylate) in divided doses.

How Supplied: Each tablet or 5 mL of liquid contains: *Antidiarrheal:* Diphenoxylate HCl, 2.5 mg. *Anticholinergic:* Atropine sulfate, 0.025 mg.

Side Effects: *GI:* N&V, anorexia, abdominal discomfort, paralytic ileus, megacolon. *Allergic:* Pruritus, ***angioneurotic edema,*** swelling of gums. *CNS:* Dizziness, drowsiness, malaise, restlessness, headache, depression, numbness of extremities, ***respiratory depression, coma.*** *Topical:* Dry skin and mucous membranes, flushing. *Other:* Tachycardia, urinary retention, hyperthermia.

OD Overdose Management: *Symptoms:* Dry skin and mucous membranes, flushing, ***hyperthermia,*** mydriasis, restlessness, tachycardia followed by miosis, lethargy, hypotonic reflexes, nystagmus, ***coma, severe (and possibly fatal) respiratory depression.*** *Treatment:*

Gastric lavage, induce vomiting, establish a patent airway, and assist respiration. Activated charcoal (100 g) given as a slurry. IV administration of a narcotic antagonist. Administration may be repeated after 10–15 min. Observe patient and readminister antagonist if respiratory depression returns.

Drug Interactions

Alcohol / Additive CNS depression
Antianxiety agents / Additive CNS depression
Barbiturates / Additive CNS depression
MAO inhibitors / ↑ Chance of hypertensive crisis
Narcotics / ↑ Effect of narcotics

EMS CONSIDERATIONS

See also *Cholinergic Blocking Agents.*

Dipyridamole
(dye-peer-ID-ah-mohl)
Pregnancy Class: B
Persantine **(Rx)**
Classification: Platelet adhesion inhibitor

Mechanism of Action: In higher doses may act by several mechanisms, including inhibition of red blood cell uptake of adenosine, itself an inhibitor of platelet reactivity; inhibition of platelet phosphodiesterase, which leads to accumulation of cAMP within platelets; direct stimulation of release of prostacyclin or prostaglandin D_2; and/or inhibition of thromboxane A_2 formation. Dipyridamole prolongs platelet survival time in patients with valvular heart disease and has maintained platelet count in open heart surgery. Also causes coronary vasodilation which may be due to inhibition of adenosine deaminase in the blood, thus allowing accumulation of adenosine which is a potent vasodilator. Vasodilation may also be caused by delaying the hydrolysis of cyclic 3',5'-adenosine monophosphate as a result of inhibition of the enzyme phosphodiesterase.

---

bold italic = life threatening side effect

Uses: PO. As an adjunct to coumarin anticoagulants in preventing postoperative thromboembolic complications of cardiac valve replacement. **IV.** As an alternative to exercise in thallium myocardial perfusion imaging for the evaluation of CAD in those who cannot exercise adequately. *Investigational:* Alone or as an adjunct to treat angina, to prevent graft occlusion in those undergoing arterial reconstructive bypass surgery, intralingual bypass grafts, and to prevent deterioration of coronary vessel patency after percutaneous transluminal angioplasty. Use with aspirin for preventing migraine headaches, MI, to reduce platelet aggregation at the carotid endarterectomy, to slow progression of peripheral occlusive arterial disease, to reduce incidence of DVT, to reduce the number of platelets deposited on dacron aortofemoral artery grafts, and TIAs.

NOTE: Not effective for the treatment of acute episodes of angina and is not a substitute for the treatment of angina pectoris.

Precautions: Use with caution in hypotension and during lactation. Safety and efficacy have not been determined in children less than 12 years of age.

Route/Dosage ———————
- **Tablets**
  Adjunct in prophylaxis of thromboembolism after cardiac valve replacement.
  Adults: 75–100 mg q.i.d. as an adjunct to warfarin therapy.
  Prevention of thromboembolic complications in other thromboembolic disorders.
  Adults: 150–400 mg/day in combination with another platelet-aggregation inhibitor (e.g., aspirin) or an anticoagulant.
- **IV**
  Adjunct to thallium myocardial perfusion imaging.
  Adjust the dose according to body weight. Recommended dose is 0.142 mg/kg/min infused over 4 min. Total dose should not exceed 60 mg.

How Supplied: *Injection:* 5 mg/mL; *Tablets:* 25 mg, 50 mg, 75 mg.

Side Effects: After PO use. *GI:* GI intolerance, N&V, diarrhea. *CNS:* Dizziness, headache, syncope. *CV:* Peripheral vasodilation, flushing. Rarely, angina pectoris or aggravation of angina pectoris (usually at the beginning of therapy). *Miscellaneous:* Weakness, rash, pruritus.

After IV use. Most common side effects (1% or greater) are listed. *GI:* Nausea, dyspepsia. *CNS:* Headache, dizziness, paresthesia, fatigue. *CV:* Chest pain, angina pectoris, ECG abnormalities (ST-T changes, extrasystoles, tachycardia), precipitation of acute myocardial ischemia in patients with CAD, hypotension, flushing, blood pressure lability, hypertension. *Miscellaneous:* Dyspnea, unspecified pain.

OD Overdose Management: *Symptoms:* Hypotension of short duration. *Treatment:* Use of a vasopressor may be beneficial. Due to the high percentage of protein binding of dipyridamole, dialysis is not likely to be beneficial.

EMS CONSIDERATIONS

None.

Disopyramide phosphate
(dye-so-PEER-ah-myd)
Pregnancy Class: C
Norpace, Norpace CR **(Rx)**
Classification: Antiarrhythmic, class IA

Mechanism of Action: Decreases the rate of diastolic depolarization (phase 4), decreases the upstroke velocity (phase 0), increases the action potential duration (of normal cardiac cells), and prolongs the refractory period (phases 2 and 3). Weak anticholinergic effects; fewer side effects than quinidine. Does not affect BP significantly; can be used in digitalized and nondigitalized patients.

Onset of Action: 30 min.

Duration of Action: average of 6 hr (range 1.5-8 hr).

Uses: Life-threatening ventricular arrhythmias (e.g., sustained ventricular tachycardia). Not been shown to improve survival in patients with ventricular arrhythmias. *Investigational:* Paroxysmal SVT.

Contraindications: Hypersensitivity to drug. Cardiogenic shock, heart failure, heart block (especially preexisting second- and third-degree AV block if no pacemaker is present), congenital QT prolongation, asymptomatic ventricular premature contractions, sick sinus syndrome, glaucoma, urinary retention, myasthenia gravis. Use of controlled-release capsules in patients with severe renal insufficiency. Lactation.

Precautions: Safe use during childhood, labor, and delivery has not been established. Use with caution in Wolff-Parkinson-White syndrome or bundle branch block. Decrease dosage in imparied hepatic function. Geriatric patients may be more sensitive to the anticholinergic effects of this drug. The drug may be ineffective in hypokalemia and toxic in hyperkalemia.

Route/Dosage

- **Immediate-Release Capsules**
  Antiarrhythmic.

Adults, initial loading dose: 300 mg of immediate-release capsule (200 mg if patient weighs less than 50 kg); **maintenance:** 400–800 mg/day in four divided doses (usual: 150 mg q 6 hr). **For patients less than 50 kg, maintenance:** 100 mg q 6 hr. **Children, less than 1 year:** 10–30 mg/kg/day in divided doses q 6 hr; **1–4 years of age:** 10–20 mg/kg/day in divided doses q 6 hr; **4–12 years of age:** 10–15 mg/kg/day in divided doses q 6 hr; **12–18 years of age:** 6–15 mg/kg/day in divided doses q 6 hr.

Severe refractory tachycardia.
Up to 400 mg q 6 hr may be required.

Cardiomyopathy.
Do not administer a loading dose; give 100 mg q 6 hr of immediate-release or 200 mg q 12 hr for controlled-release.

- **Extended-Release Capsules**
  Antiarrhythmic, maintenance only.

Adults: 300 mg q 12 hr (200 mg q 12 hr for body weight less than 50 kg).

NOTE: For all uses, decrease dosage in patients with renal or hepatic insufficiency.

Moderate renal failure or hepatic failure.
100 mg q 6 hr (or 200 mg/12 hr of sustained-release form).

Severe renal failure.
100 mg q 8–24 hr depending on severity (with or without an initial loading dose of 150 mg).

How Supplied: *Capsule:* 100 mg, 150 mg; *Capsule, Extended Release:* 100 mg, 150 mg

Side Effects: *Increased risk of death when used in patients with non-life-threatening cardiac arrhythmias. CV:* Hypotension, CHF, *worsening of arrhythmias,* edema, weight gain, cardiac conduction disturbances, SOB, syncope, chest pain, AV block, *severe myocardial depression (with hypotension and increased venous pressure). Anticholinergic:* Dry mouth, urinary retention, constipation, blurred vision, dry nose, eyes, and throat. *GU:* Urinary frequency and urgency, urinary retention, impotence, dysuria. *GI:* Nausea, pain, flatulence, anorexia, diarrhea, vomiting, severe epigastric pain. *CNS:* Headache, nervousness, dizziness, fatigue, depression, insomnia, psychoses. *Dermatologic:* Rash, dermatoses, itching. *Other:* Fever, respiratory problems, gynecomastia, *anaphylaxis,* malaise, muscle weakness, numbness, tingling, angle-closure glaucoma, hypoglycemia, reversible cholestatic jaundice, symptoms of lupus erythematosus (usually in patients switched to disopyramide from procainamide).

OD **Overdose Management:** *Symptoms:* Apnea, loss of consciousness, *cardiac arrhythmias* (widening of QRS complex and QT interval, conduction disturbances), hypotension, bradycardia, anticholinergic symptoms, *loss of spontaneous respiration,*

---

bold italic = life threatening side effect

death. *Treatment:* Induction of vomiting, gastric lavage, or a cathartic followed by activated charcoal. Monitor ECG. IV isoproterenol, IV dopamine, cardiac glycosides, diuretics, intra-aortic balloon counterpulsation, artificial respiration, hemodialysis. Use endocardial pacing to treat AV block and neostigmine to treat anticholinergic symptoms.

Drug Interactions

Anticoagulants / ↓ PT after discontinuing disopyramide

Beta-adrenergic blockers / Possible ↓ clearance of disopyramide; sinus bradycardia, hypotension

Digoxin / ↑ Serum digoxin levels (may be beneficial)

Erythromycin / ↑ Disopyramide levels → arrhythmias and ↑ QTc intervals

Phenytoin / ↓ Effect due to ↑ breakdown by liver; ↑ anticholinergic effects

Quinidine / ↑ Disopyramide serum levels or ↓ quinidine levels

Rifampin / ↓ Effect due to ↑ breakdown by liver

EMS CONSIDERATIONS

See also *Antiarrhythmic Agents.*

Disulfiram

(dye-SUL-fih-ram)

Antabuse **(Rx)**

Classification: Treatment of alcoholism

Mechanism of Action: Produces severe hypersensitivity to alcohol. Inhibits liver enzymes that participate in the normal degradation of alcohol. This results in accumulation of acetaldehyde in the blood. High levels of acetaldehyde produce a series of symptoms referred to as the disulfiram-alcohol reaction or syndrome. The specific symptoms are listed under *Side Effects.* The symptoms vary individually, are dose-dependent with respect to both alcohol and disulfiram, and persist for periods ranging from 30 min to several hours. A single dose of disulfiram may be effective for 1–2 weeks.

Onset of Action: May be delayed up to 12 hr because disulfiram is initially localized in fat stores.

Uses: To prevent further ingestion of alcohol in chronic alcoholics. Should be given only to cooperating patients fully aware of the consequences of alcohol ingestion.

Contraindications: Alcohol intoxication. Severe myocardial or occlusive coronary disease. Use of paraldehyde or alcohol-containing products such as cough syrups. If patient is exposed to ethylene dibromide.

Precautions: Use in pregnancy only if benefits outweigh risks. Use with caution in narcotic additcts or patients with diabetes, goiter, epilepsy, psychosis, hypothyroidism, hepatic cirrhosis, or nephritis.

Route/Dosage

• **Tablets**

Alcoholism.

Adults, initial (after alcohol-free interval of 12–48 hr): 500 mg/day for 1–2 weeks; **maintenance: usual,** 250 mg/day (range: 120–500 mg/day). Do not exceed 500 mg/day.

How Supplied: *Tablet:* 250 mg, 500 mg

Side Effects: In the absence of alcohol, the following symptoms have been reported: Drowsiness (most common), headache, restlessness, fatigue, psychoses, peripheral neuropathy, dermatoses, hepatotoxicity, metallic or garlic taste, arthropathy, impotence. **In the presence of alcohol,** the following symptoms may be manifested. *CV:* Flushing, chest pain, palpitations, tachycardia, hypotension, syncope, arrhythmias, *CV collapse, MI, acute CHF. CNS:* Throbbing headaches, vertigo, weakness, uneasiness, confusion, unconsciousness, *seizures, death. GI:* Nausea, severe vomiting, thirst. *Respiratory:* Respiratory difficulties, dyspnea, hyperventilation, *respiratory depression. Other:* Throbbing in head and neck, sweating. In the event of an Antabuse-alcohol interaction, measures should be undertaken to maintain BP and treat shock. Oxygen, antihistamines, ephedrine, and/or vitamin C may also be used.

Drug Interactions

Anticoagulants, oral / ↑ Effect of anticoagulants by ↑ hypoprothrombinemia

Barbiturates / ↑ Effect of barbiturates due to ↓ breakdown by liver

Chlordiazepoxide, diazepam / ↑ Effect of chlordiazepoxide or diazepam due to ↓ plasma clearance

Isoniazid / ↑ Side effects of isoniazid (especially CNS)

Metronidazole / Acute toxic psychosis or confusional state

Paraldehyde / Concomitant use produces Antabuse-like effect

Phenytoin / ↑ Effect of phenytoin due to ↓ breakdown by liver

Tricyclic antidepressants / Acute organic brain syndrome

EMS CONSIDERATIONS

None.

Divalproex sodium See Valproic Acid.
(dye-VAL-proh-ex)
Depakote **(Rx)**
How Supplied: *Enteric Coated Capsule:* 125 mg; *Enteric Coated Tablet:* 125 mg, 250 mg, 500 mg

EMS CONSIDERATIONS

None.

Dobutamine hydrochloride
(doh-BYOU-tah-meen)
Pregnancy Class: B
Dobutrex **(Rx)**
Classification: Sympathomimetic drug, direct-acting; cardiac stimulant

Mechanism of Action: Stimulates beta-1 receptors (in the heart), increasing cardiac function, CO, and SV, with minor effects on HR. Decreases afterload reduction although SBP and pulse pressure may remain unchanged or increase (due to in-

creased CO). Also decreases elevated ventricular filling pressure and helps AV node conduction.

Onset of Action: 1-2 min. **Peak effect:** 10 min.

Uses: Short-term treatment of cardiac decompensation in adults secondary to depressed contractility due to organic heart disease or cardiac surgical procedures. *Investigational:* Congenital heart disease in children undergoing diagnostic cardiac catheterization.

Contraindications: Idiopathic hypertrophic subaortic stenosis.

Precautions: Safe use during childhood or after AMI not established.

Route/Dosage
• **IV Infusion**
Adults, individualized, usual: 2.5–15 mcg/kg/min (up to 40 mcg/kg/min). Rate of administration and duration of therapy depend on response of patient, as determined by HR, presence of ectopic activity, BP, and urine flow.

How Supplied: *Injection:* 12.5 mg/mL

Side Effects: *CV:* Marked increase in HR, BP, and ***ventricular ectopic activity,*** precipitous drop in BP, premature ventricular beats, anginal and nonspecific chest pain, palpitations. *Hypersensitivity:* Skin rash, pruritus of the scalp, fever, eosinophilia, ***bronchospasm.*** *Other:* Nausea, headache, SOB, fever, phlebitis, and local inflammatory changes at the injection site.

OD **Overdose Management:** *Symptoms:* Excessive alteration of BP, anorexia N&V, tremor, anxiety, palpitations, headache, SOB, anginal and nonspecific chest pain, ***myocardial ischemia, ventricular fibrillation or tachycardia.*** *Treatment:* Reduce the rate of administration or discontinue temporarily until the condition stabilizes. Establish an airway, ensuring oxygenation and ventilation. Initiate resuscitative measures immediately. Treat severe ventricular tachyarrhythmias with propranolol or lidocaine.

---

bold italic = life threatening side effect

Drug Interactions: Additional: Concomitant use with nitroprusside causes ↑ CO and ↓ pulmonary wedge pressure.

EMS CONSIDERATIONS

See also *Sympathomimetic Drugs*.

Administration/Storage

IV 1. Reconstitute solution according to manufacturers directions; takes place in two stages.

2. Before administration, the solution is diluted further according to the fluid needs of the patient. This more dilute solution should be used within 24 hr. Solutions that can be used for further dilution include D5W, RL injection, D5/RL, and 0.9% NaCl injection.

Interventions: Monitor ECG and BP continuously during drug administration; review written parameters for SBP and titrate infusion.

Docusate calcium (Dioctyl calcium sulfosuccinate)
Docusate potassium (Dioctyl potassium sulfosuccinate)
Docusate sodium (Dioctyl sodium sulfosuccinate)

(DEW-kyou-sayt)

Pregnancy Class: C

Docusate calcium (Surfak, Surfak Liquigels **(OTC)**) Docusate potassium (Dialose, Diocto-K **(OTC)**) Docusate sodium (Colace, Diocto, Dioeze, Disonate, DOK, DOS Softgel, D-S-S, Modane Soft, Regulax SS **(OTC)**)

Classification: Laxative, emollient

Mechanism of Action: Acts by lowering the surface tension of the feces and promoting penetration by water and fat, thus increasing the softness of the fecal mass. Not absorbed systemically and does not seem to interfere with the absorption of nutrients.

Onset of Action: 24-72 hr; **onset, microenema formulation:** 15 min.

Uses: To lessen strain of defecation in persons with hernia or CV diseases or other diseases in which straining at stool should be avoided. Megacolon or bedridden patients. Constipation associated with dry, hard stools. The microemulsion formulation is indicated for relief of occasional constipation in children over the age of 3 years.

Contraindications: Nausea, vomiting, abdominal pain, and intestinal obstruction.

Route/Dosage ———————

DOCUSATE CALCIUM

• **Capsules**

Adults: 240 mg/day until bowel movements are normal; **pediatric, over 6 years:** 50–150 mg/day.

DOCUSATE POTASSIUM

• **Capsules**

Adults: 100–300 mg/day; **pediatric, over 6 years:** 100 mg at bedtime.

DOCUSATE SODIUM

• **Capsules, Oral Liquid, Syrup, Tablets**

Adults and children over 12 years: 50–500 mg; **pediatric, under 3 years:** 10–40 mg; **3–6 years:** 20–60 mg; **6–12 years:** 40–120 mg.

• **Rectal Solution**

Flushing or retention enema.

Adults: 50–100 mg.

How Supplied: Docusate calcium: *Capsule:* 240 mg. Docusate potassium: *Capsule:* 100 mg, 240 mg Docusate sodium: *Capsule:* 50 mg, 100 mg, 240 mg, 250 mg; *Oral Liquid:* 200 mg/5 mL, 150 mg/15 mL; *Powder for Reconstitution:* 283 mg; *Solution:* 100 mg/15 mL; *Syrup:* 50 mg/15 mL, 60 mg/15 mL; *Tablet:* 100 mg

Drug Interactions: Docusate may ↑ absorption of mineral oil from the GI tract.

EMS CONSIDERATIONS

See also *Laxatives*.

Donepezil hydrochloride
(dohn-EP-eh-zil)

Pregnancy Class: Pregnancy Class: C
Aricept **(Rx)**
Classification: Psychotherapeutic drug for Alzheimer's disease

Mechanism of Action: A decrease in cholinergic function may be the cause of Alzheimer's disease. Donepezil is a cholinesterase inhibitor and exerts its effect by enhancing cholinergic function by increasing levels of acetylcholine. No evidence that the drug alters the course of the underlying dementing process. Food does not affect the rate or extent of absorption.

Uses: Treatment of mild to moderate dementia of the Alzheimer's type.

Contraindications: Hypersensitivity to piperidine derivatives.

Precautions: Use with caution in patients with a history of asthma or obstructive pulmonary disease. Safety and efficacy have not been determined for use in children.

Route/Dosage

• **Tablets**
Alzheimer's disease.

Initial: 5 mg. Use of a 10-mg dose did not provide a clinical effect greater than the 5-mg dose; however, in some patients, 10 mg daily may be superior. Do not increase the dose to 10 mg until patients have been on a daily dose of 5 mg for 4 to 6 weeks.

How Supplied: *Tablet:* 5 mg, 10 mg

Side Effects: *NOTE:* Side effects with an incidence of 1% or greater are listed. *GI:* N&V, diarrhea, anorexia, fecal incontinence, GI bleeding, bloating, epigastric pain. *CNS:* Insomnia, dizziness, depression, abnormal dreams, somnolence. *CV:* Hypertension, vasodilation, atrial fibrillation, hot flashes, hypotension, bradycardia. *Body as a whole:* Headache, pain (in various locations), accident, fatigue, influenza, chest pain, toothache. *Musculoskeletal:* Muscle cramps, arthritis, bone fracture. *Dermatologic:* Diaphoresis, urticaria, pruritus. *GU:* Urinary incontinence, nocturia, frequent urination. *Respiratory:* Dyspnea, sore throat, bron-

chitis. *Ophthalmic:* Cataract, eye irritation, blurred vision. *Miscellaneous:* Dehydration, syncope, ecchymosis, weight loss.

OD **Overdose Management:** *Symptoms:* Cholinergic crisis characterized by severe N&V, salivation, sweating, bradycardia, hypotension, respiratory depression, collapse, convulsions, increased muscle weakness (may cause death if respiratory muscles are involved). *Treatment:* Atropine sulfate at an initial dose of 1–2 mg IV with subsequent doses based on the response. General supportive measures.

Drug Interactions
Anticholinergic drugs / The cholinesterase inhibitor activitiy of donepezil interferes with the activity of anticholinergics
Bethanechol / Synergistic effect
NSAIDs / ↑ Gastric acid secretion → ↑ risk of active or occult GI bleeding
Succinylcholine / ↑ Muscle relaxant effect

EMS CONSIDERATIONS
Administration/Storage: Store at controlled room temperatures from 15°C to 30°C (59°F to 86°F).
Assessment
1. Document onset/duration, other agents trialed, and the outcome.
2. Describe clinical presentation.
3. Note any history of asthma or COPD.
4. Obtain ECG and labs.

Donnatal Capsules, Elixir, Tablets
(DON-nah-tal)
Pregnancy Class: C
(Rx)
Classification: Anticholinergic

Uses: Possibly effective as an adjunct in the treatment of irritable colon, spastic colon, mucous colitis, and acute enterocolitis. Has also been used in the treatment of duodenal ulcer.

Precautions: It is not known with certainty whether or not anticholinergic drugs aid in the healing in duodenal ulcer or decrease the rate of recurrence or prevent complications.

Route/Dosage ⎯⎯⎯⎯⎯⎯

• **Tablets, Capsules, Extentabs, Elixir**

Adults, usual: 1–2 tablets or capsules t.i.d.–q.i.d. (or one Extentab q 12 hr). If the elixir is used, **adult, usual:** 5–10 mL t.i.d.–q.i.d. **Pediatric:** Use elixir as follows: **4.5–9.0 kg:** 0.5 mL q 4 hr or 0.75 mL q 6 hr; **9.1–13.5 kg:** 1.0 mL q 4 hr or 1.5 mL q 6 hr; **13.6–22.6 kg:** 1.5 mL q 4 hr or 2.0 mL q 6 hr; **22.7–33.9 kg:** 2.5 mL q 4 hr or 3.75 mL q 6 hr. **34.0–45.3 kg:** 3.75 mL q 4 hr or 5 mL q 6 hr; **45.4 kg:** 5 mL q 4 hr or 7.5 mL q 6 hr.

How Supplied: Each tablet, capsule, or 5 mL elixir contains: *Anticholinergic:* Atropine sulfate, 0.0194 mg. *Anticholinergic:* Hyoscyamine sulfate, 0.1037 mg. *Anticholinergic:* Scopolamine hydrobromide, 0.0065 mg. *Sedative:* Phenobarbital, 16.2 mg. *NOTE:* The Extentabs contain three times the amount of drugs found in tablets.

EMS CONSIDERATIONS

None.

Dopamine hydrochloride

(DOH-pah-meen)
Pregnancy Class: C
Intropin **(Rx)**
Classification: Sympathomimetic, direct- and indirect-acting; cardiac stimulant and vasopressor

Mechanism of Action: Dopamine is the immediate precursor of epinephrine in the body. Exogenously administered, it produces direct stimulation of beta-1 receptors and variable (dose-dependent) stimulation of alpha receptors (peripheral vasoconstriction). Will cause a release of norepinephrine from its storage sites . These actions result in increased myocardial contraction, CO, and SV, as well as increased re-

nal blood flow and sodium excretion. Exerts little effect on DBP and induces fewer arrhythmias than are seen with isoproterenol.

Onset of Action: 5 min.

Duration of Action: 10 min.

Uses: Cardiogenic shock due to MI, trauma, endotoxic septicemia, open heart surgery, renal failure, and chronic cardiac decompensation (as in CHF). Patients most likely to respond include those in whom urine flow, myocardial function, and BP have not deteriorated significantly. Best responses are observed when the time is short between onset of symptoms of shock and initiation of dopamine and volume correction. *Investigational:* COPD, CHF, respiratory distress syndrome in infants.

Contraindications: Additional: Pheochromocytoma, uncorrected tachycardia or arrhythmias. Pediatric patients.

Precautions: Use with caution during lactation. Safety and efficacy have not been established in children. Dosage may have to be adjusted in geriatric patients with occlusive vascular disease.

Route/Dosage ⎯⎯⎯⎯⎯⎯

• **IV Infusion**
   Shock.

Initial: 2–5 mcg/kg/min; **then,** increase in increments of 1–4 mcg/kg/min at 10–30-min intervals until desired response is obtained.
   Severely ill patients.

Initial: 5 mcg/kg/min; **then,** increase rate in increments of 5–10 mcg/kg/min up to 20–50 mcg/kg/min as needed.*NOTE:* Dopamine is a potent drug. Be sure to dilute the drug before administration. The drug should not be given as a bolus dose.

How Supplied: *Injection:* 40 mg/mL, 80 mg/mL, 160 mg/mL

Side Effects: Additional:*CV:*Ectopic heartbeats, tachycardia, anginal pain, palpitation, vasoconstriction, hypotension, hypertension. Infrequently: aberrant conduction, bradycardia, widened QRS complex. *Oth-*

*er:*Dyspnea, headache, mydriasis. Infrequently, piloerection, azotemia, polyuria. High doses may cause mydriasis and ventricular arrhythmia. Extravasation may result in necrosis and sloughing of surrounding tissue.

OD **Overdose Management:** *Symptoms:* Extravasation. *Treatment:* To prevent sloughing and necrosis, infiltrate as soon as possible with 10–15 mL of 0.9% NaCl solution containing 5–10 mg phentolamine using a syringe with a fine needle. Infiltrate liberally throughout the ischemic area.

Drug Interactions: Additional:*Diuretics*/Additive or potentiating effect.*Phenytoin*/ Hypotension and bradycardia *Propranolol*/ ↓ Effect of dopamine

EMS CONSIDERATIONS

See also *Sympathomimetic Drugs.*
Administration/Storage
IV 1. Must be diluted before use—see package insert.
2. For reconstitution use dextrose or saline solutions: 200 mg/250 mL for a concentration of 0.8 mg/mL or 800 mcg/mL; 400 mg/250 mL for a concentration of 1.6 mg/mL or 1,600 mcg/mL. Alkaline solutions such as 5% NaHCO$_3$, will inactivate drug.
3. To prevent fluid overload, may use more concentrated solutions with higher doses.
Interventions
1. Monitor VS, I&O, and ECG; titrate infusion to maintain SBP as ordered.
2. Report any ectopy, palpitations, anginal pain, or vasoconstriction.

Dornase alfa recombinant
(DOR-nace AL-fah)
Pregnancy Class: B
Pulmozyme **(Rx)**
Classification: Drug for cystic fibrosis

Mechanism of Action: This drug is a highly purified solution of recombinant human deoxyribonuclease I (rhDNase), an enzyme that selectively cleaves DNA. Cystic fibrosis (CF) patients have viscous purulent secretions in the airways that contribute to reduced pulmonary function and worsening of infection. These secretions contain high concentrations of extracellular DNA released by degenerating leukocytes that accumulate as a result of infection. Dornase alfa hydrolyzes the DNA in sputum of CF patients, thereby reducing sputum viscoelasticity and reducing infections.

Uses: In CF patients in conjunction with standard therapy to decrease the frequency of respiratory infections that require parenteral antibiotics and to improve pulmonary function.

Contraindications: Known sensitivity to dornase alfa or products from Chinese hamster ovary cells.

Precautions: Safety and effectiveness of daily use have not been demonstrated in patients with forced vital caacity (FVC) of less than 40% of predicted, or for longer than 12 months. Use with caution during lactation.

Route/Dosage
• **Inhalation Solution**
Cystic fibrosis.
One 2.5-mg single-dose ampule inhaled once daily using a recommended nebulizer (see what follows). Older patients and patients with baseline FVC above 85% may benefit from twice daily dosing.
How Supplied: *Solution:* 2.5 mg/2.5 mL

Side Effects: *Respiratory:* Pharyngitis, voice alteration, and laryngitis are the most common. Also, ***apnea,*** bronchiectasis, bronchitis, change in sputum, cough increase, dyspnea, hemoptysis, lung function decrease, nasal polyps, pneumonia, pneumothorax, rhinitis, sinusitis, sputum increase, wheezing. *Body as a whole:* Abdominal pain, asthenia, fever, flu syndrome, malaise, sepsis, weight loss. *GI:* Intestinal obstruction, gall bladder disease, liver disease, pancreatic disease. *Miscellaneous:* Rash,

bold italic = life threatening side effect

urticaria, chest pain, conjunctivitis, diabetes mellitus, hypoxia.

EMS CONSIDERATIONS
None.

D

Dorzolamide hydrochloride ophthalmic solution
(dor-ZOH-lah-myd)
Pregnancy Class: C
Trusopt **(Rx)**
Classification: Carbonic anhydrase inhibitor

Mechanism of Action: Decreases aqueous humor secretion in the ciliary processes of the eye by inhibiting carbonic anhydrase. Occurs by decreasing the formation of bicarbonate ions with a reduction in sodium and fluid transport and a subsequent decrease in intraocular pressure.

Uses: Elevated intraocular pressure (IOP) in those with ocular hypertension or open-angle glaucoma.

Contraindications: Use with severe renal impairment ($C_{CR} < 30$ mL/min) or in soft contact lens wearers as the preservative (benzalkonium chloride) may be absorbed by the lenses. Lactation.

Precautions: Dorzolamide is a sulfonamide and, as such, may cause similar systemic reaction, including side effects and allergic reactions, as sulfonamides. Use with caution in hepatic impairment. Due to additive effects, concurrent use of dorzolamide with systemic carbonic anhydrase inhibitors is not recommended. Safety and efficacy have not been determined in children. It is possible geriatric patients may show greater sensitivity to the drug.

Route/Dosage
• **Ophthalmic Solution**
  Increased intraocular pressure.
Adults: 1 gtt in the affected eye(s) t.i.d.
How Supplied: *Solution:* 2%
Side Effects: *Ophthalmic:* Conjunctivitis, lid reactions, bacterial keratitis (due to contamination by concurrent corneal disease). Ocular burning, stinging, or discomfort immediately following administration. Also, superficial punctate keratitis, ocular allergic reaction, blurred vision, tearing, dryness, photophobia, iridocyclitis (rare). *Miscellaneous:* Acid-base and electrolyte disturbances (i.e., similar to systemic use of carbonic anhydrase inhibitors). Also, bitter taste following instillation, headache, nausea, asthenia, fatigue. Rarely, skin rashes, urolithiasis.

EMS CONSIDERATIONS
None.

————COMBINATION DRUG————

Dorzolamide hydrochloride and Timolol maleate
(dor-ZOH-lah-myd/TIE-moh-lohl)
Pregnancy Class: C
Cosopt **(Rx)**
Classification: Topical carbonic anhydrase inhibitor and a topical beta-adrenergic blocking agent

Mechanism of Action: Both drugs decrease elevated IOP by reducing aqueous humor production. Inhibition of carbonic anhydrase by dorzolamide decreases aqueous humor secretion by slowing formation of bicarbonate ions with subsequent reduction in sodium and fluid transport. Timolol is a nonspecific beta-receptor blocking agent.

Uses: To reduce elevated IOP in open-angle glaucoma or ocular hypertension in those inadequately controlled with beta-blockers.

Contraindications: Use in bronchial asthma or history thereof, severe COPD, sinus bradycardia, second or third degree AV block, overt cardiac failure, cardiogenic shock. Lactation.

Precautions: Use beta-blockers with caution in diabetics receiving insulin or oral hypoglycemic drugs or in those subject to spontaneous hypoglycemia. Timolol may mask signs and symptoms of hypoglycemia or hyperthyroidism. Safety and efficacy have not been determined in children.

Route/Dosage
• **Ophthalmic Solution**
Elevated IOP.
Adults: 1 gtt of Cosopt in the affected eye(s) b.i.d.
How Supplied: *Ophthalmic Solution:* Dorzolamide 2%, Timolol .5%
Side Effects: See individual drugs. *Ophthalmic:* Conjunctival hyperemia, ocular burning and/or stinging, blurred vision, superficial punctate keratitis, eye itching, blepharitis, cloudy vision, conjunctival discharge, conjunctival edema, conjunctival follicles, conjunctival injections, corneal erosion, corneal staining, cortical lens opacity, dryness of eyes, eye debris, eye discharge, eye pain, eye tearing, eyelid edema, eyelid erythema, eyelid exudate/scales, eyelid pain or discomfort, foreign body sensation, glaucomatous cupping, lens nucleus coloration, lens opacity, nuclear lens opacity, postsubcapsular cataract, visual field defect, vitreous detachment. *GI:* Taste perversion (bitter, sour, or unusual taste), abdominal pain, dyspepsia, nausea. *Respiratory:* Bronchitis, cough, pharyngitis, sinusitis, URI. *Miscellaneous:* Back pain, dizziness, headache, hypertension, influenza, UTI.
Drug Interactions: See individual drugs.

EMS CONSIDERATIONS

See also *Dorzolamide hydrochloride.*

Doxazosin mesylate
(dox-AYZ-oh-sin)
Pregnancy Class: B
Cardura **(Rx)**
Classification: Antihypertensive

Mechanism of Action: Blocks the alpha-1 (postjunctional) adrenergic receptors resulting in a decrease in systemic vascular resistance and a corresponding decrease in BP.
Onset of Action: Peak effect: 2-6 hr.

Uses: Alone or in combination with diuretics, calcium channel blockers, or beta blockers to treat hypertension. Treatment of BPH.
Contraindications: Patients allergic to prazosin or terazosin.
Precautions: Use with caution during lactation, in impaired hepatic function, or in those taking drugs known to influence hepatic metabolism. Safety and effectiveness have not been demonstrated in children. Due to the possibility of severe hypotension, do not use the 2-, 4-, and 8-mg tablest for initial therapy.

Route/Dosage
• **Tablets**
Hypertension.
Adults: initial, 1 mg once daily at bedtime; **then,** depending on the response (patient's standing BP both 2–6 hr and 24 hr after a dose), the dose may be increased to 2 mg/day. A maximum of 16 mg/day may be required to control BP.
Benign prostatic hyperplasia.
Initial: 1 mg once daily. **Maintenance:** Depending on the urodynamics and symptoms, dose may be increased to 2 mg daily and then 4–8 mg once daily (maximum recommended dose). The recommended titration interval is 1–2 weeks.
How Supplied: *Tablet:* 1 mg, 2 mg, 4 mg, 8 mg
Side Effects: *CV:* Dizziness (most frequent), syncope, vertigo, lightheadedness, edema, palpitation, arrhythmia, postural hypotension, tachycardia, peripheral ischemia. *CNS:* Fatigue, headache, paresthesia, kinetic disorders, ataxia, somnolence, nervousness, depression, insomnia. *Musculoskeletal:* Arthralgia, arthritis, muscle weakness, muscle cramps, myalgia, hypertonia. *GU:* Polyuria, sexual dysfunction, urinary incontinence, urinary frequency. *GI:* Nausea, diarrhea, dry mouth, constipation, dyspepsia, flatulence, abdominal pain, vomiting. *Respiratory:* Fatigue or malaise, rhinitis, epistaxis, dyspnea. *Miscellaneous:* Rash, pruritus, flushing,

D

abnormal vision, conjunctivitis, eye pain, tinnitus, chest pain, asthenia, facial edema, generalized pain, slight weight gain.

OD **Overdose Management:** *Symptoms:* Hypotension. *Treatment:* IV fluids.

D

EMS CONSIDERATIONS

None.

Doxepin hydrochloride
(DOX-eh-pin)
Classification: Antidepressant, tricyclic

Mechanism of Action: Moderate anticholinergic effects and orthostatic hypotension; high sedative effects.

Uses: Psychoneurotic patients with depression or anxiety. Depression or anxiety due to organic disease or alcoholism. Psychotic depressive disorders with associated anxiety, including involutional depression and manic-depressive disorders. Chronic, severe neurogenic pain. PUD. Dermatologic disorders including chronic urticaria, angioedema, and nocturnal pruritus due to atopic eczema.

Contraindications: Use in children less than 12 years of age. Glaucoma or a tendency for urinary retention.

Precautions: Safety has not been determined in pregnancy.

Route/Dosage ⎯⎯⎯⎯⎯⎯⎯⎯
• **Capsules, Oral Concentrate**
Antidepressant, mild to moderate anxiety or depression.
Adults: 25 mg t.i.d. (or up to 150 mg can be given at bedtime); **then,** adjust dosage to individual response (usual optimum dosage: 75–150 mg/day).
Geriatric patients, initially: 25–50 mg/day; dose can be increased as needed and tolerated.
Severe symptoms.
Initial: 50 mg t.i.d.; **then,** gradually increase to 300 mg/day.
Emotional symptoms with organic disease.
25–50 mg/day.
Antipruritic.

10–30 mg at bedtime.
• **Cream 5%**
Apply a thin film q.i.d. with at least a 3–4 hr interval between applications.

How Supplied: *Capsule:* 10 mg, 25 mg, 50 mg, 75 mg, 100 mg, 150 mg; *Concentrate:* 10 mg/mL; *Cream:* 5%

Side Effects: Additional: Doxepin has a high incidence of side effects, including a high degree of sedation, decreased libido, extrapyramidal symptoms, dermatitis, pruritus, fatigue, weight gain, edema, paresthesia, breast engorgement, insomnia, tremor, chills, tinnitus, and photophobia.

EMS CONSIDERATIONS

See also *Antidepressants, Tricyclic.*

Doxercalciferol
Pregnancy Class: A
Hectorol **(Rx)**
Classification: Vitamin

Mechanism of Action: A vitamin D analog that acts on the parathyroid gland to suppress parathyroid hormone synthesis and secretion.

Uses: Management of secondary hyperparathyroidism in patients undergoing chronic dialysis.

Contraindications: Hypercalcemia, hypervitamin osis D, hypersensitivity to other vitamin D analogs or doxercalciferol, hyperphosphatemia.

Route/Dosage ⎯⎯⎯⎯⎯⎯⎯⎯
Initial dose: **10 mcg three times weekly at dialysis.** Dose titration: **Increase at 8-week intervals as needed by 2.5 mcg to decrease serum parathyroid hormone levels to the range of 150-300 pg/mL. If serum parathyroid hormone levels fall below 150 pg/mL, stop doxercalciferol for 1 week and restart at a dose that is at least 2.5 mcg lower than the last administered dose.**

How Supplied: Capsule, 2.5 mcg.

Side Effects: *Respiratory:* Dyspnea; *CV:* edema; *CNS:* headache, malaise; *Endocrine:* hypercalcemia, hypercalciuria, hyperphosphatemia.

OD **Overdose Management:**
Symptoms: Anorexia, nausea, weakness, headache, vomiting, somnolence, dry mouth, metallic taste, ataxia, hypotonia, osteoporosis, calccification of soft tissues. **Treatment:** Hydration, furosemide, dialysis.

Drug Interactions: *Cholestyramine /* ↓ absorption of doxercalciferol. *Mineral oil /* ↓ absorption of doxercalciferol.

EMS CONSIDERATIONS

None.

Doxycycline calcium
Doxycycline hyclate
Doxycycline
monohydrate

(dox-ih-SYE-kleen)
Pregnancy Class: D
Doxycycline calcium (Vibramycin **(Rx)**) Doxycycline hyclate (Vibramycin, Vibramycin IV, Vibra-Tabs, Vibra-Tabs C, Vivox **(Rx)**) Doxycycline monohydrate (Monodox, Vibramycin **(Rx)**)
Classification: Antibiotic, tetracycline

Mechanism of Action: More slowly absorbed, and thus more persistent, than other tetracyclines. Preferred for patients with impaired renal function for treating infections outside the urinary tract.

Uses: Additional: Orally for uncomplicated gonococcal infections in adults (except anorectal infections in males); acute epididymo-orchitis caused by *Neisseria gonorrhoeae* and *Chlamydia trachomatis;* gonococcal arthritis-dermatitis syndrome; nongonococcal urethritis caused by *C. trachomatis* and *Ureaplasma urealyticum.* Prophylaxis of malaria due to *Plasmodium falciparum* in shortterm travelers (< 4 months) to areas with chloroquine- or pyrimethamine-sulfadoxine-resistant strains.

Contraindications: Prophylaxis of malaria in pregnant individuals and in children less than 8 years old. Use during the last half of pregnancy and in children up to 8 years of age (tetracycline may cause permanent discoloration of the teeth). Lactation.

Precautions: Safety for IV use in children less than 8 years of age has not been established.

Route/Dosage

D

• **Capsules, Delayed-Release Capsules, Oral Suspension, Syrup, Tablets, IV**
Infections.

Adult: First day, 100 mg q 12 hr; **maintenance:** 100–200 mg/day, depending on severity of infection. **Children, over 8 years (45 kg or less): First day,** 4.4 mg/kg in 1–2 doses; **then,** 2.2–4.4 mg/kg/day in divided doses depending on severity of infection. Children over 45 kg should receive the adult dose.

Acute gonorrhea.
200 mg at once given PO; **then,** 100 mg at bedtime on first day, followed by 100 mg b.i.d. for 3 days. Alternatively, 300 mg immediately followed in 1 hr with 300 mg.

Syphilis (primary/secondary).
300 mg/day in divided PO doses for 10 days.

C. trachomatis infections.
100 mg b.i.d. PO for minimum of 7 days.

Prophylaxis of "traveler's diarrhea."
100 mg/day given PO.

Prophylaxis of malaria.
Adults: 100 mg PO once daily; **children, over 8 years of age:** 2 mg/kg/day up to 100 mg/day.

• **IV**
Endometritis, parametritis, peritonitis, salpingitis.
100 mg b.i.d. with 2 g cefoxitin, IV, q.i.d. continued for at least 4 days or 2 days after improvement observed. This is followed by doxycycline, PO, 100 mg b.i.d. for 10–14 days of total therapy.

NOTE: The Centers for Disease Control have established treatment schedules for STDs.

How Supplied: Doxycycline calcium: *Syrup:* 50 mg/5 mL. Doxycyline hyclate: *Capsule:* 50 mg, 100 mg; *Enteric Coated Capsule:* 100 mg; *Powder for injection:* 100 mg; *Tablet:* 100 mg. Doxycycline monohydrate: *Capsule:* 50 mg, 100 mg; *Powder for Reconstitution:* 25 mg/5 mL

Drug Interactions: Additional: Carbamazepine, phenytoin, and barbiturates ↓ effect of doxycycline by ↑ breakdown of doxycycline by the liver.

EMS CONSIDERATIONS

See also *Anti-Infectives* and *Tetracyclines.*

Dronabinol (Delta-9-tetrahydro-cannabinol)

(droh-NAB-ih-nohl)
Pregnancy Class: C
Marinol **(C-II) (Rx)**
Classification: Antinauseant

Mechanism of Action: As the active component in marijuana, significant psychoactive effects may occur. (See *Side Effects.*) In therapeutic doses, the drug also causes conjunctival injection and an increased HR. Antiemetic effect may be due to inhibition of the vomiting center in the medulla. Cumulative toxicity using clinical doses may occur.

Uses: Nausea and vomiting associated with cancer chemotherapy, especially in patients who have not responded to other antiemetic treatment. To stimulate appetite and prevent weight loss in AIDS patients.

Contraindications: Nausea and vomiting from any cause other than cancer chemotherapy. Lactation. Hypersensitivity to sesame oil.

Precautions: Monitor pediatric and geriatric patients carefully due to an incrreased risk of psychoactive effects. Use with caution in patients with hypertension, occasional hypotension, syncope, tachycardia; those with a history of substance abuse, including alcohol abuse or dependence; patients with mania, depression, or schizophrenia (the drug may exacerbate these illnesses); patients receiving sedatives, hypnotics,

or other psychoactive drugs (due to the potential for additive or synergistic CNS effects).

Route/Dosage —————————
• **Capsules**
  Antiemetic.
Adults and children, initial: 5 mg/m^2 1–3 hr before chemotherapy; **then,** 5 mg/m^2 q 2–4 hr for a total of four to six doses/day. If ineffective, this dose may be increased by 2.5 mg/m^2 to a maximum of 15 mg/m^2/dose. However, the incidence of serious psychoactive side effects increases dramatically at these higher dose levels.

  Appetite stimulation.
Initial: 2.5 mg b.i.d. before lunch and dinner. If unable to tolerate 5 mg/day, reduce the dose to 2.5 mg/day as a single evening or bedtime dose. If side effects are absent or minimal and an increased effect is desired, the dose may be increased to 2.5 mg before lunch and 5 mg before dinner (or 5 mg at lunch and 5 mg after dinner). The dose may be increased to 20 mg/day in divided doses. The incidence of side effects increases at higher doses.

How Supplied: *Capsule:* 2.5 mg, 5 mg, 10 mg

Side Effects: *CNS:* Side effects are due mainly to the psychoactive effects of the drug and, in addition to those listed in the preceding, include dizziness, muddled thinking, coordination difficulties, irritability, weakness, headache, ataxia, cannabinoid "high," paresthesia, hallucinations, visual distortions, depersonalization, confusion, nightmares, disorientation, and confusion. *CV:* Palpitations, tachycardia, vasodilation, facial flush, hypotension. *GI:* Abdominal pain, N&V, diarrhea, dry mouth, fecal incontinence, anorexia. *Respiratory:* Cough, rhinitis, sinusitis. *Other:* Asthenia, conjunctivitis, myalgias, tinnitus, speech difficulty, vision difficulties, chills, headache, malaise, sweating, elevated hepatic enzymes.

  Symptoms of Abstinence Syndrome: An abstinence syndrome has been reported following discontinuation of doses greater than 210 mg/day for 12–16 days. Symptoms include irritability, insomnia, and restlessness within 12 hr; within 24 hr, symptoms include "hot flashes," sweating, rhinorrhea, loose stools, hiccoughs, and anorexia. Disturbed sleep may occur for several weeks.

OD Overdose Management: *Symptoms:* Extension of the pharmacologic effects. Symptoms of mild overdose include: drowsiness, euphoria, heightened sensory awareness, altered time perception, reddened conjunctiva, dry mouth, and tachycardia. Symptoms of moderate toxicity include impaired memory, depersonalization, mood alteration, urinary retention, and reduced bowel motility. Severe intoxication includes decreased motor coordination, lethargy, slurred speech, and postural hypotension. Seizures may occur in patients with existing seizure disorders. Hallucinations, psychotic episodes, ***respiratory depression,*** and ***coma*** have been reported. *Treatment:* Patients with depressive, hallucinatory, or psychotic reactions should be placed in a quiet environment and provided supportive treatment, including reassurance. Diazepam (5–10 mg PO) may be used for extreme agitation. Hypotension usually responds to IV fluids and Trendelenburg position. In unconscious patients with a secure airway, administer activated charcoal (30–100 g in adults and 1–2 g/kg in children); this may be followed by a saline cathartic.

Drug Interactions
Amphetamine / Additive hypertension, tachycardia, possibly cardiotoxicity
Anticholinergics / Additive or super-additive tachycardia; drowsiness
CNS depressants / Additive CNS depressant effects
Cocaine / See *Amphetamine*
Antidepressants, tricyclic / Additive tachycardia, hypertension, drowsiness
Ethanol / During subchronic dronabinol use, lower and delayed peak alcohol blood levels
Sympathomimetics / See *Amphetamine*
Theophylline / Possible increased metabolism of theophylline

EMS CONSIDERATIONS
None.

Edetate disodium (EDTA)
(ED-eh-tayt)
Pregnancy Class: C
Disotate, Endrate **(Rx)**
Classification: Heavy metal chelator.

Mechanism of Action: Forms a soluble calcium chelate in the blood which is excreted through the urine. This leads to a lowering of serum calcium and a mobilization of calcium stores, especially from bone. When used to treat digitalis toxicity, edetate disodium exerts a negative inotropic effect on the heart and thus the chronotropic and inotropic effects of digitalis on the heart are antagonized. Also forms chelates with magnesium, zinc, and other trace elements. When used ophthalmically, calcified corneal deposits are dissolved from the conjunctiva, corneal epithelium, and anterior layers of the stroma.

Uses: Hypercalcemia. Ventricular arrhythmias associated with digitalis toxicity. *Investigational:* Ophthalmically to treat corneal calcium deposits, eye burns from calcium hydroxide, and eye injury by zinc chloride.

---

bold italic = life threatening side effect

Contraindications: Anuria. Ventricular arrhythmias. To treat arteriosclerosis, atherosclerotic vascular disease, lead poisoning, or renal calculi by retrograde irrigation.

Precautions: Use during pregnancy only if the benefits clearly outweigh the risks. Use with extreme caution in digitalized patients as EDTA and calcium may reverse the desired effect of digitalis. Use with caaution in patients with heart disease (e.g., CHF) or hypokalemia.

Route/Dosage ─────────

• **IV**

Hypercalcemia, digitalis toxicity.
Individualized and depending on degree of hypercalcemia. **Adults, usual:** 50 mg/kg over 24 hr (up to 3 g/day may be prescribed); dose may be repeated for 5 consecutive days followed by a 2-day rest period with repeated courses, if needed, up to 15 doses. **Pediatric:** 40 mg/kg over 24 hr up to a maximum of 70 mg/kg/day. An alternative dosing regimen is 15–50 mg/kg/day, to a maximum of 3 g/day followed by a 5-day rest period between courses.

• **Ophthalmic**

Calcium deposits, calcium hydroxide burns.
Adults and children: 0.35%–1.85% solution as an irrigation for 15–20 min.

Zinc chloride injury.
Adults and children: 1.7% solution as an irrigation for 15 min.

How Supplied: *Injection:* 150 mg/mL

Side Effects: *Metabolic:* Electrolyte imbalance including hypocalcemia, hypokalemia, hypomagnesemia, hyperuricemia may occur during treatment. *CV:* Decrease in both systolic and diastolic pressure, thrombophlebitis, anemia. *GI:* N&V, diarrhea. *CNS:* Headache, numbness, circumoral paresthesia, fever. *Other:* Exfoliative dermatitis, nephrotoxicity, ***reticuloendothelial system damage with hemorrhagic tendencies. Rapid injection may produce hypocalcemic tetany and convulsions, respiratory arrest, and severe arrhythmias.***

OD **Overdose Management:** *Symptoms:* Precipitous drop in calcium. *Treatment:* IV calcium gluconate which should be available at all times.

EMS CONSIDERATIONS
None.

──────COMBINATION DRUG──────

Edrophonium chloride
Edrophonium chloride and Atropine sulfate
(ed-roh-FOH-nee-um)
Pregnancy Class: C
Edrophonium chloride (Enlon, Reversol, Tensilon **(Rx)**) Edrophonium chloride and Atropine sulfate (Enlon-Plus **(Rx)**)
Classification: Cholinesterase inhibitor, indirectly-acting

Mechanism of Action: Atropine counteracts the muscarinic side effects that will occur due to edrophonium (e.g., increased secretions, bradycardia, bronchoconstriction).
Onset of Action: IV: < 1 min.
Duration of Action: IV: 10 min.
Uses: Edrophonium: Adjunct to treat respiratory depression due to curare and similar nondepolarizing agents such as gallamine, pancuronium, and tubocurarine.

Edrophonium and Atropine: To antagonize or reverse nondepolarizing neuromuscular blocking agents. Adjunct to treat respiratory depression caused by overdosage of curare.
Precautions: Edrophonium combined with atropine is not effective against depolarizing neuromuscular blocking agents.

Route/Dosage ─────────
Curare antagonist.
Slow IV: 10 mg over 30–45 sec to detect onset of cholinergic reaction; repeat if necessary to maximum of 40 mg. Should not be given before use of curare, gallamine, or tubocurarine.
How Supplied: Edrophonium chloride: *Injection:* 10 mg/mL. Edrophonium chloride and Atropine sulfate: *Injection:* 10 mg-0.14 mg/mL

EMS CONSIDERATIONS

See also *Neostigmine* and *Atropine sulfate.*

Administration/Storage

IV 1. Have IV atropine sulfate available to use as an antagonist.

2. When atropine is combined with edrophonium, monitor carefully; assisted or controlled ventilation should be undertaken.

Interventions

1. Monitor closely during administration; effects last up to 30 min.

2. Monitor VS.

3. Document any increased salivation, bronchial spasm, bradycardia, and cardiac arrhythmia; especially important with the elderly.

4. Evaluate respiratory effort and provide assisted ventilation prn.

5. During cholinergic crisis, monitor state of consciousness closely.

Efavirenz

(eh-FAH-vih-rehnz)
Pregnancy Class: C
Sustiva **(Rx)**
Classification: Antiviral drug

Mechanism of Action: A non-nucleoside reverse transcriptase inhibitor of HIV-1. Action is mainly by non-competitive inhibition of HIV-1.

Uses: In combination with other antiretroviral drugs to treat HIV-1 infection.

Contraindications: Use as a single agent to treat HIV or added on as a sole agent to a failing regimen.

Precautions: HIV-infected mothers should not breastfeed to avoid risking postnatal transmission of HIV infection. Use with caution in impaired hepatic function.

Route/Dosage ————————

• **Capsules**

HIV-1 infections.

Adults: 600 mg once daily in combination with a protease inhibitor or nucleoside analog reverse transcriptase inhibitors. **Children, 3 years and older. 10–< 15 kg:** 200 mg

once daily; **15–< 20 kg:** 250 mg once daily; **20–< 25 kg:** 300 mg once daily; **25–< 32.5 kg:** 350 mg once daily; **32.5–< 40 kg:** 400 mg once daily; **40 kg or more:** 600 mg once daily.

How Supplied: *Capsules:* 50 mg, 100 mg, 200 mg

Side Effects: *CNS:* Delusions, inappropriate behavior (especially in those with a history of mental illness or substance abuse), severe acute depression with suicidal ideation/attempts, dizziness, impaired con-centration, somnolence, abnormal dreams, insomnia, fatigue, headache, hypoesthesia, depression, anorexia, nervousness, ataxia, confusion, convulsions, impaired coordination, migraine headaches, neuralgia, paresthesia, peripheral neuropathy, speech disorder, tremor, vertigo, aggravated depression, agitation, amnesia, anxiety, apathy, emotional lability, euphoria, hallucinations, psychosis. *Dermatologic:* Skin rash, including moist or dry desquamation, ulceration, erythema, pruritus, diffuse maculopapular rash, vesiculation, erythema multiforme. Increased sweating, alopecia, eczema, folliculitis, urticaria. Rarely, ***Stevens-Johnson syndrome, toxic epidermal necrolysis,*** necrosis requiring surgery, exfoliative dermatitis. *GI:* N&V, diarrhea, dyspepsia, abdominal pain, flatulence, dry mouth, pancreatitis. *GU:* Hematuria, renal calculus. *CV:* Flushing, palpitations, tachycardia, thrombophlebitis. *Musculoskeletal:* Arthralgia, myalgia. *Ophthalmic:* Abnormal vision, diplopia. *Miscellaneous:* Parosmia, taste perversion, alcohol intolerance, allergic reaction, asthenia, fever, hot flushes, malaise, pain, peripheral edema, syncope, tinnitus, hepatitis, asthma.

OD **Overdose Management:** *Symptoms:* Increased nervous system symptoms. *Treatment:* General supportive measures, including monitoring of vital signs.

Drug Interactions

Astemizole / Inhibition of the metabolism of astemizole → possible

---

cardiac arrhythmias, prolonged sedation, or respiratory depression
Cisapride / Inhibition of the metabolism of cisapride → possible cardiac arrhythmias, prolonged sedation, or respiratory depression
Clarithromycin / ↓ Clarithromycin plasma levels and ↑ levels of metabolite; use alternative therapy such as azithromycin
CNS depressants / Additive CNS depression
Ergot derivatives / Inhibition of the metabolism of ergot derivatives → possible cardiac arrhythmias, prolonged sedation, or respiratory depression
Midazolam / Inhibition of the metabolism of midazolam → possible cardiac arrhythmias, prolonged sedation, or respiratory depression
Ritonavir / Higher frequency of dizziness, nausea, paresthesia, and elevated liver enzymes
Triazolam / Inhibition of the metabolism of triazolam → possible cardiac arrhythmias, prolonged sedation, or respiratory depression

EMS CONSIDERATIONS

See also *Antiviral Agents*.

Emedastine difumarate
(em-eh-DAS-teen)
Pregnancy Class: Pregnancy Class: B
Emadine **(Rx)**
Classification: Antihistamine, ophthalmic

Mechanism of Action: Selective H_1 antagonist which inhibits histamine–stimulated vascular permeability in the conjunctiva. Very little reaches the systemic circulation.
Uses: Relieve signs and symptoms of allergic conjunctivitis.
Contraindications: Parenteral or oral use. Use to treat contact lens-related irritation.
Precautions: Use with caution during lactation. Safety and efficacy have not been established in children less than 3 years of age.

Route/Dosage —————————
• **Solution**

Allergic conjunctivitis.
One drop in the affected eye(s) up to q.i.d.
How Supplied: *Solution:* 0.05%
Side Effects: *Ophthalmic:* Blurred vision, burning or stinging, corneal infiltrates, corneal staining, dry eyes, foreign body sensation, hyperemia, keratitis, tearing. *CNS:* Headache, abnormal dreams. *Respiratory:* Pruritus, rhinitis, sinusitis. *Miscellaneous:* Asthenia, bad taste, dermatitis, discomfort.

EMS CONSIDERATIONS

See also *Antihistamines*.
Administration/Storage: Store at 4°C–30°C (39°F–86°F).
Assessment: Note time of year and events/triggers that surround symptoms.

Enalapril maleate
(en-AL-ah-prill)
Pregnancy Class: D
Vasotec, Vasotec I.V. **(Rx)**
Classification: Angiotensin-converting enzyme inhibitor

Onset of Action: PO: 1 hr; **IV:** 15 min. **Time to peak action, PO:** 4-6 hr; **IV:** 1-4 hr.
Duration of Action: PO: 24 hr; **IV:** About 6 hr.
Uses: Alone or in combination with a thiazide diuretic for the treatment of hypertension (step I therapy). As adjunct with digitalis and diuretic in acute and chronic CHF. *Investigational:* Hypertension in children, hypertension related to scleroderma renal crisis, diabetic nephropathy, asymptomatic left ventricular dysfunction following MI. Enalaprilat may be used for hypertensive emergencies (effect is variable).
Precautions: Use with caution during lactation. Safety and effectiveness have not been determined in children.

Route/Dosage —————————
• **Tablets (Enalapril)**
Antihypertensive in patients not taking diuretics.

Initial: 5 mg/day; **then,** adjust dosage according to response (range: 10–40 mg/day in one to two doses).

Antihypertensive in patients taking diuretics.

Initial: 2.5 mg. Since hypotension may occur following the initiation of enalapril, the diuretic should be discontinued, if possible, for 2–3 days before initiating enalapril. If BP is not maintained with enalapril alone, diuretic therapy may be resumed.

Adjunct with diuretics and digitalis in heart failure.

Initial: 2.5 mg 1–2 times/day; **then,** depending on the response, 5–20 mg/day in two divided doses. Dose should not exceed 40 mg/day. Dosage must be adjusted in patients with renal impairment or hyponatremia.

In patients with impaired renal function.

Initial: 5 mg/day if C_{CR} ranges between 30 and 80 mL/min and serum creatinine is less than 3 mg/dL; 2.5 mg/day if C_{CR} is less than 30 mL/min and serum creatinine is more than 3 mg/dL and in dialysis patients on dialysis days.

Renal impairment or hyponatremia.

Initial: 2.5 mg/day if serum sodium is less than 130 mEq/L and serum creatinine is more than 1.6 mg/dL. The dose may be increased to 2.5 mg b.i.d. and then 5 mg b.i.d. or higher if required; dose is given at intervals of 4 or more days. Maximum daily dose is 40 mg.

Asymptomatic LV dysfunction following MI.

2.5–20 mg/day beginning 72 hr or longer after onset of MI. Therapy is continued for 1 year or longer.

NOTE: Dosage should be decreased in patients with a C_{CR} less than 30 mL/min and a serum creatinine level greater than 3 mg/dL.

• **IV (Enalaprilat)**

Hypertension.

1.25 mg over a 5-min period; repeat q 6 hr.

Antihypertensive in patients taking diuretics.

Initial: 0.625 mg over 5 min; if an adequate response is seen after 1 hr, administer another 0.625-mg dose. Thereafter, 1.25 mg q 6 hr.

Patients with impaired renal function.

Give enalaprit, 1.25 mg q 6 hr for patients with a C_{CR} more than 30 mL/min and an initial dose of 0.625 mg for patients with a C_{CR} less than 30 mL/min. If there is an adequate response, an additional 0.625 mg may be given after 1 hr; thereafter, additional 1.25-mg doses can be given q 6 hr. For dialysis patients, the initial dose is 0.625 mg q 6 hr.

How Supplied: *Tablet:* 2.5 mg, 5 mg, 10 mg, 20 mg; *Injection:* 1.25 mg/mL

Side Effects: *CV:* Palpitations, hypotension, chest pain, angina, **CVA, MI,** orthostatic hypotension, disturbances in rhythm, tachycardia, **cardiac arrest,** orthostatic effects, atrial fibrillation, tachycardia, bradycardia, Raynaud's phenomenon. *GI:* N&V, diarrhea, abdominal pain, alterations in taste, anorexia, dry mouth, constipation, dyspepsia, glossitis, ileus, melena, stomatitis. *CNS:* Insomnia, headache, fatigue, dizziness, paresthesias, nervousness, sleepiness, ataxia, confusion, depression, vertigo, abnormal dreams. *Hepatic:* Hepatitis, hepatocellular or cholestatic jaundice, pancreatitis, elevated liver enzymes, hepatic failure. *Respiratory:* Bronchitis, cough, dyspnea, bronchospasm, URI, pneumonia, pulmonary infiltrates, asthma, **pulmonary embolism and infarction, pulmonary edema.** *Renal:* Renal dysfunction, oliguria, UTI, transient increases in creatinine and BUN. *Hematologic:* Rarely, neutropenia, thrombocytopenia, bone marrow depression, decreased H&H in hypertensive or CHF patients. Hemolytic anemia, including hemolysis, in patients with G6PD deficiency. *Dermatologic:* Rash, pruritus, alopecia, flushing, erythema multiforme, exfoliative dermatitis, photosensitivity, urticaria, increased sweating, pemphi-

---

bold italic = life threatening side effect

gus, **Stevens-Johnson syndrome,** herpes zoster, toxic epidermal necrolysis. *Other:* Angioedema, asthenia, impotence, blurred vision, fever, arthralgia, arthritis, vasculitis, eosinophilia, tinnitus, syncope, myalgia, muscle cramps, rhinorrhea, sore throat, hoarseness, conjunctivitis, tearing, dry eyes, loss of sense of smell, hearing loss, peripheral neuropathy, anosmia, myositis, flank pain, gynecomastia.

EMS CONSIDERATIONS

None.

————COMBINATION DRUG————

Enalapril maleate and Hydrochlorothiazide

(en-AL-ah-prill, high-droh-KLORoh-THIGH-ah-zyd)
Pregnancy Class: D
Vaseretic **(Rx)**
Classification: Antihypertensive

Uses: Combination therapy for hypertension.
Contraindications: Use for initial therapy of hypertension. Anuria or severe renal dysfunction. History of angioedema related to use of ACE inhibitors. Lactation.
Precautions: Excessive hypotension may be observed in patients with severe salt or volume depletion such as those treated with diuretics or on dialysis. Significant hypotension may also be seen with severe CHF, with or without associated renal insufficiency. A significant fall in BP may result in MI or CVA in patients with ischemic heart or cerebrovascular disease. Safety and effectiveness have not been established in children.

Route/Dosage ————————
• **Tablets**
Adults: 1–2 tablets once daily.
How Supplied: *ACE inhibitor:* Enalapril, 5 mg or 10 mg. *Diuretic:* Hydrochlorothiazide, 12.5 mg or 25 mg.

EMS CONSIDERATIONS

See also *Enalapril maleate.*

Enoxacin

(ee-NOX-ah-sin)
Pregnancy Class: C
Penetrex **(Rx)**
Classification: Antibacterial, fluoroquinolone derivative

Uses: To treat uncomplicated urethral or cervical gonorrhea due to *Neisseria gonorrhoeae.* To treat uncomplicated UTIs due *Escherichia coli, Staphylococcus epidermidis,* or *S. saprophyticus;* for complicated UTIs due to *E. coli, Klebsiella pneumoniae, Proteus mirabilis, Pseudomonas aeruginosa, S. epidermidis,* or *Enterobacter cloacae.* Not effective for syphilis.
Contraindications: Lactation.
Precautions: Safety and efficacy have not been determined in children less than 18 years of age. dosage adjustment is not required in elderly patients with normal renal function. Not efficiently removed by hemodialysis or peritoneal dialysis.

Route/Dosage ————————
• **Tablets**
Uncomplicated gonorrhea.
Adults: 400 mg for one dose.
Uncomplicated UTIs, cystitis.
Adults: 200 mg q 12 hr for 7 days.
Complicated UTIs.
Adults: 400 mg q 12 hr for 14 days.
How Supplied: *Tablet:* 200 mg, 400 mg
Side Effects: Additional: *GI:* Anorexia, bloody stools, gastritis, stomatitis. *CNS:* Confusion, nervousness, anxiety, tremor, agitation, myoclonus, depersonalization, hypertonia. *Dermatologic:* Toxic epidermal necrolysis, **Stevens-Johnson syndrome,** urticaria, hyperhidrosis, mycotic infection, erythema multiforme. *CV:* Palpitation, tachycardia, vasodilation, *Respiratory:* Dyspnea, cough, epistaxis. *GU:* Vaginal moniliasis, urinary incontinence, renal failure. *Hematologic:* Eosinophilia, leukipenia, increased or decreased platelets, decreased hemoglobin, leukocytosis. *Miscellaneous:* Glucosuria, pyuria, increased or decreased potassium, asthenia, back or chest pain, myalgia,

arthralgia, purpura, vertigo, unusual taste, tinnitus, conjunctivitis.

Drug Interactions: Additional: *Bismuth subsalicylate/* Bioavailability of enoxacin is ↓ when bismuth subsalicylate is given within 1 hr; should not use together. *Digoxin/* ↓ Serum digoxin levels.

EMS CONSIDERATIONS

None.

Enoxaparin injection

(ee-nox-ah-PAIR-in)
Pregnancy Class: B
Lovenox, Lovenox Easy Injector **(Rx)**
Classification: Anticoagulant, low molecular weight heparin

Uses: Acute (in the hospital) and extended (at home for up to three weeks) prophylaxis of DVT, which may lead to pulmonary embolism, after hip or knee replacement surgery or abdominal surgery in those at risk for thromboembolic complications. With aspirin to prevent ischemic complications of unstable angina and non-Q-wave MI. *Investigational:* Systemic anticoagulation, secondary prophylaxis for thromboembolic recurrence.

Contraindications: In patients with active major bleeding; thrombocytopenia associated with a positive in vitro test for antiplatelet antibody in the presence of enoxaparin; or in those with hypersensitivity to enoxaparin, heparin, or pork products. IM use. Interchangeable (unit for unit) use with unfractionated heparin or other low molecular weight heparins.

Precautions: Use with caution during lactation and in patients with a bleeding diathesis, uncontrolled arterial hypertension, a history of recent GI ulceration and hemorrhage, or in patients receiving oral anticoagulants and/or platelet inhibitors. Use with extreme caution in patients with a history of heparin-induced thrombocytopenia and in conditions with increased risk of hemorrhage

(e.g., bacterial endocarditis, congenital or acquired bleeding disorders, active ulcer and angiodysplastic GI disease, hemorrhagic stroke, or shortly after brain, spinal, or ophthalmic surgery). Elderly patients and those with renal insufficiency may have delayed elimination of the drug. Safety and efficacy have not been determined in children.

E

Route/Dosage
• **SC**
Patients undergoing hip or knee replacement.
Adults: 30 mg b.i.d. with the initial dose given not more than 24 hr after surgery for 7–10 days (usually).
Abdominal surgery.
Adults: 40 mg once daily, with the initial dose given 2 hr prior to surgery.
Duration: 7–10 days, up to 12 days.
Systemic anticoagulation.
1 mg/kg b.i.d.
Thromboembolic recurrence/prophylaxis.
40 mg once daily.
Long-term prophylaxis of DVT following hip replacement
40 mg once daily.
How Supplied: *Injection:* 30 mg/ 0.3 mL, 40 mg/0.4 mL, 60 mg/0.6 mL, 80 mg/0.8 mL, 100 mg/mL

Side Effects: *Hematologic:* Thrombocytopenia, thrombocythemia, *hemorrhage,* hypochromic anemia, ecchymosis. *At site of injection:* Mild local irritation, pain, hematoma, erythema. *GI:* Nausea. *CNS:* Confusion. *Miscellaneous:* Fever, pain, edema, peripheral edema, spinal hematoma.

OD Overdose Management: *Symptoms: Hemorrhagic complications. Treatment:* Slow IV injection of protamine sulfate (1% solution). Give 1 mg protamine sulfate to neutralize 1 mg enoxaparin injection. A second infusion of 0.5 mg protamine sulfate may be given if the APTT measured 2–4 hr after the first infusion remains prolonged. However, even with higher doses of protamine sulfate, the APTT may remain more prolonged than under normal condi-

---

bold italic = life threatening side effect

tions. Take care to avoid overdosage with protamine sulfate.

EMS CONSIDERATIONS

See also *Anticoagulants*.

Entacapone
(en-TAH-kah-pohn)
Pregnancy Class: C
Comtan (Rx)
Classification: Antiparkinson drug

Mechanism of Action: A selective and reversible catechol-O-methyltransferase (COMT) inhibitor. COMT eliminates catechols (e.g., dopa, dopamine, norepinephrine, epinephrine) and in the presence of a decarboxylase inhibitor (e.g., carbidopa), COMT becomes the major metabolizing enzyme for dopa. Thus, in the presence of a COMT inhibitior, levels of dopa and dopamine increase. When entacapone is given with levodopa and carbidopa, plasma levels of levodopa are greater and more sustained than after levodopa/carbidopa alone. This leads to more constant dopaminergic stimulation in the brain resulting in improvement of the signs and symptoms of Parkinson's disease.

Uses: As an adjunct to levodopa/carbidopa to treat idiopathic Parkinsonism patients who experience signs and symptoms of end-of-dose "wearing-off."

Contraindications: Concomitant use with a nonselective MAO inhibitor (e.g., phenelzine, tranylcypromine).

Precautions: Use with caution during lactation and in patients with biliary obstruction. At the present, there is no potential use in children. Use with caution with drugs known to be metabolized by COMT (e.g., apomorphine, bitolterol, dobutamine, dopamine, epinephrine, isoetharine, isoproterenol, methyldopa, norepinephrine) due to the possibility of increased HRs, arrhythmias, and excessive changes in BP.

Route/Dosage
• **Tablets**

Parkinsonism.
200 mg given concomitantly with each levodopa/carbidopa dose up to a maximum of 8 times/day (i.e., 1,600 mg/day).

How Supplied: *Tablets:* 200 mg

Side Effects: *CNS:* Dyskinesia, hyperkinesia, hypokinesia, dizziness, anxiety, somnolence, agitation, hallucinations. *GI:* Nausea, diarrhea, abdominal pain, constipation, vomiting, dry mouth, dyspepsia, flatulence, gastritis, GI disorder. *Body as a whole:* Fatigue, asthenia, increased sweating, bacterial infection. *Miscellaneous:* Urine discoloration, back pain, dsypnea, purpura, taste perversion, rhabdomyolysis.

OD Overdose Management: *Symptoms:* Abdominal pain, loose stools. *Treatment:* Symptomatic with supportive care. Consider hospitalization. Monitor respiratory and circulatory systems. Review for possible drug interactions.

Drug Interactions
Ampicillin / ↓ Biliary excretion of entacapone
Apomorphine / Possible ↑ HR, arrhythmias, and excessive changes in BP
Bitolterol / Possible ↑ HR, arrhythmias, and excessive changes in BP
Chloramphenicol / ↓ Biliary excretion of entacapone
Cholestyramine / ↓ Biliary excretion of entacapone
Dobutamine / Possible ↑ HR, arrhythmias, and excessive changes in BP
Dopamine / Possible ↑ HR, arrhythmias, and excessive changes in BP
Epinephrine / Possible ↑ HR, arrhythmias, and excessive changes in BP
Erythromycin / ↓ Biliary excretion of entacapone
Isoetharine / Possible ↑ HR, arrhythmias, and excessive changes in BP
Isoproterenol / Possible ↑ HR, arrhythmias, and excessive changes in BP
MAO inhibitors (phenylzine, tranylcypromine) / Significant ↑ levels of catecholamines

Methyldopa / Possible ↑ HR, arrhythmias, and excessive changes in BP

Norepinephrine / Possible ↑ HR, arrhythmias, and excessive changes in BP

Probenecid / ↓ Biliary excretion of entacapone

Rifamipicin / ↓ Biliary excretion of entacapone

EMS CONSIDERATIONS
None.

Ephedrine sulfate
(eh-FED-rin)
Pregnancy Class: C
Nasal decongestants: Kondon's Nasal, Pretz-D, Vatronol Nose Drops
(OTC). Systemic: Ephed II (**RX:** injection; **OTC:** Oral dosage forms)
Classification: Adrenergic agent, direct- and indirect-acting

Mechanism of Action: Releases norepinephrine from synaptic storage sites. Has direct effects on alpha, beta-1, and beta-2 receptors, causing increased BP due to arteriolar constriction and cardiac stimulation, bronchodilation, relaxation of GI tract smooth muscle, nasal decongestion, mydriasis, and increased tone of the bladder trigone and vesicle sphincter. It may also increase skeletal muscle strength, especially in myasthenia patients. Significant CNS effects include stimulation of the cerebral cortex and subcortical centers. Hepatic glycogenolysis is increased, but not as much as with epinephrine. More stable and longer-lasting than epinephrine.

Onset of Action: IM: 10-20 min; **PO:** 15-60 min; **SC:** < 20 min.

Duration of Action: IM, SC: 30-60 min; **PO:** 3-5 hr.

Uses: Bronchial asthma and reversible bronchospasms associated with obstructive pulmonary diseases. Nasal congestion in vasomotor rhinitis, acute sinusitis, hay fever, and acute coryza. Parenterally to treat narcolepsy and depression and as a vasopressor to treat shock. In acute hypotension states, especially that associated with spinal anesthesia and Stokes-Adams syndrome with complete heart block.

Contraindications: Additional: Angle closure glaucoma, anesthesia with cyclopropane or halothane, thyrotoxicosis, diabetes, obstetrics where maternal BP is greater than 130/80. Lactation.

Precautions: Geriatric patients may be at higher risk to develop prostatic hypertrophy. May cause hypertension resulting in intracranial hemorrhage or anginal pain in patients with coronary insufficiency or ischemic heart disease.

Route/Dosage
- **Capsules**
  Bronchodilator, systemic nasal decongestant, CNS stimulant.
Adults: 25–50 mg q 3–4 hr. **Pediatric:** 3 mg/kg (100 mg/m^2) daily in four to six divided doses.
- **SC, IM, Slow IV**
  Bronchodilator.
Adults: 12.5–25 mg; subsequent doses determined by patient response. **Pediatric:** 3 mg/kg (100 mg/m^2) daily divided into four to six doses SC or IV.
  Vasopressor.
Adults: 25–50 mg (IM or SC) or 5–25 mg (by slow IV push) repeated at 5- to 10-min intervals, if necessary. Absorption following IM is more rapid than following SC use. **Pediatric (IM):** 16.7 mg/m^2 q 4–6 hr.
- **Topical (0.25% Spray)**
  Nasal decongestant.
Adults and children over 6 years: 2–3 gtt of solution or small amount of jelly in each nostril q 4 hr. Do not use topically for more than 3 or 4 consecutive days. Do not use in children under 6 years of age unless ordered by provider.

How Supplied: *Capsule:* 24.3 mg, 25 mg, 50 mg; *Injection:* 50 mg/mL; *Spray:* 0.25%

Side Effects: Additional: *CNS:* Nervousness, shakiness, confusion, delir-

E

---

bold italic = life threatening side effect

ium, hallucinations. Anxiety and nervousness following prolonged use. *CV:* Precordial pain, **excessive doses may cause hypertension sufficient to result in cerebral hemorrhage.** *GU:* Difficult and painful urination, urinary retention in males with prostatism, decrease in urine formation. *Miscellaneous:* Pallor, respiratory difficulty, hypersensitivity reactions. *Abuse:* Prolonged abuse can cause an anxiety state, including symptoms of paranoid schizophrenia, tachycardia, poor nutrition and hygiene, dilated pupils, cold sweat, and fever.

Drug Interactions: Additional: *Dexamethasone/* Ephedrine ↓ effect of dexamethasone*Diuretics/* Diuretics ↓ response to sympathomimetics*Furazolidone/* ↑ Pressor effect → possible hypertensive crisis and intracranial hemorrhage*Guanethidine/* ↓ Effect of guanethidine by displacement from its site of action*Halothane/* Serious arrhythmias due to sensitization of the myocardium to sympathomimetics by halothane*MAO Inhibitors/* ↑ Pressor effect → possible hypertensive crisis and intracranial hemorrhage*Methyldopa/* Effect of ephedrine ↓ in methyldopa-treated patients*Oxytocic drugs/* Severe persistent hypertension

EMS CONSIDERATIONS

See also *Sympathomimetic Drugs.*
Administration/Storage
IV 1. May administer 10 mg IV undiluted over at least 1 min.
2. Use only clear solutions. Protect against exposure to light.
Assessment: Assess mental status and pulmonary function; monitor ECG and VS. If administered for hypotension, monitor BP until stabilized.

Epinephrine
Epinephrine bitartrate
Epinephrine borate
Epinephrine hydrochloride
(ep-ih-NEF-rin)

Pregnancy Class: C
Epinephrine (Adrenalin Chloride Solution, Bronkaid Mist, Epi E-Z Pen, Epi E-Z Pen Jr., Epipen, Epipen Jr., Primatene Mist Solution, Sus-Phrine (Both **Rx** and **OTC**)) Epinephrine bitartrate (Asthmahaler Mist, Bronitin Mist, Bronkaid Mist Suspension, Epitrate, Primatene Mist Suspension **(OTC)**) Epinephrine hydrochloride (Adrenalin Chloride, AsthmaNefrin, Epifrin, Glaucon, microNefrin, Nephron, S-2 Inhalant, Vaponefrin (Both **Rx** and **OTC**))
Classification: Adrenergic agent, direct-acting

Mechanism of Action: Causes marked stimulation of alpha, beta-1, and beta-2 receptors, causing sympathomimetic stimulation, pressor effects, cardiac stimulation, bronchodilation, and decongestion. **Extreme caution must be taken never to inject 1:100 solution intended for inhalation—injection of this concentration has caused death.**
Onset of Action: SC: 6-15 min, **IM:** variable, **Inhalation:** 1-5 min.
Duration of Action: SC: <1-4 hr, **IM:** <1-4 hr, **Inhalation:** 1-3 hr.
Uses: Cardiac arrest, Stokes-Adams syndrome, low CO following ECB. To prolong the action of local anesthetics. As a hemostatic during ocular surgery; treatment of conjunctival congestion during surgery; to induce mydriasis during surgery; treat ocular hypertension during surgery. Topically to control bleeding. Acute bronchial asthma, bronchospasms due to emphysema, chronic bronchitis, or other pulmonary diseases. Treatment of anaphylaxis, angioedema, anaphylactic shock, drug-induced allergic reactions, transfusion reactions, insect bites or stings. As an adjunct in the treatment of open-angle glaucoma (may be used with miotics, beta blockers, hyperosmotic agents, or carbonic anhydrase inhibitors). To produce mydriasis; to treat conjunctivitis. *NOTE:* Autoinjectors are available for emergency self-administration of first aid for anaphylactic reactions due to insect stings or bites, foods, drugs, and other allergens as well as idiopathic or exercise-induced anaphylaxis.

Contraindications: Additional: Narrow-angle glaucome. Use when wearing soft contact lenses (may discolor lenses). Aphakia. Lactation.
Precautions: May cause anoxia in the fetus. Safety and efficacy of ophthalmic products have not been determined in children; administer parenteral epinephrine to children with caution. Syncope may occur if epinephrine is given to asthmatic children. Administeration of the SC injection by the IV route may cause severe or fatal hypertension or cerbrovascular hemorrhage. Epinephrine may temporarily increase the rigidity and tremor of parkinsonism. Use with caution and in small quantities in the toes, fingers, nose, ears, and genitals or in the presence of peripheral vascular disease as vasoconstriction-induced tissue sloughing may occur.

Route/Dosage
• **Metered Dose Inhaler**
Bronchodilation.
Adults and children over 4 years of age: 0.2–0.275 mg (1 inhalation) of the Aerosol or 0.16 mg (1 inhalation) of the Bitartrate Aerosol; may be repeated after 1–2 min if needed. At least 3 hr should elapse before subsequent doses. Dosage not established in children less than 4 years of age.
• **Inhalation Solution**
Bronchodilation.
Adults and children over 6 years of age: 1 inhalation of the 1% solution (of the base); may be repeated after 1–2 min.
• **IM, IV, SC**
Bronchodilation using the solution (1:1,000).
Adults: 0.3–0.5 mg SC or IM repeated q 20 min–4 hr as needed; dose may be increased to 1 mg/dose. **Infants and children (except premature infants and full-term newborns):** 0.01 mg/kg (0.3 mg/m²) SC up to a maximum of 0.5 mg/dose; may be repeated q 15 min for two doses and then q 4 hr as needed.

Bronchodilation using the sterile suspension (1:200).
Adults: 0.5–1.5 mg SC. **Infants and children, 1 month–12 years:** 0.025 mg/kg SC; **children less than 30 kg:** 0.75 mg as a single dose.
Anaphylaxis.
Adults: 0.2–0.5 mg SC q 10–15 min as needed, up to a maximum of 1 mg/dose if needed. **Pediatric:** 0.01 mg/kg (0.3 mg/m²) up to a maximum of 0.5 mg/dose; may be repeated q 15 min for two doses and then q 4 hr as needed.
• **Autoinjector, IM**
First aid for anaphylaxis.
The autoinjectors deliver a single dose of either 0.3 mg or 0.15 mg (for children) of epinephrine. In cases of a severe reaction, repeat injections may be necessary.
Vasopressor.
Adults, IM or SC, initial: 0.5 mg repeated q 5 min if needed; **then,** give 0.025–0.050 mg IV q 5–15 min as needed. **Adults, IV, initial:** 0.1–0.25 mg given slowly. May be repeated q 5–15 min as needed. Or, use IV infusion beginning with 0.001 mg/min and increasing the dose to 0.004 mg/min if needed. **Pediatric, IM, SC:** 0.01 mg/kg, up to a maximum of 0.3 mg repeated q 5 min if needed. **Pediatric, IV:** 0.01 mg/kg/5–15 min if an inadequate response to IM or SC administration is observed.
Cardiac stimulant.
Adults, intracardiac or IV: 0.1–1 mg repeated q 5 min if needed. **Pediatric, intracardiac or IV:** 0.005–0.01 mg/kg (0.15–0.3 mg/m²) repeated q 5 min if needed; this may be followed by IV infusion beginning at 0.0001 mg/kg/min and increased in increments of 0.0001 mg/kg/min up to a maximum of 0.0015 mg/kg/min.
Adjunct to local anesthesia.
Adults and children: 0.1–0.2 mg in a 1:200,000–1:20,000 solution.
Adjunct with intraspinal anesthetics.
Adults: 0.2–0.4 mg added to the anesthetic spinal fluid.

E

---
bold italic = life threatening side effect

- **Solution**

Antihemorrhagic, mydriatic.

Adults and children, intracameral or subconjunctival: 0.01%–0.1% solution.

Topical antihemorrhagic.

Adults and children: 0.002%–0.1% solution.

Nasal decongestant.

Adults and children over 6 years of age: Apply 0.1% solution as drops or spray or with a sterile swab as needed.

- **Borate Ophthalmic Solution, Hydrochloride Ophthalmic Solution**

Glaucoma.

Adults: 1–2 gtt into affected eye(s) 1–2 times/day. Determine frequency of use by tonometry. Dosage has not been established in children.

How Supplied: Epinephrine: *Metered dose inhaler:* 0.22 mg/inh; *Injection:* 1 mg/mL, 5 mg/mL; *Kit:* 0.5 mg/mL, 1 mg/mL; Epinephrine bitartrate: *Metered dose inhaler:* 0.3 mg/inh; Epinephrine hydrochloride: *Injection:* 0.1 mg/mL, 1 mg/mL; *Solution:* 1:100, 1:1000; *Ophthalmic solution:* 0.5%, 1%, 2%

Side Effects: Additional: *CV:* **Fatal ventricular fibrillation, cerebral or subarachnoid hemorrhage,** obstruction of central retinal artery. **A rapid and large increase in BP may cause aortic rupture, cerebral hemorrhage, or angin pectoris.** *GU:* Decreased urine formation, urinary retention, painful urination. *CNS:* Anxiety, fear, pallor. Parenteral use may cause or aggravate disorientation, memory impairment, psychomotor agitation, panic, hallucinations, **suicidal or homicidal tendencies,** schizophrenic-type behavior. *Miscellaneous:* Prolonged use or overdose may cause elevated serum lactic acid with severe metabolic acidosis. *At injection site:* Bleeding, urticaria, wheal formation, pain. Repeated injections at the same site may cause necrosis from vascular constriction. *Ophthalmic:* Transient stinging or burning when administered, conjunctival hyperemia, brow ache, headache, blurred vision, photophobia, allergic lid reaction, ocular hypersensitivity, poor night vision, eye ache, eye pain. Prolonged ophthalmic use may cause deposits of pigment in the cornea, lids, or conjunctiva. When used for glaucoma in aphakic patients, reversible cystoid macular edema.

Drug Interactions: Additional: *Beta-adrenergic blocking agents/* Initial effectiveness in treating glaucoma of this combination may ↓ over time- *Chymotrypsin /* Epinephrine, 1:100, will inactivate chymotrypsin in 60 min.

EMS CONSIDERATIONS

See also *Sympathomimetic Drugs.*
Administration/Storage
1. Briskly massage site of SC or IM injection to hasten drug action. Do not expose to heat, light, or air, as this causes deterioration of the drug.
2. Discard solution if reddish brown and after expiration date.
IV 3. *Never administer* 1:100 solution IV. Use 1:1,000 solution for IV administration.
4. Use a tuberculin syringe to measure.
5. For direct IV administration to adults, the drug must be well diluted as a 1:1,000 solution; inject quantities of 0.05–0.1 mL of solution cautiously taking about 1 min for each injection; note response (BP and pulse). Dose may be repeated several times if necessary. May be further diluted in D5W or NSS.
Assessment
1. During IV therapy, continuously monitor ECG, BP, and pulse until desired effect achieved. Then take VS every 2–5 min until condition has stabilized; once stable, monitor BP q 15–30 min.
2. Note any symptoms of shock such as cold, clammy skin, cyanosis, and loss of consciousness.

Epoetin alfa recombinant
(ee-POH-ee-tin)
Pregnancy Class: C

Epogen, Procrit **(Rx)**
Classification: Recombinant human erythropoietin

Mechanism of Action: A 165-amino-acid glycoprotein made by recombinant DNA technology; it has the identical amino acid sequence and same biologic effects as endogenous erythropoietin (which is normally synthesized in the kidney and stimulates RBC production). Epoetin alfa will elevate or maintain the RBC level, decreasing the need for blood transfusions.

Uses: Treatment of anemia associated with chronic renal failure, including patients on dialysis (end-stage renal disease) or not on dialysis. AZT-induced anemia in HIV-infected patients. Treatment of anemia in patients with nonmyeloid malignancies (Procrit only). Reduce allogeneic blood transfusions in surgery patients. *Investigational:* Pruritus associated with renal failure.

Contraindications: Uncontrolled hypertension. Hypersensitivity to mammalian cell-derived products or to human albumin. Use in chronic renal failure patients who need severe anemia corrected. To treat anemia in HIV-infected or cancer patients due to factors such as iron or folate deficiencies, hemolysis, or GI bleeding. Anemic patients willing to donate autologous blood.

Precautions: Safety and efficacy have not been established in children or in patients with a history of seizures or underlying hematologic disease (e.g., hypercoagulable disorders, myelodysplastic syndromes, sickle cell anemia). Use with caution in patients with porphyria, during lactation, and preexisting vascular disease. Increased anticoagulation with heparin may be required in patients on epoetin alfa undergoing hemodialysis.

Route/Dosage

• **IV, SC**
  Chronic renal failure.

IV, initial (dialysis or nondialysis patients), SC (nondialysis patients), initial: 50–100 U/kg 3 times/week. The rate of increase of hematocrit depends on both dosage and patient variation. **Maintenance:** Individualize (usual: 25 U/kg 3 times/week). However, doses of 75–150 U/kg/week have maintained hematocrits of 36%–38% for up to 6 months in nondialysis patients.

AZT-treated, HIV infections.

IV, SC, initial: 100 U/kg 3 times/week for 8 weeks (in patients with serum erythropoietin levels less than or equal to 500 mU/mL who are receiving less than or equal to 4,200 mg/week of AZT). If a satisfactory response is obtained, the dose can be increased by 50–100 U/kg 3 times/week. Evaluate the response q 4–8 weeks thereafter with dosage adjusted by 50–100 U/kg increments 3 times/week. If patients have not responded to 300 U/kg 3 times/week, it is likely they will not respond to higher doses.

Cancer patients on chemotherapy (Procrit only).

Initial, SC: 150 units/kg 3 times/week. Treatment of patients with highly elevated erythropoetin levels (> 200 mU/mL) is not recommended. If response is not satisfactory after 8 wks, the dose may be increased up to 300 units/kg 3 times/week. Patients not responding at this level are not likely to respond at higher levels. If the hematocrit exceeds 40%, withhold the dose until the hematocrit falls to 36%. When treatment is resumed, reduce the dose by 25%.

NOTE: Individualize the dose for patients on dialysis. The median dose is 75 units/kg 3 times/week (range 12.5–525 units/kg 3 times/week).

Surgery to reduce allogeneic blood transfusions.

SC: 300 U/kg/day for 10 days before surgery, on the day of surgery, and for 4 days after surgery. Alternative: 600 U/kg SC once a week 21, 14, and 7 days before surgery plus a fourth dose on the day of surgery. Iron

E

---

bold italic = life threatening side effect

supplementation is required at the time of epoetin therapy and continuing throughout the course of therapy.

How Supplied: *Injection:* 2,000 U/mL, 3,000 U/mL, 4,000 U/mL, 10,000 U/mL, 20,000 U/mL

Side Effects: In Chronic Renal Failure Patients (symptoms may be due to the disease). *CV:* Hypertension, tachycardia, edema, *MI, CV accident,* TIA, clotted vascular access. *CNS:* Headache, fatigue, dizziness, *seizures. GI:* Nausea, diarrhea, vomiting, worsening of porphyria. *Allergic reactions:* Skin rashes, urticaria, *anaphylaxis. Miscellaneous:* SOB, hyperkalemia, arthralgias, myalgia, chest pain, skin reaction at administration site, asthenia.

In AZT-Treated HIV-Infected Patients. *CNS:* Pyrexia, headache, dizziness, *seizures. Respiratory:* Cough, respiratory congestion, SOB. *GI:* Diarrhea, nausea. *Miscellaneous:* Rash, asthenia, reaction at injection site, allergic reactions.

In Cancer Patients. *CNS:* Pyrexia, fatigue, dizziness. *GI:* Diarrhea, nausea, vomiting. *Musculoskeletal:* Asthenia, paresthesia, trunk pain. *Miscellaneous:* Edema, SOB, URI.

In Surgery Patients. *CNS:* Pyrexia, insomnia, headache, dizziness, anxiety. *GI:* N&V, constipation, diarrhea, dyspepsia. *CV:* Hypertension, DVT, edema. *Miscellaneous:* Reaction at injection site, skin pain, pruritus, UTI.

OD **Overdose Management:** *Symptoms:* Polycythemia. *Treatment:* Withhold drug until hematocrit returns to the target range.

EMS CONSIDERATIONS

None.

Epoprostenol sodium
(eh-poh-PROST-en-ohl)
Pregnancy Class: B
Flolan **(Rx)**
Classification: Antihypertensive, miscellaneous

Mechanism of Action: Acts by direct vasodilation of pulmonary and systemic arterial vascular beds and by inhibition of platelet aggregation. IV infusion in patients with pulmonary hypertension results in increases in cardiac index and SV and decreases in pulmonary vascular resistance, total pulmonary resistance, and mean systemic arterial pressure.

Uses: Long-term IV treatment of primary pulmonary hypertension in New York Heart Association Class III and Class IV patients.

Contraindications: Chronic use in those with CHF due to severe LV systolic dysfunction and in those who develop pulmonary edema during dose ranging.

Precautions: Abrupt withdrawal or sudden large decreases in the dose may cause rebound pulmonary hypertension. Use caution in dose selection in the elderly due to the greater frequency of decreased hepatic, renal, or cardiac function, as well as concomitant disease or other drug therapy. Use with caution during lactation. Safety and efficacy have not been determined in children.

Route/Dosage ─────────
* **Chronic IV Infusion**
  Pulmonary hypertension.

Acute dose ranging: The initial chronic infusion rate is first determined. The mean maximum dose that did not elicit dose-limiting pharmacologic effects was 8.6 ng/kg/min. **Continuous chronic infusion, initial:** 4 ng/kg/min less than the maximum-tolerated infusion rate determined during acute dose ranging. If the maximum-tolerated infusion rate is less than 5 ng/kg/min, start the chronic infusion at one-half the maximum-tolerated infusion rate.

Dosage adjustments: Changes in the chronic infusion rate are based on persistence, recurrence, or worsening of the symptoms of primary pulmonary hypertension. If symptoms require an increase in infusion rate, increase by 1–2 ng/kg/min at intervals (at least 15 min) sufficient to allow assessment of the clinical response. If a decrease in infusion rate is necessary, gradually make 2-ng/kg/min decrements every 15 min or longer until the dose-limiting effects resolve. Avoid abrupt withdrawal or sudden large reductions in infusion rates.

How Supplied: *Powder for injection:* 0.5 mg, 1.5 mg

Side Effects: Side effects have been classified as those occurring during acute dose ranging, those as a result of the drug delivery system, and those occurring during chronic dosing.

Those occurring during acute dose ranging. *CV:* Flushing, hypotension, bradycardia, tachycardia. *GI:* N&V, abdominal pain, dyspepsia. *CNS:* Headache, anxiety, nervousness, agitation, dizziness, hypesthesia, paresthesia. *Miscellaneous:* Chest pain, musculoskeletal pain, dyspnea, back pain, sweating.

Those occurring as a result of the drug delivery system. *Due to the chronic indwelling catheter:* Local infection, pain at the injection site, sepsis, infections.

Those occurring during chronic dosing. *CV:* Flushing, tachycardia. *GI:* N&V, diarrhea. *CNS:* Headache, anxiety, nervousness, tremor, dizziness, hypesthesia, hyperesthesia, paresthesia. *Musculoskeletal:* Jaw pain, myalgia, nonspecific musculoskeletal pain. *Miscellaneous:* Flu-like symptoms, chills, fever, sepsis.

OD **Overdose Management:** *Symptoms:* Flushing, headache, hypotension, tachycardia, nausea, vomiting, diarrhea. *Treatment:* Reduce dose of epoprostenol.

Drug Interactions
Anticoagulants / Possible ↑ risk of bleeding
Antiplatelet drugs / Possible ↑ risk of bleeding
Diuretics / Additional ↓ in BP
Vasodilators / Additional ↓ in BP

EMS CONSIDERATIONS

See also *Antihypertensive Agents.*

Eprosartan mesylate
(eh-proh-SAR-tan)

Pregnancy Class: C (first trimester), D (second and third trimesters)

Teveten (Rx)

Classification: Antihypertensive, angiotensin II receptor antagonist

E

Mechanism of Action: Acts by blocking the vasoconstrictor and aldosterone-secreting effects of angiotensin II by blocking selectively the binding of angiotensin II to angiotensin II receptors located in the vascular smooth muscle and adrenal gland.

Uses: Used alone or with other antihypertensives (diuretics, calcium channel blockers) to treat hypertension.

Precautions: Drugs that act on the renin-angiotensin system directly during the second and third trimesters of pregnancy may cause fetal and neonatal injury. Symptomatic hypotension may be seen in patients who are volume- and/or salt-depleted (e.g., those taking diuretics). Safety and efficacy have not been determined in children.

Route/Dosage
• **Tablets**
Hypertension.

Adults, initial: 600 mg once daily as monotherapy in patients who are not volume-depleted. Can be given once or twice daily with total daily doses ranging from 400–800 mg.

How Supplied: *Tablets:* 400 mg, 600 mg

Side Effects: *GI:* Abdominal pain, diarrhea, dyspepsia, anorexia, constipation, dry mouth, esophagitis, flatulence, gastritis, gastroenteritis, gingivitis, nausea, peridontitis, toothache, vomiting. *CNS:* Depression, headache, dizziness, anxiety, ataxia, insomnia, migraine, neuritis, nervousness, paresthesia, somnolence, tremor, vertigo. *CV:* Angina pectoris, bradycardia, abnormal ECG, extrasystoles, atrial fibrillation, hypotension, tachycardia, palpitations, pe-

---

bold italic = life threatening side effect

ripheral ischemia. *Respiratory:* URTI, sinusitis, bronchitis, chest pain, rhinitis, pharyngitis, coughing, asthma, epistaxis. *Musculoskeletal:* Arthralgia, myalgia, arthritis, aggravated arthritis, arthrosis, skeletal pain, tendonitis, back pain. *GU:* UTI, albuminuria, cystitis, hematuria, frequent micturition, polyuria, renal calculus, urinary incontinence. *Metabolic:* Diabetes mellitus, gout. *Body as a whole:* Viral infection, injury, fatigue, alcohol intolerance, asthenia, substernal chest pain, peripheral edema, dependent edema, fatigue, fever, hot flushes, flu-like symptoms, malasie, rigors, pain, leg cramps, herpes simplex. *Hematologic:* Anemia, purpura, leukopenia, neutropenia, thrombocytopenia. *Dermatologic:* Eczema, furunculosis, pruritus, rash, maculopapular rash, increased sweating. *Ophthalmic:* Conjunctivitis, abnormal vision, xerophthalmia. *Otic:* Otitis externa, otitis media, tinnitus.

EMS CONSIDERATIONS

See also *Antihypertensive Agents.*

Equagesic
(eh-kwah-JEE-sik)
(Rx)
Classification: Analgesic

Uses: Short-term treatment of pain due to musculoskeletal disease accompanied by anxiety and tension.
Contraindications: Additional: Pregnancy. Children under 12 years of age. Use for longer than 4 months.

Route/Dosage

• **Tablets**
Pain due to musculoskeletal disease.
Adults: 1–2 tablets t.i.d.–q.i.d.
How Supplied: *Nonnarcotic Analgesic:* Aspirin, 325 mg. *Antianxiety agent:* Meprobamate, 200 mg. See also information on individual components.

EMS CONSIDERATIONS

None.

Erythromycin base
(eh-rih-throw-MY-sin)
Pregnancy Class: B (A/T/S, Erymax, Staticin, and T-Stat are C)
Capsules/Tablets: E-Base, E-Mycin, Eryc, Ery-Tab, Erythromycin Base Film-Tabs, PCE Dispertab; **Gel, topical:** A/T/S, Erygel; **Ointment, topical:** Akne-mycin; **Ointment, ophthalmic:** Ilotycin Ophthalmic, **Pledgets:** Erycette, T-Stat; **Solution:** DelMycin, Eryderm 2%, Erymax, ErythraDerm, Staticin, Theramycin Z, T-Stat **(Rx)**
Classification: Antibiotic, erythromycin

Mechanism of Action: Erythromycins are macrolide antibiotics. They inhibit protein synthesis of microorganisms by binding reversibly to a ribosomal subunit (50S), thus interfering with the transmission of genetic information and inhibiting protein synthesis. The drugs are effective only against rapidly multiplying organisms.
Uses
1. Mild to moderate upper respiratory tract infections due to *Streptococcus pyogenes* (group a beta-hemolytic streptococci), *Streptococcus pneumoniae,* and *Haemophilus influenzae* (combined with sulfonamides).
2. Mild to moderate lower respiratory tract infections due to *S. pyogenes* (group a beta-hemolytic streptococci) and *S. pneumoniae.* Respiratory tract infections due to *Mycoplasma pneumoniae.*
3. Pertussis (whooping cough) caused by *Bordetella pertussis;* may also be used as prophylaxis of pertussis in exposed individuals.
4. Mild to moderate skin and skin structure infections due to *S. pyogenes* and *Staphylococcus aureus.*
5. As an adjunct to antitoxin in diphtheria (caused by *Corynebacterium diphtheriae*), to prevent carriers, and to eradicate the organism in carriers.
6. Intestinal amebiasis due to *Entamoeba histolytica* (PO erythromycin only).
7. Acute pelvic inflammatory disease due to *Neisseria gonorrhoeae.*

8. Erythrasma due to *Corynebacterium minutissimum.*

9. *Chlamydia trachomatis* infections causing urogenital infections during pregnancy, conjunctivitis in the newborn, or pneumonia during infancy. Also, uncomplicated chlamydial infections of the urethra, endocervix, or rectum in adults (when tetracyclines are contraindicated or not tolerated).

10. Nongonococcal urethritis caused by *Ureaplasma urealyticum* when tetracyclines are contraindicated or not tolerated.

11. Legionnaires' disease due to *Legionella pneumophilia.*

12. PO as an alternative to penicillin (in penicillin-sensitive patients) to treat primary syphilis caused by *Treponema pallidum.*

13. Prophylaxis of initial or recurrent attacks of rheumatic fever in patients allergic to penicillin or sulfonamides.

14. Infections due to *Listeria monocytogenes.*

15. Bacterial endocarditis due to alpha-hemolytic streptococci, Viridans group, in patients allergic to penicillins.

Investigational: Severe or prolonged diarrhea due to *Campylobacter jejuni.* Genital, inguinal, or anorectal infections due to *Lymphogranuloma venereum.* Chancroid due to *Haemophilus ducreyi.* Primary, secondary, or early latent syphilis due to *T. pallidum.* Erythromycin base used with PO neomycin prior to elective colorectal surgery to reduce wound complications. As an alternative to penicillin to treat anthrax, Vincent's gingivitis, erysipeloid, actinomycosis, tetanus, with a sulfonamide to treat *Nocardia* infections, infections due to *Eikenella corrodens,* and *Borrelia* infections (including early Lyme disease).

Ophthalmic solution: Treatment of ocular infections (along with PO therapy) due to *Streptococcus pneumoniae, Staphylococcus aureus, S. pyogenes, Corynebacterium* species, *Haemophilus influenzae,* and *Bacteroides* infections. Also prophylaxis of ocular infections due to *Neisseria gonorrhoeae* and *Chlamydia trachomatis.* **Topical solution:** Acne vulgaris. **Topical ointment:** Prophylaxis of infection in minor skin abrasions; treatment of superficial infections of the skin. Acne vulgaris.

Contraindications: Hypersensitivity to erythromycin; in utero syphilis. Use of topical preparations in the eye or near the nose, mouth, or any mucous membrane. Ophthalmic use in dendritic keratitis, vaccinia, varicella, myobacterial infections of the eye, fungal diseases of the eye. Use with steroid combinations following uncomplicated removal of a corneal foreign body.

Precautions: Use with caution in liver disease and during lactation. Use may result in bacterial and fungal overgrowth (i.e., superinfection). Use of other drugs for acne may result in a cumulative irritant effect.

Route/Dosage

Note: Doses are listed as erythromycin base.

• **Delayed-Release Capsules, Enteric-Coated Tablets, Delayed-Release Tablets, Film-Coated Tablets, Suspension**

Respiratory tract infections due to Mycoplasma pneumoniae.

500 mg q 6 hr for 5–10 days (up to 3 weeks for severe infections).

Upper respiratory tract infections (mild to moderate) due to S. pyogenes and S. pneumoniae.

Adults: 250–500 mg q.i.d. for 10 days. **Children:** 20–50 mg/kg/day in divided doses, not to exceed the adult dose, for 10 days.

URTIs due to H. influenzae.

Erythromycin ethylsuccinate, 50 mg/kg/day for children, plus sulfisoxazole, 150 mg/kg/day, given together for 10 days.

Lower respiratory tract infections (mild to moderate) due to S. pyogenes and S. pneumoniae.

250–500 mg q.i.d. (or 20–50 mg/kg/day in divided doses) for 10 days.

Intestinal amebiasis due to Entamoeba histolytica.

Adults: 250 mg q.i.d. for 10–14 days; **pediatric:** 30–50 mg/kg/day in divided doses for 10 days.

Legionnaire's disease.

1–4 g/day in divided doses for 10–14 days.

Bordetella pertussis.

500 mg q.i.d. for 10 days (or for children, 40–50 mg/kg/day in divided doses for 5–14 days).

Infections due to Corynebacterium diphtheriae.

500 mg q 6 hr for 10 days.

Primary syphilis.

20–40 g in divided doses over 10 days.

Conjunctivitis of the newborn, pneumonia of infancy, urogenital infections during pregnancy due to Chlamydia trachomatis.

Infants: 50 mg/kg/day in four divided doses for 14 (conjunctivitis) to 21 (pneumonia) days; **adults:** 500 mg q.i.d. for 7 days or 250 mg q.i.d. for 14 days for urogenital infections.

Mild to moderate skin and skin structure infections due to S. pyogenes *and* S. aureus.

250–500 mg q 6 hr (or 20–50 mg/kg/day for children, in divided doses—to a maximum of 4 g/day) for 10 days.

Listeria monocytogenes *infections.*

Adults: 500 mg q 12 hr (or 250 mg q 6 hr), up to maximum of 4 g/day.

Pelvic inflammatory disease, acute N. gonorrhoeae.

Erythromycin lactobionate, 500 mg IV q 6 hr for 3 days; **then,** 250 mg erythromycin base 250 mg PO q 6 hr for 7 days. Alternatively for pelvic inflammatory disease, 500 mg PO q.i.d. for 10–14 days.

Prophylaxis of initial or recurrent rheumatic fever.

250 mg b.i.d.

Bacterial endocarditis due to alpha-hemolytic streptococcus.

Adults: 1 g 1–2 hr prior to the procedure; **then,** 500 mg 6 hr after the in-

itial dose. **Pediatric,** 20 mg/kg 2 hr prior to the procedure; **then,** 10 mg/kg 6 hr after the initial dose.

Uncomplicated urethral, endocervical, or rectal infections due to C. trachomatis.

500 mg q.i.d. for 7 days (or 250 mg q.i.d. for 14 days).

Nongonococcal urethritis due to Ureaplasma urealyticum.

500 mg q.i.d. for at least 7 days or 250 mg q.i.d. for 14 days if patient can not tolerate high doses of erythromycin.

Erythrasma due to Corynebacterium minutissimum.

250 mg t.i.d. for 21 days.

• **Ophthalmic Ointment**
  Mild to moderate infections.
0.5-in. ribbon b.i.d.–t.i.d.
  Acute infections.
0.5 in. q 3–4 hr until improvement is noted.
  Prophylaxis of neonatal gonococcal or chlamydial conjunctivitis.
0.2–0.4 in. into each conjunctival sac.

• **Topical Gel (2%), Ointment (2%), Solution (2%)**
Clean the affected area and apply, using fingertips or applicator, morning and evening, to affected areas. If no improvement is seen after 6 to 8 weeks, discontinue therapy.

• **Investigational Uses.**
  Diarrhea due to Campylobacter enteritis or enterocolitis. Chancroid due to Haemophilus ducreyi.
500 mg q.i.d. for 7 days.
  Genital, inguinal, or anorectal Lymphogranuloma venereum.
  Early syphilis due to Treponema palliduim.
500 mg q.i.d. for 14 days.
  Tetanus due to Clostridium tetani.
500 mg q 6 hr for 10 days.
  Granuloma inguinale due to Calymmatobacterium granulomatis.
500 mg PO q.i.d. for 21 or more days.

How Supplied: *Enteric Coated Capsule:* 250 mg; *Enteric Coated Tablet:* 250 mg, 333 mg, 500 mg; *Gel/Jelly:* 2%; *Ointment:* 2%; *Ophthalmic ointment:* 5 mg/g; *Pad:* 2%; *Solution:* 1.5%, 2%; *Swab:* 2%; *Tablet:* 250 mg,

500 mg; *Tablet, Coated Particles:* 333 mg, 500 mg

Side Effects: *GI:* Abdominal discomort or pain, anorexia, diarrhea or loose stools, dyspepsia, flatulence, GI disorder, N&V, pseudomembranous colitis, hepatotoxicity. *CV:* Ventricular arrhythmias, including *ventricular tachycardia and torsades de pointes in patients with prolonged QT intervals.* *Dermatologic:* Pruritus, rash, urticaria, bullous eruptions, eczema, erythema multiforme, *Stevens-Johnson syndrome, toxic epidermal necrolysis.* *CNS:* Dizziness, headche, insomnia. *Miscellaneous:* Asthenia, dyspnea, increased cough, non-specific pain, vaginitis, allergic reaction, *anaphylaxis.* Reversible hearing loss in those with renal or hepatic insufficiency, in the elderly, and after doses greater than 4 g/day.

Following IV use: Venous irritation, thrombophlebitis. *Following IM use:* Pain at the injection site, with development of necrosis or sterile abscesses. *Following topical use:* Itching, burning, irritation, stinging of skin; dry, scaly skin. *When used topically:* Erythema, desquamation, burning sensation, eye irritation, tenderness, dryness, pruritus, oily skin, generalized urticaria.

OD **Overdose Management:** *Symptoms:* N&V, diarrhea, epigastric distress, acute pancreatitis (mild), hearing loss (with or without tinnitus and vertigo). *Treatment:* Induce vomiting. General supportive measures. Allergic reactions should be controlled with conventional therapy.

Drug Interactions
Alfentanil / ↓ Excretion of alfentanil → ↑ effect
Anticoagulants / ↑ Anticoagulant effect → possible hemorrhage
Astemizole / Serious CV side effects, including torsades de pointes and other ventricular arrhythmias (including QT interval prolongation), cardiac arrest, and death
Antacids / Slight ↓ in elimination rate of erythromycin

Benzodiazepines (Alprazolam, Diazepam, Midazolam, Triazolam) / ↑ Plasma levels of benzodiazepine → ↑ CNS depressant effects
Bromocriptine / ↑ Serum levels of bromocriptine → ↑ pharmacologic and toxic effects
Buspirone / ↑ Plasma levels of buspirone → ↑ pharmacologic and toxic effects
Carbamazepine / ↑ Effect (and toxicity requiring hospitalization and resuscitation) of carbamazepine due to ↓ breakdown by liver
Clindamycin / Antagonism of effect if used together topically
Cisapride / Possible serious cardiac arrhythmias, including ventricular tachycardia, ventricular fibrillation, torsades de pointes, and prolonged QT interval
Cyclosporine / ↑ Effect of cyclosporine due to ↓ excretion (possibly with renal toxicity)
Digoxin / ↑ Serum digoxin levels due to effect on gut flora
Disopyramide / ↑ Plasma levels of disopyramide → arrhythmias and ↑ QTc intervals
Ergot alkaloids / Acute ergotism manifested by peripheral ischemia and dysesthesia
Felodipine / ↑ Plasma levels of felodipine → ↑ pharmacologic and toxic effects
Grepafloxacin / ↑ Risk of life-threatening cardiac arrhythmias, including torsades de pointes
HMG-CoA Reductase inhibitors / ↑ Risk of myopathy or rhabdomyolysis
Lincosamides / Drugs may each other
Methylprednisolone / ↑ Effect of methylprednisolone due to ↓ breakdown by liver
Penicillin / Erythromycins either ↓ or ↑ effect of penicillins
Pimozide / Possibility of sudden death; do not use together
Rifabutin, Rifambin / ↓ Effect of erythromycin; ↑ risk of GI side effects

E

---

bold italic = life threatening side effect

Sodium bicarbonate / ↑ Effect of erythromycin in urine due to alkalinization

Sparfloxacin / ↑ Risk of life-threatening cardiac arrhythmias, including torsades de pointes

Tacrolimus / ↑ Serum levels of tacrolimus → ↑ risk of nephrotoxicity

Terfenadine / Serious CV side effects, including torsades de pointes and other ventricular arrhythmias (including QT interval prolongation), cardiac arrest, and death

Theophyllines / ↑ Effect of theophylline due to ↓ breakdown in liver; ↓ erythromycin levels may also occur

Vinblastine / ↑ Risk of vinblastine toxicity (constipation, myalgia, neutropenia)

EMS CONSIDERATIONS

See also *Anti-Infective Agents.*

Erythromycin estolate
(eh-rih-throw-MY-sin)
Pregnancy Class: B
Ilosone **(Rx)**
Classification: Antibiotic, erythromycin

Uses: See Erythromycin Base.
Contraindications: Additional: Cholestatic jaundice or preexisting liver dysfunction. Treatment of chronic disorders such as acne, furunculosis, or prophylaxis of rheumatic fever.

Route/Dosage ————————
• **Capsules, Suspension, Tablets**
See *Erythromycin base.* Similar blood levels are achieved using erythromycin base, estolate, or stearate.
How Supplied: *Capsule:* 250 mg; *Suspension:* 125 mg/5 mL, 250 mg/5 mL

EMS CONSIDERATIONS

See also *Erythromycin Base.*

Erythromycin ethylsuccinate
(eh-rih-throw-MY-sin)

Pregnancy Class: B
Apo-Erythro-ES, E.E.S. 200 and 400, E.E.S. Granules, EryPed, EryPed 200, EryPed 400, EryPed Drops **(Rx)**
Classification: Antibiotic, erythromycin

Uses: See Erythromycin Base.
Contraindications: Additional: Preexisting liver disease.

Route/Dosage ————————
• **Oral   Suspension,   Tablets, Chewable Tablets**
See *Erythromycin base.* NOTE: 400 mg of erythromycin ethylsuccinate will achieve the same blood levels of erythromycin as 250 mg of the base, estolate, or stearate forms.

Hemophilus influenzae infections. Erythromycin ethylsuccinate, 50 mg/kg/day with sulfisoxazole, 150 mg/kg/day, both for a total of 10 days.

How Supplied: *Chew Tablet:* 200 mg; *Granule for Reconstitution:* 100 mg/2.5 mL, 200 mg/5 mL, 400 mg/5 mL; *Suspension:* 200 mg/5 mL, 400 mg/5 mL; *Tablet:* 400 mg

EMS CONSIDERATIONS

See also *Erythromycin Base.*

Erythromycin lactobionate
(eh-rih-throw-MY-sin)
Pregnancy Class: B
Erythrocin **(Rx)**
Classification: Antibiotic, erythromycin

Uses: See Erythromycin Base.

Route/Dosage ————————
• **IV**
Adults   and   children: 15–20 mg/kg/day up to 4 g/day in severe infections.

Acute pelvic inflammatory disease caused by gonorrhea.
500 mg q 6 hr for 3 days followed by 250 mg erythromycin stearate, **PO,** q 6 hr for 7 days.

Legionnaire's disease.
1–4 g/day in divided doses. Change to PO therapy as soon as possible.
How Supplied: *Powder for injection:* 500 mg, 1 g

Drug Interactions: Additional: Do not add durgs to IV solutions of erythromycin lactobionate.

EMS CONSIDERATIONS

See also *Erythromycin Base.*

Erythromycin stearate
(eh-rih-throw-MY-sin)
Pregnancy Class: B
Erythrocin Stearate **(Rx)**
Classification: Antibiotic, erythromycin

Uses: See *Erythromycins Base.*

Route/Dosage
• **Tablets, Film Coated**
See *Erythromycin base.* Similar blood levels are achieved using erythromycin base, estolate, or stearate forms.
How Supplied: *Tablet:* 250 mg, 500 mg
Side Effects: Additional: Causes more allergic reactions (e.g., skin rash and urticaria) than other erythromycins.

EMS CONSIDERATIONS

See also *Erythromycin Base.*

Esmolol hydrochloride
(EZ-moh-lohl)
Pregnancy Class: C
Brevibloc **(Rx)**
Classification: Beta-adrenergic blocking agent

Mechanism of Action: Preferentially inhibits beta-1 receptors. Rapid onset (<5 min) and a short duration of action. Has no membrane-stabilizing or intrinsic sympathomimetic activity.
Uses: Supraventricular tachycardia or arrhythmias, sinus tachycardia.
Precautions: Dosage has not been established in children.

Route/Dosage
• **IV Infusion**
SVT.
Initial: 500 mcg/kg/min for 1 min; **then,** 50 mcg/kg/min for 4 min. If after 5 min an adequate effect is not

achieved, repeat the loading dose followed by a maintenance infusion of 100 mcg/kg/min for 4 min. This procedure may be repeated, increasing the maintenance infusion by 50 mcg/kg/min increments (for 4 min) until the desired HR or lowered BP is approached. **Then,** omit the loading infusion and reduce incremental infusion rate from 50 to 25 mcg/kg/min or less. The interval between titrations may be increased from 5 to 10 min.

Once the HR has been controlled, the patient may be transferred to another antiarrhythmic agent. Reduce the infusion rate of esmolol by 50% 30 min after the first dose of the alternative antiarrhythmic agent. If satisfactory control is observed for 1 hr after the second dose of the alternative agent, the esmolol infusion may be stopped.
How Supplied: *Injection:* 10 mg/mL, 250 mg/mL
Side Effects: Additional: *Dermatologic:* Inflammation at site of infusion, flushing, pallor, induration, erythema, burning, skin discoloration, edema. *Other:* Urinary retention, midscapular pain, asthenia, changes in taste.
Drug Interactions: Additional: *Digoxin/* Esmolol ↑ digoxin blood levels*Morphine/* Morphine ↑ esmolol blood levels.

EMS CONSIDERATIONS

See also *Beta-Adrenergic Blocking Agents.*

Estazolam
(es-TAYZ-oh-lam)
Pregnancy Class: X
ProSom **(C-IV) (Rx)**
Classification: Hypnotic, benzodiazepine

Uses: Short-term use for insomnia characterized by difficulty in falling asleep, frequent awakenings, and/or early morning awakenings.
Contraindications: Pregnancy. Use during labor and delivery and during lactation.

bold italic = life threatening side effect

Precautions: Use with caution in geriatric or debilitated patients, in those with impaired renal or hepatic function, in those with compromised respiratory function, and in those with depression or who show suicidal tendencies. Safety and efficacy have not been determined in children less than 18 years of age.

Route/Dosage
• **Tablets**
Adults: 1 mg at bedtime (although some patients may require 2 mg). The initial dose in small or debilitated geriatric patients is 0.5 mg. Prolonged use is not recommended or necessary.
How Supplied: *Tablet:* 1 mg, 2 mg

EMS CONSIDERATIONS

See also *Tranquilizers, Antimanic Drugs, and Hypnotics.*

Esterified estrogens
(es-TER-ih-fyd ES-troh-jens)
Pregnancy Class: X
Estratab, Menest **(Rx)**
Classification: Estrogen, natural

Mechanism of Action: This product is a mixture of sodium salts of sulfate esters of natural estrogenic substances: 75%–85% estrone sodium sulfate and 6%–15% equilin sodium sulfate.

Uses: Replacement therapy in primary ovarian failure, following castration, or hypogonadism. Inoperable, progressing prostatic or breast carcinoma (in postmenopausal women and selected men). Moderate to severe vasomotor symptoms, atrophic vaginitis, and kraurosis vulvae due to menopause. Prophylaxis of osteoporosis (0.3 mg tablet).

Route/Dosage
• **Tablets**
Moderate to severe vasomotor symptoms, atrophic vaginitis, or kraurosis vulvae due to menopause.
0.3–1.25 mg/day given cyclically for short-term use. Adjust dose to the lowest effective level and discontinue as soon as possible.

Hypogonadism.
2.5–7.5 mg/day in divided doses for 20 days, followed by a 10-day rest period. If menses does not occur by the end of this period of time, repeat dosage schedule. The number of courses of estrogen required to produce bleeding varies, depending on the responsiveness of the endometrium. If bleeding occurs before the end of the 10-day period, a 20-day estrogen-progestin cycle should be started with 2.5–7.5 mg/day of estrogen with a progestin added the last 5 days. If bleeding occurs before the end of this regimen, discontinue therapy and resume on day 5 of bleeding.
Primary ovarian failure, castration.
1.25 mg/day given cyclically.
Prostatic carcinoma, inoperable and progressing.
1.25–2.5 mg t.i.d. Effectiveness can be determined using phosphatase determinations and symptomatic improvement.
Breast carcinoma, inoperable and progressing, in selected men and postmenopausal women.
10 mg t.i.d. for at least 3 months.
Prophylaxis of osteoporosis.
0.3 mg daily.
How Supplied: *Tablet:* 0.3 mg, 0.625 mg, 1.25 mg, 2.5 mg

EMS CONSIDERATIONS
None.

Estradiol hemihydrate
(ess-trah-DYE-ohl)
Pregnancy Class: X
Vagifem **(Rx)**
Classification: Estrogen

Uses: Treatment of atrophic vaginitis.

Route/Dosage
• **Vaginal Tablets**
Atrophic vaginitis.
Initial: 1 tablet, inserted vaginally, once daily for 2 weeks; **maintenance:** 1 tablet, inserted vaginally, twice a week.

How Supplied: *Tablets, Vaginal:* 25 mcg

EMS CONSIDERATIONS

None.

Estradiol transdermal system

(ess-trah-DYE-ohl)
Pregnancy Class: X
Alora, Climara, Esclim, Estraderm, FemPatch, Vivelle **(Rx)**
Classification: Estrogen

Mechanism of Action: This transdermal system allows a constant low dose of estradiol to directly reach the systemic circulation.

Uses: Vasomotor symptoms due to menopause, including hot flashes, night sweats, and vaginal burning, itching, and dryness. Female hypogonadism or castration; atrophic vaginitis or kraurosis vulvae due to deficient endogenous estrogen production; primary ovarian failure; prevention of osteoporosis. Abnormal uterine bleeding due to hormonal imbalance in the absence of organic pathology and only when associated with a hypoplastic or atrophic endometrium.

Route/Dosage
• **Dermal System**
Menopausal symptoms.
Initial: Lowest dose needed to control symptoms: One 0.025- or 0.05-mg system applied to the skin twice weekly (if using Alora, Estraderm, Esclim, or Vivelle) or once a week (if using Climara or FemPatch). Adjust dose as necessary to control symptoms. Taper or discontinue dose at 3- to 6-month intervals. Alora is available in strengths to release 0.05-, 0.075-, and 0.1-mg/24 hr. Climara and Estraderm are available in strengths to release 0.05- or 0.1-mg/24 hr. Esclim is available in strengths to release 0.025-, 0.0375-, 0.05-, 0.075-, or 0.1-mg/24 hr. FemPatch is available to release 0.025-mg/24 hr. Vivelle is available in

strengths to release 0.0375-, 0.05-, 0.075-, or 0.1-mg/24 hr.
Prevention of osteoporosis.
Initial: 0.05 mg/day as soon as possible after menopause. Adjust dosage to control concurrent menopausal symptoms.

How Supplied: *Film, Extended Release:* 0.025 mg/24 hr, 0.0375 mg/24 hr, 0.05 mg/24 hr, 0.075 mg/24 hr, 0.1 mg/24 hr; *Insert, Controlled Release:* 0.0075 mg/24 hr

Side Effects: Skin irritation, URTI, headache, breast tenderness.

EMS CONSIDERATIONS

None.

Estramustine phosphate

(es-trah-MUS-teen)
Emcyt **(Rx)**
Classification: Antineoplastic, hormonal agent, alkylating agent

Mechanism of Action: Water-soluble drug that combines estradiol and mechlorethamine (a nitrogen mustard). Estradiol facilitates uptake into cells containing the estrogen receptor while the nitrogen mustard acts as an alkylating agent.

Uses: Palliative treatment of metastatic and/or progressive prostatic carcinoma.

Contraindications: Active thrombophlebitis or thromboembolic disease unless the tumor mass is causing the thromboembolic disorder. Allergy to nitrogen mustard or estrogen.

Precautions: Use with caution in presence of cerebrovascular disease, CAD, diabetes, hypertension, CHF, impaired liver or kidney function, and metabolic bone diseases associated with hypercalcemia.

Route/Dosage
• **Capsules**
14 mg/kg/day in three to four divided doses (range: 10–16 mg/kg/day) or 600 mg (base)/m² daily in three divided doses. One 140-mg capsule is taken for each 10 kg or 22 lb of body weight. Treat for 30–90 days

E

bold italic = life threatening side effect

before assessing beneficial effects; continue therapy as long as the drug is effective. Some patients have taken doses from 10 to 16 mg/kg/day for more than 3 years.

How Supplied: *Capsule:* 140 mg

Side Effects: Additional: *CV:* **MI, CVA,** thrombosis, CHF, increased BP, thrombophlebitis, leg cramps, edema. *Respiratory:* **Pulmonary embolism,** dyspnea, upper respiratory discharge, hoarseness. *GI:* Flatulence, burning sensation of throat, thirst. *CNS:* Emotional lability, insomnia, anxiety, lethargy, headache. *Dermatologic:* Easy bruising, flushing, peeling of skin or fingertips. *Miscellaneous:* Chest pain, tearing of eyes, leg cramps, breast tenderness or enlargement, decreased glucose tolerance.

OD **Overdose Management:** *Symptoms:* Extensions of the side effects. *Treatment:* Gastric lavage; treat symptoms. Monitor blood counts and liver profiles for at least 6 weeks.

Drug Interactions: Drugs or food containing calcium may ↓ absorption of estramustine phosphate sodium.

EMS CONSIDERATIONS

None.

Estrogens conjugated, oral (conjugated estrogenic substances)
Estrogens conjugated, parenteral
Estrogens conjugated, vaginal

(ES-troh-jens)

Pregnancy Class: X

Estrogens conjugated, oral (Premarin **(Rx)**) Estrogens conjugated, parenteral (Premarin IV **(Rx)**) Estrogens conjugated, vaginal (Premarin **(Rx)**)

Classification: Estrogen, natural

Mechanism of Action: Contains 50%–65% sodium estrone sulfate and 20%–35% sodium equilin sulfate.

Uses: PO: Moderate to severe vasomotor symptoms due to menopause, atrophic vaginitis, kraurosis vulvae, female hypogonadism, primary ovarian failure, female castration. Palliation in mammary cancer in men or postmenopausal women; prostatic carcinoma (inoperable and progressive). Prophylaxis of osteoporosis.

Parenteral: Abnormal bleeding due to imbalance of hormones and in the absence of disease.

Vaginal: Atrophic vaginitis and kraurosis vulvae associated with menopause.

Precautions: Use of estrogen replacement therapy for prolonged periods of time may increase the risk of fatal ovarian cancer and may also have a higher risk of breast cancer.

Route/Dosage —————————

• **Tablets**

Moderate to severe vasomotor symptoms due to menopause.

1.25 mg/day given cyclically. If the patient has not menstruated in 2 or more months, begin therapy on any day; if, however, the patient is menstruating, begin therapy on day 5 of bleeding.

Primary ovarian failure, female castration.

1.25 mg/day given cyclically (3 weeks on, 1 week off). Adjust dose to lowest effective level.

Atrophic vaginitis or kraurosis vulvae associated with menopause.

0.3–1.25 mg/day (higher doses may be necessary, depending on the response) given cyclically (3 weeks on, 1 week off).

Hypogonadism in females.

2.5–7.5 mg/day in divided doses for 20 days, followed by a 10-day rest period. If menses does not occur by the end of this period of time, repeat the dosage schedule. The number of courses of estrogen required to produce bleeding varies, depending on the responsiveness of the endometrium. If bleeding occurs before the end of the 10-day period, start a 20-

day estrogen-progestin cycle with 2.5–7.5 mg/day of estrogen with a progestin added the last 5 days. If bleeding occurs before the end of this regimen, discontinue therapy and resume on day 5 of bleeding.

Palliation of mammary carcinoma in men or postmenopausal women.

10 mg t.i.d. for at least 90 days.

Palliation of prostatic carcinoma.

1.25–2.5 mg t.i.d. Effectiveness can be measured by phosphatase determinations and symptomatic improvement.

Prophylaxis of osteoporosis.

0.625 mg/day given cyclically (3 weeks on, 1 week off). Mainstays of therapy include calcium; exercise and nutrition may be important adjuncts.

- **IM, IV**

Abnormal bleeding.

25 mg; repeat after 6–12 hr if necessary.

- **Vaginal Cream**

½–2 g daily given for 3 weeks on and 1 week off. Repeat as needed. Attempt to taper the dose or discontinue the medication at 3- to 6-month intervals.

How Supplied: Estrogens conjugated, oral: *Tablet:* 0.3 mg, 0.625 mg, 0.9 mg, 1.25 mg, 2.5 mg. Estrogens conjugated, parenteral: *Powder for injection:* 25 mg. Estrogens conjugated, vaginal: *Cream:* 0.625 mg/g

EMS CONSIDERATIONS

None.

Estropipate (Piperazine estrone sulfate)

(es-troh-PIE-payt)
Pregnancy Class: X
Ogen, Ogen Vaginal Cream, OrthoEst **(Rx)**
Classification: Estrogen, semisynthetic

Uses: PO: Moderate to severe vasomotor symptoms associated with menopause. Vulval and vaginal atrophy. Primary ovarian failure, female castration, female hypogonadism. Prevention of osteoporosis.

Vaginal: Atrophic vaginitis and kraurosis vulvae associated with menopause.

Contraindications: Use during pregnancy.

Route/Dosage

- **Tablets**

Moderate to severe vasomotor symptoms; atrophic vaginitis or kraurosis vulvae due to menopause.

0.75–6 mg/day for short-term therapy (give cyclically). May also be used continuously. The lowest dose that will control symptoms should be selected. Attempt to discontinue or taper the dose at 3– to 6–month intervals.

Hypogonadism, primary ovarian failure, castration.

1.5–9 mg/day (calculated as 0.625 to 5 mg estrone sulfate) for first 3 weeks; **then,** rest period of 8–10 days. A PO progestin can be given during the third week if withdrawal bleeding does not occur.

Prevention of osteoporosis.

0.625 mg/day for 25 days of a 31-day cycle per month. Mainstays of therapy include calcium; exercise and nutrition may be important adjuncts.

- **Vaginal Cream**

2–4 g (containing 3–6 mg estropipate) daily (depending on severity of condition) for 3 weeks followed by a 1-week rest period. Attempt to taper the dose or discontinue the medication at 3- to 6-month intervals.

How Supplied: *Vaginal cream:* 1.5 mg/g; *Tablet:* 0.75 mg, 1.5 mg, 3 mg

EMS CONSIDERATIONS

None.

Etanercept

(eh-TAN-er-sept)
Pregnancy Class: B

Enbrel **(Rx)**
Classification: Antiarthritic drug

Mechanism of Action: Binds specifically to tumor necrosis factor (TNF) and blocks its interaction with cell surface TNF receptors. TNF is a cytokine that is involved in normal inflammatory and immune responses. Thus, the drug renders TNF biologically inactive. It is possible for etanercept to affect host defenses against infections and malignancies since TNF mediates inflammation and modulates cellular immune responses.

Uses: Reduce signs and symptoms of moderately to severely active rheumatoid arthritis in those who have had an inadequate response to one or more antirheumatic drugs. May be used in combination with methotrexate in those who do not respond adequately to methotrexate alone.

Contraindications: Use in patients with sepsis. Administration of live vaccines given concurrently with etanercept. Lactation.

Precautions: Safety and efficacy have not been determined in those with immunosuppression or chronic infections or in children less than 4 years of age.

Route/Dosage ──────────
• **SC**
   Treat rheumatoid arthritis.
Adults: 25 mg twice weekly SC.
How Supplied: *Single-Use Vial:* 25 mg

Side Effects: *Injection site reactions:* Erythema and/or itching, pain, swelling. *GI:* Abdominal pain, dyspepsia, cholecystitis, pancreatitis, *GI hemorrhage. CNS:* Headache, dizziness, depression. *CV: Heart failure, MI,* myocardial ischemia, cerebral ischemia, hypertension, hypotension. *Respiratory:* URI, sinusitis, rhinitis, pharyngitis, cough, respiratory disorder, dyspnea. *Miscellaneous:* Formation of autoimmune antibodies, non-URI, rash, asthenia, bursitis.

EMS CONSIDERATIONS

None.

Ethacrynate sodium
Ethacrynic acid

(eth-ah-KRIH-nayt)(eth-ah-KRIH-nik AH-sid)
Pregnancy Class: B
Ethacrynate sodium (Sodium Edecrin **(Rx)**) Ethacrynic acid (Edecrin **(Rx)**)
Classification: Diuretics, loop

Mechanism of Action: Inhibits the reabsorption of sodium and chloride in the loop of Henle; it also decreases reabsorption of sodium and chloride and increases potassium excretion in the distal tubule. Also acts directly on the proximal tubule to enhance excretion of electrolytes. Large quantities of sodium and chloride and smaller amounts of potassium and bicarbonate ion are excreted during diuresis. Careful monitoring of the diuretic effects is necessary.
Onset of Action: PO: 30 min; **IV:** Within 5 min: **Peak: PO,** 2 hr; **IV:** 15-30 min.
Duration of Action: PO: ,6-8 hr; **IV:** 2 hr.
Uses: Of value with resistance to less potent diuretics. CHF, acute pulmonary edema, edema associated with nephrotic syndrome, ascites due to idiopathic edema, lymphedema, malignancy. Short-term use for ascites as a result of malignancy, lymphedema, or idiopathic edema; also, for short-term use in pediatric patients (except infants) with congenital heart disease. *Investigational.* **Ethacrynic acid:** Single injection into the eye to treat glaucoma (effective for a week or more). **Ethacrynate sodium:** Hypercalcemia, bromide intoxication, and with mannitol in ethylene glycol poisoning.
Contraindications: Pregnancy (usually), lactation, use in neonates. Anuria and severe renal damage.
Precautions: Geriatric patients may be more sensitive to the usual adult dose. Use with caution in diabetics and in those with hepatic cirrhosis (who are particularly susceptible to electrolyte imbalance). Monitor gout patients carefully. Safety and efficacy

of oral use in infants and IV use in children have not been established.

Route/Dosage

ETHACRYNATE SODIUM

• **IV**

Adults: 50 mg (base) (or 0.5–1 mg/kg); may be repeated in 2–4 hr, although only one dose is usually needed. A single 100-mg dose IV has also been used.

ETHACRYNIC ACID

• **Tablets**

Adults, initial: 50–200 mg/day in single or divided doses to produce a gradual weight loss of 2.2–4.4 kg/day (1–2 lb/day). The dose can be increased by 25–50 mg/day if needed. **Maintenance:** Usually 50–200 mg (up to a maximum of 400 mg) daily may be required in severe, refractory edema. If used with other diuretics, the initial dose should be 25 mg with increments of 25 mg. **Pediatric, initial:** 25 mg/day; can increase by 25 mg/day if needed. **Maintenance:** Adjust dose to needs of patient. Dosage for infants has not been determined.

How Supplied: Ethacrynate Sodium: *Powder for injection:* 50 mg. Ethacrynic Acid: *Tablet:* 25 mg, 50 mg

Side Effects: *Electrolyte imbalance:* Hypokalemia, hyponatremia, hypochloremic alkalosis, hypomagnesemia, hypocalcemia. *GI:* Anorexia, nausea, vomiting, diarrhea (may be sudden watery, profuse diarrhea), acute pancreatitis, abdominal discomfort or pain, jaundice, *GI bleeding or hemorrhage,* dysphagia. *Hematologic:* Severe neutropenia, thrombocytopenia, *agranulocytosis,* rarely Henoch-Schoenlein purpura in patients with rheumatic heart disease. *CNS:* Apprehension, confusion, vertigo, headache. *Body as a whole:* Fever, chills, fatigue, malaise. *Otic:* Sense of fullness in the ears, tinnitus, irreversible hearing loss. *Miscellaneous:* Hematuria, acute gout, abnormal liver function tests in seriously ill patients on multiple drug therapy including

ethacrynic acid, blurred vision, rash, local irritation and pain following parenteral use, hyperuricemia, hyperglycemia.

Ethacrynic acid may cause death in critically ill patients refractory to other diuretics. These include (a) patients with severe myocardial disease who also received digitalis and who developed acute hypokalemia with fatal arrhythmias and (b) those with severely decompensated hepatic cirrhosis with ascites, with or without encephalopathy, who had electrolyte imbalances with death due to intensification of the electrolyte effect.

OD **Overdose Management:** *Symptoms:* Profound water loss, electrolyte depletion (causes dizziness, weakness, mental confusion, vomiting, anorexia, lethargy, cramps), dehydration, reduction of blood volume, *circulatory collapse (possibility of vascular thrombosis and embolism). Treatment:* Replace electrolytes and fluid and monitor urine output and serum electrolyte levels. Induce emesis or perform gastric lavage. Artificial respiration and oxygen may be needed. Treat other symptoms.

EMS CONSIDERATIONS

See also *Loop Diuretics.*

Ethambutol hydrochloride
(eh-THAM-byou-tohl)
Myambutol **(Rx)**
Classification: Primary antitubercular agent

Mechanism of Action: Inhibits the synthesis of metabolites resulting in impairment of cell metabolism, arrest of multiplication, and ultimately cell death. Is active against *Mycobacterium tuberculosis,* but not against fungi, other bacteria, or viruses.

Uses: Pulmonary tuberculosis in combination with other tuberculostatic drugs. Use only in conjunction with at least one other antituberculostatic.

---

bold italic = life threatening side effect

Contraindications: Hypersensitivity to ethambutol, preexisting optic neuritis, and in children under 13 years of age.

Precautions: Use with caution and in reduced dosage in patients with gout and impaired renal function and in pregnant women.

Route/Dosage
• **Tablets**
Adults, initial treatment: 15 mg/kg/day until maximal improvement noted; **for retreatment:** 25 mg/kg/day as a single dose with at least one other tuberculostatic drug; **after 60 days:** 15 mg/kg/day.

How Supplied: *Tablet:* 100 mg, 400 mg

Side Effects: *Ophthalmologic:* Optic neuritis, decreased visual acuity, loss of color (green) discrimination, temporary loss of vision or blurred vision. *GI:* N&V, anorexia, abdominal pain. *CNS:* Fever, headache, dizziness, confusion, disorientation, malaise, hallucinations. *Allergic:* Pruritus, dermatitis, **anaphylaxis.** *Miscellaneous:* Peripheral neuropathy (numbness, tingling), precipitation of gout, thrombocytopenia, joint pain, toxic epidermal necrolysis. Renal damage. Also **anaphylactic shock,** peripheral neuritis (rare), hyperuricemia, and decreased liver function. Adverse symptoms usually appear during the early months of therapy and disappear thereafter. Periodic renal and hepatic function tests as well as uric acid determinations are recommended.

Drug Interactions: Aluminum may delay and decrease the absorption of ethambutol.

EMS CONSIDERATIONS

None.

Ethosuximide
(eth-oh-SUCKS-ih-myd)
Zarontin (Rx)
Classification: Anticonvulsant, succinimide type

Uses: Absence (petit mal) seizures.

Route/Dosage
• **Capsules, Syrup**
Absence seizures.
Adults and children over 6 years, initial: 250 mg b.i.d.; the dose may be increased by 250 mg/day at 4–7-day intervals until seizures are controlled or until total daily dose reaches 1.5 g.
Children under 6 years, initial: 250 mg/day; dosage may be increased by 250 mg/day every 4–7 days until control is established or total daily dose reaches 1 g.

How Supplied: *Capsule:* 250 mg; *Syrup:* 250 mg/5 mL

Drug Interactions: Additional: Both isoniazid and valproic acid may ↑ the effects of ethosuximide.

EMS CONSIDERATIONS

See also *Anticonvulsants* and *Succinimides.*

Etidronate disodium (oral)
Etidronate disodium (parenteral)
(eh-tih-DROH-nayt)
Pregnancy Class: Etidronate disodium (oral): B
Etidronate disodium (parenteral): C
Etidronate disodium (oral): Didronel **(Rx)** Etidronate disodium (parenteral): Didronel IV **(Rx)**
Classification: Bone growth regulator, antihypercalcemic

Mechanism of Action: Slows bone metabolism, thereby decreasing bone resorption, bone turnover, and new bone formation; it also reduces bone vascularization.

Uses: PO: Paget's disease. Heterotopic ossification due to spinal cord injury or total hip replacement. **Parenteral:** Hypercalcemia of malignancy inadequately managed by dietary modification or oral hydration or which persists after adequate hydration is restored. *Investigational:* Postmenopausal osteoporosis and prevention of bone loss in early menopause.

Contraindications: Enterocolitis, fracture of long bones, hypercalcemia of hyperparathyroidism. Serum creatinine greater than 5 mg/dL.

Precautions: Use with caution in the presence of renal dysfunction, in active UGI problems, and during lactation. Safety and efficacy have not been established in children.

Route/Dosage ————————

- **Tablets**

  Paget's disease.

  Adults, initial: 5–10 mg/kg/day for 6 months or less; or, 11–20 mg/kg for a maximum of 3 months. Reserve doses above 10 mg/kg when lower doses are ineffective, when there is a need for suppression of increased bone turnover, or when a prompt decrease in CO is needed. Do not exceed doses of 20 mg/kg/day. Another course of therapy may be instituted after rest period of 3 months if there is evidence of active disease process. Monitor every 3 to 6 months.

  Heterotopic ossification due to spinal cord injury.

  Adults: 20 mg/kg/day for 2 weeks; **then** 10 mg/kg/day for 10 weeks. Treatment should be initiated as soon as possible after the injury, preferably before evidence of heterotopic ossification.

  Heterotopic ossification complicating total hip replacement.

  Adults: 20 mg/kg/day for 30 days preoperatively; **then,** 20 mg/kg/day for 90 days postoperatively.

- **IV Infusion**

  Hypercalcemia due to malignancy.

  7.5 mg/kg/day for 3 successive days. If necessary, a second course of treatment may be instituted after a 7-day rest period. The safety and effectiveness of more than two courses of therapy has not been determined. Reduce the dose in those with renal impairment. Etidronate tablets may be started the day after the last infusion at a dose of 20 mg/kg/day for 30 days (treatment may be extended to 90 days if serum calcium levels are

normal). Use for more than 90 days is not recommended.

How Supplied: Etidronate disodium (oral): *Tablet:* 200 mg, 400 mg. Etidronate disodium (parenteral): *Injection:* 50 mg /mL

Side Effects: *GI:* Nausea, diarrhea, constipation, ulcerative stomatitis. *Bones:* Increased incidence of bone fractures and increased or recurrent bone pain. Drug should be discontinued if fracture occurs and not restarted until healing takes place. *Allergy:* Angioedema, rash, pruritus, urticaria. *Electrolytes:* Hypophosphatemia, hypomagnesemia. *Miscellaneous:* Metallic taste, chest pain, abnormal hepatic function, fever, fluid overload, dyspnea, convulsions. Symptoms of rachitic syndrome have been reported in children receiving 10 mg or more/kg daily for long periods (up to 1 year) to treat heterotopic ossification or soft tissue calcification.

OD Overdose Management: *Symptoms:* Following PO ingestion, hypocalcemia may occur. Rapid IV administration may cause renal insufficiency. *Treatment:* Gastric lavage following PO ingestion. Treat hypocalcemia by giving calcium IV.

Drug Interactions: Products containing calcium or other multivalent cations ↓ absorption of etidronate

EMS CONSIDERATIONS

None.

Etoposide (VP-16-213)

(eh-TOH-poh-syd)

Pregnancy Class: D

Etopophos, VePesid **(Rx)**, Etoposide Phosphate

Classification: Antineoplastic, miscellaneous

Mechanism of Action: Acts as a mitotic inhibitor at the G_2 portion of the cell cycle to inhibit DNA synthesis. At high doses, cells entering mitosis are lysed, whereas at low doses, cells will not enter prophase.

E

Uses: With combination therapy to treat refractory testicular tumors and small cell lung cancer. *Investigational:* Alone or in combination to treat acute monocytic leukemia, non-Hodgkin's lymphoma, Hodgkin's disease, AIDS-associated Kaposi's sarcoma, Ewing's sarcoma. Also, choriocarcinoma; hepatocellular carcinoma; nonsmall cell lung, breast, endometrial, and gastric cancers; acute lymphocytic leukemia; soft tissue carcinoma; rhabdomyosarcoma.

Contraindications: Lactation.

Precautions: Safety and efficacy in children have not been established. Severe myelosuppression may occur.

Route/Dosage ───────
* **IV**
  Testicular carcinoma.
  50–100 mg/m²/day on days 1–5 or 100 mg/m²/day on days 1, 3, and 5 q 3–4 weeks (i.e., after recovery from toxic effects). Used in combination with other agents.
  Small cell lung carcinoma.
  35 mg/m²/day for 4 days to 50 mg/m²/day for 5 days, repeated q 3–4 weeks.
* **Capsules**
  Small cell lung carcinoma.
  70 mg/m² (rounded to the nearest 50 mg) daily for 4 days to 100 mg/m² (rounded to the nearest 50 mg) daily for 5 days; repeat q 3–4 weeks.
  NOTE: Etopophos is given in higher concentrations than VePesid. Doses above are for VePesid.

How Supplied: *Capsule:* 50 mg; *Injection:* 20 mg/mL; *Powder for Injection:* 100 mg

Side Effects: Additional: Anaphylactic-type reactions, hypotension, peripheral neuropathy, somnolence.

EMS CONSIDERATIONS
None.

Exemestane
(ex-eh-MESS-tayn)
Pregnancy Class: D

Aromasin **(Rx)**
Classification: Antineoplastic, hormone

Mechanism of Action: Irreversible, steroidal aromatase inactivator. Acts as a false substrate for the aromatase enzyme, which is the principal enzyme that converts androgens to estrogens. Drug is processed to an intermediate that binds irreversibly to the active enzyme site causing its inhibition (called "suicide inhibition"). Significantly lowers circulating estrogen levels in postmenopausal women; has no detectable effect on adrenal biosynthesis of corticosteroids or aldosterone.

Uses: Treatment of advanced breast cancer in postmenopausal women where the disease has progressed following tamoxifen therapy. *Investigational:* Prevention of prostate cancer.

Contraindications: Administration to premenopausal women.

Precautions: Safety and efficacy have not been established in children.

Route/Dosage ───────
* **Tablets**
  Treatment of breast cancer.
  25 mg once daily after a meal.

How Supplied: *Tablets:* 25 mg

Side Effects: *GI:* N&V, abdominal pain, anorexia, constipation, diarrhea, increased appetite, dyspepsia. *CNS:* Depression, insomnia, anxiety, dizziness, headache, hypoesthesia, confusion. *Respiratory:* Dyspnea, coughing, bronchitis, sinusitis, chest pain, URTI, pharyngitis, rhinitis. *Body as a whole:* Fatigue, edema, fever, generalized weakness, paresthesia, asthenia, peripheral edema, leg edema, flu-like symptoms, increased sweating, rash, itching, infection. *Miscellaneous:* Hypertension, hot flashes, pain, pathological fracture, UTI, lymphedema, pain at tumor site, arthralgia, back pain, skeletal pain, alopecia, lymphocytopenia.

EMS CONSIDERATIONS
None.

F

Factor IX Complex (Human)
(FAK-tor 9)
Pregnancy Class: C
AlphaNine SD, Benefix, Konyne 80, Hemonyne, Mononine, Profilnine SD, Proplex T **(Rx)**
Classification: Hemostatic, systemic

Mechanism of Action: Causes an increase in factor IX levels, thus minimizing hemorrhage in those with factor IX deficiency. Factors II, VII, and X may also be increased.
Uses: To prevent or control bleeding in patients with factor IX deficiency, especially hemophilia B and Christmas disease. Factor VII deficiency (Proplex T only). Hemophilia A with inhibitors to factor VIII.
Contraindications: Factor VII deficiency, except for Proplex T. Use when fresh frozen plasma is effective. Liver disease with suspected intravascular coagulation or fibrinolysis. Hypersensitivity to mouse proteins.
Precautions: Assess benefit versus risk prior to use in liver disease or elective surgery.

Route/Dosage
- **IV**
    Factor IX deficiency.
Individualized, depending on severity of bleeding, degree of deficiency, body weight, and level of factor required. Minimum factor IX level required in surgery or following trauma is 25% of normal, which is maintained for 1 week after surgery. As a guide in determining the units required to raise blood level percentages of factor IX, use the following formula for human-derived factor IX:

1 unit/kg × body weight (kg) × desired increase (% of normal).
For recombinant factor IX, use the following formula:

1.2 IU/kg × body weight (kg) × desired increase (% of control).
    Factor VII deficiency (Proplex T only).
To determine the units needed to raise blood level percentages, use the following:

0.5 unit/kg × body weight (kg) × desired increase (% of normal). The dose may be repeated q 4–6 hr. The package insert should be checked carefully as a guideline for doses for various factor deficiencies.
    Factor VII deficiency (hemophilia A) — Proplex T or Konyne 80 only.
Use dosage levels approximating 75 IU/kg.
    Bleeding in hemophilia A with factor VIII inhibitors.
75 IU/kg.
How Supplied: *Powder for injection*
Side Effects: *CV: **DIC, thrombosis. High doses may cause MI, venous or pulmonary thrombosis.** Miscellaneous:* Chills, fever. *Symptoms due to rapid infusion:* N&V, headache, fever, chills, tingling, flushing, urticaria, and changes in BP or pulse rate. Most of these side effects disappear when rate of administration is slowed.

The preparation also contains trace amounts of blood groups A and B and isohemagglutinins, which may cause intravascular hemolysis when administered in large amounts to patients with blood groups A, B, and AB.

Although careful screening is undertaken, both hepatitis and AIDS may be transmitted using factor IX Complex since it is derived from pooled human plasma.
Drug Interactions: ↑ Risk of thrombosis if administered with aminocaproic acid.

EMS CONSIDERATIONS

None.

Famciclovir
(fam-SY-kloh-veer)
Pregnancy Class: B
Famvir **(Rx)**
Classification: Antiviral agent

Mechanism of Action: Inhibits viral DNA synthesis and therefore replication in HSV types 1 (HSV-1) and 2 (HSV-2) and varicella-zoster virus.

Uses: Management of acute herpes zoster (shingles). Treatment of recurrent herpes simplex (genital herpes and cold sores), including those infected with HIV. To prevent outbreaks of recurrent genital herpes.

Contraindications: Use during lactation.

Precautions: The dose should be ajusted in patients with C_{cr} less than 60 mL/min. Safety and efficacy have not been determined in children less than 18 years of age.

Route/Dosage
• **Tablets**

Herpes zoster infections.
500 mg q 8 hr for 7 days. Dosage reduction is recommended in patients with impaired renal function: for C_{CR} of 40–59 mL/min, the dose should be 500 mg q 12 hr; for C_{CR} of 20–39 mL/min, the dose should be 500 mg q 24 hr; for C_{CR} less than 20 mL/min, the dose should be 250 mg q 48 hr. For hemodialysis patients, the recommended dose is 250 mg given after each dialysis treatment.

Recurrent genital herpes.
125 mg b.i.d. for 5 days. Should be taken within 6 hr of symptoms or lesion onset. Dosage reduction is as follows for those with impaired renal function: for C_{CR} of 40 mL/min or greater, use the recommended dose of 125 mg b.i.d.; for C_{CR} of 20–39 mL/min, the dose should be 125 mg q 24 hr; for C_{CR} less than 20 mL/min, the dose should be 125 mg q 48 hr. For hemodialysis patients, the recommended dose is 125 mg given after each dialysis treatment.

Recurrent orolabial or genital herpes infection in HIV-infected patients.
500 mg b.i.d. for 7 days.

Prevent outbreaks of genital herpes.
250 mg b.i.d.

How Supplied: *Tablet:* 125 mg, 250 mg, 500 mg

Side Effects: *GI:* N&V, diarrhea, constipation, anorexia, abdominal pain, dyspepsia, flatulence. *CNS:* Headache, dizziness, paresthesia, somnolence, insomnia. *Body as a whole:* Fatigue, fever, pain, rigors. *Musculoskeletal:* Back pain, arthralgia. *Respiratory:* Pharyngitis, sinusitis, upper respiratory infection. *Dermatologic:* Pruritus; signs, symptoms, and complications of zoster and genital herpes.

Drug Interactions
Digoxin / ↑ Levels of digoxin
Probenecid / Probenecid ↑ plasma levels of penciclovir
Theophylline / ↑ Levels of penciclovir

EMS CONSIDERATIONS

See also *Antiviral Agents.*

Famotidine
(fah-MOH-tih-deen)
Pregnancy Class: B
Pepcid, Pepcid AC Acid Controller, Pepcid IV, Pepcid RPD **(Rx)** (Pepcid AC is OTC)
Classification: Histamine H_2 receptor antagonist

Mechanism of Action: Competitive inhibitor of histamine H_2 receptors leading to inhibition of gastric acid secretion.

Onset of Action: 1 hr.

Duration of Action: 10-12 hr.

Uses: Rx: Treatment of active duodenal ulcers. Maintenance therapy for duodenal ulcer, at reduced dosage, after active ulcer has healed. Pathologic hypersecretory conditions such as Zollinger-Ellison syndrome or multiple endocrine adenomas. GERD, including erosive esophagitis. Treatment of benign gastric ulcer. *Investigational:* Prevent aspiration pneumonitis, for prophylaxis of stress ulcers, prevent acute upper GI bleeding, as part of multidrug therapy to eradicate *Helicobacter pylori*.

OTC: Relief of and prevention of the symptoms of heartburn, acid indigestion, and sour stomach.

Contraindications: Cirrhosis of the liver, impaired renal or hepatic function, lactation.

Precautions: Safety and efficacy in children have not been established.

Route/Dosage
• **Oral Suspension, Tablets**
Duodenal ulcer, acute therapy.
Adults: 40 mg once daily at bedtime or 20 mg b.i.d. Most ulcers heal within 4 weeks and it is rarely necessary to use the full dosage for 6–8 weeks.

Duodenal ulcer, maintenance therapy.
Adults: 20 mg once daily at bedtime.

Benign gastric ulcers, acute therapy.
Adults: 40 mg at bedtime.

Hypersecretory conditions.
Adults, individualized, initial: 20 mg q 6 hr; **then,** adjust dose to response, although doses of up to 160 mg q 6 hr may be required for severe cases.

Gastroesophageal reflux disease.
Adults: 20 mg b.i.d. for 6 weeks. For esophagitis with erosions and ulcerations, give 20 or 40 mg b.i.d. for up to 12 weeks.

Prophylaxis of upper GI bleeding.
Adults: 20 mg b.i.d.

Prophylaxis of stress ulcers.
Adults: 40 mg/day.

Relief of and prevention of heartburn, acid indigestion, and sour stomach (OTC).
Adults and children over 12 years of age, for relief: 10 mg (1 tablet) with water. **For prevention:** 10 mg 1 hr before eating a meal that may cause symptoms. **Maximum dose:** 20 mg/24 hr. Not to be used continuously for more than 2 weeks unless medically prescribed.

• **IM, IV, IV Infusion**

Hospitalized patients with hypersecretory conditions, duodenal ulcers, gastric ulcers; patients unable to take PO medication.
Adults: 20 mg IV q 12 hr.

Before anesthesia to prevent aspiration of gastric acid.
Adults: 40 mg IM or PO.

How Supplied: *Injection:* 10 mg/mL; *Powder for Reconstitution:* 40 mg/5 mL; *Tablet:* 10 mg, 20 mg, 40 mg; *Sublingual Tablet*

Side Effects: *GI:* Constipation, diarrhea, N&V, anorexia, dry mouth, abdominal discomfort. *CNS:* Dizziness, headache, paresthesias, depression, anxiety, confusion, hallucinations, insomnia, fatigue, sleepiness, agitation, ***grand mal seizure,*** psychic disturbances. *Skin:* Rash, acne, pruritus, alopecia, urticaria, dry skin, flushing. *CV:* Palpitations. *Musculoskeletal:* Arthralgia, asthenia, musculoskeletal pain. *Hematologic:* Thrombocytopenia. *Other:* Fever, orbital edema, conjunctival injection, bronchospasm, tinnitus, taste disorders, decreased libido, impotence, pain at injection site (transient).

Drug Interactions
Antacids / ↓ Absorption of famotidine from the GI tract
Diazepam / ↓ Absorption of diazepam from the GI tract

EMS CONSIDERATIONS

See also *Histamine H₂Antagonists*.

Felbamate
(FELL-bah-mayt)
Pregnancy Class: C
Felbatol **(Rx)**
Classification: Anticonvulsant, miscellaneous (second-line therapy)

Mechanism of Action: Mechanism not known. Felbamate may reduce seizure spread and increase seizure threshold.

Uses: Alone or as part of adjunctive therapy for the treatment of partial seizures with and without generalization in adults with epilepsy. As an adjunct in the treatment of partial

---

bold italic = life threatening side effect

and generalized seizures associated with Lennox-Gastaut syndrome in children. The drug should be used only as second-line therapy.

Contraindications: History of hepatic dysfunction or blood dyscrasia. Hypersensitivity to carbamates.

Precautions: Aplastic anemia and acute liver failure have been observed in a few patients. Use with caution during lactation. Safety and efficacy have not been established in children other than those with Lennox-Gastaut syndrom.*NOTE:* In August 1994 it was recommended that felbamate treatment be discontinued for epilepsy patients due to several cases of aplastic anemia. Revised labeling states, "... Felbatol should only be used in patients whose epilepsy is so severe that the risk of aplastic anemia is deemed acceptable in light of the benefits conferred by ist use..."

Route/Dosage

* **Suspension, Tablets**
  Monotherapy, initial therapy.
  Adults over 14 years of age, initial: 1,200 mg/day in divided doses t.i.d.–q.i.d. The dose may be increased in 600-mg increments q 2 weeks to 2,400 mg/day based on clinical response and thereafter to 3,600 mg/day, if needed.
  Conversion to monotherapy.
  Adults: Initiate at 1,200 mg/day in divided doses t.i.d.–q.i.d. Reduce the dose of concomitant antiepileptic drugs by ⅓ at initiation of felbamate therapy. At week 2, the felbamate dose should be increased to 2,400 mg/day while reducing the dose of other antiepileptic drugs up to another ⅓ of the original dose. At week 3, increase the felbamate dose to 3,600 mg/day and continue to decrease the dose of other antiepileptic drugs as indicated by response.
  Adjunctive therapy.
  Adults: Add felbamate at a dose of 1,200 mg/day in divided doses t.i.d.–q.i.d. while reducing current antiepileptic drugs by 20%. Further decreases of concomitant antiepileptic drugs may be needed to mini-

mize side effects due to drug interactions. The dose of felbamate can be increased by 1,200-mg/day increments at weekly intervals to 3,600 mg/day.

Lennox-Gastaut syndrome in children, aged 2–14 years.
As an adjunct, add felbamate at a dose of 15 mg/kg/day in divided doses t.i.d.–q.i.d. while decreasing present antiepileptic drugs by 20%. Further decreases in antiepileptic drug dosage may be needed to minimize side effects due to drug interactions. The dose of felbamate may be increased by 15-mg/kg/day increments at weekly intervals to 45 mg/kg/day.

How Supplied: *Suspension:* 600 mg/5 mL; *Tablet:* 400 mg, 600 mg

Side Effects: May differ depending on whether the drug is used as monotherapy or adjunctive therapy in adults or for Lennox-Gastaut syndrome in children. *CNS:* Insomnia, headache, anxiety, somnolence, dizziness, nervousness, tremor, abnormal gait, depression, paresthesia, ataxia, stupor, abnormal thinking, emotional lability, agitation, psychologic disturbance, aggressive reaction, hallucinations, euphoria, **suicide attempt,** migraine. *GI:* Dyspepsia, vomiting, constipation, diarrhea, dry mouth, nausea, anorexia, abdominal pain, hiccoughs, esophagitis, increased appetite. *Respiratory:* Upper respiratory tract infection, rhinitis, sinusitis, pharyngitis, coughing. *CV:* Palpitation, tachycardia, SVT. *Body as a whole:* Fatigue, weight decrease or increase, facial edema, fever, chest pain, pain, asthenia, malaise, flu-like symptoms, **anaphylaxis.** *Ophthalmologic:* Miosis, diplopia, abnormal vision. *GU:* Urinary incontinence, intramenstrual bleeding, UTI. *Hematologic:* **Aplastic anemia,** purpura, leukopenia, lymphadenopathy, leukocytosis, thrombocytopenia, granulocytopenia, positive antinuclear factor test, **agranulocytosis,** qualitative platelet disorder. *Dermatologic:* Acne, rash, pruritus, urticaria, bullous eruption, buccal mucous membrane swelling, **Stevens-Johnson**

syndrome. Miscellaneous: Otitis media, *acute liver failure,* taste perversion, hypophosphatemia, myalgia, photosensitivity, substernal chest pain, dystonia, allergic reaction.

Drug Interactions
Carbamazepine / Felbamate ↓ steady-state carbamazepine levels and ↑ steady-state carbamazepine epoxide (metabolite) levels. Also, carbamazepine → 50% ↑ in felbamate clearance
Methsuximide / ↑ Normethsuxide levels; decrease methsuximide dose
Phenobarbital / ↑ Phenobarbital plasma levels and a ↓ in felbamate levels
Phenytoin / Felbamate ↑ steady-state phenytoin levels necessitating a 40% decrease in phenytoin dose. Also, phenytoin ↑ felbamate clearance
Valproic acid / Felbamate ↑ steady-state valproic acid levels

EMS CONSIDERATIONS

See also *Anticonvulsants.*

Felodipine
(feh-LOHD-ih-peen)
Pregnancy Class: C
Plendil **(Rx)**
Classification: Calcium channel blocking agent

Onset of Action: PO: 120-300 min.
Uses: Treatment of mild to moderate hypertension, alone or with other antihypertensives.
Contraindications: Lactation.
Precautions: Use with caution in patients with CHF or compromised ventricular function, especially in combination with a beta-adrenergic blocking agent. Use with caution in impaired hepatic function or reduced hepatic blood flow. May cause a greater hypotensive effect in geriatric patients. Safety and effectiveness have not been determined in children.

Route/Dosage
• **Tablets, Extended Release**

Hypertension.
Initial: 5 mg once daily (2.5 mg in patients over 65 years of age and in those with impaired liver function); **then:** adjust dose according to response, usually at 2-week intervals with the usual dosage range being 2.5–10 mg once daily. Doses greater than 10 mg increase the rate of peripheral edema and other vasodilatory side effects.
How Supplied: *Tablet, Extended Release:* 2.5 mg, 5 mg, 10 mg
Side Effects: *CV:* Significant hypotension, syncope, angina pectoris, peripheral edema, palpitations, AV block, *MI, arrhythmias,* tachycardia. *CNS:* Dizziness, lightheadedness, headache, nervousness, sleepiness, irritability, anxiety, insomnia, paresthesia, depression, amnesia, paranoia, psychosis, hallucinations. *Body as a whole:* Asthenia, flushing, muscle cramps, pain, inflammation, warm feeling, influenza. *GI:* Nausea, abdominal discomfort, cramps, dyspepsia, diarrhea, constipation, vomiting, dry mouth, flatulence. *Dermatologic:* Rash, dermatitis, urticaria, pruritus. *Respiratory:* Rhinitis, rhinorrhea, pharyngitis, sinusitis, nasal and chest congestion, SOB, wheezing, dyspnea, cough, bronchitis, sneezing, respiratory infection. *Miscellaneous:* Anemia, gingival hyperplasia, sexual difficulties, epistaxis, back pain, facial edema, erythema, urinary frequency or urgency, dysuria.
Drug Interactions: Additional: *Cimetidine/* ↑ Bioavailability of felodipine*Digoxin/* ↑ Peak plasma levels of digoxin*Fentanyl/* Possible severe hypotension or ↑ fluid volume*Ranitidine/* ↑ Bioavailability of felodipine

EMS CONSIDERATIONS

See also *Calcium Channel Blocking Agents.*

Fenofibrate
(fee-noh-FY-brayt)
Pregnancy Class: C

TRICOR **(Rx)**
Classification: Antihyperlipidemic
drug

Mechanism of Action: Is converted to the active fenofibric acid, which lowers plasma triglycerides. Probable mechanism is to inhibit triglyceride synthesis, resulting in a reduction of VLDL released into the circulation, and by stimulating catabolism of triglyceride-rich lipoprotein. Also increases urinary excretion of uric acid.

Uses: Adjunct to diet to treat Types IV and V hyperlipidemia in adults who are at risk of pancreatitis and who do not respond to diet alone.

Contraindications: Hepatic or severe renal dysfunction (including primary biliary cirrhosis), those with unexplained, persistent abnormal liver function, and preexisting gallbladder disease. Lactation.

Precautions: Due to similarity to clofibrate and gemfibrozil, side effects, including death, are possible. Safety and efficacy have not been determined in children.

Route/Dosage
• **Capsules**
  Hypertriglyceridemia.
Initial: 67 mg/day given with meals to optimize bioavailability. Then, individualize based on patient response. Increase, if necessary, at 4–8–week intervals. **Maximuim daily dose:** 201 mg/day (i.e., 3 capsules). If C_{CR} is less than 50 mL/min, start with 67 mg/day; increase dose only after evaluation of effects on renal function and triglyceride levels. In the elderly, limit the initial dose to 67 mg/day.

How Supplied: *Capsules:* 67 mg

Side Effects: *GI:* Pancreatitis, cholelithiasis, dyspepsia, N&V, diarrhea, abdominal pain, constipation, flatulence, eructation, hepatitis, cholecystitis, hepatomegaly. *CNS:* Decreased libido, dizziness, increased appetite, insomnia, paresthesia. *Respiratory:* Rhinitis, cough, sinusitis, allergic pulmonary alveolitis. *GU:* Polyuria, vaginitis. *Musculoskeletal:* Myopathy, myositis, arthralgia, myalgia, myasthenia, rhabdomyolysis. *Hypersensitivity:* Severe skin rashes, urticaria. *Ophthalmic:* Eye irritation, blurred vision, conjunctivitis, eye floaters. *Miscellaneous:* Infections, pain, headache, asthenia, fatigue, flu syndrome, arrhythmia, photosensitivity, eczema.

Drug Interactions
Anticoagulants / Prolongation of PT
Bile acid sequestrants / ↓ Absorption of fenofibrate due to binding
Cyclosporine / ↑ Risk of nephrotoxicity
HMG-CoA reductase inhibitors / Possibility of rhabdomyolysis, myopathy, and acute renal failure

EMS CONSIDERATIONS
None.

Fenoldopam mesylate
(feh-NOL-doh-pam)
Pregnancy Class: B
Corlopam **(Rx)**
Classification: Drug for hypertensive emergency

Mechanism of Action: Rapid-acting vasodilator that is an agonist for D_1-like dopamine receptors and α_2-adrenoreceptors. Causes vasodilation in coronary, renal, mesenteric, and peripheral arteries; vascular beds do not respond uniformly.

Uses: Hypertensive emergencies.

Contraindications: Use with beta-blockers or in those with sulfite sensitivity.

Precautions: Use with caution during lactation and in those with glaucoma or intraocular hypertension. Safety and efficacy have not been determined in children.

Route/Dosage
• **Constant IV infusion**
  Hypertensive emergency.
Rate of infusion is individualized according to body weight and to desired speed and extent of effect. See package insert for table of infusion rates. Doses range from 0.025 mcg/kg/min–0.3 mcg/kg/min for a body weight of 40 kg to 0.094 mcg/kg/min–1.13mcg/kg/min for a body weight of 150 kg.

How Supplied: *Injection concentrate:* 10 mg/mL
Side Effects: *CV:* Tachycardia, hypotension, flushing, ST-T abnormalities, postural hypotension, extrasystoles, palpitations, bradycardia, **heart failure, ischemic heart disease, MI,** angina pectoris. *Body as a whole:* Headache, sweating, back pain, nonspecific chest pain, pyrexia, limb cramp. *CNS:* Nervousness, anxiety, insomnia, dizziness. *GI:* N&V, abdominal pain or fullness, constipation, diarrhea. *Respiratory:* Nasal congestion, dyspnea, upper respiratory disorder. *Hematologic:* Leukocytosis, bleeding. *Miscellaneous:* Reaction at injection site, urinary tract infection, oliguria.

EMS CONSIDERATIONS
Administration/Storage
IV 1. Do not use a bolus dose.
2. Most of the effect of a given infusion is reached in 15 min.
3. Initial dose is titrated up or down no more often than every 15 min, and less frequently as desired BP is approached. Recommended increments for titration are 0.05–0.1 mcg/kg/min.
4. Dilute ampule concentrate in 0.9% NaCl or D5W injection for a final concentration of 40 mcg/mL (i.e., add 4 mL of the concentrate to 1,000 mL; 2 mL of the concentrate to 500 mL; or, 1 mL of the concentrate to 250 mL). Each mL of concentrate contains 10 mg of drug. Each ampule is for single use only.
Assessment: Monitor VS.

Fenoprofen calcium
(fen-oh-PROH-fen)
Pregnancy Class: B
Nalfon **(Rx)**
Classification: Nonsteroidal antiinflammatory analgesic

Onset of Action: Peak effect: 2-3 hr, **As antiarthritic:** Within 2 days; **maximum effect:** 2-3 weeks.
Duration of Action: 4-6 hr.

Uses: Rheumatoid arthritis, osteoarthritis, mild to moderate pain. *Investigational:* Juvenile rheumatoid arthritis, prophylaxis of migraine, migraine due to menses, sunburn.
Contraindications: Use in pregnancy and children less than 12 years of age. Renal dysfunction.
Precautions: Safety and efficacy in children have not been established.

Route/Dosage
• **Capsules, Tablets**
  Rheumatoid and osteoarthritis.
Adults: 300–600 mg t.i.d.–q.i.d. Adjust dose according to response of patient.
  Mild to moderate pain.
Adults: 200 mg q 4–6 hr. Maximum daily dose for all uses: 3,200 mg.
How Supplied: *Capsule:* 200 mg, 300 mg; *Tablet:* 600 mg
Side Effects: Additional: *GU:* Dysuria, hematuria, cystitis, interstitial nephritis, nephrotic syndrome. Overdosage has caused tachycardia and hypotension.

EMS CONSIDERATIONS
None.

Fentanyl Transdermal System
(FEN-tah-nil)
Pregnancy Class: C
Duragesic-25, -50, -75, and -100 **(C-II) (Rx)**
Classification: Narcotic analgesic, morphine type

Mechanism of Action: The system provides continuous delivery of fentanyl for up to 72 hr. Following application of the system, the skin under the system absorbs fentanyl, resulting in a depot of the drug in the upper skin layers, which is then available to the general circulation. After the system is removed, the residual drug in the skin continues to be absorbed.
Uses: Restrict use for the management of severe chronic pain that cannot be managed with less powerful drugs. Only use on patients al-

bold italic = life threatening side effect

ready on and tolerant to narcotic analgesics and who require continuous narcotic administration.

Contraindications: Use for acute or postoperative pain (including outpatient surgeries). To manage mild or intermittent pain that can be managed by acetaminophen-opioid combinations, NSAIDs, or short-acting opioids. Hypersensitivity to fentanyl or adhesives. ICP, impaired consciousness, coma, medical conditions causing hypoventilation. Use during labor and delivery. Use of initial doses exceeding 25 mcg/hr, use in children less than 12 years of age and patients under 18 years of age who weigh less than 50 kg. Lactation.

Precautions: Use with caution in patients with brain tumors and bradyarrhythmias, as well as in elderly, cachectic, or debilitated individuals. Safety and efficacy have not been determined in children.

Route/Dosage
• **Transdermal System**
   Analgesia.

Adults, usual initial: 25 mcg/hr unless the patient is tolerant to opioids (Duragesic-50, -75, and -100 are intended for use only in patients tolerant to opioids).

How Supplied: *Film, Extended Release:* 25 mcg/hr, 50 mcg/hr, 75 mcg/hr, 100 mcg/hr

Side Effects: Additional: Sustained hypoventilation.

EMS CONSIDERATIONS

See also *Narcotic Analgesics.*

Ferrous fumarate
(FAIR-us FYOU-mar-ayt)
Ferniron, Feostat, Feostat Drops and Suspension, Hemocyte, Ircon, Nephro-Fer **(OTC)**
Classification: Antianemic, iron

Mechanism of Action: Better tolerated than ferrous gluconate or ferrous sulfate. Contains 33% elemental iron.

Route/Dosage
• **Extended-Release Capsules**
   Prophylaxis.

Adults: 325 mg/day.
   Anemia.

Adults: 325 mg b.i.d. Capsules are not recommended for use in children.

• **Oral Solution, Oral Suspension, Tablets, Chewable Tablets**
   Prophylaxis.

Adults: 200 mg/day. **Pediatric:** 3 mg/kg/day.
   Anemia.

Adults: 200 mg t.i.d.–q.i.d. **Pediatric:** 3 mg/kg t.i.d., up to 6 mg/kg/day, if needed.

How Supplied: *Chew Tablet:* 100 mg; *Liquid:* 45 mg/0.6 mL; *Suspension:* 100 mg/5 mL; *Tablet:* 63 mg, 200 mg, 325 mg, 350 mg; *Extended Release Capsules* 100–150 mg, 300 mg

EMS CONSIDERATIONS

None.

Ferrous gluconate
(FAIR-us GLUE-kon-ayt)
Fergon **(OTC)**
Classification: Antianemic, iron

Mechanism of Action: Contains about 11% elemental iron.
Uses: Particularly indicated for patients who cannot tolerate ferrous sulfate because of gastric irritation.

Route/Dosage
• **Capsules, Tablets**
   Prophylaxis.

Adults: 325 mg/day. **Pediatric, 2 years and older:** 8 mg/kg/day.
   Anemia.

Adults: 325 mg q.i.d. Can be increased to 650 mg q.i.d. if needed and tolerated. **Pediatric, 2 years and older:** 16 mg/kg t.i.d.
• **Elixir, Syrup**
   Prophylaxis.

Adults: 300 mg/day. **Pediatric, 2 years and older:** 8 mg/kg/day.
   Anemia.

Adults: 300 mg q.i.d. Can be increased to 600 mg q.i.d. as needed and tolerated. **Pediatric, 2 years and older:** 16 mg/kg t.i.d. The provider must determine dosage for children less than 2 years of age.

How Supplied: *Capsule:* 225 mg and 324 mg; *Extended Release Capsule:* 150 mg, 159 mg, 250 mg; *Drops:* 75 mg/0.6 mL, 25 mg/mL; *Elixir:* 220 mg/5 mL, 300 mg/5 mL; *Oral Liquid/Solution:* 300 mg/5 mL; *Tablet:* 200 mg, 300 mg, 324 mg, 325 mg; *Enteric-Coated Tablet:* 200 mg, 325 mg

EMS CONSIDERATIONS

None.

Ferrous sulfate
Ferrous sulfate, dried
(FAIR-us SUL-fayt)

Ferrous sulfate: Feosol, Fergen-sol, Fer-in-Sol, Fer-iron **(OTC) Ferrous sulfate, dried:** Fe50, Feosol, Feratab, Slow FE **(OTC)**
Classification: Antianemic, iron

Mechanism of Action: Least expensive, most effective iron salt for PO therapy. Ferrous sulfate products contain 20% elemental iron, whereas ferrous sulfate dried products contain 30% elemental iron.

Route/Dosage

FERROUS SULFATE

• **Extended-Release Capsules**
Adults: 150–250 mg 1–2 times/day. This dosage form is not recommended for children.

• **Elixir, Oral Solution, Tablets, Enteric-coated Tablets**
Prophylaxis.
Adults: 300 mg/day. **Pediatric:** 5 mg/kg/day.
Anemia.
Adults: 300 mg b.i.d. increased to 300 mg q.i.d. as needed and tolerated. **Pediatric:** 10 mg/kg t.i.d. The enteric-coated tablets are not recommended for use in children.

• **Extended-Release Tablets**
Adults: 525 mg 1–2 times/day. This dosage form is not recommended for use in children.

FERROUS SULFATE, DRIED
• **Capsules**
Prophylaxis.

Adults: 300 mg/day. **Pediatric:** 5 mg/kg/day.
Anemia.
Adults: 300 mg b.i.d. up to 300 mg q.i.d. as needed and tolerated. **Pediatric:** 10 mg/kg t.i.d.

• **Tablets**
Prophylaxis.
Adults: 200 mg/day. **Pediatric:** 5 mg/kg/day.
Anemia.
Adults: 200 mg t.i.d. up to 200 mg q.i.d. as needed and tolerated. **Pediatric:** 10 mg/kg t.i.d.

• **Extended-Release Tablets**
Adults: 160 mg 1–2 times/day. This dosage form is not recommended for use in children.

How Supplied: Ferrous sulfate: *Capsule:* 250 mg, 324 mg; *Capsule, Extended Release:* 250 mg; *Elixir:* 220 mg/5 mL; *Enteric Coated Tablet:* 325 mg; *Liquid:* 25 mg/mL, 75 mg/0.6 mL, 300 mg/5 mL; *Solution:* 300 mg/5 mL; *Syrup:* 90 mg/5 mL; *Tablet:* 195 mg, 300 mg, 324 mg, 325 mg; *Tablet, Extended Release:* 250 mg, 525 mg Ferrous sulfate, dried: *Capsule, Extended Release:* 150 mg, 159 mg; *Enteric Coated Tablet:* 200 mg; *Tablet:* 200 mg; *Tablet, Extended Release:* 152 mg, 159 mg, 160 mg

EMS CONSIDERATIONS

None.

Fexofenadine hydrochloride
(fex-oh-FEN-ah-deen)
Pregnancy Class: C
Allegra **(Rx)**
Classification: Antihistamine

Mechanism of Action: Is an H_1-histamine receptor blocker. Low to no sedative or anticholinergic effects.
Onset of Action: Rapid.
Uses: Seasonal allergic rhinitis, including sneezing; rhinorrhea; itchy nose, throat, or palate; and itchy, watery, and red eyes in adults and children 12 years of age and older.

Precautions: Use with care during lactation. Safety and efficacy have not been determined in children less than 12 years of age.

Route/Dosage
• **Capsules**
Seasonal allergic rhinitis.
Adults and children over 12 years of age: 60 mg b.i.d. In patients with decreased renal function, the initial dose should be 60 mg once daily.
How Supplied: *Capsule:* 60 mg
Side Effects: *CNS:* Drowsiness, fatigue, headache. *GI:* Nausea, dyspepsia. *Respiratory:* Sinusitis, throat irritation, pharyngitis. *Miscellaneous:* Viral infection (flu, colds), dysmenorrhea.
Drug Interactions: No differences in side effects or the QTc interval were observed when fexofenadine was given with either erythromycin or ketoconazole.

EMS CONSIDERATIONS

See also *Antihistamines.*

Filgrastim
(fill-GRASS-tim)
Pregnancy Class: C
Neupogen **(Rx)**
Classification: Human granulocyte colony-stimulating factor (G-CSF)

Mechanism of Action: Is a human granulocyte colony stimulating factor (G-CSF) produced by recombinant DNA technology by *Escherichia coli* that has been inserted with the human G-CSF gene. Endogenous G-CSF is a glycoprotein that is produced by monocytes, fibroblasts, and other endothelial cells and that regulates the production of neutrophils in the bone marrow.
Uses: To decrease the incidence of infection, as manifested by febrile neutropenia, in patients with non-myeloid malignancies who are receiving myelosuppressive anticancer drugs, which are associated with severe neutropenia with fever. To reduce the duration of neutropenia in patients with nonmyeloid malignancies undergoing myeloablative che-

motherapy followed by bone marrow transplantation. To reduce infection in severe chronic neutropenia (e.g., congenital, cyclical, or idiopathic neutropenia) after other diseases have been ruled out. For the mobilization of hematopoietic progenitor cells into the peripheral blood for leukapheresis collection. To reduce the time to neutrophil recovery and the duration of fever in patients being treated for acute myelogenous leukemia. *Investigational:* Use in AIDS, aplastic anemia, hairy cell leukemia, myelodysplasia, drug-induced and congenital agranulocytosis, and alloimmune neonatal neutropenia.
Contraindications: Hypersensitivity to proteins derived from *E. coli.* The safety and effectiveness of filgrastim given simultaneously with cytotoxic chemotherapy have not been determined; thus, filgrastim should not be given 24 hr before to 24 hr after cytotoxic chemotherapy.
Precautions: Use with caution during lactation. Use with caution in any malignancy with myeloid characteristics since the drug may act as a growth factor for any tumor type. Filgrastim does not cause any greater incidence of toxicity in children than in adults. Safety and efficacy have not been determined in neonates and patients with autoimmune neutropenia of infancy. The safety and effectiveness of chronic filgrastim therapy have not been determined. Hypersensitivity reactions usually occur within 30 min after administration and are more frequent in patients receiving the drug IV.

Route/Dosage
• **SC, IV**
Myelosuppressive chemotherapy.
Initial: 5 mcg/kg/day as a single injection, either as a SC bolus, by short IV infusion (15–30 min), or by continuous SC or IV infusion (over a 24-hr period). The dose may be increased in increments of 5 mcg/kg for each chemotherapy cycle depending on the duration and severity of the absolute neutrophil count (ANC) nadir.

The dose should be given daily for up to 2 weeks, until ANC has reached 10,000/mm³ following the expected chemotherapy-induced neutrophil nadir.

Severe chronic neutropenia.
5 mcg/kg/day SC for idiopathic and cyclic disease; 6 mcg/kg/day SC for congenital disease.

Bone marrow transplantation.
10 mcg/kg/day given as an IV infusion of 4 or 24 hr or as a continuous 24-hr SC infusion.

NOTE: During the period of neutrophil recovery, the daily dose should be titrated against the neutrophil response as follows:
1. When ANC is greater than 1,000/mm³ for 3 consecutive days, reduce the dose of filgrastim to 5 mcg/kg/day. If ANC decreases to less than 1,000/mm³ at any time during the 5-mcg/kg/day dosage, increase filgrastim to 10 mcg/kg/day.
2. If ANC remains greater than 1,000/mm³ for 3 more consecutive days, discontinue filgrastim.
3. If ANC decreases to less than 1,000/mm³, resume filgrastim at 5 mcg/kg/day.

Peripheral blood progenitor cell collection.
10 mcg/kg/day SC, either as a bolus or a continuous infusion. Filgrastim should be given at least 4 days before the first leukapheresis procedure and continued until the last leukapheresis.

How Supplied: *Injection:* 300 mcg/mL

Side Effects: When used for myelosuppressive therapy. *Musculoskeletal:* Medullary bone pain, skeletal pain. *GI:* N&V, diarrhea, anorexia, stomatitis, constipation, peritonitis. *Hypersensitivity:* Skin rash, facial edema, wheezing, dyspnea, hypotension, tachycardia. *Hematologic:* Leukocytosis; greater risk of thrombocytopenia and anemia. *Respiratory:* Dyspnea, cough, chest pain, sore throat. *Body as a whole:* Alopecia, neutropenic fever, fever, fatigue, headache, skin rash, mucositis, generalized weakness, unspecified pain. *CV:* Decreased BP (transient), cutaneous vasculitis, hypertension, ***arrhythmias, MI.***

When used for severe chronic neutropenia. *Musculoskeletal:* Mild to moderate bone pain, abdominal/flank pain, arthralgia, osteoporosis. *Hematologic:* Thrombocytopenia, epistaxis (associated with thrombocytopenia), anemia, myelodysplasia or myeloid leukemia. *Dermatologic:* Exacerbation of certain skin conditions (e.g., psoriasis), rash, alopecia. *Miscellaneous:* Palpable splenomegaly, hepatomegaly, monosomy, reaction at injection site, cutaneous vasculitis, hematuria, proteinuria.

When used for bone marrow transplantation. *GI:* N&V, stomatitis, peritonitis. *CV:* Hypertension, capillary leak syndrome (rare). *Miscellaneous:* Rash, renal insufficiency, erythema nodosum.

When used for peripheral blood progenitor cell collection. *Hematologic:* Decreased platelet counts, anemia, increase in neutrophil count, WBC count greater than 100,000/mm³. *Miscellaneous:* Mild to moderate musculoskeletal symptoms, medullary bone pain, headache, increases in alkaline phosphatase.

EMS CONSIDERATIONS

None.

Finasteride

(fin-AS-teh-ride)
Pregnancy Class: X
Propecia, Proscar **(Rx)**
Classification: Androgen hormone inhibitor

Mechanism of Action: Is a specific inhibitor of 5-α-reductase, the enzyme that converts testosterone to the active 5-α-dihydrotestosterone (DHT). Thus, there are significant decreases in serum and tissue DHT levels, resulting in rapid regression of prostate tissue and an increase in urine flow and symptomatic im-

F

---

bold italic = life threatening side effect

provement. Is also a decrease in scalp DHT levels.

Uses: Treatment of symptomatic benign prostatic hyperplasia. Male pattern baldness (vertex and anterior midscalp). *Investigational:* Adjuvant monotherapy following radical prostatectomy, prevention of the progression of first-stage prostate cancer, acne, and hirsutism.

Contraindications: Hypersensitivity to finasteride or any excipient in the product. Use in women and in children. Lactation.

Precautions: Use with caution in patients with impaired liver function.

Route/Dosage
• **Tablets**
Benign prostatic hyperplasia.
5 mg/day, with or without meals.
Androgenetic alopecia.
Males: 1 mg once a day with or without meals.

How Supplied: *Tablet:* 1 mg, 5 mg

Side Effects: *GU:* Impotence, decreased libido, decreased volume of ejaculate. *Miscellaneous:* Breast tenderness and enlargement, hypersensitivity reactions (including skin rash and swelling of the lips).

EMS CONSIDERATIONS
None.

————COMBINATION DRUG————
Fiorinal
Fiorinal with Codeine
Fiorinal (fee-OR-in-al) Fiorinal with Codeine (fee-OR-in-al, KOH-deen)
Pregnancy Class: Fiorinal with Codeine: C
Fiorinal **(Rx)** Fiorinal with Codeine **(C-III) (Rx)**
Classification: Analgesic

Uses: Fiorinal: Treat tension headaches. Fiorinal with Codeine: Analgesic for all types of pain.

Route/Dosage
• **Capsules, Tablets**
FIORINAL
1–2 tablets or capsules q 4 hr, not to exceed 6 tablets or capsules/day.

FIORINAL WITH CODEINE
Initial: 1–2 capsules; **then,** dose may be repeated, if necessary, up to maximum of 6 capsules/day.

How Supplied: Each Fiorinal capsule or tablet contains:
Nonnarcotic analgesic: Aspirin, 325 mg.
Sedative barbiturate: Butalbital, 50 mg.
CNS stimulant: Caffeine, 40 mg.
In addition to the above, Fiorinal with Codeine capsules contain codeine phosphate, 7.5 mg (No. 1), 15 mg (No. 2), or 30 mg (No. 3).

EMS CONSIDERATIONS
See also *Narcotic Analgesics, Acetylsalicylic acid,* and *Barbiturates.*

Flavoxate hydrochloride
(flay-VOX-ayt)
Pregnancy Class: B
Urispas **(Rx)**
Classification: Urinary tract antispasmodic

Mechanism of Action: Relieves muscle spasms of the urinary tract by relaxing the detrusor muscle by cholinergic blockade and also by a direct effect. Also has local anesthetic and analgesic effects.

Uses: Symptomatic relief of urinary tract irritation, dysuria, urgency, nocturia, suprapubic pain, incontinence associated with cystitis, prostatitis, urethritis, urethrocystitis, and other urinary tract disorders. Compatible for use with urinary tract germicides.

Contraindications: Obstructive disorders of urinary tract, including pyloric or duodenal obstructions, obstructive intestinal lesions, ileus, achalasia, obstructive uropathies of the lower urinary tract, and GI hemorrhage.

Precautions: Use with caution in glaucoma and during lactation. Confusion is more likely to occur in geriatric patients. Safety and effectiveness have not been determined in children less than 12 years of age.

Route/Dosage
• **Tablets**

Adults and children over 12 years: 100 or 200 mg t.i.d.–q.i.d. Reduce dose when symptoms improve.

How Supplied: *Tablet:* 100 mg

Side Effects: *GI:* N&V, xerostomia. *CNS:* Drowsiness, headache, vertigo, nervousness, mental confusion (especially in the elderly). *CV:* Tachycardia, palpitations. *Hematologic:* Eosinophilia, leukopenia. *Ophthalmologic:* Blurred vision, increased ocular tension, accommodation disturbances. *Other:* Urticaria and other dermatoses, fever, dysuria.

EMS CONSIDERATIONS

See also *Cholinergic Blocking Agents.*

Flecainide acetate
(fleh-KAY-nyd)
Pregnancy Class: C
Tambocor **(Rx)**
Classification: Antiarrhythmic, class IC

Mechanism of Action: The antiarrhythmic effect is due to a local anesthetic action, especially on the His-Purkinje system in the ventricle. Drug decreases single and multiple PVCs and reduces the incidence of ventricular tachycardia.

Uses: Life-threatening arrhythmias manifested as sustained ventricular tachycardia. Prevention of paroxysmal supraventricular tachycardias (PSVT) and paroxysmal atrial fibrillation or flutter (PAF) associated with disabling symptoms but not structural heart disease. Antiarrhythmic drugs have not been shown to improve survival in patients with ventricular arrhythmias.

Contraindications: Cardiogenic shock, preexisting second- or third-degree AV block, right bundle branch block when associated with bifascicular block (unless pacemaker is present to maintain cardiac rhythm). Recent MI. Cardiogenic shock. Chronic atrial fibrillation. Frequent premature ventricular complexes and sympto-

matic nonsustained ventricular arrhythmias. Lactation.

Precautions: Use with caution in sick sinus syndrome, in patients with a history of CHF or MI, in disturbances of potassium levels, in patients with permanent pacemakers or temporary pacing electrodes, renal and liver impairment. Safety and efficacy in children less than 18 years of age are not established. The incidence of proarrhythmic effects may be increased in geriatric patients.

Route/Dosage ————
• **Tablets**
    Sustained ventricular tachycardia.
Initial: 100 mg q 12 hr; **then,** increase by 50 mg b.i.d. q 4 days until effective dose reached. **Usual effective dose:** 150 mg q 12 hr, not to exceed 400 mg/day.
    PSVT, PAF.
Initial: 50 mg q 12 hr; **then,** dose may be increased in increments of 50 mg b.i.d. q 4 days until effective dose reached. Maximum recommended dose: 300 mg/day. *NOTE:* For PAF patients, increasing the dose from 50 to 100 mg b.i.d. may increase efficacy without a significant increase in side effects.
    NOTE: For patients with a C_{CR} less than 35 mL/min/1.73 m^2, the starting dose is 100 mg once daily (or 50 mg b.i.d.). For less severe renal disease, the initial dose may be 100 mg q 12 hr.

How Supplied: *Tablet:* 50 mg, 100 mg, 150 mg

Side Effects: *CV: **New or worsened ventricular arrhythmias, increased risk of death in patients with non-life-threatening cardiac arrhythmias,** new or worsened CHF, palpitations, chest pain, sinus bradycardia, sinus pause, sinus arrest, **ventricular fibrillation, ventricular tachycardia that cannot be resuscitated,** second- or third-degree AV block, tachycardia, hypertension, hypotension, bradycardia, angina pectoris. *CNS:* Dizziness, faintness, syncope, lightheadedness, neuropathy, unsteadiness, headache, fatigue, paresthesia, paresis, hypoesthesia, insomnia, anxiety, malaise, vertigo, depression, **seizures,** euphoria, confusion, depersonalization, apathy, morbid dreams, speech disorders, stupor, amnesia, weakness, somnolence. *GI:* Nausea, constipation, abdominal pain, vomiting, anorexia, dyspepsia, dry mouth, diarrhea, flatulence, change in taste. *Ophthalmic:* Blurred vision, difficulty in focusing, spots before eyes, diplopia, photophobia, eye pain, nystagmus, eye irritation, photophobia. *Hematologic:* Leukopenia, thrombocytopenia. *GU:* Decreased libido, impotence, urinary retention, polyuria. *Musculoskeletal:* Asthenia, tremor, ataxia, arthralgia, myalgia. *Dermatologic:* Skin rashes, urticaria, exfoliative dermatitis, pruritus, alopecia. *Other:* Edema, dyspnea, fever, **bronchospasm,** flushing, sweating, tinnitus, swollen mouth, lips, and tongue.

OD Overdose Management: *Symptoms:* Lengthening of PR interval; increase in QRS duration, QT interval, and amplitude of T wave; decrease in HR and contractility; conduction disturbances; hypotension; *respiratory failure* or *asystole. Treatment:* Charcoal will remove unabsorbed drug up to 90 min after drug ingestion. Administration of dopamine, dobutamine, or isoproterenol. Artificial respiration. Intra-aortic balloon pumping, transvenous pacing (to correct conduction block). Acidification of the urine may be beneficial, especially in those with an alkaline urine. Due to the long duration of action of the drug, treatment measures may have to be continued for a prolonged period of time.

Drug Interactions
Acidifying agents / ↑ Renal excretion of flecainide
Alkalinizing agents / ↓ Renal excretion of flecainide
Amiodarone / ↑ Plasma levels of flecainide
Cimetidine / ↑ Bioavailability and renal excretion of flecainide
Digoxin / ↑ Digoxin plasma levels
Disopyramide / Additive negative inotropic effects

Propranolol / Additive negative inotropic effects; also, ↑ plasma levels of both drugs
Smoking (Tobacco) / ↑ Plasma clearance of flecainide
Verapamil / Additive negative inotropic effects

EMS CONSIDERATIONS
See also *Antiarrhythmic Agents.*

Fluconazole
(flew-KON-ah-zohl)
Pregnancy Class: C
Diflucan **(Rx)**
Classification: Antifungal agent

Mechanism of Action: Inhibits the enzyme cytochrome P-450 in the organism, which results in a decrease in cell wall integrity and extrusion of intracellular material, leading to death.

Uses: Oropharyngeal and esophageal candidiasis. Serious systemic candidal infection (including UTIs, peritonitis, and pneumonia). Cryptococcal meningitis. Maintenance therapy to prevent cryptococcal meningitis in AIDS patients. Vaginal candidiasis. To decrease the incidence of candidiasis in patients undergoing a bone marrow transplant who receive cytotoxic chemotherapy or radiation therapy. Treatment of cryptococcal meningitis and candidal infections in children.

Contraindications: Hypersensitivity to fluconazole.

Precautions: Use with caution during lactation and if patient shows hypersensitivity to other azoles. Efficacy has not been adequately assessed in children.

Route/Dosage
• **Tablets, Oral Suspension, IV**
  Vaginal candidiasis.
150 mg as a single oral dose.
  Oropharyngeal or esophageal candidiasis.
Adults, first day: 200 mg; **then,** 100 mg/day for a minimum of 14 days (for oropharyngeal candidiasis) or 21 days (for esophageal candidiasis). Up to 400 mg/day may be required

for esophageal candidiasis. **Children, first day:** 6 mg/kg; **then,** 3 mg/kg once daily for a minimum of 14 days (for oropharyngeal candidiasis) or 21 days (for esophageal candidiasis).

Candidal UTI and peritonitis. 50–200 mg/day.

Systemic candidiasis (e.g., candidemia, disseminated candidiasis, and pneumonia).
Optimal dosage and duration in adults have not been determined although doses up to 400 mg/day have been used. **Children:** 6–12 mg/kg/day.

Acute cryptococcal meningitis.
Adults, first day: 400 mg; **then,** 200 mg/day (up to 400 mg may be required) for 10 to 12 weeks after CSF culture is negative. **Children, first day:** 12 mg/kg; **then,** 6 mg/kg once daily for 10 to 12 weeks after CSF culture is negative.

Maintenance to prevent relapse of cryptococcal meningitis in AIDS patients.
Adults: 200 mg once daily. **Pediatric:** 6 mg/kg once daily.

Prevention of candidiasis in bone marrow transplant.
400 mg once daily. In patients expected to have severe granulocytopenia (less than 500 neutrophils/mm3), start fluconazole several days before the anticipated onset of neutropenia and continue for 7 days after the neutrophil count rises about 1,000 cells/mm3. In patients with renal impairment, an initial loading dose of 50–400 mg can be given; daily dose is based then on C_{CR}.

How Supplied: *Injection:* 2 mg/mL, 200 mg/100 mL, 400 mg/200 mL; *Powder for Reconstitution:* 50 mg/5mL, 200 mg/5mL; *Tablet:* 50 mg, 100 mg, 150 mg, 200 mg

Side Effects: Following single doses. *GI:* Nausea, abdominal pain, diarrhea, dyspepsia, taste perversion. *CNS:* Headache, dizziness. *Other:* Angioedema, ***anaphylaxis (rare).***

Following multiple doses. Side effects are more frequently reported in HIV-infected patients than in non-HIV-infected patients. *GI:* N&V, abdominal pain, diarrhea, ***serious hepatic reactions.*** *CNS:* Headache, ***seizures.*** *Dermatologic:* Skin rash, exfoliative skin disorders (including ***Stevens-Johnson syndrome,*** and toxic epidermal necrolysis), alopecia. *Hematologic:* Leukopenia, thrombocytopenia. *Other:* Hypercholesterolemia, hypertriglyceridemia, hypokalemia.

Drug Interactions
Cimetidine / ↓ Plasma levels of fluconazole
Cisapride / ↑ Risk of serious cardiac arrhythmias
Cyclosporine / Fluconazole may ↑ cyclosporine levels in renal transplant patients with or without impaired renal function
Hydrochlorothiazide / ↑ Plasma levels of fluconazole due to ↓ renal clearance
Glipizide / ↑ Plasma levels of glipizide due to ↓ breakdown by the liver
Glyburide / ↑ Plasma levels of glyburide due to ↓ breakdown by the liver
Phenytoin / Fluconazole ↑ plasma levels of phenytoin
Rifampin / ↓ Plasma levels of fluconazole due to ↑ breakdown by the liver
Theophylline / ↑ Plasma levels of theophylline
Tolbutamide / ↑ Plasma levels of tolbutamide due to ↓ breakdown by the liver
Warfarin / ↑ PT
Zidovudine / ↑ Plasma levels of AZT

EMS CONSIDERATIONS
None.

Flucytosine
(flew-SYE-toe-seen)
Pregnancy Class: C
Ancobon **(Rx)**
Classification: Antibiotic, antifungal

Mechanism of Action: Appears to penetrate the fungal cell membrane and, after metabolism, acts as an antimetabolite interfering with nucleic acid and protein synthesis.

Uses: Serious systemic fungal infections by susceptible strains of *Candida* (e.g., endocarditis, septicemia, UTIs) or *Cryptococcus* (pulmonary or UTIs, meningitis, septicemia).

Contraindications: Hypersensitivity to drug. Lactation.

Precautions: Safety and effectiveness have not been determined in children. Use with extreme caution in patients with kidney disease or history of bone marrow depression. The bone marrow depressant effects may cause an increased incidence of microbial infection, gingival bleeding, and delayed healing.

Route/Dosage
• **Capsules**
Adult and children: 50–150 mg/kg/day in four divided doses. Use lower doses in renal impairment.

How Supplied: *Capsule:* 250 mg, 500 mg

Side Effects: *GI:* N&V, diarrhea, abdominal pain, dry mouth, anorexia, duodenal ulcer, GI hemorrhage, ulcerative colitis. *Hematologic:* Anemia, leukopenia, thrombocytopenia, *aplastic anemia, agranulocytosis,* pancytopenia, eosinophilia. *CNS:* Headache, vertigo, confusion, sedation, hallucinations, paresthesia, parkinsonism, psychosis, pyrexia. *Hepatic:* Hepatic dysfunction, jaundice, elevation of hepatic enzymes, increase in bilirubin. *GU:* Increase in BUN and creatinine, azotemia, crystalluria, renal failure. *Respiratory:* Chest pain, dyspnea, *respiratory arrest. Dermatologic:* Pruritus, rash, urticaria, photosensitivity. *Other:* Ataxia, hearing loss, peripheral neuropathy, weakness, hypoglycemia, fatigue, *cardiac arrest,* hypokalemia.

OD Overdose Management: *Symptoms (serum levels > 100 mcg/mL):* N&V, diarrhea, leukopenia, thrombocytopenia, hepatitis. *Treatment:* Prompt induction of vomiting or gastric lavage. Adequate fluid intake (by IV if necessary). Monitor blood, liver, and kidney parameters frequently. Hemodialysis will quickly decrease serum levels.

Drug Interactions
Amphotericin B / ↑ Effect and toxicity of flucytosine due to kidney impairment
Cytosine / Inactivates antifungal effect of flucytosine

EMS CONSIDERATIONS

See also *Anti-Infectives.*

Fludrocortisone acetate
(flew-droh-KOR-tih-sohn)
Pregnancy Class: C
Florinef **(Rx)**
Classification: Mineralocorticoid

Mechanism of Action: Produces marked sodium retention and inhibits excess adrenocortical secretion. Supplementary potassium may be indicated.

Uses: Addison's disease and adrenal hyperplasia.

Contraindications: Use systemically as an anti-inflammatory.

Route/Dosage
• **Tablets**
   Addison's disease.
0.1–0.2 mg/day to 0.1 mg 3 times/week, usually in conjunction with hydrocortisone or cortisone.
   Salt-losing adrenogenital syndrome.
0.1–0.2 mg/day.

How Supplied: *Tablet:* 0.1 mg

EMS CONSIDERATIONS

See also *Corticosteroids.*

Flumazenil
(floo-MAZ-eh-nill)
Pregnancy Class: C
Romazicon **(Rx)**
Classification: Benzodiazepine receptor antagonist

Mechanism of Action: Antagonizes the effects of benzodiazepines on the CNS by competitively inhibiting their action at the benzodiazepine recognition site on the GABA/benzodiazepine receptor complex. Does not antagonize the CNS effects of ethanol, general anesthetics, barbiturates, or opiates. Depending on the dose, there will be partial or complete antagonism of sedation, impaired recall, and psychomotor impairment.

Onset of Action: Onset of reversal: 1-2 min. **Peak effect:** 6-10 min. The duration of reversal is related to the plasma levels of the benzodiazepine and the dose of flumazenil.

Uses: Complete or partial reversal of benzodiazepine-induced depression of the ventilatory responses to hypercapnia and hypoxia. Situations include cases where general anesthesia has been induced or maintained by benzodiazepines, where sedation has been produced by benzodiazepines for diagnostic and therapeutic procedures, and for the management of benzodiazepine overdosage.

Contraindications: Use in patients given a benzodiazepine for control of intracranial pressure or status epilepticus. In patients manifesting signs of serious cyclic antidepressant overdose. Use during labor and delivery or in children as the risks and benefits are not known. To treat benzodiazepine dependence or for the management of protracted benzodiazepine abstinence syndrome. Use until the effects of neuromuscular blockade have been fully reversed.

Precautions: The reversal of benzodiazepine effects may be associated with the onset of seizures in certain high-risk patients (e.g., concurrent major sedative-hypnotic drug withdrawaal, recent therapy with repeated doses of parenteral benzodiazepines, myoclonic jerking or seizure activity prior to administration of flumazenil in cases of overdose, and concurrent cyclic antidepressant overdosage). Use with caution in patients with head injury as the drug may precipitate seizures or alter cerebral blood flow in patients receiving benzodiazepines. Use with caution in patients with alcoholism and other drug dependencies due to the increased frequency of benzodiazepine tolerance and dependence. Use with caution during lactation. Flumazenil may precipitate a withdrawal syndrome if the patient is dependent on benzodiazepines. Flumazenil may cause panic attacks in patient with a history of panic disorder. Use with caution in mixed-drug overdosage as toxic effects (e.g., cardiac dysrhythmias, convulsions) may occur (especially with cyclic antidepressants).

Route/Dosage
- **IV Only**
  To reverse conscious sedation or in general anesthesia.

Adults, initial: 0.2 mg (2 mL) given IV over 15 sec. If the desired level of consciousness is not reached after waiting an additional 45 sec, a second dose of 0.2 mg (2 mL) can be given and repeated at 60-sec intervals, up to a maximum total dose of 1 mg (10 mL). Most patients will respond to doses of 0.6–1 mg. To treat resedation, give no more than 1 mg (given as 0.2 mg/min) at any one time and give no more than 3 mg in any 1 hr.

  Management of suspected benzodiazepine overdose.

Adults, initial: 0.2 mg (2 mL) given IV over 30 sec; a second dose of 0.3 mg (3 mL) can be given over another 30 sec. Further doses of 0.5 mg (5 mL) can be given over 30 sec at 1-min intervals up to a total dose of 3 mg (although some patients may require up to 5 mg given slowly as described). If the patient has not responded 5 min after receiving a cumulative dose of 5 mg, the major cause of sedation is probably not due to benzodiazepines and additional doses of flumazenil are likely to have no effect. For resedation, repeated doses may be given at 20-min intervals; no more than 1 mg (given as 0.5 mg/min) at any one time and no more than 3 mg in any 1 hr should be administered.

How Supplied: *Injection:* 0.1 mg/mL

Side Effects: ***Deaths*** have occurred in patients receiving flumazenil, especially in those with serious underlying disease or in those who have ingested large amounts of nonbenzodiazepine drugs (usually cyclic antidepressants) as part of an overdose. ***Seizures*** are the most common serious side effect noted.

CNS: Dizziness, vertigo, ataxia, anxiety, nervousness, tremor, palpitations, insomnia, dyspnea, hyperventilation, abnormal crying, depersonalization, euphoria, increased tears, depression, dysphoria, paranoia, delirium, difficulty concentrating, ***seizures,*** somnolence, stupor, speech disorder. *GI:* N&V, hiccoughs, dry mouth. *CV:* Sweating, flushing, hot flushes, ***arrhythmias (atrial, nodal, ventricular extrasystoles),*** bradycardia, tachycardia, hypertension, chest pain. *At injection site:* Pain, thrombophlebitis, rash, skin abnormality. *Body as a whole:* Headache, increased sweating, asthenia, malaise, rigors, shivering, paresthesia. *Ophthalmologic:* Abnormal vision including visual field defect and diplopia; blurred vision. *Otic:* Transient hearing impairment, tinnitus, hyperacusis.

EMS CONSIDERATIONS

Administration/Storage

IV 1. Give only the smallest amount that is effective.

2. A major risk is resedation; the duration of effect of a long-acting or a large dose of a short-acting benzodiazepine may exceed that of flumazenil. If there is resedation, give repeated doses at 20-min intervals as needed.

3. Give through a freely running IV infusion into a large vein to minimize pain at the injection site.

4. Doses larger than a total of 3 mg do not reliably produce additional effects.

5. Flumazenil is compatible with D5W, RL, and NSS solutions.

6. Before administering, have a secure airway and IV access; awaken patients gradually.

Assessment

1. Note any history of seizure disorder.

2. Determine type, time, and amount of drug ingested; especially note any TCA or mixed-drug overdose.

3. Assess for evidence of head injury or increased ICP.

4. Note evidence of sedative or benzodiazepine dependence, alcohol abuse, or recent use of either; drug may precipitate withdrawal symptoms.

Interventions

1. Observe closely for resedation, depressed respirations, or other residual benzodiazepine effects for up to 2 hr after administration.

2. Flumazenil is intended as an adjunct to, not a substitute for, proper management of the airway, assisted breathing, circulatory access and support, use of lavage and charcoal, and adequate clinical evaluation. Prior to giving flumazenil, proper measures should be undertaken to secure an airway for ventilation and IV access. Be prepared for patients attempting to withdraw ET tubes or IV lines due to confusion and agitation following awakening; awakening should be gradual.

3. Use seizure precautions; increased risk for seizures with large overdoses of cyclic antidepressants and with long-term benzodiazepine sedation.

4. Drug-associated convulsions may be treated with benzodiazepines.

Flunisolide

(flew-NISS-oh-lyd)

Pregnancy Class: C

Inhalation: AeroBid **(Rx); Intranasal:** Nasalide, Nasarel **(Rx)**

Classification: Corticosteroid

Mechanism of Action: Minimal systemic effects with intranasal use.

Uses: Inhalation: Prophylaxis and treatment of bronchial asthma in combination with other therapy. Not used when asthma can be relieved by other drugs, in patients where systemic corticosteroid treatment is infrequent, and in nonasthmatic bronchitis. **Intranasal:** Seasonal or perennial rhinitis, especially if other treatment has proven unsatisfactory. **Contraindications:** Active or quiescent TB, especially of the respiratory tract. Untreated fungal, bacterial, systemic viral infections. Ocular herpes simplex. Use until healing occurs following recent ulceration of nasal septum, nasal surgery, or trauma. Lactation.

Precautions: Safety and effectiveness in children less than 6 years of age have not been determined.

Route/Dosage ─────────
• **Inhalation**
Bronchial asthma.
Adults: 2 inhalations (total of 500 mcg flunisolide) in a.m. and p.m., not to exceed 4 inhalations b.i.d. (i.e., total daily dose of 2,000 mcg). **Pediatric, 6–15 years:** 2 inhalations in the morning and evening, with total daily dose not to exceed 1,000 mcg.

• **Intranasal**
Rhinitis.
Adults, initial: 50 mcg (2 sprays) in each nostril b.i.d.; may be increased to 2 sprays t.i.d. up to maximum daily dose of 400 mcg (i.e., 8 sprays in each nostril). **Pediatric, 6–14 years, initial:** 25 mcg (1 spray) in each nostril t.i.d. or 50 mcg (2 sprays) in each nostril b.i.d., up to maximum daily dose of 200 mcg (i.e., 4 sprays in each nostril). **Maintenance, adults, children:** Smallest dose necessary to control symptoms. Some patients (approximately 15%) are controlled on 1 spray in each nostril daily.

How Supplied: *Metered Dose Inhaler:* 0.25 mg/inh; *Nasal Spray:* 0.025 mg/inh

Side Effects: Additional: *Respiratory:* Hoarseness, coughing, throat irritation; *Canidida* infections of nose, larynx, and pharynx. *After intranasal use:* Nasopharyngeal irritation, stinging, burning, dryness, headache. *GI:* Dry mouth. Systemic corticosteroid

effects, especially if recommended dose is exceeded.

EMS CONSIDERATIONS
See also *Corticosteroids.*

Fluorouracil (5-Fluorouracil, 5-FU)
(flew-roh-YOUR-ah-sill)
Pregnancy Class: X
Adrucil, Efudex, Fluoroplex (Abbreviation: 5-FU) **(Rx)**
Classification: Antineoplastic, antimetabolite

Mechanism of Action: Pyrimidine antagonist that inhibits the methylation reaction of deoxyuridylic acid to thymidylic acid. Thus, synthesis of DNA and, to a lesser extent, RNA is inhibited. Highly toxic; initiate use in hospital. When used topically, the following response occurs:
• Early inflammation: erythema for several days (minimal reaction)
• Severe inflammation: burning, stinging, vesiculation
• Disintegration: erosion, ulceration, necrosis, pain, crusting, reepithelialization
• Healing: within 1–2 weeks with some residual erythema and temporary hyperpigmentation

Uses: Systemic: Palliative management of certain cancers of the rectum, stomach, colon, pancreas, and breast. In combination with levamisole for Dukes' stage C colon cancer after surgical resection. In combination with leucovorin for metastatic colorectal cancer. *Investigational:* Cancer of the bladder, ovaries, prostate, cervix, endometrium, lung, liver, head, and neck. Also, malignant pleural, peritoneal, and pericardial effusions. **Topical (as solution or cream):** Multiple actinic or solar keratoses. Superficial basal cell carcinoma. *Investigational:* Condylomata acuminata (1% solution in 70% ethanol or the 5% cream).

Contraindications: Additional: Patients in poor nutritional state, with severe bone marrow depression, severe infection, or recent (4-week-old) surgical intervention. Lactation. To be used with caution in patients with hepatic or liver dysfunction.

Precautions: Safety and efficacy of topical products have not been established in children. Occlusive dressings may result in increased inflammation in adjacent normal skin when topical products are used.

Route/Dosage

• **IV**

Palliative management of selected carcinomas.

Individualize dosage. Initial: 12 mg/kg/day for 4 days, not to exceed 800 mg/day. If no toxicity seen, administer 6 mg/kg on days 6, 8, 10, and 12. Discontinue therapy on day 12 even if there are no toxic symptoms. **Maintenance:** Repeat dose of first course q 30 days or when toxicity from initial course of therapy is gone; or, give 10–15 mg/kg/week as a single dose. Do not exceed 1 g/week. **If patient is debilitated or is a poor risk:** 6 mg/kg/day for 3 days; if no toxicity, give 3 mg/kg on days 5, 7, and 9 (daily dose should not exceed 400 mg).

Metastatic colorectal cancer.

Leucovorin, **IV,** 200 mg/m²/day for 5 days followed by fluorouracil, **IV,** 370 mg/m²/day for 5 days. Repeat q 28 days to maximize response and to prolong survival.

Dukes' stage C colon cancer after surgical resection.

See *Levamisole.*

• **Cream, Topical Solution**

Actinic or solar keratoses.

Apply 1%–5% cream or solution to cover lesion 1–2 times/day for 2–6 weeks.

Superficial basal cell carcinoma.

Apply 5% cream or solution to cover lesion b.i.d. for 3–6 weeks (up to 10–12 weeks may be required).

How Supplied: *Cream:* 1%, 5%; *Injection:* 50 mg/mL; *Solution:* 1%, 2%, 5%

Side Effects: Additional: System-ic: Esophagopharyngitis, myocardial ischemia, angina, acute cerebellar syndrome, photophobis, lacrimation, decreased vision. Also, arterial thrombosis, arteial ischemia, arterial aneurysm, bleeding or infection at site of catheter, thrombophlebitis, embolism, fibromyositis, abscesses.**Topical:** *Dermatologic:* Pain, pruritus, hyperpigmentation, irrtation, inflammation, burning at site of application, scarring, soreness, allergic contact dermatitis, tenderness, scaling, swelling, suppuration, alopecia, photosensitivity, urticaria. *GI:* Stomatitis, medicinal taste. *Miscellaneous:* Lacrimation, telangiectasia, toxic granulation.

OD Overdose Management: *Symptoms:* N&V, diarrhea, GI ulceration, GI bleeding, thrombocytopenia, *agranulocytosis,* leukopenia. *Treatment:* Monitor hematologically for at least 4 weeks.

Drug Interactions: Leucovorin calcium ↑ toxicity of fluorouracil.

EMS CONSIDERATIONS

None.

Fluoxetine hydrochloride

(flew-OX-eh-teen)
Pregnancy Class: B
Prozac **(Rx)**
Classification: Antidepressant, miscellaneous

Mechanism of Action: Not related chemically to tricyclic, tetracyclic, or other antidepressants. Effect thought to be due to inhibition of uptake of serotonin into CNS neurons. Slight to no anticholinergic, sedative, or orthostatic hypotensive effects. Also binds to muscarinic, histaminergic, and alpha-1-adrenergic receptors, accounting for many of the side effects.

Uses: Depression, obsessive-compulsive disorders (as defined in the current edition of DSM), bulimia nervosa. *Investigational:* Many (see *Dosage*).

Contraindications: Use with or within 14 days of discontinuing an MAO inhibitor.

Precautions: Use with caution during lactation and in patients with impaired liver or kidney function. Safety and efficacy have not been determined in children. A lower initial dose may be necessary in geriatric patients. Use in hospitalized patients, use for longer than 5-6 weeks for depression, or use for more than 13 weeks for obsessive-compulsive disorder has not been studied adequately.

Route/Dosage

• **Capsules, Liquid**

Antidepressant.

Adults, initial: 20 mg/day in the morning. If clinical improvement is not observed after several weeks, the dose may be increased to a maximum of 80 mg/day in two equally divided doses.

Obsessive-compulsive disorder.

Initial: 20 mg/day in the morning. If improvement is not significant after several weeks, the dose may be increased. **Usual dosage range:** 20–60 mg/day; the total daily dosage should not exceed 80 mg.

Treatment of bulimia nervosa.

60 mg/day given in the morning. May be necessary to titrate up to this dose over several days.

Alcoholism.

40–80 mg/day.

Anorexia nervosa, bipolar II affective disorder, trichotillomania.

20–80 mg/day.

Attention deficit hyperactivity disorder, obesity, schizophrenia.

20–60 mg/day.

Borderline personality disorder.

5–80 mg/day.

Cataplexy and narcolepsy, Tourette's syndrome.

20–40 mg/day.

Kleptomania.

60–80 mg/day.

Migraine, chronic daily headaches, tension headaches.

20 mg every other day to 40 mg/day.

Posttraumatic stress disorder.

10–80 mg/day.

Premenstrual syndrome, recurrent syncope.

20 mg/day.

Levodopa-induced dyskinesia.

40 mg/day.

Social phobia.

10–60 mg/day.

How Supplied: *Capsule:* 10 mg, 20 mg; *Solution:* 20 mg/5 mL

Side Effects: A large number of side effects have been reported for this drug. Listed are those with a reported frequency of greater than 1%. *CNS:* Headache (most common), activation of mania or hypomania, insomnia, anxiety, nervousness, dizziness, fatigue, sedation, decreased libido, drowsiness, lightheadedness, decreased ability to concentrate, tremor, disturbances in sensation, agitation, abnormal dreams. Although less frequent than 1%, *some patients may experience seizures or attempt suicide.* *GI:* Nausea (most common), diarrhea, vomiting, constipation, dry mouth, dyspepsia, anorexia, abdominal pain, flatulence, alteration in taste, gastroenteritis, increased appetite. *CV:* Hot flashes, palpitations. *GU:* Sexual dysfunction, impotence, anorgasmia, frequent urination, UTI, dysmenorrhea. *Respiratory:* URTI, pharyngitis, cough, dyspnea, rhinitis, bronchitis, nasal congestion, sinusitis, sinus headache, yawn. *Skin:* Rash, pruritus, excessive sweating. *Musculoskeletal:* Muscle, joint, or back pain. *Miscellaneous:* Flu-like symptoms, asthenia, fever, chest pain, allergy, visual disturbances, blurred vision, weight loss, bacterial or viral infection, limb pain, chills.

Drug Interactions

Alprazolam / ↑ Alprazolam levels and ↓ psychomotor performance

Buspirone / ↓ Effects of buspirone; worsening of obsessive-compulsive disorder

Carbamazepine / ↑ Serum levels of carbamazepine → toxicity

Clozapine / ↑ Serum clozapine levels

---

bold italic = life threatening side effect

Dextromethorphan / Possibility of hallucinations

Diazepam / Fluoxetine ↑ half-life of diazepam → excessive sedation or impaired psychomotor skills

Haloperidol / ↑ Serum levels of haloperidol

Lithium / ↑ Serum levels of lithium → possible neurotoxicity

MAO inhibitors / MAO inhibitors should be discontinued 14 days before initiation of fluoxetine therapy due to the possibility of symptoms resembling a neuroleptic malignant syndrome or fatal reactions

Phenytoin / Fluoxetine may ↑ phenytoin levels

Tricyclic antidepressants / ↑ Pharmacologic and toxicologic effects of tricyclics due to ↓ breakdown by liver

Tryptophan / Symptoms of CNS toxicity (headache, sweating, dizziness, agitation, aggressiveness) or peripheral toxicity (N&V)

Warfarin / ↑ Bleeding diathesis with unaltered PT

EMS CONSIDERATIONS

None.

Fluphenazine decanoate
Fluphenazine enanthate
Fluphenazine hydrochloride

(flew-FEN-ah-zeen)

Fluphenazine decanoate (Prolixin Decanoate **(Rx)**) Fluphenazine enanthate (Prolixin Enanthate **(Rx)**) Fluphenazine hydrochloride (Permitil, Prolixin **(Rx)**)

Classification: Antipsychotic, piperazine-type phenothiazine

Mechanism of Action: High incidence of extrapyramidal symptoms and a low incidence of sedation, anticholinergic effects, antiemetic effects, and orthostatic hypotension. The enanthate and decanoate esters dramatically increase the duration of action.

Fluphenazine hydrochloride can be cautiously administered to patients with known hypersensitivity to other phenothiazines.

Fluphenazine enanthate may replace fluphenazine hydrochloride if desired response occurs with hypersensitivity reaction to fluphenazine.

Onset of Action: *Decanoate:* 24-72 hr; *Enanthate:* 24-72 hr

Duration of Action: *Decanoate:* up to 4 weeks; *Enanthate:* 1-3 weeks.

Uses: Psychotic disorders. Adjunct to tricyclic antidepressants for chronic pain states (e.g., diabetic neuropathy, and patients trying to withdraw from narcotics).

Route/Dosage ─────────────

Fluphenazine hydrochloride is administered **PO and IM.** Fluphenazine enanthate or decanoate are administered **SC and IM.**

Hydrochloride.
• **Elixir, Oral Solution, Tablets**
Psychotic disorders.

Adults and adolescents, initial: 0.5–10 mg/day in divided doses q 6–8 hr; **then,** reduce gradually to maintenance dose of 1–5 mg/day (usually given as a single dose, not to exceed 20 mg/day). **Geriatric, emaciated, debilitated patients, initial:** 1–2.5 mg/day; **then,** dosage determined by response. **Pediatric:** 0.25–0.75 mg 1–4 times/day.

Hydrochloride.
• **IM**
Psychotic disorders.

Adults and adolescents: 1.25–2.5 mg q 6–8 hr as needed. Maximum daily dose: 10 mg. Elderly, debilitated, or emaciated patients should start with 1–2.5 mg/day.

Decanoate.
• **IM, SC**
Psychotic disorders.

Adults, initial: 12.5–25 mg; **then,** the dose may be repeated or increased q 1–3 weeks. The usual maintenance dose is 50 mg/1–4 weeks. Maximum adult dose: 100 mg/dose. **Pediatric, 12 years and older:** 6.25–18.75 mg/week; the dose can be increased to 12.5–25 mg given q 1–3 weeks. **Pediatric, 5–12 years:** 3.125–12.5 mg with this dose being repeated q 1–3 weeks.

Enanthate.
- **IM, SC**
  Psychotic disorders.
  Adults and adolescents: 12.5–25 mg; dose can be repeated or increased q 1–3 weeks. For doses greater than 50 mg, increases should be made in increments of 12.5 mg. Maximum adult dose: 100 mg.
  How Supplied: Fluphenazine decanoate: *Injection:* 25 mg/mL Fluphenazine enanthate: *Injection:* 25 mg/mL Fluphenazine hydrochloride: *Elixir:* 2.5 mg/5 mL; *Injection:* 2.5 mg/mL; *Tablet:* 1 mg, 2.5 mg, 5 mg, 10 mg

EMS CONSIDERATIONS

See also *Antipsychotic Agents, Phenothiazines.*

Flurazepam hydrochloride
(flur-AYZ-eh-pam)
Dalmane, Durapam **(C-IV) (Rx)**
Classification: Benzodiazepine sedative-hypnotic

Mechanism of Action: Combines with benzodiazepine receptors, which are part of the benzodiazepine-GABA receptor-chloride ionophore complex. Results in enhanced inhibitory action of GABA leading to interference of transmission of nerve impulses in the reticular activating system. Exceeding the recommended dose may result in development of tolerance and dependence.
Onset of Action: 17 min.
Duration of Action: 7-8 hr. **Maximum effectiveness:** 2-3 days.
Uses: Insomnia (all types). Is increasingly effective on the second or third night of consecutive use and for one or two nights after the drug is discontinued.
Contraindications: Hypersensitivity. Pregnancy or in women wishing to become pregnant. Depression, renal or hepatic disease, chronic pulmonary insufficiency, children under 15 years.
Precautions: Use during the last few weeks of pregnancy may result in

CNS depression of the neonate. Use during lactation may cause sedation and feeding problems in the infant. Geriatric patients may be more sensitive to the effects of flurazepam.

Route/Dosage
- **Capsules**
Adults: 15–30 mg at bedtime; 15 mg for geriatric and/or debilitated patients.
How Supplied: *Capsule:* 15 mg, 30 mg
Side Effects: *CNS:* Ataxia, dizziness, drowsiness/sedation, headache, disorientation. Symptoms of stimulation including nervousness, apprehension, irritability, and talkativeness. *GI:* N&V, diarrhea, gastric upset or pain, heartburn, constipation. *Miscellaneous:* Arthralgia, chest pains, or palpitations. Rarely, symptoms of allergy, SOB, jaundice, anorexia, blurred vision.
Drug Interactions
Cimetidine / ↑ Effect of flurazepam due to ↓ breakdown by liver
CNS depressants / Addition or potentiation of CNS depressant effects—drowsiness, lethargy, stupor, respiratory depression or collapse, coma, and possible death
Disulfiram / ↑ Effect of flurazepam due to ↓ breakdown by liver
Ethanol / Additive depressant effects up to the day following flurazepam administration
Isoniazid / ↑ Effect of flurazepam due to ↓ breakdown by liver
Oral contraceptives / Either ↑ or ↓ effect of benzodiazepines due to effect on breakdown by liver
Rifampin / ↓ Effect of benzodiazepines due to ↑ breakdown by liver

EMS CONSIDERATIONS

See also *Tranquilizers, Antimanic Drugs, and Hypnotics.*

Flurbiprofen
Flurbiprofen sodium
(flur-BIH-proh-fen)
Pregnancy Class: Flurbiprofen: B

F

Flurbiprofen sodium: C
Flurbiprofen (Ansaid **(Rx)**) Flurbiprofen sodium (Flurbiprofen Sodium Ophthalmic, Ocufen **(Rx)**)
Classification: Nonsteroidal anti-inflammatory drug, ophthalmic and systemic use.

Mechanism of Action: By inhibiting prostaglandin synthesis, flurbiprofen reverses prostaglandin-induced vasodilation, leukocytosis, increased vascular permeability, and increased intraocular pressure. Also inhibits miosis occurring during cataract surgery.

Uses: Ophthalmic: Prevention of intraoperative miosis. **PO:** Rheumatoid arthritis, osteoarthritis. *Investigational:* Inflammation following cataract surgery, uveitis syndromes. Topically to treat cystoid macular edema. Primary dysmenorrhea, sunburn, mild to moderate pain.

Contraindications: Dendritic keratitis.

Precautions: Use with caution in patients hypersensitive to aspirin or other NSAIDs and during lactation. Wound healing may be delayed with use of the ophthalmic product. Acetylcholine chloride and carbachol may be ineffective when used with ophthalmic flubiprofen. Safety and efficacy in children have not been established.

Route/Dosage —————
• **Ophthalmic Drops**
Beginning 2 hr before surgery, instill 1 gtt q 30 min (i.e., total of 4 gtt of 0.03% solution).
• **Tablets**
Rheumatoid arthritis, osteoarthritis.
Adults, initial: 200–300 mg/day in divided doses b.i.d.–q.i.d.; **then,** adjust dose to patient response. Doses greater than 300 mg/day are not recommended.
Dysmenorrhea.
50 mg q.i.d.
How Supplied: Flurbiprofen: *Tablet:* 50 mg, 100 mg Flurbiprofen sodium: *Ophthalmic solution:* 0.03%

Side Effects: Additional: *Ophthalmic:*Ocular irritation, transient stinging or burning flollowing use, delay in

wound healing. Increased bleeding of ocular tissues in conjunction with ocular surgery.

EMS CONSIDERATIONS
None.

Flutamide
(FLOO-tah-myd)
Pregnancy Class: D
Eulexin **(Rx)**
Classification: Antineoplastic, hormonal agent

Mechanism of Action: Acts either to inhibit uptake of androgen or to inhibit nuclear binding of androgen in target tissues. Thus, the effect of androgen is decreased in androgen-sensitive tissues.

Uses: In combination with leuprolide acetate (i.e., a LHRH agonist) to treat stage D_2 metastatic prostatic carcinoma as well as locally confined stage B_2-C prostate cancer. In combination with goserelin acetate depots (Zoladex) to treat locally confined stage B_2-C prostate cancer.

Contraindications: Use during pregnancy.

Route/Dosage —————
• **Capsules**
Locally confined stage B_2-C and stage D_2 metastatic cancer of the prostate.
250 mg (2 capsules) t.i.d. q 8 hr for a total daily dose of 750 mg.

How Supplied: *Capsule:* 125 mg

Side Effects: Side effects are listed for treatment of flutamide with LHRH agonist. *GU:* Loss of libido, impotence. *CV:* Hot flashes, hypertension. *GI:* N&V, diarrhea, GI disturbances, anorexia. *CNS:* Confusion, depression, drowsiness, anxiety, nervousness. *Hematologic:* Anemia, leukopenia, thrombocytopenia, ***hemolytic anemia,*** macrocytic anemia, methemoglobinemia. *Hepatic:* Hepatitis, cholestatic jaundice, hepatic encephalopathy, ***hepatic necrosis.*** *Dermatologic:* Rash, injection site irritation, erythema, ulceration, bullous eruptions, ***epidermal necrolysis.*** *Miscellaneous:* Gynecomastia, edema, neuromuscular symptoms, pulmonary symptoms, GU symptoms, malignant breast tumors.

OD **Overdose Management:** *Symptoms:* Breast tenderness, gynecomastia, increases in AST. Also possible are ataxia, anorexia, vomiting, decreased respiration, lacrimation, sedation, hypoactivity, and piloerection. *Treatment:* Induce vomiting if patient is alert. Frequently monitor VS and observe closely.

EMS CONSIDERATIONS

None.

Fluticasone propionate
(flu-TIH-kah-sohn)
Pregnancy Class: C
Flonase, Flovent (Rx)
Classification: Corticosteroid

Mechanism of Action: Following intranasal use, a small amount is absorbed into the general circulation. **Onset of Action:** Approximately 12 hr. **Maximum effect:** May take several days.

Uses: Preventive and maintenance treatment of asthma in adults and children over four years of age. To manage seasonal and perennial allergic rhinitis in adults and children over four years of age.

Contraindications: Use for nonallergic rhinitis. Use following nasal septal ulcers, nasal surgery, or nasal trauma until healing has occurred.

Precautions: Patients on immunosuppressant drugs, such as corticosteroids, are more susceptible to infections. Use with caution, if at all, in active or quiescent tuberculosis infections; untreated fungal, bacterial, or systemic viral infections; or ocular herpes simplex. Use with caution during lactation.

Route/Dosage
• **Metered Dose Inhaler**
   Treatment of asthma.
Adults and children over 4 years of age, initial: 100 mcg b.i.d. For oral steroid sparing, the recommended dose is 1,000 mcg b.i.d.

• **Rotadisk Inhaler**
   Prevention of asthma.
Children over 4 years of age: 50–100 mcg. b.i.d.
• **Nasal Spray**
   Allergic rhinitis.
Adults and children over 4 years of age, initial: One 50-mcg spray in each nostril once a day, for a total daily dose of 100 mcg/day. Maximum dose is two sprays (200 mcg) in each nostril once a day.
• **Ointment, Cream**
Apply sparingly to affected area 2–4 times daily.

How Supplied: *Cream:* 0.05%; *Metered Dose Inhaler:* 0.11 mg/inh, 0.22 mg/inh, 0.44 mg/inh; *Nasal spray:* 0.05 mg/inh; *Powder for Inhalation:* 0.044/inh, 0.088/inh, 0.22/inh; *Ointment:* 0.005%; *Rotadisk:* 50 mcg, 100 mcg, 250 mcg

Side Effects: *Allergic:* Rarely, immediate hypersensitivity reactions or contact dermatitis. *Respiratory:* Epistaxis, nasal burning, blood in nasal mucus, pharyngitis, irritation of nasal mucous membranes, sneezing, runny nose, nasal dryness, sinusitis, nasal congestion, bronchitis, nasal ulcer, nasal septum excoriation. *CNS:* Headache, dizziness. *Ophthalmologic:* Eye disorder, cataracts, glaucoma, increased intraocular pressure. *GI:* N&V, xerostomia. *Miscellaneous:* Unpleasant taste, urticaria. High doses have resulted in hypercorticism and adrenal suppression.

EMS CONSIDERATIONS

See also *Corticosteroids*.

Fluvastatin sodium
(flu-vah-STAH-tin)
Pregnancy Class: X
Lescol (Rx)
Classification: Antihyperlipidemic agent

Uses: Adjunct to diet for the reduction of elevated total and LDL cholesterol levels in patients with primary hypercholesterolemia. The lipid-lowering effects of fluvastatin are enhanced when it is combined with a bile-acid binding resin or with niacin. To slow the progression of coronary atherosclerosis in coronary heart disease.

Contraindications: Lactation.

Precautions: Use with caution in patients with severe renal impariment.

Route/Dosage
• **Capsules**
Treat primary hypercholesterolemia. Antihyperlipidemic to slow progression of coronary atherosclerosis.
Adults: 20 mg once daily at bedtime. **Dose range:** 20–40 mg/day as a single dose in the evening. Splitting the 40-mg dose into a twice-daily regimen results in a modest improvement in LDL cholesterol.

How Supplied: *Capsule:* 20 mg, 40 mg

Side Effects: Side effects listed are those most common with fluvastatin. A complete list of possible side effects is provided under *Antihyperlipidemic Agents—HMG-CoA Reductase Inhibitors. GI:* N&V, diarrhea, abdominal pain or cramps, constipation, flatulence, dyspepsia, tooth disorder. *Musculoskeletal:* Myalgia, back pain, arthralgia, arthritis. *CNS:* Headache, dizziness, insomnia. *Respiratory:* URI, rhinitis, cough, pharyngitis, sinusitis. *Miscellaneous:* Rash, pruritus, fatigue, influenza, allergy, accidental trauma.

Drug Interactions
Alcohol / ↑ Fluvastatin absorbed
Digoxin / ↓ Bioavailability of fluvastatin
Rifampin / ↓ Fluvastatin clearance

EMS CONSIDERATIONS
None.

Fluvoxamine maleate
(flu-VOX-ah-meen)
Pregnancy Class: C
Luvox **(Rx)**
Classification: Selective serotonin-uptake inhibitor

Mechanism of Action: Mechanism in obsessive-compulsive disorders is likely due to inhibition of serotonin reuptake in the CNS. Produces few if any anticholinergic, sedative, or orthostatic hypotensive effects.

Uses: Obsessive-compulsive disorder (as defined in DSM-III-R) for adults, adolescents, and children. *Investigational:* Treatment of depression.

Contraindications: Concomitant use with astemizole or terfenadine. Alcohol ingestion. Use with MAO inhibitors or within 14 days of discontinuing treatment with a MAO inhibitor. Lactation.

Precautions: Use with caution in patients with a history of mania, seizure disorders, and liver dysfunction and in those with diseases that could affect hemodynamic responses or metabolism. Safety and efficacy have not been determined in children less than 18 years of age.

Route/Dosage
• **Tablets**
Obsessive-compulsive disorder.
Adults, initial: 50 mg at bedtime; **then,** increase the dose in 50-mg increments q 4–7 days, as tolerated, until a maximum benefit is reached, not to exceed 300 mg/day. **Children and adolescents, 8 to 17 years:** 25 mg at bedtime; **then,** increase the dose in 25-mg increments q 4–7 days until a maximum benefit is reached, not to exceed 200 mg/day.

How Supplied: *Tablet:* 25 mg, 50 mg, 100 mg

Side Effects: Side effects listed occur at an incidence of 0.1% or greater. *CNS:* Somnolence, insomnia, nervousness, dizziness, tremor, anxiety, hypertonia, agitation, decreased libido, depression, CNS stimulation, amnesia, apathy, hyperkinesia, hypokinesia, manic reaction, myoclonus, psychoses, fatigue, malaise, agoraphobia, akathisia, ataxia, ***convulsion,*** delirium, delusion, depersonalization, drug dependence, dyskinesia, dystonia, emotional lability, euphoria, extrapyramidal syndrome, unsteady gait, hallucinations, hemiplegia, hostility, hypersomnia, hypochondriasis, hypotonia, hysteria, incoordination, increased libido, neuralgia, paralysis, paranoia, phobia, sleep disorders, stupor, twitching, vertigo. *GI:* Nausea, dry mouth, diarrhea, constipation, dyspepsia, anorexia, vomiting, flatulence, toothache, tooth caries, dysphagia, colitis, eructation, esophagitis, gastritis, gastroenteritis, *GI hemorrhage,* GI ulcer, gingivitis, glossitis, hemorrhoids, melena, rectal hemorrhage, stomatitis. *CV:* Palpitations, hypertension, postural hypotension, vasodilation, syncope, tachycardia, angina pectoris, bradycardia, *cardiomyopathy,* CV disease, cold extremities, conduction delay, *heart failure, MI,* pallor, irregular pulse, ST segment changes. *Respiratory:* URI, dyspnea, yawn, increased cough, sinusitis, asthma, bronchitis, epistaxis, hoarseness, hyperventilation. *Body as a whole:* Headache, asthenia, flu syndrome, chills, malaise, edema, weight gain or loss, dehydration, hypercholesterolemia, allergic reaction, neck pain, neck rigidity, photosensitivity, *suicide attempt.* Dermatologic: Excessive sweating, acne, alopecia, dry skin, eczema, exfoliative dermatitis, furunculosis, seborrhea, skin discoloration, urticaria. *Musculoskeletal:* Arthralgia, arthritis, bursitis, generalized muscle spasm, myasthenia, tendinous contracture, tenosynovitis. *GU:* Delayed ejaculation, urinary frequency, impotence, anorgasmia, urinary retention, anuria, breast pain, cystitis, delayed menstruation, dysuria, female lactation, hematuria, menopause, menorrhagia, metrorrhagia, nocturia, polyuria, PMS, urinary incontinence, UTI, urinary urgency, impaired urination, *vaginal hemorrhage,* vaginitis. *Hematologic:* Anemia, ecchymosis, leukocytosis, lymphadenopathy, thrombocytopenia. *Ophthalmic:* Amblyopia, abnormal accommodation, conjunctivitis, diplopia, dry eyes, eye pain, mydriasis, photophobia, visual field defect. *Otic:* Deafness, ear pain, otitis media. *Miscellaneous:* Taste perversion or loss, parosmia, hypothyroidism, hypercholesterolemia, dehydration.

OD **Overdose Management:** *Treatment:* Establish an airway and maintain respiration as needed. Monitor VS and ECG. Activated charcoal may be as effective as emesis or lavage in removing the drug from the GI tract. Since absorption in overdose may be delayed, measures to reduce absorption may be required for up to 24 hr.

Drug Interactions

Astemisole / ↑ Risk of severe cardiovascular effects, including QT prolongation, ventricular tachycardia, and torsades de pointes (may be fatal)

Beta-adrenergic blockers / Possible ↑ effects on BP and HR

Carbamazepine / ↑ Risk of carbamazepine toxicity

Cloxapine / ↑ Risk of orthostatic hypotension and seizures

Diazepam / ↑ Effect of diazepam due to ↓ clearance

Diltiazem / ↑ Risk of bradycardia

Haloperidol / ↑ Serum levels of haloperidol

Lithium / ↑ Risk of seizures

MAO inhibitors / Serious and possibly fatal reactions, including hyperthermia, rigidity, myoclonus, rapid fluctuations of VS, changes in mental status (agitation, delirium, coma)

Methadone / ↑ Risk of methadone toxicity

Midazolam / ↑ Effect of midazolam due to ↓ clearance

Sumatriptan / ↑ Risk of weakness, hyperreflexia, incoordination

Terfenadine / ↑ Risk of severe cardiovascular effects, including QT prolongation, ventricular tachycardia, and torsades de pointes (may be fatal)

Theophylline / ↑ Risk of theophylline toxicity (decrease dose by one-third the usual daily maintenance dose)

Triazolam / ↑ Effect of triazolam due to ↓ clearance

Tricyclic antidepressants / Significant ↑ in plasma levels of tricyclic antidepressants

F

---

bold italic = life threatening side effect

Tryptophan / ↑ Risk of central toxicity (headache, sweating, dizziness, agitation, aggressiveness, worsening of obsessive-compulsive disorder) or peripheral toxicity (N&V)

Warfarin / ↑ Plasma levels of warfarin

EMS CONSIDERATIONS

None.

Folic acid
(FOH-lik AH-sid)
Pregnancy Class: A
Folvite **(Rx) (OTC)**
Classification: Vitamin B complex

Mechanism of Action: Folic acid (which is converted to tetrahydrofolic acid) is necessary for normal production of RBCs and for synthesis of nucleoproteins. Tetrahydrofolic acid is a cofactor in the biosynthesis of purines and thymidylates of nucleic acids. Megaloblastic and macrocytic anemias in folic acid deficiency are believed to be due to impairment of thymidylate synthesis. Natural sources of folic acid include liver, dried beans, peas, lentils, whole-wheat products, asparagus, beets, broccoli, brussels sprouts, spinach, and oranges.

Uses: Treatment of megaloblastic anemias due to folic acid deficiency (e.g., tropical and nontropical sprue, pregnancy, infancy or childhood, nutritional causes). Diagnosis of folate deficiency.

Contraindications: Use in aplastic, normocytic, or pernicious anemias (is ineffective). Folic acid injection that contains benzyl alcohol should not be used in neonates or immature infants.

Precautions: Daily folic acid doses of 0.1 mg or greater may obscure pernicious anemia. Prolonged folic acid therapy may cause decreased vitamin B_{12} levels.

Route/Dosage
• **Tablets**
   Dietary supplement.
Adults and children: 100 mcg/day (up to 1 mg in pregnancy); may be increased to 500–1,000 mcg if requirements increase.

Treatment of deficiency.
Adults, initial: 250–1,000 mcg/day until a hematologic response occurs; **maintenance:** 400 mcg/day (800 mcg during pregnancy and lactation). **Pediatric, initial:** 250–1,000 mcg/day until a hematologic response occurs. **Maintenance, infants:** 100 mcg/day; **children up to 4 years:** 300 mcg/day; **children 4 years and older:** 400 mcg/day.
• **IM, IV, Deep SC**
   Treatment of deficiency.
Adults and children: 250–1,000 mcg/day until a hematologic response occurs.

Diagnosis of folate deficiency.
Adults, IM: 100–200 mcg/day for 10 days plus low dietary folic acid and vitamin B_{12}.

How Supplied: *Injection:* 5 mg/mL; *Tablet:* 0.4 mg, 0.8 mg, 1 mg

Side Effects: *Allergic:* Skin rash, itching, erythema, general malaise, respiratory difficulty due to bronchospasm. *GI:* Nausea, anorexia, abdominal distention, flatulence, bitter or bad taste (in those taking 15 mg/day for 1 month). *CNS:* In doses of 15 mg daily, altered sleep patterns, irritability, excitement, difficulty in concentration, overactivity, depression, impaired judgment, confusion.

Drug Interactions
Aminosalicylic acid / ↓ Serum folate levels
Corticosteroids (chronic use) / ↑ Folic acid requirements
Methotrexate / Is a folic acid antagonist
Oral contraceptives / ↑ Risk of folate deficiency
Phenytoin / Folic acid ↑ seizure frequency; also, phenytoin ↓ serum folic acid levels.
Pyrimethamine / Folic acid ↓ effect of pyrimethamine in toxoplasmosis; also, pyrimethamine is a folic acid antagonist
Sulfonamides / ↓ Absorption of folic acid
Triamterene / ↓ Utilization of folic acid as it is a folic acid antagonist

Trimethoprim / ↓ Utilization of folic acid as it is a folic acid antagonist

EMS CONSIDERATIONS
None.

Follitropin alfa
Follitropin beta
(fol-ih-TROH-pin AL-fah)(fol-ih-TROH-pin BAY-tah)
Pregnancy Class: X
Follitropin alfa (Gonal-F **(Rx)**)Follitropin beta (Follistim **(Rx)**)
Classification: Ovarian stimulant, gonadotropin

Mechanism of Action: Both products are human FSH prepared by recombinant DNA technology. When given with HCG, products stimulate ovarian follicular growth in women who do not have primary ovarian failure. Increased risk of multiple births.

Uses: Induction of ovulation and pregnancy in anovulatory infertile patients where cause of infertility is functional. To stimulate development of multiple follicles in ovulatory patients undergoing in-vitro fertilization.

Contraindications: Use in primary ovarian failure; uncontrolled thyroid or adrenal dysfunction; in presence of any cause of infertility other than anovulation; tumor of ovary, breast, uterus, hypothalamus, or pituitary gland; abnormal vaginal bleeding of undetermined origin; ovarian cysts or enlargement not due to polycystic ovary syndrome; pregnancy; use in children; hypersensitivity to products.

Precautions: Use with caution during lactation.

Route/Dosage
FOLLITROPIN ALFA
• **SC only**
Ovulation induction.
Initial, first cycle: 75 IU/day. An incremental adjustment up to 37.5 IU may be considered after 14 days; further increases can be made, if

needed, every 7 days. To complete follicular development and effect ovulation in absence of an endogenous LH surge, give 5,000 units of HCG 1 day after last dose of follitropin alfa. Withold HCG if serum estradiol is greater than 2,000 pg/mL. Base initial dose in subsequent cycles on response in the preceding cycle. Doses greater than 300 IU/day are not recommended routinely. As in initial cycle, HCG at a dose of 5,000 is given 1 day after last dose of follitropin alfa.
Follicle stimulation.
Initiate on day 2 or 3 of the follicular phase at a dose of 150 IU/day, until sufficient follicular development is achieved. Usually, therapy does not exceed 10 days. In those undergoing in vitro fertilization whose endogenous gonadotropin levels are suppressed, initiate follitropin alfa at a dose of 225 IU/day. Consider dosage adjustments after 5 days based on patient response; adjust subsequent dosage every 3 to 4 days and by less than 75 to 150 IU additional drug at each adjustment, not to exceed 450 IU/day. Once follicular development is achieved, give HCG, 5,000–10,000 units, to cause final follicular maturation in preparation for oocyte retrieval.
FOLLITROPIN BETA
• **SC, IM**
Ovulation induction.
Use stepwise, gradually increasing dosage regimen. **Initial:** 75 IU/day for up to 14 days; increase by 37.5 IU at weekly intervals until follicular growth or serum estradiol levels indicate response. Maximum daily dose: 300 IU. Treat until ultrasonic visualization or serum estradiol levels indicate pre-ovulatory conditions greater than or equal to normal values. Then, give HCG 5,000–10,000 IU.
Follicle stimulation.
Initial: 150–225 IU for first 4 days of treatment. Dose may be adjusted based on ovarian response. Daily maintenance doses from 75–300 IU (however, doses from 375–600 IU

have been used) for 6 to 12 days are usually sufficient. Maximum daily dose: 600 IU. When sufficient number of follicles of adequate size are present, induce final maturation by giving HCG, 5,000–10,000 IU. Oocyte retrieval is undertaken 34–36 hr later.
How Supplied: Follitropin alfa: *Powder for injection:* 75 IU, 150. IU; Follitropin beta: *Powder for injection:* 75 IU
Side Effects: *CV:* Intravascular thrombosis and embolism causing venous thrombophlebitis, **pulmonary embolism,** pulmonary infarction, stroke, arterial occlusion (leading to loss of limb). *Pulmonary:* Atelectasis, ARDS, exacerbation of asthma. *Ovarian hyperstimulation syndrome:* Ovarian enlargement, abdominal pain/distention, N&V, diarrhea, dyspnea, oliguria, ascites, pleural effusion, hypovolemia, electrolyte imbalance, hemoperitoneum, thromboembolic events. *Hypersensitivity:* Febrile reaction, chills, musculoskeletal aches, joint pains, malaise, headache, fatigue. *GI:* N&V, diarrhea, abdominal cramps, bloating. *Dermatologic:* Dry skin, body rash, hair loss, hives. *Miscellaneous:* Ovarian cysts, pain, swelling, headache, irritation at site of injection, breast tenderness.

EMS CONSIDERATIONS

None.

Fosfomycin tromethamine
(fos-fah-MY-sin)
Pregnancy Class: B
Monurol **(Rx)**
Classification: Anti-infective, antibiotic

Mechanism of Action: Bactericidal drug that inactivates enzyme enolpyruvyl transferase, irreversibly blocking condensation of uridine diphosphate-N-acetylglucosamine with p-enolpyruvate. This is one of first steps in bacterial wall synthesis. Also reduces adherence of bacteria to uroepithelial cells.

Uses: Treatment of uncomplicated urinary tract infections (acute cystitis) in women due to *Escherichia coli* and Enterococcus faecalis.
Contraindications: Lactation.
Precautions: Safety and efficacy have not been determined in children 12 years of age and younger.

Route/Dosage
• **Sachet**
  Acute cystitis.
Women, 18 years and older: One sachet of fosfomycin mixed with water before ingesting.
How Supplied: *Granules for Reconstitution:* 3 g
Side Effects: *GI:* Diarrhea, nausea, dyspepsia, abdominal pain, abnormal stools, anorexia, constipation, dry mouth, flatulence, vomiting. *CNS:* Headache, dizziness, insomnia, migraine, nervousness, paresthesia, somnolence. *GU:* Vaginitis, dysmenorrhea, dysuria, hematuria, menstrual disorder. *Respiratory:* Rhinitis, pharyngitis. *Miscellaneous:* Asthenia, back pain, pain, rash, ear disorder, fever, flu syndrome, infection, lymphadenopathy, myalgia, pruritus, skin disorder.
Drug Interactions
Metoclopramide / ↓ serum levels and urinary excretion of fosfomycin.

EMS CONSIDERATIONS

See also *Anti-Infective Agents.*

Fosinopril sodium
(foh-SIN-oh-prill)
Pregnancy Class: D
Monopril **(Rx)**
Classification: Angiotensin-converting enzyme inhibitor

Uses: Alone or in combination with other antihypertensive agents (especially thiazide diuretics) for the treatment of hypertension. Adjunct in treating CHF in patients not responding adequately to diuretics and digitalis. Diabetic hypertensive patients show a reduction in major CV events.
Contraindications: Use during lactation.

Route/Dosage
- **Tablets**

Hypertension.

Initial: 10 mg once daily; **then,** adjust dose depending on BP response at peak (2–6 hr after dosing) and trough (24 hr after dosing) blood levels. **Maintenance:** Usually 20–40 mg/day, although some patients manifest beneficial effects at doses up to 80 mg.

In patients taking diuretics.

Discontinue diuretic 2–3 days before starting fosinopril. If diuretic cannot be discontinued, use an initial dose of 10 mg fosinopril.

Congestive heart failure.

Initial: 10 mg once daily; **then,** following initial dose, observe the patient for at least 2 hr for the presence of hypotension or orthostasis (if either is present, monitor until BP stabilizes). An initial dose of 5 mg is recommended in heart failure with moderate to severe renal failure or in those who have had significant diuresis. The dose is increased over several weeks, not to exceed a maximum of 40 mg daily (usual effective range is 20–40 mg once daily).

How Supplied: *Tablet:* 10 mg, 20 mg, 40 mg

Side Effects: *CV:* Orthostatic hypotension, chest pain, hypotension, palpitations, angina pectoris, *CVA, MI,* rhythm disturbances, TIA, tachycardia, *hypertensive crisis,* claudication, bradycardia, hypertension, conduction disorder, *sudden death, cardiorespiratory arrest, shock. CNS:* Headache, dizziness, fatigue, confusion, memory disturbance, depression, behavior change, tremors, drowsiness, mood change, insomnia, vertigo, sleep disturbances. *GI:* N&V, diarrhea, abdominal pain, constipation, dry mouth, dysphagia, taste disturbance, abdominal distention, flatulence, heartburn, appetite changes, weight changes. *Hepatic:* Hepatitis, pancreatitis, hepatomegaly, *hepatic failure. Respiratory:* Cough, sinusitis, dyspnea, URI, *bronchospasm,* asthma, pharyngitis, laryngitis, tracheobronchitis, abnormal breathing, sinus abnormalities. *Hematologic:* Leukopenia, eosinophilia, decreases in hemoglobin (mean of 0.1 g/dL) or hematocrit, neutropenia. *Dermatologic:* Diaphoresis, photosensitivity, flushing, exfoliative dermatitis, pruritus, rash, urticaria. *Body as a whole:* Angioedema, muscle cramps, fever, syncope, influenza, cold sensation, pain, myalgia, arthralgia, arthritis, edema, weakness, musculoskeletal pain. *GU:* Decreased libido, sexual dysfunction, renal insufficiency, urinary frequency, abnormal urination, kidney pain. *Miscellaneous:* Paresthesias, tinnitus, gout, lymphadenopathy, rhinitis, epistaxis, vision disturbances, eye irritation, swelling/weakness of extremities, abnormal vocalization, pneumonia, muscle ache.

EMS CONSIDERATIONS
None.

Fosphenytoin sodium
(FOS-fen-ih-toyn)
Pregnancy Class: D
Cerebyx **(Rx)**
Classification: Anticonvulsant

Mechanism of Action: Fosphenytoin is a prodrug of phenytoin; thus, its anticonvulsant effects are due to phenytoin. For every millimole of fosphenytoin administered, 1 mmol of phenytoin is produced. Fosphenytoin is better tolerated at the infusion site than is phenytoin (i.e., pain and burning associated with IV phenytoin is decreased). The IV infusion rate for fosphenytoin is three times faster than for IV phenytoin. IM use results in systemic phenytoin concentrations that are similar to PO phenytoin, thus allowing interchangeable use.

Uses: Short-term parenteral use for the control of generalized convulsive status epilepticus and prophylaxis and treatment of seizures occurring during neurosurgery. It can be substituted, short term, for PO phenytoin

bold italic = life threatening side effect

when PO administration is not possible.

Contraindications: Hypersensitivity to fosphenytoin, phenytoin, or other hydantoins. Use in patients with sinus bradycardia, SA block, second- and third-degree AV block, and Adams-Stokes syndrome. Use to treat absence seizures. Use during lactation.

Precautions: The safety and efficacy of fosphenytoin have not been determined for longer than 5 days. The safety has not been determined in pediatric patients. After administration of fosphenytoin to those with renal and/or hepatic dysfunction or in those with hypoalbuminemia, fosphenytoin clearance to phenytoin may be increased without a similar increase in phenytoin clearance, thus increasing the potential for serious side effects.

Route/Dosage —————
NOTE: Doses of fosphenytoin are expressed as phenytoin sodium equivalents (PE = phenytoin sodium equivalent). Thus, adjustments in the recommended doses should not be made when substituting fosphenytoin for phenytoin sodium or vice versa.

• **IV**
Status epilepticus.
Loading dose: 15–20 mg PE/kg given at a rate of 100–150 mg PE/min. The loading dose is followed by maintenance doses of either fosphenytoin or phenytoin, either PO or parenterally.

• **IM, IV**
Nonemergency loading and maintenance dosing.
Loading dose: 10–20 mg PE/kg given at a rate of 100–150 mg PE/min.
Maintenance: 4–6 mg PE/kg/day.
Temporary substitution for PO phenytoin.
Use the same daily PO dose of phenytoin in milligrams given at a rate not to exceed 150 mg PE/min.

How Supplied: *Injection:* 75 mg/mL

Side Effects: See *Phenytoin*. The most common side effects include ataxia, dizziness, headache, nystagmus, paresthesia, pruritus, and somnolence.

Drug Interactions: See *Phenytoin*.

EMS CONSIDERATIONS

See also *Anticonvulsants* and *Phenytoin*.

Administration/Storage

1. Do not use IM fosphenytoin to treat status epilepticus because therapeutic phenytoin concentrations may not be reached as quickly as with IV administration.

2. Do not use vials that develop particulate matter.

IV 3. Prior to IV infusion fosphenytoin must be diluted in D5W or NSS solution to obtain a concentration ranging from 1.5 to 25 mg/PE (phenytoin sodium equivalents)/mL.

4. Due to risk of hypotension, do not administer at a rate greater than 150 PE/min.

Assessment

1. Monitor ECG. During IV administration, continuously monitor ECG, BP, and respirations.

2. Do not use with bradycardia or heart block; may cause atrial and ventricular conduction depression.

Furosemide
(fur-OH-seh-myd)
Pregnancy Class: C
Lasix **(Rx)**
Classification: Loop diuretic

Mechanism of Action: Inhibits the reabsorption of sodium and chloride in the proximal and distal tubules as well as the ascending loop of Henle; this results in the excretion of sodium, chloride, and, to a lesser degree, potassium and bicarbonate ions. Has a slight antihypertensive effect.

Onset of Action: PO, IM: 30-60 min; **IV:** 5 min. **Peak: PO, IM:** 1-2 hr; **IV:** 20-60 min.

Duration of Action: PO, IM: 6-8 hr; **IV:** 2 hr.

Uses: Edema associated with CHF, nephrotic syndrome, hepatic cirrhosis, and ascites. IV for acute pulmonary edema. PO to treat hypertension in

conjunction with spironolactone, triamterene, and other diuretics *except* ethacrynic acid. *Investigational:* Hypercalcemia.
Contraindications: Never use with ethacrynic acid. Anuria, hypersensitivity to drug, severe renal disease associated with azotemia and oliguria, hepatic coma associated with electrolyte depletion. Lactation.
Precautions: Use with caution in premature infants and neonates due to prolonged half-life in these patients (dosing interval must be extended). Geriatric patients may be more sensitive to the usual adult dose. Allergic reactions may be seen in patients who show hypersensitivity to sulfonamides.

Route/Dosage
• **Oral Solution, Tablets**
   Edema.
Adults, initial: 20–80 mg/day as a single dose. For resistant cases, dosage can be increased by 20–40 mg q 6–8 hr until desired diuretic response is attained. Maximum daily dose should not exceed 600 mg. **Pediatric, initial:** 2 mg/kg as a single dose; **then,** dose can be increased by 1–2 mg/kg q 6–8 hr until desired response is attained (up to 5 mg/kg may be required in children with nephrotic syndrome; maximum dose should not exceed 6 mg/kg). A dose range of 0.5–2 mg/kg b.i.d. has also been recommended.
   Hypertension.
Adults, initial: 40 mg b.i.d. Adjust dosage depending on response.
   CHF and chronic renal failure.
Adults: 2–2.5 g/day.
   Antihypercalcemic.
Adults: 120 mg/day in one to three doses.
• **IV, IM**
   Edema.
Adults, initial: 20–40 mg; if response inadequate after 2 hr, increase dose in 20-mg increments.
Pediatric, initial: 1 mg/kg given slowly; if response inadequate after 2 hr, increase dose by 1 mg/kg. Doses

greater than 6 mg/kg should not be given.
   Antihypercalcemic.
Adults: 80–100 mg for severe cases; dose may be repeated q 1–2 hr if needed.
• **IV**
   Acute pulmonary edema.
Adults: 40 mg slowly over 1–2 min; if response inadequate after 1 hr, give 80 mg slowly over 1–2 min. Concomitant oxygen and digitalis may be used.
   CHF, chronic renal failure.
Adults: 2–2.5 g/day. For IV bolus injections, the maximum should not exceed 1 g/day given over 30 min.
   Hypertensive crisis, normal renal function.
Adults: 40–80 mg.
   Hypertensive crisis with pulmonary edema or acute renal failure.
Adults: 100–200 mg.
How Supplied: *Injection:* 10 mg /mL; *Solution:* 10 mg/ mL, 40 mg/5 mL; *Tablet:* 20 mg, 40 mg, 80 mg
Side Effects: *Electrolyte and fluid effects:* Fluid and electrolyte depletion leading to dehydration, hypovolemia, thromboembolism. Hypokalemia and hypochloremia may cause metabolic alkalosis. Hyperuricemia, azotemia, hyponatremia. *GI:* Nausea, oral and gastric irritation, vomiting, anorexia, diarrhea (especially in children) or constipation, cramps, pancreatitis, jaundice, ischemic hepatitis. *Otic:* Tinnitus, hearing impairment (may be reversible or permanent), reversible deafness. Usually following rapid IV or IM administration of high doses. *CNS:* Vertigo, headache, dizziness, blurred vision, restlessness, paresthesias, xanthopsia. *CV:* Orthostatic hypotension, thrombophlebitis, chronic aortitis. *Hematologic:* Anemia, thrombocytopenia, neutropenia, leukopenia, **_agranulocytosis,_** purpura. **_Rarely, aplastic anemia._** *Allergic:* Rashes, pruritus, urticaria, photosensitivity, exfoliative dermatitis, vasculitis, erythema multiforme. *Miscellaneous:* Interstitial nephritis, fever, weakness, hypergly-

cemia, glycosuria, exacerbation of, aggravation of or worsening of SLE, increased perspiration, muscle spasms, urinary bladder spasm, urinary frequency.

Following IV use: Thrombophlebitis, **cardiac arrest.** *Following IM use:* Pain and irritation at injection site, **cardiac arrest.**

Because this drug is resistant to the effects of pressor amines and potentiates the effects of muscle relaxants, it is recommended that the PO drug be discontinued 1 week before surgery and the IV drug 2 days before surgery.

OD **Overdose Management:** *Symptoms:* Profound water loss, electrolyte depletion (manifested by weakness, anorexia, vomiting, lethargy, cramps, mental confusion, dizziness), decreased blood volume, *circulatory collapse (possibly vascular thrombosis and embolism).* *Treatment:* Replace fluid and electrolytes. Monitor urine electrolyte output and serum electrolytes. Induce emesis or perform gastric lavage. Oxygen or artificial respiration may be needed. Treat symptoms.

EMS CONSIDERATIONS

See also *Diuretics, Loop.*

Assessment: With rapid diuresis, observe for dehydration and circulatory collapse; monitor BP and pulse.
IV Give IV injections slowly over 1–2 min.

Gabapentin
(gab-ah-PEN-tin)
Pregnancy Class: C
Neurontin **(Rx)**
Classification: Anticonvulsant

Uses: In adults as an adjunct in the treatment of partial seizures with and without secondary generalization.

Precautions: Use during lactation only if benefits outweigh risks. Plasma clearance is reduced in geriatric patients and in those with impaired renal function. Safety and efficacy have not been determined in children less than 12 years of age.

Route/Dosage
- **Capsules**
  Anticonvulsant.
Adults: Dose range of 900–1,800 mg/day in three divided doses. Titration to an effective dose can begin on day 1 with 300 mg followed by 300 mg b.i.d. on day 2 and 300 mg t.i.d. on day 3. If necessary, the dose may be increased to 300–400 mg t.i.d., up to 1,800 mg/day. In patients with a C_{CR} of 30–60 mL/min, the dose is 300 mg b.i.d.; if the C_{CR} is 15–30 mL/min, the dose is 300 mg/day; if the C_{CR} is less than 15 mL/min, the dose is 300 mg every other day.

How Supplied: *Capsule:* 100 mg, 300 mg, 400 mg

Side Effects: Side effects listed are those with an incidence of 0.1% or greater.

CNS: Most commonly: somnolence, ataxia, dizziness, and fatigue. Also, nystagmus, tremor, nervousness, dysarthria, amnesia, depression, abnormal thinking, twitching, abnormal coordination, headache, *convulsions (including the possibility of precipitation of status epilepticus),* confusion, insomnia, emotional lability, vertigo, hyperkinesia, paresthesia, decreased/increased/absent reflexes, anxiety, hostility, CNS tumors, syncope, abnormal dreaming, aphasia, hypesthesia, *intracranial hemorrhage,* hypotonia, dysesthesia, paresis, dystonia, hemiplegia, facial paralysis, stupor, cerebellar dysfunction, positive Babinski sign, decreased position sense, subdural hematoma, apathy, hallucinations, decreased or loss of libido, agitation depersonalization, euphoria, "doped-up" sensation, *suicidal tendencies,* psychoses. *GI:* Most commonly:

N&V. Also, dyspepsia, dry mouth and throat, constipation, dental abnormalities, increased appetite, abdominal pain, diarrhea, anorexia, flatulence, gingivitis, glossitis, gum hemorrhage, thirst, stomatitis, taste loss, unusual taste, increased salivation, gastroenteritis, hemorrhoids, bloody stools, fecal incontinence, hepatomegaly. *CV:* Hypertension, vasodilation, hypotension, angina pectoris, peripheral vascular disorder, palpitation, tachycardia, migraine, murmur. *Musculoskeletal:* Myalgia, fracture, tendinitis, arthritis, joint stiffness or swelling, positive Romberg test. *Respiratory:* Rhinitis, pharyngitis, coughing, pneumonia, epistaxis, dyspnea, apnea. *Dermatologic:* Pruritus, abrasion, rash, acne, alopecia, eczema, dry skin, increased sweating, urticaria, hirsutism, seborrhea, cyst, herpes simplex. *Body as a whole:* Weight increase, back pain, peripheral edema, asthenia, facial edema, allergy, weight decrease, chills. *GU:* Hematuria, dysuria, frequent urination, cystitis, urinary retention, urinary incontinence, vaginal hemorrhage, amenorrhea, dysmenorrhea, menorrhagia, breast cancer, inability to climax, abnormal ejaculation, impotence. *Hematologic:* Leukopenia, decreased WBCs, purpura, anemia, thrombocytopenia, lymphadenopathy. *Ophthalmologic:* Diplopia, amblyopia, abnormal vision, cataract, conjunctivitis, dry eyes, eye pain, visual field defect, photophobia, bilateral or unilateral ptosis, eye hemorrhage, hordeolum, eye twitching. *Otic:* Hearing loss, earache, tinnitus, inner ear infection, otitis, ear fullness.

OD **Overdose Management:** *Symptoms:* Double vision, slurred speech, drowsiness, lethargy, diarrhea. *Treatment:* Hemodialysis.

Drug Interactions
Antacids / Antacids ↓ bioavailability of gabapentin
Cimetidine / Cimetidine ↓ renal excretion of gabapentin

EMS CONSIDERATIONS
See also *Anticonvulsants.*

Ganciclovir sodium (DHPG)
(gan-SYE-kloh-veer)
Pregnancy Class: C
Cytovene, Vitrasert **(Rx)**
Classification: Antiviral

Mechanism of Action: Upon entry into viral cells infected by CMV, ganciclovir is converted to ganciclovir triphosphate by the CMV. Ganciclovir triphosphate inhibits viral DNA synthesis by competitive inhibition of viral DNA polymerases and direct incorporation into viral DNA; this results in eventual termination of viral DNA elongation. Ganciclovir is active against CMV, herpes simplex virus-1 and -2, Epstein-Barr virus, and varicella zoster virus. Use of the intraocular implant causes a significantly slower disease progression than did those treated with IV ganciclovir.

Uses: **IV:** Immunocompromised patients with CMV retinitis, including AIDS patients. Diagnosis may be confirmed by culture of CMV from the blood, urine, or throat; note that a negative CMV culture does not rule out CMV retinitis. Prevention of CMV disease in transplant patients at risk; duration of treatment depends on duration and degree of immunosuppression. *Investigational:* Treatment of CMV infections (e.g., gastroenteritis, hepatitis, pneumonitis) in immunocompromised patients.

PO: Alternative to IV for maintenance treatment of CMV retinitis in immunocompromised (including AIDS) patients. Prevention of CMV disease in patients with advanced HIV infection at risk for developing CMV disease.

Intraocular implant: CMV retinitis in those with AIDS.

Contraindications: Hypersensitivity to acyclovir or ganciclovir. Lactation. Use when the absolute neutrophil count is less than 500/mm³ or the platelet count is less than 25,000/mm³.

Precautions: Safety and effectiveness of ganciclovir have not been established for nonimmunocompromised patients, treatment of other CMV infections such as pneumonitis or colitis, or congenital or neonatal CMV disease. Use with caution in impaired renal function, in elderly patients, or with preexisting cytopenias or with a history of cytopenic reactions to other drugs, chemicals, or irradiation. Use in children only if potential benefits outweigh potential risks, including carcinogenicity and reproductive toxicity. Not a cure for CMV retinitis and progression of the disease may continue in immunocompromised patients. Treatment with AZT and ganciclovir (e.g., in AIDS patients) will likely not be tolerated and lead to severe granulocytopenia.

Route/Dosage ─────────────
• **IV Infusion, Capsules**
  CMV retinitis.
Induction treatment: 5 mg/kg over 1 hr q 12 hr for 14–21 days in patients with normal renal function. Do not use PO treatment for induction. **Maintenance, IV:** 5 mg/kg over 1 hr by IV infusion daily for 7 days or 6 mg/kg/day for 5 days each week. Dosage must be reduced in patients with renal impairment. **Maintenance, PO:** 1,000 mg t.i.d. with food. Or, 500 mg 6 times/day q 3 hr with food during waking hours.
  Prevention of CMV retinitis in those with advanced HIV infection and normal renal function.
1,000 mg t.i.d. with food.
  Prophylaxis of CMV disease in transplant patients.
Initial dose, IV: 5 mg/kg over 1 hr q 12 hr for 7–14 days. **Maintenance:** 5 mg/kg/day on 7 days each week (or 6 mg/kg/day on 5 days each week).
How Supplied: *Powder for injection:* 500 mg; *Capsules:* 250 mg, 500 mg; *Implant:* 4.5 mg
Side Effects: *Hematologic:* Granulocytopenia, thrombocytopenia, neu-

tropenia (may be irreversible), eosinophilia, leukopenia, anemia, hypochromic anemia, bone marrow depression, pancytopenia, *leukemia, lymphoma. CNS:* Ataxia, *coma,* neuropathy, confusion, abnormal dreams or thoughts, dizziness, headache, paresthesia, psychosis, nervousness, somnolence, tremor, agitation, amnesia, anxiety, depression, euphoria, hypertonia, hypesthesia, insomnia, manic reaction, *seizures,* trismus, emotional lability. *GI:* N&V, aphthous stomatitis, diarrhea, anorexia, dry mouth, *GI hemorrhage, pancreatitis,* abdominal pain, flatulence, dyspepsia, constipation, dysphagia, esophagitis, eructation, fecal incontinence, melena, mouth ulceration, tongue disorder, hepatitis, weight loss. *CV:* Hypertension or hypotension, arrhythmias, phlebitis, deep thrombophlebitis, *cardiac arrest, intracranial hypertension, MI, stroke,* pericarditis, vasodilation, migraine. *Body as a whole:* Fever (most common), chills, edema, infections, malaise, *sepsis, multiple organ failure,* asthenia, enlarged abdomen, abscess, back pain, cellulitis, chest pain, facial edema, neck pain or rigidity. *Dermatologic:* Rash (most common), alopecia, pruritus, urticaria, sweating, acne, dry skin, fixed eruption, herpes simplex, maculopapular rash, skin discoloration, vesiculobullous rash, photosensitivity, phototoxicity. *GU:* Hematuria, breast pain, kidney failure, abnormal kidney function, urinary frequency, UTI. *At injection site:* Catheter infection, catheter sepsis, inflammation or pain, abscess, edema, hemorrhage, phlebitis. *Musculoskeletal:* Arthralgia, bone pain, leg cramps, myalgia, myasthenia. *Ophthalmologic:* Abnormal vision, amblyopia, blindness, conjunctivitis, eye pain, glaucoma, retinitis, photophobia, cataracts, vitreous disorder. *Respiratory:* Dyspnea, increased cough, pneumonia. *Hepatic:* Cholestasis, cholangitis. *Miscellaneous:* Abnormal gait, decreased libido, deafness, *anaphylaxis,* taste perversion, tinnitus, acidosis, congenital anomaly, encephalopathy, impotence, transverse myelitis, infertility, splenomegaly, **Stevens-Johnson syndrome, unexplained death,** retinal detachment in CMV retinitis patients.

OD Overdose Management: *Symptoms:* Neutropenia. Possibility of hypersalivation, anorexia, vomiting, bloody diarrhea, inactivity, cytopenia, testicular atrophy, increased BUN and LFT results. *Treatment:* Hydration, hemodialysis.

Drug Interactions

Adriamycin / Additive cytotoxicity in rapidly dividing cells

Amphotericin B / Additive cytotoxicity in rapidly dividing cells; also, ↑ serum creatinine levels

Cyclosporine / ↑ Serum creatinine levels

Dapsone / Additive cytotoxicity in rapidly dividing cells

Flucytosine / Additive cytotoxicity in rapidly dividing cells

Imipenem/Cilastatin combination / Possibility of seizures

Pentamidine / Additive cytotoxicity in rapidly dividing cells

Probenecid / ↑ Effect of ganciclovir due to ↓ renal excretion

Sulfamethoxazole/Trimethoprim combinations / Additive cytotoxicity in rapidly dividing cells

Vinblastine / Additive cytotoxicity in rapidly dividing cells

Vincristine / Additive cytotoxicity in rapidly dividing cells

AZT / ↑ Risk of granulocytopenia and anemia

EMS CONSIDERATIONS

See also *Antiviral Agents.*

Ganirelix acetate
(gan-ih-REL-icks)
Pregnancy Class: X
Antagon **(Rx)**
Classification: Infertility drug

Mechanism of Action: Synthetic decapeptide that antagonizes gonadotropin-releasing hormone (GnRH). Acts by competitively blocking GnRH receptors in the pituitary gland leading to a rapid, rever-

sible suppression of gonadotropin secretion. When discontinued, pituitary LH and FSH levels fully recover within 48 hr.

Uses: Infertility treatment to inhibit premature LH surges in women undergoing controlled ovarian stimulation.

Contraindications: Hypersensitivity to ganirelix or any of its components, hypersensitivity to GnRH or GnRH analogs, known or suspected pregnancy. Lactation.

Precautions: Use with caution in hypersensitivity to GnRH. Packaging of the product contains natural rubber latex, which may cause allergic reactions.

Route/Dosage

• **Injection**
   Infertility treatment.
Initiate FSH therapy on day 2 or 3 of the cycle (may reduce exogenous FSH requirement). Give ganirelix, 250 mcg, SC once daily during the early to mid follicular phase. Continue ganirelix treatment daily until the day of chorionic gonadotropion (HCG) treatment. When a sufficient number of follicles of adequate size are present (assess by ultrasound), give HCG to finalize maturation of follicles.

How Supplied: *Injection:* 250 mcg/ 0.5 mL

Side Effects: Abdominal pain (gynecological), fetal death, headache, ovarian hyperstimulation syndrome, vaginal bleeding, injection site reaction, nausea, abdominal pain (GI).

Drug Interactions: Because ganirelix suppresses secretion of pituitary gonadotropins, dosage adjustments of exogenous gonadotropins may be necessary when used during controlled ovarian hyperstimulation.

EMS CONSIDERATIONS

None.

Gatifloxacin
(gat-ih-FLOX-ah-sin)

---

bold italic = life threatening side effect

Pregnancy Class: C
Tequin **(Rx)**
Classification: Antibiotic, quinolone

Uses: (1) Acute bacterial exacerbation of chronic bronchitis due to *Streptococcus pneumoniae, Haemophilus influenzae, Haemophilus parainfluenzae, Moraxella catarrhalis,* or *Staphylococcus aureus.* (2) Acute sinusitis due to *S. pneumoniae* or *H. influenzae.* (3) Community-acquired pneumonia due to *S. pneumoniae, H. influenze, H. parainfluenzae, M. catarrhalis, S. aureus, Mycoplasma pneumoniae, Chlamydia pneumoniae,* or *Legionella pneumoniae.* (4) Uncomplicated UTIs (cystitis) or complicated UTIs due to *Escherichia coli, Klebsiella pneumoniae,* or *Proteus mirabilis.* (5) Pyelonephritis due to *E. coli.* (6) Uncomplicated urethral and cervical gonorrhea due to *Neisseria gonorrhoeae.* (7) Acute, uncomplicated rectal infections due to *N. gonorrhoeae.*

Contraindications: Use with drugs that prolong the QTc interval, in patients with uncorrected hypokalemia, and in those receiving Class IA (e.g., quinidine, procainamide) or Class III (e.g., amiodarone, sotalol) antiarrhythmics.

Precautions: Reduce dosage in patients with a C_{CR} less than 40 mL/min, including those requiring hemodialysis or continuous ambulatory peritoneal dialysis. Use with caution with antidepressants, antipsychotics, cisapride, or erythromycin or in those with bradycardia or acute myocardial ischemia. Safety and efficacy in children, adolescents (less than 18 years of age), pregnant women, and lactating women have not been established.

Route/Dosage

• **IV infusion, Tablets**

Acute bacterial exacerbation of chronic bronchitis, complicated UTIs, acute pyelonephritis.

Adults: 400 mg once daily for 7–10 days.

Acute sinusitis.

Adults: 400 mg once daily for 10 days.

Community-acquired pneumonia.

Adults: 400 mg once daily for 7–14 days.

Uncomplicated UTIs (cystitis).

Adults: 400 mg as a single dose or 200 mg daily for 3 days.

Uncomplicated urethral gonorrhea in men, endocervical and rectal gonorrhea in women.

Single dose of 400 mg.

Adjust dosage as follows in patients with impaired renal function. C_{CR} less than 40 mL/min: Initial, **400 mg;** then, **200 mg every day.** Hemodialysis: Initial, **400 mg;** then, **200 mg every day.** Continuous peritoneal dialysis: Initial, **400 mg;** then, **200 mg every day.**

How Supplied: *IV Solution:* 10 mg/mL; *IV Solution, Premix Bags:* 2 mg/mL; *Tablets:* 200 mg, 400 mg

Side Effects: *CNS:* Tremors, restlessness, lightheadedness, confusion, hallucinations, paranoia, depression, nightmares, insomnia, paresthesia, vertigo. *GI:* Abdominal pain, constipation, dyspepsia, glossitis, oral moniliasis, stomatitis, mouth ulcer, vomiting, pseudomembranous colitis, hepatitis, jaundice, *acute hepatic necrosis or failure. Body as a whole:* Fever, chills, back pain, chest pain. *CV:* Vasculitis, palpitation, vasodilation. *Respiratory:* Dyspnea, pharyngitis, allergic pneumonitis. *Hypersensitivity: Anaphylaxis, CV collapse, angioedema, acute respiratory distress, bronchospasm, shock,* hypotension, seizure, loss of consciousness, tingling, shortness of breath, dyspnea, urticaria, itching, serious skin reactions. *Hematologic:* Hemolytic or aplastic anemia, thrombotic thrombocytopenic purpura, leukopenia, agranulocytosis, pancytopenia. *Dermatologic:* Rash, sweating, *toxic epidermal necrolysis, Stevens-Johnson syndrome. Musculoskeletal:* Arthralgia, myalgia. *GU:* Dysuria, hematuria, interstitial nephritis, acute renal insufficiency or failure. *Miscellaneous:* Serum sickness, peripheral edema, abnormal vision, taste perversion, tinnitus.

Drug Interactions

Aluminum- or magnesium-containing antacids / ↓ Absorption of gatifloxacin

Digoxin / ↑ Risk of digoxin toxicity

Ferrous sulfate / ↓ Bioavailability of gatifloxacin

NSAIDs / ↑ Risk of CNS stimulation and convulsions

Probenecid / ↓ Bioavailability of gatifloxacin

EMS CONSIDERATIONS

See also *Anti-Infective Drugs.*

Gemcitabine hydrochloride (Gemzar)

jem-SIGHT-ah-been

Pregnancy Class: D

Gemzar **(Rx)**

Classification: Antineoplastic, miscellaneous

Mechanism of Action: A nucleoside analog that kills cells undegoing DNA synthesis (S-phase) and by blocking the progression of cells through the G1/S-phase boundary. Metabolized within cells by nucleoside kinases to the active gemcitabine diphosphate and triphosphate nucleosides. The diphosphate inhibits ribonucleotide reductase, which is responsible for catalyzing reactions that generate the deoxynucleoside triphosphate for DNA synthesis. Inhibition of the reductase enzyme causes a decrease in the levels of deoxynucleotides. The triphosphate competes with triphosphate nucleosides for incorporation into DNA, resulting in inhibition of DNA synthesis. DNA polymerase is not able to remove the gemcitabine nucleoside and repair the growing DNA strands. The metabolite of gemcitabine nucleoside is excreted through the urine.

Uses: First-line treatment for locally advanced (nonresectable Stage II or Stage III) or metastatic (Stage IV) adenocarcinoma of the pancreas. The drug is indicated for those who have been treated previously with 5-fluorouracil. First-line therapy, with cisplatin, for treatment of inoperable, locally advanced, or metastatic non-small cell lung cancer.

Contraindications: Lactation.

Route/Dosage

• **IV Only**

Adenocarcinoma of the pancreas.

Adults: 1,000 mg/m² given over 30 min once a week for up to 7 weeks (or until toxicity necessitates reducing or holding a dose). This is followed by a 1-week rest period. Subsequent cycles should consist of infusions once a week for 3 consecutive weeks out of 4. Those who complete the entire 7 weeks of initial therapy or a subsequent 3-week cycle at the 1,000-mg/m² dose may have the dose for subsequent cycles increased by 25% to 1,250 mg/m² provided that the absolute neutrophil count nadir exceeds 1,500 × 10⁶/L and the platlet nadir exceeds 100,000 × 10⁶/L and if nonhematologic toxicity has not been greater than World Health Organization Grade 1. If patients tolerate a dose of 1,250 mg/m² once weekly, the dose for the next cycle can be increased to 1,500 mg/m² provided the absolute neutrophil count and platelet nadirs are as defined above.

The dose should be reduced to 75% of the full dose if the absolute granulocyte count is 500–999 × 10⁶/L and the platelet count is 50,000–99,000 × 10⁶/L. The dose should be held if the absolute granulocyte count falls below 500 × 10⁶/L and the platelet count falls below 50,000 × 10⁶/L.

How Supplied: *Powder for injection:* 200 mg, 1 g

Side Effects: *GI:* N&V, diarrhea, constipation, stomatitis. *CNS:* Somnolence, mild to severe paresthesias, insomnia. *CV:* Arrhythmia, hypertension, *MI, CVA. Hematologic:* Anemia, leukopenia, neutropenia, thrombocytopenia. *Respiratory:* Dyspnea, bronchospasm, cough, parenchymal lung toxicity (rare). *Dermatologic:* Alopecia,

G

---

bold italic = life threatening side effect

macular or finely granular maculopapular pruritic eruptions, pruritus. *Body as a whole:* Pain, fever, peripheral edema, flu syndrome (including fever), asthenia, chills, myalgia, sweating, malaise. *Miscellaneous:* **Hemorrhage, sepsis,** hemolytic uremic syndrome, infections, petechiae, rhinitis, **anaphylaxis (rare).**

OD **Overdose Management:** *Symptoms:* Myelosuppression, paresthesias, severe rash. *Treatment:* Monitor with appropriate blood counts. Supportive therapy as needed.

EMS CONSIDERATIONS

See also *Nursing Considerations* for *Antineoplastic Agents.*

Administration/Storage

IV 1. To reconstitute the drug, use 0.9% NaCl injection without preservatives. The maximum concentration upon reconstitution is 40 mg/mL; greater concentrations may cause incomplete dissolution.

2. Prolonging the infusion time beyond 60 min and more frequent administration than once weekly increases toxicity.

3. To reconstitute, add 5 mL of 0.9% NaCl injection to the 200-mg vial or 25 mL of 0.9% NaCl injection to the 1-g vial. Shake to dissolve. This results in a concentration of 40 mg/mL which may be further diluted, if needed, with 0.9% NaCl injection to concentrations as low as 0.1 mg/mL.

4. Do not refrigerate reconstituted gemcitabine as crystallization may occur. Store the diluted product at controlled room temperatures of 20°C–25°C (68°F–77°F). Reconstituted solutions are stable at these temperatures for 24 hr.

Assessment

1. Document disease stage, onset, duration of symptoms, organ(s) involved, and other agents trialed.

2. Obtain CBC, liver and renal function studies. Monitor CBC prior to each dose and liver and renal function tests periodically; causes thrombocytopenia and myelosuppression. Nadir: 1 week.

Gemfibrozil

(jem-FIH-broh-zill)
Pregnancy Class: B
Lopid **(Rx)**
Classification: Antihyperlipidemic

Mechanism of Action: Gemfibrozil, which resembles clofibrate, decreases triglycerides, cholesterol, and VLDL and increases HDL; LDL levels either decrease or do not change. Also, decreases hepatic triglyceride production by inhibiting peripheral lipolysis and decreasing extraction of free fatty acids by the liver. Also, gemfibrozil decreases VLDL synthesis by inhibiting synthesis of VLDL carrier apolipoprotein B as well as inhibits peripheral lipolysis and decreases hepatic extraction of free fatty acids (thus decreasing hepatic triglyceride production). May be beneficial in inhibiting development of atherosclerosis.

Onset of Action: 2-5 days.

Uses: Hypertriglyceridemia (type IV and type V hyperlipidemia) unresponsive to dietary control or in patients who are at risk of pancreatitis and abdominal pain. Reduce risk of coronary heart disease in patients with type IIb hyperlipidemia who have not responded to diet, weight loss, exercise, and other drug therapy.

Contraindications: Gallbladder disease, primary biliary cirrhosis, hepatic or renal dysfunction.

Precautions: Use with caution during lactation. Safety and efficacy have not been established in children. The dose may have to be reduced in geriatric patients due to age-related decreases in renal function.

Route/Dosage
• **Tablets**
Adults: 600 mg b.i.d. 30 min before the morning and evening meal. Dosage has not been established in children. Discontinue if significant improvement not observed within 3 months.

How Supplied: *Tablet:* 600 mg

Side Effects: *GI:* Cholelithiasis, abdominal or epigastric pain, N&V, diarrhea, dyspepsia, constipation, acute appendicitis, colitis, pancreatitis, cholestatic jaundice, hepatoma. *CNS:* Dizziness, headache, fatigue, vertigo, somnolence, paresthesia, hypesthesia, depression, confusion, syncope, **seizures.** *CV:* Atrial fibrillation, extrasystole, peripheral vascular disease, **intracerebral hemorrhage.** *Hematopoietic:* Anemia, leukopenia, eosinophilia, thrombocytopenia, bone marrow hypoplasia. *Musculoskeletal:* Painful extremities, arthralgia, myalgia, myopathy, myasthenia, rhabdomyolysis, synovitis. *Allergic:* Urticaria, lupus-like syndrome, angioedema, **laryngeal edema,** vasculitis, **anaphylaxis.** *Dermatologic:* Eczema, dermatitis, pruritus, skin rashes, exfoliative dermatitis, alopecia. *Ophthalmic:* Blurred vision, retinal edema, cataracts. *Miscellaneous:* Increased chance of viral and bacterial infections, taste perversion, impotence, decreased male fertility, weight loss.

Drug Interactions
Anticoagulants, oral / ↑ Effect of anticoagulants; dosage adjustment necessary
Lovastatin / Possible rhabdomyolysis
Simvastatin / Possible rhabdomyolysis

EMS CONSIDERATIONS
None.

Gentamicin sulfate
(jen-tah-MY-sin)
Pregnancy Class: C
Garamycin, Garamycin Cream or Ointment, Garamycin IV Piggyback, Garamycin Ophthalmic Ointment, Garamycin Ophthalmic Solution, Genoptic Ophthalmic Liquifilm, Genoptic S.O.P. Ophthalmic, Gentacidin Ophthalmic, Gentafair, Gentak Ophthalmic, Gentamicin, Gentamicin Ophthalmic, Gentamicin Sulfate IV Piggyback, Gentrasul Ophthalmic, G-myticin Cream or Ointment, Pediatric Gentamicin Sulfate **(Rx)**
Classification: Antibiotic, aminoglycoside

Uses: Systemic: Serious infections caused by *Pseudomonas aerugino-*

sa, Proteus, Klebsiella, Enterobacter, Serratia, Citrobacter, and *Staphylococcus.* Infections include bacterial neonatal sepsis, bacterial septicemia, and serious infections of the skin, bone, soft tissue (including burns), urinary tract, GI tract (including peritonitis), and CNS (including meningitis). Should be considered as initial therapy in suspected or confirmed gram-negative infections. In combination with carbenicillin for treating life-threatening infections due to *P. aeruginosa.* In combination with penicillin for treating endocarditis caused by group D streptococci. In combination with penicillin for treating suspected bacterial sepsis or staphylococcal pneumonia in the neonate. Intrathecal administration is used in combination with systemic gentamicin for treating meningitis, ventriculitis, or other serious CNS infections due to *Pseudomonas. Investigational:* Pelvic inflammatory disease.

Ophthalmic: Ophthalmic infections due to *Staphylococcus, S. aureus, Streptococcus pneumoniae,* beta-hemolytic streptococci, *Corynebacterium* species, *Streptococcus pyogenes, Escherichia coli, Haemophilus influenzae, H. aegyptius, H. ducreyi, Klebsiella pneumoniae, Neisseria gonorrhoeae, Proteus* species, *Acinetobacter calcoaceticus, Enterobacter aerogenes, P. aeruginosa, Serratia marcescens, Moraxella lacunata.*

Topical: Prevention of infections following minor cuts, wounds, burns, and skin abrasions. Treatment of primary or secondary skin infections. Treatment of infected skin cysts and other skin abscesses when preceded by incision and drainage to permit adequate contact between the drug and the infecting bacteria, infected stasis and other skin ulcers, infected superficial burns, paronychia, infected insect bites and stings, infected lacerations and abrasions and wounds from minor surgery.

Contraindications: Ophthalmic use to treat dendritic keratitis, vaccinia, varicella, mycobacterial infections of

G

---

bold italic = life threatening side effect

the eye, fungal diseases of the eye, use with steroids after uncomplicated removal of a corneal foreign body.

Precautions: Use with caution in premature infants and neonates. Ophthalmic ointments may retard corneal epithelial healing.

Route/Dosage ———————

• **IM (usual), IV**

Adults with normal renal function.

Infections.

1 mg/kg q 8 hr, up to 5 mg/kg/day in life-threatening infections; **children:** 2–2.5 mg/kg q 8 hr; **infants and neonates:** 2.5 mg/kg q 8 hr; **premature infants or neonates less than 1 week of age:** 2.5 mg/kg q 12 hr. Therapy may be required for 7–10 days.

Prevention of bacterial endocarditis, dental or respiratory tract procedures.

Adults: 1.5 mg/kg gentamicin (not to exceed 80 mg) plus 1 g ampicillin, each IM or IV, 30–60 min before the procedure; one additional dose of each can be given 8 hr later (alternative: penicillin V, 1 g PO, 6 hr after initial dose).

Prophylaxis of bacterial endocarditis in GI or GU tract procedures or surgery.

Adults: 1.5 mg/kg gentamicin (not to exceed 80 mg) plus 2 g ampicillin, each IM or IV, 30–60 min before procedure; dose should be repeated 8 hr later. **Children:** 2 mg/kg gentamicin plus penicillin G, 30,000 units/kg, or ampicillin, 50 mg/kg in same dosage interval as for adults. Pediatric dosage should not exceed single or 24-hr adult doses.

NOTE: In patients allergic to penicillin, vancomycin, 1 g IV given slowly over 1 hr, may be substituted; the dose of vancomycin should be repeated 8–12 hr later. **Adults with impaired renal function:** To calculate interval (hr) between doses, multiply serum creatinine level (mg/100 mL) by 8.

• **IV**

Septicemia.

Initially: 1–2 mg/kg infused over 30–60 min; **then,** maintenance doses may be administered.

• **Intrathecal**

Meningitis.

Use only the intrathecal preparation. Adults, usual: 4–8 mg/day; **children and infants 3 months and older:** 1–2 mg/day

Pelvic inflammatory disease.

Initial: 2 mg/kg IV; **then,** 1.5 mg/kg t.i.d. plus clindamycin, 500 mg IV q.i.d. Continue for at least 4 days and at least 48 hr after patient improves. Continue clindamycin, 450 mg PO q.i.d. for 10–14 days.

• **Ophthalmic Solution (0.3%)**

Acute infections.

Initially: 1–2 gtt in conjunctival sac q 15–30 min; **then,** as infection improves, reduce frequency.

Moderate infections.

1–2 gtt in conjunctival sac 4–6 times/day.

Trachoma.

2 gtt in each eye b.i.d.–q.i.d.; treatment should be continued for up to 1–2 months.

• **Ophthalmic Ointment (0.3%)**

Depending on the severity of infection, ½-in. ribbon from q 3–4 hr to 2–3 times/day.

• **Topical Cream/Ointment (0.1%)**

Apply 3–4 times/day to affected area. The area may be covered with a sterile bandage.

How Supplied: *Cream:* 0.1%; *Injection:* 10 mg/mL, 40 mg/mL; *Ointment:* 1%; *Ophthalmic ointment:* 3 mg/g; *Ophthalmic Solution:* 3 mg/mL

Side Effects: Additional: Muscle twitching, numbness, **seizures,** increased BP, alopecia, purpura, pseudotumor cerebri. Photosensitivity when used topically. *After ophthalmic use:* Transient irritation, burning, stinging, itching, inflammation, angioneurotic edema, urticaria, vesicular and maculopapular dermatitis, mydriasis, conjunctival paresthesia, conjunctival hyperemia, nonspecific conjunctivitis, conjunctival epithelial defects, lid itching and swelling, bacterial/fungal corneal ulcers.

Drug Interactions: Additional: With cargenicillin or ticarcillin, gentamicin may result in increased effect when used for *Pseudomonas* infections.

EMS CONSIDERATIONS

None.

Glatiramer acetate
(glah-TER-ah-mer)
Pregnancy Class: B
Copaxone **(Rx)**
Classification: Drug for multiple sclerosis

Mechanism of Action: May act by modifying immune processes responsible for pathology of multiple sclerosis. Some of drug enters lymphatic circulation reaching regional lymph nodes.

Uses: Reduce frequency of relapsing-remitting multiple sclerosis.

Contraindications: Hypersensitivity to glatiramer or mannitol.

Precautions: Use with caution during lactation. Safety and efficacy have not been determined in children less than 18 years of age. May interfere with useful immune function.

Route/Dosage
• **SC**
Multiple sclerosis.
Adults: 20 mg/day SC.
How Supplied: *Powder for Injection:* 20 mg

Side Effects: Side effects listed are those with incidence of 1% or more. *Immediate-post injection reaction:* Flushing, chest pain, palpitations, anxiety, dyspnea, laryngeal constriction, urticaria. *CNS:* Anxiety, hypertonia, tremor, vertigo, agitation, foot drop, nervousness, nystagmus, speech disorder, confusion, abnormal dreams, emotional lability, stupor, migraine. *GI:* Nausea, diarrhea, anorexia, vomiting, GI disorder, abdominal pain, gastroenteritis, bowel urgency, oral moniliasis, salivary gland enlargement, tooth caries, ulcerative stomatitis. *CV:* Vasodilation, palpita-

tions, tachycardia, syncope, hypertension. *Body as a whole:* Infection, asthenia, pain, transient chest pain, flu syndrome, back pain, fever, neck pain, face edema, bacterial infection, chills, cyst, headache, injection site ecchymosis, accidental injury, neck rigidity, malaise, injection site edema or atrophy, abscess, peripheral edema, edema, weight gain. *Dermatologic:* Rash, pruritus, sweating, herpes simplex, erythema, urticaria, skin nodule, eczema, herpes zoster, pustular rash, skin atrophy and warts. *GU:* Urinary urgency, vaginal moniliasis, dysmenorrhea, amenorrhea, hematuria, impotence, menorrhagia, suspicious Pap smear, vaginal hemorrhage. *Hematologic:* Ecchymosis, lymphadenopathy. *Respiratory:* Dyspnea, allergic rhinitis, bronchitis, laryngismus, hyperventilation. *At injection site:* Pain, erythema, inflammation, pruritus, mass, induration, welt, hemorrhage, urticaria. *Miscellaneous:* Ear pain, eye disorder, arthralgia.

EMS CONSIDERATIONS

None.

Glimepiride
(GLYE-meh-pye-ride)
Pregnancy Class: C
Amaryl **(Rx)**
Classification: Antidiabetic agent, sulfonylurea

Mechanism of Action: Lowers blood glucose by stimulating the release of insulin from functioning pancreatic beta cells and by increasing the sensitivity of peripheral tissues to insulin.
Onset of Action: Time to maximum effect: 2-3 hr.
Uses: As an adjunct to diet and exercise to lower blood glucose in non-insulin-dependent diabetes mellitus (Type II diabetes mellitus). In combination with insulin to decrease blood glucose in those whose hyperglycemia cannot be controlled by diet and exercise in combination with an oral hypoglycemic drug.

Contraindications: Diabetic ketoacidosis with or without coma. Use during lactation.

Precautions: The use of oral hypoglycemic drugs has been associated with increased CV mortality compared with treatment with diet alone or diet plus insulin. Safety and efficacy have not been determined in children.

Route/Dosage

• **Tablets**

Non-insulin-dependent diabetes mellitus (Type II diabetes).

Adults, initial: 1–2 mg once daily, given with breakfast or the first main meal. The initial dose should be 1 mg in those sensitive to hypoglycemic drugs, in those with impaired renal or hepatic function, and in elderly, debilitated, or malnourished patients. The maximum initial dose is 2 mg or less daily. **Maintenance:** 1–4 mg once daily up to a maximum of 8 mg once daily. After a dose of 2 mg is reached, increase the dose in increments of 2 mg or less at 1- to 2-week intervals (determined by the blood glucose response). **When combined with insulin therapy:** 8 mg once daily with the first main meal with low-dose insulin. The fasting glucose level for beginning combination therapy is greater than 150 mg/dL glucose in the plasma or serum.

Type II diabetes—transfer from other hypoglycemic agents

When transferring patients to glimepiride, no transition period is required. However, observe patients closely for 1 to 2 weeks for hypoglycemia when being transferred from longer half-life sulfonylureas (e.g., chlorpropamide) to glimepiride.

How Supplied: *Tablet:* 1 mg, 2 mg, 4 mg

Side Effects: The most common side effect is hypoglycemia. *GI:* N&V, GI pain, diarrhea, cholestatic jaundice (rare). *CNS:* Dizziness, headache. *Dermatologic:* Pruritus, erythema, urticaria, morbilliform or maculopapular eruptions. *Hematologic:* Leukopenia, agranulocytosis, thrombocytopenia, hemolytic anemia, aplastic anemia, pancytopenia. *Miscellaneous:* Hyponatremia, increased release of ADH, changes in accommodation and/or blurred vision.

Drug Interactions: See *Hypoglycemic Agents,* .

EMS CONSIDERATIONS

See also *Hypoglycemic Agents.*

Glipizide
(GLIP-ih-zyd)
Pregnancy Class: C
Glucotrol, Glucotrol XL **(Rx)**
Classification: Sulfonylurea (anti-diabetic), second-generation

Mechanism of Action: Also has mild diuretic effects.
Onset of Action: 1-1.5 hr.
Duration of Action: 10-16 hr.
Uses: Adjunct to diet for control of hyperglycemia in patients with non-insulin-dependent diabetes.

Route/Dosage

• **Tablets, Extended Release Tablets**

Diabetes.

Adults, initial: 5 mg 30 min before breakfast; **then,** adjust dosage by 2.5–5 mg every few days, depending on the blood glucose response, until adequate control is achieved. **Maintenance:** 15–40 mg/day. Older patients should begin with 2.5 mg. The Extended Release Tablets are taken once daily (usually at breakfast) in doses of either 5 or 10 mg.

How Supplied: *Tablet:* 5 mg, 10 mg; *Tablet, Extended Release:* 5 mg, 10 mg

Drug Interactions: Additional: Cimetidine may ↑ effect of glipizide due to ↓ breakdown by liver.

EMS CONSIDERATIONS

See also *Antidiabetic Agents.*

Glucagon
(GLOO-kah-gon)
Pregnancy Class: B
(Rx)
Classification: Insulin antagonist

Mechanism of Action: Produced by the alpha islet cells of the pancreas, glucacon accelerates liver glycogenolysis by stimulating synthesis of cyclic AMP and increasing phosphorylase kinase activity. Increased blood glucose levels result from increased breakdown of glycogen to glucose and inhibition of glycogen synthetase. Glucagon stimulates hepatic gluconeogenesis by increasing the uptake of amino acids and converting them to glucose precursors. Also, lipolysis is increased, resulting in free fatty acids and glycerol for gluconeogenesis. Effective in overcoming hypoglycemia only if the liver has a glycogen reserve. Also relaxes smooth muscle of the GI tract and decreases gastric and pancreatic secretions; increases myocardial contractility.

Onset of Action: Hypoglycemia: 5-20 min.; **Maximum effect:** 30 min.

Duration of Action: 1-2 hr.

Uses: Used to terminate insulin-induced shock in diabetic or psychiatric patients. Patient usually regains consciousness 5–20 min after the parenteral administration of glucagon. The drug should only be used under medical supervision or in accordance with strict instructions received from the physician. Failure to respond may be an indication for IV administration of glucose—especially true in juvenile diabetics. As a diagnostic aid in radiologic examination of the GI tract when a hypotonic state is desirable. *Investigational:* Treatment of propranolol overdose and cardiovascular emergencies.

Precautions: Use with caution during lactation, in patients with renal or hepatic disease, in those who are undernourished and emaciated, and in patients with a history of pheochromocytoma or insulinoma.

Route/Dosage
• **IM, IV, SC**
Hypoglycemia.
Children < 20 kg: 0.5; **Adults and children > 20 kg:** 1 mg; one to two

additional doses may be given at 20-min intervals, if necessary.

Insulin shock therapy.
IM, IV, SC: 0.5–1 mg after 1 hr of coma; the patient will usually awaken in 10–25 min. The dose may be repeated if there is no response.

Diagnostic aid for GI tract.
Dose dependent on desired onset of action and duration of effect necessary for the examination. **IV:** 0.25–0.5 mg (onset: 1 min; duration: 9–17 min); 2 mg (onset: 1 min; duration 22–25 min). **IM:** 1 mg (onset: 8–10 min; duration: 12–27 min); 2 mg (onset: 4–7 min; duration: 21–32 min).

For colon examination.
IM: 2 mg 10 min prior to procedure.

Treatment of toxicity of beta-adrenergic blocking agents.
Adults, IV, initial: 2–3 mg given over 30 sec; may be repeated at the rate of 5 mg/hr until patient is stabilized.

How Supplied: *Powder for injection:* 1 mg

Side Effects: *GI:* N&V. *Allergy:* Respiratory distress, urticaria, hypotension. ***Stevens-Johnson syndrome when used as diagnostic aid.***

OD Overdose Management: *Symptoms:* N&V, hypokalemia. *Treatment:* Symptomatic.

Drug Interactions
Anticoagulants, oral / ↑ Effect of anticoagulants by ↑ hypoprothrombinemia
Antidiabetic agents / Hyperglycemic effect of glucagon antagonizes hypoglycemic effect of antidiabetics
Corticosteroids, Epinephrine, Estrogens, Phenytoin / Additive hyperglycemic effect of drugs listed

EMS CONSIDERATIONS
Administration/Storage
1. Once patient with hypoglycemia responds, give supplemental carbohydrates to prevent secondary hypoglycemia.
IV 2. Reconstitute doses higher than 2 mg with sterile water for injection and use immediately.

---

bold italic = life threatening side effect

3. With direct IV administration, inject at a rate not exceeding 1 mg/min.
4. Administer with dextrose solutions. A precipitate may form if saline solutions are used.

Glyburide
(GLYE-byou-ryd)
Pregnancy Class: B
Diabeta, Prestab **(Rx)**
Classification: Sulfonylurea (anti-diabetic), second-generation

Mechanism of Action: Has a mild diuretic effect.
Onset of Action: Nonmicronized: 2-4 hr; **micronized:** 1 hr.
Duration of Action: Both forms: 24 hr.

Route/Dosage —————————
• **Tablets, Nonmicronized (Dia-Beta/Micronase)**
  Diabetes.
Adults, initial: 2.5–5 mg/day given with breakfast (or the first main meal); **then,** increase by 2.5 mg at weekly intervals to achieve the desired response. **Maintenance:** 1.25–20 mg/day. Patients sensitive to sulfonylureas should start with 1.25 mg/day.
• **Tablets, Micronized (Glynase)**
  Diabetes.
Adults, initial: 1.5–3 mg/day given with breakfast (or the first main meal); **then,** increase by no more than 1.5 mg at weekly intervals to achieve the desired response. **Maintenance:** 0.75–12 mg/day.
How Supplied: *Tablet:* 1.25 mg, 1.5 mg, 2.5 mg, 3 mg, 5 mg, 6 mg

EMS CONSIDERATIONS

See also *Antidiabetic Agents.*

Gold sodium thiomalate (Sodium aurothiomalate)
(gold SO-dee-um thigh-ah-MAH-layt)
Pregnancy Class: C
Myochrysine **(Rx)**
Classification: Antirheumatic

Mechanism of Action: Exact mechanism not known. May inhibit lysoso-mal enzyme activity in macrophages and decrease macrophage phagocytic activity. Other mechanisms may include alteration of the immune response and alteration of biosynthesis of collagen. Gold salts suppress, but do not cure, arthritis and synovitis. Beneficial effects may not be seen for 3–12 months. Most experience transient side effects, although serious effects may be manifested in some.
Uses: Adjunct to the treatment of active, early rheumatoid arthritis in children and adults who have insufficient response to or are intolerant of full doses of one or more NSAIDs.
Contraindications: Hepatic disease, CV problems such as hypertension or CHF, severe diabetes, debilitated patients, renal disease, blood dyscrasias, agranulocytosis, hemorrhagic diathesis, patients receiving radiation treatments, colitis, lupus erythematosus, pregnancy, lactation, children under 6 years of age. Patients with eczema or urticaria.

Route/Dosage —————————
• **IM**
  Rheumatoid arthritis.
Adults: w*eek 1:* 10 mg as a single injection; *week 2:* 25 mg as a single dose. Then, 25–50 mg/week until 0.8–1 g total has been given. Thereafter according to individual response. *Usual maintenance:* 25–50 mg every other week for up to 20 weeks. If condition remains stable, the dose can be given every third or fourth week indefinitely. **Pediatric, initial:** w*eek 1,* 10 mg; **then,** usual dose is 1 mg/kg, not to exceed 50 mg/injection using the same spacing of doses as for adults.
How Supplied: *Injection:* 50 mg/mL
Side Effects: *Skin:* Dermatitis (most common), pruritus, erythema, dermatoses, gray to blue pigmentation of tissues, alopecia, loss of nails. *GI:* Stomatitis (second most common), metallic taste, gastritis, colitis, gingivitis, glossitis, N&V, diarrhea (may be persistent), colic, anorexia, cramps, enterocolitis. *Hematologic:* Anemia, thrombocytopenia, granu-

locytopenia, leukopenia, eosinophilia, hemorrhagic diathesis. *Allergic:* Flushing, fainting, sweating, dizziness, **anaphylaxis,** syncope, bradycardia, angioneurotic edema, respiratory difficulties. *Other:* Interstitial pneumonitis, pulmonary fibrosis, nephrotic syndrome, glomerulitis (with hematuria), proteinuria, hepatitis, fever, headache, arthralgia, ophthalmologic problems including corneal ulcers, iritis, gold deposits, EEG abnormalities, peripheral neuritis. Corticosteroids may be used to treat symptoms such as stomatitis, dermatitis, GI, renal, hematologic, or pulmonary problems. Also, if symptoms are severe and do not respond to corticosteroids, a chelating agent such as dimercaprol may be used. Patients should be monitored carefully.

OD **Overdose Management:** *Symptoms:* Hematuria, proteinuria, thrombocytopenia, granulocytopenia, N&V, diarrhea, fever, papulovesicular lesions, urticaria, exfoliative dermatitis, severe pruritus. *Treatment:* Discontinue use of the drug immediately. Give dimercaprol. Provide supportive treatment for hematologic or renal complications.

Drug Interactions: Concomitant use contraindicated with drugs known to cause blood dyscrasias (e.g., antimalarials, cytotoxic drugs, pyrazolone derivatives, immunosuppressive drugs).

EMS CONSIDERATIONS

None.

Goserelin acetate
(GO-seh-rel-in)
Pregnancy Class: X (when used for endometriosis); D (when used for breast cancer)
Zoladex **(Rx)**
Classification: Antineoplastic, hormonal agent

Mechanism of Action: Goserelin acetate is a synthetic decapeptide analog of LHRH (or GnRH) which is a potent inhibitor of gonadotropin secretion from the pituitary gland. Initially, there is actually an increase in serum luteinizing hormone and FSH. This is followed by a long-term suppression of pituitary gonadotropins with serum levels of testosterone decreasing to those seen in surgically castrated males. When used for endometriosis, the drug controls the secretion of hormones required for the ovary to synthesize estrogen resulting in plasma estrogen levels seen in menopause.

Uses: Implant, 3.6 mg or 10.8 mg: Palliative treatment of advanced prostatic carcinoma as an alternative to orchiectomy or estrogen administration when these are either unacceptable to the patient or not indicated. With flutamide (Eulexin) prior to (start 8 weeks before) and during radiation therapy to treat Stage B2-C prostatic carcinoma. **Implant, 3.6 mg only:** Endometriosis, including pain relief and reduction of endometriotic lesions. Palliative treatment of advanced breast cancer in premenopausal and postmenopausal women. For endometrial thinning prior to ablation for dysfunctional uterine bleeding.

Contraindications: Pregnancy, lactation, nondiagnosed vaginal bleeding, hypersensitivity to LHRH or LHRH agonist analogs. Use of the 10.8-mg implant in women.

Precautions: Safety and effectiveness have not been determined in patients less than 18 years of age. There may be transient worsening of symptoms during the first few weeks of therapy. Use with caution in males who are at particular risk of developing ureteral obstruction or spinal cord compression.

Route/Dosage
• **SC Implant, 3.6 mg**
  Prostatic carcinoma, endometriosis, advanced breast cancer, thinning prior to endometrial ablation for dysfunctional uterine bleeding.

---

bold italic = life threatening side effect

3.6 mg q 28 days into the upper abdominal wall using sterile technique under the direction of a physician.

- **SC Implant, 10.8 mg**
  Advanced prostatic carcinoma.
  10.8 mg q 12 weeks into the upper abdominal wall using sterile technique under the direction of a physician.
  With flutamide to treat Stage B2-C prostatic carcinoma.
  One goserelin 3.6 mg depot followed in 28 days by one 10.8 mg depot.

How Supplied: *Implant:* 3.6 mg, 10.8 mg

Side Effects: In males. *GU:* Sexual dysfunction, decreased erections, lower urinary tract symptoms, gynecomastia, renal insufficiency, urinary obstruction, UTI, bladder neoplasm, hematuria, impotence, urinary frequency, incontinence, urinary tract disorder, impaired urination. *CV:* CHF, ***CVA, MI, heart failure, pulmonary embolus,*** arrhythmia, hypertension, peripheral vascular disorder, chest pain, angina pectoris, cerebral ischemia, varicose veins. *CNS:* Lethargy, dizziness, insomnia, asthenia, anxiety, depression, headache, paresthesia. *GI:* N&V, diarrhea, constipation, ulcer, anorexia, hematemesis. *Respiratory:* URI, COPD, increased cough, dyspnea, pneumonia. *Metabolic:* Gout, hypercalcemia, weight increase, diabetes mellitus. *Miscellaneous:* Pelvic or bone pain, anemia, chills, fever, breast pain, breast swelling or tenderness, abdominal or back pain, flu syndrome, sepsis, aggravation reaction, herpes simplex, pruritus, peripheral edema, injection site reaction, hot flashes, rash, sweating, complications of surgery, hypersensitivity, pain, edema.

In females. *GU:* Vaginitis, decreased or increased libido, pelvic symptoms, dyspareunia, dysmenorrhea, urinary frequency, UTI, vaginal bleeding (during the first 2 months) of varying duration and intensity. *CV:* ***Hemorrhage,*** hypertension, palpitations, migraine, tachycardia. *CNS:* Emotional lability, depression, headache, insomnia, dizziness, nervousness, anxiety, paresthesia, somnolence, abnormal thinking, malaise, fatigue, lethargy. *GI:* N&V, abdominal pain, increased appetite, anorexia, constipation, diarrhea, dry mouth, dyspepsia, flatulence. *Musculoskeletal:* Asthenia, back pain, myalgia, hypertonia, arthralgia, joint disorder, decrease of vertebral trabecular bone mineral density. *Dermatologic:* Sweating, acne, seborrhea, hirsutism, pruritus, alopecia, dry skin, ecchymosis, rash, skin discoloration, hair disorders. *Respiratory:* Pharyngitis, bronchitis, increased cough, epistaxis, rhinitis, sinusitis. *Ophthalmic:* Amblyopia, dry eyes. *Miscellaneous:* Hot flashes, breast atrophy or enlargement, breast pain, tumor flare, pain, infection, application site reaction, flu syndrome, voice alterations, weight gain, allergic reaction, chest pain, fever, peripheral edema, hypercalcemia, osteoporosis, hypersensitivity.

EMS CONSIDERATIONS
None.

Granisetron hydrochloride
(gran-ISS-eh-tron)
Pregnancy Class: B
Kytril **(Rx)**
Classification: Antinauseant and antiemetic

Mechanism of Action: Selective 5-HT$_3$ (serotonin) receptor antagonist with little or no affinity for other 5-HT, beta-adrenergic, dopamine, or histamine receptors. During chemotherapy-induced vomiting, mucosal enterochromaffin cells release serotonin, which stimulates 5-HT$_3$ receptors. The stimulation of 5-HT$_3$ receptors by serotonin causes vagal discharge resulting in vomiting.
Uses: Prevention of N&V associated with initial and repeat cancer chemotherapy, including high-dose cisplatin. *Investigational:* Acute N&V following surgery.
Contraindications: Known hypersensitivity to the drug.

Precautions: Use with caution during lactation. Safety and efficacy in children less than 2 years of age have not been established.

Route/Dosage ─────────────
- **IV**
    Antiemetic during cancer chemotherapy.
Adults and children over 2 years of age: 10 mcg/kg infused over 5 min beginning 30 min before initiation of chemotherapy.
    Antiemetic following surgery.
1–3 mg.
- **Tablets**
    Protection from chemotherapy-induced nausea and vomiting.
Adults: 1 mg b.i.d. with the first 1 mg-tablet given 1 hr before chemotherapy and the second 1-mg tablet given 12 hr after the first tablet only on days chemotherapy is given. Alternatively, 2 mg once daily taken 1 hr before chemotherapy. Data are not available for PO use in children.
How Supplied: *Injection:* 1 mg/mL; *Tablet:* 1 mg

Side Effects: After IV use. *CNS:* Headache, somnolence, agitation, anxiety, CNS stimulation, insomnia, extrapyramidal syndrome. *GI:* Diarrhea, constipation, taste disorder. *CV:* Hypertension, hypotension, arrhythmias (e.g., sinus bradycardia, atrial fibrillation, *AV block,* ventricular ectopy including nonsustained tachycardia, ECG abnormalities). *Allergic:* **Hypersensitivity reactions (anaphylaxis),** skin rashes. *Miscellaneous:* Asthenia, fever.

After PO use. *CNS:* Headache, dizziness, insomnia, anxiety, somnolence. *GI:* N&V, diarrhea, constipation, abdominal pain. *CV:* Hypertension, hypotension, angina, atrial fibrillation, syncope (rare). *Hypersensitivity:* Rarely, hypersensitivity reactions; *severe anaphylaxis,* shortness of breath, hypotension, urticaria. *Miscellaneous:* Fever, leukopenia, decreased appetite, anemia, alopecia, thrombocytopenia.

Drug Interactions: Because granisetron is metabolized by hepatic cytochrome P-450 drug-metabolizing enzymes, agents that induce or inhibit these enzymes may alter the clearance (and thus the half-life) of granisetron.

EMS CONSIDERATIONS
None.

Griseofulvin microsize
Griseofulvin ultramicrosize
(griz-ee-oh-FULL-vin)

Pregnancy Class: C
Griseofulvin microsize (Fulvicin-U/F, Grifulvin V, Grisactin 250, Grisactin 500 **(Rx)**) Griseofulvin ultramicrosize (Fulvicin-P/G, Grisactin Ultra, Gris-PEG **(Rx)**)
Classification: Antibiotic, antifungal

Mechanism of Action: Derived from a species of *Penicillium.* Believed to interfere with cell division (metaphase) or DNA replication. When taken systemically, the drug is deposited in the newly formed skin and nails, which are then resistant to reinfection by the tinea.

Uses: Tinea (ringworm) infections of skin (including athlete's foot), scalp, groin, and nails. Effective against tinea corporis, tinea pedis, tinea barbae, tinea unguium, tinea cruris, tinea capitis due to *Trichophyton* species, *Microsporum audouinii, M. canis, M. gypseum,* and *Epidermophyton floccosum.* It is the only PO drug effective against dermatophytid (tinea ringworm) infections. Not effective against *Candida.* Establish susceptibility of the infectious agent before treatment is begun.

Contraindications: Pregnancy. Porphyria or history thereof, hepatocellular failure, and hypersensitivity to drug. Exposure to artificial light or sunlight. Use for infections due to bacteria, candidiasis, actinomycosis, sporotrichosis, tinea versicolor, histoplasmosis, chromoblastomycosis,

G

─────────────────────────────
bold italic = life threatening side effect

coccidioidomycosis, cryptococcosis, and North American blastomycosis.
Precautions: Cross sensitivity with penicillin is possible.

Route/Dosage
• **Capsules, Oral Suspension, Tablets**
Tinea corporis, cruris, or capitis.
Adults: 0.5 g griseofulvin microsize daily in a single dose or divided dose (or 330–375 mg ultramicrosize).
Tinea pedis or unguium.
Adults: 0.75–1 g/day of griseofulvin microsize (or 660–750 mg ultramicrosize). After response, decrease dose of microsize to 0.5 g/day. **Pediatric, 13.6–22.7 kg:** 125–250 mg griseofulvin microsize daily (or 82.5–165 mg ultramicrosize); **pediatric, over 22.7 kg:** 250–500 mg microsize daily (or 165–330 mg ultramicrosize). *NOTE:* Dose has not been determined in children less than 2 years of age.
How Supplied: Griseofulvin microsize: *Capsule:* 250 mg; *Suspension:* 125 mg/5 mL; *Tablet:* 250 mg, 500 mg. Griseofulvin ultramicrosize: *Tablet:* 125 mg; 165 mg; 250 mg; 330 mg
Side Effects: *Hypersensitivity:* Rashes, urticaria, *angioneurotic edema,* allergic reactions. *GI:* N&V, diarrhea, epigastric pain, *GI bleeding. CNS:* Dizziness, headache, confusion, mental fatigue, insomnia. *Miscellaneous:* Oral thrush, acute intermittent porphyria, paresthesias of extremities after long-term therapy, proteinuria, leukopenia, photosensitivity, worsening of lupus erythematosus, menstrual irregularities, hepatic toxicity, granulocytopenia.
Drug Interactions
Alcohol, ethyl / Tachycardia and flushing
Anticoagulants, oral / ↓ Effect of anticoagulants due to ↑ breakdown in liver
Barbiturates / ↓ Effect of griseofulvin due to ↓ absorption from GI tract

Cyclosporine / ↓ Plasma levels of cyclosporine → ↓ pharmacologic effect
Oral contraceptives / ↓ Effect of contraceptives → breakthrough bleeding, pregnancy, or amenorrhea
Salicylates / ↓ Serum salicylate levels

EMS CONSIDERATIONS
See also *Anti-Infectives.*

Guaifensesin (Glyceryl guaiacolate)
(gwye-FEN-eh-sin)
Pregnancy Class: C
Allfen, Anti-Tuss, Breonesin, Fenesin, Gee-Gee, Genatuss, GG-Cen, Glyate, Glycotuss, Glytuss, Halotussin, Humibid L.A., Humibid Sprinkle, Hytuss, Hytuss-2X, Mytussin, Naldecon Senior EX, Robitussin, Scot-tussin, Sinumist-SR Capsulets, Touro EX, Unitussin **(OTC)**
Classification: Expectorant

Mechanism of Action: May increase the output of fluid of the respiratory tract by reducing the viscosity and surface tension of respiratory secretions, thereby facilitating their expectoration. Data on efficacy are lacking.
Uses: Dry, nonproductive cough due to colds and minor upper respiratory tract infections when there is mucus in the respiratory tract.
Contraindications: Chronic cough (e.g., due to smoking, asthma, or emphysema), cough accompanied by excess secretions. Use in children under age 12 for persistent or chronic cough due to asthma or cough accompanied by excessive mucus (unless prescribed by a provider).
Precautions: Persistent cough may indicate a serious infection; thus, the provider should be consulted if cough lasts for more than 1 week, is recurring, or is accompanied by high fever, rash, or persistent headache.

Route/Dosage
• **Capsules, Tablets, Oral Liquid, Syrup**
Expectorant.

Adults and children over 12 years: 100–400 mg q 4 hr, not to exceed 2.4 g/day; **pediatric, 6–12 years:** 100–200 mg q 4 hr, not to exceed 1.2 g/day; **pediatric, 2–6 years:** 50–100 mg q 4 hr, not to exceed 600 mg/day. If less than 2 years of age, individualize the dosage.

• **Sustained-Release Capsules, Sustained-Release Tablets**
Expectorant.
Adults and children over 12 years: 600–1,200 mg q 12 hr, not to exceed 2.4 g/day; **pediatric, 6–12 years:** 600 mg q 12 hr, not to exceed 1.2 g/day; **pediatric, 2–6 years:** 300 mg q 12 hr, not to exceed 600 mg/day. *NOTE:* The liquid dosage forms may be more suitable for children less than 6 years of age.
How Supplied: *Capsule:* 200 mg; *Capsule, Extended Release:* 300 mg; *Liquid:* 100 mg/5 mL, 200 mg/5 mL; *Syrup:* 50 mg/5 mL, 100 mg/5 mL; *Tablet:* 100 mg, 200 mg; *Tablet, Extended Release:* 575 mg, 600 mg, 800 mg, 1000 mg, 1200 mg

Side Effects: *GI:* N&V, GI upset. *CNS:* Dizziness, headache. *Dermatologic:* Rash, urticaria.

OD Overdose Management: *Symptoms:* N&V. *Treatment:* Treat symptomatically.

Drug Interactions: Inhibition of platelet adhesiveness by guaifenesin may result in bleeding tendencies.

EMS CONSIDERATIONS

None.

Guanabenz acetate
(GWON-ah-benz)
Pregnancy Class: C
Wytensin **(Rx)**
Classification: Antihypertensive, centrally acting antiadrenergic

Mechanism of Action: Stimulates alpha-2-adrenergic receptors in the CNS, resulting in a decrease in sympathetic impulses and in sympathetic tone. It also decreases the pulse rate, but postural hypotension has not been manifested.

Onset of Action: 60 min; **Peak effect:** 2-4 hr.
Duration of Action: 8-12 hr.
Uses: Hypertension, alone or as adjunct with thiazide diuretics.
Contraindications: Lactation, children under 12 years of age.
Precautions: Use with caution in severe coronary insufficiency, cerebrovascular disease, recent MI, hepatic or renal disease. Geriatric patients may be more sensitive to the hypotensive and sedative effects; dose reduction may be necessary due to age-related decreases in renal function. Sudden cessation may result in an increase in catecholamines and, rarely, "overshoot" hypertension.

Route/Dosage
• **Tablets**
Hypertension.
Adults, initial: 4 mg b.i.d. alone or with a thiazide diuretic; **then,** increase by 4–8 mg/day q 1–2 weeks until control achieved. Maximum recommended dose: 32 mg b.i.d.
How Supplied: *Tablet:* 4 mg, 8 mg
Side Effects: *CNS:* Drowsiness and sedation (common), dizziness, weakness, headache, ataxia, depression, disturbances in sleep, excitement. *GI:* Dry mouth (common), N&V, diarrhea, constipation, abdominal discomfort, epigastric pain. *CV:* Palpitations, chest pain, arrhythmias, AV dysfunction or block. *Dermatologic:* Rash, pruritus. *Miscellaneous:* Edema, blurred vision, muscle aches, dyspnea, nasal congestion, urinary frequency, gynecomastia, disturbances of sexual function, taste disorders, aches in extremities.

OD Overdose Management: *Symptoms:* Hypotension, sleepiness, irritability, miosis, lethargy, bradycardia. *Treatment:* Supportive treatment. VS and fluid balance should be monitored. Syrup of ipecac or gastric lavage followed by activated charcoal; administration of fluids, pressor agents, and atropine. Maintain an adequate airway; artificial respiration may be required.

G

---

bold italic = life threatening side effect

Drug Interactions: Use with CNS depressants may result in additive sedation.

EMS CONSIDERATIONS
See also *Antihypertensive Agents*.

Guanadrel sulfate
(GWON-ah-drell)
Pregnancy Class: B
Hylorel **(Rx)**
Classification: Antihypertensive, peripherally acting antiadrenergic

Mechanism of Action: Similar to that of guanethidine. Inhibits vasoconstriction by blocking efferent, peripheral sympathetic pathways by depleting norepinephrine reserves and inhibiting norepinephrine release. Causes increased sensitivity to norepinephrine.
Onset of Action: 2 hr.
Duration of Action: 4-14 hr.
Uses: Hypertension in those not responding to a thiazide diuretic.
Contraindications: Pheochromocytoma, CHF, within 1 week of MAO drug use, within 2–3 days of elective surgery, lactation.
Precautions: Use with caution in bronchial asthma and peptic ulcer. Safety and efficacy not established in children. Geriatric patients may be more sensitive to the hypotensive effects.

Route/Dosage ⸺
• **Tablets**
  Hypertension.
Individualized. Initial: 5 mg b.i.d.; **then,** increase dosage to maintenance level of 20–75 mg/day in two to four divided doses. With a C_{CR} of 30–60 mL/min, use an initial dose of 5 mg q 24 hr. If the C_{CR} is less than 30 mL/min, increase the dosing interval to q 48 hr. Make dose changes carefully q 7 or more days for moderate renal insufficiency and q 14 or more days for severe insufficiency.
How Supplied: *Tablet:* 10 mg
Side Effects: *CNS:* Fainting, fatigue, headache, drowsiness, paresthesias, confusion, psychological problems, depression, syncope, sleep disor-

ders, visual disturbances. *CV:* Chest pain, orthostatic hypotension, palpitations, peripheral edema. *Respiratory:* Exertional or resting SOB, coughing. *GI:* Increase in number of bowel movements, constipation, anorexia, indigestion, flatus, glossitis, N&V, dry mouth and throat, abdominal distress or pain. *GU:* Difficulty in ejaculation, impotence, nocturia, hematuria, urinary urgency or frequency. *Miscellaneous:* Leg cramps during both the day and night, excessive weight gain or loss, backache, neckache, joint pain or inflammation, aching limbs.
OD **Overdose Management:** *Symptoms:* Postural hypotension, syncope, dizziness, blurred vision. *Treatment:* Administration of a vasoconstrictor (e.g., phenylephrine) if hypotension persists. If used, monitor carefully as patient may be hypersensitive.
Drug Interactions
Beta-adrenergic blocking agents / Excessive hypotension, bradycardia
Phenothiazines / Reverses effect of guanadrel
Phenylpropanolamine / ↓ Effect of guanadrel
Reserpine / Excessive hypotension, bradycardia
Sympathomimetics / Hypotensive effect of guanadrel may be reversed; also, guanadrel may ↑ the effects of directly acting sympathomimetics
Tricyclic antidepressants / Reverses effect of guanadrel
Vasodilators / ↑ Risk of orthostatic hypotension

EMS CONSIDERATIONS
See also *Antihypertensive Agents*.

Guanethidine monosulfate
(gwon-ETH-ih-deen)
Pregnancy Class: C
Ismelin Sulfate **(Rx)**
Classification: Antihypertensive, peripherally acting antiadrenergic

Mechanism of Action: Produces selective adrenergic blockade of efferent, peripheral sympathetic pathways by depleting norepinephrine reserve and inhibiting norepinephrine release. Induces a gradual, prolonged drop in both SBP and DBP, usually associated with bradycardia, decreased pulse pressure, a decrease in peripheral resistance, and small changes in CO. Is not a ganglionic blocking agent and does not produce central or parasympathetic blockade. With depleted catecholamines, guanethidine can directly depress the myocardium and can cause an increase in the sensitivity of tissues to catecholamines.

Onset of Action: Peak effect: 6-8 hr; **Maximum effect:** 1-3 weeks.

Duration of Action: 24-48 hr; 7-10 days after discontinuation.

Uses: Moderate to severe hypertension—used alone or in combination. *NOTE:* The use of a thiazide diuretic may increase the effectiveness of guanethidine and reduce the incidence of edema. Also used for renal hypertension, including that secondary to pyelonephritis, renal artery stenosis, and renal amyloidosis.

Contraindications: Mild, labile hypertension; pheochromocytoma, CHF not due to hypertension, use of MAO inhibitors, lactation.

Precautions: Administer with caution and at a reduced rate to patients with impaired renal function, coronary disease, CV disease especially when associated with encephalopathy, or severe cardiac failure or to those who have suffered a recent MI. Use with caution in hypertensive patients with renal disease and nitrogen retention or increasing BUN levels. Fever decreases dosage requirements. During prolonged therapy, cardiac, renal, and blood tests should be performed. Used with caution in peptic ulcer. Geriatric patients may be more sensitive to the hypotensive effects of guanethidine; also, it may be necessary to decrease the dose in these patients due to age-related decreases in renal function. Safety and efficacy have not been determined in children.

Route/Dosage
• **Tablets**
Ambulatory patients.
Initial: 10–12.5 mg/day; increase in 10–12.5-mg increments q 5–7 days; **maintenance:** 25–50 mg/day.
Hospitalized patients.
Initial: 25–50 mg; increase by 25 or 50 mg/day or every other day; **maintenance:** approximately one-seventh of loading dose. **Pediatric, initial:** 0.2 mg/kg/day (6 mg/m²) given in one dose; **then,** dose may be increased by 0.2 mg/kg/day q 7–10 days to maximum of 3 mg/kg/day.

How Supplied: *Tablet:* 10 mg, 25 mg

Side Effects: *CNS:* Dizziness, weakness, lassitude. Rarely, fatigue, psychic depression. *CV:* Syncope due to exertional or postural hypotension, bradycardia, fluid retention and edema with possible CHF. Less commonly, angina. *Respiratory:* Dyspnea, nasal congestion, asthma in susceptible individuals. *GI:* Persistent diarrhea (may be severe enough to cause discontinuation of use), increased frequency of bowel movements. N&V, dry mouth, and parotid tenderness are less common. *GU:* Inhibition of ejaculation, nocturia, urinary incontinence, priapism, impotence. *Hematologic:* Anemia, thrombocytopenia, leukopenia (rare). *Miscellaneous:* Dermatitis, scalp hair loss, blurred vision, myalgia, muscle tremors, chest paresthesia, weight gain, ptosis of the lids.

OD **Overdose Management:** *Symptoms:* Bradycardia, postural hypotension, diarrhea (may be severe). *Treatment:* If the patient was previously normotensive, keep in a supine position (symptoms usually subside within 72 hr). If the patient was previously hypertensive (especially with impaired cardiac reserve or other CV problems or renal disease), intensive treatment may be needed. Vasopressors may be required. Treat severe diarrhea.

Drug Interactions
Alcohol, ethyl / Additive orthostatic hypotension

---

bold italic = life threatening side effect

Amphetamines / ↓ Effect of guanethidine by ↓ uptake of the drug to its site of action

Anesthetics, general / Additive hypotension

Antidepressants, tricyclic / ↓ Effect of guanethidine by ↓ uptake of the drug to its site of action

Antidiabetic drugs / Additive effect ↓ in blood glucose

Cocaine / ↓ Effect of guanethidine by ↓ uptake of the drug at its site of action

Digitalis / Additive slowing of HR

Ephedrine / ↓ Effect of guanethidine by ↓ uptake of the drug at its site of action

Epinephrine / Guanethidine ↑ effect of epinephrine

Haloperidol / ↓ Effect of guanethidine by ↓ uptake of the drug at its site of action

Levarterenol / See *Norepinephrine*

MAO inhibitors / Reverse effect of guanethidine

Metaraminol / Guanethidine ↑ effect of metaraminol

Methotrimeprazine / Additive hypotensive effect

Methoxamine / Guanethidine ↑ effect of methoxamine

Methylphenidate / ↓ Effect of guanethidine

Minoxidil / Profound drop in BP

Norepinephrine / ↑ Effect of norepinephrine probably due to ↑ sensitivity of norepinephrine receptor and ↓ uptake of norepinephrine by the neuron

Oral contraceptives / ↓ Effect of guanethidine by ↓ uptake of the drug to its site of action

Phenothiazines / ↓ Effect of guanethidine by ↓ uptake of the drug to its site of action

Phenylephrine / ↑ Response to phenylephrine in guanethidine-treated patients

Phenylpropanolamine / ↓ Effect of guanethidine by ↓ uptake of the drug to its site of action

Procainamide / Additive hypotensive effect

Procarbazine / Additive hypotensive effect

Propranolol / Additive hypotensive effect

Pseudoephedrine / ↓ Effect of guanethidine by ↓ uptake of the drug at its site of action

Quinidine / Additive hypotensive effect

Reserpine / Excessive bradycardia, postural hypotension, and mental depression

Sympathomimetics / ↓ Effect of guanethidine; also, guanethidine potentiates the effects of directly acting sympathomimetics

Thiazide diuretics / Additive hypotensive effect

Thioxanthenes / ↓ Effect of guanethidine by ↓ uptake of the drug at its site of action

Tricyclic antidepressants / Inhibition of the effects of guanethidine

Vasodilator drugs, peripheral / Additive hypotensive effect

Vasopressor drugs / ↑ Effect of vasopressor agents probably due to ↑ sensitivity of norepinephrine receptor and ↓ uptake of vasopressor agent by the neuron

EMS CONSIDERATIONS

See also *Antihypertensive Agents*.

Guanfacine hydrochloride
(GWON-fah-seen)

Pregnancy Class: B
Tenex **(Rx)**
Classification: Antihypertensive, centrally acting

Mechanism of Action: Thought to act by central stimulation of alpha-2 receptors. Causes a decrease in peripheral sympathetic output and HR resulting in a decrease in BP. May also manifest a direct peripheral alpha-2 receptor stimulant action. **Onset of Action:** 2 hr; **Peak effect:** 6-12 hr.

Duration of Action: 24 hr.

Uses: Hypertension alone or with a thiazide diuretic. *Investigational:* Withdrawal from heroin use, to reduce the frequency of migraine headaches.

Contraindications: Hypersensitivity to guanfacine. Acute hypertension associated with toxemia. Children less than 12 years of age.

Precautions: Use with caution during lactation and in patients with recent MI, cerebrovascular disease, chronic renal or hepatic failure, or severe coronary insufficiency. Geriatric patients may be more sensitive to the hypotensive and sedative effects. Safety and efficacy in children less than 12 years of age have not been determined.

Route/Dosage
• **Tablets**
Hypertension.
Initial: 1 mg/day alone or with other antihypertensives; if satisfactory results are not obtained in 3–4 weeks, dosage may be increased by 1 mg at 1–2-week intervals up to a maximum of 3 mg/day in one to two divided doses.
Heroin withdrawal.
0.03–1.5 mg/day.
Reduce frequency of migraine headaches.
1 mg/day for 12 weeks.
How Supplied: *Tablet:* 1 mg, 2 mg
Side Effects: *GI:* Dry mouth, constipation, nausea, abdominal pain, diarrhea, dyspepsia, dysphagia, taste perversion or alterations in taste. *CNS:* Sedation, weakness, dizziness, headache, fatigue, insomnia, amnesia, confusion, depression, vertigo, agitation, anxiety, malaise, nervousness, tremor. *CV:* Bradycardia, substernal pain, palpitations, syncope, chest pain, tachycarida, cardiac fibrillation, CHF, heart block, MI (rare), cardiovascular accident (rare). *Ophthalmic:* Visual disturbances, conjunctivitis, iritis, blurred vision. *Dermatologic:* Pruritus, dermatitis, purpura, sweating, skin rash with exfoliation, alopecia, rash. *GU:* Decreased libido, impotence, urinary incontinence or frequency, urinary incontinence or frequency, testicular disorder, nocturia, acute renal failure. *Musculoskeletal:* Leg cramps, hypokinesia, arthralgia, leg pain, myalgia. *Other:* Rhinitis, tinnitus, dyspnea, paresthesias, paresis, asthenia, edema, abnormal LFTs.

OD **Overdose Management:** *Symptoms:* Drowsiness, bradycardia, lethargy, hypotension. *Treatment:* Gastric lavage. Supportive therapy, as needed. The drug is not dialyzable.
Drug Interactions: Additive sedative effects when used concomitantly with CNS depressants.

EMS CONSIDERATIONS

See also *Antihypertensive Agents.*

H

Haloperidol
(hah-low-PAIR-ih-dohl)
Pregnancy Class: C
Haldol **(Rx)**
Classification: Antipsychotic, butyrophenone

Mechanism of Action: Precise mechanism not known. Competitively blocks dopamine receptors in the tuberoinfundibular system to cause sedation. Also causes alpha-adrenergic blockade, decreases release of growth hormone, and increases prolactin release by the pituitary. Causes significant extrapyramidal effects, as well as a low incidence of sedation, anticholinergic effects, and orthostatic hypotension. Narrow margin between the therapeutically effective dose and that causing extrapyramidal symptoms. Also has antiemetic effects.

Uses: Psychotic disorders including manic states, drug-induced psychoses, and schizophrenia. Severe behavior problems in children (those with combative, explosive hyperexcitability not accounted for by immediate provocation). Short-term treat-

bold italic = life threatening side effect

ment of hyperactive children who show excessive motor activity with accompanying conduct consisting of impulsivity, poor attention, aggression, mood lability, or poor frustration tolerance. Control of tics and vocal utterances associated with Gilles de la Tourette's syndrome in adults and children. The decanoate is used for prolonged therapy in chronic schizophrenia.

Investigational: Antiemetic for cancer chemotherapy, phencyclidine (PCP) psychosis, intractable hiccoughs, infantile autism. IV for acute psychiatric conditions.

Contraindications: Use with extreme caution, or not at all, in patients with parkinsonism. Lactation.

Precautions: PO dosage has not been determined in children less than 3 years of age; IM dosage is not recommended in children. Geriatric patients are more likely to exhibit orthostatic hypotension, anticholinergic effects, sedation, and extrapyramidal side effects (such as parkinsonism and tardive dyskinesia).

Route/Dosage

• **Oral Solution, Tablets**
Psychoses.
Adults: 0.5–2 mg b.i.d.–t.i.d. up to 3–5 mg b.i.d.–t.i.d. for severe symptoms; **maintenance:** reduce dosage to lowest effective level. Up to 100 mg/day may be required in some. **Geriatric or debilitated patients:** 0.5–2 mg b.i.d.–t.i.d. **Pediatric, 3–12 years or 15–40 kg:** 0.5 mg/day in two to three divided doses; if necessary the daily dose may be increased by 0.5-mg increments q 5–7 days for a total of 0.15 mg/kg/day for psychotic disorders.
Tourette's syndrome.
Adults, initial: 0.5–1.5 mg t.i.d., up to 10 mg daily. Adjust dose carefully to obtain the optimum response. **Children, 3 to 12 years:** 0.05–0.075 mg/kg/day. Higher doses may be needed for those severely disturbed.
Behavioral disorders/hyperactivity in children.
Children, 3 to 12 years: 0.05–0.075 mg/kg/day. Higher doses may be needed for those severely disturbed.

Intractable hiccoughs (investigational).
1.5 mg t.i.d.
Infantile autism (investigational).
0.5–4 mg/day.
• **IM, Lactate**
Acute psychoses.
Adults and adolescents, initial: 2–5 mg to control acute agitation; may be repeated if necessary q 4–8 hr to a total of 100 mg/day. Switch to **PO** therapy as soon as possible.
• **IM, Decanoate**
Chronic therapy.
Adults, initial dose: 10–15 times the daily PO dose, not to exceed 100 mg initially, regardless of the previous oral antipsychotic dose; **then,** repeat q 4 weeks (decanoate is not to be given IV).

How Supplied: Haloperidol: *Tablet:* 0.5 mg, 1 mg, 2 mg, 5 mg, 10 mg, 20 mg. Haloperidol decanoate: *Injection:* 50 mg/mL, 100 mg/mL. Haloperidol lactate: *Concentrate:* 2 mg/mL; *Injection:* 5 mg/mL; *Solution:* 1 mg/mL

Side Effects: Extrapyramidal symptoms, especially akathisia and dystonias, occur more frequently than with the phenothiazines. Overdosage is characterized by severe extrapyramidal reactions, hypotension, or sedation. The drug does not elicit photosensitivity reactions like those of the phenothiazines.

OD Overdose Management: *Symptoms:* CNS depression, hypertension or hypotension, extrapyramidal symptoms, agitation, restlessness, fever, hypothermia, hyperthermia, *seizures, cardiac arrhythmias,* changes in the ECG, autonomic reactions, *coma. Treatment:* Treat symptomatically. Antiparkinson drugs, diphenhydramine, or barbiturates can be used to treat extrapyramidal symptoms. Fluid replacement and vasoconstrictors (either norepinephrine or phenylephrine) can be used to treat hypotension. Ventricular arrhythmias can be treated with phenytoin. To treat seizures, use pentobarbital or diazepam. A saline cathartic can be used to hasten the excretion of sustained-release products.

Drug Interactions

Amphetamine / ↓ Effect of amphetamine by ↓ uptake of drug at its site of action

Anticholinergics / ↓ Effect of haloperidol

Antidepressants, tricyclic / ↑ Effect of antidepressants due to ↓ breakdown by liver

Barbiturates / ↓ Effect of haloperidol due to ↑ breakdown by liver

Guanethidine / ↓ Effect of guanethidine by ↓ uptake of drug at site of action

Lithium / ↑ Toxicity of haloperidol

Methyldopa / ↑ Toxicity of haloperidol

Phenytoin / ↓ Effect of haloperidol due to ↑ breakdown by liver

EMS CONSIDERATIONS
Administration/Storage
1. Give the decanoate by deep IM injection using a 21-gauge needle. Do not exceed a volume of 3 mL/site.
2. Do not give decanoate IV.

Heparin calcium
Heparin sodium and sodium chloride
Heparin sodium lock flush solution
(HEP-ah-rin)

Pregnancy Class: C

Heparin sodium and sodium chloride (Heparin Sodium and 0.45% Sodium Chloride, Heparin Sodium and 0.9% Sodium Chloride **(Rx)**) Heparin sodium lock flush solution (Heparin lock flush, Hep-Lock, HepLock U/P **(Rx)**)

Classification: Anticoagulant

Mechanism of Action: Heparin potentiates the inhibitory action of antithrombin III on various coagulation factors including factors IIa, IXa, Xa, XIa, and XIIa. This occurs due to the formation of a complex with and causing a conformational change in the antithrombin III molecule. Inhibition of factor Xa results in interference with thrombin generation; thus, the action of thrombin in coagulation is inhibited. Heparin also increases the rate of formation of antithrombin III–thrombin complex causing inactivation of thrombin and preventing the conversion of fibrinogen to fibrin. By inhibiting the activation of fibrin-stabilizing factor by thrombin, heparin also prevents formation of a stable fibrin clot. Therapeutic doses of heparin prolong thrombin time, whole blood clotting time, activated clotting time, and PTT. Heparin also decreases the levels of triglycerides by releasing lipoprotein lipase from tissues; the resultant hydrolysis of triglycerides causes increased blood levels of free fatty acids.

Onset of Action: IV: Immediate; **Deep SC:** 20-60 min.

Uses: Pulmonary embolism, peripheral arterial embolism, prophylaxis, and treatment of venous thrombosis and its extension. Atrial fibrillation with embolization. Diagnosis and treatment of disseminated intravascular coagulation. Low doses to prevent deep venous thrombosis and pulmonary embolism in pregnant patients with a history of thromboembolism, urology patients over 40 years of age, patients with stroke or heart failure, AMI or pulmonary infection, high-risk surgery patients, moderate and high-risk gynecologic patients with no malignancy, neurology patients with extracranial problems, and patients with severe musculoskeletal trauma. Prophylaxis of clotting in blood transfusions, extracorporeal circulation, dialysis procedures, blood samples for lab tests, and arterial and heart surgery. *Investigational:* Prophylaxis of post-MI, CVAs, and LV thrombi. By continuous infusion to treat myocardial ischemia in unstable angina refractory to usual treatment. Adjunct to treat coronary occlusion with AMI. Prophylaxis of cerebral thrombosis in evolving stroke.

Heparin lock flush solution: Dilute solutions are used to maintain pa-

---

tency of indwelling catheters used for IV therapy or blood sampling. Not to be used therapeutically.

Contraindications: Active bleeding, blood dyscrasias (or other disorders characterized by bleeding tendencies such as hemophilia), purpura, thrombocytopenia, liver disease with hypoprothrombinemia, suspected intracranial hemorrhage, suppurative thrombophlebitis, inaccessible ulcerative lesions (especially of the GI tract), open wounds, extensive denudation of the skin, and increased capillary permeability (as in ascorbic acid deficiency). IM use.

Do not administer during surgery of the eye, brain, or spinal cord or during continuous tube drainage of the stomach or small intestine. Use is also contraindicated in subacute endocarditis, shock, advanced kidney disease, threatened abortion, severe hypertension, or hypersensitivity to drug. Premature neonates due to the possibility of a fatal "gasping syndrome."

Precautions: NaCl, 0.9%, is effective in maintaining patency of peripheral (noncentral) intermittent infusion devices and in reducing added medical costs. The following procedure has been recommended:
• Determine patency by aspirating lock.
• Flush with 2 mL NSS.
• Administer medication therapy. (Flush between drugs.)
• Flush with 2 mL NSS.
• Frequency of flushing to maintain patency when not actively in use varies from every 8 hr to every 24–48 hr.
• This does *NOT* apply to any central venous access devices.

Route/Dosage ─────────────
NOTE: Adjusted for each patient on the basis of laboratory tests.
• **Deep SC**
General heparin dosage.
Initial loading dose: 10,000–20,000 units; **maintenance:** 8,000–10,000 units q 8 hr or 15,000–20,000 units q 12 hr. *Use concentrated solution.*

Prophylaxis of postoperative thromboembolism.
5,000 units of concentrated solution 2 hr before surgery and 5,000 units q 8–12 hr thereafter for 7 days or until patient is ambulatory.
• **Intermittent IV**
General heparin dosage.
Initial loading dose: 10,000 units undiluted or in 50–100 mL saline; **then,** 5,000–10,000 units q 4–6 hr undiluted or in 50–100 mL saline.
• **Continuous IV Infusion**
General heparin dosage.
Initial loading dose: 20,000–40,000 units/day in 1,000 mL saline (preceded initially by 5,000 units IV).
• **Special Uses**
Surgery of heart and blood vessels.
Initial, 150–400 units/kg to patients undergoing total body perfusion for open heart surgery. *NOTE:* 300 units/kg may be used for procedures less than 60 min while 400 units/kg is used for procedures lasting more than 60 min. To prevent clotting in the tube system, add heparin to fluids in pump oxygenator.
Extracorporeal renal dialysis.
See instructions on equipment.
Blood transfusion.
400–600 units/100 mL whole blood. 7,500 units should be added to 100 mL 0.9% sodium chloride injection; from this dilution, add 6–8 mL/100 mL whole blood.
Laboratory samples.
70–150 units/10- to 20-mL sample to prevent coagulation.
Heparin lock sets.
To prevent clot formation in a heparin lock set, inject 10–100 units/mL heparin solution through the injection hub in a sufficient quantity to fill the entire set to the needle tip.
How Supplied: Heparin sodium injection: *Injection:* 1,000 U/mL, 2,000 U/mL, 2,500 U/mL, 5,000 U/mL, 7,500 U/mL, 10,000 U/mL, 20,000 U/mL. Heparin sodium and sodium chloride: *Injection:* 200 U/100 mL-0.9%, 5,000 U/100 mL-0.45%, 10,000 U/100 mL-0.45%; *Pack:* 10U/mL-0.9%, 100 U/mL-0.9%. Heparin sodium lock flush solution: *Kit:* 10 U/mL, 100 U/mL

Side Effects: *CV: Hemorrhage ranging from minor local ecchymoses to major hemorrhagic complications from any organ or tissue.* Higher incidence is seen in women over 60 years of age. Hemorrhagic reactions are more likely to occur in prophylactic administration during surgery than in the treatment of thromboembolic disease. White clot syndrome. *Hematologic:* Thrombocytopenia (both early and late). *Hypersensitivity:* Chills, fever, urticaria are the most common. Rarely, asthma, lacrimation, headache, N&V, rhinitis, ***shock, anaphylaxis.*** Allergic vasospastic reaction within 6–10 days after initiation of therapy (lasts 4–6 hr) including painful, ischemic, cyanotic limbs. Use a test dose of 1,000 units in patients with a history of asthma or allergic disease. *Miscellaneous:* Hyperkalemia, cutaneous necrosis, osteoporosis (after long-term high doses), delayed transient alopecia, priapism, suppressed aldosterone synthesis. Discontinuance of heparin has resulted in rebound hyperlipemia. *Following IM (usual), SC:* Local irritation, erythema, mild pain, ulceration, hematoma, and tissue sloughing.

OD **Overdose Management:** *Symptoms:* Nosebleeds, hematuria, tarry stools, petechiae, and easy bruising may be the first signs. *Treatment:* Drug withdrawal is usually sufficient to correct heparin overdosage. Protamine sulfate (1%) solution; each mg of protamine neutralizes about 100 USP heparin units.

Drug Interactions
Alteplase, recombinant / ↑ Risk of bleeding, especially at arterial puncture sites
Anticoagulants, oral / Additive ↑ PT
Antihistamines / ↓ Effect of heparin
Aspirin / Additive ↑ PT
Cephalosporins / ↑ Risk of bleeding due to additive effect
Dextran / Additive ↑ PT
Digitalis / ↓ Effect of heparin
Dipyridamole / Additive ↑ PT

Hydroxychloroquine / Additive ↑ PT
Ibuprofen / Additive ↑ PT
Indomethacin / Additive ↑ PT
Insulin / Heparin antagonizes effect of insulin
Nicotine / ↓ Effect of heparin
Nitroglycerin / ↓ Effect of heparin
NSAIDs / Additive ↑ PT
Penicillins / ↑ Risk of bleeding due to possible additive effects
Salicylates / ↑ Risk of bleeding
Streptokinase / Relative resistance to effects of heparin
Tetracyclines / ↓ Effect of heparin
Ticlopidine / Additive ↑ PT

EMS CONSIDERATIONS
See also *Anticoagulants.*
Administration/Storage
1. Do *not* administer IM.
2. Administer by deep SC injection to minimize local irritation, hematoma, and tissue sloughing and to prolong action of drug.
  Do not administer within 2 in. of the umbilicus; due to increased vascularity of area.
3. Do not massage site.
4. Rotate sites of administration.

Histrelin acetate
(hiss-TREL-in)
Pregnancy Class: X
Supprelin, Synarel **(Rx)**
Classification: Gonadotropin-releasing hormone

Mechanism of Action: Histrelin contains a synthetic nonapeptide agonist of the naturally occurring GnRH. Initially the drug stimulates release of GnRH; however, chronic use desensitizes responsiveness of the pituitary gonadotropin, causing a reduction in ovarian and testicular steroidogenesis. Decreases in LH, FSH, and sex steroid levels are observed within 3 months of initiation of therapy.
Uses: To control the biochemical and clinical symptoms of central precocious puberty (either idiopathic or neurogenic) occurring before 8

years of age in girls or 9.5 years of age in boys.

Contraindications: Hypersensitivity to the product or any of its components. Lactation.

Precautions: Acute, serious hypersensitivity reactions may occur that require emergency medical treatment. Safety and efficacy in children less than 2 years of age have not been determined.

Route/Dosage
- **SC**

  Central precocious puberty.

10 mcg/kg given as a single, daily SC injection. Doses greater than 10 mcg/kg/day have not been evaluated.

How Supplied: *Kit:* 0.5 mg/mL, 1 mg/mL

Side Effects: *Acute hypersensitivity reaction:* Angioedema, urticaria, *CV collapse,* hypotension, tachycardia, loss of consciousness, *bronchospasm,* dyspnea, flushing, pruritus. *CV:* Vasodilation (common), edema, palpitations, tachycardia, epistaxis, hypertension, migraine headache, pallor. *GI:* GI or abdominal pain, N&V, diarrhea, flatulence, decrease appetite, dyspepsia, GI cramps or distress, constipation, decreased appetite, thirst, gastritis. *CNS:* Headache (common), nervousness, dizziness, depression, changes in libido, mood changes, insomnia, anxiety, paresthesia, syncope, somnolence, cognitive changes, lethargy, impaired consciousness, tremor, hyperkinesia, convulsions (increased frequency), hot flashes or flushes, conduct disorder. *Endocrine:* Vaginal dryness, leukorrhea, metrorrhagia, breast pain, breast edema, decreased breast size, breast discharge, tenderness of female genitalia, anemia, goiter, hyperlipidemia, glycosuria. *Musculoskeletal:* Arthralgia, joint stiffness, muscle cramp or stiffness, myalgia, hypotonia, pain. *Respiratory:* Cough, URI, pharyngitis, respiratory congestion, asthma, breathing disorder, rhinorrhea, bronchitis, sinusitis, hyperventilation. *Dermatologic:* Commonly, redness, itching, and swelling at the injection site. Also, urticaria, sweating, keratoderma, pruritus, pain, dyschromia, alopecia, erythema. *Ophthalmologic:* Visual disturbances, abnormal pupillary function, polyopia, photophobia. *Otic:* Otalgia, hearing loss. *GU:* Vaginal bleeding (most often one episode within 1–3 weeks after starting therapy and lasting several days). Also, vaginitis, dysmenorrhea, and problems of the female genitalia including pruritus, irritation, odor, pain, infections, and hypertrophy. Dyspareunia, polyuria, dysuria, incontinence, urinary frequency, hematuria, nocturia. *Miscellaneous:* Pyrexia (common), weight gain, fatigue, viral infection, chills, various body pains, malaise, purpura.

EMS CONSIDERATIONS

None.

Hycodan Syrup and Tablets
(HY-koh-dan)
Pregnancy Class: C
(Rx) (C-III)
Classification: Antitussive

Uses: Relief of symptoms of cough.
Precautions: May be habit-forming. Use with caution in children with croup, in geriatric or debilitated patients, impaired renal or hepatic function, hyperthyroidism, asthma, narrow-angle glaucoma, prostatic hypertrophy, urethral stricture, Addison's disease. Safety and effectiveness in children less than 6 years of age have not been determined.

Route/Dosage
- **Tablets, Syrup**
Adults and children over 12 years: 1 tablet or 5 mL q 4–6 hr as needed, not to exceed 6 tablets or 30 mL in 24 hr. Pediatric, 6–12 years: ½ tablet or 2.5 mL q 4–6 hr as needed, not to exceed 3 tablets or 15 mL in 24 hr.

How Supplied: Each tablet or 5 mL contains: *Antitussive, narcotic:* Hydrocodone bitartrate, 5 mg. *Anticholinergic:* Homatropine methylbromide, 1.5 mg.

EMS CONSIDERATIONS

See also *Narcotic Analgesics* and *Cholinergic Blocking Agents.*

Hydralazine hydrochloride

(hy-DRAL-ah-zeen)
Pregnancy Class: C
Apresoline **(Rx)**
Classification: Antihypertensive, direct action on vascular smooth muscle

Mechanism of Action: Exerts a direct vasodilating effect on vascular smooth muscle. Also alters cellular calcium metabolism that interferes with calcium movement within the vascular smooth muscle responsible for initiating or maintaining contraction. Preferentially dilates arterioles compared with veins; this minimizes postural hypotension and increases CO. Increases renin activity in the kidney, leading to an increase in angiotensin II, which then causes stimulation of aldosterone and thus sodium reabsorption. Because there is a reflex increase in cardiac function, hydralazine is commonly used with drugs that inhibit sympathetic activity (e.g., beta blockers, clonidine, methyldopa).
Onset of Action: PO: 45 min; **IM:** 10-30 min; **IV:** 10-20 min; **maximum effect:** 10-80 min.
Duration of Action: PO: 3-8 hr; **IM:** 2-4 hr; **IV:** 2-4 hr.
Uses: PO: In combination with other drugs for essential hypertension. **Parenteral:** Severe essential hypertension when PO use is not possible or when there is an urgent need to lower BP. Hydralazine is the drug of choice for eclampsia. *Investigational:* To reduce afterload in CHF, severe aortic insufficiency, and after valve replacement.
Contraindications: Coronary artery disease, angina pectoris, advanced renal disease (as in chronic renal hypertension), rheumatic heart disease (e.g., mitral valvular) and chronic glomerulonephritis.
Precautions: Use with caution in stroke patients, in those with pulmonary hypertension, during lactation, in patients with advanced renal disease, and in patients with tartrazine sensitivity. Safety and efficacy have not been established in children. Geriatric patients may be more sensitive to the hypotensive and hypothermic effects of hydralazine; also, a decrease in dose may be necessary in these patients due to age-related decreases in renal function.

Route/Dosage ———————
• **Tablets**
Hypertension.
Adult, initial: 10 mg q.i.d for 2–4 days; **then,** increase to 25 mg q.i.d. for rest of first week. For second and following weeks, increase to 50 mg q.i.d. **Maintenance:** individualized to lowest effective dose; do not exceed a maximum daily dose of 300 mg. **Pediatric, initial:** 0.75 mg/kg/day (25 mg/m²/day) in two to four divided doses; dosage may be increased gradually up to 7.5 mg/kg/day (or 300 mg/day). Food increases the bioavailability of the drug.
• **IV, IM**
Hypertensive crisis.
Adults, usual: 20–40 mg, repeated as necessary. BP may fall within 5–10 min, with maximum response in 10–80 min. Usually switch to PO medication in 1–2 days. Decrease dosage in patients with renal damage. **Pediatric:** 0.1–0.2 mg/kg q 4–6 hr as needed.
Eclampsia.
5–10 mg q 20 min as an IV bolus. If no effect after 20 mg, another drug should be tried.
How Supplied: *Injection:* 20 mg/mL; *Tablet:* 10 mg, 25 mg, 50 mg, 100 mg
Side Effects: *CV:* Orthostatic hypotension, hypotension, *MI,* angina pectoris, palpitations, paradoxical pressor reaction, tachycardia. *CNS:* Head-

---

bold italic = life threatening side effect

ache, dizziness, psychoses, tremors, depression, anxiety, disorientation. *GI:* N&V, diarrhea, anorexia, constipation, paralytic ileus. *Allergic:* Rash, urticaria, fever, chills, arthralgia, pruritus, eosinophilia. Rarely, hepatitis, obstructive jaundice. *Hematologic:* Decrease in hemoglobin and RBCs, purpura, agranulocytosis, leukopenia. *Other:* Peripheral neuritis (paresthesias, numbness, tingling), dyspnea, impotence, nasal congestion, edema, muscle cramps, lacrimation, flushing, conjunctivitis, difficulty in urination, lupus-like syndrome, lymphadenopathy, splenomegaly. Side effects are less severe when dosage is increased slowly. *NOTE:* Hydralazine may cause symptoms resembling SLE (e.g., arthralgia, dermatoses, fever, splenomegaly, glomerulonephritis). Residual effects may persist for several years and long-term treatment with steroids may be necessary.

OD **Overdose Management:** *Symptoms:* Hypotension, tachycardia, skin flushing, headache. Also, *cardiac arrhythmias, MI, and severe shock.* *Treatment:* If the CV status is stable, induce vomiting or perform gastric lavage followed by activated charcoal. Treat shock with volume expanders, without vasopressors; if a vasopressor is necessary, one should be used that is least likely to cause or aggravate tachycardia and cardiac arrhythmias. Monitor renal function.

Drug Interactions
Beta-adrenergic blocking agents / ↑ Effect of both drugs
Indomethacin / ↓ Effect of hydralazine
Methotrimeprazine / Additive hypotensive effect
Procainamide / Additive hypotensive effect
Quinidine / Additive hypotensive effect
Sympathomimetics / ↑ Risk of tachycardia and angina

EMS CONSIDERATIONS

See also *Antihypertensive Agents.*

Hydrochlorothiazide
(hy-droh-klor-oh-THIGH-ah-zyd)
Pregnancy Class: B
Esidrex, Ezide, HydroDiuril, Hydro-Par, Microzide, Oretic **(Rx)**
Classification: Diuretic, thiazide type

Onset of Action: 2 hr; **Peak effect:** 4-6 hr.
Duration of Action: 6-12 hr.
Uses: **Additional:** Microzide is available for once-daily, low-dose treatment for hypertension.
Precautions: Geriatric patients may be more sensitive to the usual adult dose.

Route/Dosage
• **Oral Solution, Tablets**
Diuretic.
Adults, initial: 25–200 mg/day for several days until dry weight is reached; **then,** 25–100 mg/day or intermittently. Some patients may require up to 200 mg/day.
Antihypertensive.
Adults, initial: 25 mg/day as a single dose. The dose may be increased to 50 mg/day in one to two doses. Doses greater than 50 mg may cause significant reductions in serum potassium. **Pediatric, under 6 months:** 3.3 mg/kg/day in two doses; **up to 2 years of age:** 12.5–37.5 mg/day in two doses; **2–12 years of age:** 37.5–100 mg/day in two doses.
How Supplied: *Capsule:* 12.5 mg; *Solution:* 50 mg/5 mL; *Tablet:* 25 mg, 50 mg, 100 mg
Side Effects: Additional: *CV:* Allergic myocarditis, hypotension. *Dermatologic:* Alopecia, exfoliative dermatitis, **toxic epidermal necrolysis,** erythema multiforme, **Stevens-Johnson syndrome.** *Miscellaneous:* **Anaphylactic reactions, respiratory distress including pneumonitis and pulmonary edema.**

EMS CONSIDERATIONS

See also *Diuretics, Thiazide.*

———*COMBINATION DRUG*———
Hydrocodone bitartrate and Acetaminophen
(high-droh-KOH-dohn, ah-seat-ah-MIN-oh-fen)

Pregnancy Class: C
Anexia 5/500, Anexia 7.5/650, Anexsia 10 mg Hydrocodone bitartrate, Anexsia 660 mg Acetaminophen, Lorcet 10/650, Lorcet Plus, Lortab 10/500 10 mg Hydrocodone bitartrate, Lortab 500 mg Acetaminophen **(Rx) (C-III)**
Classification: Analgesic

Mechanism of Action: Hydrocodone produces its analgesic activity by an action on the CNS via opiate receptors. The analgesic action of acetaminophen is produced by both peripheral and central mechanisms.
Uses: Relief of moderate to moderately severe pain.
Contraindications: Hypersensitivity to acetaminophen or hydrocodone. Lactation.
Precautions: Use with caution, if at all, in patients with head injuries as the CSF pressure may be increased further. Use with caution in geriatric or debilitated patients; in those with impaired hepatic or renal function; in hypothyroidism, Addison's disease, prostatic hypertrophy, or urethral stricture; and in patients with pulmonary disease. Use shortly before delivery may cause respiratory depression in the newborn. Safety and efficacy have not been determined in children.

Route/Dosage —————————
• **Tablets**
 Analgesia.
1 tablet of Anexia 7.5/650, Lorcet 10/650, or Lorcet Plus q 4–6 hr as needed for pain. The total 24-hr dose should not exceed 6 tablets. 1–2 tablets of Anexsia 5/500 q 4–6 hr as needed for pain. The total 24-hr dose should not exceed 8 tablets.
How Supplied: Anexia 5/500: *Narcotic analgesic:* Hydrocodone bitartrate, 5 mg, and *Nonnarcotic analgesic:* Acetaminophen, 500 mg.
 Anexia 10/650 and Lorcet 10/650: *Narcotic analgesic:* Hydrocodone bitartrate, 10 mg, and *Nonnarcotic analgesic:* Acetaminophen, 650 mg. Anexia 7.5/650 and Lorcet Plus: *Narcotic analgesic:* Hydrocodone bitar-

trate, 7.5 mg, and *Nonnarcotic analgesic:* Acetaminophen, 650 mg. Lortab 10/500: *Narcotic analgesic:* Hydrocodone bitartrate, 10 mg, and *Nonnarcotic analgesic:* Acetaminophen, 500 mg.
Side Effects: *CNS:* Lightheadedness, dizziness, sedation, drowsiness, mental clouding, lethargy, impaired mental and physical performance, anxiety, fear, dysphoria, psychologic dependence, mood changes. *GI:* N&V. *Respiratory:* Respiratory depression (dose-related), irregular and periodic breathing. *GU:* Ureteral spasm, spasm of vesical sphincters, urinary retention.
OD Overdose Management: *Symptoms: Acetaminophen overdose may result in potentially fatal hepatic necrosis.* Also, renal tubular necrosis, hypoglycemic coma, and thrombocytopenia. Symptoms of hepatotoxic overdose include N&V, diaphoresis, and malaise. Symptoms of hydrocodone overdose include respiratory depression, somnolence progressing to stupor or *coma,* skeletal muscle flaccidity, cold and clammy skin, bradycardia, and hypotension. *Severe overdose may cause apnea, circulatory collapse, cardiac arrest, and death.* Treatment (Acetaminophen):
• Empty stomach promptly by lavage or induction of emesis with syrup of ipecac.
• Serum acetaminophen levels should be determined as early as possible but no sooner than 4 hr after ingestion.
• Determine liver function initially and at 24-hr intervals.
• The antidote, *N*-acetylcysteine, should be given within 16 hr of overdose for optimal results.

Treatment (Hydrocodone):
• Reestablish adequate respiratory exchange with a patent airway and assisted or controlled ventilation.
• Respiratory depression can be reversed by giving naloxone IV.
• Oxygen, IV fluids, vasopressors, and other supportive measures may be instituted as required.

—————————————————————
bold italic = life threatening side effect

Drug Interactions

Anticholinergics / ↑ Risk of paralytic ileus

CNS depressants, including other narcotic analgesics, antianxiety agents, antipsychotics, alcohol / Additive CNS depression

MAO inhibitors / ↑ Effect of either the narcotic or the antidepressant

Tricyclic antidepressants / ↑ Effect of either the narcotic or the antidepressant

EMS CONSIDERATIONS

See also *Narcotic Analgesics* and *Acetaminophen*.

Hydrocodone bitartrate and Ibuprofen

(high-droh-KOH-dohn/eye-byou-PROH-fen)

Pregnancy Class: C

Vicoprofen **(Rx) (C-III)**

Classification: Narcotic analgesic and nonsteroidal anti-inflammatory drug

Uses: Short-term (less than 10 days) for management of acute pain.

Contraindications: Additional: Use for osteoartharitis or rheumatoid arthritis. Use during labor and delivery or during lacatation.

Precautions: Use with caution and at reduced doses in geriatric patients. Safety and efficacy have not been determined in children.

Route/Dosage ────────

• **Tablets**

Analgesic.

Adults: 1 tablet q 4–6 hr, as needed. Dosage should not exceed 5 tablets in a 24–hr period. Adjust dose and frequency of dosing to patient needs.

How Supplied: Each tablet contains *Narcotic:* Hydrocodone bitartrate, 7.5 mg and *NSAID:* Ibuprofen, 200 mg.

EMS CONSIDERATIONS

See also *Hydrocodone bitartrate* and *Ibuprofen*.

Hydrocortisone (Cortisol)
Hydorcortisone acetate
Hydrocortisone butyrate
Hydrocortisone cypionate
Hydrocortisone probutate
Hydrocortisone sodium phosphate
Hydrocortisone sodium succinate
Hydrocortisone valerate

(hy-droh-KOR-tih-zohn)

Pregnancy Class: C

Cortisol: **Parenteral:** Sterile Hydrocortisone Suspension, **Rectal:** Dermolate Anal-Itch, Proctocort, Procto-Cream.HC 2.5%, **Retention Enema:** Cortenema, **Roll-on Applicator:** Cortaid FastStick, Maximum Strength Cortaid Faststick, **Tablets:** Cortef, Hydrocortone, **Topical Cream:** AlaCort, Allercort, Alphaderm, Bactine, Cort-Dome, Cortifair, Dermacort, Dermi-Cort, Dermolate Anti-Itch, Dermtex HC, H₂Cort, Hi-Cor 1.0 and 2.5, Hydro-Tex, Hytone, Nutracort, Penecort, Synacort, **Topical Gel:** Extra Strength CortaGel, **Topical Liquid:** Scalpicin, T/Scalp, **Topical Lotion:** Acticort 100, Ala-Cort, Ala-Scalp, Allercort, Cetacort, Cort-Dome, Delacort, Dermacort, Dermolate Scalp-Itch, Gly-Cort, Hytone, LactiCare-HC, Lemoderm, Lexocort Forte, My Cort, Nutracort, Pentacort, Rederm, **Topical Ointment:** Allercort, Cortril, Hytone, Lemoderm, Penecort, **Topical Solution:** Penecort, Emo-Cort Scalp Solution, Texacort Scalp Solution, **Topical Spray:** Cortaid, Dermolate Anti-Itch, Maximum Strength Coraid, Procort, **(OTC) (Rx)** Acetate: **Dental Paste:** Orabase-HCA, **Intra-rectal Foam:** Cortifoam, **Peranteral:** Hydrocortone Acetate, **Rectal:** Cort-Dome High Potency, Cortenema, Corti-caine, Cortifoam, **Topical Cream:** CaldeCort Light, Carmol-HC, Cortaid, Cortef Feminine Itch, Corti-caine, FoilleCort, Gynecort, Gynecort Female Cream, Lanacort, Lanacort 10, Lanacort 5, Maximum Strength Cortaid, Pharma-Cort, Rhulicort, **Topical Lotion:** Cortaid, Rhulicort, **Topical Ointment:** Anusol HC-1, Cortef Acetate, Lanacort, Lanacort 5, Nov-Hydrocort, Maximum Strength Cortaid **(OTC) (Rx)** Butyrate: **Topical Cream/Ointment/Solution:** Locoid **(Rx)** Cypionate: **Oral Suspension:** Cortef **(Rx)** Probutate: **Topical Cream:** Pandel **(Rx)** Sodium phosphate: **Parenteral:** Hydrocortone Phosphate **(Rx)** Sodium succinate: **Parenteral:** A-hydroCort, Solu-Cortef **(Rx)** Valerate: **Topical Cream/Ointment:** Westcort **(Rx)**

Classification: Corticosteroid, naturally occurring; glucocorticoid-type

Mechanism of Action: Short-acting. Topical products are available without a prescription in strengths of 0.5% and 1%.

Route/Dosage

HYDROCORTISONE

• **Tablets**

20–240 mg/day, depending on disease.

• **IM Only**

One-third to one-half the PO dose q 12 hr.

• **Rectal**

100 mg in retention enema nightly for 21 days (up to 2 months of therapy may be needed; discontinue gradually if therapy exceeds 3 weeks).

• **Topical Ointment, Cream, Gel, Lotion, Solution, Spray**

Apply sparingly to affected area and rub in lightly t.i.d.–q.i.d.

HYDROCORTISONE ACETATE

• **Intralesional, Intra-articular, Soft Tissue**

5–50 mg, depending on condition.

• **Intrarectal Foam**

1 applicatorful (90 mg) 1–2 times/day for 2–3 weeks; **then** every second day.

• **Topical**

See *Hydrocortisone*.

HYDROCORTISONE BUTYRATE

• **Topical Cream, Ointment, Solution**

Apply a thin film to the affected area b.i.d.–t.i.d.

HYDROCORTISONE PROBUTATE

• **Topical Cream**

Apply a thin film to the affected area 1–2 times/day.

HYDROCORTISONE CYPIONATE

• **Suspension**

20–240 mg/day, depending on the severity of the disease.

HYDROCORTISONE SODIUM PHOSPHATE

• **IV, IM, SC**

General uses.

Initial: 15–240 mg/day depending on use and on severity of the disease. Usually, one-half to one-third of the PO dose is given q 12 hr.

Adrenal insufficiency, acute.

Adults, initial: 100 mg IV; **then,** 100 mg q 8 hr in an IV fluid; **older children, initial:** 1–2 mg/kg by IV bolus; **then,** 150–250 mg/kg/day **IV** in divided doses; **infants, initial:** 1–2 mg/kg by IV bolus; **then,** 25–150 mg/kg/day in divided doses.

HYDROCORTISONE SODIUM SUCCINATE

• **IM, IV**

Initial: 100–500 mg; **then,** may be repeated at 2-, 4-, and 6-hr intervals depending on response and severity of condition.

HYDROCORTISONE VALERATE

• **Topical Cream**

See *Hydrocortisone*.

How Supplied: Hydrocortisone Cortisol: *Balm:* 1%; *Cream:* 0.5%, 1%, 2.5%; *Enema:* 100 mg/60 mL; *Gel/jelly:* 1%; *Liquid:* 1%; *Lotion:* 0.25%, 0.5%, 1%, 2%, 2.5%; *Ointment:* 0.5%, 1%, 2.5%; *Pad:* 0.5%, 1%; *Solution:* 1%, 2.5%; *Spray:* 1%; *Tablet:* 5 mg, 10 mg, 20 mg. Hydrocortisone acetate: *Cream:* 0.5%, 1%; *Foam:* 10%; *Injection:* 50 mg/mL; *Ointment:* 0.5%, 1%; *Spray:* 0.5%; *Suppository:* 25 mg, 30 mg. Hydrocortisone butyrate: *Cream:* 0.1%; *Ointment:* 0.1%; *Solution:* 0.1%. Hydrocortisone cypionate: *Suspension:* 10 mg/5 mL. Hydrocortisone probutate: *Cream:* 0.1%. Hydrocortisone sodium phosphate: *Injection:* 50 mg/mL. Hydrocortisone sodium succinate: *Powder for injection:* 100 mg, 250 mg, 500 mg, 1 g. Hydrocortisone valerate: *Cream:* 0.2%; *Ointment:* 0.2%.

EMS CONSIDERATIONS

See also *Corticosteroids.*

Administration/Storage

IV 1. Check label of parenteral hydrocortisone because IM and IV preparations are not necessarily interchangeable.

2. Give reconstituted direct IV solution at a rate of 100 mg over 30 sec. Doses larger than 500 mg should be infused over 10 min. Drug may be further diluted in 50–100 mL of dextrose or saline solutions and administered as ordered within 24 hr.

Hydromorphone hydrochloride

(hy-droh-MOR-fohn)
Pregnancy Class: C
Dilaudid, Dilaudid-HP, **(C-II) (Rx)**
Classification: Narcotic analgesic, morphine type

Mechanism of Action: Hydromorphone is 7–10 times more analgesic than morphine, with a shorter duration of action. It manifests less sedation, less vomiting, and less nausea than morphine, although it induces pronounced respiratory depression. Give rectally for prolonged activity. **Onset of Action:** 15-30 min; **Peak effect:** 30-60 min.

Duration of Action: 4-5 hr.

Uses: Analgesia for moderate to severe pain (e.g., surgery, cancer, biliary colic, burns, renal colic, MI, bone trauma). Dilaudid-HP is a concentrated solution intended for those tolerant to narcotics.

Contraindications: Additional: Migraine headaches. Use in children. Status asthmaticus, obstetrics, respiratory depression in absence of resuscitative equipment. Lactation.

Precautions: Do not confuse Dilaudid-HP with standard parenteral solutions of Dilaudid or with other narcotics as overdose and death can result. Use Dilaudid-HP with caution in patients with circulatory shock.

Route/Dosage —————

• **Tablets, Liquid**
  Analgesia.

Adults: 2 mg q 4–6 hr as necessary. For severe pain, 4 or more mg q 4–6 hr.

• **Suppositories**
  Analgesia.
Adults: 3 mg q 6–8 hr.

• **SC, IM, IV**
  Analgesia.
Adults: 1–2 mg q 4–6 hr. For severe pain, 3–4 mg q 4–6 hr.

How Supplied: *Injection:* 1 mg/mL, 2 mg/mL, 4 mg/mL, 10 mg/mL; *Liquid:* 1 mg/mL; *Powder for injection:* 250 mg/vial; *Suppository;* 3 mg; *Tablet:* 2 mg, 4 mg, 8 mg

EMS CONSIDERATIONS

See also *Narcotic Analgesics.*

Hydroxychloroquine sulfate

(hy-drox-ee-KLOR-oh-kwin)
Plaquenil Sulfate **(Rx)**
Classification: 4-Aminoquinoline, antimalarial, and antirheumatic

Uses: Prophylaxis and treatment of acute attacks of malaria due to *Plasmodium vivax, P. malariae, P. ovale,* and susceptible strains of *P. falciparum.* Acute or chronic rheumatoid arthritis (not a drug of choice; discontinue after 6 months if no beneficial effects noted). Discoid and SLE. Not used as a first line of therapy.

Contraindications: Additional: Long-term therapy in children, ophthalmologic changes due to 4-aminoquinolines. Pregnency.

Precautions: Use with caution in alcoholism or liver disease. Use in psoriasis may precipitate an acute attack.

Route/Dosage —————

• **Tablets**
  Acute malarial attack.
Adults, initial: 800 mg; **then,** 400 mg after 6–8 hr and 400 mg/day for next 2 days. **Children:** A total of 32 mg/kg given over a 3-day period as follows: **initial:** 12.9 mg/kg (not to exceed a single dose of 800 mg); **then,** 6.4 mg/kg (not to exceed a single

dose of 400 mg) 6, 24, and 48 hr after the first dose.

Suppression of malaria.
Adults: 400 mg q 7 days. If therapy has not been initiated 14 days prior to exposure, an initial loading dose of 800 mg may be given in two divided doses 6 hr apart. **Children:** 6.4 mg/kg (not to exceed the adult dose) q 7 days. If therapy has not been initiated 14 days prior to exposure, an initial loading dose of 12.9 mg/kg may be given in two doses 6 hr apart.

Rheumatoid arthritis.
Adults: 400–600 mg/day taken with milk or meals; **maintenance** (usually after 4–12 weeks): 200–400 mg/day. Use in children is limited, but if use is warranted, a dose of 3–5 mg/kg, up to a maximum of 400 mg/day (given once or twice daily), may be used. (*NOTE:* Several months may be required for a beneficial effect to be seen in adults and children.)

Lupus erythematosus.
Adults, usual: 400 mg once or twice daily; **prolonged maintenance:** 200–400 mg/day.

How Supplied: *Tablet:* 200 mg

Side Effects: Additional: The appearances of skin eruptions or of misty vision and visual halos are indications for withdrawal. Patients on long-term therapy should be examined thoroughly at regular intervals for knee and ankle reflexes and hematopoietic studies.

Drug Interactions
Digoxin / Hydroxychloroquine ↑ serum digoxin levels
Gold salts / Dermatitis and ↑ risk of severe skin reactions
Phenylbutazone / Dermatitis and ↑ risk of severe skin reactions

EMS CONSIDERATIONS

None.

Hydroxyurea
(hy-DROX-ee-you-ree-ah)
Pregnancy Class: D

Droxia, Hydrea (Abbreviation: HYD) **(Rx)**
Classification: Antineoplastic, antimetabolite

Mechanism of Action: Inhibits DNA synthesis but not synthesis of RNA or protein. As an antimetabolite, it interferes with the conversion of ribonucleotides to deoxyribonucleotides due to blockade of the ribonucleotide reductase system. May also inhibit incorporation of thymidine into DNA. Effectiveness in sickle cell anemia may be due to increases in hemoglobin F levels in RBCs, decrease in neutrophils, increases in the water content of RBCs, increases the deformability of sickled cells, and altered adhesion of RBCs to the endothelium. Rapidly absorbed from GI tract.

Uses: Chronic, resistant, myelocytic leukemia. Carcinoma of the ovary (recurrent, inoperable, or metastatic). Melanoma. With irradiation to treat primary squamous cell carcinoma of the head and neck (but not the lip). Sickle cell anemia (Droxia). *Investigational:* Thrombocytopenia, HIV, psoriasis.

Contraindications: Leukocyte count less than 2,500/mm³ or thrombocyte count less than 100,000/mm³. Severe anemia.

Precautions: Use during pregnancy only if benefits clearly outweigh risks. Give with caution to patients with marked renal dysfunction. Geriatric patients may be more sensitive to the effects of hydroxyurea necessitating a lower dose. Dosage has not been established in children.

Route/Dosage
• **Capsules**
Solid tumors, intermittent therapy or when used together with irradiation.
Dose individualized. Usual: 80 mg/kg as a single dose every third day. Intermittent dosage offers advantage of reduced toxicity. If effective, maintain patient on drug indefinitely unless toxic effects preclude such a regimen.

---

bold italic = life threatening side effect

Solid tumors, continuous therapy.
20–30 mg/kg/day as a single dose.
Resistant chronic myelocytic leukemia.
20–30 mg/kg/day in a single dose or two divided daily doses.
Concomitant therapy with irradiation for carinoma of the head and neck.
80 mg/kg as a single dose every third day.
Sickle cell anemia.
Initial: 15 mg once daily. Base dosage on the smaller of ideal or actual body weight. Increase dose gradually to the maximum tolerated dose or to 35 mg/kg/day.
How Supplied: *Capsule:* 200 mg, 300 mg, 400 mg, 500 mg
Side Effects: Additional: Erythrocyte abnormalities including megaloblastic erythropoiesis. Constipation, redness of the face, maculopapular rash.

EMS CONSIDERATIONS
None.

Hydroxyzine hydrochloride
(hy-DROX-ih-zeen)
Atarax, Atarax 100, Vistaril, Vistazine 50 **(Rx)**
Classification: Nonbenzodiazepine antianxiety agent

Mechanism of Action: Manifests anticholinergic, antiemetic, antispasmodic, local anesthetic, antihistaminic, and skeletal relaxant effects. Has mild antiarrhythmic activity and mild analgesic effects. High sedative and antiemetic effects and moderate anticholinergic activity.
Onset of Action: 15-30 min.
Duration of Action: 4-6 hr.
Uses: PO: Symptomatic relief of anxiety and tension associated with psychoneurosis. Anxiety observed in organic disease. Prior to dental procedures, in acute emotional problems, in alcoholism, allergic conditions with strong emotional overlay (e.g., chronic urticaria and pruritus). Beneficial to the cardiac patient to allay

anxiety and apprehension occurring with certain types of heart disease. Pruritus caused by allergic conditions. **IM:** Acute hysteria or agitation, withdrawal symptoms (including delirium tremens) in the acute or chronic alcoholic. Pre- and postoperative and pre- and postpartum adjunct to allay anxiety, to control emesis or to allow a decrease in dosage of narcotics.
Contraindications: Pregnancy (especially early) or lactation; treatment of morning sickness during pregnancy or as sole agent for treatment of psychoses or depression. Hypersensitivity to drug. IV, SC, or intra-arterially.
Precautions: Possible increased anticholinergic and sedative effects in geriatric patients.

Route/Dosage
• **Capsules, Oral Suspension, Syrup, Tablets. Hydroxyzine hydrochloride and hydroxyzine pamoate**
Antianxiety.
Adults: 50–100 mg q.i.d.; **pediatric under 6 years:** 50 mg/day in divided doses; **over 6 years:** 50–100 mg/day in divided doses.
Pruritus.
Adults: 25 mg t.i.d.–q.i.d.; **children under 6 years:** 50 mg/day in divided doses; **children over 6 years:** 50–100 mg/day in divided doses.
Preoperative or post–general anesthetic sedative.
Adults: 50–100 mg; **children:** 0.6 mg/kg.
• **IM. Hydroxyzine Hydrochloride**
Acute anxiety, including alcohol withdrawal.
Adults: 50–100 mg q.i.d.
Antiemetic/analgesia, adjunctive therapy.
Adults: 25–100 mg; **pediatric,** 1.1 mg/kg. Switch to **PO** as soon as possible.
Pruritus.
Adults: 25 mg t.i.d. or q.i.d.
Sedative, as premedication and following general anesthesia.
Adults: 50–100 mg. **Children:** 0.6 mg/kg.

How Supplied: Hydroxyzine hydrochloride: *Injection:* 25 mg/mL, 50 mg/mL; *Syrup:* 10 mg/5 mL; *Tablet:* 10 mg, 25 mg, 50 mg, 100 mg. Hydroxyzine pamoate: *Capsule:* 25 mg, 50 mg, 100 mg; *Suspension:* 25 mg/5 mL

Side Effects: Low incidence at recommended dosages. Drowsiness, dryness of mouth, involuntary motor activity (rarely, tremors and convulsions), ECG abnormalities (e.g., alterations in T-waves), dizziness, urticaria, skin reactions, hypersensitivity. Worsening of porphyria. Marked discomfort, induration, and even gangrene at site of IM injection.

OD **Overdose Management:** *Symptoms:* Oversedation. *Treatment:* Immediate induction of vomiting or performance of gastric lavage. General supportive care with monitoring of VS. Control hypotension with IV fluids and either norepinephrine or metaraminol (epinephrine should not be used).

Drug Interactions: Additive effects when used with other CNS depressants. See *Drug Interactions for Tranquilizers.*

EMS CONSIDERATIONS

See also *Tranquilizers.*

Hyoscyamine sulfate (Levsin)

high-oh-SIGH-ah-meen

Pregnancy Class: C

Anaspaz, Cystospaz-M, Espasmotex, Levbid, Levsin, Levsinex, Levsin SL, Spasdel **(Rx)**

Classification: Cholinergic blocking agent

Mechanism of Action: One of the belladonna alkaloids; acts by blocking the action of acetylcholine at the postganglionic nerve endings of the parasympathetic nervous system. **t^1/$_2$:** 3^1/$_2$ hr for tablets, 7 hr for extended-release capsules, and 9 hr for extended-release tablets. Majority of the drug is excreted in the urine unchanged.

Uses: To control gastric secretion, visceral spasm, and hypermotilitiy in spastic colitis, spastic bladder, cystitis, pylorospasm, and associated abdominal cramps. Adjunctive therapy to treat irritable bowel syndrome and functional GI disorders. Adjunctive therapy in neurogenic bladder and neurogenic bowel disturbances. Treat infant colic (use elixir or solution). Use with morphine or other narcotics for symptomatic relief of biliary and renal colic. In Parkinsonism to reduce rigidity and tremors and to control sialorrhea and hyperhidrosis. To treat poisoning by anticholinesterase agents. To reduce GI motility to facilitate diagnostic procedures, such as endoscopy or hypersecretion in pancreatitis. To treat selected cases of partial heart block associated with vagal activity. Used as a preoperative medication to reduce salivary, tracheobronchial, and pharyngeal secretions.

Route/Dosage
• **Extended-Release Capsules (0.375 mg) or Extended-Release Tablets (0.375 mg)**
Adults and children over 12 years of age: 0.375–0.750 mg q 12 hr, not to exceed 1.5 mg in 24 hr.
• **Tablets (0.125 mg)**
Adults and children over 12 years of age: 0.125–0.25 mg q 4 hr or as needed, not to exceed 1.5 mg in 24 hr.
• **Elixir (0.125 mg/5 mL)**
Adults and children over 12 years of age: 0.125 mg–0.25 mg (5–10 mL) q 4 hr, not to exceed 1.5 mg (60 mL) in 24 hr. **Children, 2 to 12 years of age:** 10 kg: 1.25 mL (0.031 mg) q 4 hr; 20 kg: 2.5 mL (0.062 mg) q 4 hr; 40 kg: 3.75 mL (0.093 mg) q 4 hr; 50 kg: 5 mL (0.125 mg) q 4 hr.
• **Drops (0.125 mg/mL)**
Adults and children over 12 years of age: 0.125–0.25 mg 5–10 mL q 4 hr, not to exceed 1.5 mg (12 mL) in 24 hr. **Children, 2 to 12 years of age:** 0.031–0.125 mg (0.251 mL)q 4 hr or as needed, not to exceed 0.75 mg (6 mL) in 24 hr. **Children, under 2 years of age:** 3.4 kg: 4 drops q 4 hr,

H

---

bold italic = life threatening side effect

not to exceed 24 drops in 24 hr; 5 kg: 5 drops q 4 hr, not to exceed 30 drops in 24 hr; 7 kg: 6 drops q 4 hr, not to exceed 36 drops in 24 hr; 10 kg: 8 drops q 4 hr, not to exceed 48 drops in 24 hr.

• **Injection (0.5 mg/mL)**
   GI disorders.

Adults: 0.25–0.5 mg (0.5–1 mL). Some patients need only one dose while others require doses 2, 3, or 4 times a day at 4 hr intervals.
   Diagnostic procedures.

Adults: 0.25–0.5 mg (0.5–1 mL) given IV 5 to 10 min prior to the procedure.
   Preanesthetic medication.

Adults and children over 2 years of age: 0.005 mg/kg 30–60 min prior to the time of induction of anesthesia. May also be given at the time the preanesthetic sedative or narcotic is given.
   During surgery to reduce drug-induced bradycardia.

Adults and children over 2 years of age: Increments of 0.125 mg (0.25 mL) IV repeated as needed.
   Reverse neuromuscular blockade.

Adults and children over 2 years of age: 0.2 mg (0.4 mL) for every 1 mg neostigmine or equivalent dose of physostigmine or pyridostigmine.

How Supplied: *Capsule, Extended Release:* 0.375 mg; *Elixir:* 0.125 mg/5 mL; *Injection:* 0.5 mg/mL; *Liquid:* 0.125 mg/mL; *Tablet:* 0.125 mg; *Tablet, Extended Release:* 0.375 mg.

Side Effects: See *Cholinergic Blocking Agents.*

EMS CONSIDERATIONS

Administration/Storage

1. May take hyoscyamine SL tablets sublingually, PO, or chewed. May take hyoscyamine tablets PO or sublingually.
2. Depending on the use, give the injection SC, IM, or IV.
3. Visually inspect the injectable form for particulate matter/discoloration.

Assessment

1. Document indications for therapy, type, onset, and duration of symptoms.
2. List other agents trialed and the outcome.
3. Determine any evidence of glaucoma, bladder neck or GI tract obstruction.

Ibuprofen
(eye-byou-PROH-fen)

Pregnancy Class: B (first two trimesters); D (third trimester)

(Rx): Children's Advil, Children's Motrin, IBU, Ibuprohm, Motrin, Saleto-400, -600, and -800 **(OTC):** Advil Caplets and Tablets, Bayer Select Pain Relief Formula Caplets, Children's Advil Suspension, Children's Motrin Liquid Suspension, Children's Motrin Drops, Genpril Caplets and Tablets, Haltran, Ibuprin, Ibuprohm Caplets and Tablets, Junior Strength Motrin Caplets, Menadol, Midol IB, Motrin-IB Caplets and Tablets, Nuprin Caplets and Tablets, PediaCare Fever Drops, Saleto-200

Classification: Nonsteroidal anti-inflammatory drug (NSAID)

Onset of Action: 30 min for analgesia and approximately 1 week for anti-inflammatory effect; **Time to peak levels:** 1-2 hr.

Duration of Action: 4-6 hr for analgesia and 1-2 weeks for anti-inflammatory effect.

Uses: Rx: Analgesic for mild to moderate pain. Primary dysmenorrhea, rheumatoid arthritis, osteoarthritis, antipyretic. *Investigational:* Resistant acne vulgaris (with tetracyclines); inflammation due to ultraviolet-B exposure (sunburn), juvenile rheumatoid arthritis. High doses to treat progressive lung deterioration in cystic fibrosis. **OTC:** Relief of fever and minor aches and pains due to colds, flu, sore throats, headaches, and toothaches.

Contraindications: Pregnancy, especially during the last trimester.

Precautions: Individualize dosage for children less than 12 years of age as safety and effectiveness have not been established.

Route/Dosage

• **Suspension, Chewable Tablets, Tablets**

Rheumatoid arthritis, osteoarthritis.
Either 300 mg q.i.d. or 400, 600, or 800 mg t.i.d.–q.i.d.; adjust dosage according to patient response. Full therapeutic response may not be noted for 2 or more weeks.

Juvenile arthritis.
30–70 mg/kg/day in three to four divided doses (20 mg/kg/day may be adequate for mild cases).

Mild to moderate pain.
Adults: 400 mg q 4–6 hr, as needed.

Antipyretic.
Pediatric, 2–12 years of age: 5 mg/kg if baseline temperature is 102.5°F (39.1°C) or below or 10 mg/kg if baseline temperature is greater than 102.5°F (39.1°C). Maximum daily dose: 40 mg/kg.

Primary dysmenorrhea.
Adults: 400 mg q 4 hr, as needed.

• **Tablets for OTC Use**

Mild to moderate pain, antipyretic, dysmenorrhea.
200 mg q 4–6 hr; dose may be increased to 400 mg if pain or fever persist. Dose should not exceed 1,200 mg/day.

• **Suspension for OTC Use**

Pain, fever.
Children, 2–11 years: 7.5 mg/kg, up to q.i.d., to a maximum of 30 mg/kg/day.

How Supplied: *Chew Tablet:* 50 mg, 100 mg; *Suspension:* 50 mg/1.25 mL, 100 mg/5 mL; *Tablet:* 50 mg, 100 mg, 200 mg, 300 mg, 400 mg, 600 mg, 800 mg

Side Effects: Additional: Dermatitis (maculopapular type), rash. Hypersensitivity reaction consisting of abdominal pain, fever, headache, **men-**

ingitis, N&V, signs of liver damage; especially seen in patients with SLE.

Drug Interactions: Additional: *Furosemide/* Ibuprofen ↓ diuretic effect of furosemide due to ↓ renal prostaglandin synthesis. *Lithium/* Ibuprofen ↑ plasma levels of lithium. *Thiazide diuretics/* Ibuprofen ↓ diuretic effect of furosemide due to ↓ renal prostaglandin synthesis.

EMS CONSIDERATIONS

None.

Ibutilide fumarate

(ih-BYOU-tih-lyd)
Pregnancy Class: C
Corvert **(Rx)**
Classification: Antiarrhythmic agent

Mechanism of Action: Class III antiarrhythmic agent. Delays repolarization by activation of a slow, inward current (mostly sodium), rather than by blocking outward potassium currents (the way other class III antiarrhythmics act). This results in prolongation in the duration of the atrial and ventricular action potential and refractoriness. Also a dose-related prolongation of the QT interval.

Uses: For rapid conversion of atrial fibrillation or atrial flutter of recent onset to sinus rhythm. Determination of patients to receive ibutilide should be based on expected benefits of maintaining sinus rhythm and whether this outweighs both the risks of the drug and of maintenance therapy.

Contraindications: Use of certain class Ia antiarrhythmic drugs (e.g., disopyramide, quinidine, procainamide) and certain class III drugs (e.g., amiodarone and sotalol) concomitantly with ibutilide or within 4 hr of postinfusion.

Precautions: May cause potentially fatal arrhythmias, especially sustained polymorphic ventricular tachycardia, usually in association with QT prolongation (torsades de pointes). Effectiveness has not been determined in patients with arrhythmias of more than 90 days in duration. Breast feed-

---

bold italic = life threatening side effect

ing should be discouraged during therapy. Safety and efficacy have not been determined in children less than 18 years of age.

Route/Dosage
- **IV Infusion**
  Atrial fibrillation or atrial flutter of recent onset.

Patients weighing 60 kg or more, initial: 1 mg (one vial) infused over 10 min. **Patients weighing less than 60 kg, initial:** 0.01 mg/kg infused over 10 min. If the arrhythmia does not terminate within 10 min after the end of the initial infusion (regardless of the body weight), a second 10-min infusion of equal strength may be given 10 min after completion of the first infusion.

How Supplied: *IV Solution:* 0.1 mg/mL.

Side Effects: *CV: **Life-threatening arrhythmias, either sustained or nonsustained polymorphic ventricular tachycardia (torsades de pointes).*** Induction or worsening of ventricular arrhythmias. Nonsustained monomorphic ventricular extrasystoles, nonsustained monomorphic ventricular tachycardia, sinus tachycardia, SVT, hypotension, postural hypotension, bundle branch block, AV block, bradycardia, QT-segment prolongation, hypertension, palpitation, supraventricular extrasystoles, nodal arrhythmia, CHF, idioventricular rhythm, sustained monomorphic VT. *Miscellaneous:* Headache, nausea, syncope, renal failure.

OD Overdose Management: *Symptoms:* Increased ventricular ectopy, monomorphic ventricular tachycardia, AV block, nonsustained polymorphic VT. *Treatment:* Treat symptoms.

Drug Interactions
Amiodarone / ↑ Risk of prolonged refractoriness
Antidepressants, tricyclic and tetracyclic / ↑ Risk of proarrhythmias
Digoxin / Supraventricular arrhythmias, due to ibutilide, may mask the cardiotoxicity due to high digoxin levels
Disopyramide / ↑ Risk of prolonged refractoriness

Histamne H₁ receptor antagonists / ↑ *Risk of proarrhythmias*
Quinidine / ↑ Risk of prolonged refractoriness
Phenothiazines / ↑ Risk of proarrhythmias
Procainamide / ↑ Risk of prolonged refractoriness
Sotalol / ↑ Risk of prolonged refractoriness

EMS CONSIDERATIONS

Administration/Storage: **IV** May give undiluted or diluted in 50 mL of 0.9% NaCl or D5W injection before infusion. One vial (1 mg) mixed with 50 mL of diluent forms an admixture of approximately 0.017 mg/mL of ibutilide; administer infusion over 10 min.

Assessment
1. Monitor VS and ECG.
2. Ibutilide must be given in a setting with continuous ECG monitoring.
3. Document conversion to NSR. Drug infusion should cease: when arrhythmia is terminated or in the event of sustained or nonsustained ventricular tachycardia or marked prolongation of QT interval.

Idoxuridine (IDU)
(eye-dox-YOUR-deen)
Pregnancy Class: C
Herplex Liquifilm **(Rx)**
Classification: Antiviral agent, ophthalmic

Mechanism of Action: Resembles thymidine; inhibits thymidylic phosphorylase and specific DNA polymerases required for incorporation of thymidine into viral DNA. Idoxuridine, instead of thymidine, is incorporated into viral DNA, resulting in faulty DNA and the inability of the virus to infect tissue or reproduce.

Uses: Herpes simplex keratitis, especially for initial epithelial infections characterized by the presence of thread-like extensions. *NOTE:* Idoxuridine will control infection but will not prevent scarring, loss of vision, or vascularization. Alternative form of therapy must be instituted if no improvement is noted after 7 days or if complete reepithelialization fails to occur after 21 days of therapy.

Contraindications: Hypersensitivity; deep ulcerations involving stromal layers of cornea. Lactation. Concomitant use of corticosteroids in herpes simplex keratitis (corticosteroids may accelerate the spread of the viral infection).

Precautions: May be sensitizing, especially with dermal use. Safety and efficacy have not been determined in children.

Route/Dosage

• **Ophthalmic (0.1%) Solution.**
Initially: 1 gtt every hour during the day and q 2 hr during the night until definite improvement is noted (usually within 7 days). **Following improvement:** 1 gtt q 2 hr during the day and q 4 hr at night. Continue for 3–7 days after healing is complete. Alternate dosing schedule: 1 gtt q min for 5 min; repeat q 4 hr, day and night.

How Supplied: *Solution:* 0.1%

Side Effects: Localized to eye. Temporary visual haze, irritation, pain, pruritus, inflammation, sensitivity to bright light, follicular conjunctivitis with preauricular adenopathy, mild edema of eyelids and cornea, allergic reactions (rare), photosensitivity, corneal clouding and stippling, small punctate defects. *NOTE:* Squamous cell carcinoma has been reported at the site of application.

OD Overdose Management: *Symptoms (frequent administration):* Defects on corneal epithelium. *Treatment:* If an excess amount of drug is instilled in the eye, flush with water or normal saline.

Drug Interactions: Concurrent use of boric acid may cause irritation.

EMS CONSIDERATIONS

See also *Antiviral Agents.*

Imipenem-Cilastatin sodium
(em-ee-PEN-em, sigh-lah-STAT-in)

Pregnancy Class: C
Primaxin I.M., Primaxin I.V. **(Rx)**
Classification: Antibiotic combined with inhibitor of dehydropeptidase I

Mechanism of Action: Inhibits cell wall synthesis. Is bactericidal against a wide range of gram-positive and gram-negative organisms. Stable in the presence of beta-lactamases. Addition of cilastatin prevents the metabolism of imipenem in the kidneys by dehydropeptidase I, thus ensuring high levels of the imipenem in the urinary tract.

Uses: IV: To treat the following serious infections: lower respiratory tract, urinary tract (complicated and uncomplicated), gynecologic, skin and skin structures, bone and joint, endocarditis, intra-abdominal, bacterial septicemia, and infections caused by more than one agent. Infections resistant to aminoglycosides, cephalosporins, or penicillins have responded to imipenem. Bacterial eradication may not be achieved in patients with cystic fibrosis, chronic pulmonary disease, and lower respiratory tract infections caused by *Pseudomonas aeruginosa.*

IM: This route of administration is not intended for severe or life-threatening infections (including endocarditis, or bacterial sepsis). Used for lower respiratory tract infections (including pneumonia and bronchitis), intra-abdominal infections, skin and skin structure infections, gynecologic infections.

Contraindications: IM use in patients allergic to local anesthetics of the amide type and use in patients with heart block (due to the use of lidocaine HCl diluent) or severe shock. Use in patients with a C_{CR} of less than or equal to 5 mL/min/1.73 m². unless hemodialysis is begun within 48 hr. IV use in children with CNS infections due to the risk of seizures and in children less than 30 kg with impaired renal function.

Precautions: Use with caution in pregnancy and lactation. Due to cross sensitivity, use with caution in patients with penicillin allergy. Safety and effectiveness have not been determined for use IM in children less than 12 years of age.

Route/Dosage

- **IV**

  Fully susceptible gram-positive organisms, gram-negative organisms, anaerobes.

  Mild: 250 mg q 6 hr; *moderate:* 500 mg q 6 hr or q 8 hr; *severe/life-threatening:* 500 mg q 6 hr.

  Urinary tract infections due to fully susceptible organisms.

  Uncomplicated: 250 mg q 6 hr; *complicated:* 500 mg q 6 hr.

  Moderately susceptible organisms (especially some strains of P. aeruginosa*).*

  Mild: 500 mg q 6 hr; *moderate,* 500 mg q 6 hr to 1 g q 6 hr; *severe/life-threatening,* 1 g q 6 or 8 hr.

  Urinary tract infections due to moderately susceptible organisms.

  Uncomplicated: 250 mg q 6 hr; *complicated:* 500 mg q 6 hr.

  The total daily dose should not exceed 50 mg/kg or 4 g, whichever is lower.

  Pediatric, non-CNS infections.

  Children, 3 months of age or older: 15–25 mg/kg/dose q 6 hr, up to a maximum of dose of 2 g/day for treating infections with fully susceptible organisms and up to a maximum of 4 g/day for infections with moderately susceptible organisms. Doses as high as 90 mg/kg/day have been used in older children with cystic fibrosis. **Children, three months of age or less (weighing 1,500 g or more):** Less than 1 week of age, 25 mg/kg q 12 hr; 1–4 weeks of age, 25 mg/kg q 8 hr; 4 weeks to 3 months of age, 25 mg/kg q 6 hr. Give doses less than or equal to 500 mg by IV infusion over 15 to 20 min; give doses greater than 500 mg by IV infusion over 40 to 60 min.

- **IM**

  Lower respiratory tract, skin and skin structure, or gynecologic infections: mild to moderate.

  500 or 750 mg q 12 hr depending on severity.

  Intra-abdominal infections: mild to moderate.

  750 mg q 12 hr. The total daily dose should not exceed 1.5 g.

  Pediatric, 3 months to 3 years, all uses: 15–25 mg/kg q 6 hr, to a maximum of 2 g/day. **Pediatric, over 3 years, all uses:** 15 mg/kg q 6 hr.

How Supplied: The Powder for IV injection and the Powder for IM injection contain: imipenem, 500 mg, and cilastatin sodium, 500 mg, or imipenem, 750 mg, and cilastatin sodium, 750 mg.

Side Effects: *GI:* **Pseudomembranous colitis,** nausea, diarrhea, vomiting, abdominal pain, heartburn, increased salivation, **hemorrhagic colitis,** gastroenteritis, glossitis, pharyngeal pain, tongue papillar hypertrophy, hepatitis, jaundice, staining of the teeth or tongue. *CNS:* Fever, confusion, **seizures,** dizziness, sleepiness, myoclonus, headache, vertigo, paresthesia, encephalopathy, tremor, psychic disturbances (including hallucinations). *CV:* Hypotension, tachycardia, palpitations. *Dermatologic:* Rash, urticaria, pruritus, flushing, cyanosis, facial edema, erythema multiforme, skin texture changes, hyperhidrosis, angioneurotic edema, *toxic epidermal necrolysis,* **Stevens-Johnson syndrome.** *CV:* Hypotension, palpitations, tachycardia. *Respiratory:* Chest discomport, dyspnea, hyperventilation. *GU:* Pruritus vulvae, anuria/oliguria, acute renal failure, polyuria, urine discoloration. *Hematologic:* Pancytopenia, bone marrow depression, thrombocytopenia, neutropenia, leukopenia, hemolytic anemia. *Miscellaneous:* Candidiasis, superinfection, tinnitus, polyarthralgia, asthenia, muscle weakness, transient hearing loss in patients with existing hearing impairment, taste perversion, thoracic spine pain.

Children, 3 months and older: Diarrhea, rash, phlebitis, gastroenteritis, vomiting, IV site irritation, urine discoloration. *Children, newborn to 3 months:* Convulsions, diarrhea, oliguria, anuria, oral candidiasis, rash, tachycardia.

The following side effects may occur at the injection site: Thrombophlebitis, phlebitis, pain, erythema, vein induration, infused vein infection.

Drug Interactions

Cyclosporine / ↑ CNS side effects of both drugs

Ganciclovir / ↑ Risk of generalized seizures

Probenecid / ↑ Imipenem levels and half-life; do not use together

EMS CONSIDERATIONS

See also *Anti-Infectives*.

Imipramine hydrochloride
Imipramine pamoate
(im-IHP-rah-meen)
Pregnancy Class: B
Imipramine hydrochloride (Tofranil **(Rx)**) Imipramine pamoate (Tofranil-PM **(Rx)**)
Classification: Antidepressant, tricyclic (tertiary amine)

Mechanism of Action: Moderate anticholinergic and sedative effects; high orthostatic hypotensive effects.

Uses: Symptoms of depression. Enuresis in children. Chronic, severe neurogenic pain. Bulimia nervosa.

Route/Dosage ——————

• **Tablets, Capsules**
  Depression.

Hospitalized patients: 50 mg b.i.d.–t.i.d. Can be increased by 25 mg every few days up to 200 mg/day. After 2 weeks, dosage may be increased gradually to maximum of 250–300 mg/day at bedtime. **Outpatients:** 75–150 mg/day. Maximum dose for outpatients is 200 mg. Decrease when feasible to maintenance dosage: 50–150 mg/day at bedtime.

Adolescent and geriatric patients: 30–40 mg/day up to maximum of 100 mg/day. **Pediatric:** 1.5 mg/kg/day in three divided doses; can be increased 1–1.5 mg/kg/day q 3–5 days to a maximum of 5 mg/kg/day.
  Childhood enuresis.

Age 5 years and over: 25 mg/day 1 hr before bedtime. Dose can be increased to 50 mg/day up to 12 years of age and to 75 mg/day in children over 12 years of age. Dose should not exceed 2.5 mg/kg/day.

• **IM**
  Antidepressant.

Adults: Up to 100 mg/day in divided doses. IM route not recommended for use in children less than 12 years of age.

How Supplied: Imipramine hydrochloride: *Tablet:* 10 mg, 25 mg, 50 mg. Imipramine pamoate: *Capsule:* 75 mg, 100 mg, 125 mg, 150 mg

Side Effects: Additional: High therapeutic dosage may increase frequency of seizures in epileptic patients and cause seizures in nonepileptic patients. Elderly and adolescent patients may have low tolerance to the drug.

EMS CONSIDERATIONS

See also *Antidepressants, Tricyclic.*

Imiquimod
(ih-MIH-kwih-mod)
Pregnancy Class: B
Aldara **(Rx)**
Classification: Drug for genital and perianal warts

Mechanism of Action: May induce cytokines, including interferon-alpha and others, to modify immune response. Minimal percutaneous absorption.

Uses: External genital and perianal warts/condyloma acuminata in adults.

Contraindications: Use in urethral, intravaginal, cervical, rectal, or intra-anal human papilloma viral disease.

Precautions: Safety and efficacy have not been determined in patients less than 18 years of age. Use with caution during lactation.

Route/Dosage ——————

• **Cream**
  Genital/perianal warts.

Adults: Apply 3 times/week prior to normal sleeping hours; leave on skin for 6–10 hr. Following treatment, remove by washing the area

---

bold italic = life threatening side effect

with mild soap and water. Continue treatment until there is total clearance of warts (16 weeks or less).

How Supplied: *Topical Cream:* 5%

Side Effects: *Dermatologic:* Erythema, itching, erosion, burning, excoriation/flaking, edema, pain, induration, ulceration, scabbing, vesicles, soreness. *Systemic:* Fungal infection, fatigue, fever, flu-like symptoms, headache, diarrhea, myalgia.

EMS CONSIDERATIONS
None.

Immune globulin IV (Human)
(im-MYOUN GLOH-byou-lin)

Pregnancy Class: C

Gamimune N 5% and 10%, Gammagard S/D, Gammar-P I.V., Iveegam, Polygam, Polygam S/D, Sandoglobulin, Venoglobulin-I, Venoglobulin-S Solvent Detergent Treated **(Rx)**

Classification: Immunoglobulin G antibody product. *NOTE:* The available products differ significantly with respect to the process by which they are made (e.g., donor pool and fractionation/purification) as well as isotonicity. Thus, information on each product should be carefully read before use. *NOTE:* Gammagard has been replaced by Gammagard S/D. Also, Gammagard S/D is a higher concentration than Gammagard; thus, the drug can be infused more quickly. Certain products have been treated by compounds that are capable of inactivating several bloodborne viruses.

Mechanism of Action: Derived from a human volunteer pool. Contains the various IgG antibodies normally occurring in humans. The products may also contain traces of IgA and IgM. Plasma in the manufacturing pool has been found nonreactive for hepatitis B antigen. Have been no documented cases of viral transmission. Antibodies present in the products will cause both opsonization and neutralization of microbes and toxins. Reconstituted products may contain sucrose, maltose, protein, and/or small amounts of sodium chloride. Immune globulin IV provides immediate antibody levels. The percentage of IgG in the products is over 90%.

Uses: *All products:* Severe combined immunodeficiency and primary immunoglobulin deficiency syndromes, including congenital agammaglobulinemia, X-linked agammaglobulinemia with or without hyper IgM, combined immunodeficiency, and Wiskott-Aldrich syndrome. *Investigational:* Chronic fatigue syndrome, quinidine-induced thrombocytopenia.

Gamimune N, Gammagard S/D, Polygam S/D, Sandoglobulin, Venoglobulin-I and Venoglobulin-S: Acute and chronic ITP in both children and adults.

Gammagard S/D, Polygam S/D: B-cell CLL in those with hypogammaglobulinemia or recurrent associated bacterial infections.

Iveegam: Kawasaki syndrome (given with aspirin within 10 days of onset of the disease).

Gamimune N: Prophylactic use to decrease infections and the incidence of graft-versus-host-disease in bone marrow patients and in HIV-infected children to prevent bacterial infections.

Contraindications: Patients with selective IgA deficiency who have antibodies to IgA (the products contain IgA). Sensitivity to human immune globulin.

Precautions: The various products are used for different conditions and at different doses; thus, check information carefully.

Route/Dosage

NOTE: Due to differences in products, dosage must be listed separately for each product.

• **IV Only for All Products**

GAMIMUNE N

Immunodeficiency syndrome.

100–200 mg/kg given once a month; if response is satisfactory, dose can be increased to 400 mg/kg or infusion may be repeated more frequently than once a month. Rate of infusion for all uses: 0.01–0.02 mL/kg/min for

30 min; if no discomfort is experienced, the rate can be increased up to 0.08 mL/kg/min.

ITP.

400 mg/kg for 5 consecutive days or 1,000 mg/kg/day for 1 day or 2 consecutive days. **Maintenance:** If platelet count falls to less than 30,000/mm³ or if bleeding occurs, 400 mg/kg may be given as a single infusion. If an adequate response is not seen, the dose can be increased to 800–1,000 mg/kg given as a single infusion. Maintenance infusions are given, as needed, to maintain platelet counts greater than 30,000/mm³.

Bone marrow transplantation.

500 mg/kg beginning on days 7 and 2 pretransplant or at the time conditioning therapy for transplantation is initiated; then, give weekly throughout the 90-day post-transplant period.

Pediatric HIV infection.

400 mg/kg q 28 days.

GAMMAGARD S/D

Immunodeficiency syndrome.

200–400 mg/kg (minimum of 100 mg/kg/month).

B-cell CLL.

400 mg/kg q 3–4 weeks.

ITP.

1,000 mg/kg; additional doses depend on platelet count (up to three doses can be given on alternate days). Rate of infusion: 0.5 mL/kg/min initially; may be increased gradually, not to exceed 4 mL/kg/hr if there is no patient distress.

GAMMAR-P I.V.

Immunodeficiency syndrome.

200–400 mg/kg q 3–4 weeks. An alternative is a loading dose of at least 200 mg/kg at more frequent intervals and then 200–600 mg/kg at 3-week intervals once a therapeutic plasma level has been reached. Rate of infusion: 0.01 mL/kg/min, increasing to 0.02 mL/kg/min after 15 to 30 min. Most patients will tolerate a gradual increase to 0.03–0.06 mL/kg/min.

IVEEGAM

Immunodeficiency syndrome.

200 mg/kg/month. If desired effect not achieved, the dose may be increased up to fourfold (i.e., up to 800 mg/kg/month) or the intervals between doses shortened. Rate of infusion for all uses: 1 mL/min to a maximum of 2 mL/min of the 5% solution. The product may be further diluted with saline or 5% dextrose.

Kawasaki syndrome.

400 mg/kg/day for 4 consecutive days or a single dose of 2,000 mg/kg given over a 10-hr period. Treatment should be initiated within 10 days of onset and should include aspirin, 100 mg/kg each day through the 14th day of illness; then, aspirin is given at a dose of 3–5 mg/kg/day for 5 weeks.

POLYGAM S/D

Immunodeficiency syndrome.

Initial: 200–400 mg/kg may be given; **then,** 100 mg/kg/month. Rate of administration for all uses: Initially, 0.5 mL/kg/hr. If there is no distress, the rate can be gradually increased, not to exceed 4 mL/kg/hr. Those who tolerate the 5% solution at a rate of 4 mL/kg/hr can receive the 10% solution starting at 0.5 mL/kg/hr.

B-cell CLL.

400 mg/kg q 3 to 4 weeks.

ITP.

1 g/kg. Depending on response, additional doses can be given—three separate doses on alternate days can be given, if needed.

SANDOGLOBULIN

Immunodeficiency syndrome.

200 mg/kg/month; increase to 300 mg/kg if patient response satisfactory (i.e., IgG serum level of 300 mg/dL). Rate of administration for all uses: 3% solution at an initial rate of 0.5–1 mL/min; after 15–30 min can increase to 1.5–2.5 mL/min (subsequent infusions at a rate of 2–2.5 mL/min). If the 6% solution is used, the initial infusion rate should be 1–1.5 mL/min and increased after 15–30 min to a maximum of 2.5 mL/min.

ITP.

400 mg/kg for 2–5 consecutive days.

VENOGLOBULIN-I

Immunodeficiency disease.

200 mg/kg/month by IV infusion; can increase to 300–400 mg/kg if response is insufficient or can repeat infusion more frequently than once monthly. Rate of infusion for all uses: 0.01 to 0.02 mL/kg/min for the first 30 min; if no distress is noted, the rate may be increased to 0.04 mL/kg/min. Higher rates may be used if tolerated. The drug can be given sequentially into a primary IV line containing normal saline; it is not compatible with 5% dextrose solution.

ITP.

Induction: Up to 2,000 mg/kg for 2 to 7 consecutive days; those who respond to induction therapy (platelet count of 30,000/mm³–50,000/mm³) may be discontinued after two to seven daily doses. **Maintenance:** Single infusion of 2,000 mg/kg q 2 weeks, as needed to maintain a platelet count of 30,000/mm³ in children and 20,000/mm³ in adults or to prevent bleeding episodes between infusions.

VENOGLOBULIN-S

Immunodeficiency disease.

200 mg/kg/month; can increase to 300–400 mg/kg if response is insufficient or can repeat infusion more frequently than once monthly. Rate of infusion for all uses: Initially, 0.01–0.02 mL/kg/min or 1.2 mL/kg/hr for the first 30 min. If no discomfort is noted, the rate for the 5% solution may be increased to 0.04 mL/kg/min or 2.4 mL/kg/hr and the rate for the 10% solution may be increased to 0.05 mL/kg/min or 3 mL/kg/hr.

ITP.

Induction: 2,000 mg/kg over a maximum of 5 days. **Maintenance:** 1,000 mg/kg as needed to maintain platelet counts of 30,000/mm³ for children and 20,000/mm³ for adults or to prevent bleeding episodes between infusions.

How Supplied: *Injection:* 50 mg/mL, 100 mg/mL; *Powder for injection:* 1 g, 2.5 g, 3 g, 5 g, 6 g, 10 g, 12 g

Side Effects: *CNS:* Headache, malaise, feeling of faintness. Aseptic meningitis syndrome, including symptoms of severe headache, nuchal rigidity, drowsiness, fever, photophobia, painful eye movements, N&V. *Allergic:* Hypersensitivity or ***anaphylactic reactions.*** *Body as a whole:* Fever, chills. *GI:* Headache, nausea, vomiting. *Miscellaneous:* Chest tightness, dyspnea; chest, back, or hip pain; mild erythema following infiltration; burning sensation in the head; tachycardia.

Agammaglobulinemic and hypogammaglobulinemic patients never having received immunoglobulin therapy or where the time from the last treatment is more than 8 weeks may manifest side effects if the infusion rate exceeds 1 mL/min. Symptoms include flushing of the face, hypotension, tightness in chest, chills, fever, dizziness, diaphoresis, and nausea.

EMS CONSIDERATIONS

None.

Indapamide
(in-DAP-ah-myd)
Pregnancy Class: B
Lozol **(Rx)**
Classification: Diuretic, thiazide type

Onset of Action: 1-2 weeks after multiple doses.

Duration of Action: Up to 8 weeks with multiple doses.

Uses: Alone or in combination with other drugs for treatment of hypertension. Edema in CHF.

Precautions: Dosage has not been established in children. Geriatric patients may be more sensitive to the hypotensive and electrolyte effects.

Route/Dosage
• **Tablets**
  Edema of CHF.
Adults: 2.5 mg as a single dose in the morning. If necessary, may be increased to 5 mg/day after 1 week.
  Hypertension.
Adults: 1.25 mg as a single dose in the morning. If the response is not sat-

isfactory after 4 weeks, the dose may be increased to 2.5 mg taken once daily. If the response to 2.5 mg is not satisfactory after 4 weeks, the dose may be increased to 5 mg taken once daily (however, consideration should be given to adding another antihypertensive).

How Supplied: *Tablet:* 1.25 mg, 2.5 mg

EMS CONSIDERATIONS

See also *Diuretics, Thiazide.*

Indinavir sulfate

(in-DIN-ah-veer)
Pregnancy Class: C
Crixivan **(Rx)**
Classification: Antiviral drug, protease inhibitor

Mechanism of Action: Binds to active sites on the HIV protease enzyme resulting in inhibition of enzyme activity. Inhibition prevents cleavage of the viral polyproteins resulting in the formation of immature noninfectious viral particles. Varying degrees of cross resistance have been noted between indinavir and other HIV-protease inhibitors.

Uses: Treatment of HIV infection in adults when antiretroviral therapy is indicated. May be used with other anti-HIV drugs.

Contraindications: Lactation. Use with astemizole, cisapride, midazolam, rifampin, terfenadine, and triazolam. Mild to moderate liver or kidney disease.

Precautions: Not a cure for HIV infections; patients may continue to develop opportunistic infections and other complications of HIV disease. Not been shown to reduce the risk of transmission of HIV through sexual contact or blood contamination. No data on the effect of indinavir therapy on clinical progression of HIV infection, including survival or the incidence of opportunistic infections. Hemophiliacs treated for HIV infections with protease inhibitors may manifest spontaneous bleeding epi-

sodes. Safety and efficacy have not been determined in children.

Route/Dosage
• **Capsules**
HIV infections.
Adults: 800 mg (two 400-mg capsules) q 8 hr ATC. The dosage is the same whether the drug is used alone or in combination with other retroviral agents. Reduce the dose to 600 mg q 8 hr with mild to moderate hepatic insufficiency due to cirrhosis.

How Supplied: *Capsules:* 200 mg, 400 mg.

Side Effects: *GI:* N&V, diarrhea, abdominal pain, abdominal distention, acid regurgitation, anorexia, dry mouth, aphthous stomatitis, cheilitis, cholecystitis, cholestasis, constipation, dyspepsia, eructation, flatulence, gastritis, gingivitis, glossodynia, gingival hemorrhage, increased appetite, infectious gastroenteritis, jaundice, liver cirrhosis. *CNS:* Headache, insomnia, dizziness, somnolence, agitation, anxiety, bruxism, decreased mental acuity, depression, dream abnormality, dysesthesia, excitement, fasciculation, hypesthesia, nervousness, neuralgia, neurotic disorder, paresthesia, peripheral neuropathy, sleep disorder, tremor, vertigo. *CV:* CV disorder, palpitation. *Musculoskeletal:* Back pain, arthralgia, leg pain, myalgia, muscle cramps, muscle weakness, musculoskeletal pain, shoulder pain, stiffness. *Body as a whole:* Asthenia, fatigue, flank pain, malaise, chest pain, chills, fever, flu-like illness, fungal infection, malaise, pain, syncope. *Hematologic:* Anemia, lymphadenopathy, spleen disorder. *Respiratory:* Cough, dyspnea, halitosis, pharyngeal hyperemia, pharyngitis, pneumonia, rales, rhonchi, ***respiratory failure,*** sinus disorder, sinusitis, URI. *Dermatologic:* Body odor, contact dermatitis, dermatitis, dry skin, flushing, folliculitis, herpes simplex, herpes zoster, night sweats, pruritus, seborrhea, skin disorder, skin infection, sweating, urticaria. *GU:* Nephrolithiasis, dysuria, hematuria, hydro-

---

bold italic = life threatening side effect

nephrosis, nocturia, PMS, proteinuria, renal colic, urinary frequency, UTI, uterine abnormality, urine sediment abnormality, urolithiasis. *Ophthalmic:* Accommodation disorder, blurred vision, eye pain, eye swelling, orbital edema. *Miscellaneous:* Asymptomatic hyperbilirubinemia, food allergy, taste disorder.

Drug Interactions

Astemizole / ↓ Metabolism of astemizole → possibility of cardiac arrhythmias and prolonged sedation

Cisapride / ↓ Metabolism of cisapride → possibility of cardiac arrhythmias and prolonged sedation

Clarithromycin / ↑ Plasma levels of both indinavir and clarithromycin

Didanosine / pH Dependent ↓ in absorption

Fluconazole / ↓ Plasma levels of indinavir

Isoniazid / ↑ Plasma levels of isoniazid

Ketoconazole / ↑ Plasma levels of indinavir

Midazolam / ↓ Metabolism of midazolam → possibility of cardiac arrhythmias and prolonged sedation

Oral contraceptives / ↑ Plasma levels of both estrogen and progestin components of the oral contraceptive product

Quinidine / ↑ Plasma levels of indinavir

Rifabutin / ↑ Plasma levels of rifabutin; ↓ dose by 50%

Rifampin / ↓ Plasma levels of indinavir

Stavudine / ↑ Plasma levels of stavudine

Terfenadine / ↓ Metabolism of terfenadine → possibility of cardiac arrhythmias and prolonged sedation

Triazolam / ↓ Metabolism of triazolam → possibility of cardiac arrhythmias and prolonged sedation

Trimethoprim/Sulfamethoxazole / ↑ Plasma levels of trimethoprim (no change in levels of sulfamethoxazole

AZT / ↑ Plasma levels of both indinavir and AZT

EMS CONSIDERATIONS

See also *Antiviral Drugs.*

Indomethacin
Indomethacin sodium trihydrate
(in-dah-METH-ah-sin)

Indomethacin (Indochron E-R **(Rx)**)
Indomethacin sodium trihydrate (Indocin I.V. **(Rx)**)
Classification: Nonsteroidal antiinflammatory drug, analgesic, antipyretic

Onset of Action: PO: 30 min for analgesia and up to 1 week for antiinflammatory effect.**Peak action for gout:** 24-36 hr; swelling gradually disappears in 3-5 days. **Peak activity for antirheumatic effect:** About 4 weeks.

Duration of Action: 4-6 hr for analgesia and 1-2 weeks for anti-inflammatory effect.

Uses: Not a simple analgesic; use only for the conditions listed. Moderate to severe rheumatoid arthritis, osteoarthritis, and ankylosing spondylitis (drug of choice). Acute gouty arthritis and acute painful shoulder (tendinitis, bursitis). *IV:* Pharmacologic closure of persistent patent ductus arteriosus in premature infants. *Investigational:* Topically to treat cystoid macular edema (0.5% and 1% drops), sunburn, primary dysmenorrhea, prophylaxis of migraine, cluster headache, polyhydramnios.

Contraindications: Additional: Pregnancy and lactation. PO indomethacin in children under 14 years of age. GI lesions or history of recurrent GI lesions. *IV use:* GI or intracranial bleeding, thrombocytopenia, renal disease, defects of coagulation, necrotizing enterocolitis. *Suppositories:* Recent rectal bleeding, history of proctitis.

Precautions: Restrict use in children to those unresponsive to or intolerant of other anti-inflammatory agents; efficacy has not been determined in children less than 14 years of age. Geriatric patients are at greater risk of developing CNS side effects, especially confusion. Use with caution in patients with history of epilepsy, psychiatric illness, or parkinsonism and in the elderly. Use with extreme caution in the presence of existing, controlled infections.

Route/Dosage

• **Capsules, Oral Suspension**

Moderate to severe arthritis, osteoarthritis, ankylosing spondylitis.

Adults, initial: 25 mg b.i.d.–t.i.d.; may be increased by 25–50 mg at weekly intervals, according to condition and, if tolerated, until satisfactory response is obtained. With persistent night pain or morning stiffness, a maximum of 100 mg of the total daily dose can be given at bedtime. **Maximum daily dosage:** 150–200 mg. In acute flares of chronic rheumatoid arthritis, the dose may need to be increased by 25–50 mg/day until the acute phase is under control.

Acute gouty arthritis.

Adults, initial: 50 mg t.i.d. until pain is tolerable; **then,** reduce dosage rapidly until drug is withdrawn. Pain relief usually occurs within 2–4 hr, tenderness and heat subside in 24–36 hr, and swelling disappears in 3–4 days.

Acute painful shoulder (bursitis/tendinitis).

75–150 mg/day in three to four divided doses for 1–2 weeks.

• **Sustained-Release Capsules**

Antirheumatic, anti-inflammatory.

Adults: 75 mg, of which 25 mg is released immediately, 1–2 times/day.

• **Suppositories**

Anti-inflammatory, antirheumatic, antigout.

Adults: 50 mg up to q.i.d. **Pediatric:** 1.5–2.5 mg/kg/day in three to four divided doses (up to a maximum of 4 mg/kg or 250–300 mg/day, whichever is less).

How Supplied: Indomethacin: *Capsule:* 25 mg, 50 mg; *Capsule, Extended Release:* 75 mg; *Suppository:* 50 mg; *Suspension:* 25 mg/5 mL Indomethacin sodium trihydrate: *Powder for injection:* 1 mg

Side Effects: Additional: Reactivation of latent infections may mask signs of infection. More marked CNS mani-

festations than for other drugs of this group. Aggravation of depression or other psychiatric problems, epilepsy, and parkinsonism.

Drug Interactions: Additional: *Captopril/* Indomethacin ↓ effect of captopril, probably due to inhibition of prostaglandin synthesis.*Diflunisal/* ↑ Plasma levels of indomethacin; also, possible fatal GI hemorrhage.*Diuretics (loop, potassium-sparing, thiazide)/* Indomethacin may reduce the antihypertensive and natriuretic action of diuretics.*Lisinopril/* Possible ↓ effect of lisinopril.*Prazosin/* Indomethacin ↓ antihypertensive effects of prazosin.

EMS CONSIDERATIONS

See also *Nonsteroidal Anti-Inflammatory Drugs.*

Insulin injection (crystalline zinc insulin, unmodified insulin, regular insulin)

(IN-sue-lin)

Pork: Regular Iletin II, Regular Purified Pork Insulin, **Beef/Pork:** Regular Iletin I, **Human:** Novolin R, Novolin R PenFill, Novolin R Prefilled, Velosulin Human BR **(OTC)**

Classification: Rapid-acting insulin

Mechanism of Action: Rarely administered as the sole agent due to its short duration of action. Injections of 100 units/mL are clear; cloudy, colored solutions should not be used. Regular insulin is the only preparation suitable for IV administration. Available only as 100 units/mL. *Note:* Regular beef/pork insulins are being phased out.

Onset of Action: SC: 30-60 min; **IV:** 10-30 min; **Peak, SC:** 2-4 hr; **IV:** 15-30 min.

Duration of Action: SC: 6-8 hr; **IV:** 30-60 min.

Uses: Suitable for treatment of diabetic coma, diabetic acidosis, or other emergency situations. Especially suitable for the patient suffering from la-

---

bold italic = life threatening side effect

bile diabetes. During acute phase of diabetic acidosis or for the patient in diabetic crisis, patient is monitored by serum glucose and serum ketone levels.

Route/Dosage
• **SC**
   Diabetes.
Adults, individualized, usual, initial: 5–10 units; **pediatric:** 2–4 units. Injection is given 15–30 min before meals and at bedtime.
   Diabetic ketoacidosis.
Adults: 0.1 unit/kg/hr given by continuous IV infusion.
How Supplied: *Injection:* 100 U/mL

EMS CONSIDERATIONS
See also *Insulins.*

Insulin injection, concentrated

(IN-sue-lin)
Pregnancy Class: C
Regular (Concentrated) Iletin II U-500 **(Rx)**
Classification: Insulin, concentrated

Mechanism of Action: Concentrated insulin injection (500 U/mL). Depending on response, may be given SC or IM as a single or as two or three divided doses.
Uses: Insulin resistance requiring more than 200 units insulin/day.
Contraindications: Allergy to pork or mixed pork/beef insulin (unless patient has been desensitized). IV use due to possible allergic or anaphylactoid reactions.
Precautions: Use with caution during lactation.

Route/Dosage
• **SC, IM**
   Individualized, depending on severity of condition. Patients must be kept under close observation until dosage is established.
How Supplied: *Injection:* 500 U/mL
Side Effects: Additional: Deep secondary hypoglycemia 18-24 hr after administration.
Drug Interactions: Do not use together with PO hypoglycemic agents.

EMS CONSIDERATIONS
See also *Insulins.*

Insulin lispro injection (rDNA origin)

(IN-sue-lin LYE-sproh)
Pregnancy Class: B
Humalog **(Rx)**
Classification: Insulin, rDNA origin

Mechanism of Action: Rapid-acting insulin derived from *Escherichia coli* that has been genetically altered by the addition of the gene for insulin lispro. Is a human insulin analog created when the amino acids at positions 28 and 29 on the insulin B-chain are reversed. Absorbed faster than regular human insulin. Compared with regular insulin, has a more rapid onset of glucose-lowering activity, an earlier peak for glucose lowering, and a shorter duration of glucose-lowering activity. However, is equipotent to human regular insulin (i.e., one unit of insulin lispro has the same glucose-lowering capacity as one unit of regular insulin). May lower the risk of nocturnal hypoglycemia in patients with type I diabetes.
Onset of Action: 15 min; **Peak effect:** 30-90 min.
Duration of Action: 5 hr or less.
Uses: Diabetes mellitus.
Contraindications: Use during episodes of hypoglycemia. Hypersensitivity to insulin lispro.
Precautions: Since insulin lispro has a more rapid onset and shorter duration of action than regular insulin, patients with type I diabetes also require a longer acting insulin to maintain glucose control. Requirements may be decreased in impaired renal or hepatic function. Use with caution during lactation. Safety and efficacy have not been determined in children less than 12 years of age.

Route/Dosage
• **SC**
   Diabetes.
Individualized, depending on severity of the condition.
How Supplied: *Injection:* 100 U/mL

Side Effects: See *Insulins*.
Drug Interactions: See *Insulins*.

EMS CONSIDERATIONS

See also *Insulins*.

Insulin zinc suspension (Lente)

(IN-sue-lin)
Pork: Lente Iletin II, Lente L,
Beef/Pork: Lentin Iletin I, **Human:** Humulin L, Novolin L **(OTC)**
Classification: Intermediate-acting insulin

Mechanism of Action: Contains 70% crystalline and 30% amorphous insulin suspension. Considered intermediate-acting. Principal advantage is the absence of a sensitizing agent such as protamine. *Note:* Lente beef/pork insulins are being phased out.
Onset of Action: 1–2.5 hr; **Peak:** 7–15 hr.
Duration of Action: About 22 hr.
Uses: Allergy to other types of insulin and in patients disposed to thrombotic phenomena in which protamine may be a factor. Not a replacement for regular insulin and is not suitable for emergency use.

Route/Dosage
• **SC**
  Diabetes.
Adults, initial: 7–26 units 30–60 min before breakfast. Dosage is then increased by daily or weekly increments of 2–10 units until satisfactory readjustment is established. A second smaller dose may be given prior to the evening meal or at bedtime. Patients on NPH can be transferred to insulin zinc suspension on a unit-for-unit basis. Patients being transferred from regular insulin should begin zinc insulin at two-thirds to three-fourths the regular insulin dosage. If the patient is being transferred from protamine zinc insulin, the dose of zinc insulin should be about 50% of that required for protamine zinc insulin.
How Supplied: *Injection:* 100 U/mL

EMS CONSIDERATIONS

See also *Insulins*

Insulin zinc suspension, extended (Ultralente)

(IN-sue-lin)
Humulin U Ultralente **(OTC)**
Classification: Long-acting insulin

Mechanism of Action: Large crystals of insulin and a high content of zinc are responsible for the slow-acting properties of this preparation.
Onset of Action: 4–8 hr; **Peak:** 10–30 hr.
Duration of Action: 36 hr or longer.
Uses: Mild to moderate hyperglycemia in stabilized diabetics.
Contraindications: Use to treat diabetic coma or emergency situations

Route/Dosage
• **SC**
  Individualized.
Usual, initial: 7–26 units as a single dose 30–60 min before breakfast.
Do not administer IV.
How Supplied: *Injection:* 100 U/mL

EMS CONSIDERATIONS

See also *Insulin*.

Interferon alfa-2a recombinant (rI FN-A; IFLrA)

(in-ter-FEER-on AL-fah)
Pregnancy Class: C
Roferon-A **(Rx)**
Classification: Antineoplastic, miscellaneous agent

Mechanism of Action: Interferon alfa-2a is the product of recombinant DNA technology using strains of genetically engineered *Escherichia coli*. Activity is expressed as International Units, which are determined by comparing the antiviral activity of recombinant interferons with the activity of the international reference standard of human leukocyte interferon. Interferons bind to specific receptors on the cell sur-

---

bold italic = life threatening side effect

face, resulting in inhibition of virus replication in virus-infected cells, suppression of cell proliferation, increase in the phagocytic activity of macrophages, and enhancement of the toxic effects of leukocytes for target cells.

Uses: Hairy cell leukemia in patients older than 18 years of age. Can be used in splenectomized and nonsplenectomized patients. AIDS-related Kaposi's sarcoma in patients older than 18 years of age. Chronic myelogenous leukemia. Chronic hepatitis C. *Investigational:* The drug has been used for a large number of other conditions. Significant activity has been noted against the following neoplastic diseases: locally for superficial bladder tumors, carcinoid tumor, cutaneous T-cell lymphoma, essential thrombocythemia, low-grade non-Hodgkin's lymphoma. Limited activity has been noted in acute leukemias, cervical carcinoma, chronic lymphocytic leukemia, Hodgkin's disease, malignant gliomas, melanoma, multiple myeloma, mycosis fungoides/Sézary syndrome, nasopharyngeal carcinoma, osteosarcoma, ovarian carcinoma, renal carcinoma. Interferon alfa-2a also has significant activity against the following viral infections: chronic non-A, non-B hepatitis, condylomata acuminata, cutaneous warts, cytomegaloviruses, herpes keratoconjunctivitis; limited activity is seen against herpes simplex, HIV infection to slow progression, papillomaviruses, rhinoviruses, vaccinia virus, varicella zoster, and viral hepatitis B.

Contraindications: Lactation.
Precautions: Use with caution in patients with a history of unstable angina, uncontrolled CHF, COPD, diabetes mellitus prone to ketoacidosis, thrombophlebitis, pulmonary embolism, seizure disorders, severe renal and hepatic disease, compromised CNS function, and severe myelosuppression. Safety and efficacy in individuals less than 18 years of age have not been established.

Route/Dosage
• **IM, SC**

Hairy cell leukemia.
Induction: 3 million IU/day for 16–24 weeks; **maintenance,** 3 million IU 3 times/week. Doses higher than 3 million IU are not recommended.
AIDS-related Kaposi's sarcoma.
Induction: 36 million IU/day for 10–12 weeks; or, 3 million IU/day on days 1–3; 9 million IU/day on days 4–6; and 18 million IU/day on days 7–9 followed by 36 million IU/day for the remainder of the 10 to 12-week induction period. **Maintenance:** 36 million IU 3 times/week. If severe side effects occur, the dose can be withheld or reduced by one-half.
Chronic myelogenous leukemia.
Induction: 9 million IU/day. The dose can be graded during the first week of therapy to improve short-term tolerance by giving 3 million IU/day for 3 days to 6 million IU/day for 3 days and then to the target dose of 9 million IU/day. **Maintenance:** Optimal dose and duration of therapy have not been determined. Continue the regimen until the disease progresses.
Chronic hepatitis C.
3 million IU, SC or IM, 3 times/week for 12 months.

How Supplied: *Injection:* 3 million IU/0.5 mL, 3 million IU/mL, 6 million IU/0.5 mL, 6 million IU/mL, 9 million IU/0.5 mL, 9 million IU/0.9 mL, 36 million IU/mL

Side Effects: *Flu-like symptoms:* Fever, headache, fatigue, arthralgia, myalgias, chills, weight loss, dizziness. *CV:* Hypotension, **arrhythmias,** syncope, hypertension, edema, palpitations, transient ischemic attacks, pulmonary edema, CHF, cardiac murmur, **MI, stroke, cardiomyopathy,** hot flashes, Raynaud's phenomenon, thrombophlebitis. *Respiratory:* Coughing, dyspnea, dryness or inflammation of oropharynx, chest pain or congestion, **bronchospasm,** pneumonia, tachypnea, rhinitis, rhinorrhea, sinusitis. *CNS:* Depression, confusion, dizziness, headache, paresthesia, anxiety, ataxia, aphasia, aphonia, dysarthria, amnesia, weakness, nervousness, emotional lability, impotence, numbness, lethargy, sleep disturbances, visual disturbances, vertigo, decreased mental status, memory loss, disturbances of libido, involuntary movements, *suicidal ideation, seizures,* forgetfulness, neuropathy, tremor. *GI:* Anorexia, N&V, diarrhea, emesis, abdominal pain, hypermotility, abdominal fullness, abdominal pain, flatulence, constipation, gastric distress. *Hematologic:* Thrombocytopenia, neutropenia, leukopenia, decreased hemoglobin, severe anemia, severe cytopenias, coagulopathy, Coombs' positive hemolytic anemia, aplastic anemia. *Musculoskeletal:* Joint or bone pain, arthritis, polyarthritis, poor coordination, muscle contractions, gait disturbances. *Dermatologic:* Rash, pruritus, dry skin, ecchymosis, petechiae, skin flushing, alopecia, urticaria, diaphoresis, cyanosis, bruising. *Miscellaneous:* Generalized pain, back pain, inflammation at injection site, epistaxis, bleeding gums, weight loss, alteration of taste, altered hearing, edema, night sweats, earache, eye irritation, hypothyroidism, hypertriglyceridemia.

Drug Interactions

Interleukin-2 / ↑ Risk of renal failure

Theophylline / ↓ Clearance of theophylline

EMS CONSIDERATIONS

None.

Interferon alfa-2b recombinant (rI FN-α2; α-2-interferon)

(in-ter-FEER-on AL-fah)
Pregnancy Class: C
Intron A **(Rx)**
Classification: Antineoplastic, miscellaneous agent

Mechanism of Action: A product of recombinant DNA technology using strains of genetically engineered *Escherichia coli.* The activity is expressed as International Units, which are determined by comparing the antiviral activity of the recombinant interferon with the activity of the international reference standard of human leukocyte interferon. Interferons bind to specific receptors on the cell surface, resulting in inhibition of virus replication in virus-infected cells, suppression of cell proliferation, increase in the phagocytic activity of macrophages, and enhancement of the toxic effects of leukocytes for target cells.

Uses: Hairy cell leukemia in patients older than 18 years of age (in both splenectomized and nonsplenectomized patients). Intralesional use for genital or venereal warts (*Condylomata acuminata.*) AIDS-related Kaposi's sarcoma in patients over 18 years of age. Chronic hepatitis C in patients at least 18 years of age with compensated liver disease and a history of blood or blood product exposure or who are HCV antibody positive. Chronic hepatitis B in patients over 18 years of age with compensated liver disease and HBV replication (patients must be serum HBsAg positive for at least 6 months and have HBV replication with elevated serum ALT). Adjunct therapy for malignant melanoma in those who are 18 years of age or older who are free of the disease but at a high risk for recurrence within 56 days of surgery. With an anthracycline drug for the initial treatment of clinically aggressive non-Hodgkin's lymphoma.

Investigational: The drug has been used for a large number of conditions. Significant activity has been noted against the following neoplastic diseases: locally for superficial bladder tumors, carcinoid tumor, chronic myelogenous leukemia, cutaneous T-cell lymphoma, essential thrombocythemia, low-grade non-Hodgkin's lymphoma, and chronic granulocytic leukemia. Limited activity has been noted in acute leukemias, cervical carcinoma, chronic lymphocytic leukemia, Hodgkin's disease, malignant gliomas, melanoma, multiple myeloma, nasopharyngeal carcinoma, osteosarcoma, ovarian carcinoma, renal carcinoma, and chronic granulomatous disease. Interferon alfa-2b has also been used to treat the following viral infections: Significant activity has been seen against cutaneous warts, CMVs, herpes keratoconjunctivitis, and herpes simplex. Limited activity has been noted against papillomaviruses, rhinoviruses, vaccinia virus, varicella zoster, and HIV (used with foscarnet/AZT). It has also been used to treat multiple sclerosis.

Contraindications: Lactation. Use to treat rapidly progressive visceral disease in AIDS-related Kaposi's sarcoma. Use in patients with decompensated liver disease, autoimmune hepatitis, history of autoimmune disease, or immunosuppressed transplant patients.

Precautions: Use with caution in patients with a history of unstable angina, uncontrolled CHF, COPD, diabetes mellitus prone to ketoacidosis, thrombophlebitis, pulmonary embolism, seizure disorders, severe renal and hepatic disease, compromised CNS function, and severe myelosuppression. Safety and efficacy in individuals less than 18 years of age have not been established.

Route/Dosage

• **IM, SC**

Hairy cell leukemia.
2 million IU/m² 3 times/week. Higher doses are not recommended. May require 6 or more months of therapy for improvement. Do not use the 50-million-IU strength of the powder for injection for treating hairy cell leukemia.

AIDS-related Kaposi's sarcoma
30 million IU/m² 3 times/week SC or IM using only the 50-million-IU vial. Using this dose, patients should tolerate an average dose of 110 million IU/week at the end of 12 weeks of therapy and 75 million IU/week at the end of 24 weeks of therapy.

Chronic hepatitis C.
3 million IU 3 times/week for 16 weeks. At 16 weeks, extend treatment to 18 to 24 months at 3 million IU 3 times/week to improve the sustained response of normalization of

ALT. Discontinue therapy if there is no response after 16 weeks.

Chronic hepatitis B.
30–35 million IU/week SC or IM, given as either 5 million IU/day or 10 million IU 3 times/week for 16 weeks. If serious side effects occur, the dose may be decreased by 50%.

• **IV**

Malignant melanoma.
20 million IU/m² IV on 5 consecutive days/week for 4 weeks. **Maintenance:** 10 million IU/m² SC 3 times/week for 48 weeks.

• **Intralesional**

Condylomata acuminata (genital or venereal warts).
1 million IU/lesion 3 times/week for 3 weeks. For this purpose, use only the vial containing 10 million units and reconstitute using no more than 1 mL diluent. To reduce side effects, give in the evening with acetaminophen. Maximum response usually occurs within 4–8 weeks. If results are unsatisfactory after 12–16 weeks, a second course may be started.

How Supplied: *Solution for Injection:* 3 million IU/0.2 mL, 3 million IU/0.5 mL, 5 million IU/0.2 mL, 5 million IU/0.5 mL, 6 million IU/mL, 10 million IU/0.2 mL, 10 million IU/0.5 mL; *Kit:* 3 million IU/0.5 mL, 5 million IU/0.5 mL, 10 million IU/mL; *Powder for injection:* 3 million IU, 5 million IU, 10 million IU, 18 million IU, 25 million IU, 50 million IU

Side Effects: *Flu-like symptoms:* Fever, headache, fatigue, myalgia, chills. *CV:* Hypotension, *arrhythmias,* tachycardia, syncope, hypertension, coagulation disorders, chest pain, palpitations, flushing, atrial fibrillation, bradycardia, *cardiac failure, cardiomyopathy,* extrasystoles, postural hypotension. *CNS:* Depression, confusion, somnolence, migraine, dizziness, ataxia, insomnia, irritability, paresthesia, anxiety, nervousness, emotional lability, amnesia, impaired concentration, weakness, tremor, syncope, abnormal coordination, hypoesthesia, hypesthesia, abnormal coordination, aggravated depression, aggressive reaction, hypertonia, hypokinesia, impaired consciousness, neuropathy, agitation, apathy, aphasia, dysphonia, extrapyramidal disorder, hot flashes, hyperesthesia, hyperkinesia, neurosis, paresis, paroniria, parosmia, personality disorder, *seizures, coma,* polyneuropathy, *suicide attempt. GI:* N&V, diarrhea, stomatitis, weight loss, anorexia, flatulence, thirst, dehydration, constipation, eructation, abdominal pain, loose stools, abdominal distention, dysphagia, esophagitis, gastric ulcer, *GI hemorrhage,* GI mucosal discoloration, gum hyperplasia, gingival bleeding, gingivitis, increased saliva, increased appetite, melena, oral leukoplakia, rectal bleeding after stool, *rectal hemorrhage,* ulcerative stomatitis, ascites, gallstones, gastroenteritis, halitosis. *Hematologic:* Thrombocytopenia, granulocytopenia, anemia, *hemolytic anemia,* leukopenia. *Musculoskeletal:* Arthralgia, leg cramps, asthenia, arthrosis, arthritis, muscle pain or weakness, back pain, bone pain, rigors, CTS. *Respiratory:* Pharyngitis, coughing, dyspnea, sinusitis, rhinitis, epistaxis, nasal congestion, dry mouth, *bronchospasm,* pleural pain, pneumonia, rhinorrhea, sneezing, wheezing, bronchitis, cyanosis, lung fibrosis. *EENT:* Alteration or loss of taste, tinnitus, hearing disorders, conjunctivitis, photophobia, vision disorders, eye pain, diplopia, dry eyes, earache, lacrimal gland disorder, periorbital edema, vertigo, speech disorder. *Dermatologic:* Rash, pruritus, alopecia, urticaria, dry skin, dermatitis, purpura, photosensitivity, acne, nail disorder, facial edema, moniliasis, reaction at injection site, abnormal hair texture, cold/clammy skin, cyanosis of the hand, epidermal necrolysis, dermatitis lichenoides, furunculosis, increased hair growth, erythema, melanosis, nonherpetic cold sores, peripheral ischemia, skin depigmentation or discoloration, vitiligo, folliculitis, lipoma, psoriasis. *GU:* Amenorrhea, hematuria, impotence, leukorrhea, menorrhagia, urinary frequency, nocturia, polyuria, uterine bleeding, increased BUN, in-

continence, pelvic pain. *Endocrine:* Gynecomastia, thyroid disorder, aggravation of diabetes mellitus, virilism. *Hepatic:* Jaundice, upper right quadrant pain, *hepatic encephalopathy, hepatic failure. Other:* Pain, increased sweating, malaise, decreased libido, herpes simplex, lymphadenopathy, chest pain, abscess, cachexia, hypercalcemia, peripheral edema, stye, substernal chest pain, weakness, sepsis, dehydration, fungal infection, herpes zoster, viral infection, trichomoniasis.

Drug Interactions
Aminophylline / ↓ Clearance of aminophylline due to ↓ breakdown by the liver
AZT / ↑ Risk of neutropenia

EMS CONSIDERATIONS
None.

Interferon alfacon-1
(in-ter-FEER-on AL-fah-kon)
Pregnancy Class: C
Infergen **(Rx)**
Classification: Drug for chronic hepatitis

Mechanism of Action: Prepared by recombinant technology. Has antiviral, antiproliferative, and immunomodulatory effects.

Uses: Treatment of chronic hepatitis C infections in those over 18 years of age with compensated liver disease. *Investigational:* With G-CSF therapy to treat hairy-cell leukemia.

Contraindications: Hypersensitivity to alpha interferons or to products derived from *E. coli*. Use in autoimmune hepatitis or in decompensated hepatic disease.

Precautions: Use with caution during lactation and in preexisting cardiac disease, in depression, in those with abnormally low peripheral blood cell counts, in those receiving myelosuppressive agents, and in autoimmune disorder. Safety and efficacy have not been determined in children less than 18 years of age.

Route/Dosage

• **SC Injection**

Chronic hepatitis C infection.

Adults over 18 years of age: 9 mcg SC as a single injection three times a week for 24 weeks. At least 48 hr should elapse between doses. Those who tolerate therapy but did not respond or relapsed following discontinuation may be subsequently treated with 15 mcg three times a week for 6 months.

How Supplied: *Injection:* 30 mcg/mL

Side Effects: *Flu-like symptoms:* Headache, fatigue, fever, myalgia, rigors, arthralgia, increased sweating. *Body as a whole:* Body pain, hot flushes, non-cardiac chest pain, malaise, asthenia, peripheral edema, access pain, allergic reactions, weight loss. *Hypersensitivity:* Urticaria, angioedema, bronchoconstriction, **anaphylaxis.** *CNS:* Insomnia, dizziness, paresthesia, amnesia, hypoesthesia, hypertonia, nervousness, depression, anxiety, emotional lability, abnormal thinking, agitation, decreased libido. *GI:* Abdominal pain, N&V, diarrhea, anorexia, dyspepsia, constipation, flatulence, toothache, hemorrhoids, decreased saliva, tender liver. *CV:* Hypertension, palpitation. *Hematologic:* Granulocytopenia, thrombocytopenia, leukopenia, ecchymosis, lymphadenopathy, lymphocytosis. *Respiratory:* Pharyngitis, URI, cough, sinusitis, rhinitis, respiratory tract congestion, upper respiratory tract congestion, epistaxis, dyspnea, bronchitis. *Dermatologic:* Alopecia, pruritus, rash, erythema, dry skin. *Musculoskeletal:* Back, limb, neck, or skeletal pain. *GU:* Dysmenorrhea, vaginitis, menstrual disorder. *Ophthalmic:* Conjunctivitis, eye pain. *Otic:* Tinnitus, earache.

EMS CONSIDERATIONS

See also *Interferon alfa-2a* and *Interferon alfa-*2b, .

Interferon alfa-n1 lymphoblastoid

(in-ter-FEER-on AL-fah)

Pregnancy Class: C

Wellferon (Rx)

Classification: Interferon for hepatitis C

Mechanism of Action: A mixture of alpha interferons isolated from a human cell line. Natural alpha interferons are derived from leukocytes. They bind to a high-affinity type I receptor and produce immunomodulatory, antiviral, and antiproliferative effects. After binding to the cell membrane, interferon initiates a complex sequence of intracellular events that cause induction of certain enzymes, inhibition of virus replication, suppression of cell proliferation, enhancement of macrophage phagocytic activity, and enhancement of lymphocyte cytotoxicity. The mechanism in the treatment of chronic hepatitis C is not known.

Uses: Treatment of chronic hepatitis C in patients 18 years and older without decompensated liver disease.

Contraindications: Hypersensitivity to alpha interferons, history of anaphylaxis to bovine or ovine immunoglobulins, egg protein, polymyxin B, or neomycin sulfate. Use in patients with decompensated liver disease or autoimmune hepatitis because of the potential for worsening of disease symptoms. Lactation.

Precautions: Use with caution in the elderly; in preexisting cardiac disease; clinically significant, preexisting depressive disorders; severe, preexisting autoimmune, renal, or hepatic disease; seizure disorders or compromised CNS function; leukopenia or thrombocytopenia or in those receiving myelosuppressive drugs; pulmonary dysfunction, including unstable asthma or other conditions. Safety and efficacy have not been determined in children.

Route/Dosage

• **IM, SC**

Chronic hepatitis C virus.

Adults: 3 MU SC or IM 3 times a week for 48 weeks.

How Supplied: *Solution:* 3 MU/mL

Side Effects: *Flu-like symptoms:* Asthenia, headache, fever, myalgia, chills, nausea. *GI:* Nausea, diarrhea, abdominal pain, anorexia, vomiting, weight loss, cholecystitis, abnormal liver function, liver tenderness, hepatotoxicity, peritonitis, ruptured spleen. *CNS:* Nervousness, agitation, hostility, emotional lability, insomnia, somnolence, sleep disorder, depression, dizziness (including vertigo), confusion, abnormal thinking, amnesia, paresthesia, convulsions, hallucinations, migraine, suicidal ideation/attempts, decrease in mental status, dizziness, impaired memory, manic behavor, psychotic reactions. *Hematologic:* Thrombocytopenia, decreased WBC count and absolute neutrophil count, leukopenia, myelosuppression, leukocytosis. *CV:* Arrhythmia, angina, hypotension, hypertension, myocardial ischemia, atrial fibrillation. *Hypersensitivity:* Urticaria, angioedema, ***bronchoconstriction, anaphylaxis.*** *Respiratory:* Cough, bronchitis, dyspnea, pneumonia, rhinitis, pharyngitis; respiratory, lung, and pleural disorders. *Musculoskeletal:* Myalgia, arthralgia. *Dermatologic:* Alopecia, rash, pruritus, dry skin, urticaria, sweating, herpes simplex, photosensitivity, psoriasis, worsening of cellulitis and dermatitis. *GU:* Abnormal ejaculation, UTI, decreased libido, menstrual irregularities, renal hemorrhage. *Endocrine:* Thyroid carcinoma, altered hormone levels, hyperglycemia, hypothyroidism, hyperthyroidism, development or exacerbation of preexisting diabetes mellitus. *Injection site reaction:* Pain, edema, hemorrhage, inflammation of injection site. *Autoimmunity disease:* Vasculitis, Raynaud's disease, rheumatoid arthritis, lupus erythematosus, rhabdomyolysis. *Ophthalmic:* Amblyopia, retinal vein thrombosis, retinal artery or vein obstruction. *Miscellaneous:* Pain, back pain, cyst, peripheral edema, accidental injury, cotton-wool spots.

OD **Overdose Management:** *Symptoms:* Profound lethargy, prostration, coma, neurotoxicity, EEG abnormalities, seizures. Transient abnormalities in serum LFTs, hyperkalemia, elevations of serum BUN and creatinine, proteinuria, nephrotic syndromes, renal insufficiency, renal failure. *Treatment:* Symptomatic, supportive treatment.

Drug Interactions: Use with caution when giving interferon alfa-n1 with other drugs metabolized by the cytochrome P450 enzyme system (e.g., vinblastine, zidovudine, theophylline).

EMS CONSIDERATIONS
None.

Interferon beta-1a
Interferon beta-1b
(f1FN-B)
(in-ter-FEER-on BAY-tah)
Pregnancy Class: C
Avonex (Interferon beta-1a), Betaseron (Interferon beta-1b) **(Rx)**
Classification: Drug for multiple sclerosis (MS)

Mechanism of Action: Interferon beta-1a is produced by mammalian cells into which the human interferon beta gene has been introduced. Interferon beta-1b is made by bacterial fermentation of a strain of *Escherichia coli* that is a genetically engineered plasmid containing the gene for human interferon beta$_{ser17}$. Interferon betas have antiviral, antiproliferative, and immunoregulatory effects. Mechanism for the beneficial effect in MS is unknown, although the effects are mediated through combination with specific cell receptors located on the cell membrane. The receptor-drug complex induces the expression of a number of interferon-induced gene products that are thought to be the mediators of the biologic effects of interferon beta-1a and beta-1b.

Uses: Interferon beta-1a: Treatment of relapsing forms of MS to slow the appearance of physical disability and decrease the frequency

---

bold italic = life threatening side effect

of clinical exacerbations. **Interferon beta-1b:** Treatment of ambulatory patients with relapsing-remitting MS to reduce the frequency of clinical exacerbations. Remitting-relapsing MS is manifested by recurrent attacks of neurologic dysfunction followed by complete or incomplete recovery. *Investigational:* Treatment of AIDS, AIDS-related Kaposi's sarcoma, metastatic renal cell carcinoma, herpes of the lips or genitals, malignant melanoma, cutaneous T-cell lymphoma, and acute non-A/non-B hepatitis.

Contraindications: Hypersensitivity to natural or recombinant interferon beta or human albumin. Lactation.

Precautions: The safety and efficacy for use in chronic progressive MS and in children less than 18 years of age have not been studied. Depression and attempted suicide and suicide have occurred. Potential to be an abortifacient. Use with caution in those with preexisting seizure disorder.

Route/Dosage

• **Interferon beta-1a: IM**
  Relapsing forms of MS.
  30 mcg IM once a week.
• **Inteferon beta-1b: SC**
  Relapsing-remitting MS patients.
  0.25 mg (8 mIU) every other day.
How Supplied: *Kit:* 33 mcg; *Powder for injection:* 0.3 mg

Side Effects: Side effects common to interferon beta-1a and beta-1b. *Body as a whole:* Headache, fever, flu-like symptoms, pain, asthenia, chills, reaction at injection site (including necrosis/inflammation), malaise. *GI:* Abdominal pain, diarrhea, dry mouth, *GI hemorrhage,* gingivitis, hepatomegaly, intestinal obstruction, periodontal abscess, proctitis. *CV:* Arrhythmia, hypotension, postural hypotension. *CNS:* Dizziness, speech disorder, convulsion, suicide attempt, abnormal gait, depersonalization, facial paralysis, hyperesthesia, neurosis, psychosis. *Respiratory:* Sinusitis, dyspnea, hemoptysis, hyperventilation. *Musculoskeletal:* Myalgia, ar-

thritis. *Dermatologic:* Contact dermatitis, furunculosis, seborrhea, skin ulcer. *GU:* Epididymitis, gynecomastia, hematuria, kidney calculus, nocturia, vaginal hemorrhage, ovarian cyst. *Miscellaneous:* Abscess, ascites, cellulitis, hernia, hypothyroidism, *sepsis,* hiccoughs, thirst, leukorrhea.

Interferon beta-1a. *Body as a whole:* Infection. *GI:* Nausea, dyspepsia, anorexia, blood in stool, colitis, constipation, diverticulitis, gall bladder disorder, gastritis, gum hemorrhage, hepatoma, increased appetite, *intestinal perforation,* periodontitis, tongue disorder. *CV:* Syncope, vasodilation, arteritis, *heart arrest, hemorrhage, pulmonary embolus,* palpitation, pericarditis, peripheral ischemia, peripheral vascular disorder, spider angioma, telangiectasia. *CNS:* Sleep difficulty, muscle spasm, ataxia, amnesia, Bell's palsy, clumsiness, drug dependence, increased libido. *Respiratory:* URTI, emphysema, laryngitis, pharyngeal edema, pneumonia. *Musculoskeletal:* Arthralgia, bone pain, myasthenia, osteonecrosis, synovitis. *Dermatologic:* Urticaria, alopecia, nevus, herpes zoster, herpes simplex, basal cell carcinoma, blisters, cold clammy skin, erythema, genital pruritus, skin discoloration. *GU:* Vaginitis, breast fibroadenosis, breast mass, dysuria, fibrocystic change of the breast, fibroids, kidney pain, menopause, pelvic inflammatory disease, penis disorder, Peyronie's disease, polyuria, postmenopausal hemorrhage, prostatic disorder, pyelonephritis, testis disorder, urethral pain, urinary urgency, urinary retention, urinary incontinence. *Hematologic:* Anemia, ecchymosis at injection site, eosinophils greater than 10%, hematocrit less than 37%, increased coagulation time, ecchymosis, lymphadenopathy, petechia. *Metabolic:* Dehydration, hypoglycemia, hypomagnesemia, hypokalemia. *Ophthalmic:* Abnormal vision, conjunctivitis, eye pain, vitreous floaters. *Miscellaneous:* Otitis media, decreased hearing, facial edema, fibrosis at injection site, hypersensitivity at injection site, lipoma, neoplasm, photosensitivity, toothache, sinus headache, chest pain.

Interferon beta-1b. *Body as a whole:* Generalized edema, hypothermia, **anaphylaxis, shock,** adenoma, sarcoma. *GI:* Constipation, vomiting, GI disorder, aphthous stomatitis, cardiospasm, cheilitis, cholecystitis, cholelithiasis, duodenal ulcer, enteritis, esophagitis, fecal impaction or incontinence, flatulence, gastritis, glossitis, hematemesis, hepatic neoplasia, hepatitis, ileus, increased salivation, melena, nausea, oral leukoplakia, oral moniliasis, **pancreatitis, rectal hemorrhage,** salivary gland enlargement, stomach ulcer, peritonitis, tenesmus. *CV:* Migraine, palpitation, hypertension, tachycardia, peripheral vascular disorder, **hemorrhage,** angina pectoris, atrial fibrillation, cardiomegaly, **cardiac arrest, cerebral hemorrhage, heart failure, MI, pulmonary embolus, ventricular fibrillation** cerebral ischemia, endocarditis, pericardial effusion, spider angioma, subarachnoid hemorrhage, syncope, thrombophlebitis, thrombosis, varicose veins, vasospasm, venous pressure increase, ventricular extrasystoles. *CNS:* Mental symptoms, hypertonia, somnolence, hyperkinesia, acute/chronic brain syndrome, agitation, apathy, aphasia, ataxia, brain edema, **coma,** delirium, delusions, dementia, dystonia, encephalopathy, euphoria, hallucinations, hemiplegia, hypalgesia, incoordination, intracranial hypertension, decreased libido, manic reaction, meningitis, neuralgia, neuropathy, paralysis, paranoid reaction, decreased reflexes, stupor, subdural hematoma, torticollis, tremor. *Respiratory:* Laryngitis, apnea, asthma, atelectasis, lung carcinoma, hypoventilation, interstitial pneumonia, lung edema, pleural effusion, pneumothorax. *Musculoskeletal:* Myasthenia, arthrosis, bursitis, leg cramps, muscle atrophy, myopathy, myositis, ptosis, tenosynovitis. *Dermatologic:* Sweating, alopecia, erythema nodosum, exfoliative dermatitis, hirsutism, leukoderma, lichenoid dermatitis, maculopapular rash, photosensitivity, psoriasis, benign skin neoplasm, skin carcinoma, skin hypertrophy, skin necrosis, urticaria, vesiculobullous rash. *GU:* Dysmenorrhea, menstrual disorder, metrorrhagia, cystitis, breast pain, menorrhagia, urinary urgency, fibrocystic breast, breast neoplasm, urinary retention, anuria, balanitis, breast engorgement, cervicitis, impotence, kidney failure, tubular disorder, nephritis, oliguria, polyuria, salpingitis, urethritis, urinary incontinence, enlarged uterine fibroids, uterine neoplasm. *Hematologic:* Lymphocytes less than 1500/mm³, active neutrophil count less than 1500/mm³, WBCs less than 3000/mm³, lymphadenopathy, chronic lymphocytic leukemia, petechia, hemoglobin less than 9.4 g/dL, platelets less than 75,000/mm³, splenomegaly. *Metabolic:* Weight gain, weight loss, goiter, glucose less than 55 mg/dL or greater than 160 mg/dL, AST or ALT greater than 5 times baseline, total bilirubin greater than 2.5 times baseline, urine protein greater than 1+, alkaline phosphatase greater than 5 times baseline, BUN greater than 40 mg/dL, calcium greater than 11.5 mg/dL, cyanosis, edema, glycosuria, hypoglycemic reaction, hypoxia, ketosis. *Ophthalmic:* Conjunctivitis, abnormal vision, diplopia, nystagmus, oculogyric crisis, papilledema, blepharitis, blindness, dry eyes, iritis, keratoconjunctivitis, mydriasis, photophobia, retinitis, visual field defect. *Miscellaneous:* Pelvic pain, hydrocephalus, alcohol intolerance, otitis externa, otitis media, parosmia, taste loss, taste perversion.

EMS CONSIDERATIONS

None.

Interferon gamma-1b
(in-ter-FEER-on GAM-uh)
Pregnancy Class: C
Actimmune **(Rx)**
Classification: Interferon

Mechanism of Action: Consists of a single-chain polypeptide of 140 ami-

---

bold italic = life threatening side effect

no acids. Produced by fermentation of a genetically engineered *Escherichia coli* bacterium containing the DNA that encodes for the human protein. Manifests potent phagocyte-activating effects including generation of toxic oxygen metabolites within phagocytes. Such metabolites result in the death of microorganisms such as *Staphylococcus aureus, Toxoplasma gondii, Leishmania donovani, Listeria monocytogenes,* and *Mycobacterium avium intracellulare.* Since interferon gamma regulates activity of immune cells, it is characterized as a lymphokine of the interleukin type. Interferon gamma interacts functionally with other interleukin molecules (e.g., interleukin-2) and all interleukins form part of a complex, lymphokine regulatory network. As an example, interferon gamma and interleukin-4 may interact reciprocally to regulate murine IgE levels; interferon gamma can suppress IgE levels and inhibit the production of collagen at the transcription level in humans.

Uses: Decrease the frequency and severity of serious infections associated with chronic granulomatous disease.

Contraindications: Hypersensitivity to interferon gamma or *E. coli*-derived products. Lactation.

Precautions: Safety and effectiveness have not been determined in children less than 1 year of age. Use with caution in patients with preexisting cardiac disease, including symptoms of ischemia, arrhythmia, or CHF, and in patients with myelosuppression, seizure disorders, or compromised CNS function.

Route/Dosage

• **SC**
  Chronic granulomatous disease.
  50 mcg/m² (1.5 million units/m²) for patients whose body surface is greater than 0.5 m². If the body surface is less than 0.5 m², the dose of interferon gamma should be 1.5 mcg/kg/dose. The drug is given 3 times/week (e.g., Monday, Wednesday, Friday).

How Supplied: *Injection:* 3 million U/0.5 mL

Side Effects: The following side effects were noted in patients with chronic granulomatous disease receiving the drug SC. *GI:* Diarrhea, vomiting, nausea, abdominal pain, anorexia. *CNS:* Fever (over 50%), headache, fatigue, depression. *Miscellaneous:* Rash, chills, erythema or tenderness at injection site, pain at injection site, weight loss, myalgia, arthralgia, back pain.

When used in patients other than those with chronic granulomatous disease, in addition to the preceding, the following side effects were reported. *GI:* **GI bleeding,** pancreatitis, hepatic insufficiency. *CV:* Hypotension, heart block, **heart failure,** syncope, **tachyarrhythmia, MI.** *CNS:* Confusion, disorientation, symptoms of parkinsonism, gait disturbance, **seizures,** hallucinations, transient ischemic attacks. *Hematologic:* **Deep venous thrombosis, pulmonary embolism.** *Respiratory:* **Bronchospasm,** tachypnea, interstitial pneumonitis. *Metabolic:* Hyperglycemia, hyponatremia. *Miscellaneous:* Reversible renal insufficiency, worsening of dermatomyositis.

EMS CONSIDERATIONS

None.

Ipecac syrup
(IP-eh-kak)
Pregnancy Class: C
(OTC)
Classification: Emetic

Mechanism of Action: Acts both locally on the gastric mucosa as an irritant and centrally to stimulate the CTZ. The central effect is caused by emetine and cephaeline, which are two alkaloids in the product. **Ipecac syrup must not be confused with ipecac fluid extract, which is 14 times as potent.** Syrup of ipecac can be purchased without a prescription.

Onset of Action: 20 min.
Duration of Action: 20-25 min.
Uses: To empty the stomach promptly and completely after oral poisoning or drug overdose.

Contraindications: With corrosives or petroleum distillates, in individuals who are unconscious or semicomatose, severely inebriated, or in shock. Infants under 6 months of age.

Precautions: Use with caution during lactation. If used in children less than 12 months of age, there is an increased risk of aspiration of vomitus. Abuse may occur in anorexic or bulemic patients and its use in these groups has been associated with severe cardiomyopathies and death.

Route/Dosage
• **Syrup**
  Emetic.

Adults and children over 12 years: 15–30 mL followed by 240 mL of water; **infants up to 1 year:** 5–10 mL followed by one-half to one glass of water; **pediatric, 1–12 years:** 15 mL followed by one to two glasses of water.

How Supplied: *Syrup*

Side Effects: Diarrhea, drowsiness, coughing, or choking with emesis, mild CNS depression, GU upset (may last several hours) after emesis. Can be cardiotoxic if not vomited and allowed to be absorbed. Cardiotoxic effects include heart conduction disturbances, atrial fibrillation, or fatal myocarditis.

OD Overdose Management: *Symptoms:* If absorbed into the general circulation, symptoms may include cardiac conduction disturbances, bradycardia, atrial fibrillation, hypotension, or *fatal myocarditis. Treatment:* Activated charcoal to absorb ipecac syrup. Gastric lavage. Support the CV system with symptomatic treatment.

Drug Interactions: Activated charcoal adsorbs ipecac syrup, thus decreasing its effect.

EMS CONSIDERATIONS
Administration/Storage
1. Dosage may be repeated in children over 1 year of age and adults once if vomiting does not occur within 30 min. Consider gastric lavage

if vomiting does not occur within 15 min of second dose.
2. Administer ipecac syrup with 200–300 mL of water.

Assessment
1. Estimate amount and time of ingestion.
2. Do not use if intoxicant is a convulsant (i.e., TCAs); may trigger seizures abruptly.
3. Do not use for petroleum-based or caustic substances such as kerosene, lye, Drano, or gasoline.
4. Assess respiratory status and level of consciousness; do not use if there is no gag reflex or if semicomatose.

Ipratropium bromide
(eye-prah-TROH-pee-um)
Pregnancy Class: B
Atrovent **(Rx)**
Classification: Anticholinergic, quaternary ammonium compound

Mechanism of Action: Chemically related to atropine. Antagonizes the action of acetylcholine. Prevents the increase in intracellular levels of cyclic guanosine monophosphate, which is caused by the interaction of acetylcholine with muscarinic receptors in bronchial smooth muscle; this leads to bronchodilation which is primarily a local, site-specific effect.

Uses: Aerosol or solution: Bronchodilation in COPD, including chronic bronchitis and emphysema. **Nasal spray:** Symptomatic relief (using 0.03%) of rhinorrhea associated with allergic and nonallergic perennial rhinitis in patients over 6 years of age. Symptomatic relief (using 0.03%) of rhinorrhea associated with the common cold in those over 12 years of age. *NOTE:* The use of ipratropium with sympathomimetic bronchodilators, methylxanthines, steroids, or cromolyn sodium (all of which are used in treating COPD) are without side effects.

Contraindications: Hypersensitivity to atropine, ipratropium, or derivatives. Hypersensitivity to soya lecithin or related food products, including soy bean or peanut (inhalation aerosol).

Precautions: Use with caution in patients with narrow-angle glaucoma, prostatic hypertrophy, or bladder neck obstruction and during lactation. Safety and efficacy have not been determined in children. Use of ipratropium as a single agent for the relief of bronchospasm in acute COPD has not been studied adequately.

Route/Dosage

- **Respiratory Aerosol**
  Treat bronchospasms.
Adults: 2 inhalations (36 mcg) q.i.d. Additional inhalations may be required but should not exceed 12 inhalations/day.
- **Solution for Inhalation**
  Treat bronchospasms.
Adults: 500 mcg (1-unit-dose vial) administered t.i.d.–q.i.d. by oral nebulization with doses 6–8 hr apart.
- **Nasal Spray, 0.03%**
  Perennial rhinitis.
2 sprays (42 mcg) per nostril b.i.d.–t.i.d. for a total daily dose of 168–252 mcg/day.
- **Nasal Spray, 0.06%**
  Rhinitis due to the common cold.
2 sprays (84 mcg) per nostril t.i.d.–q.i.d. for a total daily dose of 504–672 mcg/day. The safety and efficacy for use for the common cold for more than 4 days have not been determined.

How Supplied: *Aerosol:* 0.018 mg/inh; *Nasal Spray:* 0.03%; *Solution for Inhalation:* 0.02%

Side Effects: *Inhalation aerosol. CNS:* Cough, nervousness, dizziness, headache, fatigue, insomnia, drowsiness, difficulty in coordination, tremor. *GI:* Dryness of oropharynx, GI distress, dry mouth, nausea, constipation. *CV:* Palpitations, tachycardia, flushing. *Dermatologic:* Itching, hives, alopecia. *Miscellaneous:* Irritation from aerosol, worsening of symptoms, rash, hoarseness, blurred vision, difficulty in accommodation, drying of secretions, urinary difficulty, paresthesias, mucosal ulcers.

Inhalation solution. CNS: Dizziness, insomnia, nervousness, tremor, headache. *GI:* Dry mouth, nausea, constipation. *CV:* Hypertension, aggravation of hypertension, tachycardia, palpitations. *Respiratory:* Worsening of COPD symptoms, coughing, dyspnea, bronchitis, bronchospasm, increased sputum, URI, pharyngitis, rhinitis, sinusitis. *Miscellaneous:* Urinary retention, UTIs, urticaria, pain, flu-like symptoms, back or chest pain, arthritis.

Nasal spray. CNS: Headache, dizziness. *GI:* Nausea, dry mouth, taste perversion. *CV:* Palpitation, tachycardia. *Respiratory:* URI, epistaxis, pharyngitis, nasal dryness, miscellaneous nasal symptoms, nasal irritation, blood-tinged mucus, dry throat, cough, nasal congestion, nasal burning, coughing. *Ophthalmic:* Ocular irritation, blurred vision, conjunctivitis. *Miscellaneous:* Hoarseness, thirst, tinnitis, urinary retention.

All products. Allergic: Skin rash; angioedema of the tongue, throat, lips, and face; urticaria, laryngospasm, **anaphylaxis.** *Anticholinergic reactions:* Precipitation or worsening of narrow angle glaucoma, prostatic disorders, tachycardia, urinary retention, constipation, and bowel obstruction.

EMS CONSIDERATIONS

See also *Cholinergic Blocking Agents.*

Ipratropium bromide and Albuterol sulfate

(eye-prah-TROH-pee-um/al-BYOU-ter-ohl)
Pregnancy Class: C
Combivent **(Rx)**
Classification: Drug for chronic obstructive pulmonary disease

Uses: Treatment of COPD in those who are on regular aerosol bronchodilator therapy and who require a second bronchodilator.

Contraindications: History of hypersensitivity to soya lecithin or related food products, such as soybean and peanuts. Lactation.

Precautions: Use with caution in CV disorders, especially coronary insufficiency, cardiac arrhythmias, and hypertension. Use with caution in narrow-angle glaucoma, prostatic hypertrophy, bladder-neck obstruction, convulsive disorders, hyperthyroidism, diabetes mellitus, in those unusually responsive to sympathomimetic amines, and renal or hepatic disease. Safety and efficacy have not been determined in children.

Route/Dosage
- **Inhalation**
  COPD.
2 inhalations q 6 hr not to exceed 12 inhalations/24-hr.

How Supplied: Each actuation of metered dose inhaler delivers: *Cholinergic blocking drug:* Iptratropium bromide, 18 mcg; and *Sympathomimetic:* Albuterol sulfate, 103 mcg.

Side Effects: *Respiratory:* **Paradoxical bronchospasm,** bronchitis, dyspnea, coughing, respiratory disorders, pneumonia, URTI, pharyngitis, sinusitis, rhinitis. *CV:* ECG changes including flattening of T wave, prolongation of QTc interval, and ST segment depression. Also, arrhythmias, palpitation, tachycardia, angina, hypertension. *Hypersensitivity, immediate:* Urticaria, **angioedema, bronchospasm, anaphylaxis, oropharyngeal edema.** *Body as a whole:* Headache, pain, flu, chest pain, edema, fatigue. *GI:* N&V, dry mouth, diarrhea, dyspepsia. *CNS:* Dizziness, nervousness, paresthesia, tremor, dysphonia, insomnia. *Miscellaneous:* Arthralgia, increased sputum, taste perversion, UTI, dysuria.

Drug Interactions: See individual drugs.

EMS CONSIDERATIONS

See also *Ipratropium bromide* and *Aalbuterol sulfate.*

Irbesartan
(ihr-beh-SAR-tan)
Pregnancy Class: C (first trimester), D (second and third trimesters)

Avapro **(Rx)**
Classification: Antihypertensive, angiotensin II receptor antagonist

Mechanism of Action: By binding to AT_1 angiotensin II receptor, blocks vasoconstrictor and aldosterone-secreting effects of angiotensin II.

Uses: Treat hypertension alone or in combination with other antihypertensives. *Investigational:* Heart failure, reduce rate of progression of renal disease and adverse clinical sequelae in hypertensives with diabetic nephropathy.

Precautions: Safety and efficacy have not been determined in children.

Route/Dosage
- **Tablets**
  Hypertension.
150 mg once daily, up to 300 mg once daily. Lower initial dose of 75 mg is recommended for patients with depleted intravascular volume or salt. If BP is not controlled by irbesartan alone, hydrochlorothiazide may have an additive effect. Patients not adequately treated by 300 mg irbesartan are unlikely to get benefit from higher dose or b.i.d. dosing.

How Supplied: *Tablet:* 75 mg, 150 mg, 300 mg

Side Effects: *GI:* Diarrhea, dyspepsia, heartburn, abdominal pain, N&V, constipation, oral lesion, gastroenteritis, flatulence, abdominal distention. *CV:* Tachycardia, syncope, orthostatic hypotension, hypotension (especially in volume- or salt-depletion), flushing, hypertension, cardiac murmur, **MI, cardio-respiratory arrest, heart failure, hypertensive crisis, CVA,** angina pectoris, arrhythmias, conduction disorder, transient ischemic attack. *CNS:* Sleep disturbance, anxiety, nervousness, dizziness, numbness, somnolence, emotional disturbance, depression, paresthesia, tremor. *Musculoskeletal:* Extremity swelling, muscle cramp, arthritis, muscle ache, musculoskeletal pain, musculoskeletal chest pain, joint stiffness, bursitis, muscle weakness. *Respiratory:* Epistaxis, tracheo-

---

bold italic = life threatening side effect

bronchitis, congestion, pulmonary congestion, dyspnea, wheezing, upper respiratory infection, rhinitis, pharyngitis, sinus abnormality. *GU:* Abnormal urination, prostate disorder, UTI, sexual dysfunction, libido change. *Dermatologic:* Pruritus, dermatitis, ecchymosis, facial erythema, urticaria. *Ophthalmic:* Vision disturbance, conjunctivitis, eyelid abnormality. *Otic:* Hearing abnormality, ear infection, ear pain, ear abnormality. *Miscellaneous:* Gout, fever, fatigue, chills, facial edema, upper extremity edema, headache, influenza, rash, chest pain.

EMS CONSIDERATIONS

See also *Antihypertensive Drugs.*

Isoetharine hydrochloride
(eye-so-ETH-ah-reen)
Pregnancy Class: C
(Rx)
Classification: Adrenergic agent, bronchodilator

Mechanism of Action: Has a greater stimulating activity on beta-2 receptors of the bronchi than on beta-1 receptors of the heart. Causes relief of bronchospasms.
Onset of Action: Inhalation: 1-6 min; **Peak effect:** 15-60 min.
Duration of Action: 1-3 hr.
Uses: Bronchial asthma, bronchospasms due to chronic bronchitis or emphysema, bronchiectasis, pulmonary obstructive disease.
Precautions: Dosage has not been established in children less than 12 years of age.

Route/Dosage —————————
• **Inhalation Solution**
   Hand nebulizer.
Adults: 3–7 inhalations (use undiluted) of the 0.5% or 1% solution.
   Oxygen aerosolization or IPPB.
Adults: Dose depends on strength of solution used (range: 0.062%–1%) and whether the solution is used undiluted or diluted according to the following: **1%:** 0.25–1 mL by IPPB or 0.25–0.5 mL by oxygen aerosolization diluted 1:3 with saline or other

diluent. **0.2–0.5%:** 2 mL used undiluted; **0.2%:** 1.25–2.5 mL used undiluted; **0.167 or 0.17%:** 3 mL used undiluted; **0.125%:** 2–4 mL used undiluted; **0.1%:** 2.5-5 mL used undiluted; **0.08%:** 3 mL used undiluted; **0.062%:** 4 mL used undiluted.
How Supplied: Isoetharine hydrochloride: *Solution:* 1%

EMS CONSIDERATIONS

See also *Sympathomimetic Drugs.*

Isoniazid (INH, Isonicotinic acid hydrazide)
(eye-so-NYE-ah-zid)
Pregnancy Class: C
Laniazid, Laniazid C.T., Nydrazid Injection **(Rx)**
Classification: Primary antitubercular agent

Mechanism of Action: The most effective tuberculostatic agent. Probably interferes with lipid and nucleic acid metabolism of growing bacteria, resulting in alteration of the bacterial wall. Is tuberculostatic.
Uses: Tuberculosis caused by human, bovine, and BCG strains of *Mycobacterium tuberculosis.* Not to be used as the sole tuberculostatic agent. Prophylaxis of tuberculosis. *Investigational:* To improve severe tremor in patients with multiple sclerosis.
Contraindications: Severe hypersensitivity to isoniazid or in patients with previous isoniazid-associated hepatic injury or side effects.
Precautions: Severe and sometimes fatal hepatitis may occur even after several months of therapy; incidence is age-related and current alcohol use increases the risk. Increased risk of fatal hepatitis in minority women, especially Blacks and Hispanics; also increased risk postpartum. Extreme caution should be exercised in patients with convulsive disorders, in whom the drug should be administered only when the patient is adequately controlled by anticonvul-

sant medication. Also, use with caution for the treatment of renal tuberculosis and, in the lowest dose possible, in patients with impaired renal function and in alcoholics.

Route/Dosage
• **Syrup, Tablets**
Active tuberculosis.
Adults: 5 mg/kg/day (up to 300 mg/day) as a single dose; **children and infants:** 10–20 mg/kg/day (up to 300 mg total) in a single dose.
Prophylaxis.
Adults: 300 mg/day in a single dose; **children and infants:** 10 mg/kg/day (up to 300 mg total) in a single dose.
• **IM**
Active tuberculosis.
Adults: 5 mg/kg (up to 300 mg) once daily. **Pediatric:** 10–20 mg/kg (up to 300 mg) once daily.
Prophylaxis.
Adults/adolescents: 300 mg/day.
Pediatric: 10 mg/kg/day.
NOTE: Pyridoxine, 6–50 mg/day, is recommended in the malnourished and those prone to neuropathy (e.g., alcoholics, diabetics).
How Supplied: *Syrup:* 50 mg/5 mL; *Tablet:* 100 mg, 300 mg
Side Effects: *Neurologic:* Peripheral neuropathy characterized by symmetrical numbness and tingling of extremities (dose-related). Rarely, toxic encephalopathy, optic neuritis, optic atrophy, *seizures,* impaired memory, toxic psychosis. *GI:* N&V, epigastric distress, xerostomia. *Hypersensitivity:* Fever, skin rashes and eruptions, vasculitis, lymphadenopathy. *Hepatic:* Liver dysfunction, jaundice, bilirubinemia, bilirubinuria, *serious and sometimes fatal hepatitis (especially in patients over 50 years of age).* Increases in serum AST and ALT. *Hematologic: Agranulocytosis,* eosinophilia, thrombocytopenia, *hemolytic, sideroblastic, or aplastic anemia.* *Metabolic/Endocrine:* Metabolic acidosis, pyridoxine deficiency, pellagra, hyperglycemia, gynecomastia. *Miscellaneous:* Tinnitus, urinary reten-

tion, rheumatic syndrome, lupus-like syndrome, arthralgia.
NOTE: Pyridoxine, 10–50 mg/day, may be given concomitantly with isoniazid to decrease CNS side effects. Ophthalmologic and liver function tests are recommended periodically.
OD Overdose Management: *Symptoms:* N&V, dizziness, blurred vision, slurred speech, visual hallucinations within 30–180 min. Severe overdosage may cause respiratory distress, *CNS depression (coma can occur), severe seizures,* metabolic acidosis, acetonuria, hyperglycemia. *Treatment:* Maintain respiration and undertake gastric lavage (within first 2–3 hr providing seizures are not present). To control seizures, give diazepam or a short-acting IV barbiturate followed by pyridoxine (1 mg IV/1 mg isoniazid ingested). Sodium bicarbonate, IV, to correct metabolic acidosis. Forced osmotic diuresis; monitor fluid I&O. For severe cases, consider hemodialysis or peritoneal dialysis.
Drug Interactions
Aluminum salts / ↓ Effect of isoniazid due to ↓ absorption from GI tract
Anticoagulants, oral / ↓ Anticoagulant effect
Atropine / ↑ Side effects of isoniazid
Benzodiazepines / ↑ Effect of benzodiazepines that undergo oxidative metabolism (e.g., diazepam, triazolam)
Carbamazepine / ↑ Risk of both carbamazepine and isoniazid toxicity
Cycloserine / ↑ Risk of cycloserine CNS side effects
Disulfiram / ↑ Risk of acute behavioral and coordination changes
Enflurane / Isoniazid may produce high levels of hydrazine, which increases defluorination of enflurane
Ethanol / ↑ Chance of isoniazid-induced hepatitis
Halothane / ↑ Risk of hepatotoxicity and hepatic encephalopathy

Hydantoins (phenytoin) / ↑ Effect of hydantoins due to ↓ breakdown in liver

Ketoconazole / ↓ Serum levels of ketoconazole → ↓ effect

Meperidine / ↑ Risk of hypotension or CNS depression

PAS / ↑ Effect of isoniazid by ↑ blood levels

Rifampin / Additive liver toxicity

EMS CONSIDERATIONS

None.

Isophane insulin suspension (NPH)

(EYE-so-fayn IN-sue-lin)

Pork: NPH-N, NPH Iletin II, **Beef/Pork:** NPH Iletin I, **Human:** Humulin N, Novolin N, Novolin N PenFill, Novolin N Prefilled **(OTC)**

Classification: Intermediate-acting insulin

Mechanism of Action: Contains zinc insulin crystals modified by protamine, appearing as a cloudy or milky suspension. Not recommended for emergency use. Not suitable for IV administration or in the presence of ketosis. *Note:* NPH beef/pork insulins are being phased out.

Onset of Action: 1-1.5 hr; **Peak:** 4-12 hr.

Duration of Action: Up to 24 hr.

Route/Dosage
• **SC**
  Diabetes.

Adult, individualized, usual, initial: 7–26 units as a single dose 30–60 min before breakfast. A second smaller dose may be given, if needed, prior to the evening meal or at bedtime. If necessary, the daily dose may be increased in increments of 2–10 units at daily or weekly intervals until desired control is achieved.

Patients on insulin zinc may be transferred directly to isophane insulin on a unit-for-unit basis. If patient is being transferred from regular insulin, the initial dose of isophane should be from two-thirds to three-fourths the dose of regular insulin.

How Supplied: *Injection:* 100 U/mL

EMS CONSIDERATIONS

See also *Insulins.*

Isophane insulin suspension and insulin injection

(EYE-so-fayn IN-sue-lin)

Human: Humulin 50/50, Humulin 70/30, Novolin 70/30, Novolin 70/30 Penfill, Novolin 70/30 Prefilled **(OTC)**

Classification: Mixture of insulins to achieve variable duration of action

Onset of Action: 30-60 min; **Peak effect:** 4-8 hr.

Duration of Action: 24 hr.

Route/Dosage
• **SC**
  Diabetes.

Adults: Individualized and given once daily 15–30 min before breakfast, or as directed. **Children:** Individualized according to patient size.

How Supplied: Contains from 10% to 50% insulin injection and from 50% to 70% isophane insulin. Except for Humulin 50/50 and Novolin ge 50/50, the larger number in the product refers to the percentage of isophane insulin suspension.

EMS CONSIDERATIONS

See also *Insulins.*

Isoproterenol hydrochloride Isoproterenol sulfate

(eye-so-proh-TER-ih-nohl)

Pregnancy Class: C

Hydrochloride (Dispos-a-Med Isoproterenol HCl, Isuprel, Isuprel Mistometer, Norisodrine Aerotrol **(Rx)**) Sulfate (Medihaler-Iso **(Rx)**)

Classification: Sympathomimetic, direct-acting

Mechanism of Action: Produces pronounced stimulation of both beta-1 and beta-2 receptors of the heart, bronchi, skeletal muscle vasculature, and the GI tract. Has both positive inotropic and chronotropic activity; systolic BP may increase while diastolic BP may decrease.

Thus, mean arterial BP may not change or may be decreased. Causes less hyperglycemia than epinephrine, but produces bronchodilation and the same degree of CNS excitation.

Onset of Action: Inhalation: 2-5 min; **peak effect:** 3-5 min; **IV:** immediate; **SL:** 15-30 min.

Duration of Action: Inhalation: 30-120 min; **IV:** less than 1 hr; **SL:** 1-2 hr.

Uses: Bronchodilator in asthma, chronic pulmonary emphysema, bronchiectasis, bronchitis, and other conditions involving bronchospasms (e.g., during surgery). Treat bronchospasms during anesthesia. Cardiac arrest, heart block, syncope due to complete heart block, Adams-Stokes syndrome. Certain cardiac arrhythmias including ventricular tachycardia, ventricular arrhythmias; syncope due to carotid sinus hypersensitivity. Hypoperfusion shock syndrome. Hypovolemic and septic shock as an adjunct to fluid and electrolyte replacement. Use in cardiac arrest until electric shock or pacemaker therapy are available.

Contraindications: Tachyarrhythmias, tachycardia, or heart block caused by digitalis intoxication, ventricular arrhythmias that require inotropic therapy, and angina pectoris.

Precautions: Use with caution during lactation and in the presence of tuberculosis. Safety and effectiveness have not been determined in children less than 12 years of age.

Route/Dosage ──────────────

ISOPROTERENOL HYDROCHLORIDE

• **IV Infusion**

Shock.

5 mcg/min (1.25 mL/min of solution prepared by diluting 10 mL of 1:5,000 solution in 500 mL of D5W or 5 mL of 1:5,000 solution in 250 mL of D5W).

Cardiac standstill and cardiac arrhythmias.

Adults: 5 mcg/min (1.25 mL of either 1.25 mL/min of solution prepared by

diluting 10 mL of 1:5,000 solution in 500 mL of D5W or 5 mL of 1:5,000 solution in 250 mL of D5W).

• **IV**

Cardiac standstill and cardiac arrhythmias.

1–3 mL (0.02–0.06 mg) of solution prepared by diluting 1 mL of 1:5,000 solution to 10 mL with NaCl or 5% dextrose solution. Dosage range: 0.01–0.2 mg.

Bronchospasm during anesthesia.

Adults: Dilute 1 mL of the 1:5,000 solution to 10 mL with NaCl injection or D5 solution and given an initial dose of 0.01–0.02 mg IV; repeat when necessary.

• **IM, SC**

Cardiac standstill and cardiac arrhythmias.

Adults: 1 mL (0.2 mg) of 1:5,000 solution (range: 0.02–1 mg).

Intracardiac (in extreme emergencies): 0.1 mL (0.02 mg) of 1:5,000 solution.

• **Hand Bulb Nebulizer**

Acute bronchial asthma.

Adults and children: 5–15 deep inhalations of the 1:200 solution. In adults 3–7 inhalations of the 1:100 solution may be useful. If there is no relief after 5–10 min, the doses may be repeated one more time. Repeat treatment up to 5 times/day may be necessary if there are repeat attacks.

Bronchospasm in chronic obstructive lung disease.

Adults and children: 5–15 deep inhalations of the 1:200 solution (in patients with severe attacks, 3–7 inhalations of the 1:100 solution may be useful). An interval of 3–4 hr should elapse between uses.

• **Metered-Dose Inhalation**

Acute bronchial asthma.

Adults, usual: 1–2 inhalations beginning with 1 inhalation, and if no relief occurs within 2–5 min, a second inhalation may be used. **Maintenance:** 1–2 inhalations 4–6 times/day. No more than 2 inhalations at any one time or more than 6 inhalations in 1 hr should be taken.

Bronchospasm in COPD.

Adults and children: 1–2 inhalations repeated at no less than 3–4 hr intervals (i.e., 4–6 times/day).

- **Nebulization by Compressed Air or Oxygen**
  Bronchospasms in COPD.

Adults and children: 0.5 mL of the 1:200 solution is diluted to 2–2.5 mL (for a concentration of 1:800–1:1,000). The solution is delivered over 15–20 min and may be repeated up to 5 times/day.

- **IPPB**
  Bronchospasms in COPD.

Adults and children: 0.5 mL of a 1:200 solution diluted to 2–2.5 mL with water or isotonic saline. The solution is delivered over 10–20 min and may be repeated up to 5 times/day.

ISOPROTERENOL SULFATE

Dispensed from metered aerosol inhaler for bronchospasms. See preceding dosage for *Hydrochloride.*

How Supplied: Isoproterenol Hydrochloride: *Metered dose inhaler:* 0.131 mg/inh; *Injection:* 0.02 mg/mL, 0.2 mg/mL; *Solution:* 0.25%, 0.5%, 1% Isoproterenol Sulfate: *Metered dose inhaler:* 0.08 mg/inh

Side Effects: Additional: *CV:* **Cardiac arrest,** Adams-Stokes attack, hypotension, precordial pain or distress. *CNS:* Hyperactivity, hyperkinesia. *Respiratory:* Wheezing, bronchitis, increase in sputum, **bronchial edema and inflammation, pulmonary edema, paradoxical airway resistance.** Excessive inhalation causes refractory bronchial obstruction. *Miscellaneous:* Flushing, sweating, swelling of the parotid gland. Sublingual administration may cause buccal ulceration. Side effects of drug are less severe after inhalation.

Drug Interactions

Bretylium / Possibility of arrhythmias

Guanethidine / ↑ Pressor response of isoproterenol

Halogenated hydrocarbon anesthetics / Sensitization of the heart to catecholamines which may cause serious arrhythmias

Oxytocic drugs / Possibility of severe, persistent hypertension

Tricyclic antidepressants / Potentiation of pressor effect

EMS CONSIDERATIONS

See also *Sympathomimetic Drugs.*

Administration/Storage: **IV** Do not use the injection if it is pinkish to brownish in color. Protect from light and store at 15°C–30°C (59°F–86°F).

Isosorbide dinitrate chewable tablets
Isosorbide dinitrate extended-release capsules
Isosorbide dinitrate extended-release tablets
Isosorbide dinitrate sublingual tablets
Isodorbide dinitrate tablets

(eye-so-SOR-byd)

Pregnancy Class: C
Chewable tablets (Sorbitrate **(Rx)**) Extended-release capsules (Dilatrate-SR, Isordil Tembids **(Rx)**) Extended-release tablets (Tembids **(Rx)**) Sublingual tablets (Isordil, Sorbitrate **(Rx)**) Tablets (Isordil Titradose, Sorbitrate **(Rx)**)

Classification: Coronary vasodilator, antianginal drug

Onset of Action: Sublingual, chewable: 2-5 min; **Capsules/Tablets:** 20-40 min; **Extended-release:** up to 4 hr.

Duration of Action: Sublingual, chewable: 1-3 hr; **Capsules/Tablets:** 4-6 hr; **Extended-release:** 6-8 hr.

Uses: Additional: Diffuse esophageal spasm. Oral tablets are only for prophylaxis while sublingual and chewable forms may be used to terminate acute attacks of angina.

Precautions: Use with caution during lactation. Safety and efficacy have not been established in children.

Route/Dosage
- **Tablets**

Antianginal.
Initial: 5–20 mg q 6 hr; **maintenance:** 10–40 mg q 6 hr (usual: 20–40 mg q.i.d.
- **Chewable Tablets**
  Antianginal, acute attack.
Initial: 5 mg q 2–3 hr. The dose can be titrated upward until angina is relieved or side effects occur.
  Prophylaxis.
5–10 mg q 2–3 hr.
- **Extended-Release Capsules**
  Antianginal.
Initial: 40 mg; **maintenance:** 40–80 mg q 8–12 hr.
- **Extended-Release Tablets**
  Antianginal.
Initial: 40 mg; **maintenance:** 40–80 mg q 8–12 hr.
- **Sublingual**
  Acute attack.
2.5–5 mg q 2–3 hr as required. The dose can be titrated upward until angina is relieved or side effects occur.
  Prophylaxis.
5–10 mg q 2–3 hr.
How Supplied: *Chew Tablet:* 5 mg; *Capsule, Extended Release:* 40 mg; *Tablet, Extended Release:* 40 mg; *Sublingual tablet:* 2.5 mg, 5 mg, 10 mg; *Tablet:* 2.5 mg, 5 mg, 20 mg, 30 mg, 40 mg
Side Effects: Additional: Vascular headaches occur frequently.
Drug Interactions: Additional: *Acetylcholine/* Isosorbide antagonizes the effect of acetylcholine.*Norepinephrine/* Isosorbide antagonizes the effect of norepinephrine.

EMS CONSIDERATIONS

See also *Antianginal Drugs, Nitrates/Nitrites.*

Isosorbide mononitrate, oral
(eye-so-SOR-byd)
Pregnancy Class: C
Imdur, ISMO, Monoket **(Rx)**
Classification: Coronary vasodilator, antianginal drug

Onset of Action: 30-60 min.
Uses: Prophylaxis of angina pectoris.
Contraindications: To abort acute anginal attacks. Use in acute MI or CHF.
Precautions: Use with caution during lactation and in patients who may be volume depleted or who are already hypotensive. Safety and effectiveness have not been determined in children. The benefits have not been established in acute MI or CHF.

Route/Dosage ————————
IMDUR TABLETS
  Prophylaxis of angina.
Initial: 30 mg (given as one-half of the 60-mg tablet) or 60 mg once daily; **then,** dosage may be increased to 120 mg given as 2–60-mg tablets once daily. Rarely, 240 mg daily may be needed.
ISMO, MONOKET TABLETS
  Prevention and treatment of angina.
Adults: 20 mg b.i.d. with the doses 7 hr apart (it is preferable that first dose be given on awakening). An initial dose of 5 mg may be best for patients of small stature; increase the dose to at least 10 mg by the second or third day of therapy.
How Supplied: *Tablet:* 10 mg, 20 mg; *Tablet, Extended Release:* 30 mg, 60 mg, 120 mg
Side Effects: *CV:* Hypotension (may be accompanied by paradoxical bradycardia and increased angina pectoris). *CNS:* Headache, lightheadedness, dizziness. *GI:* N&V. *Miscellaneous:* Possibility of methemoglobinemia.
OD Overdose Management: *Symptoms:* Increased intracranial pressure manifested by throbbing headache, confusion, moderate fever. Also, vertigo, palpitations, visual disturbances, N&V, syncope, air hunger, dyspnea (followed by reduced ventilatory effort), diaphoresis, skin either flushed or cold and clammy, heart block, bradycardia, paralysis, ***coma, seizures, death.*** *Treatment:* Direct therapy toward an

---

bold italic = life threatening side effect

increase in central fluid volume. Do *not* use vasoconstrictors.

Drug Interactions

Ethanol / Additive vasodilation
Calcium channel blockers / Severe orthostatic hypotension
Organic nitrates / Severe orthostatic hypotension

EMS CONSIDERATIONS

See also *Antianginal Drugs, Nitrates/Nitrites,* and *Isosorbide dinitrate.*

Isotretinoin

(eye-so-TRET-ih-noyn)
Pregnancy Class: X
Accutane **(Rx)**
Classification: Vitamin A metabolite (antiacne, keratinization stabilizer)

Mechanism of Action: Reduces sebaceous gland size, decreases sebum secretion, and inhibits abnormal keratinization.

Uses: Severe recalcitrant cystic acne unresponsive to other therapy. *Investigational:* Cutaneous disorders of keratinization, cutaneous T-cell lymphoma (mycosis fungoides), leukoplakia, prevention of secondary primary tumors in those treated for squamous-cell carcinoma of the head and neck.

Contraindications: Due to the possibility of fetal abnormalities or spontaneous abortion, women who are pregnant or intend to become pregnant should not use the drug. Certain conditions for use should be met in women with childbearing potential (see package insert). Use during lactation and in children.

Precautions: Intolerance to contact lenses may develop.

Route/Dosage ————————
• **Capsules**
Recalcitrant cystic acne.
Adults, individualized, initial: 0.5–1 mg/kg/day (range: 0.5–2 mg/kg/day) divided in two doses for 15–20 weeks. Adjust dose based on toxicity and clinical response; if cyst count decreases by 70% or more, drug may be discontinued. If neces-

sary, a second course of therapy may be instituted after a rest period of 2 months. Doses of 0.05–0.5 mg/kg/day are effective but result in higher frequency of relapses.

Keratinization disorders.
Doses up to 4 mg/kg/day have been used.

Prevent second tumors in squamous-cell carcinoma of the head and neck.
50–100 mg/m^2.

How Supplied: *Capsule:* 10 mg, 20 mg, 40 mg

Side Effects: *Skin:* Cheilitis, skin fragility, pruritus, dry skin, desquamation of facial skin, drying of mucous membranes, brittle nails, photosensitivity, rash, hypo- or hyperpigmentation, urticaria, erythema nodosum, hirsutism, excess granulation of tissues as a result of healing, petechiae, peeling of palms and soles, skin infections, paronychia, thinning of hair, nail dystrophy, pyogenic granuloma, bruising. *CNS:* Headache, fatigue, pseudotumor cerebri (i.e., headaches, papilledema, disturbances in vision), depression. *Ocular:* Conjunctivitis, optic neuritis, corneal opacities, dry eyes, decrease in acuity of night vision, photophobia, eyelid inflammation, cataracts, visual disturbances. *GI:* Dry mouth, N&V, abdominal pain, nonspecific GI symptoms, inflammatory bowel disease (including regional enteritis), anorexia, weight loss, inflammation and bleeding of gums. *Neuromuscular:* Arthralgia, muscle pain, bone and joint pain and stiffness, skeletal hyperostosis. *CV:* Flushing, palpitation, tachycardia. *GU:* White cells in urine, proteinuria, nonspecific urogenital findings, microscopic or gross hematuria, abnormal menses. *Other:* Epistaxis, dry nose and mouth, respiratory infections, disseminated herpes simplex, edema, transient chest pain, development of diabetes, hepatitis, hepatotoxicity, vasculitis, anemia, lymphadenopathy, flushing, palpitations.

OD Overdose Management: *Symptoms:* Abdominal pain, ataxia, cheilosis, dizziness, facial flushing, headache, vomiting. Symptoms are transient. *Treatment:* Symptoms are quickly resolved with drug cessation or decrease in dose.

Drug Interactions

Alcohol / Potentiation of ↑ in serum triglycerides

Benzoyl peroxide / ↑ Drying effects of isotretinoin

Carbamazepine / ↓ Carbamazepine plasma levels

Minocycline / ↑ Risk of development of pseudotumor cerebri or papilledema

Tetracycline / ↑ Risk of development of pseudotumor cerebri or papilledema

Tretinoin / ↑ Drying effects of isotretinoin

Vitamin A / ↑ Risk of toxicity

EMS CONSIDERATIONS

None.

Isradipine
(iss-RAD-ih-peen)
Pregnancy Class: C
DynaCirc, DynaCirc CR (Rx)
Classification: Calcium channel blocking agent

Mechanism of Action: Binds to calcium channels resulting in the inhibition of calcium influx into cardiac and smooth muscle and subsequent arteriolar vasodilation. Reduced systemic resistance leads to a decrease in BP with a small increase in resting HR. In patients with normal ventricular function, the drug reduces afterload leading to some increase in CO.

Onset of Action: 2-3 hr.

Uses: Alone or with thiazide diuretics in the management of essential hypertension. *Investigational:* Chronic stable angina.

Contraindications: Lactation.

Precautions: Safety and effectiveness have not been determined in children. Use with caution in patients with CHF, especially those taking a beta-adrenergic blocking agent. Bioavailability increases in those over 65 years of age, in impaired hepatic function, and in mild renal impairment.

Route/Dosage

• **Capsules**
  Hypertension.
  Adults, initial: 2.5 mg b.i.d. alone or in combination with a thiazide diuretic. If BP is not decreased satisfactorily after 2–4 weeks, the dose may be increased in increments of 5 mg/day at 2 to 4-week intervals up to a maximum of 20 mg/day. Adverse effects increase at doses above 10 mg/day.

• **Tablets, Controlled-Release**
  Hypertension.
  Adults: 5–10 mg once daily.

How Supplied: *Capsule:* 2.5 mg, 5 mg; *Tablet, Extended Release:* 5 mg, 10 mg

Side Effects: *CV:* Palpitations, edema, flushing, tachycardia, SOB, hypotension, transient ischemic attack, ***stroke,*** atrial fibrillation, ***ventricular fibrillation, MI,*** CHF, angina. *CNS:* Headache, dizziness, fatigue, drowsiness, insomnia, lethargy, nervousness, depression, syncope, amnesia, psychosis, hallucinations, weakness, jitteriness, paresthesia. *GI:* Nausea, abdominal discomfort, diarrhea, vomiting, constipation, dry mouth. *Respiratory:* Dyspnea, cough. *Dermatologic:* Pruritus, urticaria. *Miscellaneous:* Chest pain, rash, pollakiuria, cramps of the legs and feet, nocturia, polyuria, hyperhidrosis, visual disturbances, numbness, throat discomfort, leukopenia, sexual difficulties.

Drug Interactions: Severe hypotension has been observed during fentanyl anesthesia with concomitant use of a beta-blocker and a calcium channel blocking agent.

EMS CONSIDERATIONS

See also *Calcium Channel Blocking Agents.*

Itraconazole
(ih-trah-KON-ah-zohl)

---

bold italic = life threatening side effect

Pregnancy Class: C
Sporanox **(Rx)**
Classification: Antifungal

Mechanism of Action: Believed to inhibit cytochrome P-450-dependent synthesis of ergosterol, a necessary component of fungal cell membranes. Absorption appears to increase when taken with a cola beverage.

Uses: Treatment of blastomycosis (pulmonary and extrapulmonary) and histoplasmosis (including chronic cavitary pulmonary disease and disseminated, nonmeningeal histoplasmosis) in both immunocompromised and nonimmunocompromised patients. To treat aspergillus infections (pulmonary and extrapulmonary) in patients intolerant or refractory to amphotericin B. Onychomycosis due to tinea unguium of the toenail with or without fingernail involvement. The drug is effective against *Blastomyces dermatitidis, Histoplasma capsulatum* and *H. duboisii, Aspergillus flavus* and *A. fumigatis,* and *Cryptococcus neoformans.* Oropharyngeal and esophageal candidiasis. In vitro activity has also been found for a number of other organisms, including *Sporothirx scheneckii, Trochophyton* species, *Candida albicans,* and *Candida species. Investigational:* (1) Superficial mycoses including dermatophytoses (tinea capitis, tinea corporis, tinea cruris, tinea pedis, and tinea manuum), pityriasis versicolor, candidiasis (vaginal, oral, chronic mucocutaneous), and seborpsoriasis. (2) Systemic mycoses including dimorphic infections (paracoccidioidomycosis, coccidioidomycosis), cryptococcal infections (meningitis, disseminated), and candidiasis. (3) Miscellaneous mycoses including fungal keratitis, alternariosis, leishmaniasis (cutaneous), subcutaneous mycoses (chromomycosis, sporotrichosis), and zygomycosis.

Contraindications: Concomitant use of astemizole, cisapride, triazolam, oral midazolam, or terfenadine. Hypersensitivity to the drug or its excipients. Lactation. Use for the treatment of onychomycosis in pregnant women or in women wishing to become pregnant.

Precautions: Safety and efficacy have not been determined in children although pediatric patients have been treated for systemic fungal infections.

Route/Dosage

• **Capsules**
Blastomycosis or histoplasmosis.
Adults: 200 mg once daily. If there is no improvement or the disease is progressive, the dose may be increased in 100-mg increments to a maximum of 400 mg/day. **Children, 3–16 years of age:** 100 mg/day (for systemic fungal infections).
Aspergilliosis.
200–400 mg daily.
Life-threatening infections.
Adults: A loading dose of 200 mg t.i.d. for the first 3 days should be given.
Onychomycosis.
200 mg once a day for 12 consecutive weeks. Alternatively, for fingernail fungus, 200 mg b.i.d. for 1 week, followed by a 3-week rest and then a second 1-week pulse of 200 mg b.i.d.
Unlabeled uses.
Adults: 50–400 mg/day for 1 day to more than 6 months, depending on the condition and the response.

• **Oral Solution**
Oropharyngeal candidiasis.
200 mg/day for 1–2 weeks.
Esophageal candidiasis.
100 mg/day for a minimum of 3 weeks.

How Supplied: *Capsule:* 100 mg; *Oral Solution:* 10 mg/mL

Side Effects: *GI:* N&V, diarrhea, abdominal pain, anorexia, general GI disorders, flatulence, constipation, gastritis. *CNS:* Headache, dizziness, vertigo, insomnia, decreased libido, somnolence, depression. *CV:* Hypertension, orthostatic hypotension, vasculitis. *Dermatologic:* Rash (occurs more frequently in immunocompromised patients also taking immunosuppressant drugs), pruritus. *Allergic:* Rash, pruritus, urticaria, angioedema, and rarely, ***anaphylaxis and Stevens-Johnson syndrome.*** *Miscellaneous:* Edema, fatigue, fever, malaise, abnormal hepatic function, hypokalemia, albuminuria, tinnitus, impotence, adrenal insufficiency, gynecomastia, breast pain in males, menstrual disorder, hepatitis (rare), neuropathy (rare).

OD **Overdose Management:** *Symptoms:* Extension of side effects. *Treatment:* Use supportive measures, including gastric lavage and sodium bicarbonate. Dialysis will not remove itraconazole.

Drug Interactions

Astemizole / ↑ Astemizole levels → serious CV toxicity including ventricular tachycardia, torsades de pointes, and death.

Calcium blockers (especially amlodipine and nifedipine) / Development of edema

Cisapride / Cisapride levels serious CV toxicity including ventricular tachycardia, torsades de pointes, and death.

Cyclosporine and HMG-CoA reductase inhibitors / Possible development of rhabdomyolysis. ↑ Cyclosporine levels (dose of cyclosporine should be ↓ by 50% if itraconazole doses are much greater than 100 mg/day)

Digoxin / ↑ Digoxin levels

H₂ Antagonists / ↓ *Plasma levels of itraconazole*

Midazolam, oral / ↑ Levels of oral midazolam → potentiation of sedative and hypnotic effects

Isoniazid / ↓ Plasma levels of itraconazole

Phenytoin / ↓ Plasma levels of itraconazole; also, metabolism of phenytoin may be altered

Rifampin / ↓ Plasma levels of itraconazole

Quinidine / Tinnitus and decreased hearing

Sulfonylureas / ↑ Risk of hypoglycemia

Tacrolimus / ↑ Levels of tacrolimus

Terfenadine / ↑ Terfenadine levels → serious CV toxicity including

ventricular tachycardia, torsades de pointes, and death

Triazolam / Levels of triazolam potentiation of sedative and hypnotic effects

Warfarin / ↑ Anticoagulant effect of warfarin

EMS CONSIDERATIONS
None.

Ivermectin
(eye-ver-MEK-tin)
Pregnancy Class: C
Stromectol **(Rx)**
Classification: Anthelmintic

Mechanism of Action: Binds selectively to glutamate-gated chloride channels that occur in invertebrate nerve and muscle cells. This leads to increase in permeability of cell membrane to chloride ions and hyperpolarization of nerve or muscle cell, resulting in paralysis and death of parasite.

Uses: Intestinal strongyloidiasis due to *Strongyloides stercoralis.* Onchocerciasis due to Onchocerca volvulus.

Precautions: Use during lactation only if benefits outweigh risks. Those with hyperreactive onchodermatitis (sowdah) may be more likely to have severe side effects. Control of extraintestinal strongyloidiasis is difficult in immunocompromised patients.

Route/Dosage
- **Tablets**
    Strongyloidiasis.
Single oral dose to provide about 200 mcg/kg: **15–24 kg:** 0.5 tablet; **25–35 kg:** 1 tablet; **36–50 kg:** 1.5 tablets; **51–65 kg:** 2 tablets; **66–79 kg:** 2.5 tablets.
    Onchocerciasis.
Single oral dose to provide about 150 mcg/kg: **15–25 kg:** 0.5 tablet; **26–44 kg:** 1 tablet; **45–64 kg:** 1.5 tablets; **65–84 kg:** 2 tablets.

How Supplied: *Tablet:* 6 mg

Side Effects: When used to treat strongyloidiasis. *GI:* Diarrhea,

---

bold italic = life threatening side effect

nausea, anorexia, constipation, vomiting, abdominal pain. *CNS:* Dizziness, somnolence, tremor, vertigo. *Dermatologic:* Pruritus, rash, urticaria. *Miscellaneous:* Asthenia, fatigue.

When used to treat onchocerciasis. *Mazzotti reaction:* Pruritus, edema, papular and pustular or frank urticarial rash, fever, inguinal lymph node enlargement and tenderness, axillary lymph node enlargement and tenderness, arthralgia, synovitis, cervical lymph node enlargement and tenderness. *Ophthalmic:* Limbitis, punctate opacity, abnormal sensation in the eyes, anterior uveitis, chorioretinitis, choroiditis, conjunctivitis, eyelid edema, keratitis. *Miscellaneous:* Tachycardia, peripheral edema, facial edema, orthostatic hypotension, headache, myalgia, worsening of bronchial asthma.

OD **Overdose Management:** *Symptoms:* Asthenia, diarrhea, dizziness, edema, headache, nausea, rash, vomiting, abdominal pain, ataxia, dyspnea, paresthesia, seizure, urticaria. *Treatment:* Supportive therapy, including parenteral fluids and electrolytes, respiratory support, and pressor agents (if significant hypotension). Induce emesis or gastric lavage as soon as possible, followed by laxatives and other anti-poison measures.

EMS CONSIDERATIONS
None.

K

Kanamycin sulfate
(kan-ah-MY-sin)
Pregnancy Class: D
Kantrex, Klebcil **(Rx)**
Classification: Aminoglycoside antibiotic and antitubercular agent (tertiary)

Mechanism of Action: Activity resembles that of neomycin and streptomycin.

Uses: Parenteral: Initial therapy for infections due to *Escherichia coli, Proteus, Enterobacter aerogenes, Klebsiella pneumoniae, Serratia marcescens,* and *Acinetobacter.* May be combined with a penicillin or cephalosporin before knowing results of susceptibility tests. *Investigational:* As part of a multiple-drug regimen for *Mycobacterium avium* complex in AIDS patients.

PO: Adjunct to mechanical cleansing of large bowel for suppression of intestinal bacteria; hepatic coma.

Precautions: Use with caution in premature infants and neonates.

Route/Dosage ———————
• **Capsules**
  Intestinal bacteria suppression.
1 g every hour for 4 hr; **then,** 1 g q 6 hr for 36–72 hr.
  Hepatic coma.
8–12 g/day in divided doses.
• **IM, IV**
Adults and children: 15 mg/kg/day in two to three equal doses. Maximum daily dose should not exceed 1.5 g regardless of route of administration.

For calculating dosage interval (in hr) in patients with impaired renal function, multiply serum creatinine (mg/100 mL) by 9.
• **IM**
  Tuberculosis.
Adults: 15 mg/kg/day. Not recommended for use in children.
• **Intraperitoneal**
500 mg diluted in 20 mL sterile distilled water.
• **Inhalation**
250 mg in saline—nebulize b.i.d.–q.i.d.
  Irrigation of abscess cavities, pleural space, ventricular cavities.
0.25% solution.

How Supplied: *Capsule:* 500 mg; *Injection:* 1 g/3 mL, 75 mg/2 mL, 500 mg/2 mL

Side Effects: Additional: Sprue-like syndrome with steatorrhea, malabsorption, and electrolyte imbalance.
Drug Interactions: Additional: Procainamide ↑ muscle relaxation.

EMS CONSIDERATIONS

See also *Anti-Infectives*.

Ketoconazole

(kee-toe-KON-ah-zohl)
Pregnancy Class: C
name>Nizoral **(Rx)**,Nizoral !B(Ketoconazole)!B> Nizoral AD **(OTC)**
Classification: Broad-spectrum antifungal

Mechanism of Action: Inhibits synthesis of sterols (e.g., ergosterol), damaging the cell membrane and resulting in loss of essential intracellular material. Also inhibits biosynthesis of triglycerides and phospholipids and inhibits oxidative and peroxidative enzyme activity. When used to treat *Candida albicans,* it inhibits transformation of blastospores into the invasive mycelial form. Use in Cushing's syndrome is due to its ability to inhibit adrenal steroidogenesis.
Uses: PO: Candidiasis, chronic mucocutaneous candidiasis, candiduria, histoplasmosis, chromomycosis, oral thrush, blastomycosis, coccidioidomycosis, paracoccidioidomycosis. Recalcitrant cutaneous dermatophyte infections not responding to other therapy. **Cream:** Tinea pedis. Tinea corporis and tinea cruris due to *Trichophyton rubrum, T. mentagrophytes,* and *Epidermophyton floccosum.* Tinea versicolor caused by *Microsporum furfur;* cutaneous candidiasis caused by *Candida* species; seborrheic dermatitis. **Shampoo:** To reduce scaling due to dandruff and tinea versicolor. *Investigational:* Onychomycosis due to *Candida* and *Trichophyton.* High doses to treat CNS fungal infections. Advanced prostate cancer, Cushing's syndrome.
Contraindications: Hypersensitivity, fungal meningitis. Topical product not for ophthalmic use. Use during lactation.
Precautions: Use tablets with caution in children less than 2 years of age. The safety and effectiveness of the shampoo and cream have not been determined in children. Use with caution during lactation.

Route/Dosage
• **Tablets**
Fungal infections.
Adults: 200 mg once daily; in serious infections or if response is not sufficient, increase to 400 mg once daily.
Pediatric, over 2 years: 3.3–6.6 mg/kg once daily. Dosage has not been established for children less than 2 years of age.
CNS fungal infections.
Adults: 800–1,200 mg/day.
Advanced prostate cancer.
400 mg q 8 hr.
Cushing's syndrome.
800–1,200 mg/day.
• **Topical Cream (2%)**
Tinea corporis, tinea cruris, tinea versicolor, tinea pedis, cutaneous candidiasis.
Cover the affected and immediate surrounding areas once daily (twice daily for more resistant cases). Duration of treatment is usually 2 weeks.
Seborrheic dermatitis.
Apply to affected area b.i.d. for 4 weeks or until symptoms clear.
• **Shampoo (1%, 2%)**
Use twice a week for 4 weeks with at least 3 days between each shampooing. **Then,** use as required to maintain control.
How Supplied: *Cream:* 2%; *Shampoo:* 2%; *Tablet:* 200 mg
Side Effects: *GI:* N&V, abdominal pain, diarrhea. *CNS:* Headache, dizziness, somnolence, fever, chills, suicidal tendencies, depression (rare). *Hematologic:* Thrombocytopenia, leukopenia, **hemolytic anemia.** *Miscellaneous:* Hepatotoxicity, photophobia, pruritus, gynecomastia, impotence, bulging fontanelles, urticaria, decreased serum testosterone levels, anaphylaxis (rare). *Topical cream:* Stinging, irritation, pruritus. *Sham-*

K

---

bold italic = life threatening side effect

poo: Increased hair loss, irritation, abnormal hair texture, itching, oiliness or dryness of the scalp and hair, scalp pustules.

Drug Interactions

Antacids / ↓ Absorption of ketoconazole due to ↑ pH induced by these drugs

Anticoagulants / ↑ Effect of anticoagulants

Anticholinergics / ↓ Absorption of ketoconazole due to ↑ pH induced by these drugs

Astemizole / ↑ Plasma levels of astemizole → serious CV effects

Cisapride / ↑ Risk of serious cardiac arrhythmias

Corticosteroids / ↑ Risk of corticosteroid toxicity due to ↑ bioavailability

Cyclosporine / ↑ Levels of cyclosporine (may be used therapeutically to decrease the dose of cyclosporine)

Histamine H$_2$ antagonists / ↓ *Absorption of ketoconazole due to ↑ pH induced by these drugs*

Isoniazid / ↓ Bioavailability of ketoconazole

Rifampin / ↓ Serum levels of both drugs

Terfenadine / ↑ Plasma levels of terfenadine → serious CV effects

Theophyllines / ↓ Serum levels of theophylline

EMS CONSIDERATIONS

See also *Anti-Infectives.*

Ketoprofen

(kee-toe-PROH-fen)
Pregnancy Class: B
Orudis, Orudis KT **(Rx)**
Classification: Nonsteroidal anti-inflammatory drug

Mechanism of Action: Possesses anti-inflammatory, antipyretic, and analgesic properties. Known to inhibit both prostaglandin and leukotriene synthesis, to have antibradykinin activity, and to stabilize lysosomal membranes.

Onset of Action: 15-30 min.

Duration of Action: 4-6 hr.

Uses: Rx: Acute or chronic rheumatoid arthritis and osteoarthritis (both capsules and sustained-release capsules). Primary dysmenorrhea. Analgesic for mild to moderate pain.

OTC: Temporary relief of aches and pains associated with the common cold, toothache, headache, muscle aches, backache, menstrual cramps, reduction of fever, and minor pain of arthritis.

Investigational: Juvenile rheumatoid arthritis, sunburn, prophylaxis of migraine, migraine due to menses.

Contraindications: Use during late pregnancy, in children, and during lactation. Use of the extended-release product for acute pain in any patient or for initial therapy in patients who are small, elderly, or who have renal or hepatic impairment.

Precautions: Safety and effectiveness have not been established in children. Geriatric patients may manifest increased and prolonged serum levels due to decreased protein binding and clearance. Use with caution in patients with a history of GI tract disorders, in fluid retention, hypertension, and heart failure.

Route/Dosage

• **Rx: Extended Release Capsules, Capsules**

Rheumatoid arthritis, osteoarthritis.
Adults, initial: 75 mg t.i.d. or 50 mg q.i.d.; **maintenance:** 150–300 mg in three to four divided doses daily. Doses above 300 mg/day are not recommended. Alternatively, 200 mg once daily using the sustained-release formulation (Oruvail). Decrease dose by one-half to one-third in patients with impaired renal function or in geriatric patients.

Mild to moderate pain, dysmenorrhea.
Adults: 25–50 mg q 6–8 hr as required, not to exceed 300 mg/day. Reduce dose in smaller or geriatric patients and in those with liver or renal dysfunction. Doses greater than 75 mg do not provide any added therapeutic effect.

• **OTC: Tablets**

Adults, over 16 years of age: 12.5 mg with a full glass of liquid every 4 to 6 hr. If pain or fever persists after 1 hr follow with an additional 12.5

mg. Experience may determine that an initial dose of 25 mg gives a better effect. Do not exceed a dose of 25 mg in a 4- to 6-hr period or 75 mg in a 24-hr period.

How Supplied: *Capsule:* 25 mg, 50 mg, 75 mg; *Capsule, Extended Release:* 100 mg, 150 mg, 200 mg; *Tablet:* 12.5 mg

Side Effects: Additional: *GI:* Peptic ulcer, **GI bleeding,** dyspepsia, nausea, diarrhea, constipation, abdominal pain, flatulence, anorexia, vomiting, stomatitis. *CNS:* Headache, *CV:* Peripheral edema, fluid retention.

Drug Interactions: Additional: *Acetylsalicylic acid/* ↑ Plasma ketoprofen levels due to ↓ plasma protein binding. *Hydrochlorothiazide/* ↓ Chloride and potassium excretion. *Methotrexate/* Concomitant use → toxic plasma levles of methotrexate. *Probenecid/* ↓ Plasma clearance of ketoprofen and ↓ plasma protein binding. *Warfarin/* Additive effect to cause bleeding.

EMS CONSIDERATIONS

See also *Nonsteroidal Anti-Inflammatory Drugs.*

Ketorolac tromethamine
(kee-toh-ROH-lack)
Pregnancy Class: C
Acular, Acular PF, Toradol, Toradol IM **(Rx)**
Classification: Nonsteroidal anti-inflammatory drug

Mechanism of Action: Possesses anti-inflammatory, analgesic, and antipyretic effects.
Onset of Action: Within 30 min; **Maximum effect:** 1-2 hr after IV or IM dosing.
Duration of Action: 4-6 hr.
Uses: PO: Short-term (up to 5 days) management of severe, acute pain that requires analgesia at the opiate level. Always initiate therapy with IV or IM followed by PO only as continuation treatment, if necessary.
IM/IV: Ketorolac has been used with morphine and meperidine and shows an opioid-sharing effect. The combination can be used for break through pain. **Ophthalmic:** Relieve itching caused by seasonal allergic conjunctivitis. Reduce ocular pain and photophobia following incisional refractive surgery (Acular PF).

Contraindications: Hypersensitivity to the drug, incomplete or partial syndrome of nasal polyps, angioedema, and bronchospasm due to aspirin or other NSAIDs. Use in patients with advanced renal impairment or in those at risk for renal failure due to volume depletion. Use in suspected or confirmed cardiovascular bleeding, hemorrhagic diathesis, or incomplete hemostasis and in those with a high risk of bleeding. Use as an obstetric preoperative medication or for obstetric analgesia. Routine use with other NSAIDs. Intrathecal or epidural administration. Use in labor and delivery. Use of the ophthalmic solution in patients wearing soft contact lenses.

Precautions: Use with caution in impaired hepatic or renal function, during lactation, in geriatric patients, and in patients on high-dose salicylate regimens. The age, dosage, and duration of therapy should receive special consideration when using this drug. Safety and effectiveness have not been determined in children.

Route/Dosage
• **IM**
  Analgesic, single dose.
Adults: less than 65 years of age: One 60-mg dose. **Adults, over 65 years of age, in renal impairment, or weight less than 50 kg:** One 30-mg dose.
  Analgesic, multiple dose.
Adults, less than 65 years of age: 30 mg q 6 hr, not to exceed 120 mg daily. **Adults, over 65 years of age, in renal impairment, or weight less than 50 kg:** 15 mg q 6 hr, not to exceed 60 mg daily.
• **IV**
  Analgesic, single dose.
Adults, less than 65 years of age: One 30-mg dose. **Adults, over 65**

K

years of age, in renal impairment, or weight less than 50 kg:
One 15-mg dose.

• **Tablets**

Transition from IV/IM to PO.

Adults less than 65 years of age: 20 mg as a first PO dose for patients who received 60 mg IM single dose, 30 mg IV single dose, or 30 mg multiple dose IV/IM; **then,** 10 mg q 4–6 hr, not to exceed 40 mg in a 24-hr period. **Adults, over 65 years of age, in renal impairment, or weight less than 50 kg:** 10 mg as a first PO dose for those who received a 30-mg IM single dose, a 15-mg IV single dose, or a 15-mg multiple dose IV/IM; **then,** 10 mg q 4–6 hr, not to exceed 40 mg in a 24-hr period.

• **Ophthalmic Solution**

Seasonal allergic conjunctivitis.

1 gtt (0.25 mg) q.i.d. Efficacy has not been determined beyond 1 week of use.

Following cataract extraction.

1 gtt to the affected eye(s) q.i.d. beginning 24 hr after surgery and continuing for 2 weeks postoperatively.

Ocular pain and photophobia after incisional refractive surgery.

1 gtt (0.25 mg) q.i.d. for up to 3 days after surgery.

How Supplied: *Injection:* 15 mg/mL, 30 mg/mL; *Ophthalmic solution:* 0.5%; *Tablet:* 10 mg

Side Effects: Additional: *CV:* Vasodilation, pallor. *GI:* GI pain, peptic ulcers, nausea, dyspepsia, flatulence, GI fullness, somatitis, excessive thirst, GI bleeding (higher risk in geriatric patients), **perforation.** *CNS:* Headache, nervousness, abnormal thinking, depression, euphoria. *Hypersensitivity:* **Bronchospasm, anaphylaxis.** *Miscellaneous:* Purpura, asthma, abnormal vision, abnormal liver function. *Ophthalmic solution:* Transient stinging and burning following instillation, ocular irritation, allergic reactions, superficial ocular infections, superficial keratitis.

Drug Interactions: Ketorolac may ↑ plasma levels of salicylates due to ↓ plasma protein binding.

EMS CONSIDERATIONS

See also *Nonsteroidal Anti-Inflammatory Drugs.*

Administration/Storage

IV 1. When used IM/IV, the IV bolus must be given over no less than 15 sec. Give IM slowly and deeply into the muscle.

2. Protect the injection from light.

Ketotifen fumarate

(kee-TOHT-ih-fen)
Pregnancy Class: C
Zaditor **(Rx)**
Classification: Ophthalmic decongestant

Mechanism of Action: Selective, non-competitive histamine H_1 receptor antagonist and mast cell stabilizer. Inhibits release of mediators from cells involved in hypersensitivity reactions. Decreased chemotaxis and activation of eosinophils. Rapid acting; effect seen within minutes of administration.

Uses: Temporary prophylaxis of itching of the eye due to allergic conjunctivitis.

Contraindications: Use orally or by injection. Use to treat contact lens-related irritation.

Precautions: Use with caution during lactation. Safety and efficacy have not been determined in children less than 3 years of age.

Route/Dosage

• **Solution, Ophthalmic**

Allergic conjunctivitis.

1 gtt in the affected eye(s) q 8–12 hr.

How Supplied: *Solution:* 0.025%

Side Effects: *Ophthalmic:* Burning, stinging, conjunctivitis, conjunctival injection, discharge, dry eyes, eye pain, eyelid disorder, itching, keratitis, lacrimation disorder, mydriasis, photophobia. *Miscellaneous:* Headache, rhinitis, allergic reactions, rash, flu syndrome, pharyngitis.

EMS CONSIDERATIONS

None.

L

Labetalol hydrochloride
(lah-BET-ah-lohl)
Pregnancy Class: C
Normodyne, Trandate **(Rx)**
Classification: Alpha- and beta-
adrenergic blocking agent

Mechanism of Action: Decreases BP by blocking both alpha- and beta-adrenergic receptors. Standing BP is lowered more than supine. Significant reflex tachycardia and bradycardia do not occur although AV conduction may be prolonged. **Onset of Action: PO:** 2-4 hr; **IV:** 5 min. **Peak effect, PO:** 2-4 hr. **Duration of Action: PO:** 8-12 hr. **Uses: PO:** Alone or in combination with other drugs for hypertension. **IV:** Hypertensive emergencies. *Investigational:* Pheochromocytoma, clonidine withdrawal hypertension.

Contraindications: Cardiogenic shock, cardiac failure, bronchial asthma, bradycardia, greater than first-degree heart block.

Precautions: Use with caution during lactation, in impaired renal and hepatic function, in chronic bronchitis and emphysema, and in diabetes (may prevent premonitory signs of acute hypoglycemia). Safety and efficacy in children have not been established.

Route/Dosage
• **Tablets**
  Hypertension.
Individualize. Initial: 100 mg b.i.d. alone or with a diuretic; **maintenance:** 200–400 mg b.i.d. up to 1,200–2,400 mg/day for severe cases.
• **IV**
  Hypertension.
Individualize. Initial: 20 mg slowly over 2 min; **then,** 40–80 mg q 10 min until desired effect occurs or a total of 300 mg has been given.
• **IV Infusion**
  Hypertension.

Initial: 2 mg/min; **then,** adjust rate according to response. **Usual dose range:** 50–300 mg.
  Transfer from IV to PO therapy.
Initial: 200 mg; **then,** 200–400 mg 6–12 hr later, depending on response. Thereafter, dosage based on response.
How Supplied: *Injection:* 5 mg/mL; *Tablet:* 100 mg, 200 mg, 300 mg
Side Effects: See also *Beta-Adrenergic Blocking Agents.* **After PO Use.** *GI:* Diarrhea, cholestasis with or without jaundice. *CNS:* Fatigue, drowsiness, paresthesias, headache, syncope (rare). *GU:* Impotence, priapism, ejaculation failure, difficulty in micturition, Peyronie's disease, acute urinary bladder retention. *Respiratory:* Dyspnea, bronchospasm. *Musculoskeletal:* Muscle cramps, asthenia, toxic myopathy. *Dermatologic:* Generalized maculopapular, lichenoid, or urticarial rashes; bullous lichen planus, psoriasis, facial erythema, reversible alopecia. *Ophthalmic:* Abnormal vision, dry eyes. *Miscellaneous:* SLE, positive antinuclear factor, antimitochondrial antibodies, fever, edema, nasal stuffiness.

After parenteral use. *CV:* Ventricular arrhythmias. *CNS:* Numbness, somnolence, yawning. *Miscellaneous:* Pruritus, flushing, wheezing.

After PO or parenteral use. *GI:* N&V, dyspepsia, taste distortion. *CNS:* Dizziness, tingling of skin or scalp, vertigo. *Miscellaneous:* Postural hypotension, increased sweating.

OD Overdose Management: *Symptoms:* Excessive hypotension and bradycardia. *Treatment:* Induce vomiting or perform gastric lavage. Place patients in a supine position with legs elevated. If required, the following treatment can be used:
• Epinephrine or a beta-2 agonist (aerosol) to treat bronchospasm.
• Atropine or epinephrine to treat bradycardia.

L

---

bold italic = life threatening side effect

- Digitalis glycoside and a diuretic for cardiac failure; dopamine or dobutamine may also be used.
- Diazepam to treat seizures.
- Norepinephrine (or another vasopressor) to treat hypotension.
- Administration of glucagon (5–10 mg rapidly over 30 sec), followed by continuous infusion of 5 mg/hr, may be effective in treating severe hypotension and bradycardia.

Drug Interactions
Beta-adrenergic bronchodilators / Labetalol ↓ bronchodilator effect of these drugs
Cimetidine / ↑ Bioavailability of PO labetalol
Glutethimide / ↓ Effects of labetalol due to ↑ breakdown by liver
Halothane / ↑ Risk of severe myocardial depression → hypotension
Nitroglycerin / Additive hypotension
Tricyclic antidepressants / ↑ Risk of tremors

EMS CONSIDERATIONS

See also *Beta-Adrenergic Blocking Agents* and *Antihypertensive Agents*.
Administration/Storage
IV 1. Not compatible with 5% sodium bicarbonate injection.
2. May give IV undiluted (20 mg over 2 min) or reconstituted with dextrose or saline solutions (infuse at a rate of 2 mg/min).

Lactulose
(LAK-tyou-lohs)
Pregnancy Class: B
Cephulac, Cholac, Chronulac, Constilac, Constulose, Duphalac, Enulose, Evalose, Heptalac **(Rx)**
Classification: Ammonia detoxicant, laxative

Mechanism of Action: A disaccharide containing both lactose and galactose; causes a decrease in the blood concentration of ammonia in patients suffering from portal-systemic encephalopathy. Due to bacteria-induced degradation of lactulose in the colon, resulting in an acid medium. Ammonia will then migrate from the blood to the colon to form ammonium ion, which is trapped and cannot be absorbed. A laxative action due to increased osmotic pressure from lactic, formic, and acetic acids then expels the trapped ammonium. The decrease in blood ammonia concentration improves the mental state, EEG tracing, and diet protein tolerance of patients. The increased osmotic pressure also results in a laxative effect, which may take up to 24 hr.

Onset of Action: 24-48 hr.

Uses: Prevention and treatment of portal-systemic encephalopathy, including hepatic and prehepatic coma (Cephylac, Cholac, Enulose, Evalose, Heptalac are used). Chronic constipation (Chronulac, Constilac, Duphalac are used).

Contraindications: Patients on galactose-restricted diets.

Precautions: Safe use during lactation and in children has not been established. Infants who have been given lactulose have developed hyponatremia and dehydration. Use with caution in presence of diabetes mellitus.

Route/Dosage ————————
- **Syrup, Oral Solution**
  Encephalopathy.
Adults, initial: 30–45 mL (20–30 g) t.i.d.–q.i.d.; adjust q 2–3 days to obtain two or three soft stools daily. Long-term therapy may be required in portal-systemic encephalopathy; **infants:** 2.5–10 mL/day (1.6–6.6 g/day) in divided doses; **older children and adolescents:** 40–90 mL/day (26.6–60 g/day) in divided doses.
  During acute episodes of constipation.
30–45 mL (20–30 g) q 1–2 hr to induce rapid initial laxation.
  Chronic constipation.
Adults and children: 15–30 mL/day (10–20 g/day) as a single dose after breakfast (up to 60 mL/day may be required).

How Supplied: *Oral Solution:* 10g/15 mL ; *Syrup:* 10 g/15 mL

Side Effects: *GI:* N&V, diarrhea, cramps, flatulence, gaseous distention, belching.

Drug Interactions

Antacids / May inhibit the drop in pH of the colon required for lactulose activity

Neomycin / May cause ↓ degradation of lactulose due to neomycin-induced ↑ in elimination of certain bacteria in the colon

EMS CONSIDERATIONS

None.

Lamivudine (3TC)

(lah-MIH-vyou-deen)

Pregnancy Class: C

Epivir **(Rx)**

Classification: Antiviral drug

Mechanism of Action: Synthetic nucleoside analog effective against HIV. Converted to active 5'-triphosphate (L-TP) metabolite which inhibits HIV reverse transcription via viral DNA chain termination. L-TP also inhibits the RNA- and DNA-dependent DNA polymerase activities of reverse transcriptase.

Uses: In combination with AZT for the treatment of HIV infection, based on clinical or immunologic evidence of progression of the disease. There are no data on the effect of lamivudine and AZT on clinical progression of HIV infection, such as the incidence of opportunistic infections or survival.

Contraindications: Lactation.

Precautions: Patients taking lamivudine and AZT may continue to develop opportunistic infections and other complications of HIV infection. Use with caution and at a reduced dose in those with impaired renal function. Data on the use of lamivudine and AZT in pediatric patients are lacking; however, use the combination with extreme caution in children with pancreatitis.

Route/Dosage

• **Oral Solution, Tablets**

HIV infection.

Adults and adolescents, aged 12–16 years: 150 mg b.i.d. in combination with AZT. For adults with low body weight (less than 50 kg), the recommended dose is 2 mg/kg b.i.d. in combination with AZT. **Children, 3 months to 12 years of age:** 4 mg/kg b.i.d. (up to a maximum of 150 mg b.i.d.) in combination with AZT. In patients over 16 years of age, adjust the dose as follows in impaired renal function: C_{CR} less than 50 mL/min: 150 mg b.i.d.; C_{CR} 30–49 mL/min: 150 mg once daily; C_{CR} 15–29 mL/min: 150 mg for the first dose followed by 100 mg once daily; C_{CR} 5–14 mL/min: 150 mg for the first dose followed by 50 mg once daily; C_{CR} less than 5 mL/min: 50 mg for the first dose followed by 25 mg once daily.

How Supplied: *Tablet:* 150 mg; Solution 10 mg/mL

Side Effects: Side effects are for the combination of lamivudine plus AZT. *GI:* N&V, diarrhea, anorexia, or decreased appetite, abdominal pain, abdominal cramps, dyspepsia. *CNS:* Neuropathy, insomnia or other sleep disorders, dizziness, depressive disorders, paresthesias, peripheral neuropathies. *Respiratory:* Nasal signs and symptoms, cough. *Musculoskeletal:* Musculoskeletal pain, myalgia, arthralgia. *Body as a whole:* Headache, malaise, fatigue, fever or chills, skin rashes. *NOTE:* Pediatric patients have an increased risk to develop ***pancreatitis.***

Drug Interactions: Use of lamivudine with trimethoprim-sulfamethoxazole resulted in a significant increase in lamivudine levels.

EMS CONSIDERATIONS

See also *Antiviral Drugs.*

————*COMBINATION DRUG*————

Lamivudine/Zidovudine

(lah-MIH-vyou-deen, zye-DOH-vyou-deen)

Pregnancy Class: C

Combivir **(Rx)**

Classification: Antiviral drug combination

Mechanism of Action: Both drugs are reverse transcriptase inhibitors

L

with activity against HIV. Combination results in synergistic antiretroviral effect.

Uses: Treatment of HIV infection.

Contraindications: Use in patients requiring dosage reduction, children less than 12 years of age, C_{CR} less than 50 mL/min, body weight less than 50 kg, and in those experiencing dose-limiting side effects.

Route/Dosage ———————————
• **Tablets**
  HIV infection.
Adults and children over 12 years of age: One combination tablet—150 mg lamivudine/300 mg zidovudine—b.i.d.

How Supplied: Each Combivir tablet contains: *Antiviral:* Lamivudine, 150 mg and *Antiviral:* Zidovudine, 300 mg.

Side Effects: See individual drugs.

EMS CONSIDERATIONS

See also *Antiviral Drugs.*

Lamotrigine
(lah-MAH-trih-jeen)
Pregnancy Class: C
Lamictal **(Rx)**
Classification: Anticonvulsant

Mechanism of Action: Mechanism of anticonvulsant action not known. May act to inhibit voltage-sensitive sodium channels. This effect stabilizes neuronal membranes and modulates presynaptic transmitter release of excitatory amino acids such as glutamate and aspartate.

Uses: Adjunct in the treatment of partial seizures in adults with epilepsy. For add-on treatment of generalized seizures in adults and children with Lennox-Gastaut syndrome. *Investigational:* Adults with generalized clonic-tonic, absence, atypical absence, and myoclonic seizures.

Contraindications: Use during lactation and in children less than 16 years of age.

Precautions: Use with caution in patients with diseases or conditions that could affect metabolism or elimination of the drug, such as in im-paired renal, hepatic, or cardiac function.

Route/Dosage ———————————
• **Tablets**
  Treatment of partial seizures.
Adults and children over 16 years of age who are taking enzyme-inducing antiepileptic drugs, but not valproate: 50 mg once a day for weeks 1 and 2, followed by 100 mg/day in two divided doses for weeks 3 and 4. **Maintenance dose:** 300–500 mg/day given in two divided doses. The dose should be increased by 100 mg/day every week until maintenance levels are reached. **Adults and children over 16 years of age who are taking enzyme-inducing antiepileptic drugs plus valproic acid:** 25 mg every other day for weeks 1 and 2, followed by 25 mg once daily for weeks 3 and 4. **Maintenance dose:** 100–150 mg/day in two divided doses. The dose should be increased by 25–50 mg/day every 1–2 weeks.

How Supplied: *Chewable Tablet:* 5 mg, 25 mg; *Tablet:* 25 mg, 100 mg, 150 mg, 200 mg

Side Effects: Side effects listed are those with an incidence of 0.1% or greater. *CNS:* Dizziness, ataxia, somnolence, headache, incoordination, insomnia, tremor, depression, anxiety, irritability, decreased memory, speech disorder, confusion, disturbed concentration, sleep disorder, emotional lability, vertigo, mind racing, amnesia, nervousness, abnormal thinking, abnormal dreams, agitation, akathisia, aphasia, CNS depression, depersonalization, dyskinesia, dysphoria, euphoria, faintness, hallucinations, hostility, hyperkinesia, hypesthesia, myoclonus, panic attack, paranoid reaction, personality disorder, psychosis, stupor. *GI:* N&V, diarrhea, dyspepsia, constipation, tooth disorder, anorexia, dry mouth, abdominal pain, dysphagia, flatulence, gingivitis, gum hyperplasia, increased appetite, increased salivation, abnormal liver function tests, mouth ulceration, stomatitis, thirst. *CV:* Hot flashes, palpitations, flushing, migraine, syncope, tachycardia, vasodilation. *Musculoskeletal:* Arthralgia, joint disorder, myasthenia, dysarthria, muscle spasm, twitching. *Hematologic:* Anemia, ecchymosis, leukocytosis, leukopenia, lymphadenopathy, petechiae. *Respiratory:* Rhinitis, pharyngitis, increased cough, dyspnea, epistaxis, hyperventilation. *Dermatologic:* **Stevens-Johnson syndrome, toxic epidermal necrolysis,** pruritus, alopecia, acne, dry skin, eczema, erythema, hirsutism, maculopapular rash, sweating, urticaria. *Ophthalmologic:* Diplopia, blurred vision, nystagmus, abnormal vision, abnormal accommodation, conjunctivitis, oscillopsia, photophobia. *GU:* Dysmenorrhea, vaginitis, amenorrhea, female lactation, hematuria, polyuria, urinary frequency or incontinence, UTI, vaginal moniliasis. *Body as a whole:* **Possibility of sudden unexplained death in epilepsy,** flu syndrome, fever, infection, neck pain, malaise, **seizure exacerbation,** chills, halitosis, facial edema, weight gain or loss, peripheral edema, hyperglycemia. *Miscellaneous:* Ear pain, tinnitus, taste perversion.

OD **Overdose Management:** *Symptoms:* Possibility of dizziness, headache, somnolence, coma. *Treatment:* Hospitalization with general supportive care. If indicated, induce emesis or perform gastric lavage. Protect the airway.

Drug Interactions
Acetaminophen / ↓ Serum lamotrigine levels
Carbamazepine / Lamotrigine concentration is ↓ by about 40%
Phenobarbital / Lamotrigine concentration is ↓ by about 40%
Phenytoin / Lamotrigine concentration is ↓ by 45%–54%
Primidone / Lamotrigine concentration is ↓ by about 40%
Valproic acid / Lamotrigine concentration is ↑ twofold while valproic acid concentration is ↓ by 25%

EMS CONSIDERATIONS

See also *Anticonvulsants.*

Lansoprazole
(lan-SAHP-rah-zohl)
Pregnancy Class: B
Prevacid (Rx)
Classification: GI drug, proton pump inhibitor

Mechanism of Action: Suppresses gastric acid secretion by inhibition of the (H^+, K^+)-ATPase system located at the secretory surface of the parietal cells in the stomach. Drug is a gastric acid (proton) pump inhibitor in that it blocks the final step of acid production. Both basal and stimulated gastric acid secretion are inhibited, regardless of the stimulus. May have antimicrobial activity against *Helicobacter pylori.*

Uses: Short-term treatment (up to 4 weeks) for healing and symptomatic relief of active duodenal ulcer. Maintain healing of duodenal ulcer. With clarithromycin and/or amoxicillin to eradicate *Helicobacter pylori* infection in active or recurrent duodenal ulcers. Short-term treatment (up to 8 weeks) for healing and symptomatic relief of benign gastric ulcer. Short-term treatment (up to 8 weeks) for healing and symptomatic relief of all grades of erosive esophagitis. Maintain healing of erosive esophagitis. Long-term treatment of pathologic hypersecretory conditions, including Zollinger-Ellison syndrome. Short-term treatment of symptomatic GERD.

Contraindications: Lactation.

Precautions: Reduce dosage in impaired hepatic function. Symptomatic relief does not preclude the presence of gastric malignancy. Safety and efficacy have not been determined in children less than 18 years of age.

Route/Dosage
• **Capsules, Delayed Release**
   Treatment of duodenal ulcer.
Adults: 15 mg once daily before breakfast for 4 weeks.
   Maintenance of healed duodenal ulcer.
Adults: 15 mg once daily.

Duodenal ulcers associated with H. pylori.

Triple therapy: Lansoprazole, 30 mg, plus clarithromycin, 500 mg, and amoxicilin, 1 g, b.i.d. for 10 to 14 days. **Double therapy:** Lansoprazole, 30 mg, plus amoxicillin, 1 g, t.i.d. for 14 days in those intolerant or resistant to clarithromycin.

Treatment of gastric ulcer.

30 mg once daily for up to 8 weeks.

Treatment of erosive esophagitis.

30 mg before eating for up to 8 weeks. If the patient does not heal in 8 weeks, an additional 8 weeks of therapy may be given. If there is a recurrence, an additional 8-week course may be considered.

Maintenance of healed erosive esophagitis.

15 mg once daily for up to 12 months.

Pathologic hypersecretory conditions.

Initial: 60 mg once daily. Adjust the dose to patient need. Dosage may be continued as long as necessary. Doses up to 90 or 120 mg (in divided doses) daily have been given.

Treatment of GERD.

15 mg once daily.

How Supplied: *Enteric-coated capsule:* 15 mg, 30 mg

Side Effects: *GI:* Diarrhea, abdominal pain, nausea, melena, anorexia, bezoar, cardiospasm, cholelithiasis, constipation, dry mouth, thirst, dyspepsia, dysphagia, eructation, esophageal stenosis, esophageal ulcer, esophagitis, fecal discoloration, flatulence, gastric nodules, fundic gland polyps, gastroenteritis, *GI hemorrhage, rectal hemorrhage,* hematemesis, increased appetite, increased salivation, stomatitis, tenesmus, vomiting, ulcerative colitis. *CV:* Angina, hypertension or hypotension, *CVA, MI, shock,* palpitations, vasodilation. *CNS:* Headache, agitation, amnesia, anxiety, apathy, confusion, depression, syncope, dizziness, hallucinations, hemiplegia, aggravated hostility, decreased libido, nervousness, paresthesia, abnormal thinking. *GU:* Abnormal menses, breast enlargement, gynecomastia, breast tenderness, hematuria, albuminuria, glycosuria, impotence, kidney calculus. *Respiratory:* Asthma, bronchitis, increased cough, dyspnea, epistaxis, hemoptysis, hiccoughs, pneumonia, upper respiratory inflammation or infection. *Endocrine:* Diabetes mellitus, goiter, hypoglycemia or hyperglycemia. *Hematologic:* Anemia, eosinophilia, hemolysis. *Musculoskeletal:* Arthritis, arthralgia, musculoskeletal pain, myalgia. *Dermatologic:* Acne, alopecia, pruritus, rash, urticaria. *Ophthalmologic:* Amblyopia, eye pain, visual field defect. *Otic:* Deafness, otitis media, tinnitus. *Miscellaneous:* Gout, weight loss or gain, taste perversion, asthenia, candidiasis, chest pain, edema, fever, flu syndrome, halitosis, infection, malaise.

Drug Interactions

Ampicillin / ↓ Effect of ampicillin due to ↓ absorption

Digoxin / ↓ Effect of digoxin due to ↓ absorption

Iron salts / ↓ Effect of iron salts due to ↓ absorption

Ketoconazole / ↓ Effect of ketoconazole due to ↓ absorption

Sucralfate / Delayed absorption of lansoprazole

EMS CONSIDERATIONS

None.

Latanoprost

(lah-TAH-noh-prost)
Pregnancy Class: C
Xalatan **(Rx)**
Classification: Prostaglandin agonist

Mechanism of Action: A prostaglandin $F_2\alpha$ analog that decreases intraocular pressure by increasing the outflow of aqueous humor.

Onset of Action: 3-4hr. **Maximum effect:** 8-12 hr.

Uses: To reduce intraocular pressure in open-angle glaucoma and ocular hypertension in patients who are intolerant of other drugs to reduce intraocular pressure or who have been unresponsive to other drug therapy.

Contraindications: Use while wearing contact lenses.

Precautions: May gradually change eye color by increasing the amount of brown pigment in the iris; the resultant color changes may be permanent. Use with caution during lactation. The drug product contains benzalkonium chloride, which may be absorbed by contact lenses. Safety and efficacy have not been determined in children.

Route/Dosage
- **Solution, 0.005%**
  Elevated intraocular pressure.
1 gtt (1.5 mcg) in the affected eye(s) once daily in the evening. More frequent use may decrease the intraocular pressure lowering effect.

How Supplied: *Ophthalmic solution:* 0.005%

Side Effects: *Ophthalmic:* Blurred vision, burning, stinging, conjunctival hyperemia, foreign body sensation, itching, increased pigmentation of the iris, punctate epithelial keratopathy, dry eye, excessive tearing, eye pain, lid crusting, lid edema, lid erythema, lid discomfort or pain, photophobia, conjunctivitis, diplopia, discharge from the eye, retinal artery embolus, retinal detachment, vitreous hemorrhage from diabetic retinopathy (rare). *Systemic:* URTI (e.g., cold, flu), pain in muscles/joints/back, chest pain/angina pectoris, rash, allergic skin reactions.

Drug Interactions: A precipitate may form if lanatoprost is used with eye drops containing thimerosal.

EMS CONSIDERATIONS
None.

Leflunomide
(leh-FLOON-ah-myd)
Pregnancy Class: X
Arava **(Rx)**
Classification: Anti-arthritic drug

Mechanism of Action: Inhibits dihydroorotate dehydrogenase, an enzyme involved in de novo pyrimidine synthesis; has antiproliferative activity and an anti-inflammatory effect.

Uses: Treatment of active rheumatoid arthritis in adults, including to retard structural damage.

Contraindications: Use in pregnancy, lactation, in children less than 18 years of age, in hepatic insufficiency, or positive hepatitis B or C. Also, use in those with severe immunodeficiency, bone marrow dysplasia, severe uncontrolled infections, or vaccination with live vaccines.

Precautions: Use with caution in those with renal insufficiency.

Route/Dosage
- **Tablets**
  Rheumatoid arthritis.
Loading dose: 100 mg/day PO for 3 days. **Maintenance:** 20 mg/day; if this dose is not well tolerated, decrease to 10 mg/day. Doses greater than 20 mg/day are not recommended due to increased risk of side effects.

How Supplied: *Tablets:* 10 mg, 20 mg, 100 mg

Side Effects: *GI:* Diarrhea, N&V, dyspepsia, abnormal liver enzymes, GI/abdominal pain, anorexia, dry mouth, gastroenteritis, mouth ulcer, cholelithiasis, colitis, constipation, esophagitis, flatulence, gastritis, gingivitis, melena, oral moniliasis, pharyngitis, enlarged salivary gland, stomatitis or aphthous stomatitis, tooth disorder. *CNS:* Headache, dizziness, paresthesia, anxiety, depression, insomnia, neuralgia, neuritis, sleep disorder, sweat, vertigo. *CV:* Hypertension (as pre-existing condition was over represented in drug treatment groups), chest pain, angina pectoris, migraine, palpitation, tachycardia, vasculitis, vasodilation, varicose vein. *Dermatologic:* Alopecia, rash, pruritus, eczema, dry skin, acne, contact dermatitis, fungal dermatitis, hair discoloration, hematoma, herpes simplex, herpes zoster, nail disorder, skin nodule, subcutaneous nodule, maculopapular rash, skin disorder, skin discoloration, skin ulcer. *Mus-*

L

culoskeletal: Joint disorder, tenosynovitis, synovitis, arthralgia, leg cramps, arthrosis, bursitis, muscle cramps, myalgia, bone necrosis, bone pain, tendon rupture. *Respiratory:* Respiratory infection, bronchitis, increased cough, pharyngitis, pneumonia, rhinitis, sinusitis, asthma, dyspnea, epistaxis, lung disorder. *GU:* Albuminuria, cystitis, dysuria, hematuria, menstrual disorder, vaginal moniliasis, prostate disorder, urinary frequency, UTI. *Hematologic:* Anemia, including iron deficiency anemia; ecchymosis. *Metabolic:* Weight loss, hypokalemia, peripheral edema, hyperglycemia, hyperlipidemia. *Ophthalmic:* Blurred vision, cataract, conjunctivitis, eye disorder. *Miscellaneous:* Diabetes mellitus, hyperthyroidism, taste perversion, back pain, injury accident, infection, asthenia, allergic reaction, flu syndrome, pain, abscess, cyst, fever, hernia, malaise, neck pain, pelvic pain.

OD Overdose Management: *Symptoms:* See Side Effects. *Treatment:* Give cholestyramine or charcoal. Dose of cholestyramine is 8 g t.i.d. PO for 24 hr. Dose of charcoal is 50 g made into a suspension for PO or NGT given q 6 hr for 24 hr.

Drug Interactions
Charcoal / Rapid and significant ↓ in active M1 metabolite of leflunomide
Cholestyramine / Rapid and significant ↓ in active M1 metabolite of leflunomide
Hepatotoxic drugs / ↑ Side effects
Rifampin / ↑ M1 peak levels

EMS CONSIDERATIONS
None.

Letrozole
(LET-roh-zohl)
Pregnancy Class: D
Femara **(Rx)**
Classification: Antineoplastic, hormone

Mechanism of Action: A nonsteroidal competitive inhibitor of aromatase, resulting in inhibition of conversion of androgens to estrogens. It acts by competitively binding to heme of cytochrome P450 subunit of aromatase, leading to decreased biosynthesis of estrogen in all tissues. Does not cause increase in serum FSH and does not affect synthesis of adrenocorticosteroids, aldosterone, or thyroid hormones.

Uses: Advanced breast cancer in postmenopausal women with disease progression following antiestrogen therapy.

Precautions: Use with caution during lactation and in those with severely impaired hepatic function. Safety and efficacy have not been determined in children.

Route/Dosage
• **Tablets**
 Advanced breast cancer.
Adults and elderly: 2.5 mg once/day. Continue until tumor progression is evident. Dosage adjustment is not needed in renal impairment if C_{CR} is greater than or equal to 10 mL/min.

How Supplied: *Tablet:* 2.5 mg

Side Effects: *CNS:* Headache, somnolence, dizziness, vertigo, depression, anxiety. *GI:* N&V, constipation, diarrhea, abdominal pain, anorexia, dyspepsia. *Body as a whole:* Fatigue, viral infections, peripheral edema, asthenia, decreased weight. *Dermatologic:* Hot flashes, rash, pruritus, alopecia, increased sweating. *Respiratory:* Dyspnea, coughing, pleural effusion. *Miscellaneous:* Chest pain, hypertension, arthralgia, fracture.

EMS CONSIDERATIONS
None.

Leucovorin calcium (Citrovorum factor, Folinic acid)
(loo-koh-VOR-in)
Pregnancy Class: C
Wellcovorin **(Rx)**
Classification: Folic acid derivative

Mechanism of Action: Derivative of folic acid; is a mixture of the diasterioisomers of the 5-formyl derivative of tetrahydrofolic acid. Does not require reduction by dihydrofolate reductase to be active in intracellular metabolism; thus, it is not affected by dihydrofolate inhibitors. Leucovorin can counteract the therapeutic and toxic effects of methotrexate (acts by inhibiting dihydrofolate reductase) but can enhance the effects of 5-fluorouracil (5-FU). Is rapidly absorbed.

Onset of Action: PO: 20-30 min; **IM:** 10-20 min; **IV:** <5 min.

Duration of Action: 3-6 hr.

Uses: PO and Parenteral: Prophylaxis and treatment of toxicity due to methotrexate and folic acid antagonists (e.g., pyrimethamine and trimethoprim). Leucovorin rescue following high doses of methotrexate for osteosarcoma. **Parenteral:** Megaloblastic anemias due to nutritional deficiency, sprue, pregnancy, and infancy when oral folic acid is not appropriate. Adjunct with 5-FU to prolong survival in the palliative treatment of metastatic colorectal carcinoma. *Note:* It is recommended for megaloblastic anemia caused by pregnancy even though the drug is pregnancy category C.

Contraindications: Pernicious anemia or megaloblastic anemia due to vitamin B_{12} deficiency.

Precautions: Use with caution during lactation. May increase the frequency of seizures in susceptible children. When leucovorin is used with 5-FU for advanced colorectal cancer, the dosage of 5-FU must be lower than usual as leucovorin enhances the toxicity of 5-FU. The benzyl alcohol in the parenteral form may caues a fatal gasping syndrome in premature infants.

Route/Dosage ────────────
• **IM, IV, Tablets**
  Advanced colorectal cancer.
Either leucovorin, 200 mg/m² by slow IV over a minimum of 3 min followed by 5-FU, 370 mg/m² IV **or** leucovorin 20 mg/m² IV followed by 5-FU, 425 mg/m² IV. Treatment is re-

peated daily for 5 days with the 5-day treatment course repeated at 28-day intervals for two courses and then repeated at 4- to 5-week intervals as long as the patient has recovered from the toxic effects.

Leucovorin rescue after high-dose methotrexate therapy.
The dose of leucovorin is based on a methotrexate dose of 12–15 mg/m² given by IV infusion over 4 hr. The dose of leucovorin is 15 mg (10 mg/m²) PO, IM, or IV q 6 hr for 10 doses starting 24 hr after the start of the methotrexate infusion. Give leucovorin parenterally if there is nausea, vomiting, or GI toxicity. If serum methotrexate levels are greater than 0.2 µM at 72 hr and greater than 0.05 µM at 96 hr after administration, leucovorin should be continued at a dose of 15 mg PO, IM, or IV q 6 hr until methotrexate levels are less than 0.05 µM. If serum methotrexate levels are equal to or greater than 50 µM at 24 hr or equal to or greater than 5 µM at 48 hr after administration or if there is a 100% or greater increase in serum creatinine levels at 24 hr after methotrexate administration, the dose of leucovorin should be 150 mg IV q 3 hr until methotrexate levels are less than 1 µM; **then,** give leucovorin, 15 mg IV q 3 hr until methotrexate levels are less than 0.05 µM. If significant clinical toxicity is seen following methotrexate, leucovorin rescue should total 14 doses over 84 hr in subsequent courses of methotrexate therapy.

Impaired methotrexate elimination or accidental overdose.
Start leucovorin rescue as soon as the overdose is discovered and within 24 hr of methotrexate administration when excretion is impaired. Give leucovorin, 10 mg/m² PO, IM, or IV q 6 hr until serum methotrexate levels are less than 10^{-8} M. If the 24-hr serum creatinine has increased 50% over baseline or if the 24- or 48-hr methotrexate level is more than 5×10^{-6} M or greater than 9×10^{-7} M, respectively, the dose of leucovorin should

be increased to 100 mg/m² IV q 3 hr until the methotrexate level is less than 10⁻⁸ M. Urinary alkalinization with sodium bicarbonate solution (to maintain urine pH at 7 or greater) and hydration with 3 L/day should be undertaken at the same time.

Overdosage of folic acid antagonists.

5–15 mg/day.

Megaloblastic anemia due to folic acid deficiency.

Adults and children: Up to 1 mg/day.

How Supplied: *Injection:* 10 mg/mL; *Powder for injection:* 50 mg, 100 mg, 200 mg, 350 mg; *Tablet:* 5 mg, 10 mg, 15 mg, 25 mg

Side Effects: Leucovorin alone. Allergic reactions, including urticaria and *anaphylaxis.*

Leucovorin and 5-FU. *GI:* N&V, diarrhea, stomatitis, constipation, anorexia. *Hematologic:* Leukopenia, thrombocytopenia. *CNS:* Fatigue, lethargy, malaise. *Miscellaneous:* Infection, alopecia, dermatitis.

Drug Interactions

5-FU / ↑ Toxicity of 5-FU

Methotrexate / High doses of leucovorin ↓ effect of intrathecally administered methotrexate

PAS / ↓ Serum folate levels → folic acid deficiency

Phenobarbital / ↓ Effect of phenobarbital → ↑ frequency of seizures, especially in children

Phenytoin / ↓ Effect of phenytoin due to ↑ rate of breakdown by liver; also, phenytoin may ↓ plasma folate levels

Primidone / ↓ Effect of primidone → ↑ frequency of seizures, especially in children

Sulfasalazine / ↓ Serum folate levels → folic acid deficiency

EMS CONSIDERATIONS
None.

Leuprolide acetate
(loo-PROH-lyd)
Pregnancy Class: X
Lupron, Lupron Depot, Lupron Depot —3 Month, Lupron Depot — 4 Month, Lupron Depot-Ped, Lupron for Pediatric Use **(Rx)**
Classification: Antineoplastic agent, hormonal

Mechanism of Action: Related to the naturally occurring GnRH. By desensitizing GnRH receptors, gonadotropin secretion is inhibited. Initially, however, LH and FSH levels increase, leading to increases of sex hormones. However, decreases in these hormones will be observed within 2–4 weeks.

Uses: Palliative treatment in advanced prostatic cancer when orchiectomy or estrogen treatment are not appropriate. Endometriosis (use depot form). Central precocious puberty (use depot-PED form). In combination with iron supplements for the presurgical treatment of anemia caused by uterine fibroid tumors (use depot form). *Investigational:* With flutamide for metastatic prostatic cancer.

Contraindications: Pregnancy, in women who may become pregnant while receiving the drug, and during lactation. Sensitivity to benzyl alcohol (found in leuprolide injection). Undiagnosed abnormal vaginal bleeding. Hypersensitivity to GnRH or GnRH agonist analogs. The 30-mg depot in women.

Precautions: Safety and efficacy have not been determined in children (except depot-PED). May cause increased bone pain and difficulty in urination during the first few weeks of therapy for prostatic cancer.

Route/Dosage ————————

• **Depot, Injection**
Advanced prostatic cancer.
Injection: 1 mg/day SC using the syringes provided. Depot (IM): 7.5 mg monthly, 22.5 mg q 3 months, or 30 mg q 4 months.
Central precocious puberty.
Injection: **Initial:** 50 mcg/kg/day SC as a single dose. Dose may increased by 10 mcg/kg/day, which is the maintenance dose. Depot-Ped: **Initial:** 0.3 mg/kg/4 weeks (minimum 7.5 mg) as a single IM dose.
Endometriosis, uterine fibroids.

3.75 mg IM once a month for at least 6 months for endometriosis and 3 months or less for uterine fibroids. If further treatment is contemplated, assess bone density prior to beginning therapy.

How Supplied: *Injection:* 5 mg/mL; *Kit:* 5 mg/mL, 7.5 mg, 11.25 mg, 15 mg, 22.5 mg; *Powder for injection:* 3.75 mg, 7.5 mg. 11.5 mg, 15 mg, 30 mg

Side Effects: Injection and Depot. *GI:* N&V, anorexia, diarrhea, constipation, taste disorders/perversion, gingivitis, dysphagia, hepatic dysfunction. *CNS:* Pain, depression, emotional lability, insomnia, headache, dizziness, nervousness, paresthesias, anxiety, memory disorder, syncope, personality disorder, somnolence, spinal fracture/paralysis. *CV:* Peripheral edema, angina, *cardiac arrhythmias, TIA/stroke,* hypotension, vasodilation. *GU:* Hematuria, urinary frequency or urgency, dysuria, testicular pain, incontinence, cervix disorder, penile swelling, prostate pain. *Respiratory:* Dyspnea, hemoptysis, pneumonia, epistaxis, pulmonary infiltrates. *Endocrine:* Gynecomastia, breast tenderness, impotency, hot flashes, sweating, decreased testicular size, increased or decreased libido. *Musculoskeletal:* Myalgia, bone pain, pelvic fibrosis, ankylosing spondylosis. *Dermatologic:* Dermatitis, skin reactions, acne, seborrhea, hair growth, ecchymosis, hair loss, skin striae, erythema multiforme and other rashes, androgen-like effects. *Ophthalmic:* Ophthalmic disorder, abnormal vision. *Other:* Asthenia, diabetes, fever, chills, tinnitus, infection, body odor, hard nodule in throat, accelerated sexual maturation, hearing disorder, peripheral neuropathy.

Injection. *CV: MI, pulmonary emboli. GI: GI bleeding,* rectal polyps, peptic ulcer. *CNS:* Lethargy, mood swings, numbness, blackouts, fatigue. *Respiratory:* Cough, *pulmonary fibrosis,* pleural rub. *Dermatologic:* Carcinoma of the skin/ear, itching, dry skin, pigmentation, skin lesions. *GU:* Bladder spasms, urinary obstruction. *Miscellaneous:* Enlarged thyroid, inflammation, temporal bone swelling, blurred vision.

Depot. *CV:* Tachycardia, bradycardia, *heart failure,* varicose vein, palpitations. *GI:* Dysphagia, gingivitis. *CNS:* Delusions, confusion, hypesthesia. *GI:* Duodenal ulcer, dry mouth, thirst, appetite changes. *Respiratory:* Rhinitis, pharyngitis, pleural effusion. *Endocrine:* Lactation, menstrual disorder. *GU:* Penis disorder, testis disorder. *Ophthalmic:* Conjunctivitis, amblyopia, dry eyes. *Miscellaneous:* Nail disorder, flu syndrome, enlarged abdomen, lymphedema, dehydration, lymphadenopathy.

EMS CONSIDERATIONS
None.

Levalbuterol hydrochloride
(lehv-al-BYOU-ter-all)
Xopenex **(Rx)**
Classification: Sympathomimetic, bronchodilator

Uses: Treatment or prevention of bronchospasms in adults and adolescents 12 years and older with reversible obstructive airway disease.

Route/Dosage ────────────
• **Inhalation Solution: Nebulization**
Bronchospasms.
Adults and adolescents over 12 years of age, initial: 0.63 mg t.i.d. (q 6–8 hr) by nebulization. Those with severe asthma or who do not respond to the 0.63 mg dose may benefit from a dose of 1.25 mg t.i.d.
How Supplied: *Inhalation Solution:* 0.63 mg/3 mL, 1.25 mg/3 mL

EMS CONSIDERATIONS
See also *Sympathomimetics.*

Levamisole hydrochloride
(lee-VAM-ih-sohl)

---

bold italic = life threatening side effect

Pregnancy Class: C
Ergamisol **(Rx)**
Classification: Antineoplastic, adjunct

Mechanism of Action: Used in combination with fluorouracil; considered to be an immunomodulator. It restores depressed immune function. As such, it stimulates formation of antibodies, stimulates T-cell activation and proliferation, potentiates monocyte and macrophage function (including phagocytosis and chemotaxis), and increases mobility adherence and chemotaxis of neutrophils.
Uses: In combination with fluorouracil to treat patients with Dukes' stage C colon cancer following surgical resection.
Contraindications: Lactation.
Precautions: Safety and effectiveness have not been demonstrated in children. Agranulocytosis, caused by levamisole, may be accompanied by a flu-like syndrome, or it may be asymptomatic. Thus, hematologic monitoring is required.

Route/Dosage
• **Tablets**
Adults, initial: Levamisole, 50 mg q 8 hr for 3 days (starting 7–30 days after surgery) given together with fluorouracil, 450 mg/m²/day by IV push for 5 days (starting 21–34 days after surgery). **Maintenance:** Levamisole, 50 mg q 8 hr for 3 days q 2 weeks for 1 year; fluorouracil, 450 mg/m²/day by IV push once a week beginning 28 days after the beginning of the 5-day course and continuing for 1 year.
How Supplied: *Tablet:* 50 mg
Side Effects: *GI:* Commonly nausea and diarrhea; vomiting, stomatitis, anorexia, abdominal pain, constipation, flatulence, dyspepsia. *Hematologic:* Leukopenia, thrombocytopenia, anemia, granulocytopenia. *Dermatologic:* Commonly: dermatitis and pruritus; alopecia, skin discoloration. *CNS:* Dizziness, headache, inability to concentrate, weakness, memory loss, paresthesia, ataxia, somnolence, depression, insomnia, confusion, nervousness, anxiety, forgetfulness. *Musculoskeletal:* Arthralgia, myalgia.

Ophthalmologic: Abnormal tearing, conjunctivitis, blurred vision. *Miscellaneous:* Fatigue, fever, rigors, chest pain, edema, taste perversion, altered sense of smell, infection, hyperbilirubinemia, epistaxis.
Drug Interactions
Ethanol / Disulfiram-like reaction when used with levamisole
Phenytoin / ↑ Phenytoin plasma levels

EMS CONSIDERATIONS
None.

Levarterenol bitartrate (Norepinephrine bitartrate)
(lee-var-TER-ih-nohl)
Pregnancy Class: C
Levophed **(Rx)**
Classification: Adrenergic agent, direct-acting

Mechanism of Action: Produces vasoconstriction (increase in BP) by stimulating alpha-adrenergic receptors. Also causes a moderate increase in contraction of heart by stimulating beta-1 receptors. Minimal hyperglycemic effect.
Onset of Action: Immediate.
Duration of Action: 1-2 min.
Uses: Hypotensive states caused by trauma, septicemia, blood transfusions, drug reactions, spinal anesthesia, poliomyelitis, central vasomotor depression, and MIs. Adjunct to treatment of cardiac arrest and profound hypotension.
Contraindications: Additional: Hypotension due to blood volume deficiency (except in emergencies), mesenteric or peripheral vascular thrombosis, in halothane or cyclopropane anesthesia (due to possibilities of fatal arrhythmias). Pregnancy (may cause fetal anoxia or hypoxia).
Precautions: Use with caution in patients taking MAO inhibitors or tricyclic antidepressants.

Route/Dosage
• **IV Infusion Only**

Effect on BP determines dosage, initial: 8–12 mcg/min or 2–3 mL of a 4-mcg/mL solution/min; **maintenance,** 2–4 mcg/min with the dose determined by patient response.

How Supplied: *Injection:* 1 mg/mL

Side Effects: Additional: Bradycardia that can be abolished by atropine.

EMS CONSIDERATIONS

See also *Sympathomimetic Drugs.*
Administration/Storage
IV 1. Discard solutions that are brown or that have a precipitate.
2. Continue the infusion until BP is maintained without therapy. Avoid abrupt withdrawal of levarterenol.
3. Dilute in either D5W or 5% dextrose in saline.
4. For IV administration, use a large vein (preferably the antecubital or subclavian). Avoid veins with poor circulation.
5. Monitor the rate of flow constantly.
Assessment
1. Monitor BP.
2. Observe infusion site frequently for extravasation; ischemia and sloughing may occur. Blanching along the course of the vein may indicate permeability of the vein wall, which could allow leakage to occur.
3. Withdraw drug gradually; may experience an initial rebound drop in BP. Extra fluids parenterally may diminish rebound hypotension and help stabilize BP during withdrawal.

Levetiracetam
(lehv-ah-ter-ASS-ah-tam)
Pregnancy Class: C
Keppra (Rx)
Classification: Anticonvulsant

Mechanism of Action: Prescise mechanism unknown. May act in synaptic plasma membranes in the CNS to inhibit burst firing without affecting normal neuronal excitability. Thus, it may selectively prevent hypersynchronization of epileptiform burst firing and propagation of seizure activity.

Uses: Adjunctive treatment of partial onset seizures in adults with epilepsy.

Precautions: Reduce dosage in patients with impaired renal function. Clearance is increased in children. Half-life is prolonged in the elderly. Use with caution during lactation. Safety and efficacy have not been determined in children less than 16 years of age.

Route/Dosage ——————
• **Tablets**
  Partial onset seizures in adults.
Initial: 500 mg b.i.d. Can increase dose by 1,000 mg/day q 2 weeks up to a maximum daily dose of 3,000 mg. For impaired renal function, use the following doses: C_{CR}, 50–80 mL/min: **500–1,000 mg q 12 hr;** C_{CR}, 30–50 mL/min: **250–750 mg q 12 hr;** C_{CR}, less than 30 mL/min: **250–500 mg q 12 hr.**

How Supplied: *Tablets:* 250 mg, 500 mg, 750 mg

Side Effects: *CNS:* Somnolence, dizziness, depression, nervousness, ataxia, vertigo, amnesia, anxiety, hostility, paresthesia, emotional lability, psychotic symptoms, withdrawal seizures. *Respiratory:* Pharyngitis, rhinitis, sinusitis, increased cough. *GI:* Abdominal pain, constipation, diarrhea, dyspepsia, gastroenteritis, gingivitis, N&V. *Miscellaneous:* Asthenia, headache, infection, pain, anorexia, diplopia, coordination difficulties.

OD **Overdose Management:** *Symptom:* Drowsiness. *Treatment:* Emesis or gastric lavage; maintain airway. General supportive care. Monitor VS. Hemodialysis may be beneficial.

EMS CONSIDERATIONS
None.

Levobunolol hydrochloride
(lee-voh-BYOU-no-lohl)

L

Pregnancy Class: C
AKBeta, Betagan Liquifilm **(Rx)**
Classification: Beta-adrenergic
blocking agent

Mechanism of Action: Both beta-1-
and beta-2-adrenergic receptor agonist. May act by decreasing the formation of aqueous humor.
Onset of Action: < 60 min; **Peak effect:** 2-6 hr.
Duration of Action: 24 hr.
Uses: To decrease intraocular pressure
in chronic open-angle glaucoma or
ocular hypertension.
Precautions: Safety and effectiveness have not been determined in
children. Significant absorption in
geriatric patients may result in myocardial depression. Also, use with
caution in angle-closure glaucoma
(use with a miotic), in patients with
muscle weaknesses, and in those
with decreased pulmonary function.

Route/Dosage
• **Ophthalmic Solution (0.25%,
0.5%)**
Adults, usual: 1 gtt of 0.25% or
0.5% solution in affected eye(s) 1–2
times/day (depending on variations in
diurnal intraocular pressure).
How Supplied: *Ophthalmic Solution:* 0.25%, 0.5%
Side Effects: Additional: *Ophthalmic:* Stinging and burning (transient), decreased corneal sensitivity,
blepharoconjunctivitis. *Dermatologic:* Urticaria, pruritus.

EMS CONSIDERATIONS

See also *Beta-Adrenergic Blocking
Agents.*

Levocabastine
hydrochloride
(lee-voh-kah-BASS-teen)
Pregnancy Class: C
Livostin Nasal Spray **(Rx)**
Classification: Ophthalmic antihista-
mine

Mechanism of Action: A histamine
H_1 receptor antagonist.
Duration of Action: 2 hr.

Uses: Temporary relief of seasonal
allergic conjunctivitis.
Contraindications: Use while soft
contact lenses are being worn.
Precautions: The drug is only for
ophthalmic use. Safety and efficacy
have not been determined in children less than 12 years of age.

Route/Dosage
• **Ophthalmic Suspension**
Allergic conjunctivitis.
1 gtt instilled in affected eye(s) q.i.d.
for up to 2 weeks.
How Supplied: *Ophthalmic Suspension:* 0.05%
Side Effects: *Ophthalmologic:* Transient stinging and burning, visual
disturbances, eye pain, eye dryness,
red eyes, lacrimation, discharge from
eyes, eyelid edema. *CNS:* Headache,
fatigue, somnolence. *Miscellaneous:*
Pharyngitis, cough, nausea, rash,
erythema, dyspnea.

EMS CONSIDERATIONS
None.

Levodopa
(lee-vah-DOH-pah)
Dopar, Larodopa, L-Dopa **(Rx)**
Classification: Antiparkinson agent

Mechanism of Action: Depletion
of dopamine in the striatum of the
brain is thought to cause the symptoms of Parkinson's disease. Levodopa, a dopamine precursor, is able
to cross the blood-brain barrier to
enter the CNS. It is decarboxylated
to dopamine in the basal ganglia,
thus replenishing depleted dopamine stores.
Onset of Action: 2-3 weeks, although some patients may require
up to 6 months.
Uses: Idiopathic, arteriosclerotic, or
postencephalitic parkinsonism due
to carbon monoxide or manganese intoxication and in the elderly associated with cerebral arteriosclerosis.
Levodopa only provides symptomatic relief and does not alter the
course of the disease. When effective, it relieves rigidity, bradykinesia,
tremors, dysphagia, seborrhea, sia-

lorrhea, and postural instability. Used in combination with carbidopa. *Investigational:* Pain from herpes zoster; restless legs syndrome.

Contraindications: Concomitant use with MAO inhibitors, except MAO-B inhibitors (e.g., selegiline). History of melanoma or in patients with undiagnosed skin lesions. Lactation. Hypersensitivity to drug, narrow-angle glaucoma, blood dyscrasias, hypertension, coronary sclerosis.

Precautions: Use with extreme caution in patients with history of MIs, convulsions, arrhythmias, bronchial asthma, emphysema, active peptic ulcer, psychosis or neurosis, wide-angle glaucoma, and renal, hepatic, or endocrine diseases. Use during pregnancy only if benefits clearly outweigh risks. Safety has not been established in children less than 12 years of age. Geriatric patients may require a lower dose as they have a reduced tolerance for the drug and its side effects (including cardiac effects). Patients may experience an "on-off" phenomenon in which they experience an improved clinical status followed by loss of therapeutic effect.

Route/Dosage

• **Capsules, Tablets**
  Parkinsonism.

Adults, initial: 250 mg b.i.d.–q.i.d. taken with food; **then,** increase total daily dose by 100–750 mg/3–7 days until optimum dosage reached (should not exceed 8 g/day). Up to 6 months may be required to achieve a significant therapeutic effect.

How Supplied: *Capsule:* 250 mg; *Tablet:* 100 mg, 250 mg, 500 mg

Side Effects: The side effects of levodopa are numerous and usually dose related. Some may abate with usage. *CNS:* Choreiform and/or dystonic movements, paranoid ideation, psychotic episodes, ***depression (with possibility of suicidal tendencies),*** dementia, ***seizures (rare),*** dizziness, headache, faintness, confusion, insomnia, nightmares, hallucinations,

delusions, agitation, anxiety, malaise, fatigue, euphoria. *GI:* N&V, anorexia, abdominal pain, dry mouth, sialorrhea, dysphagia, dysgeusia, hiccups, diarrhea, constipation, burning sensation of tongue, bitter taste, flatulence, weight gain or loss, GI bleeding (rare), duodenal ulcer (rare). *CV:* Cardiac irregularities, palpitations, orthostatic hypotension, hypertension, phlebitis, hot flashes. *Ophthalmologic:* Diplopia, dilated pupils, blurred vision, development of Horner's syndrome, oculogyric crisis. *Hematologic:* **Hemolytic anemia, agranulocytosis,** leukopenia. *Musculoskeletal:* Muscle twitching (early sign of overdose), tonic contraction of the muscles of mastication, increased hand tremor, ataxia. *Miscellaneous:* Blepharospasm (early sign of overdose), urinary retention, urinary incontinence, increased sweating, unusual breathing patterns, weakness, numbness, bruxism, alopecia, priapism, hoarseness, edema, dark sweat and/or urine, flushing, skin rash, sense of stimulation. Levodopa interacts with many other drugs (see what follows) and must be administered cautiously.

OD **Overdose Management:** *Symptoms:* Muscle twitching, blepharospasm. Also see *Side Effects. Treatment:* Immediate gastric lavage for acute overdose. Maintain airway and give IV fluids carefully. General supportive measures.

Drug Interactions
Antacids / ↑ Effect of levodopa due to ↑ absorption from GI tract
Anticholinergic drugs / Possible ↓ effect of levodopa due to ↑ breakdown of levodopa in stomach (due to delayed gastric emptying time)
Antidepressants, tricyclic / ↓ Effect of levodopa due to ↓ absorption from GI tract; also, ↑ risk of hypertension
Benzodiazepines / ↓ Effect of levodopa
Clonidine / ↓ Effect of levodopa
Digoxin / ↓ Effect of digoxin
Furazolidone / ↑ Effect of levodopa due to ↓ breakdown by liver

---

bold italic = life threatening side effect

Guanethidine / ↑ Hypotensive effect of guanethidine

Hypoglycemic drugs / Levodopa upsets diabetic control with hypoglycemic agents

MAO inhibitors / Concomitant administration may result in hypertension, lightheadedness, and flushing due to ↓ breakdown of dopamine and norepinephrine formed from levodopa

Methionine / ↓ Effect of levodopa

Methyldopa / Additive effects including hypotension

Metoclopramide / ↑ Bioavailability of levodopa; ↓ effect of metoclopramide

Papaverine / ↓ Effect of levodopa

Phenothiazines / ↓ Effect of levodopa due to ↓ uptake of dopamine into neurons

Phenytoin / Antagonizes the effect of levodopa

Propranolol / May antagonize the hypotensive and positive inotropic effect of levodopa

Pyridoxine / Reverses levodopa-induced improvement in Parkinson's disease

Thioxanthines / ↓ Effect of levodopa in Parkinson patients

Tricyclic antidepressants / ↓ Absorption of levodopa → ↓ effect

EMS CONSIDERATIONS

See also *Cholinergic Blocking Agents.*

Levofloxacin
(lee-voh-FLOX-ah-sin)
Pregnancy Class: C
Levaquin **(Rx)**
Classification: Fluoroquinolone antibiotic

Uses: Acute maxillary sinusitis due to *Streptococcus pneumoniae, Haemophilus influenzae,* or *Moraxella catarrhalis.* Acute bacterial exacerbation of chronic bronchitis due to *Staphylococcus aureus, S. pneumoniae, H. influenzae, Haemophilus parainfluenzae,* or *M. catarrhalis.* Community acquired pneumonia due to *S. aureus, S. pneumoniae, H. influenzae, H. parainfluenzae, Klebsiella pneumoniae, M. catarrhalis, Chlamydia pneumoniae, Legionella pneumophila,* or *Mycoplasma pneumoniae.* Uncomplicated mild to moderate infections of the skin and skin structures, including abscesses, cellulitis, furuncles, impetigo, pyoderma, and wound infections due to *S. aureus* or *Streptococcus pyogenes.* Mild to moderate complicated UTIs due to *Enterococcus faecalis, Enterobacter cloacae, Escherichia coli, Klebsiella pneumoniae, Proteus mirabilis,* or *Pseudomonas aeruginosa.* Acute mild to moderate pyelonephritis due to *E. coli.*

Contraindications: Lactation.

Precautions: The dose must be reduced with impaired renal function. (See *Administration/Storage.*) Safety and efficacy have not been determined in those less than 18 years of age.

Route/Dosage

- **Injection, Tablets**
   Acute maxillary sinusitis.
500 mg once daily for 10–14 days.
   Acute bacterial exacerbation of chronic bronchitis.
500 mg once daily for 7 days.
   Community acquired pneumonia.
500 mg once daily for 7–14 days.
   Uncomplicated skin and skin structure infections.
500 mg once daily for 7–10 days.
   Complicated UTIs.
250 mg once daily for 10 days.
   Acute pyelonephritis.
250 mg once daily for 10 days.

How Supplied: *Injection:* 500 mg; *Injection (premix):* 250 mg, 500 mg; *Tablets:* 250 mg, 500 mg.

EMS CONSIDERATIONS

None.

Levomethadyl acetate hydrochloride
(lee-voh-METH-ah-dill)
Pregnancy Class: C
ORLAAM **(Rx)**
Classification: Narcotic analgesic only for use in opiate dependence

Uses: Treatment of opiate dependence. *NOTE:* This drug can be dispensed only by treatment programs approved by the FDA, DEA, and the designated state authority. The drug can be dispensed only in the oral form and according to treatment requirements stated in federal regulations. The drug has no approved uses outside of the treatment of opiate dependence.

Precautions: Usual dose must not be given on consecutive days due to the risk of fatal overdosage.

Route/Dosage
- **Oral Solution**
  Induction.
Initial: 20–40 mg administered at 48–72-hr intervals; **then,** dose may be increased in increments of 5–10 mg until steady state is reached (usually within 1–2 weeks). Patients dependent on methadone may require higher initial doses of levomethadyl; the suggested initial 3-times/week dose for such patients is 1.2–1.3 times the daily methadone maintenance dose being replaced. This initial dose should not exceed 120 mg with subsequent doses given at 48- or 72-hr intervals, depending on the response. If additional opioids are required, supplemental amounts of methadone should be given rather than giving levomethadyl on 2 consecutive days.
  Maintenance.
Most patients are stabilized on doses of 60–90 mg 3 times/week although the dose may range from 10 to 140 mg 3 times/week. The maximum *total* amount of levomethadyl recommended for any patient is either 140, 140, 140 mg or 130, 130, 180 mg on a thrice-weekly schedule.
  Reinduction after an unplanned lapse in dosing: following a lapse of one levomethadyl dose.
If the patient comes to the clinic the day following a missed scheduled dose (e.g., misses Monday and arrives at clinic on Tuesday), the regular Monday dose is given, with the scheduled Wednesday dose given on Thursday and the Friday dose given on Saturday. The patient's regular schedule can be resumed the following Monday. If the patient misses one dose and comes to the clinic the day of the next scheduled dose (i.e., misses Monday, comes to clinic on Wednesday), the usual dose will be well tolerated in most cases although some patients will need a reduced dose.
  Reintroduction after a lapse of more than one levomethadyl dose.
Restart the patient at an initial dose of 50%–75% of the previous dose, followed by increases of 5–10 mg every dosing day (i.e., intervals of 48–72 hr) until the previous maintenance dose is reached.
  Transfer from levomethadyl to methadone.
Transfer can be done directly, although the dose of methadone should be 80% of the levomethadyl dose being replaced. The first methadone dose should not be given sooner than 48 hr after the last levomethadyl dose. Increases or decreases of 5–10 mg may be made in the daily methadone dose to control symptoms of withdrawal or symptoms of excessive sedation.
  Detoxification from levomethadyl.
Both gradual reduction (i.e., 5%–10% a week) and abrupt withdrawal have been used successfully.

How Supplied: *Concentrate:* 10 mg/mL

Side Effects: See *Narcotic Analgesics.* Induction with levomethadyl that is too rapid for the level of tolerance of the patient may result in overdosage, including symptoms of both ***respiratory and CV depression.***

EMS CONSIDERATIONS
See also *Narcotic Analgesics.*

Levonorgestrel Implants
(lee-voh-nor-JES-trel)
Pregnancy Class: X

Norgestrel II, Norplant System **(Rx)**
Classification: Progestin, contraceptive system

Mechanism of Action: Levonorgestrel implants are marketed either in a set of six flexible Silastic capsules each containing 36 mg of levonorgestrel (Norplant) or two rods containing 150 mg of levonorgestrel (Norgestrel II); an insertion kit is provided to the provider to assist with implantation. Small amounts of the drug slowly diffuse through the wall of each capsule resulting in blood levels of levonorgestrel that are lower than those seen when levonorgestrel or norgestrel is taken as oral contraceptive. The dose released is initially 85 mcg/day, followed by a decrease to approximately 50 mcg/day after 9 months, to 35 mcg/day after 18 months, and then leveling off to 30 mcg/day thereafter. Blood levels of levonorgestrel vary over a wide range and cannot be used as the sole measure of the risk of pregnancy. If used properly, the risk of pregnancy is less than 1 for every 100 users. Does not have any estrogenic effects. The implant system lasts up to 5 years and the contraceptive effect is rapidly reversed if the system is removed from the body.

Uses: Prevention of pregnancy (system lasts for up to 5 years). A new system may be inserted after 5 years if continuing contraception is desired.

Contraindications: Active thrombophlebitis, thromboembolic disorders, undiagnosed abnormal genital bleeding, acute liver disease, benign or malignant liver tumors, known or suspected breast carcinoma, confirmed or suspected pregnancy.

Precautions: Menstrual bleeding irregularities are commonly observed. Monitor carefully women who have a family history of breast cancer or who have breast nodules. Monitor closely women being treated for hyperlipidemias because an increase in LDL levels may occur. Use with caution in individuals in whom fluid retention might be dangerous and in those with a history of depression.

Do not insert until 6 weeks after parturition in women who are breast-feeding.

Route/Dosage
• **Silastic Capsules, Rods**
Six Silastic capsules (36 mg levonorgestrel each) or two rods (150 mg levonorgestrel each) implanted subdermally in the midportion of the upper arm (8–10 cm above the elbow crease). Capsules are distributed in a fan-like pattern 15° apart (total of 75°).

How Supplied: *Kit:* 36 mg/implant, 150 mg/implant

Side Effects: *Menstrual irregularities:* Prolonged menses, spotting, irregular onset of menses, frequent menses, amenorrhea, scanty bleeding, cervicitis, vaginitis. *At implant site:* Pain or itching, infection, bruising following insertion or removal, hyperpigmentation (reversible upon removal). *GI:* Abdominal discomfort, nausea, change of appetite, weight gain. *CNS:* Headache, nervousness, dizziness. *Dermatologic:* Dermatitis, acne, hirsutism, scalp hair loss, excess hair growth. *Miscellaneous:* Breast discharge, breast pain, leukorrhea, musculoskeletal pain, fluid retention, possibility of ectopic pregnancy in long-term users, delayed follicular atresia.

OD **Overdose Management:** *Symptoms:* Overdosage can result if more than six capsules are inserted. Symptoms include fluid retention and uterine bleeding irregularities. *Treatment:* All capsules should be removed.

Drug Interactions
Carbamazepine / ↓ Effectiveness → ↑ risk of pregnancy
Phenytoin / ↓ Effectiveness → ↑ risk of pregnancy

EMS CONSIDERATIONS
None.

Levothyroxine sodium (T₄)
(lee-voh-thigh-ROX-een)

Pregnancy Class: A

Eltroxin, Euthyrox, Levo-T, Levothroid, Levoxyl, Synthroid, L-Thyroxine Sodium **(Rx)**

Classification: Thyroid preparation

Mechanism of Action: Levothyroxine is the synthetic sodium salt of the levoisomer of T_4 (tetraiodothyronine). Levothyroxine, 0.05–0.6 mg equals approximately 60 mg (1 grain) of thyroid. More active on a weight basis than thyroid. Is usually the drug of choice. *NOTE:* All levothyroxine products are not bioequivalent; thus, changing brands is not recommended.

Onset of Action: Time to peak therapeutic effect: 3-4 weeks; 9-10 days in a hypothyroid patient; 3-4 days in a hyperthyroid patient.

Duration of Action: 1-3 weeks after withdrawal of chronic therapy.

Route/Dosage

• **Tablets**

Mild hypothyroidism.

Adults, initial: 50 mcg once daily; **then,** increase by 25–50 mcg q 2–3 weeks until desired clinical response is attained; **maintenance, usual:** 75–125 mcg/day (although doses up to 200 mcg/day may be required in some patients).

Severe hypothyroidism.

Adults, initial: 12.5–25 mcg once daily; **then,** increase dose, as necessary, in increments of 25 mcg at 2- to 3-week intervals.

Congenital hypothyroidism.

Pediatric, 12 years and older: 2–3 mcg/kg once daily until the adult daily dose (usually 150 mcg) is reached. **6–12 years of age:** 4–5 mcg/kg/day or 100–150 mcg once daily. **1–5 years of age:** 5–6 mcg/kg/day or 75–100 mcg once daily. **6–12 months of age:** 6–8 mcg/kg/day or 50–75 mcg once daily. **Less than 6 months of age:** 8–10 mcg/kg/day or 25–50 mcg once daily.

• **IM, IV**

Myxedematous coma.

Adults, initial: 400 mcg by rapid IV injection, even in geriatric patients; **then,** 100–200 mcg/day, IV. **Maintenance:** 100–200 mcg/day, IV. Smaller daily doses should be given until patient can tolerate PO medication.

Hypothyroidism.

Adults: 50–100 mcg once daily; **pediatric, IV, IM:** A dose of 75% of the usual PO pediatric dose should be given.

How Supplied: *Powder for injection:* 0.2 mg, 0.5 mg; *Tablet:* 0.025 mg, 0.05 mg, 0.075 mg, 0.088 mg, 0.1 mg, 0.112 mg, 0.125 mg, 0.137 mg, 0.15 mg, 0.175 mg, 0.2 mg, 0.3 mg, 0.5 mg

Drug Interactions: Concurrent use of aluminum hydroxide and levothyroxine may result in adsorption of levothyroxine to the aluminum and increased fecal elimination of levothyroxine.

EMS CONSIDERATIONS

None.

Librax

(LIB-rax)

Pregnancy Class: DO NOT USE DURING PREGNANCY, ESPECIALLY FIRST TRIMESTER. **(Rx)**

Classification: Antianxiety agent

Uses: Possibly effective as an adjunct in the treatment of irritable colon, spastic colon, mucous colitis, and acute enterocolitis.

Contraindications: Pregnancy, glaucoma, prostatic hypertrophy.

Route/Dosage

• **Capsules**

Individualized. Adults, usual: 1–2 capsules t.i.d.–q.i.d. before meals and at bedtime.

How Supplied: *Antianxiety agent:* Chlordiazepoxide, 5 mg. *Anticholinergic agent:* Clidinium bromide, 2.5 mg. See also information on individual components.

EMS CONSIDERATIONS

See also *Tranquilizers, Antimanic Drugs* and *Hypnotics* and *Cholinergic Blocking Agents.*

bold italic = life threatening side effect

Lidocaine hydrochloride
(LYE-doh-kayn)
Pregnancy Class: B
IM: LidoPen Auto-injector **(Rx)**, **Direct IV or IV admixtures:** Lidocaine HCl for Cardiac Arrhythmias, Xylocaine HCl IV for Cardiac Arrhythmias **(Rx)**, **IV Infusion:** Lidocaine HCl in 5% Dextrose **(Rx)**
Classification: Antiarrhythmic, class IB

Mechanism of Action: Shortens the refractory period and suppresses the automaticity of ectopic foci without affecting conduction of impulses through cardiac tissue. Increases the electrical stimulation threshold of the ventricle during diastole. It does not affect BP, CO, or myocardial contractility. Since lidocaine has little effect on conduction at normal antiarrhythmic doses, use in acute situations (instead of procainamide) in instances in which heart block might occur.

Onset of Action: IV: 45-90 sec; **IM:** 5-15 min.

Duration of Action: 60-90 min.

Uses: IV: Treatment of acute ventricular arrhythmias such as those following MIs or occurring during surgery. The drug is ineffective against atrial arrhythmias. **IM:** Certain emergency situations (e.g., ECG equipment not available; mobile coronary care unit, under advice of a physician).

Investigational: IV in children who develop ventricular couplets or frequent premature ventricular beats.

Contraindications: Hypersensitivity to amide-type local anesthetics, Stokes-Adams syndrome, Wolff-Parkinson-White syndrome, severe SA, AV, or intraventricular block (when no pacemaker is present). Use of the IM autoinjector for children.

Precautions: Use with caution during labor and delivery, during lactation, and in the presence of liver or severe kidney disease, CHF, marked hypoxia, digitalis toxicity with AV block, severe respiratory depression, or shock. In geriatric patients, the rate and dose for IV infusion should be decreased by one-half and slowly

adjusted. Safety and efficacy have not been determined in children.

Route/Dosage

• **IV Bolus**
Antiarrhythmic.
Adults: 50–100 mg at rate of 25–50 mg/min. Bolus is used to establish rapid therapeutic plasma levels. Repeat if necessary after 5-min interval. Onset of action is 10 sec. **Maximum dose/hr:** 200–300 mg.

• **Infusion**
Antiarrhythmic.
20–50 mcg/kg at a rate of 1–4 mg/min. No more than 200–300 mg/hr should be given. **Pediatric, loading dose:** 1 mg/kg IV or intratracheally q 5–10 min until desired effect reached (maximum total dose: 5 mg/kg).

• **IV Continuous Infusion**
Maintain therapeutic plasma levels following loading doses.
Adults: Give at a rate of 1–4 mg/min (20–50 mcg/kg/min). Reduce the dose in patients with heart failure, with liver disease, or who are taking drugs that interact with lidocaine. **Pediatric:** 20–50 mcg/kg/min (usual is 30 mcg/kg/min).

• **IM**
Antiarrhythmic.
Adults: 4.5 mg/kg (approximately 300 mg for a 70-kg adult). Switch to IV lidocaine or oral antiarrhythmics as soon as possible although an additional IM dose may be given after 60–90 min.

How Supplied: *Dextrose/Lidocaine Hydrochloride—Injection:* 5%-0.2%, 5%-0.4%, 5%-0.8%, 7.5%-5%; *Lidocaine Hydrochloride—Injection:* 0.5%, 1%, 1.5%, 2%, 10%, 20%; *Kit:* 2%

Side Effects: *Body as a whole:* Malignant hyperthermia characterized by tachycardia, tachypnea, labile BP, metabolic acidosis, temperature elevation. *CV:* **Precipitation or aggravation of arrhythmias (following IV use),** hypotension, **bradycardia (with possible cardiac arrest), CV collapse.** *CNS:* Dizziness, apprehension, euphoria, lightheadedness, nervousness, drowsiness, confusion, changes in mood, hallucinations, twitching, "doom anxiety," **convulsions,** unconsciousness. *Respiratory:* Difficulties in breathing or swallowing, **respiratory depression or arrest.** *Allergic:* Rash, cutaneous lesions, urticaria, edema, **anaphylaxis.** *Other:* Tinnitus, blurred or double vision, vomiting, numbness, sensation of heat or cold, twitching, tremors, soreness at IM injection site, fever, **venous thrombosis or phlebitis (extending from site of injection),** extravasation. During anesthesia, CV depression may be the first sign of lidocaine toxicity. During other usage, convulsions are the first sign of lidocaine toxicity.

OD **Overdose Management:** *Symptoms:* Dependent on plasma levels. If plasma levels range from 4 to 6 mcg/mL, mild CNS effects are observed. Levels of 6 to 8 mcg/mL may result in significant CNS and CV depression while levels greater than 8 mcg/mL cause hypotension, decreased CO, respiratory depression, obtundation, **seizures, and coma.** *Treatment:* Discontinue the drug and begin emergency resuscitative procedures. Seizures can be treated with diazepam, thiopental, or thiamylal. Succinylcholine, IV, may be used if the patient is anesthetized. IV fluids, vasopressors, and CPR are used to correct circulatory depression.

Drug Interactions
Aminoglycosides / ↑ Neuromuscular blockade
Beta-adrenergic blockers / ↑ Lidocaine levels with possible toxicity
Cimetidine / ↓ Clearance of lidocaine → possible toxicity
Phenytoin / IV phenytoin → excessive cardiac depression
Procainamide / Additive cardiodepressant effects
Succinylcholine / ↑ Action of succinylcholine by ↓ plasma protein binding
Tocainide / ↑ Risk of side effects
Tubocurarine / ↑ Neuromuscular blockade

EMS CONSIDERATIONS

See also *Antiarrhythmic Agents.*

Administration/Storage
IV 1. Do not use lidocaine solutions that contain epinephrine to treat arrhythmias. Make certain that vial states, "For Cardiac Arrhythmias."
2. Use D5W to prepare solution; this is stable for 24 hr.
3. Reduce IV bolus dosage in patients over 70 years old, with CHF or liver disease, and if taking cimetidine or propranolol (i.e., where metabolism of lidocaine is reduced).

Assessment
1. Note any hypersensitivity to amide-type local anesthetics.
2. Elderly patients who have hepatic or renal disease or who weigh less than 45.5 kg will need to be watched especially closely for adverse side effects; adjust dosage as directed.
3. Document CNS status; report sudden changes in mental status, dizziness, visual disturbances, twitching, and tremors. These symptoms may precede convulsions. Note pulmonary findings; assess for respiratory depression, characterized by slow, shallow respirations. Monitor ECG; assess for hypotension and cardiac collapse.
4. View monitor strips for myocardial depression, variations of rhythm, or aggravation of arrhythmia.

Liothyronine sodium (T₃)
(lye-oh-THIGH-roh-neen)
Pregnancy Class: A
Cytomel, Sodium-L-Triicdothyronine, Triostat **(Rx)**
Classification: Thyroid preparation

Mechanism of Action: Synthetic sodium salt of levoisomer of T_3. Has more predictable effects due to standard hormone content. From 15 to 37.5 mcg is equivalent to about 60 mg of desiccated thyroid. May be preferred when a rapid effect or rapidly reversible effect is required. Has a rapid onset, which may result in difficulty in controlling the dosage as well as the possibility of cardiac side effects and changes in metabolic de-

L

mands. However, its short duration allows quick adjustment of dosage and helps control overdosage.

Contraindications: Additional: Use in children with cretinism because there is some question about whether the hormone crosses the blood-brain barrier.

Route/Dosage ——————————
• **Tablets**
  Mild hypothyroidism.

Adults, individualized, initial: 25 mcg/day. Increase by 12.5–25 mcg q 1–2 weeks until satisfactory response has been obtained. **Usual maintenance:** 25–75 mcg/day (100 mcg may be required in some patients). Use lower initial dosage (5 mcg/day) for the elderly, children, and patients with CV disease. Increase only by 5-mcg increments.

  Myxedema.

Adults, initial: 5 mcg/day increased by 5–10 mcg/day q 1–2 weeks until 25 mcg/day is reached; **then,** increase q 1–2 weeks by 12.5–50 mcg. **Usual maintenance:** 50–100 mcg/day.

  Simple (nontoxic) goiter.

Adults, initial: 5 mcg/day; **then,** increase q 1–2 weeks by 5–10 mcg until 25 mcg/day is reached; **then,** dose can be increased by 12.5–25 mcg/week until the maintenance dose of 50–100 mcg/day is reached (usual is 75 mcg/day).

  T_3 suppression test.

75–100 mcg/day for 7 days followed by a repeat of the I[131] thyroid uptake test (a 50% or greater suppression of uptake indicates a normal thyroid-pituitary axis).

  Congenital hypothyroidism.

Adults and children, initial: 5 mcg/day; **then,** increase by 5 mcg/day q 3–4 days until the desired effect is achieved. Approximately 20 mcg/day may be sufficient for infants a few months of age while children 1 year of age may require 50 mcg/day. Children above 3 years may require the full adult dose.

• **IV Only**
  Myxedema coma, precoma.

Adults, initial: 25–50 mcg. Base subsequent doses on continuous monitoring of patient's clinical status and response. Doses should be given at least 4 hr, and no more than 12 hr, apart. Total daily doses of 65 mcg in initial days of therapy are associated with a lower incidence of mortality. In cases of known CV disease, give an initial dose of 10–20 mcg.

How Supplied: *Injection:* 10 mcg/mL; *Tablet:* 5 mcg, 25 mcg, 50 mcg

EMS CONSIDERATIONS

See also *Thyroid Drugs,* and *Levothyroxine.*

Liotrix
(LYE-oh-trix)
Pregnancy Class: A
Thyrolar **(Rx)**
Classification: Thyroid preparation

Mechanism of Action: Mixture of synthetic levothyroxine sodium (T_4) and liothyronine (T_3) in a 4:1 ratio by weight and in a 1:1 ratio by biologic activity.

Route/Dosage ——————————
• **Tablets**
  Hypothyroidism.

Adults and children, initial: 50 mcg levothyroxine and 12.5 mcg liothyronine (Thyrolar); **then,** at monthly intervals, increments of like amounts can be made until the desired effect is achieved. **Usual maintenance:** 50–100 mcg of levothyroxine and 12.5–25 mcg liothyronine daily.

  Congenital hypothyroidism.

Children, 0–6 months: 8–10 mcg T_4/kg/day (25–50 mcg/day); **6–12 months:** 6–8 mcg T_4/kg/day (50–75 mcg/day); **1–5 years:** 5–6 mcg T_4/kg/day (75–100 mcg/day); **6–12 years:** 4–5 mcg T_4/kg/day (100–150 mcg/day); **over 12 years:** 2–3 mcg T_4/kg/day (over 150 mcg/day).

How Supplied: *Tablet:* 15 mg, 30 mg, 60 mg, 120 mg, 180 mg

EMS CONSIDERATIONS

None.

Lisinopril

(lie-SIN-oh-prill)
Pregnancy Class: C
Prinivil, Zestril **(Rx)**
Classification: Antihypertensive, ACE inhibitor

Mechanism of Action: Both supine and standing BPs are reduced, although the drug is less effective in blacks than in Caucasians.
Onset of Action: 1 hr.
Duration of Action: 24 hr.
Uses: Alone or in combination with a diuretic (usually a thiazide) to treat hypertension. In combination with digitalis and a diuretic for treating CHF not responding to other therapy. Use within 24 hr of acute MI to improve survival in hemodynamically stable patients (patients should receive the standard treatment, including thrombolytics, aspirin, and beta blockers).
Precautions: Use with caution during lactation. Safety and efficacy have not been established in children. Geriatric patients may manifest higher blood levels. Reduce the dosage in patients with impaired renal function.

Route/Dosage
- **Tablets**
Essential hypertension, used alone.
10 mg once daily. Adjust dosage depending on response (range: 20–40 mg/day given as a single dose). Doses greater than 80 mg/day do not give a greater effect.
Essential hypertension in combination with a diuretic.
Initial: 5 mg. The BP-lowering effects of the combination are additive. Reduce dosage in renal impairment.
CHF.
Initial: 5 mg once daily (2.5 mg/day in patients with hyponatremia) in combination with diuretics and digitalis. **Dosage range:** 5–20 mg/day as a single dose.
Acute MI.
First dose: 5 mg; **then,** 5 mg after 24 hr, 10 mg after 48 hr, and then 10 mg

daily. Continue dosing for 6 weeks. In patients with a systolic pressure less than 120 mm Hg when treatment is started or within 3 days after the infarct should be given 2.5 mg. If hypotension occurs (systolic BP less than 100 mm Hg), the dose may be temporarily reduced to 2.5 mg. If prolonged hypotension occurs, withdraw the drug.
How Supplied: *Tablet:* 2.5 mg, 5 mg, 10 mg, 20 mg, 40 mg
Side Effects: *CV:* Hypotension, orthostatic hypotension, angina, tachycardia, palpitations, rhythm disturbances, **stroke,** chest pain, orthostatic effects, peripheral edema, **MI, CVA,** worsening of heart failure, chest sound abnormalities, PVCs, TIAs, decreased blood pressure, atrial fibrillation. *CNS:* Dizziness, headache, fatigue, vertigo, insomnia, depression, sleepiness, paresthesias, malaise, nervousness, confusion, ataxia, impaired memory, tremor, irritability, hypersomnia, peripheral neuropathy, spasm. *GI:* Diarrhea, N&V, dyspepsia, anorexia, constipation, dysgeusia, dry mouth, abdominal pain, flatulence, dry mouth, gastritis, heartburn, GI cramps, weight loss/gain, taste alterations, increased salivation. *Respiratory:* Cough, dyspnea, bronchitis, upper respiratory symptoms, nasal congestion, sinusitis, pharyngeal pain, **bronchospasm, asthma,** pulmonary edema, **pulmonary embolism, pulmonary infarction,** paroxysmal nocturnal dyspnea, chest discomfort, common cold, nasal congestion, pulmonary infiltrates, pleural effusion, wheezing, painful respiration, epistaxis, laryngitis, pharyngitis, rhinitis, rhinorrhea, orthopnea. *Musculoskeletal:* Asthenia, muscle cramps, neck/hip/leg/knee/arm/joint/shoulder/back/pelvic/flank pain, myalgia, arthralgia, arthritis, lumbago. *Hepatic:* Hepatitis, hepatocellular/cholestatic jaundice, pancreatitis, hepatomegaly. *Dermatologic:* Rash, pruritus, flushing, increased sweating, urticaria, alopecia, erythema multiforme, photophobia. *GU:* Impotence, oliguria,

progressive azotemia, acute renal failure, UTI, anuria, uremia, renal dysfunction, pyelonephritis, dysuria. *Ophthalmic:* Blurred vision, visual loss, diplopia. *Miscellaneous:* **Angioedema (may be fatal if laryngeal edema occurs),** hyperkalemia, neutropenia, anemia, **bone marrow depression,** decreased libido, fever, syncope, vasculitis of the legs, gout, eosinophilia, fluid overload, dehydration, diabetes mellitus, chills, virus infection, edema, **anaphylactoid reaction,** malignant lung neoplasms, hemoptysis, breast pain.

OD **Overdose Management:** *Symptoms:* Hypotension. *Treatment:* Supportive. To correct hypotension, IV normal saline is treatment of choice. Lisinopril may be removed by hemodialysis.

Drug Interactions
Diuretics / Excess ↓ BP
Indomethacin / Possible ↓ effect of lisinopril
Potassium-sparing diuretics / Significant ↑ serum potassium

EMS CONSIDERATIONS
None.

Lisinopril and Hydrochlorothiazide
(lie-SIN-oh-pril, hy-droh-kloh-roh-THIGH-ah-zyd)
Pregnancy Class: C
Prinzide, Zestoretic **(Rx)**
Classification: Antihypertensive

Uses: Hypertension in patients in whom combination therapy is appropriate. Not for initial therapy.

Route/Dosage
• **Tablets**
Hypertension.
Individualized. Usual: 1 or 2 tablets once daily of Prinzide 12.5, Prinzide 25, Zestoretic 20–12.5, or Zestoretic 20–25.

How Supplied: Lisinopril is an ACE inhibitor and hydrochlorothiazide is a diuretic. Prinzide 12.5 and Zestoretic 20–12.5: Lisinopril, 20 mg, and hydrochlorothiazide, 12.5 mg. Prinzide

25 and Zestoretic 20–25: Lisinopril, 20 mg, and hydrochlorothiazide, 25 mg.

EMS CONSIDERATIONS
None.

Lithium carbonate
Lithium citrate
(LITH-ee-um)
Pregnancy Class: D
Carbonate (Eskalith, Eskalith CR, Lithobid, Lithonate, Lithotabs **(Rx)**) Citrate (**(Rx)**)
Classification: Antipsychotic agent, miscellaneous

Mechanism of Action: Mechanism for the antimanic effect of lithium is unknown. Various hypotheses include: (a) a decrease in catecholamine neurotransmitter levels caused by lithium's effect on Na^+–K^+ ATPase to improve transneuronal membrane transport of sodium ion; (b) a decrease in cyclic AMP levels caused by lithium which decreases sensitivity of hormonal-sensitive adenyl cyclase receptors; or (c) interference by lithium with lipid inositol metabolism ultimately leading to insensitivity of cells in the CNS to stimulation by inositol.

Affects the distribution of calcium, magnesium, and sodium ions and affects glucose metabolism. Lithium and sodium are excreted by the same mechanism in the proximal tubule. Thus, to reduce the danger of lithium intoxication, sodium intake must remain at normal levels.

Onset of Action: 5-14 days.

Uses: Control of mania in manic-depressive patients. *Investigational:* To reverse neutropenia induced by cancer chemotherapy, in children with chronic neutropenia, and in AIDs patients receiving AZT. Prophylaxis of cluster headaches. Also for premenstrual tension, alcoholism accompanied by depression, tardive dyskinesia, bulimia, hyperthyroidism, excess ADH secretion, postpartum affective psychosis, corticosteroid-induced psychosis. Lithium

succinate, in a topical form, has been used for the treatment of genital herpes and seborrheic dermatitis.
Contraindications: Cardiovascular or renal disease. Brain damage. Dehydration, sodium depletion, patients receiving diuretics. Lactation.
Precautions: Safety and efficacy have not been established for children less than 12 years of age. Use with caution in geriatric patients because lithium is more toxic to the CNS in these patients; also, geriatric patients are more likely to develop lithium-induced goiter and clinical hypothyroidism and are more likely to manifest excessive thirst and larger volumes of urine.

Route/Dosage

• **Capsules, Tablets, Extended-Release Tablets, Syrup**
Acute mania.
Adults: Individualized and according to lithium serum level (not to exceed 1.4 mEq/L) and clinical response. **Usual initial:** 300–600 mg t.i.d. or 600–900 mg b.i.d. of slow-release form; **elderly and debilitated patients:** 0.6–1.2 g/day in three doses. **Maintenance:** 300 mg t.i.d.–q.i.d.

Administration of drug is discontinued when lithium serum level exceeds 1.2 mEq/L and resumed 24 hr after it has fallen below that level.

To reverse neutropenia.
300–1,000 mg/day (to achieve serum levels of 0.5–1.0 mEq/L) for 7–10 days.

Prophylaxis of cluster headaches.
600–900 mg/day.

How Supplied: Lithium carbonate: *Capsule:* 150 mg, 300 mg, 600 mg; *Tablet:* 300 mg; *Tablet, Extended Release:* 300 mg, 450 mg; Lithium citrate: *Syrup:* 300 mg/5 mL

Side Effects: *Due to initial therapy:* Fine hand tremor, polyuria, thirst, transient and mild nausea, general discomfort. The following side effects are dependent on the serum level of lithium. *CV:* Arrhythmia, hypotension, *peripheral circulatory collapse,* bradycardia, sinus node dysfunction with severe bradycardia causing syncope; reversible flattening, isoelectricity, or inversion of T waves. *CNS:* Blackout spells, epileptiform seizures, slurred speech, dizziness, vertigo, somnolence, psychomotor retardation, restlessness, sleepiness, confusion, stupor, coma, acute dystonia, startled response, hypertonicity, slowed intellectual functioning, hallucinations, poor memory, tics, cog wheel rigidity, tongue movements. Pseudotumor cerebri leading to increased intracranial pressure and papilledema; if undetected may cause enlargement of the blind spot, constriction of visual fields, and eventual blindness. Diffuse slowing of EEG; widening of frequency spectrum of EEG; disorganization of background rhythm of EEG. *GI:* Anorexia, N&V, diarrhea, dry mouth, gastritis, salivary gland swelling, abdominal pain, excessive salivation, flatulence, indigestion, incontinence of urine or feces, dysgeusia/taste distortion, salty taste, swollen lips, denal caries. *Dermatologic:* Drying and thinning of hair, anesthesia of skin, chronic folliculitis, xerosis cutis, alopecia, exacerbation of psoriasis, acne, angioedema. *Neuromuscular:* Tremor, muscle hyperirritability (fasciculations, twitching, clonic movements), ataxia, choreoathetotic movements, hyperactive DTRs, polyarthralgia. *GU:* Albuminuria, oliguria, polyuria, glycosuria, decreased C_{CR}, symptoms of nephrogenic diabetes, impotence/sexual dysfunction. *Thyroid:* Euthyroid goiter or hypothyroidism, including myxedema, accompanied by lower T_3 and T_4. *Miscellaneous:* Fatigue, lethargy, dehydration, weight loss, transient scotomata, tightness in chest, hypercalcemia, hyperparathyroidism, thirst, swollen painful joints, fever.

The following symptoms are unrelated to lithium dosage. Transient EEG and ECG changes, leukocytosis, headache, diffuse nontoxic goiter with or without hypothyroidism, transient hyperglycemia, generalized

L

---

pruritus with or without rash, cutaneous ulcers, albuminuria, worsening of organic brain syndrome, excessive weight gain, edematous swelling of ankles or wrists, thirst or polyuria (may resemble diabetes mellitus), metallic taste, symptoms similar to Raynaud's phenomenon.

OD **Overdose Management:** *Symptoms:* Symptoms dependent on serum lithium levels. Levels less than 2 mEq/L: N&V, diarrhea, muscle weakness, drowsiness, loss of coordination.

Levels of 2–3 mEq/L: Agitation, ataxia, blackouts, blurred vision, choreoathetoid movements, confusion, dysarthria, fasciculations, giddiness, hyperreflexia, hypertonia, agitation or manic-like behavior, myoclonic twitching or movement of entire limbs, slurred speech, tinnitus, urinary or fecal incontinence, vertigo.

Levels over 3 mEq/L: Complex clinical picture involving multiple organs and organ systems. *Arrhythmias, coma,* hypotension, *peripheral vascular collapse, seizures (focal and generalized),* spasticity, stupor, twitching of muscle groups.

Treatment: Early symptoms are treated by decreasing the dose or stopping treatment for 24–48 hr:
• Use gastric lavage.
• Restore fluid and electrolyte balance (can use saline) and maintain kidney function.
• Increase lithium excretion by giving aminophylline, mannitol, or urea.
• Prevent infection. Maintain adequate respiration.
• Monitor thyroid function.
• Institute hemodialysis.

Drug Interactions
Acetazolamide / ↓ Lithium effect by ↑ renal excretion
Bumetanide / ↑ Lithium toxicity due to ↓ renal clearance
Carbamazepine / ↑ Risk of lithium toxicity
Diazepam / ↑ Risk of hypothermia
Ethacrynic acid / ↑ Lithium toxicity due to ↓ renal clearance
Fluoxetine / ↑ Serum levels of lithium
Furosemide / ↑ Lithium toxicity due to ↓ renal clearance

Haloperidol / ↑ Risk of neurologic toxicity
Iodide salts / Additive effect to cause hypothyroidism
Mannitol / ↓ Lithium effect by ↑ renal excretion
Mazindol / ↑ Chance of lithium toxicity due to ↑ serum levels
Methyldopa / ↑ Chance of neurotoxic effects with or without ↑ lithium serum levels
Neuromuscular blocking agents / Lithium ↑ effect of these agents → severe respiratory depression and apnea
NSAIDs / ↓ Renal clearance of lithium, possibly due to inhibition of renal prostaglandin synthesis
Phenothiazines / ↓ Levels of phenothiazines or ↑ lithium levels
Phenytoin / ↑ Chance of lithium toxicity
Probenecid / ↑ Chance of lithium toxicity due to ↑ serum levels
Sodium chloride / Excretion of lithium is proportional to amount of sodium chloride ingested; if patient is on salt-free diet, may develop lithium toxicity since less lithium excreted
Sympathomimetics / ↓ Pressor effect of sympathomimetics
Theophyllines, including Aminophylline / ↓ Effect of lithium due to ↑ renal excretion
Thiazide diuretics, triamterene / ↑ Chance of lithium toxicity due to ↓ renal clearance
Tricyclic antidepressants / ↑ Effect of tricyclic antidepressants
Urea / ↓ Lithium effect by ↑ renal excretion
Urinary alkalinizers / ↓ Lithium effect by ↑ renal excretion
Verapamil / ↓ Lithium levels and toxicity

EMS CONSIDERATIONS
None.

Lodoxamide tromethamine
(loh-DOX-ah-myd)

Pregnancy Class: B
Alomide **(Rx)**
Classification: Antiallergenic ophthalmic

Mechanism of Action: Mast cell stabilizer that prevents the release of mast cell inflammatory mediators, including slow-reacting substances of anaphylaxis (peptidoleukotrienes), and inhibits eosinophil chemotaxis. Beneficial effect may be due to prevention of calcium influx into mast cells upon stimulation by antigens.
Uses: To treat ocular disorders such as vernal keratoconjunctivitis, vernal conjunctivitis, and vernal keratitis.
Contraindications: Use in patients wearing soft contact lenses.
Precautions: Use with caution during lactation. The drug is for ophthalmic use only and should not be injected. Safety and efficacy have not been determined for use in children less than 2 years of age.

Route/Dosage ───────────
• **Ophthalmic Solution**
  Ocular disorders.
Adults and children over 2 years of age: 1–2 gtt in each affected eye q.i.d. for up to 3 months.
How Supplied: *Solution:* 0.1%
Side Effects: *Ophthalmologic:* Transient burning, stinging, or discomfort upon instillation. Ocular itching or pruritus, blurred vision, dry eye, tearing, discharge from eyes, hyperemia, crystalline deposits in eye, foreign body sensation, corneal erosion or ulcer, scales on lid or lash, eye pain, ocular edema or swelling, ocular warming sensation, ocular fatigue, chemosis, corneal abrasion, anterior chamber cells, keratopathy, keratitis, blepharitis, allergy, sticky sensation, epitheliopathy. *CNS:* Headache, dizziness, somnolence. *GI:* Nausea, stomach discomfort. *Miscellaneous:* Heat sensation, sneezing, dry nose, rash.

EMS CONSIDERATIONS

None.

Lomefloxacin hydrochloride
(loh-meh-FLOX-ah-sin)
Pregnancy Class: C
Maxaquin **(Rx)**
Classification: Antibacterial, fluoroquinolone derivative

Uses: Acute bacterial exacerbation of chronic bronchitis caused by *Haemophilus influenzae* or *Morazella catarrhalis.* Uncomplicated UTIs due to *Escherichia coli, Klebsiella pneumoniae, Proteus mirabilis,* or *Staphylococcus saprophyticus.* Complicated UTIs due to *E. coli, K. pneumoniae, P. mirabilis, Pseudomonas aeruginosa, Citrobacter diversus,* or *Enterobacter cloacae.* Preoperatively to decrease the incidence of UTIs 3–5 days after surgery in patients undergoing transurethral procedures. Uncomplicated gonococcal infections. Prevent infection in preoperative transrectal prostate biopsy.
Contraindications: Use in minor urologic procedures for which prophylaxis is not indicated (e.g., simply cystoscopy, retrograde pyelography). Use for the empiric treatment of acute bacterial exacerbation of chronic bronchitis due to *Streptococcus pneumoniae.* Lactation.
Precautions: Plasma clearance is reduced in the elderly. Safety and efficacy have not been determined in children less than 18 years of age. Serious hypersensitivity reactions that are occasionally fatal have occurred, even with the first dose. No dosage adjustment is needed for elderly patients with normal renal function. Not efficiently removed from the body by hemodialysis or peritoneal dialysis.

Route/Dosage ───────────
• **Tablets**
  Acute bacterial exacerbation of chronic bronchitis. Cystitis.
Adults: 400 mg once daily for 10 days.
  Complicated UTIs.
Adults: 400 mg once daily for 14 days.

L

Uncomplicated UTIs.
400 mg once daily for 3 days.

Prophylaxis of infection before surgery for transurethral procedures.
Single 400-mg dose 2–6 hr before surgery.

Uncomplicated gonococcal infections.
400 mg as a single dose (as an alternative to ciprofloxacin or ofloxacin).

How Supplied: *Tablet:* 400 mg

Side Effects: Additional: *CNS:* Confusion, tremor, vertigo, nervousness, anxiety, hyperkinesia, anorexia, agitation, increased appetite, depersonalization, paranoiaa, *coma. GI:* GI inflammation or bleeding, dysphagia, tongue discoloration, bad taste in mouth. *GU:* Dysuria, hematuria, micturition disorder, anuria, strangury, liekorrhea, intermenstrual bleeding perineal pain, vaginal moniliasis, orchitis, epididymitis, proteinuria, albuminuria. *Hypesneititvity Reactions:* Uritcaria, itching, pharyngeal or facial edema, *CV collapse,* tingling, loss of consciousness, dyspnea. *CV:* Hypotension, tachycardia, bradycardia, extrasystoles, cyanosis, *arrhythmia, cardiac failure,* angina pectoris, *MI, pulmonary embolism, cardiomyopathy,* phlebitis, cerebrovascular disorder. *Respiratory:* Dyspnea, respiratory infection, epistaxis, *bronchospasm,* cough, increased sputum, respiratory disorder, stridor. *Hematologic:* Eosinphilia, leukipenia, increase or decrease in platelets, increase in ESR, lymphocytopenia, decreased hemoglobin, anemia, bleeding, increased PT, increase in monocytes. *Dermatologic:* Urticaria, eczema, skin exfoliation, skin disorder. *Ophthalmologic:* Conjunctivitis, eye pain. *Otic:* Earache, tinnitus. *Musculoskeletal:* Back or chest pain, asthenia, leg cramps, arthralgia, myalgia. *Miscellaneous:* Increase or decrease in blood glucose, flushing, increased sweating, facial edema, influenza-like symptoms, decreased heat tolerance, purpura, lymphadenopathy, increased fibrinolysis, thirst, gout, hypoglycemia, phototoxicity.

EMS CONSIDERATIONS
See also *Anti-Infectives*

Lomustine
(loh-MUS-teen)
Pregnancy Class: D
CeeNu (Abbreviation: CCNU) **(Rx)**
Classification: Antineoplastic, alkylating agent

Mechanism of Action: Alkylating agent that inhibits DNA and RNA synthesis through DNA alkylation. It also affects other cellular processes, includling RNA, protein synthesis and the processing of ribosomal and nucleoplasmic messenger RNA; DNA base component structure; the rate of DNA synthesis and DNA polymerase activity.

Uses: Used alone or in combination to treat primary and metastatic brain tumors. Secondary therapy in Hodgkin's disease (in combination with other antineoplastics).

Contraindications: Lactation.

Route/Dosage
• **Capsules**

Adults and children, initial: 130 mg/m^2 as a single dose q 6 weeks. If bone marrow function is reduced, decrease dose to 100 mg/m^2 q 6 weeks. Subsequent dosage based on blood counts of patients (platelet count above 100,000/mm^3 and leukocyte count above 4,000/mm^3). Undertake weekly blood tests and do not repeat therapy before 6 weeks.

How Supplied: *Capsule:* 10 mg, 40 mg, 100 mg

Side Effects: Additional: High incidence of N&V 3-6 hr after administration and lasting for 24 hr. Renal and pulmonary toxicity. Dysarthria. *Delayed bone marrow suppression* may occur due to cumulative bone marrow toxicity. *Thrombocytopenia and leukopenia may lead to bleeding and overwhelming infections.* Secondary malignancies.

EMS CONSIDERATIONS
None.

Loperamide hydrochloride

(loh-PER-ah-myd)

Pregnancy Class: B

Imodium, Imodium A-D Caplets, Kaopectate II Caplets, Maalox Anti-Diarrheal Caplets, Pepto Diarrhea Control, (Imodium is Rx, all others are OTC)

Classification: Antidiarrheal agent, systemic

Mechanism of Action: Slows intestinal motility by acting on the nerve endings and/or intramural ganglia embedded in the intestinal wall. The prolonged retention of the feces in the intestine results in reducing the volume of the stools, increasing viscosity, and decreasing fluid and electrolyte loss. Reportedly more effective than diphenoxylate.

Onset of Action: Time to peak effect, capsules: 5 hr; **PO solution:** 2.5 hr.

Uses: Rx: Symptomatic relief of acute nonspecific diarrhea and of chronic diarrhea associated with inflammatory bowel disease. Decrease the volume of discharge from ileostomies.

OTC: Control symptoms of diarrhea, including traveler's diarrhea. *Investigational:* With trimethoprim-sulfamethoxazole to treat traveler's diarrhea.

Contraindications: In patients in whom constipation should be avoided. OTC if body temperature is over 101°F (38°C) and in presence of bloody diarrhea. Use in acute diarrhea associated with organisms that penetrate the intestinal mucosa, such as *E. coli, Salmonella,* and Shigella.

Precautions: Safe use in children under 2 years of age and during lactation has not been established. Fluid and electrolyte depletion may occur in patients with diarrhea. Children less than 3 years of age are more sensitive to the narcotic effects of loperamide.

Route/Dosage —————————
• **Rx Capsules, Liquid**

Acute diarrhea.

Adults, initial: 4 mg, followed by 2 mg after each unformed stool, up to maximum of 16 mg/day. **Pediatric: Day 1 doses: 8–12 years:** 2 mg t.i.d.; **6–8 years:** 2 mg b.i.d.; **2–5 years:** 1 mg t.i.d. using only the liquid. *After day 1:* 1 mg/10 kg after a loose stool (total daily dosage should not exceed day 1 recommended doses).

Chronic diarrhea.

Adults: 4–8 mg/day as a single or divided dose. Dosage not established for chronic diarrhea in children.

• **OTC Oral Solution, Tablets**

Acute diarrhea.

Adults: 4 mg after the first loose bowel movement followed by 2 mg after each subsequent bowel movement to a maximum of 8 mg/day for no more than 2 days. **Pediatric, 9–11 years:** 2 mg after the first loose bowel movement followed by 1 mg after each subsequent loose bowel movement, not to exceed 6 mg/day for no more than 2 days. **Pediatric, 6–8 years:** 1 mg after the first bowel movement followed by 1 mg after each subsequent loose bowel movement, not to exceed 4 mg/day for no more than 2 days.

How Supplied: *Capsule:* 2 mg; *Liquid:* 1 mg/5 mL; *Tablet:* 2 mg

Side Effects: *GI:* Abdominal pain, distention, or discomfort. Constipation, dry mouth, N&V, epigastric distress. Toxic megacolon in patients with acute colitis. *CNS:* Drowsiness, dizziness, fatigue. *Other:* Allergic skin rashes.

OD **Overdose Management:** *Symptoms:* Constipation, CNS depression, GI irritation. *Treatment:* Give activated charcoal (it will reduce absorption up to ninefold). If vomiting has not occurred, perform gastric lavage followed by activated charcoal, 100 g, through a gastric tube. Give naloxone for respiratory depression.

EMS CONSIDERATIONS

None.

---

bold italic = life threatening side effect

Loracarbef

(lor-ah-KAR-bef)
Pregnancy Class: B
Lorabid **(Rx)**
Classification: Beta-lactam antibiotic

Mechanism of Action: Related chemically to cephalosporins. Acts by inhibiting cell wall synthesis. Stable in the presence of certain bacterial beta-lactamases.

Uses: Secondary bacterial infections of acute bronchitis and acute bacterial exacerbations of chronic bronchitis-caused by *Streptococcus pneumoniae, Haemophilus influenzae,* or *Morazella catarrhalis* (including beta-lactamase-producing strains of both organisms). Pneumonia caused by *S. pneumoniae* or *H. influenzae* (only non-beta-lactamase-producing strains). Otitis media caused by *S. pneumoniae, Streptococcus pyogenes, H. influenzae,* or *M. catarrhalis* (including beta-lactamase-producing strains of both organisms). Acute maxillary sinusitis caused by *S. pneumoniae, H. influenzae* (only non-beta-lactamase-producing strains), or *M. catarrhalis* (including beta-lactamase-producing strains). Pharyngitis and tonsillitis caused by *S. pyogenes.* Uncomplicated skin and skin structure infections caused by *Staphylococcus aureus* (including penicillinase-producing strains) or *S. pyogenes.* Uncomplicated UTIs caused by *Escherichia coli* or *Staphylococcus saprophyticus.* Uncomplicated pyelonephritis caused by *E. coli.*

Contraindications: Hypersensitivity to loracarbef or cephalosporin-class antibiotics.

Precautions: Use during labor and delivery only if clearly needed. Pseudomembranous colitis is possible with most antibacterial agents. Use with caution and at reduced dosage in patients with impaired renal function, in those with a history of colitis, in patients receiving concurrent treatment with potent diuretics, during lactation, and in patients with known penicillin allergies. Safety and efficacy in children less than 6 months of age have not been determined.

Route/Dosage

• **Capsules, Oral Suspension**
  Secondary bacterial infection of acute bronchitis.
  Adults 13 years of age and older: 200–400 mg q 12 hr for 7 days.
  Acute bacterial exacerbation of chronic bronchitis.
  Adults 13 years of age and older: 400 mg q 12 hr for 7 days.
  Pneumonia.
  Adults 13 years of age and older: 400 q 12 hr for 14 days.
  Pharyngitis, tonsillitis.
  Adults 13 years of age and older: 200 mg q 12 hr for 10 days (longer for *S. pyogenes* infections). **Infants and children, 6 months–12 years:** 15 mg/kg/day in divided doses q 12 hr for 10 days (longer for *S. pyogenes* infections).
  Sinusitis.
  Adults 13 years of age and older: 400 mg q 12 hr for 10 days.
  Acute otitis media, Acute maxillary sinusitis.
  Infants and children, 6 months–12 years: 30 mg/kg/day in divided doses q 12 hr for 10 days. Use the suspension as it is more rapidly absorbed than the capsules, resulting in higher peak plasma levels when given at the same dose.
  Skin and skin structure infections (impetigo).
  Adults: 200 mg q 12 hr for 7 days. **Infants and children, 6 months–12 years:** 15 mg/kg/day in divided doses q 12 hr for 7 days.
  Uncomplicated cystitis.
  Adults 13 years of age and older: 200 mg q 24 hr for 7 days.
  Uncomplicated pyelonephritis.
  Adults 13 years of age and older: 400 mg q 12 hr for 14 days.

How Supplied: *Capsule:* 200 mg, 400 mg; *Powder for reconstitution:* 100 mg/5 mL, 200 mg/5 mL

Side Effects: The incidence of certain side effects is different in the pediatric population compared with the adult population. *GI:* Diarrhea, N&V, abdominal pain, anorexia, pseudomembranous colitis. *Hypersensitivity:* Skin rashes, urticaria, pruritus, erythema multiforme. *CNS:* Headache, somnolence, nervousness, insomnia, dizziness. *Hematologic:* Transient thrombocytopenia, leukopenia, eosinophilia. *Miscellaneous:* Vasodilation, vaginitis, vaginal moniliasis, rhinitis.

OD Overdose Management: *Symptoms:* N&V, epigastric distress, diarrhea. *Treatment:* Hemodialysis may be effective in increasing the elimination of loracarbef from plasma from patients with chronic renal failure.

Drug Interactions
Diuretics, potent / ↑ Risk of renal dysfunction
Probenecid / ↓ Renal excretion resulting in ↑ plasma levels of loracarbef

EMS CONSIDERATIONS

See also *Anti-Infectives.*

Loratidine
(loh-RAH-tih-deen)
Pregnancy Class: B
Claritin, Claritin Reditabs **(Rx)**
Classification: Antihistamine

Mechanism of Action: Low to no sedative and anticholinergic effects. Does not alter cardiac repolarization and has not been linked to development of torsades de pointes as seen with astemizole and terfenadine.
Uses: Relief of nasal and nonnasal symptoms of seasonal allergic rhinitis, including runny nose, itchy and watery eyes, itchy palate, and sneezing. Treatment of chronic idiopathic urticaria in patients 6 years of age and older.
Precautions: Use with caution, if at all, during lactation. Give a lower initial dose in liver impairment. Safety and efficacy have not been determined in children less than 2 years of age.

Route/Dosage
• **Syrup, Tablets**
  Allergic rhinitis, chronic idiopathic urticaria.

Adults and children over 12 years of age: 10 mg once daily on an empty stomach. **Children, 6 to 11 years of age:** 10 mg (10 mL) once daily. *In patients with impaired liver function (GFR less than 30 mL/min):* 10 mg every other day.
How Supplied: *Syrup:* 5 mg/5 mL; *Tablet:* 10 mg
Side Effects: Most commonly, headache, somnolence, fatigue, and dry mouth. *GI:* Altered salivation, gastritis, dyspepsia, stomatitis, toothache, thirst, altered taste, flatulence. *CNS:* Hypoesthesia, hyperkinesia, migraine, anxiety, depression, agitation, paroniria, amnesia, impaired concentration. *Ophthalmologic:* Altered lacrimation, conjunctivitis, blurred vision, eye pain, blepharospasm. *Respiratory:* Upper respiratory infection, epistaxis, pharyngitis, dyspnea, coughing, rhinitis, sinusitis, sneezing, bronchitis, **bronchospasm,** hemoptysis, laryngitis. *Body as a whole:* Asthenia, increased sweating, flushing, malaise, rigors, fever, dry skin, aggravated allergy, pruritus, purpura. *Musculoskeletal:* Back/chest pain, leg cramps, arthralgia, myalgia. *GU:* Breast pain, menorrhagia, dysmenorrhea, vaginitis. *Miscellaneous:* Earache, dysphonia, dry hair, urinary discoloration.

EMS CONSIDERATIONS

See also *Antihistamines.*

————*COMBINATION DRUG*————

Loratidine and Pseudoephedrine sulfate
(loh-RAH-tih-deen, soo-doh-eh-FED-rin)
Pregnancy Class: B
Claritin-D, Claritin-D 24 Hour Extended Release Tablets, Claritin-D 24 hour **(Rx)**
Classification: Antihistamine/decongestant

Uses: To relieve symptoms of seasonal allergic rhinitis, including those with asthma.
Contraindications: Patients with narrow-angle glaucoma or urinary retention and in those receiving

MAO inhibitors and within 14 days of such treatment. In patients with severe hypertension, severe CAD, hepatic insufficiency, and hypersensitivity to the components. In those who have difficulty swallowing due to possibility of upper GI tract obstruction.

Precautions: Use with caution in patients with hypertension, diabetes mellitus, ischemic heart disease, increased intraocular pressure, hyperthyroidism, renal impairment, or prostatic hypertrophy. The safety and efficacy in patients over 60 years of age and below 12 years of age have not been determined. Use with caution during lactation.

Route/Dosage —————————————
• **Tablets**
   Allergic rhinitis.
Adults and children over 12 years of age: 1 tablet q 12 hr given on an empty stomach. Patients with a GFR less than 30 mL/min should receive 1 tablet daily.
• **Extended Release Tablets**
   Allergic rhinitis.
Adults: One 24 Hour Extended Release Tablet daily.

How Supplied: Each tablet of Claritin-D contains: *Antihistamine:* Loratidine, 5 mg. *Decongestant:* Pseudoephedrine sulfate, 120 mg. The product is formulated such that loratidine is released immediately and pseudoephedrine is released both immediately and over time.

Each tablet of Claritin-D 24 Hour Extended Release contains: *Antihistamine:* Loratidine, 10 mg. *Decongestant:* Pseudoephedrine sulfate, 240 mg. Tablet Extended Relaease 10 mg-240 mg.

Side Effects: See individual components. The most common side effects for this product are: *CNS:* Headache, insomnia, somnolence, nervousness, dizziness, fatigue. *GI:* Dry mouth, dyspepsia, nausea. *Miscellaneous:* Pharyngitis, anorexia, thirst.

EMS CONSIDERATIONS

See also *Antihistamines,* and individual agents.

Lorazepam
(lor-AYZ-eh-pam)
Pregnancy Class: D
Ativan, Lorazepam intensol **(Rx)**
Classification: Antianxiety agent, benzodiazepine

Mechanism of Action: Absorbed and eliminated faster than other benzodiazepines.

Uses: PO: Anxiety, tension, anxiety with depression, insomnia, acute alcohol withdrawal symptoms. **Parenteral:** Amnesic agent, anticonvulsant, antitremor drug, adjunct to skeletal muscle relaxants, preanesthetic medication, adjunct prior to endoscopic procedures, treatment of status epilepticus, relief of acute alcohol withdrawal symptoms. *Investigational:* Antiemetic in cancer chemotherapy.

Contraindications: Additional: Narrow-angle glaucoma. Perenterally in children less than 18 years of age.

Precautions: PO dosage has not been established in children less than 12 years of age and IV dosage has not been established in children less than 18 years of age. Use cautiously in presence of renal and hepatic disease.

Route/Dosage —————————————
• **Tablets, Concentrate**
   Anxiety.
Adults: 1–3 mg b.i.d.–t.i.d.
   Hypnotic.
Adults: 2–4 mg at bedtime. **Geriatric/debilitated patients, initial:** 0.5–2 mg/day in divided doses. Dose can be adjusted as required.
• **IM**
   Preoperatively.
Adults: 0.05 mg/kg up to maximum of 4 mg 2 hr before surgery for maximum amnesic effect.
• **IV**
   Preoperatively.
Adults, initial: 0.044 mg/kg or a total dose of 2 mg, whichever is less.
   Amnesic effect.
Adults: 0.05 mg/kg up to a maximum of 4 mg administered 15–20 min prior to surgery.
   Antiemetic in cancer chemotherapy.

Initial: 2 mg 30 min before beginning chemotherapy; **then,** 2 mg q 4 hr as needed.

How Supplied: *Concentrate:* 2 mg/mL; *Injection:* 2 mg/mL, 4 mg/mL; *Tablet:* 0.5 mg, 1 mg, 2 mg

Drug Interactions: Additional: With parenteral lorazepam, scopolamine → sedation, hallucinations, and behavioral abnormalities.

EMS CONSIDERATIONS

See also *Tranquilizers, Antimanic Drugs, and Hypnotics.*
Administration/Storage
IV 1. For IV use, dilute just before use with equal amounts of either sterile water for injection, NaCl injection, or 5% dextrose injection.
2. Do not exceed an IV rate of 2 mg/min.
3. Do not use if solution is discolored or contains a precipitate.

Losartan potassium
(loh-SAR-tan)
Pregnancy Class: C (first trimester), D (second and third trimesters)
Cozaar **(Rx)**
Classification: Antihypertensive, angiotensin II receptor antagonist

---

Mechanism of Action: Angiotensin II, a potent vasoconstrictor, is the primary vasoactive hormone of the renin-angiotensin system; it is involved in the pathophysiology of hypertension. Angiotensin II increases systemic vascular resistance, causes sodium and water retention, and leads to increased heart rate and vasoconstriction. Losartan competitively blocks the angiotensin AT_1 receptor located in vascular smooth muscle and the adrenal glands, which is involved in mediating the effects of angiotensin II. Thus, BP is reduced. No significant effects on heart rate, has minimal orthostatic effects, and does not affect potassium levels significantly. Also, losartan does act on the AT_2 receptor. Maximum effects are usually seen within 1 week, although from 3 to 6 weeks may be required in some patients.

Uses: Treatment of hypertension, alone or in combination with other antihypertensive agents. *Investigational:* Treatment of heart failure.

Contraindications: Lactation. Use after pregnancy is discouraged.

Precautions: When used alone, the effect to decease BP in blacks was less than in non-blacks. Dosage adjustments are not required in patients with renal impairment, unless they are volume depleted. In patients with severe CHF, there is a risk of oliguria and/or progressive azotemia with acute renal failure and/or death (which are rare). In those with unilateral or bilateral renal artery stenosis, there is a risk of increased serum creatinine or BUN. Lower doses are recommended in those with hepatic insufficiency. Safety and efficacy have not been determined in children less than 18 years of age.

Route/Dosage ————
• **Tablets**
Hypertension.
Adults: 50 mg once daily with or without food. Total daily doses range from 25 to 100 mg. In those with possible depletion of intravascular volume (e.g., patients treated with a diuretic), use 25 mg once daily. If the antihypertensive effect (measured at trough) is inadequate, a twice-a-day regimen, using the same dose, may be tried; or an increase in dose may give a more satisfactory result. If BP is not controlled by losartan alone, a diuretic (e.g., hydrochlorothiazide) may be added.

How Supplied: *Tablet:* 25 mg, 50 mg

Side Effects: *GI:* Diarrhea, dyspepsia, anorexia, constipation, dental pain, dry mouth, flatulence, gastritis, vomiting, taste perversion. *CV:* Angina pectoris, second-degree AV block, ***CVA, MI, ventricular tachycardia, ventricular fibrillation,*** hypotension, palpitation, sinus bradycardia, tachycardia, orthostatic effects. *CNS:* Dizziness, insomnia, anxiety, anxiety disor-

---

bold italic = life threatening side effect

der, ataxia, confusion, depression, abnormal dreams, hypesthesia, decreased libido, impaired memory, migraine, nervousness, paresthesia, peripheral neuropathy, panic disorder, sleep disorder, somnolence, tremor, vertigo. *Respiratory:* URI, cough, nasal congestion, sinus disorder, sinusitis, dyspnea, bronchitis, pharyngeal discomfort, epistaxis, rhinitis, respiratory congestion. *Musculoskeletal:* Muscle cramps, myalgia, joint swelling, musculoskeletal pain, stiffness, arthralgia, arthritis, fibromyalgia, muscle weakness; pain in the back, legs, arms, hips, knees, shoulders. *Dermatologic:* Alopecia, dermatitis, dry skin, ecchymosis, erythema, flushing, photosensitivity, pruritus, rash, sweating, urticaria. *GU:* Impotence, nocturia, urinary frequency, UTI. *Ophthalmologic:* Blurred vision, burning/stinging in the eye, conjunctivitis, decrease in visual acuity. *Miscellaneous:* Gout, anemia, tinnitus, facial edema, fever, syncope.

OD **Overdose Management:** *Symptoms:* Hypotension, tachycardia, bradycardia (due to vagal stimulation). *Treatment:* Supportive treatment. Hemodialysis is not indicated.

Drug Interactions: Administration of losartan and phenobarbital resulted in a decreased plasma level (20%) of losartan.

EMS CONSIDERATIONS

See also *Antihypertensive Agents.*

──────COMBINATION DRUG──────

Losartan potassium and Hydrochlorothiazide

(loh-SAR-tan, hy-droh-klor-oh-THIGH-ah-zyd)
Pregnancy Class: C (first trimester), D (second and third trimesters)
Hyzaar **(Rx)**
Classification: Antihypertensive

Mechanism of Action: Maximum effects are usually seen within 1 week, although from 3 to 6 weeks may be required in some patients.
Onset of Action: Peak effects, hydrochlorothiazide: 4 hr.

Duration of Action: Hydrochlorothiazide: 6-12 hr.
Uses: Treatment of hypertension. Not indicated for initial therapy. Use the combination of losartan potassium and hydrochlorothiazide when BP is not controlled adequately with losartan potassium alone. Also used for patients whose BP is inadequately controlled by 25 mg/day of hydrochlorothiazide or is controlled but experiences hypokalemia.
Contraindications: Use in pregnancy, especially during the second and third trimesters. In those with anuria or hypersensitivity to sulfonamide-derived drugs (e.g., hydrochlorothiazide). In severe renal impairment. Lactation.
Precautions: Use with caution in patients with impaired hepatic function or progressive liver disease. Hypersensitivity reactions to hydrochlorothiazide may occur in those with or without a history of allergy or bronchial asthma, although such reactions are more likely in these patients. Thiazides may worsen or activate systemic lupus erythematosus. Safety and efficacy have not been determined in children.

Route/Dosage ──────────
• **Tablets**
  Hypertension.
Adults: One tablet (losartan, 50 mg, and hydrochlorothiazide, 12.5 mg) daily. If BP is not controlled after approximately 3 weeks of therapy, the dose may be increased to 2 tablets daily. The total daily dose should not exceed 2 tablets.
How Supplied: Each tablet contains *Antihypertensive:* Losartan potassium, 50 mg, and *Diuretic:* Hydrochlorothiazide, 12.5 mg.
Side Effects: See individual drug entries.
Drug Interactions: See individual drug entries.

EMS CONSIDERATIONS

See also *Losartan potassium,* and *Antihypertensive Agents.*

Loteprednol etabonate

(loh-teh-PRED-nohl)
Pregnancy Class: C
Alrex, Lotemax **(Rx)**
Classification: Corticosteroid, ophthalmic

Uses: 0.2% Suspension: Treat seasonal allergic conjunctivitis. **0.5% Suspension:** Treat steroid-responsive inflammatory conditions of the conjunctiva.
Contraindications: Bacterial, fungal, or viral eye infection.
Precautions: Use with caution with cataracts, diabetes mellitus, glaucoma, intraocular hypertension, use beyond 10 days. Safety and efficacy have not been determined in children.

Route/Dosage
• **Suspension, 0.2%**
Seasonal allergic conjunctivitis.
1 gtt in the affected eye(s) q.i.d.
• **Suspension, 0.5%**
Conjunctivitis, steroid-responsive.
1–2 gtt into the conjunctival sac of the affected eye q.i.d. For the first week, dose may be increased to 1 gtt every hour.
Conjunctivitis, postoperative.
1–2 gtt into the conjunctival sac of the affected eye q.i.d. beginning 24 hr after surgery and continuing for 2 weeks.
Contact lens-associated giant papillary conjunctivitis.
1 gtt q.i.d.
How Supplied: *Ophthalmic Suspension:* 0.2%, 0.5%
Side Effects: *Ophthalmic:* Increased IOP, thinning of sclera or cornea, blurred vision, discharge, dry eyes, burning on instillation.

EMS CONSIDERATIONS

See also *Corticosteroids.*

Lovastatin (Mevinolin)

(LOW-vah-STAT-in, me-VIN-oh-lin)
Pregnancy Class: X
Mevacor **(Rx)**
Classification: Antihyperlipidemic

Onset of Action: Within 2 weeks using multiple doses.
Duration of Action: 4-6 weeks after termination of therapy.
Uses: As an adjunct to diet in primary hypercholesterolemia (types IIa and IIb) in patients with a significant risk of CAD and who have not responded to diet or other measures. May also be useful in patients with combined hypercholesterolemia and hypertriglyceridemia. To slow the progression of coronary atherosclerosis in patients with CAD in order to lower total and LDL cholesterol levels. *Investigational:* Diabetic dyslipidemia, nephrotic hyperlipidemia, familial dysbetalipoproteinemia, and familial combined hyperlipidemia.
Contraindications: During pregnancy and lactation, active liver disease, persistent unexplained elevations of serum transaminases. Use in children less than 18 years of age. Use with mibefradil (Posicor).
Precautions: Use with caution in patients who have a history of liver disease or who are known heavy consumers of alcohol. Carefully monitor patients with impaired renal function.

Route/Dosage
• **Tablets**
Adults/adolescents, initial: 20 mg once daily with the evening meal. Initiate at 10 mg/day in patients on immunosuppressants. Dose range: 10–80 mg/day in single or two divided doses, not to exceed 20 mg/day if given with immunosuppressants. Adjust dose at intervals of every 4 weeks, if necessary. If C_{CR} is less than 30 mL/min, use doses greater than 20 mg/day with caution.
How Supplied: *Tablet:* 10 mg, 20 mg, 40 mg
Side Effects: See Antihyperlipidemic Agents—HMG-COA Reductase Inhibitors. *CNS:* Headache, dizziness, insomnia, paresthesia. *GI:* Flatus (most common), abdominal pain, cramps, diarrhea, constipation, dys-

L

---

bold italic = life threatening side effect

pepsia, N&V, heartburn, dysgeusia, acid regurgitation, dry mouth. *Musculoskeletal:* Myalgia, muscle cramps, pain, arthralgia, leg pain, shoulder pain, localized pain. *Miscellaneous:* Blurred vision, eye irritation, rash, pruritus, chest pain, alopecia.

Drug Interactions: Additional: *Isradipine/* ↑ Clearance of lovastatin. *Niacin/* ↑ Risk of rhabdomyolysis or severe myopathy.

EMS CONSIDERATIONS

None.

Loxapine hydrochloride
Loxapine succinate
(LOX-ah-peen)
Pregnancy Class: C
Hydrochloride (Loxitane C, Loxitane IM **(Rx)**)
Classification: Antipsychotic, tricyclic

Mechanism of Action: Thought to act by blocking dopamine at postsynaptic brain receptors. Causes significant extrapyramidal symptoms, moderate sedative effects, and a low incidence of anticholinergic effects, as well as orthostatic hypotension.
Onset of Action: 20-30 min; **Peak effects:** 1.5-3 hr.
Duration of Action: About 12 hr.
Uses: Psychotic disorders. *Investigational:* Anxiety neurosis with depression.
Contraindications: Additional: History of convulsive disorders.

Precautions: Use with caution in patients with CV disease. Use during lactation only if benefits outweigh risks. Dosage has not been established in children less than 16 years of age. Geriatric patients may be more prone to developing orthostatic hypotension, anticholinergic, sedative, and extrapyramidal side effects.

Route/Dosage
• **Capsules, Oral Solution**
   Psychoses.
Adults, initial: 10 mg (of the base) b.i.d. For severe cases, up to 50 mg/day may be required. Increase dosage rapidly over 7–10 days until symptoms are controlled. **Range:** 60–100 mg up to 250 mg/day. **Maintenance:** If possible reduce dosage to 20–60 mg/day.
• **IM**
   Psychoses.
Adults: 12.5–50 mg (of the base) q 4–6 hr; once adequate control has been established, switch to PO medication after control achieved (usually within 5 days).
How Supplied: Loxapine hydrochloride: *Concentrate:* 25 mg/mL; *Injection:* 50 mg/mL Loxapine succinate: *Capsule:* 5 mg, 10 mg, 25 mg, 50 mg
Side Effects: Additional: Tachycardia, hypertension, hypotension, lightheadedness, and syncope.

EMS CONSIDERATIONS

None.

Mafenide acetate
(MAH-fen-eyed)
Pregnancy Class: C
Sulfamylon **(Rx)**
Classification: Sulfonamide, topical

Mechanism of Action: Active against many gram-positive and gram-negative organisms and in the presence of serum and pus.

Uses: Topical application to prevent infections in second- and third-degree burns. To control bacterial infections when used under moist dressing over meshed autografts on excised burn wounds.
Contraindications: Use for established infections or in infants less than 1 month of age.

Precautions: Use with caution during lactation and in those with acute renal failure.

Route/Dosage
• **Cream**

$\frac{1}{16}$-in.-thick film applied over entire surface of burn with gloves once or twice daily until healing is progressing satisfactorily or until site is ready for grafting.

How Supplied: *Cream:* 85 mg/g; *Powder for Topical Solution:* 5%; *Topical Powder:* 50 g/packet

Side Effects: *Allergic:* Rash, itching, swelling, hives, blisters, facial edema, erythema, eosinophilia. *Dermatologic:* Pain or burning (common) on application; excoriation of new skin, bleeding (rare). *Respiratory:* Hyperventilation or tachypnea, decrease in arterial pCO_2. *Metabolic:* Acidosis, increase in serum chloride. *Miscellaneous:* **Fatal hemolytic anemia with DIC,** diarrhea.

EMS CONSIDERATIONS

See also *Anti-Infectives* and for *Sulfonamides.*

Magnesium sulfate
(mag-NEE-see-um SUL-fayt)
Pregnancy Class: A
Epsom Salts **(OTC and Rx)**
Classification: Anticonvulsant, electrolyte, saline laxative

Mechanism of Action: Magnesium is an essential element for muscle contraction, certain enzyme systems, and nerve transmission. Mg depresses the CNS and controls convulsions by blocking release of acetylcholine at the myoneural junction. Also, Mg decreases the sensitivity of the motor end plate to acetylcholine and decreases the excitability of the motor membrane.

Onset of Action: IM: 1 hr; **IV:** immediate.

Duration of Action: IM: 3-4 hr; **IV:** 30 min.

Uses: Seizures associated with toxemia of pregnancy, epilepsy, or when abnormally low levels of magnesium may be a contributing factor in convulsions, such as in hypothyroidism or glomerulonephritis. For eclampsia, IV use is restricted to control of life-threatening seizures. Acute nephritis in children to control hypertension, encephalopathy, and seizures. Replacement therapy in magnesium deficiency. Adjunct in TPN. Laxative. *Investigational:* Inhibit premature labor (not a first-line agent). IV use as an adjunct to treat acute exacerbations of moderate to severe asthma in patients who respond poorly to beta agonists. IV use to reduce early mortality in patients with acute MI (is given as soon as possible and continued for 24–48 hr).

Contraindications: In the presence of heart block or myocardial damage. In toxemia of pregnancy during the 2 hr prior to delivery.

Precautions: Use with caution in patients with renal disease because magnesium is removed from the body solely by the kidneys.

Route/Dosage
• **IM**
Anticonvulsant.
Adults: 1–5 g of a 25%–50% solution up to 6 times/day. **Pediatric:** 20–40 mg/kg using the 20% solution (may be repeated if necessary).
• **IV**
Anticonvulsant.
Adults: 1–4 g using 10%–20% solution, not to exceed 1.5 mL/min of the 10% solution.
Hypomagnesemia, mild.
Adults: 1 g as a 50% solution q 6 hr for 4 times (or total of 32.5 mEq/24 hr).
Hypomagnesemia, severe.
Adults: Up to 2 mEq/kg over 4 hr.
• **IV Infusion**
Anticonvulsant.
Adults: 4–5 g in 250 mL 5% dextrose at a rate not to exceed 3 mL/min.
Hypomagnesemia, severe.
Adults: 5 g (40 mEq) in 1,000 mL dextrose 5% or sodium chloride solu-

M

tion by **slow** infusion over period of 3 hr.

Hyperalimentation.
Adults: 8–24 mEq/day; **infants:** 2–10 mEq/day.
• **Oral Solution**
Laxative.
Adults: 10–15 g; **pediatric:** 5–10 g.

How Supplied: *Injection:* 40 mg/mL, 80 mg/mL, 100 mg/mL, 125 mg/mL, 500 mg/mL

Side Effects: Magnesium intoxication. *CNS:* Depression. *CV:* Flushing, hypotension, *circulatory collapse, depression of the myocardium. Other:* Sweating, hypothermia, muscle paralysis, CNS depression, *respiratory paralysis.* Suppression of knee jerk reflex can be used to determine toxicity. *Respiratory failure may occur if given after knee jerk reflex disappears.* Hypocalcemia with signs of tetany secondary to magnesium sulfate when used for eclampsia.

OD **Overdose Management:** *Symptoms:* Serum levels can predict symptoms of toxicity. Symptoms include *sharp decrease in BP and respiratory paralysis,* changes in ECG (increased PR interval, increased QRS complex, prolonged QT interval), *asystole, heart block.* At serum levels of 7–10 mEq/L there is hypotension, narcosis, and loss of DTRs. *Levels of 12–15 mEq/L result in respiratory paralysis; greater than 15 mEq/L cause cardiac conduction problems. Levels greater than 25 mEq/L cause cardiac arrest. Treatment:*
• Use artificial ventilation immediately.
• Have 5–10 mEq of calcium (e.g., 10–20 mL of 10% calcium gluconate) readily available for IV injection to reverse heart block and respiratory depression.
• Hemodialysis and peritoneal dialysis are effective.

Drug Interactions
CNS depressants (general anesthetics, sedative-hypnotics, narcotics) / Additive CNS depression
Digitalis / Heart block when Mg intoxication is treated with calcium in digitalized patients

Neuromuscular blocking agents / Possible additive neuromuscular blockade

EMS CONSIDERATIONS
See also *Anticonvulsants* and *Laxatives.*
Administration/Storage
IV 1. For IV injections, administer undiluted only 1.5 mL of 10% solution per minute; discontinue when convulsions cease.
2. For IV infusion, dilute 4 g in 250 mL of D5W or NSS; do not exceed 3 mL/min.
Assessment: Assess cardiac status and the ECG for evidence of any abnormality.

Mannitol
(MAN-nih-tol)
Pregnancy Class: C
Osmitrol **(Rx)**
Classification: Diuretic, osmotic

Mechanism of Action: Increases the osmolarity of the glomerular filtrate, which decreases the reabsorption of water and increases excretion of sodium and chloride. It also increases the osmolarity of the plasma, which causes enhanced flow of water from tissues into the interstitial fluid and plasma. Thus, cerebral edema, increased ICP, and CSF volume and pressure are decreased.
Onset of Action: IM: 30-60 min for diuresis and within 15 min for reduction of cerebrospinal and intraocular pressures. **Peak:** 30-60 min.
Duration of Action: 6-8 hr diuresis and 4-8 hr for reduction of intraocular pressure.
Uses: Diuretic to prevent or treat the oliguric phase of acute renal failure before irreversible renal failure occurs. Decrease ICP and cerebral edema by decreasing brain mass. Decrease elevated intraocular pressure when the pressure cannot be lowered by other means. To promote urinary excretion of toxic substances. As a urinary irrigant to prevent hemolysis and hemoglobin buildup during transurethral prostatic resection or other transurethral surgical proce-

dures. *Investigational:* Prevent hemolysis during cardiopulmonary bypass surgery.

Contraindications: Anuria, pulmonary edema, severe dehydration, active intracranial bleeding except during craniotomy, progressive heart failure or pulmonary congestion after mannitol therapy, progressive renal damage following mannitol therapy.

Precautions: Use with caution during lactation. If blood is given simultaneously with mannitol, add at least 20 mEq of sodium chloride to each liter of mannitol solution to avoid pseudoagglutination. Sudden expansion of the extracellular volume that occurs after rapid IV mannitol may lead to fulminating CHF. Mannitol may obscure and intensify inadequate hydration or hypovolemia.

Route/Dosage

• **IV Infusion Only**

Test dose (oliguria or reduced renal function).
Either 50 mL of a 25% solution, 75 mL of a 20% solution, or 100 mL of a 15% solution infused over 3–5 min. If urine flow is 30–50 mL/hr, therapeutic dose can be given. If urine flow does not increase, give a second test dose; if still no response, patient must be reevaluated.

Prevention of acute renal failure (oliguria).
Adults: 50–100 g, as a 5%–25% solution, given at a rate to maintain urine flow of at least 30–50 mL/hr.

Treatment of oliguria.
Adults: 50–100 g of a 15%–25% solution.

Reduction of intracranial pressure and brain mass.
Adults: 1.5–2 g/kg as a 15%–25% solution, infused over 30–60 min.

Reduction of intraocular pressure.
Adults: 1.5–2 g/kg as a 20% solution (7.5–10 mL/kg) or as a 15% solution (10–13 mL/kg) given over 30–60 min. When used preoperatively, the dose should be given 1–1.5 hr before surgery to maintain the maximum effect.

Antidote to remove toxic substances.
Adults: Dose depends on the fluid requirement and urinary output. IV fluids and electrolytes are given to replace losses. If a beneficial effect is not seen after 200 g mannitol, the infusion should be discontinued.

• **Irrigation Solution**
Urologic irrigation.
Adults: Use as a 2.5% irrigating solution for the bladder (this concentration minimizes the hemolytic effect of water alone).

How Supplied: *Injection:* 5%, 10%, 15%, 20%, 25%; *Irrigation solution:* 5%

Side Effects: *Electrolyte:* Fluid and electrolyte imbalance, acidosis, loss of electrolytes, dehydration. *GI:* Nausea, vomiting, dry mouth, thirst, diarrhea. *CV:* Edema, hypotension or hypertension, increase in heart rate, angina-like chest pain, CHF, thrombophlebitis. *CNS:* Dizziness, headaches, blurred vision, **seizures.** *Miscellaneous:* Pulmonary congestion, marked diuresis, rhinitis, chills, fever, urticaria, pain in arms, skin necrosis.

OD Overdose Management: *Symptoms:* Increased electrolyte excretion, especially sodium, chloride, and potassium. Sodium depletion results in orthostatic tachycardia or hypotension and decreased CVP. Potassium loss can impair neuromuscular function and cause intestinal dilation and ileus. If urine flow is inadequate, pulmonary edema or water intoxication may occur. Other symptoms include hypotension, polyuria that rapidly becomes oliguria, stupor, **seizures,** hyperosmolality, and hyponatremia. *Treatment:* Discontinue the infusion immediately and begin supportive measures to correct fluid and electrolyte imbalances. Hemodialysis is effective.

Drug Interactions: May cause deafness when used in combination with kanamycin.

EMS CONSIDERATIONS
IV Administration/Storage: Use a filter with concentrated mannitol (15%, 20%, and 25%).

M

---

bold italic = life threatening side effect

Assessment: Monitor VS and I&O. Slow infusion and report S&S of pulmonary edema manifested by dyspnea, cyanosis, rales, or frothy sputum.

Masoprocol
(mah-SOH-proh-kol)
Pregnancy Class: B
Actinex **(Rx)**
Classification: Dermatologic agent

Mechanism of Action: Mechanism of action is unknown.
Uses: Actinic (solar) keratoses.
Contraindications: Hypersensitivity to masoprocol or other ingredients in the formulation. Use with an occlusive dressing.
Precautions: Use with caution during lactation. Safety and efficacy have not been determined in children. The presence or absence of local skin reactions does not correlate with effectiveness of the drug.

Route/Dosage
• **Cream**
Following washing and drying areas where actinic keratoses are located, the drug should be gently massaged into the area, until it is evenly distributed, morning and evening for 28 days.
How Supplied: *Cream:* 10%
Side Effects: *Dermatologic:* Commonly, erythema, flaking, itching, dryness, edema, burning, soreness, allergic contact dermatitis. Also, bleeding, crusting, eye irritation, oozing, rash, soreness, skin irritation, stinging, tightness, tingling, blistering, eczema, fissuring, leathery feeling to the skin, skin roughness, wrinkling, excoriation.

EMS CONSIDERATIONS
None.

Mazindol
(MAYZ-in-dohl)
Pregnancy Class: C
Mazanor, Sanorex **(C-IV) (Rx)**
Classification: Anorexiant

Onset of Action: 30-60 min.
Duration of Action: 8-15 hr.

Uses: Short-term (8–12 weeks) treatment of exogenous obesity in conjunction with a weight reduction program including exercise, reduced caloric intake, and behavior modification.

Route/Dosage
• **Tablets**
Adults, initial: 1 mg once daily 1 hr before the first meal of the day; **then,** dose can be increased to 1 mg t.i.d. before meals or 2 mg once daily 1 hr before lunch.
How Supplied: *Tablet:* 1 mg, 2 mg
Side Effects: Additional: Testicular pain.

EMS CONSIDERATIONS

See also *Amphetamines and Derivatives.*

Mebendazole
(meh-BEN-dah-zohl)
Pregnancy Class: C
Vermox **(Rx)**
Classification: Anthelmintic

Mechanism of Action: Anthelmintic effect occurs by blocking the glucose uptake of the organisms, thereby reducing their energy until death results. It also inhibits the formation of microtubules in the helminth.
Uses: Whipworm, pinworm, roundworm, common and American hookworm infections; in single or mixed infections. Mebendazole is not effective for hydatid disease.
Contraindications: Hypersensitivity to mebendazole.
Precautions: Use with caution in children under 2 years of age and during lactation.

Route/Dosage
• **Tablets, Chewable**
Whipworm, roundworm, and hookworm.
Adults and children: 1 tablet morning and evening on 3 consecutive days.
Pinworms.
1 tablet, one time. All treatments can be repeated after 3 weeks if the patient is not cured.

How Supplied: *Chew Tablet:* 100 mg

Side Effects: *GI:* Transient abdominal pain and diarrhea. *Hematologic:* Reversible neutropenia. *Miscellaneous:* Fever.

Drug Interactions: Carbamazepine and hydantoin may ↓ effect due to ↓ plasma levels of mebendazole.

EMS CONSIDERATIONS

None.

Meclizine hydrochloride
(MEK-lih-zeen)
Pregnancy Class: B
Antivert, Antivert/25 and /50, Antivert/25 Chewable, Antrizine, Bonine, Dizmiss, Dramamine II, Meni-D, Ru-Vert-M **(OTC and Rx)**
Classification: Antihistamine (piperidine-type), antiemetic, antimotion sickness

---

Mechanism of Action: Mechanism for the antiemetic effect may be due to a central anticholinergic effect to decrease vestibular stimulation and depress labyrinthine activity. May also act on the CTZ to decrease vomiting.
Onset of Action: 30-60 min.
Duration of Action: 8-24 hr.

Uses: Nausea and vomiting, dizziness of motion sickness, vertigo associated with diseases of the vestibular system.

Precautions: Safety for use during lactation and in children less than 12 years of age has not been determined. Pediatric and geriatric patients may be more sensitive to the anticholinergic effects of meclizine.

Route/Dosage
• **Capsules, Tablets, Chewable Tablets**
Motion sickness.
Adults: 25–50 mg 1 hr before travel; may be repeated q 24 hr during travel.
Vertigo.
Adults: 25–100 mg/day in divided doses.

How Supplied: *Capsule:* 25 mg; *Chew Tablet:* 25 mg; *Tablet:* 12.5 mg, 25 mg, 30 mg, 50 mg

Side Effects: *CNS:* Drowsiness, excitation, nervousness, restlessness, insomnia, euphoria, vertigo, hallucinations (auditory or visual). *GI:* N&V, diarrhea, constipation, anorexia. *GU:* Urinary frequency or retention; difficulty in urination. *CV:* Hypotension, tachycardia, palpitations. *Miscellaneous:* Dry nose and throat, blurred or double vision, tinnitus, rash, urticaria.

EMS CONSIDERATIONS

See also *Antihistamines* and *Antiemetics.*

Meclofenamate sodium
(me-kloh-fen-AM-ayt)
Meclomen **(Rx)**
Classification: Nonsteroidal antiinflammatory drug

Uses: Acute and chronic rheumatoid arthritis and osteoarthritis. Not indicated as the initial drug for rheumatoid arthritis due to GI side effects. Has been used in combination with gold salts or corticosteroids. Mild to moderate pain. Primary dysmenorrhea, excessive menstrual blood loss. *Investigational:* Sunburn, prophylaxis of migraine, migraine due to menses.
Contraindications: Additional: Use during pregnancy, lactation, or in children less than 14 years of age.
Precautions: Safe use during lactation not established. Safety and efficacy not established in functional class IV rheumatoid arthritis.

Route/Dosage
• **Capsules**
Rheumatoid arthritis, osteoarthritis.
Adults, usual: 200–400 mg/day in three to four equal doses. Initiate at lower dose and increase to maximum of 400 mg/day if necessary. After initial satisfactory response, lower dosage to decrease severity of side effects.
Mild to moderate pain.

M

Adults: 50 mg q 4–6 hr (100 mg may be required in some patients), not to exceed 400 mg/day.

Excessive menstrual blood loss and primary dysmenorrhea.
Adults: 100 mg t.i.d. for up to 6 days, starting at the onset of menses.
How Supplied: *Capsule:* 50 mg, 100 mg

Side Effects: Additional: Severe diarrhea, nausea, headache, rash, dermatitis, abdominal pain, pyrosis, flatulence, malaise, fatigue, paresthesia, insomnia, depression, taste disturbances, nocturia, blood loss (through feces: 2 mL/day).

Drug Interactions
Aspirin / ↓ Plasma levels of meclofenamate
Warfarin / ↑ Effect of warfarin

EMS CONSIDERATIONS
None.

Medroxyprogesterone acetate

(meh-drox-see-proh-JESS-ter-ohn)
Pregnancy Class: X
Amen, Curretab, Cycrin, Depo-Provera, Depo-Provera C-150, Provera **(Rx)**
Classification: Progestational hormone, synthetic

Mechanism of Action: Synthetic progestin devoid of estrogenic and androgenic activity. Prevents stimulation of endometrium by pituitary gonadotropins. Priming with estrogen is necessary before response is noted.
Uses: Secondary amenorrhea, abnormal uterine bleeding due to hormonal imbalance (no organic pathology). Adjunct in palliative treatment of inoperable, recurrent, or metastatic endometrial or renal carcinoma. Long-acting contraceptive (injectable form). Reduce endometrial hyperplasia in postmenopausal women receiving 0.625 mg conjugated estrogen for 12 to 14 days/month; can begin on the 1st or 16th day of the cycle. *Investigational:*

Polycystic ovary syndrome, precocious puberty. With estrogen to treat menopausal symptoms and hypermenorrhea. To stimulate respiration in obesity-hypoventilation syndrome (oral).
Contraindications: Patients with or a history of thrombophlebitis, thromboembolic disease, cerebral apoplexy. Liver dysfunction. Known or suspected malignancy of the breasts or genital organs. Missed abortion; as a diagnostic for pregnancy. Undiagnosed vaginal bleeding. Use during the first 4 months of pregnancy.
Precautions: The overall risk of breast, liver, ovarian, endometrial, and cervical cancer is not thought to increase with use of the injectable long-acting contraceptive preparation. Possibility of ectopic pregnancy. Use with caution in patients with a history of depression. Due to the possibility of fluid retention, use with caution in patients with epilepsy, migraine, asthma, or cardiac or renal dysfunction.

Route/Dosage
• **Tablets**
Secondary amenorrhea.
5–10 mg/day for 5–10 days, with therapy beginning at any time during the menstrual cycle. If endometrium has been estrogen primed: 10 mg medroxyprogesterone/day for 10 days beginning any time.
Abnormal uterine bleeding with no pathology.
5–10 mg/day for 5–10 days, with therapy beginning on day 16 or 21 of the menstrual cycle. If endometrium has been estrogen primed: 10 mg/day for 10 days, beginning on day 16 of the menstrual cycle. Bleeding usually begins within 3–7 days.
• **IM**
Endometrial or renal carcinoma.
Initial: 400–1,000 mg/week; **then, if improvement noted,** 400 mg/month. Medroxyprogesterone is not intended to be the primary therapy.
Long-acting contraceptive.
150 mg of depot form q 3 months by deep IM injection given only during the first 5 days after the onset of a nor-

mal menstrual period, within 5 days postpartum if not breastfeeding, or 6 weeks postpartum if breastfeeding.
How Supplied: *Injection:* 150 mg/mL, 400 mg/mL; *Tablet:* 2.5 mg, 5 mg, 10 mg
Side Effects: *GU:* Amenorrhea or infertility for up to 18 months. *CV:* Thrombophlebitis, **pulmonary embolism.** *GI:* Nausea (rare), jaundice. *CNS:* Nervousness, drowsiness, insomnia, fatigue, dizziness, headache (rare). *Dermatologic:* Pruritus, urticaria, rash, acne, hirsutism, alopecia, angioneurotic edema. *Miscellaneous:* **Hyperpyrexia, anaphylaxis,** decrease in glucose tolerance, weight gain, fluid retention.
Drug Interactions: Aminoglutethimide may ↑ metabolism of medroxyprogesterone → ↓ effect.

EMS CONSIDERATIONS

None.

Mefenamic acid
(meh-fen-NAM-ick AH-sid)
Pregnancy Class: C
Ponstel **(Rx)**
Classification: Nonsteroidal, antiinflammatory drug

Mechanism of Action: Inhibits prostaglandin synthesis. Is an antiinflammatory, antipyretic, and analgesic.
Duration of Action: 4-6 hr.
Uses: Short-term relief (< 1 week) of mild to moderate pain (e.g., pain associated with tooth extraction and musculoskeletal disorders). Primary dysmenorrhea. *Investigational:* PMS, sunburn.
Contraindications: Ulceration or chronic inflammation of the GI tract, pregnancy or possibility thereof, children under 14, and hypersensitivity to the drug.
Precautions: Dosage has not been established in children less than 14 years of age. Use with caution in patients with impaired renal or hepatic function, asthma, or patients on anticoagulant therapy.

Route/Dosage
• **Capsules**
Analgesia, primary dysmenorrhea.
Adults and children over 14 years of age, initial: 500 mg; **then,** 250 mg q 6 hr.
How Supplied: *Capsule:* 250 mg
Side Effects: Additional:*Autoimmune hemolytic anemia if used more than 12 months.* Diarrhea maya be significant. Rash (maculopapular type).
Drug Interactions
Anticoagulants / ↑ Hypoprothrombinemia due to ↓ plasma protein binding
Insulin / ↑ Insulin requirement
Lithium / ↑ Plasma levels of lithium

EMS CONSIDERATIONS
None.

Mefloquine hydrochloride
(meh-FLOH-kwin)
Pregnancy Class: C
Loriam **(Rx)**
Classification: Antimalarial

Mechanism of Action: Related chemically to quinine and acts as a blood schizonticide. It may increase intravesicular pH in acid vesicles of parasite. It shows myocardial depressant activity with about 20% of the antifibrillatory activity of quinidine and 50% of the increase in the PR interval noted with quinine.
Uses: Mild to moderate acute malaria caused by mefloquine-susceptible strains of *Plasmodium falciparum* (both chloroquine susceptible and resistant strains) or *P. vivax.* Data are not available regarding effectiveness in treating *P. ovale* or *P. malariae.* Also, prophylaxis of *P. falciparum* and *P. vivax* infections, including prophylaxis of chloroquine-resistant strains of *P. falciparum.* *NOTE:* Patients with acute *P. vivax* malaria are at a high risk for relapse as mefloquine does not eliminate the exoe-

rythrocytic (hepatic) parasites. Thus, these patients should also be treated with primaquine. *NOTE:* Strains of *P. falciparum* are reported to be resistant to mefloquine.

Contraindications: Hypersensitivity to mefloquine or related compounds.

Precautions: Use with caution during lactation and in those with psychiatric disturbances due to the possibility of emotional reactions. Safety and effectiveness have not been determined in children.

Route/Dosage

• **Tablets**

Mild to moderate malaria caused by susceptible strains of P. falciparum *or* P. vivax.

1,250 mg (5 tablets) as a single dose with at least 8 oz of water (not to be taken on an empty stomach).

Prophylaxis of malaria.

250 mg (1 tablet) once a week for 4 weeks; **then,** 1 tablet every other week. The CDC recommends a single dose taken weekly starting 1 week before travel, continued weekly during travel, and for 4 weeks after leaving malarious areas. **Pediatric, 15–19 kg: ¼ tablet (62.5 mg) weekly; 20–30 kg: ½ tablet (125 mg) weekly; 31–45 kg: ¾ tablet (187.5 mg) weekly; over 45 kg:** 1 tablet (250 mg) weekly. The CDC recommends a similar dosing schedule for children as for adults.

How Supplied: *Tablet:* 250 mg

Side Effects: *NOTE:* At the doses used, it is difficult to distinguish side effects due to the drug from symptoms attributable to the disease itself. **When used for treatment of acute malaria.** *GI:* N&V, diarrhea, abdominal pain, loss of appetite. *CNS:* Dizziness, fever, headache, fatigue, emotional problems, *seizures.* *Miscellaneous:* Myalgia, chills, skin rash, tinnitus, bradycardia, hair loss, pruritus, asthenia. **When used for prophylaxis of malaria.** *CNS:* Dizziness, syncope, encephalopathy of unknown etiology. *Miscellaneous:* Vomiting, extrasystoles. **Postmar-**

keting surveillance. *CNS:* Vertigo, psychoses, confusion, anxiety, depression, *seizures,* hallucinations, insomnia, abnormal dreams, forgetfulness, motor and sensory neuropathy. *CV:* Hypertension, hypotension, tachycardia, palpitations. *Dermatologic:* Flushing, urticaria, Stevens-Johnson syndrome, erythema multiforme. *Miscellaneous:* Visual disturbances.

OD Overdose Management: *Symptoms:* Cardiotoxic effects, vomiting, diarrhea. *Treatment:* Induce vomiting and administer fluid therapy to treat vomiting and diarrhea.

Drug Interactions

Beta-adrenergic blocking agents / ECG abnormalities or cardiac arrest
Chloroquine / ↑ Risk of seizures
Quinidine / ↑ Risk of ECG abnormalities or cardiac arrest
Quinine / ↑ Risk of seizures, ECG abnormalities, or cardiac arrest; also, ↑ risk of convulsions
Valproic acid / Loss of seizure control and ↓ blood levels of valproic acid

EMS CONSIDERATIONS

See also *Anti-Infectives.*

Megestrol acetate
(meh-JESS-trohl)
Pregnancy Class: D
Megace **(Rx)**
Classification: Synthetic progestin

Mechanism of Action: Antineoplastic activity is due to suppression of gonadotropins (antiluteinizing effect). Has appetite-enhancing properties (mechanism unknown). Contains tartrazine, which can cause allergic-type reactions, including asthma, often occurring in aspirin sensitivity.

Uses: Tablets: Palliative treatment of advanced endometrial or breast cancer. Should not be used instead of chemotherapy, radiation, or surgery.

Oral suspension: Treatment of anorexia, cachexia, or an unexplained, significant weight loss in patients with a diagnosis of AIDS.

Contraindications: Use as a diagnostic aid test for pregnancy, in known or suspected pregnancy, or for prophylaxis to avoid weight loss. Use during the first 4 months of pregnancy.

Precautions: Use with caution in patients with a history of thromboembolic disease. Use in HIV-infected women with endometrial or breast cancer has not been widely studied. Long-term use may increase the risk of respiratory infections and may cause secondary adrenal suppression. Safety and efficacy in children have not been determined.

Route/Dosage

• **Oral Suspension**

Appetite stimulant in AIDS patients.

Adults, initial: 800 mg/day (20 mL/day). The dose should be adjusted to 400 mg/day (10 mL/day) after 1 month.

• **Tablets**

Breast cancer.

40 mg q.i.d.

Endometrial cancer.

40–320 mg/day in divided doses. To determine efficacy, treatment should be continued for at least 2 months.

How Supplied: *Suspension:* 40 mg/mL; *Tablet:* 20 mg, 40 mg

Side Effects: *GI:* Diarrhea, flatulence, nausea, dyspepsia, vomiting, constipation, dry mouth, hepatomegaly, increased salivation, abdominal pain, oral moniliasis. *CV:* Hypertension, *cardiomyopathy,* palpitation. *CNS:* Insomnia, headache, paresthesia, confusion, *seizures,* depression, neuropathy, hypesthesia, abnormal thought process. *Respiratory:* Pneumonia, dyspnea, cough, pharyngitis, chest pain, lung disorder, increased risk of respiratory infection with chronic use. *Dermatologic:* Rash, alopecia, herpes, pruritus, vesiculobullous rash, sweating, skin disorder. *GU:* Impotence, decreased libido, urinary frequency, albuminuria, urinary incontinence, UTI, gynecomastia. *Body as a whole:* Asthenia, anemia, fever, pain, moniliasis, infection, sar-

coma. *Miscellaneous:* Leukopenia, edema, peripheral edema, amblyopia.

EMS CONSIDERATIONS

None.

Melphalan (L-PAM, L-Phenylalanine mustard, L-Sarcolysin)

(MEL-fah-lan)

Pregnancy Class: D

Alkeran (Abbreviation: MPL) **(Rx)**

Classification: Antineoplastic, alkylating agent

Mechanism of Action: A bifunctional alkylating agent that forms an unstable ethylenimmonium ion that binds to or alkylates various intracellular substances including nucleic acids. It produces a cytotoxic effect by cross-linking of DNA and RNA strands as well as inhibition of protein synthesis.

Uses: Multiple myeloma. Epithelial carcinoma of ovary (nonresectable). Use IV only when PO therapy is not appropriate. *Investigational:* Cancer of the breast and testes.

Contraindications: Lactation. Known resistance to drug.

Precautions: Safety and efficacy have not been determined in children less than 12 years of age. Use with extreme caution in those with compromised bone marrow function due to prior chemotherapy or radiation. Reduce IV dosage in impaired renal function.

Route/Dosage

• **Tablets**

Multiple myeloma.

One of the following regimens may be used. (1) 6 mg given once daily for 2–3 weeks (adjust dose based on weekly blood counts). Drug is then discontinued for up to 4 weeks with blood count being monitored. When WBC and platelet counts are increasing, a maintenance dose of 2 mg/day can be started. (2) 10 mg/day

M

bold italic = life threatening side effect

for 7–10 days. Maximum leukocyte and platelet suppression occurs within 3–5 weeks with recovery within 4–8 weeks. When the WBC exceeds 4,000/mm³ and the platelet count is greater than 100,000/mm³, a maintenance dose of 2 mg/day can be started. Dose is then adjusted to 1–3 mg/day, depending on the hematologic response. Keep leukocytes in the range of 3,000–3,500 cells/mm³. (3) 0.15 mg/kg/day for 7 days followed by a rest period of at least 2 weeks (up to 5 weeks may be needed). During the rest period, the leukocyte count will decrease; when WBC and platelet counts are increasing, a maintenance dose of 0.05 mg/kg/day may be given. (4) 0.25 mg/kg/day for 4 consecutive days (or 0.2 mg/kg/day for 5 consecutive days) for a total dose of 1 mg/kg/course of therapy. The 4- to 5-day courses can be repeated q 4–6 weeks if the granulocyte and platelet counts have returned to normal.

Epithelial ovarian cancer.
0.2 mg/kg/day for 5 days repeated q 4–5 weeks (as long as blood counts return to normal).

- **IV**
  Multiple myeloma.
Adults, usual: 16 mg/m² as a single infusion over 15–20 min. Give this dose at 2-week intervals for a total of four doses. Reduce the dose up to 50% in patients with a BUN less than or equal to 30 mg/dL.

How Supplied: *Powder for injection:* 50 mg; *Tablet:* 2 mg

Side Effects: Additional: *Severe bone marrow depression (especially after IV use),* chromosomal aberrations (may be mutagenic), **leukemia (acute, nonlymphatic) in patients with multiple myeloma.** Also, hypersensitivity reactions including **anaphylaxis, pulmonary fibrosis,** interstitial pneumonia, vasulitis, **hemolytic anemia.**

OD **Overdose Management:** *Symptoms:* Severe N&V, decreased consciousness, *seizures,* muscle paralysis, cholinomimetic symptoms, diarrhea, severe mucositis, stomatitis, colitis, **hemorrhage of GI tract, bone**

marrow toxicity. *Treatment:* General supportive treatment, blood transfusions, antibiotics. Monitor hematology for up to 6 weeks. Use of filgrastim or sargramostim may decrease the period of pancytopenia.

Drug Interactions
Carmustine / ↑ Risk of lung toxicity
Cisplatin / Cisplatin-induced renal dysfunction → ↓ melphalan excretion
Cyclosporine / ↑ Risk of nephrotoxicity
Interferon alfa / ↓ Levels of melphalan
Nalidixic acid / ↑ Risk of severe hemorrhagic necrotic enterocolitis in pediatric patients

EMS CONSIDERATIONS
None.

Menotropins
(men-oh-TROH-pinz)
Pregnancy Class: X
Humegon, Pergonal, Repronex **(Rx)**
Classification: Ovarian stimulant

Mechanism of Action: Menotropins are a mixture of FSH and LH extracted from the urine of postmenopausal women. Causes growth and maturation of ovarian follicles. For ovulation to occur, HCG is administered the day following menotropins.

Uses: Females: In combination with HCG to induce ovulation in patients with anovulatory cycles not due to primary ovarian failure. **Males:** In combination with HCG to induce spermatogenesis in patients with primary or secondary hypogonadotrophic hypogonadism.

Contraindications: *Women:* Pregnancy. Primary ovarian failure as indicated by high levels of urinary gonadotropins, ovarian cysts, intracranial lesions, including pituitary tumors. Overt thyroid and adrenal dysfunction. Any cause of infertility other than anovulation. Abnormal bleeding of undetermined origin. Ovarian cysts or enlargement of the ovaries not due to polycystic ovarian syndrome. *Men:* Normal gonadotropin levels, primary testicular failure, disorders of fertility other than hypogonadotrophic hypogonadism. Thyroid or adrenal dysfunction. Absence of neoplastic disease should be established before treatment is initiated.

Route/Dosage
• **IM**

Induction of ovulation.
Individualized, initial: 75 IU of FSH and 75 IU of LH for 7–12 days (maximum), followed by 10,000 USP units of HCG 1 day after last dose of menotropins. **Subsequent courses:** Same dosage schedule for two more courses, if ovulation has occurred. **Then,** dose may be increased to 150 IU of FSH and 150 IU of LH for 7–12 days, followed by HCG as in the preceding for two or more courses.

Induction of spermatogenesis.
It may be necessary to give HCG alone, 5,000 IU 3 times/week, for 4–6 months prior to menotropins; **then,** 75 IU FSH and 75 IU LH **IM** 3 times/week and HCG 2,000 IU 2 times/week for at least 4 months. If no response after 4 months, double each dose of menotropins with the HCG dose unchanged.

How Supplied: *Powder for injection:* 75 IU, 150 IU

Side Effects: *Women. GU:* Ovarian overstimulation, hyperstimulation syndrome (maximal 7–10 days after discontinuation of drug), ovarian enlargement (20% of patients), adnexal torsion, ***ruptured ovarian cysts, ectopic pregnancy,*** multiple births (20%). *CV:* ***Hemoperitoneum, thromboembolism,*** tachycardia, pulmonary and vascular complications. *Hypersentivity:* Generalized urticaria, angioneurotic edema, facial edema, ***dyspnea indicating laryngeal edema.*** *CNS:* Headaches, malaise, dizziness. *GI:* N&V, abdominal pain, diarrhea, abdominal cramps, bloating. *At injection site:* Pain, rash, swelling, irritation. *Miscellaneous:* Fever, chills, musculoskeletal aches, joint pains, body rashes, dyspnea, tachypnea.

Men. Gynecomastia, breast pain, mastitis, nausea, abnormal lipoprotein fraction, abnormal AST and ALT.

EMS CONSIDERATIONS
None.

Meperidine hydrochloride (Pethidine hydrochloride)
(meh-PER-ih-deen)
Pregnancy Class: C
Demerol Hydrochloride **(C-II) (Rx)**
Classification: Narcotic analgesic, synthetic

Mechanism of Action: Only one-tenth as potent an analgesic as morphine. Its analgesic effect is only one-half when given PO rather than parenterally. Has no antitussive effects and does not produce miosis. Produces moderate spasmogenic effects on smooth muscle. **Duration:** Less than that of most opiates; keep in mind when establishing a dosing schedule. Produces both psychologic and physical dependence; overdosage causes severe respiratory depression (see *Narcotic Overdose*).

Onset of Action: 10–45 min; **Peak effect:** 30-60 min.

Duration of Action: 2-4 hr.

Uses: Analgesic for severe pain, hepatic and renal colic, obstetrics, preanesthetic medication, adjunct to anesthesia. Particularly useful for minor surgery, as in orthopedics, ophthalmology, rhinology, laryngology, and dentistry, and for diagnostic procedures such as cystoscopy, retrograde pyelography, and gastroscopy. Spasms of GI tract, uterus, urinary bladder. Anginal syndrome and distress of CHF.

Contraindications: Additional: Hypersensitivity to drug, convulsive states as in epilepsy, tetanus and strychnine poisoning, children under 6 months, diabetic acidosis, head injuries, shock, liver disease, respiratory depression, increased cranial pressure, and before labor during pregnancy.

M

---

bold italic = life threatening side effect

Precautions: Use with caution during lactation and in older or debilitated patients. Use with extreme caution in patients with asthma. Atropine-like effects may aggravate glaucoma, especially when given with other drugs which should be used with caution in glaucoma.

Route/Dosage

- **Tablets, Syrup, IM, SC**
  Analgesic.
Adults: 50–100 mg q 3–4 hr as needed; **pediatric:** 1.1–1.8 mg/kg, up to adult dosage, q 3–4 hr as needed.
  Preoperatively.
Adults, IM, SC: 50–100 mg 30–90 min before anesthesia; **pediatric, IM, SC:** 1–2 mg/kg 30–90 min before anesthesia.
  Obstetrics.
Adults, IM, SC: 50–100 mg q 1–3 hr.
- **IV**
  Support of anesthesia.
IV infusion: 1 mg/mL or **slow IV injection:** 10 mg/mL until patient needs met.
How Supplied: *Injection:* 10 mg/mL, 25 mg/mL, 50 mg/mL, 100 mg/mL; *Syrup:* 50 mg/5 mL; *Tablet:* 50 mg, 100 mg

Side Effects: Additional: Transient hallucinations, transient hypotension (high doses), visual distrubances. Meperidine may accumulate in patients with renal dysfunction, leading to an increased risk of CNS toxicity.

OD Overdose Management: *Symptoms:* Severe respiratory depression. See *Narcotic Analgesics. Treatment:* Naloxone 0.4 mg IV is effective in the treatment of acute overdosage. In PO overdose, gastric lavage and induced emesis are indicated. Treatment, however, is aimed at combating the progressive respiratory depression usually through artificial ventilation.

Drug Interactions: Additional: *Antidepressants, tricyclic/* Additive anticholinergic side effects.*Hydantoins/* ↓ Effect of meperidine due to ↑ breakdown by liver.*MAO inhibitors/* ↑ Risk of severe symptoms including hyperpyrexia, restlessness, hyper- or hypotension, convulsions, or coma.

EMS CONSIDERATIONS

See also *Narcotic Analgesics.*

Mephentermine sulfate
(meh-FEN-ter-meen)
Pregnancy Class: C
Wyamine Sulfate **(Rx)**
Classification: Adrenergic agent, indirectly acting; vasopressor

Mechanism of Action: Acts indirectly by releasing norepinephrine from its storage sites and directly by exerting a slight effect on alpha and beta-1 receptors and a moderate effect on beta-2 receptors mediating vasodilation. Causes increased CO; also elicits slight CNS effects.
Onset of Action: IV: immediate; **IM:** 5-15 min.
Duration of Action: IV: 15-30 min; **IM:** 1-2 hr.
Uses: Hypotension due to anesthesia, ganglionic blockade, or hemorrhage (only as emergency treatment until blood or blood substitutes can be given).
Contraindications: To treat hypotension caused by chlorpromazine. In combination with MAO inhibitors.
Precautions: Use with caution in CV disease, in chronically ill patients, and in treating shock secondary to hemorrhage. Safety and efficacy have not been demonstrated in children.

Route/Dosage

- **IV, IM**
  Hypotension during spinal anesthesia.
IV, Adults: 30–45 mg; 30-mg doses may be repeated as required; or, **IV infusion, Adults and children:** 0.1% (1 mg/mL) mephentermine in D5W with the rate of infusion and duration dependent on patient response. **IV, Pediatric:** 0.4 mg/kg (12 mg/m^2) as a single dose.
  Prophylaxis of hypotension in spinal anesthesia.

IM, Adults: 30–45 mg 10–20 min before anesthesia. **IM, Pediatric:** 0.4 mg/kg (12 mg/m²) as a single dose.
Shock following hemorrhage.
Not recommended, but IV infusion of 0.1% in D5W may maintain BP until blood volume is replaced.
How Supplied: *Injection:* 15 mg/mL, 30 mg/mL
Side Effects: Anxiety, cardiac arrhythmias, increased BP (especially in those with heart disease).

EMS CONSIDERATIONS

See also *Sympathomimetic Drugs.*

Meprobamate
(meh-proh-BAM-ayt)
Pregnancy Class: D
Equanil, Equanil Wyseals, Meprospan 200 and 400, Miltown 200, 400 and 600, Neuramate **(C-IV) (Rx)**
Classification: Nonbenzodiazepine antianxiety agent

Mechanism of Action: Also possesses muscle relaxant and anticonvulsant effects. Acts on the limbic system and the thalamus, as well as inhibits polysynaptic spinal reflexes.
Onset of Action: 1 hr.
Uses: Short-term treatment (no more than 4 months) of anxiety.
Contraindications: Hypersensitivity to meprobamate or carisoprodol. Porphyria. Children less than 6 years of age.
Precautions: Use with caution in pregnancy, lactation, epilepsy, liver and kidney disease. Geriatric patients may be more sensitive to the depressant effects of meprobamate; also, due to age-related impaired renal function, the dose of meprobamate may have to be reduced.

Route/Dosage
• **Tablets**
   Anxiety.
Adults, initial: 400 mg t.i.d.–q.i.d. (or 600 mg b.i.d.). May be increased, if necessary, up to maximum of 2.4 g/day. **Pediatric, 6–12 years of age:** 100–200 mg b.i.d.–t.i.d. (the

600-mg tablet is not recommended for use in children).
How Supplied: *Tablet:* 200 mg, 400 mg
Side Effects: *CNS:* Ataxia, drowsiness, dizziness, weakness headache, paradoxical excitement, euphoria, slurred speech, vertigo. *GI:* N&V, diarrhea. *Miscellaneous:* Visual disturbances, allergic reactions including hematologic and dermatologic symptoms, paresthesias.
OD **Overdose Management:** *Symptoms:* Drowsiness, stupor, lethargy, ataxia, *shock, coma, respiratory collapse, death.* Also, arrhythmias, tachycardia or bradycardia, reduced venous return, *profound hypotension, CV collapse.* Excessive oronasal secretions, *relaxation of pharyngeal wall leading to obstruction of airway. Treatment:* Induction of vomiting or gastric lavage if detected shortly after ingestion. It is imperative that gastric lavage be continued or gastroscopy be performed as incomplete gastric emptying can cause relapse and death.
• Give fluids to treat hypotension. Avoid fluid overload.
• Institute artificial respiration.
• Use care in treating seizures due to combined CNS depressant effects.
• Use forced diuresis and vasopressors followed by hemodialysis or hemoperfusion if condition deteriorates.
Drug Interactions: Additive depressant effects when used with CNS depressants, MAO inhibitors, and tricyclic antidepressants.

EMS CONSIDERATIONS

See also *Tranquilizers, Antimanic Drugs, and Hypnotics.*

Mercaptopurine
(6-Mercaptopurine)
(mer-kap-toe-PYOUR-een)
Pregnancy Class: D
Purinethol (Abbreviation: 6-MP) **(Rx)**
Classification: Antineoplastic, antimetabolite (purine analog)

M

---

bold italic = life threatening side effect

Mechanism of Action: Cell-cycle specific for the S phase of cell division. Converted to thioinosinic acid by the enzyme hypoxanthine-guanine phosphoribosyltransferase. Thioinosinic acid then inhibits reactions involving inosinic acid. Also, both thioinosinic acid and 6-methylthioinosinate (also formed from mercaptopurine) inhibit RNA synthesis.

Uses: Acute lymphocytic or myelocytic leukemia. Lymphoblastic leukemia, especially in children. Acute myelogenous and myelomonocytic leukemia. Effectiveness varies depending on use. The drug is not effective for leukemia of the CNS, solid tumors, lymphomas, or chronic lymphatic leukemia. *Investigational:* Inflammatory bowel disease, chronic myelocytic leukemia, polycythemia vera, non-Hodgkin's lymphoma, psoriatic arthritis.

Contraindications: Use in resistance to mercaptopurine or thioguanine. To treat CNS leukemia, chronic lymphatic leukemia, lymphomas (including Hodgkin's disease), solid tumors. Lactation.

Precautions: Use with caution in patients with impaired renal function. Use during lactation only if benefits clearly outweigh risks. Severe bone marrow depression (anemia, leukopenia, thrombocytopenia) may occur. There is an increased risk of pancreatitis when used for inflammatory bowel disease.

Route/Dosage
• **Tablets**
Highly individualized: 2.5 mg/kg/day. **Adults, usual:** 100–200 mg; **pediatric:** 50 mg. Dosage may be increased to 5 mg/kg/day after 4 weeks if beneficial effects are not noted. Dosage is increased until symptoms of toxicity appear. **Maintenance after remission:** 1.5–2.5 mg/kg/day.

How Supplied: *Tablet:* 50 mg

Side Effects: Additional: Hepatotoxicity, oral lesions, drug fever, hyperuricemia. Produces less GI toxicity than folic acid antagonists, and

side effects are less frequent in children than in adults. Pancreatitis (when used for inflammatory bowel disease).

OD Overdose Management: *Symptoms:* Immediate symptoms include N&V, diarrhea, and anorexia while delayed symptoms include myelosuppression, gastroenteritis, and liver dysfunction. *Treatment:* Induction of emesis if detected soon after ingestion. Supportive measures.

Drug Interactions
Allopurinol / ↑ Effect of methotrexate due to ↓ breakdown by liver (reduce dose of methotrexate by 25%–33%)
Trimethoprim–Sulfamethoxazole / ↑ Risk of bone marrow suppression

EMS CONSIDERATIONS

None.

Meropenem
(mer-oh-PEN-em)
Pregnancy Class: B
Merrem IV **(Rx)**
Classification: Antibiotic, miscellaneous

Mechanism of Action: Broad-spectrum carbapenem antibiotic. Acts by inhibiting cell wall synthesis in gram-positive and gram-negative bacteria.

Uses: Complicated appendicitis and peritonitis caused by *Escherichia coli, Klebsiella pneumoniae, Pseudomonas aeruginosa, Bacteroides fragilis, Bacteroides thetaiotaomicron, Peptostreptococcus* species, and viridans group streptococci. Bacterial meningitis caused by *Streptococcus pneumoniae, Haemophilus influenzae* (β-lactamase- and non-β-lactamase-producing strains), and Neisseria meningitidis.

Contraindications: Hypersensitivity to meropenem or other drugs in the same class. Those who have had anaphylactic reactions to β-lactams.

Precautions: Use with caution during lactation. Safety and efficacy have not been determined for children less than 3 months of age.

Route/Dosage
• **IV**

Bacterial infections, meningitis.
Adults: 1 g IV q 8 hr given over 15–30 min or as an IV bolus injection (5–20 mL) over 3–5 min. In patients with impaired renal function, the dose is reduced as follows: C_{CR} 26–50 mL/min, 1 g q 12 hr; C_{CR} 10–25 mL/min, one-half the recommended dose q 12 hr; C_{CR} less than 10 mL/min, one-half the recommended dose q 24 hr. **Children, 3 months or older:** 20 or 40 mg/kg (depending on the type of infection) q 8 hr, up to a maximum of 2 g q 8 hr. For pediatric patients weighing 50 kg or more, administer 1 g q 8 hr for intra-abdominal infections and 2 g q 8 hr for meningitis given over 15–30 min or as an IV bolus injection (5–20 mL) over 3–5 min.

How Supplied: *Powder for injection:* 500 mg, 1 g

Side Effects: *GI:* Diarrhea, N&V, constipation, abdominal pain, *GI hemorrhage,* pseudomembranous colitis, abdominal pain, melena, oral moniliasis, anorexia, cholestatic jaundice, jaundice, flatulence, ileus. *CNS:* Insomnia, agitation, headache, delirium, confusion, dizziness, nervousness, paresthesia, hallucinations, somnolence, anxiety, depression, *seizures.* *CV: Heart failure, cardiac arrest, MI, pulmonary embolus,* tachycardia, hypertension, bradycardia, hypotension, syncope. *Dermatologic:* Rash, pruritus, urticaria, sweating. *Body as a whole:* Pain, chest pain, *sepsis, shock, hepatic failure,* fever, abdominal enlargement, back pain. *GU:* Dysuria, kidney failure, presence of urine RBCs. *Respiratory:* Respiratory disorder, dyspnea. *At injection site:* Inflammation, phlebitis, thrombophlebitis, pain, edema. *Miscellaneous:* Anemia, peripheral edema, hypoxia, epistaxis, hemoperitoneum.

In children, the drug may cause diarrhea, rash, and vomiting when used for bacterial infections. Also, when used for meningitis in children, rash (diaper area moniliasis), diarrhea, oral moniliasis, and glossitis have been noted.

EMS CONSIDERATIONS
See also *Anti-Infectives.*

Mesalamine (5-aminosalicylic acid)
(mes-AL-ah-meen)
Pregnancy Class: B
Asacol, Mesasal, Rowasa **(Rx)**
Classification: Anti-inflammatory agent

Mechanism of Action: Chemically related to acetylsalicylic acid. Acts locally in the colon to inhibit cyclooxygenase and therefore prostaglandin synthesis, resulting in a reduction of inflammation of colitis.

Uses: PO: Maintaining remission and treatment of mild to moderate active ulcerative colitis. **Rectal:** Treatment of active mild to moderate distal ulcerative colitis, proctosigmoiditis, or proctitis.

Contraindications: Hypersensitivity to salicylates.

Precautions: Use with caution in patients with sulfasalazine sensitivity, in those with impaired renal function, and during lactation. Safety and efficacy have not been established in children. Pyloric stenosis may delay the drug in reaching the colon.

Route/Dosage
• **Suppository**
One suppository (500 mg) b.i.d.
• **Rectal Suspension Enema**
4 g in 60 mL once daily for 3–6 weeks, usually given at bedtime. For maintenance, the drug can be given every other day or every third day at doses of 1–2 g.
• **Capsules, Extended-Release**
1 g (4 capsules) q.i.d. for a total daily dose of 4 g for up to 8 weeks.
• **Tablets, Enteric-Coated**
800 mg t.i.d. for a total dose of 2.4 g/day for 6 weeks.
How Supplied: *Capsule, Extended Release:* 250 mg; *Enema:* 4 g/60 mL;

Enteric Coated Tablet: 400 mg; *Suppository:* 500 mg

Side Effects: *Sulfite sensitivity:* Hives, wheezing, itching, **anaphylaxis.** *Intolerance syndrome:* Acute abdominal pain, cramping, bloody diarrhea, rash, fever, headache. *GI:* Abdominal pain or discomfort, flatulence, cramps, dyspepsia, nausea, diarrhea, hemorrhoids, rectal pain or burning, rectal urgency, constipation, bloating, worsening of colitis, eructation, pain following insertion of enema, vomiting (after PO use). *CNS:* Headache, dizziness, insomnia, fatigue, malaise, chills, fever, asthenia. *Respiratory:* Cold, sore throat; increased cough, pharyngitis, rhinitis following PO use. *Dermatologic:* Acne, pruritus, itching, rash. *Musculoskeletal:* Back pain, hypertonia, arthralgia, myalgia, leg and joint pain, arthritis. *Miscellaneous:* Flu-like symptoms, hair loss, anorexia, peripheral edema, urinary burning, sweating, pain, chest pain, conjunctivitis, dysmenorrhea, pancreatitis.

In addition to the preceding, PO use may result in the following side effects. *GI:* Anorexia, gastritis, gastroenteritis, cholecystitis, dry mouth, increased appetite, oral ulcers, tenesmus, perforated peptic ulcer, bloody diarrhea, duodenal ulcer, dysphagia, esophageal ulcer, fecal incontinence, GI bleeding, oral moniliasis, rectal bleeding, abnormal stool color and texture. *CNS:* Anxiety, depression, hyperesthesia, nervousness, confusion, peripheral neuropathy, somnolence, emotional lability, vertigo, paresthesia, migraine, tremor, transverse myelitis, Guillain-Barré syndrome. *Dermatologic:* Dry skin, psoriasis, pyoderma gangrenosum, urticaria, erythema nodosum, eczema, photosensitivity, lichen planus, nail disorder. *CV:* Pericarditis, myocarditis, vasodilation, palpitations, **fatal myocarditis,** chest pain, T-wave abnormalities. *GU:* Nephropathy, interstitial nephritis, urinary urgency, dysuria, hematuria, menorrhagia, epididymitis, amenorrhea, hypomenorrhea, metrorrhagia, nephrotic syndrome, urinary frequency, albuminuria, nephrotoxicity. *Hematologic:* **Agranulocytosis,** anemia, eosinophilia, leukopenia, thrombocytopenia, lymphadenopathy, thrombocythemia, ecchymosis. *Respiratory:* Worsening of asthma, sinusitis, interstitial pneumonitis, pulmonary infiltrates, fibrosing alveolitis. *Ophthalmologic:* Eye pain, blurred vision. *Miscellaneous:* Ear pain, tinnitus, taste perversion, neck pain, enlargement of abdomen, facial edema, gout, hypersensitivity pneumonitis, breast pain, Kawasaki-like syndrome.

OD **Overdose Management:** *Symptoms:* Salicylate toxicity manifested by tinnitus, vertigo, headache, confusion, drowsiness, sweating, hyperventilation, vomiting, and diarrhea. Severe toxicity results in disruption of electrolyte balance and blood pH, **hyperthermia, and dehydration.** *Treatment:* Therapy to treat salicylate toxicity, including emesis, gastric lavage, fluid and electrolyte replacement (if necessary), maintenance of adequate renal function.

EMS CONSIDERATIONS

None.

Mesoridazine besylate
(mez-oh-RID-ah-zeen)
Pregnancy Class: C
Serentil **(Rx)**
Classification: Antipsychotic, piperidine-type phenothiazine

Mechanism of Action: Pronounced sedative and hypotensive effects, moderate anticholinergic effects, and a low incidence of extrapyramidal symptoms and antiemetic effects.

Uses: Schizophrenia, acute and chronic alcoholism, behavior problems in patients with mental deficiency and chronic brain syndrome, psychoneurosis.

Precautions: Use during pregnancy only if benefits clearly outweigh risks. Dosage has not been established in children less than 12 years of age. Geriatric, debilitated, and emaciated patients require a lower initial dose.

Route/Dosage
• **Oral Solution, Tablets**
Psychotic disorders.
Adults and adolescents, initial: 50 mg t.i.d.; **optimum total dose:** 100–400 mg/day.
Alcoholism.
Adults, initial: 25 mg b.i.d.; **optimum total dose:** 50–200 mg/day.
Behavior problems in mental deficiency and chronic brain syndrome.
Adults, initial: 25 mg b.i.d.; **optimum total dose:** 75–300 mg/day.
Psychoneurotic manifestations.
Adults, initial: 10 mg t.i.d.; **optimum total dose:** 30–150 mg/day.
• **IM**
Psychotic disorders.
Adults and adolescents, initial: 25 mg (base); **then,** repeat the dose in 30–60 min as needed. **Optimum total dose:** 25–200 mg/day.
How Supplied: *Concentrate:* 25 mg/mL; *Injection:* 25 mg/mL; *Tablet:* 10 mg, 25 mg, 50 mg, 100 mg

EMS CONSIDERATIONS

See also *Antipsychotic Agents, Phenothiazines.*

Metaproterenol sulfate (Orciprenaline sulfate)
(met-ah-proh-TER-ih-nohl)
Pregnancy Class: C
Alupent, Arm-A-Med Metaproterenol Sulfate, Metaprel **(Rx)**
Classification: Adrenergic agent, direct-acting; bronchodilator

Mechanism of Action: Markedly stimulates beta-2 receptors, resulting in relaxation of smooth muscles of the bronchial tree, as well as peripheral vasodilation. Minimal effects on beta-1 receptors. Similar to isoproterenol but with a longer duration of action and fewer side effects.
Onset of Action: Inhalation aerosol: within 1min; **peak effect:** 1 hr; **hand bulb nebulizer or IPPB:** 5-30 min; **PO:** 15-30 min; **peak effect:** 1 hr.
Duration of Action: Inhalation aerosol: 1-5 hr; **hand bulb nebulizer or IPPB:** 4-6 hr; **PO:** 4 hr.

Uses: Bronchodilator in asthma, bronchitis, emphysema, and other conditions associated with reversible bronchospasms. Treatment of acute asthmatic attacks in children over 6 years of age.
Precautions: Dosage of syrup or tablets not determined in children less than 6 years of age.

Route/Dosage
• **Syrup, Tablets**
Bronchodilation.
Adults and children over 27.2 kg or 9 years: 20 mg t.i.d.–q.i.d.; **children under 27.2 kg or 6–9 years of age:** 10 mg t.i.d.–q.i.d.; **children less than 6 years of age:** 1.3–2.6 mg/kg/day of the syrup has been studied.
• **Inhalation. Hand Nebulizer**
Bronchodilation.
Usual dose is 10 inhalations (range: 5–15 inhalations) of undiluted 5% solution.
• **IPPB**
Bronchodilation.
0.3 mL (range: 0.2–0.3 mL) of 5% solution diluted to 2.5 mL saline or other diluent.
• **MDI**
Bronchodilation.
2–3 inhalations (1.30–2.25 mg) q 3–4 hr. Do not exceed a total daily dose of 12 inhalations (9 mg).
How Supplied: *Metered dose inhaler:* 0.65 mg/inh; *Solution:* 0.4%, 0.6%, 5%; *Syrup:* 10 mg/5 mL; *Tablet:* 10 mg, 20 mg
Side Effects: Additional: *GI:* Diarrhea, bad taste or taste changes. *Respiratory:* Worsening of asthma, nasal congestion, hoarseness. *Miscellaneous:* Hypersensitivity reactions, rash, fatigue, backache, skin reactions.
Drug Interactions: Possible potentiation of adrenergic effects if used before or after other sympathomimetic bronchodilators.

EMS CONSIDERATIONS

See also *Adrenergic Bronchodilators* under *Sympathomimetic Drugs.*

M

---

bold italic = life threatening side effect

Metaraminol bitartrate

(met-ah-RAM-ih-nohl)
Pregnancy Class: C
Aramine **(Rx)**
Classification: Adrenergic agent,
direct-acting; vasopressor

Mechanism of Action: Indirectly releases norepinephrine from storage sites and directly stimulates primarily alpha receptors and, to a slight extent, beta-1 receptors. Causes marked increases in BP due primarily to vasoconstriction and to a slight increase in CO. Reflex bradycardia is also manifested. Increases venous tone, causes pulmonary vasoconstriction, and increases pulmonary pressure, even if CO is decreased. CNS stimulation usually does not occur.
Onset of Action: IV: 1-2 min; **IM:** 10 min; **SC:** 5-20 min.
Duration of Action: IV: 20 min; **IM, SC:** About 60 min.
Uses: Hypotension associated with surgery, spinal anesthesia, hemorrhage, trauma, infections, tumors, and adverse drug reactions. Adjunct to the treatment of either septicemia or cardiogenic shock. *Investigational:* Injected intracavernosally to treat priapism due to phentolamine, papaverine, or other causes.
Contraindications: Use with cyclopropane or halothane anesthesia (unless clinical conditions mandate such use). As a substitute for blood or fluid replacement.
Precautions: Use with caution in cirrhosis, malaria, heart or thyroid disease, hypertension, diabetes, or during lactation. Hypertension and ischemic ECG changes may occur when used to treat priapism. Use is not a substitute for the replacement of blood, plasma, fluids, and electrolytes.

Route/Dosage ————————
• **IM, SC**
   Prophylaxis of hypotension.
Adults: 2–10 mg given IM or SC; **pediatric:** 0.01 mg/kg (3 mg/m²) IM or SC.
• **IV Infusion**

Hypotension.
Adults: 15–100 mg in 250–500 mL of 0.9% NaCl injection or 5% dextrose injection by IV infusion at a rate to maintain desired BP (up to 500 mg/500 mL has been used). **Pediatric:** 0.4 mg/kg (12 mg/m²) by IV infusion in a solution containing 1 mg/25 mL 0.9% NaCl injection or 5% dextrose injection.
• **Direct IV**
   Severe shock.
Adults: 0.5–5.0 mg by direct IV followed by IV infusion of 15–100 mg in 250–500 mL fluid. **Pediatric:** 0.01 mg/kg (0.3 mg/m²) by direct IV.
• **Endotracheal Tube**
If IV access is not possible, metaraminol may be given by an ET tube. Perform five quick insufflations; forcefully expel 5 mg diluted to 10 mL into the ET tube and follow with five quick insufflations.
How Supplied: *Injection:* 10 mg/mL
Side Effects: Additional: Rapidly induced hypertension may cause acute pulmonary edema, arrhythmias, and ***cardiac arrest.*** Due to its long duration of action, cumulative effects are possible with prolonged increases in BP.
Drug Interactions
Digitalis glycosides / ↑ Risk of ectopic arrhythmias
Furazolidone / Possible hypertensive crisis and intracranial hemorrhage
Guanethidine / Antihypertensive effects of guanethidine may be partially or totally reversed
Halogenated hydrocarbons / Sensitization of the heart to catecholamines; use of metaraminol may cause serious arrhythmias
MAO Inhibitors / Possible hypertensive crisis and intracranial hemorrhage
Oxytocic drugs / Possiblity of severe, persistent hypertension
Tricyclic antidepressants / ↓ Pressor effect of metaraminol

EMS CONSIDERATIONS

See also *Sympathomimetic Drugs.*

Metformin hydrochloride
(met-FOR-min)
Pregnancy Class: B
Glucophage (Rx)
Classification: Oral antidiabetic

Mechanism of Action: Decreases hepatic glucose production, decreases intestinal absorption of glucose, and increases peripheral uptake and utilization of glucose. Does not cause hypoglycemia in either diabetic or nondiabetic patients, and it does not cause hyperinsulinemia. Insulin secretion remains unchanged, while fasting insulin levels and day-long plasma insulin response may decrease. In contrast to sulfonylureas, the body weight of patients treated with metformin remains stable or may decrease somewhat.

Uses: Alone as an adjunct to diet to lower blood glucose in patients having NIDDM whose blood glucose cannot be managed satisfactorily via diet alone. Also, metformin may be used concomitantly with a sulfonylurea when diet and metformin or a sulfonylurea alone do not result in adequate control of blood glucose.

Contraindications: Renal disease or dysfunction (serum creatinine levels greater than 1.5 mg/dL in males and greater than 1.4 mg/dL in females) or abnormal C_{CR} due to cardiovascular collapse, acute MI, or septicemia. In patients undergoing radiologic studies using iodinated contrast media, because use of such products may cause alteration of renal function, leading to acute renal failure and lactic acidosis. Acute or chronic metabolic acidosis, including diabetic ketoacidosis, with or without coma. Lactation.

Precautions: Cardiovascular collapse, acute CHF, acute MI, and other conditions characterized by hypoxia have been associated with lactic acidosis, which may also be caused by metformin. Use of oral hypoglycemic agents may increase the risk of cardiovascular mortality. Although hypoglycemia does not usually occur with metformin, it may result with deficient caloric intake, with strenuous exercise not supplemented by increased intake of calories, or when metformin is taken with sulfonylureas or alcohol. Because of age-related decreases in renal function, use with caution as age increases. Safety and efficacy have not been determined in children.

Route/Dosage
- **Tablets**
  NIDDM.
  Adults, using 500-mg tablet: Starting dose is one 500-mg tablet b.i.d. given with the morning and evening meals. Dosage increases may be made in increments of 500 mg every week, given in divided doses, up to a maximum of 2,500 mg/day. If a 2,500-mg daily dose is required, it may be better tolerated when given in divided doses t.i.d. with meals. **Adults, using 850-mg tablet:** Starting dose is 850 mg once daily given with the morning meal. Dosage increases may be made in increments of 850 mg every other week, given in divided doses, up to a maximum of 2,550 mg/day. **Usual maintenance dose:** 850 mg b.i.d. with the morning and evening meals. However, some patients may require 850 mg t.i.d. with meals.

How Supplied: *Tablet:* 500 mg, 850 mg

Side Effects: *Metabolic:* Lactic acidosis (fatal in approximately 50% of cases). *GI:* Diarrhea, N&V, abdominal bloating, flatulence, anorexia, unpleasant or metallic taste. *Hematologic:* Asymptomatic subnormal serum vitamin B_{12} levels.

OD Overdose Management: *Symptoms:* Lactic acidosis.

Drug Interactions
Alcohol / Alcohol ↑ the effect of metformin on lactate metabolism
Cimetidine / Cimetidine ↑ (by 60%) peak metformin plasma and whole blood levels

---

bold italic = life threatening side effect

Furosemide / Furosemide ↑ metformin plasma and blood levels; also, metformin ↓ the half-life of furosemide

Iodinated contrast media / ↑ Risk of acute renal failure and lactic acidosis

Nifedipine / Nifedipine ↑ the absorption of metformin, leading to ↑ plasma metformin levels

EMS CONSIDERATIONS

None.

Methadone hydrochloride
(METH-ah-dohn)
Pregnancy Class: C
Dolophine, Methadose **(C-II) (Rx)**
Classification: Narcotic analgesic, morphine type

Mechanism of Action: Produces only mild euphoria, which is the reason it is used as a heroin withdrawal substitute and for maintenance programs. Produces physical dependence; withdrawal symptoms develop more slowly and are less intense but more prolonged than those associated with morphine. Does not produce sedation or narcosis. Not effective for preoperative or obstetric anesthesia. Only one-half as potent PO as when given parenterally.
Onset of Action: 30-60 min; **Peak effects:** 30-60 min.
Duration of Action: 4-6 hr.
Uses: Severe pain. Drug withdrawal and maintenance of narcotic dependence.
Contraindications: Additional: IV use, liver disease, during pregnancy, in children, or in jobstetrics (due to long duration of action and chance of respiratory depression in the neonate).
Precautions: Use with caution during lactation.

Route/Dosage ————————
• **Tablets, Oral Solution, Oral Concentrate**
Analgesia.
Adults, individualized: 2.5–10 mg q 3–4 hr, although higher doses may

be necessary for severe pain or due to development of tolerance.
Narcotic withdrawal.
Initial: 15–20 mg/day PO (some may require 40 mg/day); **then,** depending on need of the patient, slowly decrease dosage.
Maintenance following narcotic withdrawal.
Adults, individualized, initial: 20–40 mg PO 4–8 hr after heroin is stopped; **then,** adjust dosage as required up to 120 mg/day.
How Supplied: *Oral Concentrate:* 10 mg/mL; *Oral Solution:* 5 mg/5 mL, 10 mg/5 mL; *Tablet:* 5 mg, 10 mg, 40 mg
Side Effects: Additional: Marked constipation, excessive sweating, pulmonary edema, choreic movements.
Drug Interactions: Rifampin and phenytoin ↓ plasma methadone levels by ↑ breakdown by liver; thus, possible symptoms of narcotic withdrawal may develop.

EMS CONSIDERATIONS

See also *Narcotic Analgesics.*

Methamphetamine hydrochloride
(meth-am-FET-ah-meen)
Pregnancy Class: C
Desoxyn **(Rx)**
Classification: Central nervous system stimulant, amphetamine-type

Uses: Attention-deficit disorders in children over 6 years of age. Obesity (use controversial and often not recommended).
Contraindications: Use for obesity. Attention-deficit disorders in children less than 6 years of age.

Route/Dosage ————————
• **Tablets**
ADD in children 6 years and older.
Initial: 5 mg 1–2 times/day; increase in increments of 5 mg/day at weekly intervals until optimum dose is reached (usually 20–25 mg/day).
• **Extended-Release Tablets**

ADD in children 6 years and older, maintenance.
20–25 mg once daily.
Obesity.
Either one 5-mg tablet 30 min before each meal or 10–15 mg of the long-acting form in the morning. Do not exceed more than a few weeks of treatment.
How Supplied: *Tablet:* 5 mg; *Tablet, Extended Release:* 5 mg, 10 mg, 15 mg

EMS CONSIDERATIONS

See also *Amphetamines and Derivatives.*

Methazolamide
(meth-ah-ZOH-lah-myd)
Pregnancy Class: C
Glauctabs, Neptazane **(Rx)**
Classification: Antiglaucoma drug

Mechanism of Action: Inhibition of carbonic anhdyrase decreases the secretion of aqueous humor resulting in a decrease in intraocular pressure. Has weak diuretic effects and, due to inhibition of carbonic anhydrase, produces an alkaline urine.
Onset of Action: 2-4 hr; **Peak effect:** 6-8 hr.
Duration of Action: 10-18 hr.
Uses: Treatment of chronic open-angle glaucoma, secondary glaucoma. Preoperatively in acute angle-closure glaucoma to lower IOP prior to surgery.
Contraindications: Use in marked kidney or liver disease or dysfunction, in adrenal gland failure, and in hyperchloremic acidosis. Long-term use in patients with angle-closure glaucoma, since organic closure of the angle may occur even if IOP is lowered. Lactation.
Precautions: Use with caution in those with pulmonary obstruction or emphysema as acidosis may be aggravated or precipitated. Use with caution in those with cirrhosis or hepatic insufficiency due to the possibility of hepatic coma. The safety and efficacy have not been determined for use in children.

Route/Dosage
• **Tablets**
  Glaucoma.
50–100 mg b.i.d.–t.i.d.
How Supplied: *Tablets:* 25 mg, 50 mg
Side Effects: *GI:* Taste alteration, N&V, diarrhea, melena. *CNS:* Paresthesias (especially a "tingling" feeling in the extremities), fatigue, malaise, loss of appetite, drowsiness, confusion, ***convulsions.*** *Metabolic:* Metabolic acidosis, electrolyte imbalance. *GU:* Polyuria, hematuria, glycosuria. Rarely, crystalluria and renal calculi. *Dermatologic:* Urticaria, photosensitivity. *Miscellaneous:* Hearing dysfunction or tinnitus, transient myopia, hepatic insufficiency, flaccid paralysis.

NOTE: Side effects may be observed that are due to the sulfonamide. See *Sulfonamides.*
Drug Interactions
Aspirin (high doses) / Symptoms of anorexia, tachypnea, lethargy, coma, and death are possible
Corticosteroids / ↑ Risk of hypokalemia

EMS CONSIDERATIONS

None.

Methenamine hippurate
Methenamine mandelate
(meh-THEEN-ah-meen)
Pregnancy Class: C
Hippurate: Hiprex, Urex **(Rx)) Mandelate: (Rx)**
Classification: Urinary tract anti-infective

Mechanism of Action: Converted in an acid medium into ammonia and formaldehyde (the active principle), which denatures protein. Formaldehyde levels in the urine may be bacteriostatic or bactericidal, depending on the pH; it is most effective when the urine has a pH value of 5.5 or less, which is maintained by using the hippurate or mandelate salt.
Uses: Acute, chronic, and recurrent UTIs by susceptible organisms, especially gram-negative organisms in-

M

cluding *Escherichia coli.* As a prophylactic before urinary tract instrumentation. Never used as sole agent in the treatment of acute infections.

Contraindications: Renal insufficiency, severe liver damage, severe dehydration. Concurrent use of sulfonamides as an insoluble precipitate may form with formaldehyde.

Precautions: Use with caution in gout (methenamine may cause urate crystals to precipitate in the urine).

Route/Dosage

• **Tablets**

Hippurate: **Adults and children over 12 years:** 1 g b.i.d. in the morning and evening; **children, 6–12 years:** 0.5 g b.i.d.

• **Oral Suspension, Enteric-Coated Tablets**

Mandelate: **Adults:** 1 g q.i.d. after meals and at bedtime; **children 6–12 years:** 0.5 g q.i.d.; **children under 6 years:** 0.25 g/13.6 kg q.i.d.

How Supplied: Methenanamine hippurate: *Tablet:* 1 g Methenamine mandelate: *Tablet:* 0.5 g, 1 g; *Suspension:* 0.5 g/5 mL

Side Effects: *GI:* N&V, diarrhea, anorexia, cramps, stomatitis. *GU:* Hematuria, albuminuria, crystalluria, dysuria, urinary frequency or urgency, bladder irritation. *Dermatologic:* Skin rashes, urticaria, pruritus, erythematous eruptions. *Other:* Headache, dyspnea, edema, lipoid pneumonitis.

OD Overdose Management: *Treatment:* Absorption following overdose may be minimized by inducing vomiting or by gastric lavage, followed by activated charcoal. Fluids should be forced.

Drug Interactions

Acetazolamide / ↓ Effect of methenamine due to inhibition of conversion to formaldehyde

Sodium bicarbonate / ↓ Effect of methenamine due to inhibition of conversion to formaldehyde

Sulfonamides / ↑ Chance of sulfonamide crystalluria due to acid urine produced by methenamine

Thiazide diuretics / ↓ Effect of methenamine due to ↑ alkalinity of urine produced by thiazides

EMS CONSIDERATIONS

None.

Methimazole (Thiamazole)

(meth-IM-ah-zohl)
Pregnancy Class: D
Tapazole **(Rx)**
Classification: Antithyroid drug

Onset of Action: 10-20 days; **Time to peak effect:** 2-10 weeks.

Precautions: Incidence of hepatic toxicity may be greater than for propylthiouracil.

Route/Dosage

• **Tablets**

Mild hyperthyroidism.

Adults, initial: 15 mg/day.

Moderately severe hyperthyroidism.

Adults, initial: 30–40 mg/day.

Severe hyperthyroidism.

Adults, initial: 60 mg/day. For hyperthyroidism, the daily dose is usually given in three equal doses 8 hr apart. **Maintenance:** 5–15 mg/day as a single dose or divided into two doses. **Pediatric:** 0.4 mg/kg given once daily or divided into two doses; **maintenance:** 0.2 mg/kg. Alternatively, **initial:** 0.5–0.7 mg/kg/day (15–20 mg/m²/day in three divided doses); **maintenance:** ⅓–⅔ initial dose when patient is euthyroid up to a maximum of 30 mg/day.

Thyrotoxic crisis.

Adults, 15–20 mg/4 hr during the first day as an adjunct to other treatments.

How Supplied: *Tablet:* 5 mg, 10 mg

EMS CONSIDERATIONS

None.

Methocarbamol

(meth-oh-KAR-bah-mohl)
Pregnancy Class: C
Robaxin, Robaxin-750 **(Rx)**
Classification: Centrally acting muscle relaxant

Mechanism of Action: Beneficial effect may be related to the sedative properties of the drug. Has no direct effect on the contractile mechanism of striated muscle, the motor endplate, or the nerve fiber and it does not directly relax tense skeletal muscles. Of limited usefulness. May be given IM or IV in polyethylene glycol 300 (50% solution). PO therapy should be initiated as soon as possible.

Onset of Action: 30 min; **Peak plasma levels:** 2 hr after 2 g.

Uses: Adjunct for the relief of acute, painful musculoskeletal conditions (e.g., sprains, strains). Adjunct in tetanus.

Contraindications: Hypersensitivity, when muscle spasticity is required to maintain upright position, seizure disorders, pregnancy, lactation, children under 12 years. Renal disease (parenteral dosage form only since it contains polyethylene glycol 300).

Precautions: Use with caution in epilepsy and during lactation. Use the injectable form with caution in suspected or known epileptics.

Route/Dosage ————————
- **Tablets**
  Skeletal muscle disorders.
  Adults, initial: 1.5 g q.i.d. for the first 2–3 days (for severe conditions, 8 g/day may be given); **maintenance:** 1 g q.i.d., 0.75 g q 4 hr, or 1.5 g t.i.d.
- **IM, IV**
  Skeletal muscle disorders.
  Adults, usual initial: 1 g; in severe cases, up to 2–3 g may be necessary. **IV administration should not exceed 3 days.**
  Tetanus.
  Adults: 1–2 g IV, initially, into tube of previously inserted indwelling needle. An additional 1–2 g may be added to the infusion for a total initial dose of 3 g. May be given q 6 hr (up to 24 g/day may be needed) until PO administration is feasible. **Pediatric, initial:** 15 mg/kg given into tube of previously inserted indwelling needle. Dose may be repeated q 6 hr.

How Supplied: *Injection:* 100 mg/mL; *Tablet:* 500 mg, 750 mg

Side Effects: *Following PO use. CNS:* Dizziness, drowsiness, lightheadedness, vertigo, lassitude, headache. *GI:* Nausea. *Miscellaneous:* Allergic symptoms including rash, urticaria, pruritus, conjunctivitis, nasal congestion, blurred vision, fever. *Following IV use (in addition to the preceding). CV:* Hypotension, bradycardia, syncope. *CNS:* Fainting, mild muscle incoordination. *Miscellaneous:* Metallic taste, GI upset, flushing, nystagmus, double vision, thrombophlebitis, sloughing or pain at injection site, *anaphylaxis.*

OD Overdose Management: *Symptoms:* CNS depression, including coma, is often seen when methocarbamol is used with alcohol or other CNS depressants. *Treatment:* Supportive, depending on the symptoms.

Drug Interactions: Central nervous system depressants (including alcohol) may ↑ the effect of methocarbamol.

EMS CONSIDERATIONS

See also *Skeletal Muscle Relaxants.*

Methotrexate, Methotrexate sodium
(meth-oh-TREKS-ayt)
Pregnancy Class: D (X for pregnant psoriatic or rheumatoid arthritis patients).
Amethopterin, Folex PFS, Rheumatrex Dose Pack (Abbreviation: MTX) **(Rx)**
Classification: Antineoplastic, antimetabolite (folic acid analog)

Mechanism of Action: Cell-cycle specific for the S phase of cell division. Acts by inhibiting dihydrofolate reductase, which prevents reduction of dihydrofolate to tetrahydrofolate; this results in decreased synthesis of purines and consequently DNA. The most sensitive cells are bone marrow, fetal cells, dermal epithelium, urinary bladder, buccal mucosa, intestinal mucosa, and malignant cells. When used for rheumatoid arthritis it may affect immune function.

---

bold italic = life threatening side effect

Uses: Uterine choriocarcinoma (curative), chorioadenoma destruens, hydatidiform mole, acute lymphocytic and lymphoblastic leukemia, lymphosarcoma, and other disseminated neoplasms in children; meningeal leukemia, some beneficial effect in regional chemotherapy of head and neck tumors, breast tumors, and lung cancer. In combination for advanced stage non-Hodgkin's lymphoma. Advanced mycosis fungoides. High doses followed by leucovorin rescue in combination with other drugs for prolonging relapse-free survival in nonmetastatic osteosarcoma in individuals who have had surgical resection or amputation for the primary tumor. Severe, recalcitrant, disabling psoriasis. Rheumatoid arthritis (severe, active, classical, or definite) in patients who have had inadequate response to NSAIDs and at least one or more antirheumatic drugs (disease modifying). *Investigational:* Severe corticosteroid-dependent asthma to reduce corticosteroid dosage; adjunct to treat osteosarcoma. Psoriatic arthritis and Reiter's disease.

Contraindications: Psoriasis patients with kidney or liver disease; blood dyscrasias as hypoplasia, thrombocytopenia, anemia, or leukopenia. Alcoholism, alcoholic liver disease, or other chronic liver disease. Immunodeficiency syndromes. Pregnancy and lactation.

Precautions: Use with caution in impaired renal function and elderly patients. Use with extreme caution in the presence of active infection and in debilitated patients. Safety and efficacy have not been established for juvenile rheumatoid arthritis.

Route/Dosage ————————
- **Tablets (Methotrexate). IM, IV, IA, Intrathecal (Methotrexate Sodium)**

Choriocarcinoma and similar trophoblastic diseases.
Dose individualized. PO, IM: 15–30 mg/day for 5 days. May be re-

peated 3–5 times with 1-week rest period between courses.
Acute lymphatic (lymphoblastic) leukemia.
Initial: 3.3 mg/m² (with 60 mg/m² prednisone daily); **maintenance: PO, IM,** 30 mg/m² 2 times/week or **IV,** 2.5 mg/kg q 14 days.
Meningeal leukemia.
Intrathecal: 12 mg/m² q 2–5 days until cell count returns to normal.
Lymphomas.
PO: 10–25 mg/day for 4–8 days for several courses of treatment with 7- to 10-day rest periods between courses.
Mycosis fungoides.
PO: 2.5–10 mg/day for several weeks or months; **alternatively, IM:** 50 mg once weekly or 25 mg twice weekly.
Lymphosarcoma.
0.625–2.5 mg/kg/day in combination with other drugs.
Osteosarcoma.
Used in combination with other drugs, including doxorubicin, cisplatin, bleomycin, cyclophosphamide, and dactinomycin. **Usual IV starting dose for methotrexate:** 12 g/m²; dose may be increased to 15 g/m² to achieve a peak serum level of 10⁻³ mol/L at the end of the methotrexate infusion.
Psoriasis.
Adults, usual: PO, IM, IV, 10–25 mg/week, continued until beneficial response observed. Weekly dose should not exceed 50 mg. **Alternate regimens: PO,** 2.5 mg q 12 hr for three doses or q 8 hr for four doses each week (not to exceed 30 mg/week); **or PO,** 2.5 mg daily for 5 days followed by 2 days of rest (dose should not exceed 6.25 mg/day). Once beneficial effects are noted, reduce dose to lowest possible level with longest rest periods between doses.
Rheumatoid arthritis.
Initial: Single PO doses of 7.5 mg/week or divided PO doses of 2.5 mg at 12-hr intervals for three doses given once a week; **then,** adjust dosage to achieve optimum response, not to exceed a total weekly

dose of 20 mg. Once response has been reached, reduce the dose to the lowest possible effective dose.

How Supplied: *Injection:* 25 mg/mL; *Powder for injection:* 20 mg, 1 g; *Tablet:* 2.5 mg

Side Effects: Additional: *Severe bone marrow depression.* Hepatotoxicity, fibrosis, cirrhosis. *Hemorrhagic enteritis, intestinal ulceration or perforation,* acne, ecchymosis, hematemesis, melena, increased pigmentation, diabetes, leukoencephalopathy, chronic interstitial obstructive pulmonary disease, acute renal failure. Intrathecal use may result in chemical arachnoiditis, transient paresis, or *seizures.* Concomitant exposure to sunlight may aggravate psoriasis.

OD **Overdose Management:** *Symptoms:* See *Antineoplastic Agents,* Chapter 2. *Treatment:* Leucovorin, given as soon as possible, may decrease toxic effects. The dose used is 10 mg/m^2 PO or parenterally followed by 10 mg/m^2 PO q 6 hr for 72 hr. Charcoal hemoperfusion will reduce serum levels. In massive overdosage, hydration and urinary alkalinization are needed to prevent precipitation of methotrexate and metabolites in the renal tubules.

Drug Interactions
Alcohol, ethyl / Additive hepatotoxicity; combination can result in coma
Aminoglycosides, oral / ↓ Absorption of PO methotrexate
Anticoagulants, oral / Additive hypoprothrombinemia
Chloramphenicol / ↑ Effect of methotrexate by ↓ plasma protein binding
Etretinate / Possible hepatotoxicity if used together for psoriasis
Folic acid–containing vitamin preparations / ↓ Response to methotrexate
Ibuprofen / ↑ Effect of methotrexate by ↓ renal secretion
NSAIDs / Possible fatal interaction
PABA / ↑ Effect of methotrexate by ↓ plasma protein binding

Phenylbutazone / ↑ Effect of methotrexate by ↓ renal secretion
Phenytoin / ↑ Effect of methotrexate by ↓ plasma protein binding
Probenecid / ↑ Effect of methotrexate by ↓ renal clearance
Procarbazine / Possible ↑ nephrotoxicity
Pyrimethamine / ↑ Methotrexate toxicity
Salicylates (aspirin) / ↑ Effect of methotrexate by ↓ plasma protein binding; also, salicylates ↓ renal excretion of methotrexate
Smallpox vaccination / Methotrexate impairs immunologic response to smallpox vaccine
Sulfonamides / ↑ Effect of methotrexate by ↓ plasma protein binding
Tetracyclines / ↑ Effect of methotrexate by ↓ plasma protein binding
Thiopurines / ↑ Plasma levels of thiopurines

EMS CONSIDERATIONS
None.

Methsuximide
(meth-SUCKS-ih-myd)
Pregnancy Class: C
Celontin **(Rx)**
Classification: Anticonvulsant, succinimide type

Uses: Treat absence seizures refractory to other drugs. May be given with other anticonvulsants when absence seizures coexist with other types of epilepsy.

Route/Dosage
• **Capsules**
Absence seizures.
Adults and children, initial: 300 mg/day for first week; **then,** if necessary, increase dosage by 300 mg/day at weekly intervals until control established. **Maximum daily dose:** 1.2 g in divided doses.
How Supplied: *Capsule:* 150 mg, 300 mg
Side Effects: Additional: Most common are ataxia, dizziness, and drowsiness.

---

bold italic = life threatening side effect

Drug Interactions: Additional: Methsuximide may ↑ the effect of primidone.

EMS CONSIDERATIONS

None.

Methyldopa
Methyldopa hydrochloride
(meth-ill-DOH-pah)

Pregnancy Class: Methyldopa: B (PO); Methyldopa hydrochloride: B (PO), C (IV)
Methyldopa (Aldomet **(Rx)**) Methyldopa hydrochloride (Aldomet Hydrochloride **(Rx)**)
Classification: Antihypertensive, centrally acting antiadrenergic

Mechanism of Action: The active metabolite, alpha-methylnorepinephrine, lowers BP by stimulating central inhibitory alpha-adrenergic receptors, false neurotransmission, and/or reduction of plasma renin. Little change in CO.
Onset of Action: PO: 7-12 hr; **IV:** 4-6 hr; **Full therapeutic effect:** 1-4 days.
Duration of Action: PO: 12-24 hr. All effects terminated within 48 hr; **IV:** 10-16 hr.
Uses: Moderate to severe hypertension. Particularly useful for patients with impaired renal function, renal hypertension, resistant cases of hypertension complicated by stroke, CAD, or nitrogen retention, and for hypertensive crisis (parenterally).
Contraindications: Sensitivity to drug (including sulfites), labile and mild hypertension, pregnancy, active hepatic disease, use with MAO inhibitors, or pheochromocytoma.
Precautions: Use with caution in patients with a history of liver or kidney disease. A decrease in dose in geriatric patients may prevent syncope.

Route/Dosage
• **Methyldopa. Tablets**
Hypertension.
Initial: 250 mg b.i.d.–t.i.d. for 2 days. Adjust dose q 2 days. If in-

creased, start with evening dose. **Usual maintenance:** 0.5–3.0 g/day in two to four divided doses; **maximum:** 3 g/day. Gradually transfer to and from other antihypertensive agents, with initial dose of methyldopa not exceeding 500 mg. *NOTE:* Do not use combination medication to initiate therapy. **Pediatric, initial:** 10 mg/kg/day in two to four divided doses, adjusting maintenance to a maximum of 65 mg/kg/day (or 3 g/day, whichever is less).
• **Methyldopate HCl. IV Infusion**
Hypertension.
Adults: 250–500 mg q 6 hr; **maximum:** 1 g q 6 hr for hypertensive crisis.
Switch to PO methyldopa, at same dosage level, when BP is brought under control. **Pediatric:** 20–40 mg/kg/day in divided doses q 6 hr; **maximum:** 65 mg/kg/day (or 3 g/day, whichever is less).
How Supplied: Methyldopa: *Tablet:* 125 mg, 250 mg, 500 mg. Methyldopate hydrochloride: *Injection:* 50 mg/mL
Side Effects: *CNS:* Sedation (transient), weakness, headache, asthenia, dizziness, paresthesias, Parkinson-like symptoms, psychic disturbances, symptoms of CV impairment, choreoathetotic movements, Bell's palsy, decreased mental acuity, verbal memory impairment. *CV:* Bradycardia, orthostatic hypotension, hypersensitivity of carotid sinus, worsening of angina, paradoxical hypertensive response (after IV), myocarditis, CHF, pericarditis, vasculitis. *GI:* N&V, abdominal distention, diarrhea or constipation, flatus, colitis, dry mouth, sore or "black tongue," pancreatitis, sialoadenitis. *Hematologic:* **Hemolytic anemia,** leukopenia, granulocytopenia, thrombocytopenia, **bone marrow depression.** *Endocrine:* Gynecomastia, amenorrhea, galactorrhea, lactation, hyperprolactinemia. *GU:* Impotence, failure to ejaculate, decreased libido. *Dermatologic:* Rash, **toxic epidermal necrolysis.** *Hepatic:* Jaundice, hepatitis, liver disorders, abnormal liver function tests. *Miscellaneous:* Edema, fever, lupus-like symptoms,

nasal stuffiness, arthralgia, myalgia, *septic shock-like syndrome.*

OD **Overdose Management:** *Symptoms:* CNS, GI, and CV effects including sedation, weakness, lightheadedness, dizziness, coma, bradycardia, acute hypotension, impairment of AV conduction, constipation, diarrhea, distention, flatus, N&V. *Treatment:* Induction of vomiting or gastric lavage if detected early. General supportive treatment with special attention to HR, CO, blood volume, urinary function, electrolyte imbalance, paralytic ileus, and CNS activity. In severe cases, hemodialysis is effective.

Drug Interactions

Anesthetics, general / Additive hypotension

Antidepressants, tricyclic / Tricyclic antidepressants may block hypotensive effect of methyldopa

Haloperidol / Methyldopa ↑ toxic effects of haloperidol

Levodopa / ↑ Effect of both drugs

Lithium / ↑ Possibility of lithium toxicity

MAO inhibitors / Metabolites of methyldopa, usually metabolized by MAO inhibitors, may → excessive sympathetic stimulation

Methotrimeprazine / Additive hypotensive effect

Phenothiazines / ↑ Risk of serious ↑ BP

Propranolol / Paradoxical hypertension

Sympathomimetics / Potentiation of hypertensive effect of sympathomimetics

Thiazide diuretics / Additive hypotensive effect

Thioxanthenes / Additive hypotensive effect

Tolbutamide / ↑ Hypoglycemia due to ↓ breakdown by liver

Tricyclic antidepressants / ↓ Effect of methyldopa

Vasodilator drugs / Additive hypotensive effect

Verapamil / ↑ Effect of methyldopa

EMS CONSIDERATIONS

See also *Antihypertensive Agents.*

Methyldopa and Hydrochlorothiazide

(meth-ill-DOH-pah, hy-droh-klor-oh-THIGH-ah-zyd)
Pregnancy Class: C
Aldoril 15, Aldoril 25, Aldoril D30, Aldoril D50 **(Rx)**
Classification: Antihypertensive

Uses: Hypertension (not for initial treatment).
Contraindications: Active hepatic disease.
Precautions: Use in pregnancy only if benefits outweigh risks.

Route/Dosage ─────────
• **Tablets**
Adults: 1 tablet b.i.d.–t.i.d. for first 48 hr; **then,** increase or decrease dose, depending on response, in intervals of not less than 2 days. Maximum daily dosage: methyldopa, 3.0 g; hydrochlorothiazide, 100–200 mg.
How Supplied: *Antihypertensive:* Methyldopa, 250 or 500 mg. *Diuretic/antihypertensive:* Hydrochlorothiazide, 15–50 mg.

EMS CONSIDERATIONS

None.

Methylphenidate hydrochloride

(meth-ill-FEN-ih-dayt)
Pregnancy Class: C
Ritalin, Ritalin-SR **(C-II) (Rx)**
Classification: Central nervous system stimulant

Mechanism of Action: May act by blocking the reuptake mechanism of dopaminergic neurons. In children with attention-deficit disorders, methylphenidate causes decreases in motor restlessness with an increased attention span. In narcolepsy the drug acts on the cerebral cortex and subcortical structures (e.g., thalamus) to increase motor activity and mental alertness and decrease fatigue.

Uses: Attention-deficit disorders in children as part of overall treatment regimen. Narcolepsy. *Investigation-*

M

al: Depression in elderly, cancer, and poststroke patients. Anesthesia-related hiccups.

Contraindications: Marked anxiety, tension and agitation, glaucoma. Severe depression, to prevent normal fatigue, diagnosis of Tourette's syndrome, motor tics. In children who manifest symptoms of primary psychiatric disorders (psychoses) or acute stress.

Precautions: Use with caution during lactation. Use with great caution in patients with history of hypertension or convulsive disease. Safety and efficacy in children less than 6 years of age have not been established.

Route/Dosage

• **Tablets**
   Narcolepsy.
Adults: 5–20 mg b.i.d.–t.i.d. preferably 30–45 min before meals.
   Attention-deficit disorders.
Pediatric, 6 years and older, initial: 5 mg b.i.d. before breakfast and lunch; **then,** increase by 5–10 mg/week to a maximum of 60 mg/day.

• **Extended-Release Tablets**
   Narcolepsy.
Adults: 20 mg 1–3 times/day q 8 hr, preferably on an empty stomach.
   Attention-deficit disorders.
Pediatric, 6 years and older: 20 mg 1–3 times/day.

How Supplied: *Tablet:* 5 mg, 10 mg, 20 mg; *Tablet, Extended Release:* 20 mg

Side Effects: *CNS:* Nervousness, insomnia, headaches, dizziness, drowsiness, chorea, depressed mood (transient). Toxic psychoses, dyskinesia, Tourette's syndrome. Psychologic dependence. *CV:* Palpitations, tachycardia, angina, arrhythmias, hyper- or hypotension, cerebral arteritis or occlusion. *GI:* Nausea, anorexia, abdominal pain, weight loss (chronic use). *Allergic:* Skin rashes, fever, urticaria, arthralgia, exfoliative dermatitis, erythema multiforme with necrotizing vasculitis, erythema. *Hematologic:* Thrombocytopenic purpura, leukopenia, anemia. *Miscellaneous:* Hair loss, abnormal liver function.

In children, the following side effects are more common: anorexia, abdominal pain, weight loss (chronic use), tachycardia, insomnia.

OD **Overdose Management:** *Symptoms:* Characterized by CV symptoms (hypertension, cardiac arrhythmias, tachycardia), mental disturbances, agitation, headaches, vomiting, hyperreflexia, *hyperpyrexia, convulsions, and coma. Treatment:* Symptomatic. Treat excess CNS stimulation by keeping the patient in quiet, dim surroundings to reduce external stimuli. Protect the patient from self-injury. A short-acting barbiturate may be used. Undertake emesis or gastric lavage if the patient is conscious. Adequate circulatory and respiratory function must be maintained. Hyperpyrexia may be treated by cooling the patient (e.g., cool bath, hypothermia blanket).

Drug Interactions
Anticoagulants, oral / ↑ Effect of anticoagulants due to ↓ breakdown by liver
Anticonvulsants (phenobarbital, phenytoin, primidone) / ↑ Effect of anticonvulsants due to ↓ breakdown by liver
Guanethidine / ↓ Effect of guanethidine by displacement from its site of action
MAO inhibitors / Possibility of hypertensive crisis, hyperthermia, convulsions, coma
Tricyclic antidepressants / ↑ Effect of antidepressants due to ↓ breakdown by liver

EMS CONSIDERATIONS
None.

Methylprednisolone
Methylprednisolone acetate
Methylprednisolone sodium succinate

(meth-ill-pred-NISS-oh-lohn)
Pregnancy Class: C
Methylprednisolone **Tablets:** (Medrol, Meprolone **(Rx)**) Methylprednisolone acetate **Enema:** Medrol Enpak **(Rx)**,

Parenteral: (depMedalone-40 and -80, Depoject 40 and 80, Depo-Medrol, D-Med 80, Duralone-40 and -80, Medralone-40 and -80, M-Prednisol-40 and -80 **(Rx)**)
Methylprednisolone sodium succinate **Parenteral:** A-methaPred, Solu-Medrol **(Rx)**
Classification: Glucocorticoid

Onset of Action: Slow, 12-24 hr.
Duration of Action: Long, up to 1 week. Rapid onset of sodium succinate by both IV and IM routes. Long duration of action of the acetate.
Uses: Additional: Severe hepatitis due to alcoholism. Within 8 hr of severe spinal cord injury (to improve neurologic function). Septic shock (controversial).
Precautions: Use during pregnancy only if benefits outweigh risks.

Route/Dosage ⎯⎯⎯⎯⎯⎯⎯⎯
METHYLPREDNISOLONE
• **Tablets**
Rheumatoid arthritis.
Adults: 6–16 mg/day. Decrease gradually when condition is under control. **Pediatric:** 6–10 mg/day.
SLE.
Adults, acute: 20–96 mg/day; **maintenance:** 8–20 mg/day.
Acute rheumatic fever.
1 mg/kg body weight daily. Drug is always given in four equally divided doses after meals and at bedtime.
METHYLPREDNISOLONE ACETATE
• **IM**
Adrenogenital syndrome.
40 mg q 2 weeks.
Rheumatoid arthritis.
40–120 mg/week.
Dermatologic lesions, dermatitis.
40–120 mg/week for 1–4 weeks; for severe cases, a single dose of 80–120 mg should provide relief.
Seborrheic dermatitis.
80 mg/week.
Asthma, rhinitis.
80–120 mg.
• **Intra-articular, Soft Tissue and Intralesional Injection**
4–80 mg, depending on site.
• **Retention Enema**

40 mg 3–7 times/week for 2 or more weeks.
METHYLPREDNISOLONE SODIUM SUCCINATE
• **IM, IV**
Most conditions.
Adults, initial: 10–40 mg, depending on the disease; **then,** adjust dose depending on response, with subsequent doses given either **IM, IV.**
Severe conditions.
Adults: 30 mg/kg infused IV over 10–20 min; may be repeated q 4–6 hr for 2–3 days only. **Pediatric:** not less than 0.5 mg/kg/day.
How Supplied: Methylprednisolone: *Tablet:* 2 mg, 4 mg, 8 mg, 16 mg, 24 mg, 32 mg. Methylprednisolone acetate: *Injection:* 20 mg/mL, 40 mg/mL, 80 mg/mL. Methylprednisolone sodium succinate: *Powder for injection:* 40 mg, 125 mg, 500 mg, 1 g, 2 g

EMS CONSIDERATIONS

See also *Corticosteroids.*

Methysergide maleate
(meth-ih-SIR-jyd)
Pregnancy Class: X
Sansert **(Rx)**
Classification: Prophylactic for vascular headaches

Mechanism of Action: Semisynthetic ergot alkaloid derivative. May act by directly stimulating smooth muscle leading to vasoconstriction. Blocks the effects of serotonin, a powerful vasodilator believed to play a role in vascular headaches; it also inhibits the release of histamine from mast cells and prevents the release of serotonin from platelets. Has weak emetic and oxytocic activity.
Onset of Action: 1-2 days.
Duration of Action: 1-2 days.
Uses: Prevention or reduction of the intensity and frequency of vascular headache (in patients having one or more per week or in cases where headaches are so severe preventive therapy is indicated). Prophylaxis of vascular headache.

Contraindications: Severe renal or hepatic disease, severe hypertension, CAD, peripheral vascular disease, tendency toward thromboembolic disease, cachexia (profound ill health or malnutrition), severe arteriosclerosis, pulmonary disease, phlebitis or cellulitis of lower limbs, collagen diseases or fibrotic processs, debilitated states, valvular heart disease, infectious disease, or peptic ulcer. Use to terminate acute attacks. Pregnancy, lactation, use in children.

Precautions: Geriatric patients may be more affected by peripheral vasoconstriction leading to the possibility of hypothermia.

Route/Dosage
• **Tablets**
Adults: Administer 4–8 mg/day in divided doses. Continuous administration should not exceed 6 months. May be readministered after a 3- to 4-week rest period.

How Supplied: *Tablet:* 2 mg

Side Effects: The drug is associated with a high incidence of side effects. *Fibrosis:* **Retroperitoneal fibrosis, cardiac fibrosis, pleuropulmonary fibrosis,** Peyronie's-like disease. The fibrotic condition may result in vascular insufficiency in the lower legs. *CV:* Vasoconstriction of arteries leading to paresthesia, chest pain, abdominal pain, or extremities that are cold, numb, or painful. Tachycardia, postural hypotension. *CNS:* Dizziness, ataxia, drowsiness, vertigo, insomnia, euphoria, lightheadedness, and psychic reactions such as depersonalization, depression, and hallucinations. *GI:* N&V, diarrhea, heartburn, abdominal pain, increased gastric acid, constipation. *Hematologic:* Eosinophilia, neutropenia. *Other:* Peripheral edema, flushing of face, skin rashes, transient alopecia, myalgia, arthralgia, weakness, weight gain, telangiectasia.

Drug Interactions: Narcotic analgesics are inhibited by methysergide.

EMS CONSIDERATIONS
None.

Metipranolol hydrochloride
(met-ih-PRAN-oh-lohl)
Pregnancy Class: C
OptiPranolol **(Rx)**
Classification: Beta-adrenergic blocking agent

Mechanism of Action: Blocks both beta-1- and beta-2-adrenergic receptors. Reduction in intraocular pressure may be related to a decrease in production of aqueous humor and a slight increase in the outflow of aqueous humor. A decrease from 20% to 26% in intraocular pressure may be seen if the intraocular pressure is greater than 24 mm Hg at baseline. May be absorbed and exert systemic effects. When used topically, has no local anesthetic effect and exerts no action on pupil size or accommodation.

Onset of Action: 30 min; **Maximum effect:** 1-2 hr.

Uses: To reduce IOP in patients with ocular hypertension and chronic open-angle glaucoma.

Precautions: Use with caution during lactation. Safety and effectiveness have not been determined in children.

Route/Dosage
• **Ophthalmic Solution (0.3%)**
Adults: 1 gtt in the affected eye(s) b.i.d. Increasing the dose or more frequent administration does not increase the beneficial effect.

How Supplied: *Ophthalmic solution:* 0.3%

Side Effects: *Ophthalmologic:* Local discomfort, dermatitis of the eyelid, blepharitis, conjunctivitis, browache, tearing, blurred vision, abnormal vision, photophobia, edema. Due to absorption, the following systemic side effects have been reported. *CV:* Hypertension, MI, atrial fibrillation, angina, bradycardia, palpitation. *CNS:* Headache, dizziness, anxiety, depression, somnolence, nervousness. *Respiratory:* Dyspnea, rhinitis, bronchitis, coughing. *Miscellaneous:* Allergic reaction, asthenia, nausea, epistaxis, arthritis, myalgia, rash.

EMS CONSIDERATIONS

See also *Beta-Adrenergic Blocking Agents*.

Metoclopramide
(meh-toe-kloh-PRAH-myd)
Pregnancy Class: B
Reglan **(Rx)**
Classification: Gastrointestinal stimulant

Mechanism of Action: Dopamine antagonist that acts by increasing sensitivity to acetylcholine; results in increased motility of the upper GI tract and relaxation of the pyloric sphincter and duodenal bulb. Gastric emptying time and GI transit time are shortened. No effect on gastric, biliary, or pancreatic secretions. Facilitates intubation of the small bowel and speeds transit of a barium meal. Produces sedation, induces release of prolactin, increases circulating aldosterone levels (is transient), and is an antiemetic.
Onset of Action: IV: 1-3 min; **IM:** 10-15 min; **PO:** 30-60 min.
Duration of Action: 1-2 hr.
Uses: PO: Acute and recurrent diabetic gastroparesis, gastroesophageal reflux. **Parenteral:** Facilitate small bowel intubation, stimulate gastric emptying, and increase intestinal transit of barium to aid in radiologic examination of stomach and small intestine. Prophylaxis of N&V in cancer chemotherapy and following surgery (when nasogastric suction is not desired). *Investigational:* To improve lactation. N&V due to various causes, including vomiting during pregnancy and labor, gastric ulcer, anorexia nervosa. Improve patient response to ergotamine, analgesics, and sedatives when used to treat migraine (may increase absorption). Postoperative gastric bezoars. Atonic bladder. Esophageal variceal bleeding.
Contraindications: Gastrointestinal hemorrhage, obstruction, or perforation; epilepsy; patients taking drugs likely to cause extrapyramidal symptoms, such as phenothiazines. Pheochromocytoma.
Precautions: Use with caution during lactation and in hypertension. Extrapyramidal effects are more likely to occur in children and geriatric patients.

Route/Dosage
* **Tablets, Syrup, Concentrate**
  Diabetic gastroparesis.
Adults: 10 mg 30 min before meals and at bedtime for 2–8 weeks (therapy should be reinstituted if symptoms recur).
  Gastroesophageal reflux.
Adults: 10–15 mg q.i.d. 30 min before meals and at bedtime. If symptoms occur only intermittently, single doses up to 20 mg prior to the provoking situation may be used.
  To enhance lactation.
Adults: 30–45 mg/day.
* **IM, IV**
  Prophylaxis of vomiting due to chemotherapy.
Initial: 1–2 mg/kg IV q 2 hr for two doses, with the first dose 30 min before chemotherapy; **then,** 10 mg or more q 3 hr for three doses. Inject slowly IV over 15 min.
  Prophylaxis of postoperative N&V.
Adults: 10–20 mg IM near the end of surgery.
  Facilitate small bowel intubation.
Adults: 10 mg given over 1–2 min; **pediatric, 6–14 years:** 2.5–5 mg; **pediatric, less than 6 years:** 0.1 mg/kg.
  Radiologic examinations to increase intestinal transit time.
Adults: 10 mg as a single dose given IV over 1–2 min.
How Supplied: *Concentrate:* 10 mg/mL; *Injection:* 5 mg/mL; *Tablet:* 5 mg, 10 mg
Side Effects: *CNS:* Restlessness, drowsiness, fatigue, lassitude, akathisia, anxiety, insomnia, confusion. Headaches, dizziness, extrapyramidal symptoms (especially acute dystonic reactions), Parkinson-like symptoms (including cogwheel rigidity, mask-like facies, bradykinesia, tremor),

M

---

bold italic = life threatening side effect

dystonia, myoclonus, **depression (with suicidal ideation),** tardive dyskinesia (including involuntary movements of the tongue, face, mouth, or jaw), seizures, hallucinations. *GI:* Nausea, bowel disturbances (usually diarrhea). *CV:* Hypertension (transient), hypotension, SVT, bradycardia. *Hematologic:* **Agranulocytosis,** leukopenia, neutropenia. Methemoglobinemia in premature and full-term infants at doses of 1–4 mg/kg/day IM, IV, or PO for 1–3 or more days. *Endocrine:* Galactorrhea, amenorrhea, gynecomastia, impotence (due to hyperprolactinemia), fluid retention (due to transient elevation of aldosterone). **Neuroleptic malignant syndrome: Hyperthermia, altered consciousness, autonomic dysfunction, muscle rigidity, death.** *Miscellaneous:* Incontinence, urinary frequency, porphyria, visual disturbances, flushing of the face and upper body, hepatotoxicity.

OD **Overdose Management:** *Symptoms:* Agitation, irritability, hypertonia of muscles, drowsiness, disorientation, extrapyramidal symptoms. *Treatment:* Treat extrapyramidal effects by giving anticholinergic drugs, anti-Parkinson drugs, or antihistamines with anticholinergic effects. General supportive treatment. Reverse methemoglobinemia by giving methylene blue.

Drug Interactions
Acetaminophen / ↑ GI absorption of acetaminophen
Anticholinergics / ↓ Effect of metoclopramide
Cimetidine / ↓ Effect of cimetidine due to ↓ absorption from GI tract
CNS depressants / Additive sedative effects
Cyclosporine / ↓ Absorption of cyclosporine → ↑ immunosuppressive and toxic effects
Digoxin / ↓ Effect of digoxin due to ↓ absorption from GI tract
Ethanol / ↑ GI absorption of ethanol
Levodopa / ↑ GI absorption of levodopa and levodopa ↓ effects of metoclopramide on gastric emptying and lower esophageal pressure

MAO inhibitors / ↑ Release of catecholamines → toxicity
Narcotic analgesics / ↓ Effect of metoclopramide
Succinylcholine / ↑ Effect of succinylcholine due to inhibition of plasma cholinesterase
Tetracyclines / ↑ GI absorption of tetracyclines

EMS CONSIDERATIONS
None.

Metolazone
(meh-TOH-lah-zohn)
Pregnancy Class: B
Mykrox, Zaroxolyn **(Rx)**
Classification: Diuretic, thiazide

Onset of Action: 1 hr.
Duration of Action: Rapid or slow availablity tablets: 24 hr or more.
Uses: Slow availability tablets: Edema accompanying CHF; edema accompanying renal diseases, including nephrotic syndrome and conditions of reduced renal function. Alone or in combination with other drugs for the treatment of hypertension.

Rapid availability tablets: Treatment of newly diagnosed mild to moderate hypertension alone or in combination with other drugs. The rapid availability tablets are not to be used to produce diuresis.

Investigational: Alone or as an adjunct to treat calcium nephrolithiasis, premanagement of menstrual syndrome, and adjunct treatment of renal failure.

Contraindications: Anuria, prehepatic and hepatic coma, allergy or hypersensitivity to metolazone. Routine use during pregnancy. Lactation.
Precautions: Use with caution in those with severely impaired renal function. Safety and effectiveness have not been determined in children.

Route/Dosage ——————
• **Slow Availability Tablets**

Edema due to cardiac failure or renal disease.

Adults: 5–20 mg once daily. For those who experience paroxysmal nocturnal dyspnea, a larger dose may be required to ensure prolonged diuresis and saluresis for a 24-hr period.

Mild to moderate essential hypertension.

Adults: 2.5–5 mg once daily.

• **Rapid Availability Tablets**

Mild to moderate essential hypertension.

Adults, initial: 0.5 mg once daily, usually in the morning. If inadequately controlled, the dose may be increased to 1 mg once a day. Increasing the dose higher than 1 mg does not increase the effect.

How Supplied: *Tablets:* 0.5 mg, 2.5 mg, 5 mg, 10 mg.

Side Effects: See *Diuretics, Thiazide.* The most commonly reported side effects are dizziness, headache, muscle cramps, malaise, lethargy, lassitude, joint pain/swelling, and chest pain.

EMS CONSIDERATIONS

See also *Diuretics, Thiazide.*

Metoprolol succinate
Metoprolol tartrate
(me-toe-PROH-lohl)
Pregnancy Class: Succinate:
C Tartrate: B
Succinate (Toprol XL **(Rx)**) Tartrate
(Lopressor **(Rx)**)
Classification: Beta-adrenergic
blocking agent

Mechanism of Action: Exerts mainly beta-1-adrenergic blocking activity although beta-2 receptors are blocked at high doses. Has no membrane stabilizing or intrinsic sympathomimetic effects.

Onset of Action: 15 min.

Uses: Metoprolol Succinate: Alone or with other drugs to treat hypertension. Chronic management of angina pectoris.

Metoprolol Tartrate: Hypertension (either alone or with other antihypertensive agents, such as thiazide diuretics). Acute MI in hemodynamically stable patients. Angina pectoris. *Investigational:* IV to suppress atrial ectopy in COPD, aggressive behavior, prophylaxis of migraine, ventricular arrhythmias, enhancement of cognitive performance in geriatric patients, essential tremors.

Contraindications: Additional: Myocardial infarction in patients with a HR of less than 45 beats/min, in second- or third-degree heart block, or if SBP is less than 100 mm Hg. Moderate to severe cardiac failure.

Precautions: Safety and effectiveness have not been established in children. Use with caution in impaired hepatic function and during lactation.

Route/Dosage —————————

• **Metoprolol Succinate Tablets**

Angina pectoris.

Individualized. Initial: 100 mg/day in a single dose. Dose may be increased slowly, at weekly intervals, until optimum effect is reached or there is a pronounced slowing of HR. Doses above 400 mg/day have not been studied.

Hypertension.

Initial: 50–100 mg/day in a single dose with or without a diuretic. Dosage may be increased in weekly intervals until maximum effect is reached. Doses above 400 mg/day have not been studied.

• **Metoprolol Tartrate Tablets**

Hypertension.

Initial: 100 mg/day in single or divided doses; **then,** dose may be increased weekly to maintenance level of 100–450 mg/day. A diuretic may also be used.

Aggressive behavior.

200–300 mg/day.

Essential tremors.

50–300 mg/day.

Prophylaxis of migraine.

50–100 mg b.i.d.

Ventricular arrhythmias.

200 mg/day.

M

bold italic = life threatening side effect

- **Metoprolol Tartrate Injection (IV) and Tablets**

Early treatment of MI.

3 IV bolus injections of 5 mg each at approximately 2-min intervals. If patients tolerate the full IV dose, give 50 mg q 6 hr PO beginning 15 min after the last IV dose (or as soon as patient's condition allows). This dose is continued for 48 hr followed by **late treatment:** 100 mg b.i.d. as soon as feasible; continue for 1–3 months (although data suggest treatment should be continued for 1–3 years). In patients who do not tolerate the full IV dose, begin with 25–50 mg q 6 hr PO beginning 15 min after the last IV dose or as soon as the condition allows.

How Supplied: Metoprolol succinate: *Tablet, Extended Release:* 50 mg, 100 mg, 200 mg. Metoprolol tartrate: *Injection:* 1 mg/mL; *Tablet:* 50 mg, 100 mg

Drug Interactions: Additional: *Cimetidine/* May ↑ plasma levels of metoprolol. *Contraceptives, oral/* May ↑ effects of metoprolol. *Methimazole/* May ↓ effects of metoprolol. *Phenobarbital/* ↓ Effect of metoprolol due to ↑ breakdown by liver. *Propylthiouracil/* May ↓ the effects of metoprolol. *Quinidine/* May ↑ effects of metoprolol. *Rifampin/* ↓ Effect of metoprolol due to ↑ breakdown by liver.

EMS CONSIDERATIONS

See also *Beta-Adrenergic Blocking Agents* and *Antihypertensive Agents.*

Metronidazole

(meh-troh-NYE-dah-zohl)
Pregnancy Class: B
Femazole, Flagyl, Flagyl ER, Flagyl I.V., Flagyl I. V. RTU, Metric 21, Metro-Cream Topical, MetroGel Topical, MetroGel-Vaginal, Metro I. V., Metryl, Metryl-500, Metryl I. V., Noritate Cream 1%, Protostat, Satric, Satric 500 **(Rx)**
Classification: Systemic trichomonacide, amebicide

Mechanism of Action: Effective against anaerobic bacteria and protozoa. Specifically inhibits growth of trichomonae and amoebae by binding to DNA, resulting in loss of helical structure, strand breakage, inhibition of nucleic acid synthesis, and cell death. The mechanism for its effectiveness in reducing the inflammatory lesions of acne rosacea is not known.

Uses: Systemic: Amebiasis. Symptomatic and asymptomatic trichomoniasis; to treat asymptomatic partner. Amebic dysentery and amebic liver abscess. To reduce postoperative anaerobic infection following colorectal surgery, elective hysterectomy, and emergency appendectomy. Anaerobic bacterial infections of the abdomen, female genital system, skin or skin structures, bones and joints, lower respiratory tract, and CNS. Also, septicemia, endocarditis, hepatic encephalopathy. PO for Crohn's disease and pseudomembranous colitis. *Investigational:* giardiasis, *Gardnerella vaginalis.*

Topical: Inflammatory papules, pustules, and erythema of rosacea. *Investigational:* Infected decubitus ulcers (use 1% solution prepared from oral tablets).

Vaginal: Bacterial vaginosis.

Contraindications: Blood dyscrasias, active organic disease of the CNS, trichomoniasis during the first trimester of pregnancy, lactation. Topical use if hypersensitive to parabens or other ingredients of the formulation. Consumption of alcohol during use.

Precautions: Safety and efficacy have not been established in children.

Route/Dosage
- **Capsules, Tablets**

Amebiasis: Acute amebic dysentery or amebic liver abscess.

Adult: 500–750 mg t.i.d. for 5–10 days; **pediatric:** 35–50 mg/kg/day in three divided doses for 10 days.

Trichomoniasis, female.

250 mg t.i.d. for 7 days, 2 g given on 1 day in single or divided doses, or 375 mg b.i.d. for 7 days. **Pediatric:** 5 mg/kg t.i.d. for 7 days. An interval of 4–6 weeks should elapse between courses of therapy. *NOTE:* Do not

treat pregnant women during the first trimester. *Male:* Individualize dosage; usual, 250 mg t.i.d. for 7 days.

Giardiasis.

250 mg t.i.d. for 7 days.

G. vaginalis.

500 mg b.i.d. for 7 days.

- **Tablets, Extended-Release**

Bacterial vaginosis.

One 750-mg tablet per day for 7 days.

- **IV**

Anaerobic bacterial infections.

Adults, initially: 15 mg/kg infused over 1 hr; **then,** after 6 hr, 7.5 mg/kg q 6 hr for 7–10 days (daily dose should not exceed 4 g). Treatment may be necessary for 2–3 weeks, although PO therapy should be initiated as soon as possible.

Prophylaxis of anaerobic infection during surgery.

Adults: 15 mg/kg given over a 30- to 60-min period, with completion 1 hr prior to surgery and 7.5 mg/kg infused over 30–60 min 6 and 12 hr after the initial dose.

- **Topical (0.75%, 1%)**

Rosacea.

After washing, apply a thin film and rub in well either once daily or b.i.d. in the morning and evening for 4–9 weeks.

- **Vaginal (0.75%)**

Bacterial vaginosis.

One applicatorful (5 g) in the morning and evening for 5 days. Metro-Gel Vaginal allows for once-daily dosing at bedtime.

How Supplied: *Capsule:* 375 mg; *Cream:* 0.75%, 1%; *Gel/jelly:* 0.75%; *Injection:* 500 mg/100 mL; *Tablet:* 250 mg, 500 mg; *Tablet, Extended-Release:* 750 mg

Side Effects: Systemic Use. *GI:* Nausea, dry mouth, metallic taste, vomiting, diarrhea, abdominal discomfort, constipation. *CNS:* Headache, dizziness, vertigo, incoordination, ataxia, confusion, irritability, depression, weakness, insomnia, syncope, seizures, peripheral neuropathy including paresthesias. *He-*

matologic: Leukopenia, **bone marrow aplasia.** *GU:* Burning, dysuria, cystitis, polyuria, incontinence, dryness of vagina or vulva, dyspareunia, decreased libido. *Allergic:* Urticaria, pruritus, erythematous rash, flushing, nasal congestion, fever, joint pain. *Miscellaneous:* Furry tongue, glossitis, stomatitis (due to overgrowth of *Candida*) ECG abnormalities, thrombophlebitis.

Topical Use: Watery eyes if gel applied too closely to this area; transient redness; mild burning, dryness, and skin irritation.

Vaginal Use: Symptomatic candida vaginitis, N&V.

OD **Overdose Management:** *Symptoms:* Ataxia, N&V, peripheral neuropathy, **seizures** up to 5–7 days. *Treatment:* Supportive treatment.

Drug Interactions

Barbiturates / Possible therapeutic failure of metronidazole

Cimetidine / ↑ Serum levels of metronidazole due to ↓ clearance

Disulfiram / Concurrent use may cause confusion or acute psychosis

Ethanol / Possible disulfiram-like reaction, including flushing, palpitations, tachycardia, and N&V

Hydantoins / ↑ Effect of hydantoins due to ↓ clearance

Lithium / ↑ Lithium toxicity

Warfarin / ↑ Anticoagulant effect

EMS CONSIDERATIONS

See also *Anti-Infectives.*

Mexiletine hydrochloride

(mex-ILL-eh-teen)

Pregnancy Class: C

Mexitil **(Rx)**

Classification: Antiarrhythmic, class IB

Mechanism of Action: Similar to lidocaine but is effective PO. Inhibits the flow of sodium into the cell, thereby reducing the rate of rise of the action potential. The drug decreases the effective refractory period in Purkinje fibers. BP and pulse rate are not affected following use, but there may be a small decrease in CO and an increase in peripheral vascular resistance. Also has both local anesthetic and anticonvulsant effects.

Onset of Action: 30-120 min.

Uses: Documented life-threatening ventricular arrhythmias (such as ventricular tachycardia). *Investigational:* Prophylactically to decrease the incidence of ventricular tachycardia and other ventricular arrhythmias in the acute phase of MI. To reduce pain, dysesthesia, and paresthesia associated with diabetic neuropathy.

Contraindications: Cardiogenic shock, preexisting second- or third-degree AV block (if no pacemaker is present). Use with lesser arrhythmias. Lactation.

Precautions: There is the possibility of increased risk of death when used in patients with non-life-threatening cardiac arrhythmias. Use with caution in hypotension, severe CHF, or known seizure disorders. Dosage has not been established in children.

Route/Dosage
• **Capsules**
  Antiarrhythmic.
Adults, individualized, initial: 200 mg q 8 hr if rapid control of arrhythmia not required; dosage adjustment may be made in 50- or 100-mg increments q 2–3 days, if required. **Maintenance:** 200–300 mg q 8 hr, depending on response and tolerance of patient. If adequate response is not achieved with 300 mg or less q 8 hr, 400 mg q 8 hr may be tried although the incidence of CNS side effects increases. If the drug is effective at doses of 300 mg or less q 8 hr, the same total daily dose may be given in divided doses q 12 hr (e.g., 450 mg q 12 hr). Maximum total daily dose: 1,200 mg.
  Rapid control of arrhythmias.
Initial loading dose: 400 mg followed by a 200-mg dose in 8 hr.
  Diabetic neuropathy.
Initial: 150 mg/day for 3 days; **then,** 300 mg/day for 3 days. **Maintenance:** 10 mg/kg/day.
How Supplied: *Capsule:* 150 mg, 200 mg, 250 mg

Side Effects: *CV: **Worsening of arrhythmias,** palpitations, chest pain, increased ventricular arrhythmias (PVCs), CHF, angina or angina-like pain, hypotension, bradycardia, syncope, **AV block or conduction disturbances,** atrial arrhythmias, hypertension, **cardiogenic shock,** hot flashes, edema. GI:* High incidence of upper GI distress, N&V, heartburn. Also, diarrhea or constipation, changes in appetite, dry mouth, abdominal cramps or pain, abdominal discomfort, salivary changes, dysphagia, altered taste, pharyngitis, changes in oral mucous membranes, upper GI bleeding, peptic ulcer, esophageal ulceration. *CNS:* High incidence of lightheadedness, dizziness, tremor, coordination difficulties, and nervousness. Also, changes in sleep habits, headache, fatigue, weakness, tinnitus, paresthesias, numbness, depression, confusion, difficulty with speech, short-term memory loss, hallucinations, malaise, psychosis, *seizures,* loss of consciousness. *Hematologic:* Leukopenia, neutropenia, agranulocytosis, thrombocytopenia. *GU:* Decreased libido, impotence, urinary hesitancy or retention. *Dermatologic:* Rash, dry skin. Rarely, exfoliative dermatitis, and **Stevens-Johnson syndrome.** *Miscellaneous:* Blurred vision, visual disturbances, dyspnea, arthralgia, fever, diaphoresis, loss of hair, hiccoughs, laryngeal or pharyngeal changes, syndrome of SLE, myelofibrosis.

OD Overdose Management: *Symptoms:* Nausea. CNS symptoms (dizziness, drowsiness, paresthesias, seizures) usually precede CV symptoms (hypotension, sinus bradycardia, intermittent left bundle branch block (LBBB), **temporary asystole). Massive overdoses cause coma and respiratory arrest.** *Treatment:* General supportive treatment. Give atropine to treat hypotension or bradycardia. Acidification of the urine may increase rate of excretion.

Drug Interactions
Aluminum hydroxide / ↓ Absorption of mexiletine

Atropine / ↓ Absorption of mexiletine

Caffeine / ↓ Clearance of caffeine (50%)

Cimetidine / ↑ or ↓ Plasma levels of mexiletine

Magnesium hydroxide / ↓ Absorption of mexiletine

Metoclopramide / ↑ Absorption of mexiletine

Narcotics / ↓ Absorption of mexiletine

Phenobarbital / ↓ Plasma levels of mexiletine

Phenytoin / ↑ Clearance → ↓ plasma levels of mexiletine

Rifampin / ↑ Clearance → ↓ plasma levels of mexiletine

Theophylline / ↑ Effect of theophylline due to ↑ serum levels

Urinary acidifiers / ↑ Rate of excretion of mexiletine

Urinary alkalinizers / ↓ Rate of excretion of mexiletine

EMS CONSIDERATIONS

See also *Antiarrhythmic Drugs.*

Mezlocillin sodium
(mez-low-SILL-in)
Pregnancy Class: B
Mezlin (Rx)
Classification: Antibiotic, penicillin

Mechanism of Action: Broad-spectrum (gram-negative and gram-positive organisms, including aerobic and anaerobic strains) antibiotic used parenterally.

Uses: (1) Lower respiratory tract infections, including pneumonia and lung abscess, due to *Haemophilus influenzae, Klebsiella pneumoniae, Proteus mirabilis, Pseudomonas aeruginosa, E. coli,* and *Bacteroides fragilis.* (2) Intra-abdominal infections, including acute cholecystitis, cholangitis, peritonitis, hepatic abscess, and intra-abdominal abscess due to *E. coli, P. mirabilis, Klebsiella* species (sp.), *Pseudomonas* sp., *Streptococcus faecalis, Bacteroides* sp., *Peptococcus* sp., and *Peptostreptococcus* sp. (3) UTIs due to *E. coli, P. mirabilis,*

Proteus sp. (indole-positive), *Morganella morganii, Klebsiella* sp., *Enterobacter* sp., *Serratia* sp., *Pseudomonas* sp., and *S. faecalis.* (4) Uncomplicated gonorrhea due to *Neisseria gonorrhoeae.* (5) Gynecologic infections, including endometritis, pelvic cellulitis, and PID due to *N. gonorrhoeae, Peptococcus* sp., *Peptostreptococcus* sp., *Bacteroides* sp., *E. coli, P. mirabilis, Klebsiella* sp., and *Enterobacter* sp. (6) Skin and skin structure infections due to *S. faecalis, E. coli, P. mirabilis, Proteus* sp. (indole-positive), *P. vulgaris, Providencia rettgeri, Klebsiella* sp., *Enterobacter* sp., *Pseudomonas* sp., *Peptococcus* sp., and *Bacteroides* sp. Septicemia, including bacteremia, due to *E. coli, Klebsiella* sp., *Enterobacter* sp., *Pseudomonas* sp., *Bacteroides* sp., and *Peptococcus* sp.

Streptococcal infections due to *Streptococcus* sp., including group A beta-hemolytic streptococcus and *S. pneumoniae.* However, these infections are usually treated with more narrow spectrum penicillins. Use in certain severe infections when the causative organisms are not known; give in conjunction with an aminoglycoside or a cephalosporin. In combination with an aminoglycoside to treat life-threatening *P. aeruginosa* infections. Perioperative use to decrease incidence of infection in patients undergoing surgical procedures that are classified as contaminated or potentially contaminated (e.g., vaginal hysterectomy, colorectal surgery). Caesarean section intraoperative after clamping the umbilical cord and postoperative to reduce postoperative infections.

Route/Dosage
• **IV, IM**
   Serious infections.
Adults: 200–300 mg/kg/day in four to six divided doses; **usual:** 3 g q 4 hr or 4 g q 6 hr. **Infants and children, 1 month–12 years:** 50 mg/kg q 4 hr given **IM** or **IV** over 30 min; **infants more than 2 kg and less than 1 week of age or less than 2 kg and**

M

less than 1 week of age: 75 mg/kg q 12 hr; **infants less than 2 kg and more than 1 week of age:** 75 mg/kg q 8 hr; **infants more than 2 kg and more than 1 week of age:** 75 mg/kg q 6 hr.

Life-threatening infections.
Adults: Up to 350 mg/kg/day, not to exceed 24 g/day. If C_{CR} is 10 to 30 mL/min, give 3 g q 8 hr; if C_{CR} is less than 10 mL/min, give 2 g q 8 hr.

Uncomplicated UTIs.
100–125 mg/kg/day (6 to 8 g/day); 1.5–2 g q 6 hr. If there is renal impairment, give 1.5 g q 8 hr.

Complicated UTIs.
150–200 mg/kg/day (12 g/day); 3 g q 6 hr IV. If C_{CR} is 10 to 30 mL/min, give 1.5 g q 6 hr; if C_{CR} is less than 10 mL/min, give 1.5 g q 8 hr.

Lower respiratory tract infection, intra-abdominal infection, gynecologic infection, skin and skin structure infections, septicemia.
225–300 mg/kg/day (16 to 18 g/day); 4 g q 6 hr or 3 g q 4 hr IV. If C_{CR} is 10 to 30 mL/min, give 3 g q 8 hr; if C_{CR} is less than 10 mL/min, give 2 g q 8 hr. For serious systemic infections in those undergoing hemodialysis for renal failure or peritoneal dialysis: 3–4 g after each dialysis; then q 12 hr.

Gonococcal urethritis.
Adults: Single dose of 1–2 g IV or IM with probenecid, 1 g given at time of dosing or up to 30 min before.

Prophylaxis of postoperative infection.
Adults: 4 g 30–90 min prior to start of surgery; **then,** 4 g, IV, 6 and 12 hr later.

Prophylaxis of infection in patients undergoing cesarean section.
First dose: 4 g IV when cord is clamped; **second and third doses:** 4 g IV 4 and 8 hr after the first dose.
How Supplied: *Powder for injection:* 1 g, 2 g, 3 g, 4 g, 20 g
Side Effects: Additional: Bleeding abnormalities. Decreased hemoglobin or hematocrit values.

EMS CONSIDERATIONS

See also *Anti-Infectives* and *Penicillins.*

Miconazole

(my-KON-ah-zohl)
Pregnancy Class: C
Topical: Micatin, Monistat-Derm;
Vaginal: Monistat 3, Monistat 7, M-Zole 3 Combination Pack (Rx and OTC)
Classification: Antifungal agent

Mechanism of Action: Broad-spectrum fungicide that alters the permeability of the fungal membrane by inhibiting synthesis of sterols; thus, essential intracellular materials are lost. The drug also inhibits biosynthesis of triglycerides and phospholipids and also inhibits oxidative and peroxidative enzyme activity. May be fungistatic or fungicidal, depending on the concentration.

Uses: Topical, Vaginal: Tinea pedis, tinea cruris, tinea corporis caused by *Trichophyton rubrum, T. mentagrophytes,* and *Epidermophyton floccosum* (both OTC and Rx). Moniliasis and tinea versicolor (Rx only).

Contraindications: Hypersensitivity. Use of topical products in or around the eyes.

Precautions: Safe use in children less than 1 year of age has not been established.

Route/Dosage

• **Topical, Aerosol Powder, Aerosol Solution, Cream, Lotion, Powder**
Apply to cover affected areas in morning and evening (once daily for tinea versicolor) for 7 days.

• **Vaginal Cream or Suppository**
Monistat 3: One suppository daily at bedtime for 7 days (100-mg suppositories) or 3 consecutive days (200-mg suppositories).
Monistat 7: One applicator full of cream or one suppository at bedtime daily for 7 days. Course may be repeated after presence of other pathogens has been ruled out.

• **Combination Pack**
Vaginal yeast infections, relief of external vulval itching and irritation due to yeast infection.
Three day treatment consisting of miconizole suppositories, 200 mg and miconazole nitrate cream, 2%.

How Supplied: *Topical Cream:* 2%; *Powder:* 2%; *Spray:* 2%; *Vaginal Cream:* 2%; *Suppository:* 100 mg, 200 mg; *Combination Pack:* Suppositories, 200 mg and Cream, 2%

Side Effects: Following systemic use. *GI:* N&V, diarrhea, anorexia. *Hematologic:* Thrombocytopenia, aggregation of erythrocytes, rouleaux formation on blood smears. Transient decrease in hematocrit. *Dermatologic:* Pruritus, rash, flushing, phlebitis at injection site. *CV:* Transient tachycardia or arrhythmias following rapid injection of undiluted drug. *Miscellaneous:* Fever, chills, drowsiness, transient decrease in serum sodium values. Hyperlipemia due to the vehicle (polyethylene glycol 40 and castor oil). **Following topical use:** Vulvovaginal burning, pelvic cramps, hives, skin rash, headache, itching, irritation, maceration, and allergic contact dermatitis.

Drug Interactions

Amphotericin B / ↓ Activity of miconazole of each drug

Coumarin anticoagulants / Miconazole ↑ anticoagulant effect

EMS CONSIDERATIONS

See also *Anti-Infectives.*

Midazolam hydrochloride
(my-DAYZ-oh-lam)
Pregnancy Class: D
Versed **(C-IV) (Rx)**
Classification: Benzodiazepine sedative; adjunct to general anesthesia

Mechanism of Action: Short-acting benzodiazepine with sedative–general anesthetic properties. Depresses the response of the respiratory system to carbon dioxide stimulation, which is more pronounced in patients with COPD. Possible mild to moderate decreases in CO, mean arterial BP, SV, and systemic vascular resistance. HR may rise somewhat in those with slow HRs (< 65/min) and decrease in others (especially those with HRs more than 85/min).

Onset of Action: IM: 15 min; **IV:** 2-2.5 min for induction (if combined with a preanesthetic narcotic, induction is about 1.5 min). **Maximum effect:** 30-60 min.

Duration of Action: Time to recovery: Usually within 2 hr, although up to 6 hr may be required.

Uses: IV, IM: Preoperative sedation, anxiolysis, and amnesia. **IV:** To facilitate intubation. Sedation, anxiolysis, and amnesia prior to or during short diagnostic, therapeutic, or endoscopic procedures (either alone or with other CNS depressants). Sedation of intubated and mechanically ventilated patients as a component of anesthesia or during treatment in a critical care setting. *Investigational:* Treat epileptic seizures. Alternative to terminate refractory status epilepticus.

Contraindications: Hypersensitivity to benzodiazepines. Acute narrow-angle glaucoma. Use in obstetrics, coma, shock, or acute alcohol intoxication where VS are depressed. IA injection.

Precautions: Use with caution during lactation. Pediatric patients may require higher doses than adults. Hypotension may be more common in conscious sedated patients who have received a preanesthetic narcotic. Geriatric and debilitated patients require lower doses to induce anesthesia and they are more prone to side effects. Use IV with extreme caution in severe fluid or electrolyte disturbances.

Route/Dosage ————————
• **IM**
 Preoperative sedation, anxiolysis, amnesia.
Adults: 0.07–0.08 mg/kg IM (average: 5 mg) 1 hr before surgery. **Children:** 0.1–0.15 mg/kg (up to 0.5 mg/kg may be needed for more anxious patients).
• **IV**
 Conscious sedation, anxiolysis, amnesia for endoscopic or CV proce-

M

dures in healthy adults less than 60 years of age.

Using the 1 mg/mL (can be diluted with 0.9% sodium chloride or D5W) product, titrate slowly to the desired effect (usually slurred speech); initial dose should be no higher than 2.5 mg IV (may be as low as 1 mg IV) within a 2-min period; wait an additional 2 min to evaluate the sedative effect. If additional sedation is necessary, give small increments waiting an additional 2 min or more after each increment to evaluate the effect. Total doses greater than 5 mg are usually not required. **Children:** Dosage must be individualized by the physician.

Conscious sedation for endoscopic or CV procedures in debilitated or chronically ill patients or patients aged 60 or over.

Slowly titrate to the desired effect using no more than 1.5 mg initially IV (may be as little as 1 mg IV) given over a 2-min period; wait an additional 2 min or more to evaluate the effect. If additional sedation is needed, no more than 1 mg should be given over 2 min; wait an additional 2 min or more after each increment in dose. Total doses greater than 3.5 mg are usually not needed.

Induction of general anesthesia, before use of other general anesthetics, in unmedicated patients.

Adults, unmedicated patients up to 55 years of age, IV, initial: 0.3–0.35 mg/kg given over 20–30 sec, waiting 2 min for effects to occur. If needed, increments of about 25% of the initial dose can be used to complete induction; or, induction can be completed using a volatile liquid anesthetic. Up to 0.6 mg/kg may be used but recovery will be prolonged. **Adults, unmedicated patients over 55 years of age who are good risk surgical patients, initial IV:** 0.15–0.3 mg/kg given over 20–30 sec. **Adults, unmedicated patients over 55 years of age with severe systemic disease or debilitation, initial IV:** 0.15–0.25 mg/kg given over 20–30 sec. **Pediatric:** 0.05–0.2 mg/kg IV.

Induction of general anesthesia, before use of other general anesthetics, in medicated patients.

Adults, premedicated patients up to 55 years of age, IV, initial: 0.15–0.35 mg/kg. If less than 55 years of age, 0.25 mg/kg may be given over 20–30 sec, allowing 2 min for effect. **Adults, premedicated patients over 55 years of age who are good risk surgical patients, initial, IV:** 0.2 mg/kg. **Adults, premedicated patients over 55 years of age with severe systemic disease or debilitation, initial, IV:** 0.15 mg/kg may be sufficient.

How Supplied: *Injection:* 1 mg/mL, 5 mg/mL; *Syrup:* 2 mg/mL

Side Effects: Fluctuations in VS, including decreased respiratory rate and tidal volume, apnea, variations in BP and pulse rate are common. The following are general side effects regardless of the route of administration. *CV:* Hypotension, cardiac arrest. *CNS:* Oversedation, headache, drowsiness, grogginess, confusion, retrograde amnesia, euphoria, nervousness, agitation, anxiety, argumentativeness, restlessness, emergence delirium, increased time for emergence, dreaming during emergence, nightmares, insomnia, tonic-clonic movements, ataxia, muscle tremor, involuntary or athetoid movements, dizziness, dysphoria, dysphonia, slurred speech, paresthesia. *GI:* Hiccoughs, N&V, acid taste, retching, excessive salivation. *Ophthalmologic:* Double vision, blurred vision, nystagmus, pinpoint pupils, visual disturbances, cyclic eyelid movements, difficulty in focusing. *Dermatologic:* Hives, swelling or feeling of burning, warmth or cold feeling at injection site, hive-like wheal at injection site, pruritus, rash. *Miscellaneous:* Blocked ears, loss of balance, chills, weakness, faint feeling, lethargy, yawning, toothache, hematoma.

More common following IM use: Pain at injection site, headache, induration and redness, muscle stiffness.

More common following IV use:

Respiratory: **Bronchospasm,** coughing, dyspnea, laryngospasm, hyperventilation, shallow respirations, tachypnea, airway obstruction, wheezing, respiratory depression and ***respiratory arrest*** when used for conscious sedation. *CV:* PVCs, bigeminy, bradycardia, tachycardia, vasovagal episode, nodal rhythm.*At injection site:* Tenderness, pain, redness, induration, phlebitis.

Drug Interactions

Alcohol / ↑ Risk of apnea, airway obstruction, desaturation or hypoventilation

Anesthetics, inhalation / ↓ Dose if midazolam used as an induction agent

CNS Depressants / ↑ Risk of apnea, airway obstruction, desaturation or hypoventilation

Droperidol / ↑ Hypnotic effect of midazolam when used as a premedication

Fentanyl / ↑ Hypnotic effect of midazolam when used as a premedication

Indinavir / Possible prolonged sedation and respiratory depression

Meperidine / See *Narcotics;* also, ↑ Risk of hypotension

Narcotics / ↑ Hypnotic effect of midazolam when used as premedications

Propofol / ↑ Effect of propofol

Ritonavir / Possible prolonged sedation and respiratory depression

Thiopental / ↓ Dose if midazolam used as an induction agent

EMS CONSIDERATIONS

See also *Tranquilizers, Antimanic Drugs, and Hypnotics.*

Administration/Storage

IV 1. When used for induction of general anesthesia, give the initial dose over 20–30 sec.

2. Carefully monitor all IV doses with the immediate availability of oxygen, resuscitative equipment, and personnel who are skilled in maintaining a patent airway and for support of ventilation; continue monitoring during recovery period.

3. At a concentration of 0.5 mg/mL

midazolam is compatible with D5W and 0.9% NaCl and with RL solution.

Midodrine hydrochloride

(MIH-doh-dreen)

Pregnancy Class: C

ProAmatine **(Rx)**

Classification: Treat orthostatic hypotension

Mechanism of Action: Midodrine, a prodrug, is converted to an active metabolite—desglymidodrine—that is an alpha-1 agonist. Desglymidodrine produces an increase in vascular tone and elevation of BP by activating alpha-adrenergic receptors of the arteriolar and venous vasculature. No effect on cardiac beta-adrenergic receptors. The active metabolite does not cross the blood-brain barrier; thus, there are no CNS effects. Standing systolic BP is increased by approximately 15–30 mm Hg at 1 hr after a 10-mg dose; duration: 2–3 hr.

Uses: Orthostatic hypotension in those whose lives are significantly impaired despite standard clinical care. *Investigational:* Management of urinary incontinence.

Contraindications: Use in severe organic heart disease, acute renal disease, urinary retention, pheochromocytoma, thyrotoxicosis, persistent and excessive supine hypertension.

Precautions: Use with caution in impaired renal or hepatic function, during lactation, in orthostatic hypotensive patients who are also diabetic, or in those with a history of visual problems or who are also taking fludrocortisone acetate. Safety and efficacy have not been determined in children.

Route/Dosage

• **Tablets**

Orthostatic hypotension.

10 mg t.i.d. given during the daytime hours when the patient is upright and pursuing daily activities (e.g., shortly before or upon arising in the

M

---

morning, midday, and late afternoon—not later than 6:00 p.m.). To control symptoms, dosing may be q 3 hr. Initial dose in impaired renal function: 2.5 mg t.i.d.

Urinary incontinence.
2.5–5 mg b.i.d.–t.i.d.

How Supplied: *Tablet:* 2.5 mg, 5 mg

Side Effects: *CNS:* Paresthesia, pain, headache, feeling of pressure or fullness in the head, confusion, abnormal thinking, nervousness, anxiety. Rarely, dizziness, insomnia, somnolence. *GI:* Dry mouth. Rarely, canker sore, nausea, GI distress, flatulence. *Dermatologic:* Piloerection, pruritus, rash, vasodilation, flushed face. Rarely, erythema multiforme, dry skin. *Miscellaneous:* Dysuria, supine hypertension. Rarely, visual field defect, skin hyperesthesia, impaired urination, asthenia, backache, pyrosis, leg cramps.

OD Overdose Management: *Symptoms:* Hypertension, piloerection, sensation of coldness, urinary retention. *Treatment:* Emesis and administration of an alpha-adrenergic blocking agent (e.g., phentolamine).

Drug Interactions
Alpha-adrenergic agonists / ↑ Pressor effects of midodrine
Alpha-adrenergic antagonists / Antagonism of the effects of midodrine
Beta-adrenergic blockers / ↑ Risk of bradycardia, AV block, or arrhythmias
Cardiac glycosides / ↑ Risk of bradycardia, AV block, or arrhythmias
Fludrocortisone / ↑ Intraocular pressure and glaucoma
Psychopharmacologic drugs / ↑ Risk of bradycardia, AV block, or arrhythmias

EMS CONSIDERATIONS

None.

Miglitol

(MIG-lih-tohl)
Pregnancy Class: B
Glyset **(Rx)**
Classification: Antidiabetic, oral

Mechanism of Action: Acts by delaying digestion of ingested carbohydrates resulting in smaller rise in blood glucose levels after meals. Effect is due to reversible inhibition of membrane-bound intestinal glucoside hydrolase enzymes which hydrolyze oligosaccharides and disaccharides to glucose and other monosaccharides. Reduces levels of glycosylated hemoglobin in type II diabetes. Does not enhance insulin secretion or increase insulin sensitivity. Does not cause hypoglycemia when given in fasted state.

Uses: Alone as adjunct to diet to treat non-insulin-dependent diabetes. With sulfonylurea when diet plus either miglitol or a sulfonylurea alone do not result in adequate control (effects of sulfonylurea and miglitol are additive).

Contraindications: Lactation, diabetic ketoacidosis, inflammatory bowel disease, colonic ulceration, partial intestinal obstruction, those predisposed to intestinal obstruction, chronic intestinal diseases associated with marked disorders of digestion or absorption, conditions that may deteriorate due to increased gas formation in the intestine, hypersensitivity to drug.

Precautions: When given with sulfonylurea or insulin, miglitol causes further decrease in blood sugar and increased risk of hypoglycemia. Safety and efficacy have not been determined in children.

Route/Dosage ⸻
• **Tablets**
Type II diabetes.
Individualize dosage. **Initial:** 25 mg t.i.d. with first bite of each main meal (some may benefit from starting with 25 mg once daily to minimize GI side effects). After 4 to 8 weeks of 25 mg t.i.d. dose, increase dosage to 50 mg t.i.d. for about 3 months. Measure glycosylated hemoglobin; if not satisfactory, increase dose to 100 mg t.i.d. **Maintenance:** 50 mg t.i.d., up to 100 mg t.i.d. (maximum).

How Supplied: *Tablets:* 25 mg, 50 mg, 100 mg

Side Effects: *GI:* Flatulence, diarrhea, abdominal pain, soft stools, abdominal discomfort. *Dermatologic:* Skin rash (transient).

Drug Interactions
Amylase / ↓ Effect of miglitol
Charcoal / Adsorbent effect ↓ effect of miglitol
Digoxin / May ↓ plasma levels of digoxin
Pancreatin / ↓ Effect of miglitol
Propranolol / Significant ↓ bioavailability of propranolol
Ranitidine / Significant ↓ bioavailability of ranitidine

EMS CONSIDERATIONS

See also *Antidiabetic Agents.*

Milrinone lactate
(MILL-rih-nohn)
Pregnancy Class: C
Primacor **(Rx)**
Classification: Inotropic/vasodilator

Mechanism of Action: Selective inhibitor of peak III cyclic AMP phosphodiesterase isozyme in cardiac and vascular muscle, resulting in a direct inotropic effect and a direct arterial vasodilator activity. Also improves diastolic function as manifested by improvements in LV diastolic relaxation. In patients with depressed myocardial function, produces a prompt increase in CO and a decrease in pulmonary wedge pressure and vascular resistance, without a significant increase in HR or myocardial oxygen consumption. Causes an inotropic effect in patients who are fully digitalized without causing signs of glycoside toxicity. Also, LV function has improved in patients with ischemic heart disease.

Uses: Short-term treatment of CHF, usually in patients receiving digoxin and diuretics.

Contraindications: Hypersensitivity to the drug. Use in severe obstructive aortic or pulmonic valvular disease in lieu of surgical relief of the obstruction.

Precautions: Use with caution during lactation. Safety and efficacy have not been determined in children.

Route/Dosage
• **IV Infusion**
Adults, loading dose: 50 mcg/kg administered slowly over 10 min.
Maintenance, minimum: 0.59 mg/kg/24 hr (infused at a rate of 0.375 mcg/kg/min); **maintenance, standard:** 0.77 mg/kg/24 hr (infused at a rate of 0.5 mcg/kg/min); **maintenance, maximum:** 1.13 mg/kg/24 hr (infused at a rate of 0.75 mcg/kg/min).

How Supplied: *Injection:* 1 mg/mL
Side Effects: *CV: Ventricular and supraventricular arrhythmias, including ventricular ectopic activity, nonsustained ventricular tachycardia, sustained ventricular tachycardia, and ventricular fibrillation. Infrequently, life-threatening arrhythmias associated with preexisting arrhythmias,* metabolic abnormalities, abnormal digoxin levels, and catheter insertion. Also, hypotension, angina, chest pain. *Miscellaneous:* Mild to moderately severe headaches, hypokalemia, tremor, thrombocytopenia, bronchospasm (rare).

OD Overdose Management: *Symptoms:* Hypotension. *Treatment:* If hypotension occurs, reduce or temporarily discontinue administration of milrinone until the condition of the patient stabilizes. Use general measures to support circulation.

EMS CONSIDERATIONS
None.

Minocycline hydrochloride (Minocin)
mih-no-SYE-kleen
Pregnancy Class: D
Alti-Minocyclin, Apo-Minocycline, Gen-Minocycline, Dynacin, Minocin, Novo-Minocycline, Vectrin **(Rx)**
Classification: Antibiotic, tetracycline

Mechanism of Action: In fasting adults, 90% to 100% of an oral dose

M

---

bold italic = life threatening side effect

is absorbed. **Peak plasma levels:** 1–4 hr. Absorption is less affected by milk or food than for other tetracyclines. **t½, elimination:** 11–26 hr. Metabolized in the liver.

Uses: See also *Tetracyclines.* To eliminate meningococci from the nasopharynx of asymptomatic *Neisseria meningitidis* carriers in which the risk of meningococcal meningitis is high. *Note:* Due to adverse CNS effects, use rifampin to treat meningococcus carriers when the drug susceptibility is not known or when the organism is sulfa-resistant. Use minocycline only when rifampin is contraindicated.

(1) Granulomas of the skin caused by *Mycobacterium marinum.* (2) In combination with gonococcal regimens for presumptive treatment of coexisting chlamydial infections. (3) Uncomplicated gonogocal urethritis in adult males. (4) Treatment of uncomplicated urethral, endocervical, or rectal infections caused by *Chlamydia trachomatis* or *Ureaplasma urealyticum* in adults. (5) Intrapleurally as a sclerosing agent to control pleural effusions assocated with metastatic tumors. (6) Treatment of cholera and nocardiosis. (7) Adjunctive treatment of inflammatory acne unresponsive to oral tetracycline HCl or oral erythromycin.

Route/Dosage ———————
• **Capsules, Injection, Suspension, Tablets**
Infections against which effective, including asymptomatic meningococcus carriers.
Adults, initial: 200 mg; **then,** 100 mg q 12 hr. An alternative regimen is 100–200 mg initially followed by 50 mg q 6 hr. The length of treatment is 5 days for meningococcus carriers.
Children over 8 years of age, initial: 4 mg/kg; **then,** 2 mg/kg q 12 hr.
Mycobacterial infections.
100 mg PO b.i.d. for 6–8 weeks.
Uncomplicated gongococcal urethritis in adult males.
100 mg b.i.d. for 5 days.
Uncomplicated urethral, endocervical, or rectal infections due to Chla-

mydia trachomatis *or* Ureaplasma urealyticum.
100 mg PO b.i.d. for at least 7 days.
Nongonococcal urethritis caused by C. trachomatis or Mycoplasma.
100/day PO in 1 or 2 divided doses for 1 to 3 weeks.
Sclerosing agent to control pleural effusions associated with metastatic cancer.
300 mg diluted with 40–50 mL of 0.9% NaCl injection and instilled into the pleural space through a thoracostomy tube.
Cholera in conjunction with fluid and electrolyte replacement.
Initial: 200 mg PO; **then,** 100 mg PO 12 hr for 48–72 hr.
Adjunct to treat inflammatory acne unresponsive to PO tetracycline HCl or erythromycin.
50 mg PO 1–3 times/day.
How Supplied: *Capsules:* 50 mg, 100 mg; *Powder for Injection:* 100 mg; *Syrup:* 50 mg/5 mL; *Tablets:* 100 mg.

EMS CONSIDERATIONS

See also *Nursing Considerations* for *Anti-Infectives,* and *Tetracyclines,* .
Administration/Storage
IV 1. Do not dissolve in solutions containing calcium; forms a precipitate.
2. After dissolving medication in the vial, further dilute to 500–1,000 mL with any of the following: dextrose, dextrose and NaCl injection, NaCl injection, Ringer's injection, RL injection.
3. Start administration of the final dilution immediately.
4. Discard reconstituted solutions after 24 hr at room temperature.
Assessment
1. Document onset, duration, location, and characteristics of symptoms.
2. Monitor cultures and CBC; identify contacts when treating a contagious disease.

Minoxidil, oral
(mih-NOX-ih-dil)

Pregnancy Class: C
Loniten **(Rx)**
Classification: Antihypertensive, depresses sympathetic nervous system

Mechanism of Action: Decreases elevated BP by decreasing peripheral resistance by a direct effect. Causes increase in renin secretion, increase in cardiac rate and output, and salt/water retention. Does not cause orthostatic hypotension.

Onset of Action: 30 min.

Duration of Action: 24-48 hr.

Uses: Severe hypertension not controllable by the use of a diuretic plus two other antihypertensive drugs. Usually taken with at least two other antihypertensive drugs (a diuretic and a drug to minimize tachycardia such as a beta-adrenergic blocking agent). Can produce severe side effects; reserve for resistant cases of hypertension. Close medical supervision required, including possible hospitalization during initial administration. Topically to promote hair growth in balding men.

Contraindications: Pheochromocytoma. Within 1 month after a MI. Dissecting aortic aneurysm.

Precautions: Safe use during lactation not established. Use with caution and at reduced dosage in impaired renal function. Geriatric patients may be more sensitive to the hypotensive and hypothermic effects of minoxidil; also, may be necessary to decrease the dose due to age-related decreases in renal function. BP controlled too rapidly may cause syncope, stroke, MI, and ischemia of affected organs. Experience with use in children is limited.

Route/Dosage
• **Tablets**
  Hypertension.
Adults and children over 12 years, Initial: 5 mg/day. For optimum control, dose can be increased to 10, 20, and then 40 mg in single or divided doses/day. Do not exceed 100 mg/day. **Children under 12 years: Initial,** 0.2 mg/kg/day. Effective dose range: 0.25–1.0 mg/

kg/day. Dosage must be titrated to individual response. Do not exceed 50 mg/day.

How Supplied: *Tablet:* 2.5 mg, 10 mg

Side Effects: *CV:* Edema, *pericardial effusion that may progress to tamponade* (acute compression of heart caused by fluid or blood in pericardium), CHF, angina pectoris, changes in direction of T waves, increased HR. In children, rebound hypertension following slow withdrawal. *GI:* N&V. *CNS:* Headache, fatigue. *Hypersensitivity:* Rashes, including bullous eruptions and *Stevens-Johnson syndrome.* *Hematologic:* Initially, decrease in hematocrit, hemoglobin, and erythrocyte count but all return to normal. Rarely, thrombocytopenia and leukopenia. *Other:* Hypertrichosis (enhanced hair growth, pigmentation and thickening of fine body hair 3–6 weeks after initiation of therapy), breast tenderness, darkening of skin.

OD Overdose Management: *Symptoms:* Excessive hypotension. *Treatment:* Give NSS IV (to maintain BP and urine output). Vasopressors, such as phenylephrine and dopamine, can be used but only in underperfusion of a vital organ.

Drug Interactions: Concomitant use with guanethidine may result in severe hypotension.

EMS CONSIDERATIONS

See also *Antihypertensive Agents.*

Minoxidil, topical solution

(mih-NOX-ih-dill)
Pregnancy Class: C
Rogaine, Rogaine Extra Strength for Men **(Rx) (OTC)**
Classification: Hair growth stimulant

Mechanism of Action: The topical solution stimulates vertex hair growth in patients with male pattern baldness or in women with androgenetic alopecia. Mechanism may be related to dilation of arterioles and

M

stimulation of resting hair follicles into active growth.

Onset of Action: 4 months, but is variable.

Duration of Action: New hair growth may be lost 3-4 months after withdrawal of therapy.

Uses: To treat male and female pattern baldness (alopecia androgenetica). Extra Strength (5%) is only for treatment of hereditary male pattern baldness. *Investigational:* Alopecia areata.

Contraindications: Lactation. Use of 5% solution in women.

Precautions: Use with caution in patients with hypertension, coronary heart disease, or predisposition to heart failure. Safety and efficacy in patients under 18 years of age have not been determined. Increased systemic absorption may occur if the scalp is irritated or there are abrasions.

Route/Dosage ───────────
• **Topical Solution: 2%, 5%**
  Stimulate hair growth.
Adults: Apply 1 mL b.i.d. directly onto the scalp in the hair loss area. 5% solution not to be used on women.

How Supplied: *Solution:* 2%, 5%

Side Effects: *Dermatologic:* Allergic contact dermatitis, irritant dermatitis, pruritus, dry skin, flaking of scalp, alopecia, hypertrichosis, erythema, worsening of hair loss. *Allergic:* Hives, facial swelling, allergic rhinitis. *CNS:* Dizziness, lightheadedness, headache, faintness, anxiety, depression, fatigue. *Respiratory:* Sinusitis, bronchitis, respiratory infection. *Miscellaneous:* Conjunctivitis, decreased visual acuity, vertigo. *NOTE:* The incidence of side effects due to placebos is often similar to the incidence of side effects due to the drug itself.

Drug Interactions
Corticosteroids, topical / Enhance absorption of topical minoxidil
Guanethidine / Possible ↑ risk of orthostatic hypotension
Petrolatum / Enhances absorption of topical minoxidil
Retinoids / Enhance absorption of topical minoxidil

EMS CONSIDERATIONS
None.

Mirtazapine
(mir-TAZ-ah-peen)
Pregnancy Class: C
Remeron **(Rx)**
Classification: Antidepressant, tetracyclic

Mechanism of Action: Enhances central noradrenergic and serotonergic activity, perhaps by antagonism at central presynaptic alpha-2 adrenergic inhibitory autoreceptors and heteroreceptors. Also a potent antagonist of 5-HT_2, 5-HT_3 and histamine H_1 receptors. Moderate antagonist of peripheral alpha-1 adrenergic receptors and muscarinic receptors.

Uses: Treatment of depression.

Contraindications: Use in combination with a MAO inhibitor or within 14 days of initiating or discontinuing therapy with a MAO inhibitor.

Precautions: Use with caution in those with impaired renal or hepatic disease, in geriatric patients, during lactation, in CV or cerebrovascular disease that can be exacerbated by hypotension (e.g., history of MI, angina, ischemic stroke), and in conditions that would predispose to hypotension (e.g., dehydration, hypovolemia, treatment with antihypertensive medications). The effect of mirtazapine for longer than 6 weeks has not been evaluated, although treatment is indicated for 6 months or longer. Safety and efficacy have not been determined in children.

Route/Dosage ───────────
• **Tablets**
  Treatment of depression.
Initial: 15 mg/day given as a single dose, preferably in the evening before sleep. Those not responding to the 15-mg dose may respond to doses up to a maximum of 45 mg/day. Do not make dose changes at intervals of less than 1 to 2 weeks. Consider treatment for up to 6 months.

How Supplied: *Tablet:* 15 mg, 30 mg

Side Effects: Side effects with an incidence of 0.1% or greater are listed. *CNS:* Somnolence, dizziness, activation of mania or hypomania, suicidal ideation, sedation, drowsiness, abnormal dreams, abnormal thinking, tremor, confusion, hypesthesia, apathy, depression, hypokinesia, vertigo, twitching, agitation, anxiety, amnesia, hyperkinesia, paresthesia, ataxia, delirium, delusions, depersonalization, dyskinesia, extrapyramidal syndrome, increased libido, abnormal coordination, dysarthria, hallucinations, neurosis, dystonia, hostility, increased reflexes, emotional lability, euphoria, paranoid reaction. *GI:* N&V, anorexia, dry mouth, constipation, ulcer, eructation, glossitis, cholecystitis, gum hemorrhage, stomatitis, colitis, abnormal liver function tests. *CV:* Hypertension, vasodilation, angina pectoris, **MI,** bradycardia, ventricular extrasystoles, syncope, migraine, hypotension. *Hematologic:* Agranulocytosis. *Body as a whole:* Asthenia, flu syndrome, back pain, malaise, abdominal pain, acute abdominal syndrome, chills, fever, facial edema, photosensitivity reaction, neck rigidity, neck pain, enlarged abdomen. *Respiratory:* Dyspnea, increased cough, sinusitis, epistaxis, bronchitis, asthma, pneumonia. *GU:* Urinary frequency, UTI, kidney calculus, cystitis, dysuria, urinary incontinence, urinary retention, vaginitis, hematuria, breast pain, amenorrhea, dysmenorrhea, leukorrhea, impotence. *Musculoskeletal:* Myalgia, myasthenia, arthralgia, arthritis, tenosynovitis. *Dermatologic:* Pruritus, rash, acne, exfoliative dermatitis, dry skin, herpes simplex, alopecia. *Metabolic/nutritional:* Increased appetite, weight gain, peripheral edema, edema, thirst, dehydration, weight loss. *Ophthalmic:* Eye pain, abnormal accommodation, conjunctivitis, keratoconjunctivitis, lacrimation disorder, glaucoma. *Miscellaneous:* Deafness, hyperacusis, ear pain.

OD Overdose Management: *Symptoms:* Disorientation, drowsiness, impaired memory, tachycardia. *Treatment:* General supportive measures. If the patient is unconscious, establish and maintain an airway. Consider induction of emesis or gastric lavage and administration of activated charcoal. Monitor cardiac and vital signs.

Drug Interactions
Alcohol / Additive impairment of motor skills
Diazepam / Additive impairment of motor skills

EMS CONSIDERATIONS

See also *Antidepressants.*

Misoprostol
(my-soh-PROST-ohl)
Pregnancy Class: X
Cytotec **(Rx)**
Classification: Prostaglandin

Mechanism of Action: Synthetic prostaglandin E_1 analog that inhibits gastric acid secretion, protects the gastric mucosa by increasing bicarbonate and mucous production, and decreases pepsin levels during basal conditions. May also stimulate uterine contractions that may endanger pregnancy.

Uses: Prevention of aspirin and other nonsteroidal anti-inflammatory-induced gastric ulcers in patients with a high risk of gastric ulcer complications (e.g., geriatric patients with debilitating disease) or in those with a history of ulcer. *Investigational:* Treat duodenal ulcers including those unresponsive to histamine H_2 antagonists. With cyclosporine and prednisone to decrease the incidence of acute graft rejection in renal transplant patients (the drug improves renal function). With methotrexate to induce abortion.

Contraindications: Allergy to prostaglandins, pregnancy, during lactation (may cause diarrhea in nursing infants).

Precautions: Use with caution in patients with renal impairment and in

M

bold italic = life threatening side effect

patients older than 64 years of age. Safety and efficacy have not been established in children less than 18 years of age. May cause miscarriage with potentially serious bleeding.

Route/Dosage —————————
• **Tablets**
Adults: 200 mcg q.i.d. with food. Dose can be reduced to 100 mcg if the larger dose cannot be tolerated. In renal impairment, the 200-mcg dose can be reduced if necessary.
How Supplied: *Tablet:* 100 mcg, 200 mcg
Side Effects: *GI:* Diarrhea, abdominal pain, nausea, dyspepsia, flatulence, vomiting, constipation. *Gynecologic:* Spotting, cramps, dysmenorrhea, hypermenorrhea, menstrual disorders, postmenopausal vaginal bleeding. *Miscellaneous:* Headache.

[OD] Overdose Management: *Symptoms:* Abdominal pain, diarrhea, dyspnea, sedation, tremor, fever, palpitations, bradycardia, hypotension, *seizures*. *Treatment:* Use supportive therapy.

EMS CONSIDERATIONS
None.

Mitotane (O,P'-DDD)
(MY-toe-tayn)
Pregnancy Class: C
Lysodren **(Rx)**
Classification: Antineoplastic, antihormone

Mechanism of Action: Directly suppresses activity of adrenal cortex and changes the peripheral metabolism of corticosteroids, resulting in a decrease in 17-hydroxycorticosteroids. Steroid replacement therapy may have to be instituted (i.e., increased) to correct adrenal insufficiency. Therapy is continued as long as drug seems effective. Beneficial results may not become apparent until after 3 months of therapy.
Uses: Inoperable carcinoma (both functional and nonfunctional) of the adrenal cortex. *Investigational:* Cushing's syndrome.
Contraindications: Hypersensitivity to drug. Discontinue temporarily

after shock or severe trauma. Lactation.
Precautions: Use with caution in the presence of liver disease other than metastatic lesions. Long-term usage may cause brain damage and functional impairment. Use during lactation only if benefits outweigh risks.

Route/Dosage —————————
• **Tablets**
Carcinoma of the adrenal cortex.
Adults, initial: 2–6 g/day in three to four equally divided doses (maximum tolerated dose may range from 2 to 16 g/day). Adjust dosage upward or downward according to severity of side effects or lack thereof. **Pediatric, initial:** 1–2 g/day in divided doses; **then,** dose can be increased gradually to 5–7 g/day.
Cushing's syndrome.
Initial: 3–6 g/day in three to four divided doses; **then,** 0.5 mg 2 times/week to 2 g/day.
How Supplied: *Tablet:* 500 mg
Side Effects: *CNS:* Continuous doses may result in brain damage and impairment of function. Depression, lethargy, somnolence, dizziness, vertigo. *GI:* N&V, anorexia, diarrhea. *CV:* Hypertension, orthostatic hypotension, flushing. *Dermatologic:* Transient skin rashes. *Ophthalmic:* Visual blurring, diplopia, lens opacity, toxic retinopathy. *GU:* Hematuria, hemorrhagic cystitis, albuminuria. *Miscellaneous:* Adrenal insufficiency, generalized aching, hyperpyrexia.**Additional:** Adrenal insufficiency. *CNS:* Depression, sedation, vertigo, lethargy. *Ophthalmic:* Blurring, diplopia, retinopathy, opacity of lens. *Renal:* Hemorrhagic cystitis, hematuria, proteinuria. *CV:* Flushing, orthostatic hypotension, hypertension. *Miscellaneous:* Hyperpyrexia, skin rashes, aching of body.
Drug Interactions
Corticosteroids / ↑ Metabolism of corticosteroids resulting in need for higher doses
Warfarin / Mitotane may ↑ rate of metabolism of warfarin, requiring an increase of dosage

EMS CONSIDERATIONS
None.

Modafinil (Provigil)
moh-DEH-fin-ill
Pregnancy Class: C
Provigil **(Rx)**
Classification: Analeptic

Mechanism of Action: Precise mechanism unknown. Has wake-promoting effects similar to amphetamine and methylphenidate. Produces psychoactive and euphoric effects; alterations in mood, perception, and thinking; and, feelings typical of other CNS stimulants. Rapidly absorbed. **Peak plasma levels:** 2–4 hr. Absorption may be delayed by about 1 hr if taken with food. Metabolized by the liver and excreted in the urine. After chronic use, may induce its own metabolism. Clearance may be decreased in the elderly.
Uses: Improve wakefulness in patients with excessive daytime sleepiness associated with narcolepsy.

Route/Dosage
• **Tablets**
  Narcolepsy.
Adults: 200 mg/day as a single dose in the morning. Doses of 400 mg/day are well tolerated but no data to indicate increased beneficial effect. In patients with impaired hepatic function reduce the dose by 50%. Consider lower doses in elderly patients.
How Supplied: *Tablets:* 100 mg, 200 mg
Side Effects: *CNS:* Headache, nervousness, dizziness, depression, anxiety, cataplexy, insomnia, paresthesia, oro-facial dyskinesia, hypertonia, confusion, amnesia, emotional lability, ataxia, tremor. *GI:* N&V, diarrhea, dry mouth, anorexia, mouth ulcer, gingivitis, thirst. *CV:* Hypotension, hypertension, vasodilation, arrhythmia, syncope. *Dermatologic:* Herpes simplex, dry skin. *GU:* Abnormal urine, urinary retention, abnormal ejaculation. *Respiratory:* Rhinitis, pharyngitis, lung disorder, dyspnea, asthma, epistaxis. *Ophthalmic:* Amblyopia, abnormal vision. *Miscellaneous:* Infection, chest pain, neck pain, eosinophilia, rigid neck, fever, chills, joint disorder.

OD Overdose Management: *Symptoms:* Excitation, agitation, insomnia, slight to moderate increases in hemodynamic parameters. *Treatment:* Supportive care, including CV monitoring. Consider inducing emesis or gastric lavage.

Drug Interactions
Cyclosporine / Possible ↓ blood levels of modafinil
MAO inhibitors / Use caution when taken together
Methylphenidate / Delayed absorption (by 1 hr) of modafinil
Phenytoin / Possible phenytoin toxicity
Oral contraceptives / Possible ↓ effectiveness of oral contraceptives
Tricyclic antidepressants / Possible ↑ plasma levels of clomipramine or desipramine
Warfarin / Possible ↑ effects of warfarin

EMS CONSIDERATIONS
Assessment
1. Note onset, duration, and characteristics of symptoms.
2. Reduce dose with liver dysfunction and in the elderly.
3. Obtain ECG and monitor BP; do not use with LVH, ischemic ECG changes, chest pain, or arrhythmias.
4. Observe for S&S of abuse (e.g.,drug seeking behaviors, increased useage).

Moexipril hydrochloride
(moh-EX-ih-prill)
Pregnancy Class: C (first trimester), D (second and third trimesters)
Univasc **(Rx)**
Classification: Angiotensin-converting enzyme inhibitor

Onset of Action: 1-2 hr; **Peak effect:** 3-6 hr.
Duration of Action: 24 hr.

M

---

bold italic = life threatening side effect

Uses: Treatment of hypertension alone or in combination with thiazide diuretics.

Contraindications: In those with a history of angioedema as a result of previous treatment with ACE inhibitors.

Precautions: Use with caution during lactation, in patients with impaired renal function or renal artery stenosis, hyperkalemia, CHF, severe hepatic impairment, and volume depletion. Those who are salt or volume depleted are at a greater risk of developing hypotension. Safety and efficacy have not been determined in children.

Route/Dosage ———————
• **Tablets**
  Hypertension.
Initial, adults not receiving diuretics: 7.5 mg 1 hr before meals once daily. Dose is adjusted depending on response. **Maintenance:** 7.5–30 mg daily in one or two divided doses 1 hr before meals. **Initial, adults receiving diuretics:** Discontinue diuretic 2–3 days before beginning moexipril at a dose of 7.5 mg. If BP is not controlled, diuretic therapy can be resumed. If diuretic cannot be discontinued, give moexipril in an initial dose of 3.75 mg once daily 1 hr before meals. In those with impaired renal function, start with 3.75 mg once daily if C_{CR} is less than 40 mL/min/1.73 m². The dose may be increased to a maximum of 15 mg/day.

How Supplied: *Tablet:* 7.5 mg, 15 mg

Side Effects: *GI:* Abdominal pain, N&V, diarrhea, dysgeusia, constipation, dry mouth, dyspepsia, pancreatitis, hepatitis, changes in appetite, weight changes. *CNS:* Insomnia, sleep disturbances, headache, dizziness, fatigue, drowsiness/sleepiness, malaise, nervousness, anxiety, mood changes. *CV:* Chest pain, hypotension, palpitations, angina pectoris, **CVA, MI,** orthostatic hypotension, rhythm disturbances, peripheral edema. *Respiratory:* Cough, bronchospasm, dyspnea, URI, pharyn-

gitis, rhinitis. *GU:* Oliguria, urinary frequency, renal insufficiency. *Dermatologic:* Flushing, rash, diaphoresis, photosensitivity, pruritus, urticaria, pemphigus. *Musculoskeletal:* Myalgia, arthralgia. *Miscellaneous:* Angioedema, neutropenia, syncope, anemia, tinnitus, flu syndrome, pain.

Drug Interactions
Diuretics / Excessive hypotension
Lithium / Moexipril ↑ serum levels of lithium → lithium toxicity
Potassium-sparing diuretics / ↑ Hyperkalemic effect of moexipril
Potassium supplements / ↑ Hyperkalemic effect of moexipril

EMS CONSIDERATIONS
None.

Mometasone furoate monohyrate
(moh-MET-ah-sohn)
Pregnancy Class: C
Nasonex (Rx)
Classification: Corticosteroid, nasal

Mechanism of Action: Anti-inflammatory corticosteroid. No effect on adrenal function.

Uses: Prophylaxis and treatment of the nasal symptoms of seasonal allergic rhinitis and perennial allergic rhinitis.

Contraindications: Use in those with recent nasal septum ulcers, nasal surgery, or nasal trauma until healing has occurred.

Precautions: Use with caution, if at all, in those with active or quiescent tuberculosis infection of the respiratory tract, or in untreated fungal, bacterial, systemic viral infections, or ocular herpes simplex. Use with caution during lactation. Safety and efficacy have not been determined in children less than 12 years of age.

Route/Dosage ———————
• **Nasal Spray**
  Seasonal/perennial allergic rhinitis.
Adults and children over 12 years: 2 sprays (50 mcg in each spray) in each nostril once daily

(i.e., total daily dose: 200 mcg). In those with a known seasonal allergen that precipitates seasonal allergic rhinitis, give prophylactically, 200 mcg/day, 2 to 4 weeks prior to the anticipated start of the pollen season.

How Supplied: *Nasal spray:* 50 mcg/actuation

Side Effects: *Respiratory:* Pharyngitis, epistaxis, blood-tinged mucus, coughing, URI, sinusitis, rhinitis, asthma, bronchitis. Rarely, nasal ulcers and nasal and oral candidiasis. *GI:* Diarrhea, dyspepsia, nausea. *Miscellaneous:* Headache, viral infection, dysmenorrhea, musculoskeletal pain, arthralgia, chest pain, conjunctivitis, earache, flu-like symptoms, myalgia, increased IOP.

EMS CONSIDERATIONS

See also *Corticosteroids.*

Montelukast sodium (Singulair)
mon-teh-LOO-kast
Pregnancy Class: B
Singulair **(Rx)**
Classification: Antiasthmatic

Mechanism of Action: Cysteinyl leukotrienes and leukotriene receptor occupation are associated with symptoms of asthma, including airway edema, smooth muscle contraction, and inflammation. Montelukast binds with cysteinyl leukotriene receptors thus preventing the action of cysteinyl leukotrienes. Rapidly absorbed after PO use. **Time to peak levels:** 3–4 hr for 10 mg tablet and 2–2.5 hr for 5 mg tablet. Metabolized in liver and mainly excreted in feces. **t½:** 2.7–5.5 hr.

Uses: Prophylaxis and chronic treatment of asthma in adults and children aged 6 years of age and older. *Investigational:* With loratidine for hayfever.

Contraindications: Use to reverse bronchospasm in acute asthma attacks, including status asthmaticus. Use to abruptly substitute for inhaled or oral corticosteroids. Use as monotherapy to treat and manage exercise-induced bronchospasm. Use with known aspirin or NSAID sensitivity.

Route/Dosage
• **Tablets**
Asthma.
Adolescents and adults age 15 years and older: 10 mg once daily taken in evening.
• **Chewable tablets**
Asthma.
Pediatric patients aged 6 to 14 years: 5 mg chewable tablet once daily taken in evening.
How Supplied: *Tablets:* 10 mg. *Chewable Tablets:* 5 mg.

Side Effects: *Adolescents and adults aged 15 and older. GI:* Dyspepsia, infectious gastroenteritis, abdominal pain, dental pain. *CNS:* Headache, dizziness. *Body as a whole:* Asthenia, fatigue, trauma. *Respiratory:* Influenza, cough, nasal congestion. *Dermatologic:* Rash. *Miscellaneous:* Pyuria.

Children, aged 6 to 14 years. GI: Nausea, diarrhea. *Respiratory:* Pharyngitis, laryngitis, otitis, sinusitus. *Miscellaneous:* Viral infection.

EMS CONSIDERATIONS
Administration/Storage: Take daily as prescribed, even when patient is asymptomatic. Contact provider if asthma is not well controlled.
Assessment
1. Document indications for therapy, onset, triggers, and characteristics of disease. List other agents trialed and outcome.
2. Note other agents prescribed for asthma and reinforce which should be continued.
3. Document pulmonary assessments, PFTs, and x-rays when indicated.
4. Chewable 5 mg tablet contains 0.842 mg of phenylalanine and should not be used with phenylketonurics.
5. Assist to identify and eliminate/minimize triggers.

M

Moricizine hydrochloride

(mor-IS-ih-zeen)
Pregnancy Class: B
Ethmozine **(Rx)**
Classification: Antiarrhythmic, class I

Mechanism of Action: Causes a stabilizing effect on the myocardial membranes as well as local anesthetic activity. Shortens phase II and III repolarization leading to a decreased duration of the action potential and an effective refractory period. Also, there is a decrease in the maximum rate of phase O depolarization and a prolongation of AV conduction in patients with ventricular tachycardia. Whether the patient is at rest or is exercising, has minimal effects on cardiac index, stroke index volume, systemic or pulmonary vascular resistance or ejection fraction, and pulmonary capillary wedge pressure. There is a small increase in resting BP and HR. The time, course, and intensity of antiarrhythmic and electrophysiologic effects are not related to plasma levels of the drug.

Onset of Action: 2 hr.

Duration of Action: 10-24 hr.

Uses: Documented life-threatening ventricular arrhythmias (e.g., sustained VT) where benefits of the drug are determined to outweigh the risks. *Investigational:* Ventricular premature contractions, couplets, and nonsustained VT.

Contraindications: Preexisting second- or third-degree block, right bundle branch block when associated with bifascicular block (unless the patient has a pacemaker), cardiogenic shock. Lactation.

Precautions: There is the possibility of increased risk of death when used in patients with non-life-threatening cardiac arrhythmias. Safety and effectiveness in children less than 18 years of age have not been determined. Geriatric patients have a higher rate of side effects. Increased survival rates following use of antiarrhythmic drugs have not been proven in patients with ventricular arrhythmias. Use with caution in patients with sick sinus syndrome due to

the possibility of sinus bradycardia, sinus pause, or sinus arrest. Use with caution in patients with CHF.

Route/Dosage
• **Tablets**
  Antiarrhythmic.
Adults: 600–900 mg/day in equally divided doses q 8 hr. If needed, the dose can be increased in increments of 150 mg/day at 3-day intervals until the desired effect is obtained. In patients with hepatic or renal impairment, the initial dose should be 600 mg or less with close monitoring and dosage adjustment.

How Supplied: *Tablet:* 200 mg, 250 mg, 300 mg

Side Effects: *CV: **Proarrhythmias, including new rhythm disturbances or worsening of existing arrhythmias;** ECG abnormalities, including conduction defects, sinus pause, junctional rhythm, AV block; palpitations, **sustained VT,** cardiac chest pain, CHF, **cardiac death,** hypotension, hypertension, atrial fibrillation, atrial flutter, syncope, bradycardia, **cardiac arrest, MI, pulmonary embolism,** vasodilation, thrombophlebitis, **cerebrovascular events.** CNS:* Dizziness (common), anxiety, headache, fatigue, nervousness, paresthesias, sleep disorders, tremor, anxiety, hypoesthesias, depression, euphoria, somnolence, agitation, confusion, **seizures,** hallucinations, loss of memory, vertigo, coma. *GI:* Nausea, dry mouth, abdominal pain, vomiting, diarrhea, dyspepsia, anorexia, ileus, flatulence, dysphagia, bitter taste. *Musculoskeletal:* Asthenia, abnormal gait, akathisia, ataxia, abnormal coordination, dyskinesia, pain. *GU:* Urinary retention, dysuria, urinary incontinence, urinary frequency, impotence, kidney pain, decreased libido. *Respiratory:* Dyspnea, apnea, asthma, hyperventilation, pharyngitis, cough, sinusitis. *Ophthalmologic:* Nystagmus, diplopia, blurred vision, eye pain, periorbital edema. *Dermatologic:* Rash, pruritus, dry skin, urticaria. *Miscellaneous:* Sweating, drug fever, hypothermia, temperature intolerance, swelling of the lips and tongue, speech disorder, tinnitus, jaundice.

OD **Overdose Management:** *Symptoms:* Vomiting, hypotension, lethargy, worsening of CHF, *MI, conduction disturbances, arrhythmias (e.g., junctional bradycardia, VT, ventricular fibrillation, asystole), sinus arrest, respiratory failure. Treatment:* In acute overdose, induce vomiting, taking care to prevent aspiration. Hospitalize and closely monitor for cardiac, respiratory, and CNS changes. Provide life support, including an intracardiac pacing catheter, if necessary.

Drug Interactions
Cimetidine / ↑ Plasma levels of moricizine due to ↓ excretion
Digoxin / Additive prolongation of the PR interval (but no significant increase in the rate of second- or third-degree AV block)
Propranolol / Additive prolongation of the PR interval
Theophylline / ↓ Plasma levels of theophylline due to ↑ rate of clearance

EMS CONSIDERATIONS

See also *Antiarrhythmic Agents.*

Morphine sulfate
(MOR-feen SUL-fayt)
Pregnancy Class: C
Astramorph PF, Duramorph, Infumorph, Kadian, MS Contin, MS-IR, MSIR Capsules, Oramorph SR, RMS, RMS Rectal Suppositories, Roxanol, Roxanol 100, Roxanol Rescudose, Roxanol-T, Roxanol UD **(C-II) (Rx)**
Classification: Narcotic analgesic, morphine type

Mechanism of Action: Morphine is the prototype for opiate analgesics. Oral morphine is only one-third to one-sixth as effective as parenteral products.
Onset of Action: Approximately 15-60 min, based on epidural or intrathecal use. **Peak effect:** 30-60 min.
Duration of Action: 3-7 hr.
Uses: Intrathecally, epidurally, PO (including sustained-release prod-

ucts), or by continuous IV infusion for acute or chronic pain. In low doses, morphine is more effective against dull, continuous pain than against intermittent, sharp pain. Large doses, however, will dull almost any kind of pain. Preoperative medication. To facilitate induction of anesthesia and reduce dose of anesthetic. *Investigational:* Acute LV failure (for dyspneic seizures) and pulmonary edema. Morphine should not be used with papaverine for analgesia in biliary spasms but may be used with papaverine in acute vascular occlusions.

Contraindications: Additional:
Epidural or intrathecal morphine if infection is present at injection site, in patients on anticoagulant therapy, bleeding diathesis, if patient has received parenteral corticosteroids within the past 2 weeks.
Precautions: May increase the length of labor. Patients with known seizure disorders may be at greater risk for morphine-induced seizure activity.

Route/Dosage
• **Capsules, Tablets, Oral Solution, Soluble Tablets, Syrup**
Analgesia.
5–30 mg q 4 hr.
• **Sustained-Release Tablets**
Analgesia.
30 mg q 8–12 hr, depending on patient needs and response. Kadian is indicated for once-daily dosing at doses of 20, 50, or 100 mg where analgesia is indicated for just a few days.
• **IM, SC**
Analgesia.
Adults: 5–20 mg/70 kg q 4 hr as needed; **pediatric:** 100–200 mcg/kg up to a maximum of 15 mg.
• **IV Infusion**
Analgesia.
Adults: 2.5–15 mg/70 kg in 4–5 mL of water for injection (should be administered slowly over 4–5 min).
• **IV Infusion, Continuous**
Analgesia.

M

---

bold italic = life threatening side effect

Adults: 0.1–1 mg/mL in D5W by a controlled-infusion pump.
• **Rectal Suppositories**
Adults: 10–30 mg q 4 hr.
• **Intrathecal**
Adults: 0.2–1 mg as a single daily injection.
• **Epidural**
Initial: 5 mg/day in the lumbar region; if analgesia is not manifested in 1 hr, increasing doses of 1–2 mg can be given, not to exceed 10 mg/day. For continuous infusion, 2–4 mg/day with additional doses of 1–2 mg if analgesia is not satisfactory.

How Supplied: Morphine hydrochloride: *Syrup:* 1 mg/mL, 5 mg/mL, 10 mg/mL, 20 mg/mL; *Concentrate:* 20 mg/mL, 50 mg/mL; *Suppository:* 10 mg, 20 mg, 30 mg; *Tablets:* 10 mg, 20 mg, 40 mg, 60 mg; *Slow-release tablets:* 30 mg, 60 mg. Morphine sulfate: *Capsule:* 15 mg, 30 mg; *Capsule, Extended Release:* 20 mg, 50 mg, 100 mg; *Oral Concentrate:* 20 mg/mL; *Injection:* 0.5 mg/mL, 1 mg/mL, 2 mg/mL, 4 mg/mL, 5 mg/mL, 8 mg/mL, 10 mg/mL, 15 mg/mL, 25 mg/mL, 50 mg/mL; *Solution:* 10 mg/5 mL, 20 mg/5 mL; *Suppository:* 5 mg, 10 mg, 20 mg, 30 mg; *Tablet:* 10 mg, 15 mg, 30 mg; *Tablet, Extended Release:* 15 mg, 30 mg, 60 mg, 100 mg, 200 mg

EMS CONSIDERATIONS

See also *Narcotic Analgesics.*
Administration/Storage
IV 1. For IV use, dilute 2–10 mg with at least 5 mL sterile water or NSS and administer over 4–5 min.
2. Rapid IV administration increases the risk of adverse effects; have a narcotic antagonist (e.g., naloxone) available.

Moxifloxacin hydrochloride

(mox-ee-FLOX-ah-sin)
Pregnancy Class: C
Avelox **(Rx)**
Classification: Antibiotic, fluoroquinolone

Uses: (1) Acute bacterial sinusitis due to *Streptococcus pneumoniae, Haemophilus influenzae,* or *Moraxella catarrhalis.* (2) Acute bacterial exacerbation of chronic bronchitis due to *S. pneumoniae, H. influenzae, Haemophilus parainfluenzae, Klebsiella pneumoniae, Staphylococcus aureus,* or *M. catarrhalis.* (3) Mild to moderate community acquired pneumonia due to *S. pneumoniae, H. influenzae, Mycoplasma pneumoniae, Chlamydia pneumoniae,* or *M. catarrhalis.*

Contraindications: Hypersensitivity to moxifloxacin or any quinolone antibiotic. Use with moderate to severe hepatic insufficiency. Use in patients with known prolongation of the QT interval (the drug prolongs the QT interval in some), with uncorrected hypokalemia, and in those receiving class IA (e.g., quinidine, procainamide) or Class III (e.g., amiodarone, sotalol) antiarrhythmic drugs. Lactation.

Precautions: Use with caution in those with clinically significant bradycardia or acute myocardial ischemia, in patients with known or suspected CNS disorders (e.g., severe cerebral arteriosclerosis, epilepsy), or in the presence of risk factors that predispose to seizures or lower the seizure threshold. Safety and efficacy have not been determined in children, adolescents less than 18 years of age, in pregnancy, and during lactation.

Route/Dosage ———————
• **Tablets**
Acute bacterial sinusitis, community acquired pneumonia.
Adults: 400 mg q 24 hr for 10 days.
Acute bacterial exacerbation of chronic bronchitis.
Adults: 400 mg q 24 hr for 5 days.
How Supplied: *Tablets:* 400 mg
Side Effects: *Hypersensitivity: **Anaphylaxis after the first dose, CV collapse,** loss of consciousness, tingling, pharyngeal or facial edema, dyspnea, urticaria, itching. CNS:* Dizziness, headache, convulsions, confusion, tremors, hallucinations, depres-

sion, insomnia, nervousness, anxiety, depersonalization, hypertonia, incoordination, somnolence, vertigo, paresthesia, suicidal thoughts/acts (rare). *GI:* N&V, diarrhea, abdominal pain, taste perversion, dyspepsia, dry mouth, constipation, oral moniliasis, anorexia, stomatitis, gastritis, glossitis, GI disorder, pseudomembranous colitis, cholestatic jaundice. *CV:* Palpitation, vasodilatation, tachycardia, hypertension, peripheral edema, hypotension. *Body as a whole:* Asthenia, moniliasis, pain, malaise, allergic reaction, leg pain, pelvic pain, back pain, chills, infection, chest pain, hand pain. *Hematologic:* Thrombocytopenia, thrombocythemia, eosinophilia, leukopenia. *Respiratory:* Asthma, dyspnea, increased cough, pneumonia, pharyngitis, rhinitis, sinusitis. *Musculoskeletal:* Arthralgia, myalgia. *Dermatologic:* Rash, pruritus, sweating, urticaria, dry skin. *GU:* Vaginal moniliasis, vaginitis, cystitis. *Miscellaneous:* Tinnitus, amblyopia.

Drug Interactions
Antacids / Significant ↓ bioavailability of moxifloxacin
Antidepressants, tricyclic / Potential to add to the QTC prolonging effect of moxifloxacin
Antipsychotics / Potential to add to the QTC prolonging effect of moxifloxacin
Cisapride / Potential to add to the QTC prolonging effect of moxifloxacin
Didanosine / ↓ Absorption of moxifloxacin
Erythromycin / Potential to add to the QTC prolonging effect of moxifloxacin
Iron products / Significant ↓ bioavailabilitiy of moxifloxaicn
NSAIDs / ↑ Risk of CNS stimulation and convulsions
Sucralfate / ↓ Absorption of moxifloxacin

EMS CONSIDERATIONS
None.

Mupirocin
Mupirocin Calcium
(myou-PEER-oh-sin)
Pregnancy Class: B
Mupirocin (Bactroban **(Rx)**) Mupirocin Calcium (Bactroban Cream, Bactroban Nasal **(Rx)**)
Classification: Anti-infective, topical

Mechanism of Action: Binds to bacterial isoleucyl transfer RNA synthetase, which results in inhibition of protein synthesis by the organism. Not absorbed into the systemic circulation. Serum present in exudative wounds decreases the antibacterial activity. Metabolized to the inactive monic acid in the skin which is removed by normal skin desquamation. No cross resistance with other antibiotics such as chloramphenicol, erythromycin, gentamicin, lincomycin, methicillin, neomycin, novobiocin, penicillin, streptomycin, or tetracyclines.

Uses: Topical: To treat impetigo and secondarily infected traumatic skin lesions due to *Staphylococcus aureus, Streptococcus pyogenes,* and beta-hemolytic streptococcus. **Nasal:** Eradication of nasal colonization with methicillin-resistant *S. aureus* in adult patients and health care workers.

Contraindications: Ophthalmic use. Lactation. Use if absorption of large quantities of polyethylene glycol is possible (i.e., large, open wounds). Use with other nasal products.

Precautions: Superinfection may result from chronic use. Safety and efficacy have not been established in children for mupirocin nasal.

Route/Dosage
• **Topical Cream**
Apply to affected area t.i.d. for 10 days.
• **Topical Ointment**
A small amount of ointment is applied to the affected area t.i.d. If no response is seen after 3–5 days, the patient should be reevaluated.
• **Nasal Ointment**

M

Divide about one-half of the ointment from the single-use tube between the nostrils and apply in the morning and evening for 5 days.
How Supplied: *Nasal Ointment:* 2%; *Ointment:* 2%; *Topical Cream:* 2%
Side Effects: Topical use: Superinfection, rash, burning, stinging, pain, nausea, tenderness, erythema, swelling, dry skin, contact dermatitis, and increased exudate.

Nasal use: Headache, rhinitis, respiratory disorder (including upper respiratory tract congestion), pharyngitis, taste perversion, burning, stinging, cough, pruritus, blepharitis, diarrhea, dry mouth, ear pain, epistaxis, nausea, rash.

EMS CONSIDERATIONS
None.

Mycophenolate mofetil
(my-koh-FEN-oh-layt)
Pregnancy Class: C
CellCept, CellCept IV **(Rx)**
Classification: Immunosuppressant

Mechanism of Action: Inhibits proliferative responses of T- and B-lymphocytes to both mitogenic and allospecific stimulation. MPA also suppresses antibody formation of B-lymphocytes.
Uses: With cyclosporine and corticosteroids to prevent organ rejection in those receiving allogeneic renal transplants or undergoing heart transplants.
Contraindications: Hypersensitivity to mycophenolate or MPA. Lactation.
Precautions: Patients receiving immunosuppressant drugs are at a higher risk of developing lymphomas and other malignancies, especially of the skin. Higher blood levels are seen in those with severe impaired renal function. Use with caution in active serious digestive system disease. Safety and efficacy have not been determined in children.

Route/Dosage
• **Capsules**

Prevent rejection following allogeneic renal transplantation and heart transplants.
Adults: 1 g b.i.d. in combination with corticosteroids and cyclosporine.
How Supplied: *Capsules:* 250 mg; *Powder for Injection:* 500 mg; *Tablets:* 500 mg
Side Effects: *Hematologic:* Severe neutropenia, anemia, leukopenia, thrombocytopenia, hypochromic anemia, leukocytosis. *GI:* **GI tract hemorrhage/perforations,** GI tract ulceration, diarrhea, constipation, nausea, dyspepsia, vomiting, oral moniliasis, anorexia, esophagitis, flatulence, gastritis, gastroenteritis, GI moniliasis, gingivitis, gum hyperplasia, hepatitis, ileus, infection, mouth ulceration, rectal disorder. *CNS:* Tremor, insomnia, dizziness, anxiety, depression, hypertonia, paresthesia, somnolence. *GU:* UTI, hematuria, kidney tubular necrosis, urinary tract disorder, albuminuria, dysuria, hydronephrosis, impotence, pain, pyelonephritis, urinary frequency. *CV:* Hypertension, angina pectoris, atrial fibrillation, cardiovascular disorder, hypotension, palpitation, peripheral vascular disorder, postural hypotension, tachycardia, thrombosis, vasodilation. *Respiratory:* Infection, dyspnea, increased cough, pharyngitis, bronchitis, pneumonia, asthma, lung disorder, lung edema, pleural effusion, rhinitis, sinusitis. *Dermatologic:* Acne, rash, alopecia, fungal dermatitis, hirsutism, pruritus, benign skin neoplasm, skin disorder, skin hypertrophy, skin ulcer, sweating. *Metabolic/Endocrine:* Peripheral edema, dehydration, hypercholesterolemia, hypophosphatemia, edema, hypokalemia, hyperkalemia, hyperglycemia, diabetes mellitus, parathyroid disorder. *Musculoskeletal:* Arthralgia, joint disorder, leg cramps, myalgia, myasthenia. *Ophthalmologic:* Amblyopia, cataract, conjunctivitis. *Body as a whole:* Pain, abdominal pain, fever, chills, headache, infection, malaise, **sepsis,** asthenia, chest pain, back pain. *Miscellaneous:* Increased incidence of lymphoma/lymphoproliferative disease, nonmelanoma skin carcinoma, and other malignancies. In-

creased incidence of opportunistic infections, including herpes simplex, CMV, herpes zoster, *Candida, Aspergillus/Mucor* invasive disease, and *Pneumocystis carinii*. Enlarged abdomen, accidental injury, cyst, facial edema, flu syndrome, **hemorrhage,** hernia, weight gain, pelvic pain, ecchymosis, polycythemia.

OD **Overdose Management:** *Symptoms:* Nausea, vomiting, diarrhea, hematologic abnormalities, especially neutropenia. *Treatment:* Reduce dose of the drug. Removal of MPA by bile acid sequestrants (e.g., cholestyramine).

Drug Interactions
Acyclovir / ↑ Plasma levels of both drugs due to competition for renal tubular excretion

Antacids containing aluminum/magnesium / ↓ Absorption of mycophenolate
Cholestyramine / ↓ Absorption of mycophenolate
Ganciclovir / ↑ Plasma levels of both drugs due to competition for renal tubular excretion
Phenytoin / ↓ Plasma protein binding of phenytoin
Probenecid / Significant ↑ plasma levels of MPA
Salicylates / ↑ Free fraction of MPA
Theophylline / ↓ Plasma protein binding of theophylline

EMS CONSIDERATIONS
None.

N

Nabumetone
(nah-BYOU-meh-tohn)
Pregnancy Class: B
Relafen **(Rx)**
Classification: Nonsteroidal anti-inflammatory agent

Uses: Acute and chronic treatment of osteoarthritis and rheumatoid arthritis. Has also been used to treat mild to moderate pain including postextraction dental pain, postsurgical episiotomy pain, and soft tissue athletic injuries.
Contraindications: Lactation.
Precautions: Safety and efficacy have not been determined in children.

Route/Dosage
• **Tablets**
Osteoarthritis, rheumatoid arthritis.
Adults, initial: 1,000 mg as a single dose; **maintenance:** 1,500–2,000 mg/day. Doses greater than 2,000 mg/day have not been studied.
How Supplied: *Tablet:* 500 mg, 750 mg

EMS CONSIDERATIONS
See also *Nonsteroidal Anti-Inflammatory Drugs.*

Nadolol
(NAY-doh-lohl)
Pregnancy Class: C
Corgard **(Rx)**
Classification: Beta-adrenergic blocking agent

Mechanism of Action: Manifests both beta-1- and beta-2-adrenergic blocking activity. Has no membrane stabilizing or intrinsic sympathomimetic activity.
Uses: Hypertension, either alone or with other drugs (e.g., thiazide diuretic). Angina pectoris. *Investigational:* Prophylaxis of migraine, ventricular arrhythmias, aggressive behavior, essential tremor, tremors associated with lithium or parkinsonism, antipsychotic-induced akathisia, rebleeding of esophageal varices, situational anxiety, reduce intraocular pressure.
Contraindications: Use in bronchial asthma or bronchospasm, including severe COPD.

---

bold italic = life threatening side effect

Precautions: Dosage has not been established in children.

Route/Dosage ───────────
• **Tablets**
Hypertension.
Initial: 40 mg/day; **then,** may be increased in 40- to 80-mg increments until optimum response obtained. **Maintenance:** 40–80 mg/day although up to 240–320 mg/day may be needed.
Angina.
Initial: 40 mg/day; **then,** increase dose in 40- to 80-mg increments q 3–7 days until optimum response obtained. **Maintenance:** 40–80 mg/day, although up to 160–240 mg/day may be needed.
Aggressive behavior.
40–160 mg/day.
Antipsychotic-induced akathisia.
40–80 mg/day.
Essential tremor.
120–240 mg/day.
Lithium-induced tremors.
20–40 mg/day.
Tremors associated with parkinsonism.
80–320 mg/day.
Prophylaxis of migraine.
40–80 mg/day.
Rebleeding from esophageal varices.
40–160 mg/day.
Situational anxiety.
20 mg.
Ventricular arrhythmias.
10–640 mg/day.
Reduction of intraocular pressure.
10–20 mg b.i.d.
NOTE: For all uses decrease dose in patients with renal failure.
How Supplied: *Tablet:* 20 mg, 40 mg, 80 mg, 120 mg, 160 mg

EMS CONSIDERATIONS

See also *Beta-Adrenergic Blocking Agents* and *Antihypertensive Agents.*

Nafarelin acetate
(NAF-ah-rel-in)
Pregnancy Class: X
Synarel **(Rx)**
Classification: Gonadotropin-releasing hormone

Mechanism of Action: Produced through biotechnology; differs by only one amino acid from naturally occurring GnRH. Stimulates the release of LH and FSH from the adeno-hypophysis. Causes estrogen and progesterone synthesis in the ovary, resulting in the maturation and subsequent release of an ovum. With repeated use of the drug, however, the pituitary becomes desensitized and no longer produces endogenous LH and FSH; thus endogenous estrogen is not produced, leading to a regression of endometrial tissue, cessation of menstruation, and a menopausal-like state.
Uses: Endometriosis (including reduction of endometriotic lesions) in patients aged 18 or older. Central precocious puberty in children of both sexes.
Contraindications: Hypersensitivity to GnRH or analogs. Abnormal vaginal bleeding of unknown origin. Pregnancy or possibility of becoming pregnant. Lactation.
Precautions: Rule out pregnancy before initiating therapy. Safety and effectiveness have not been established in children.

Route/Dosage ───────────
• **Nasal Spray**
Endometriosis.
200 mcg into one nostril in the morning and 200 mcg into the other nostril at night (400 mcg b.i.d. may be required by some women).
Central precocious puberty.
400 mcg (2 sprays) into each nostril in the morning (i.e., 4 sprays) and in the evening (total of 8 sprays/day). If adequate suppression is not achieved, 3 sprays (600 mcg) into alternating nostrils t.i.d. (i.e., a total of 9 sprays/day).
How Supplied: *Spray:* 0.2 mg/inh
Side Effects: *Due to hypoestrogenic effects:* Hot flashes (common), decreased libido, vaginal dryness, headaches, emotional lability, insomnia. *Due to androgenic effects:* Acne, myalgia, reduced breast size, edema, seborrhea, weight gain, increased libido, hirsutism. *Musculoskeletal:* Decrease in vertebral trabecular bone density

and total vertebral bone mass. *Miscellaneous:* Nasal irritation, depression, weight loss.

EMS CONSIDERATIONS

None.

Nafcillin sodium
(naf-SILL-in)
Pregnancy Class: B
Nallpen, Unipen **(Rx)**
Classification: Antibiotic, penicillin

Mechanism of Action: Parenteral therapy is recommended initially for severe infections.
Uses: Infections by penicillinase-producing staphylococci. As initial therapy if staphylococcal infection is suspected (i.e., until results of culture have been obtained).
Contraindications: Use for treatment of penicillin G-susceptible staphylococcus.

Route/Dosage
• **IV**
Adults: 0.5–1 g q 4 hr.
• **IM**
Adults: 0.5 g q 4–6 hr. **Children and infants, less than 40 kg:** 25 mg/kg b.i.d. **Neonates:** 10 mg/kg b.i.d. Or, for neonates weighing more than 2,000 g and less than 7 days of age, 100 mg/kg/day in 2 divided doses; for neonates older than 7 days, 100 mg/kg/day in 3 divided doses; if the weight is less than 2,000 g, 20 mg/kg q 8 hr.
• **Capsules**
Mild to moderate infections.
Adults: 250–500 mg q 4–6 hr.
Severe infections.
Adults: Up to 1 g q 4–6 hr.
Pneumonia/scarlet fever.
Children: 25 mg/kg/day in four divided doses.
Staphylococcal infections.
Children: 50 mg/kg/day in four divided doses. **Neonates:** 10 mg/kg t.i.d.–q.i.d.
Streptococcal pharyngitis.
Children: 250 mg t.i.d. for 10 days.

NOTE: IV administration is not recommended for neonates or infants.
How Supplied: *Injection:* 1 g/50 mL, 2 g/50 mL; *Powder for injection:* 500 mg, 1 g, 2 g, 10 g
Side Effects: Additional: Steril abscesses and thrombophlebitis occur frequently, expecially in the elderly.
Drug Interactions: Additional: When used with cylosporine, subtherapeutic levels of cyclosporine are possible.

EMS CONSIDERATIONS

See also *Anti-Infectives* and *Penicillins.*

Naftifine hydrochloride
(NAF-tih-feen)
Pregnancy Class: B
Naftin **(Rx)**
Classification: Antifungal agent

Mechanism of Action: Synthetic antifungal agent with a broad spectrum of activity. Thought to inhibit squalene 2,3-epoxidase, which is responsible for synthesis of sterols. The decreased levels of sterols (especially ergosterol) and the accumulation of squalene in cells result in fungicidal activity.
Uses: To treat tinea cruris, tinea pedis, and tinea corporis caused by *Candida albicans, Epidermophyton floccosum, Microsporum canis, M. audouinii, M. gypseum, Trichophyton rubrum, T. mentagrophytes,* and *T. tonsurans.*
Contraindications: Ophthalmic use.
Precautions: Discontinue nursing while using naftifine and for several days after the last application. Safety and efficacy in children have not been determined.

Route/Dosage
• **Topical Cream (1%), Topical Gel (1%)**
Massage into affected area and surrounding skin once daily if using the cream and twice daily (morning and evening) if using the gel.

N

How Supplied: *Cream:* 1%; *Gel/jelly:* 1%

Side Effects: *Topical cream:* Burning, stinging, dryness, itching, local irritation, erythema. *Topical gel:* Burning, stinging, itching, rash, tenderness, erythema.

EMS CONSIDERATIONS

See also *Anti-Infectives.*

Nalbuphine hydrochloride

(NAL-byou-feen)
Nubain **(Rx)**
Classification: Narcotic agonist/antagonist

Mechanism of Action: Synthetic compound resembling oxymorphone and naloxone. Potent analgesic with both narcotic agonist and antagonist actions. Analgesic potency is approximately equal to that of morphine, while its antagonistic potency is approximately one-fourth that of nalorphine.

Onset of Action: IV: 2-3 min; **SC or IM:** < 15 min; **Peak effect:** 30-60 min.

Duration of Action: 3-6 hr.

Uses: Moderate to severe pain. Preoperative analgesia, anesthesia adjunct, obstetric analgesia.

Contraindications: Hypersensitivity to drug. Children under 18 years.

Precautions: Safe use during pregnancy (except for delivery) and lactation not established. Use with caution in presence of head injuries and asthma, MI (if patient is nauseous or vomiting), biliary tract surgery (may induce spasms of sphincter of Oddi), renal insufficiency. Patients dependent on narcotics may experience withdrawal symptoms.

Route/Dosage
• **SC, IM, IV**
  Analgesia.

Adults: 10 mg/70 kg q 3–6 hr as needed (single dose should not exceed 20 mg q 3–6 hr; do not exceed a total daily dose of 160 mg).

How Supplied: *Injection:* 1.5 mg/mL, 10 mg/mL, 20 mg/mL

Side Effects: Additional: Even though nalbuphine is an agonist-antagonist, it may cause dependence and may precipitate withdrawal symptoms in an individual physically dependent on narcotics. *CNS:* Sedation is common. Crying, feeling of unreality, and other psychologic reactions. *GI:* Cramps, dry mouth, bitter tase, dyspepsia. *Skin:* Itching, burning, urticaria, sweaty, clammy skin. *Other:* Blurred vision, difficulty with speech, urinary frequency.

Drug Interactions: Concomitant use with CNS depressants, other narcotics, phenothiazines, may result in additive depressant effects.

EMS CONSIDERATIONS

See also *Narcotic Analgesics.*

Nalmefene hydrochloride

(NAL-meh-feen)
Pregnancy Class: B
Revex **(Rx)**
Classification: Narcotic antagonist

Mechanism of Action: Prevents or reverses respiratory depression, sedation, and hypotension due to opioids, including propoxyphene, nalbuphine, pentazocine, and butorphanol. Has a significantly longer duration of action than naloxone. Does not produce respiratory depression, psychotomimetic effects, or pupillary constriction (i.e., it has no intrinsic activity). Also, tolerance, physical dependence, or abuse potential have not been noted.

Onset of Action: IV: 2 min.

Duration of Action: Up to 8 hr.

Uses: For complete or partial reversal of the effects of opioid drugs postoperatively. Management of known or suspected overdose of opiates.

Precautions: Will precipitate acute withdrawal symptoms in those who have some degree of tolerance and dependence on opioids. Use with caution during lactation, in high CV risk patients, or in those who have received potentially cardiotoxic drugs. Reversal of buprenorphine- induced respiratory depression may be incomplete; therefore artificial respiration may be necessary. Safety and effectiveness have not been determined in children.

Route/Dosage
• **IV**
Reversal of postoperative depression due to opiates.
Adults: Titrate in 0.25-mcg/kg incremental doses at 2–5-min intervals until the desired degree of reversal is achieved (i.e., adequate ventilation and alertness without significant pain or discomfort). If patient is an increased CV risk, use an incremental dose of 0.1 mcg/kg (the drug may be diluted 1:1 with saline or sterile water). A total dose greater than 1 mcg/kg does not provide additional effects.
Management of known or suspected overdose of opiates.
Adults, initial: 0.5 mg/70 kg; **then,** 1 mg/70 kg 2–5 min later, if needed. Doses greater than 1.5 mg/70 kg do not increase the beneficial effect. If there is a reasonable suspicion of dependence on opiates, give a challenge dose of 0.1 mg/70 kg first; if there is no evidence of withdrawal in 2 min, give the recommended dose.
How Supplied: *Injection:* 1 mg/mL, 100 mcg/mL
Side Effects: *CV:* Tachycardia, hypertension, hypotension, vasodilation, bradycardia, arrhythmia. *GI:* N&V, diarrhea, dry mouth. *CNS:* Dizziness, somnolence, depression, agitation, nervousness, tremor, confusion, withdrawal syndrome, myoclonus. *Body as a whole:* Fever, headache, chills, postoperative pain. *Miscellaneous:* Pharyngitis, pruritus, urinary retention.

EMS CONSIDERATIONS

See also *Narcotic Antagonists.*
Administration/Storage
1. Give SC or IM at doses of 1 mg if IV access is lost or not readily obtainable. This dose is effective in 5–15 min.
IV 2. Treatment should follow, not precede, establishment of a patent

airway, ventilatory assistance, oxygen, and circulatory access.
3. Nalmefene is supplied in two concentrations—ampules containing 1 mL (blue label) at a concentration suitable for postoperative use (100 mcg) and ampules containing 2 mL (green label) suitable for management of overdose (1 mg/mL), i.e., **10 times as concentrated.** Follow specific guidelines, as indicated.
Assessment
1. Observe carefully for recurrent respiratory depression. Overdose with long-acting opiates (e.g., methadone, LAAM) may cause recurrence of respiratory depression.
2. Patient may experience N&V, fever, headaches, chills, pain, dizziness, and tachycardia.

Naloxone hydrochloride
(nal-OX-ohn)
Pregnancy Class: B
Narcan **(Rx)**
Classification: Narcotic antagonist

Mechanism of Action: Combines competitively with opiate receptors and blocks or reverses the action of narcotic analgesics. Since the duration of action of naloxone is shorter than that of the narcotic analgesics, the respiratory depression may return when the narcotic antagonist has worn off.
Onset of Action: IV: 2 min; **SC, IM:** < 5 min.
Duration of Action: Dependent on dose and route of administration but may be as short as 45 min.
Uses: Respiratory depression induced by natural and synthetic narcotics, including butorphanol, methadone, nalbuphine, pentazocine, and propoxyphene. Drug of choice when nature of depressant drug is not known. Diagnosis of acute opiate overdosage. Not effective when respiratory depression is induced by hypnotics, sedatives, or anesthetics and other nonnarcotic CNS depressants. Adjunct to increase BP in septic shock. *Investigational:* Treatment of

Alzheimer's dementia, alcoholic coma, and schizophrenia.

Contraindications: Sensitivity to drug. Narcotic addicts (drug may cause severe withdrawal symptoms). Use in neonates.

Precautions: Safe use during lactation and in children is not established.

Route/Dosage

• **IV, IM, SC**

Narcotic overdose.

Initial: 0.4–2 mg IV; if necessary, additional IV doses may be repeated at 2- to 3-min intervals. If no response after 10 mg, reevaluate diagnosis. **Pediatric, initial:** 0.01 mg/kg IV; **then,** 0.1 mg/kg IV, if needed. The SC or IM route may be used if an IV route is not available.

To reverse postoperative narcotic depression.

Adults: IV, initial, 0.1- to 0.2-mg increments at 2- to 3-min intervals; **then,** repeat at 1- to 2-hr intervals if necessary. Supplemental IM dosage increases the duration of reversal. **Children: Initial,** 0.005–0.01 mg IV at 2- to 3-min intervals until desired response is obtained.

Reverse narcotic-induced depression in neonates.

Initial: 0.01 mg/kg IV, IM, or SC. May be repeated using adult administration guidelines.

How Supplied: *Injection:* 0.02 mg/mL, 0.4 mg/mL, 1 mg/mL

Side Effects: N&V, sweating, hypertension, tremors, sweating due to reversal of narcotic depression. If used postoperatively, excessive doses may cause ***VT and fibrillation,*** hypo- or hypertension, pulmonary edema, and ***seizures (infrequent).***

EMS CONSIDERATIONS

See also *Narcotic Antagonists.*

IV Administration/Storage: May administer undiluted at a rate of 0.4 mg over 15 sec with narcotic overdosage. May reconstitute 2 mg in 500 mL of NSS or D5W to provide a 4 mcg/mL or 0.004 mg/mL concentration. Administration rate varies with patient response.

Naltrexone
(nal-TREX-ohn)
Pregnancy Class: C
ReVia **(Rx)**
Classification: Narcotic antagonist

Mechanism of Action: Competitively binds to opiate receptors, thereby reversing or preventing the effects of narcotics.

Duration of Action: 24-72 hr.

Uses: To prevent narcotic use in former narcotic addicts. Adjunct to the psychosocial treatment for alcoholism. *Investigational:* To treat eating disorders and postconcussional syndrome not responding to other approaches.

Contraindications: Those taking narcotic analgesics, dependent on narcotics, or in acute withdrawal from narcotics. Liver failure, acute hepatitis.

Precautions: Use with caution during lactation. Safety in children under 18 years of age has not been established.

Route/Dosage

• **Tablets**

To produce blockade of opiate actions.

Initial: 25 mg followed by an additional 25 mg in 1 hr if no withdrawal symptoms occur. **Maintenance:** 50 mg/day.

Alternate dosing schedule for blockade of opiate actions.

The weekly dose of 350 mg may be given as: (a) 50 mg/day on weekdays and 100 mg on Saturday; (b) 100 mg/48 hr; (c) 100 mg every Monday and Wednesday and 150 mg on Friday; or, (d) 150 mg q 72 hr.

Alcoholism.

50 mg once daily for up to 12 weeks. Treatment for longer than 12 weeks has not been studied.

How Supplied: *Tablet:* 50 mg

Side Effects: *CNS:* Headache, anxiety, nervousness, sleep disorders, dizziness, change in energy level, depression, confusion, restlessness, disorientation, hallucinations, nightmares, bad dreams, paranoia, fatigue, drowsiness. *GI:* N&V, diarrhea, constipation, anorexia, abdominal pain or cramps, flatulence, ulcers, increased appetite, weight gain or loss, increased thirst, xerostomia, hemorrhoids. *CV:* Phlebitis, edema, increased BP, changes in ECG, palpitations, epistaxis, tachycardia. *GU:* Delayed ejaculation, increased urinary frequency or urinary discomfort, increased or decreased interest in sex. *Respiratory:* Cough, sore throat, nasal congestion, rhinorrhea, sneezing, excess secretions, hoarseness, SOB, heaving breathing, sinus trouble. *Dermatologic:* Rash, oily skin, itching, pruritus, acne, cold sores, alopecia, athlete's foot. *Musculoskeletal:* Joint/muscle pain, muscle twitches, tremors, pain in legs, knees, or shoulders. *Ophthalmologic:* Blurred vision, aching or strained eyes, burning eyes, light-sensitive eyes, swollen eyes. *Other:* Hepatotoxicity, tinnitus, painful or clogged ears, chills, swollen glands, inguinal pain, cold feet, "hot" spells, "pounding" head, fever, yawning, side pains.

A severe narcotic withdrawal syndrome may be precipitated if naltrexone is administered to a dependent individual. The syndrome may begin within 5 min and may last for up to 2 days.

EMS CONSIDERATIONS

See also *Narcotic Antagonists.*

Naproxen
Naproxen sodium
(nah-PROX-en)
Pregnancy Class: B
Naproxen (EC-Naprosyn, Naprosyn, Napron X **(Rx)** Naproxen sodium (Anaprox, Anaprox DS, Naprelan **(Rx)**)
Classification: Nonsteroidal, antiinflammatory analgesic

Onset of Action: Immediate release for analgesia: 1-2 hr; **both immediate and delayed release:** 30 min; **anti-inflammatory effects:** up to 2 weeks.
Duration of Action: Analgesia: Approximately 7 hr; **both immediate**

and delayed release: 24 hr; **anti-inflammatory effects:** 2-4 weeks.
Uses: Rx. Mild to moderate pain. Musculoskeletal and soft tissue inflammation including rheumatoid arthritis, osteoarthritis, bursitis, tendinitis, ankylosing spondylitis. Primary dysmenorrhea, acute gout. Juvenile rheumatoid arthritis (naproxen only). *NOTE:* The delayed-release or enteric-coated products are not recommended for initial treatment of pain because, compared to other naproxen products, absorption is delayed. *Investigational:* Antipyretic in cancer patients, sunburn, acute migraine (sodium salt only), prophylaxis of migraine, migraine due to menses, PMS (sodium salt only). **OTC.** Relief of minor aches and pains due to the common cold, headache, toothache, muscular aches, backache, minor arthritis pain, pain due to menstrual cramps. Decrease fever.

Contraindications: Simultaneous use of naproxen and naproxen sodium. Lactation. Use of delayed-release product for initial treatment of acute pain.
Precautions: Safety and effectiveness of naproxen have not been determined in children less than 2 years of age; the safety and effectiveness of naproxen sodium have not been established in children. Geriatric patients may manifest increased total plasma levels of naproxen.

Route/Dosage ———————
NAPROXEN
• **Oral Suspension, Tablets**
    Rheumatoid arthritis, osteoarthritis, ankylosing spondylitis, pain, dysmenorrhea, acute tendinitis, bursitis.
Adults, individualized, usual: 250–500 mg b.i.d. May increase to 1.5 g for short periods of time. If no improvement is seen within 2 weeks, consider an additional 2-week course of therapy.
    Acute gout.
Adults, initial: 750 mg; **then,** 250 mg naproxen q 8 hr until symptoms subside.

---

bold italic = life threatening side effect

Juvenile rheumatoid arthritis.
Naproxen only, 10 mg/kg/day in two divided doses. If the suspension is used, the following dosage can be used: **13 kg:** 2.5 mL b.i.d.; **25 kg:** 5 mL b.i.d.; **38 kg:** 7.5 mL b.i.d.

• **Delayed Release Tablets**
Rheumatoid arthritis, osteoarthritis, ankylosing spondylitis, pain, dysmenorrhea, acute tendinitis, bursitis.
375–500 mg b.i.d.

NAPROXEN SODIUM
• **Tablets (Rx)**
Rheumatoid arthritis, osteoarthritis, ankylosing spondylitis, pain, dysmenorrhea, acute tendinitis, bursitis.
Adults: 275–550 mg b.i.d. in the morning and evening. May be increased to 1.65 g for short periods of time.
Acute gout.
Adults, initial: 825 mg; **then,** 275 mg q 8 hr until symptoms subside.
Mild to moderate pain, primary dysmenorrhea, acute bursitis and tendinitis.
Adults, initial: 550 mg; **then,** 275 mg q 6–8 hr as needed, not to exceed a total daily dose of 1,375 mg.

• **Controlled Release Tablets**
Rheumatoid arthritis, osteoarthritis, ankylosing spondylitis, pain, dysmenorrhea, acute tendinitis, bursitis.
Adults: 750 mg or 1,000 mg once daily, not to exceed 1,000 mg/day.
Acute gout.
Adults: 1,000 mg once daily. For short periods of time, 1,500 mg may be given.

• **Tablets (OTC)**
Adults: 200 mg q 8–12 hr with a full glass of liquid. For some patients, 400 mg initially followed by 200 mg 12 hr later will provide better relief. Do not exceed 600 mg in a 24-hr period. Do not exceed 200 mg q 12 hr for geriatric patients. Not for use in children less than 12 years of age unless directed by a physician.

How Supplied: Naproxen: *Enteric Coated Tablet:* 375 mg, 500 mg; *Suspension:* 25 mg/mL; *Tablet:* 250 mg, 375 mg, 500 mg Naproxen sodium: *Tablet:* 220 mg, 275 mg, 550 mg; *Tablet, Extended Release:* 375 mg, 500 mg

Drug Interactions
Methotrexate / Possibility of a fatal interaction
Probenecid / ↓ Plasma clearance of naproxen

EMS CONSIDERATIONS

See also *Nonsteroidal Anti-Inflammatory Drugs.*

Naratriptan hydrochloride
(NAR-ah-trip-tan)
Pregnancy Class: C
Amerge **(Rx)**
Classification: Antimigraine drug

Mechanism of Action: Binds to serotonin $5\text{-}HT_{1D}$ and $5\text{-}HT_{1B}$ receptors. Activation of these receptors located on intracranial blood vessels, including those on arteriovenous anastomoses, leads to vasoconstriction and thus relief of migraine. Another possibility is that activation of these receptors on sensory nerve endings in trigeminal system causes inhibition of pro-inflammatory neuropeptide release.

Uses: Acute treatment of migraine attacks in adults with or without aura.

Contraindications: Use for prophylaxis of migraine or for management of hemiplegic or basilar migraine. Use in patients with ischemic cardiac, cerebrovascular, or peripheral vascular syndromes; use in uncontrolled hypertension; severe renal impairment (C_{CR} less than 15 mL/min); severe hepatic impairment; within 24 hr of treatment with another $5\text{-}HT_1$ agonist, dihydroergotamine, or methysergide.

Precautions: Safety and efficacy have not been determined for use in cluster headaches or for use in children. Use with caution during lactation and with diseases that may alter the absorption, metabolism, or excretion of drugs, such as impaired renal or hepatic function.

Route/Dosage

- **Tablets**

Migraine headaches.

Adults: Either 1 mg or 2.5 mg taken with fluid. If headache returns or patient has had only partial response, dose may be repeated once after 4 hr, for maximum of 5 mg in a 24-hr period.

How Supplied: *Tablets:* 1 mg, 2.5 mg

Side Effects: Most common side effects follow. *CNS:* Paresthesia, dizziness, drowsiness, malaise, fatigue. *GI:* Nausea. *Miscellaneous:* Throat and neck symptoms, pain and pressure sensation.

Side effects that occurred in 0.1% to 1% of patients follow. *GI:* Hyposalivation, vomiting, dyspeptic symptoms, diarrhea, GI discomfort and pain, gastroenteritis, constipation. *CNS:* Vertigo, tremors, cognitive function disorders, sleep disorders, disorders of equilibrium, anxiety, depression, detachment. *CV:* Palpitations, increased BP, tachyarrhythmias, syncope, abnormal ECG (PR prolongation, QTc prolongation, ST/T wave abnormalities, premature ventricular contractions, atrial flutter, or atrial fibrillation). *Musculoskeletal:* Muscle pain, arthralgia, articular rheumatism, muscle cramps and spasms, joint and muscle stiffness, tightness, and rigidity. *Dermatologic:* Sweating, skin rashes, pruritus, urticaria. *GU:* Bladder inflammation, polyuria, diuresis. *Body as a whole:* Chills, fever, descriptions of odor or taste, edema and swelling, allergies, allergic reactions, warm/cold temperature sensations, feeling strange, burning/stinging sensation. *Respiratory:* Bronchitis, cough, pneumonia. *Ophthalmic:* Photophobia, blurred vision. *ENT:* Ear, nose, and throat infections; phonophobia, sinusitis, upper respiratory inflammation, tinnitus. *Endocrine/Metabolic:* Thirst, polydipsia, dehydration, fluid retention. *Hematologic:* Increased WBCs.

OD Overdose Management: *Symptoms:* Increased BP, chest pain. *Treat-*

ment: Standard supportive treatment. Possible use of antihypertensive therapy. Monitor ECG if chest pain presents.

Drug Interactions

Dihydroergotamine / Prolonged vasospastic reaction; effects additive
Methysergide / Prolonged vasospastic reaction; effects additive
Oral contraceptives / ↑ Mean plasma levels of naratriptan
Selective serotonin reuptake inhibitors / Possible weakness, hyperreflexia, and incoordination
Serotonin 5-HT$_1$ agonists / Additive effects

EMS CONSIDERATIONS

None.

Natamycin
(nah-tah-MY-sin)
Pregnancy Class: C
Natacyn **(Rx)**
Classification: Antifungal (ophthalmic)

Mechanism of Action: Antifungal antibiotic derived from *Streptomyces natalensis.* Binds to the fungal cell membrane, resulting in alteration of permeability and loss of essential intracellular materials. Is fungicidal.

Uses: For ophthalmic use only. Drug of choice for *Fusarium solanae* keratitis. For treatment of fungal blepharitis, conjunctivitis, and keratitis caused by susceptible organisms. It is active against a variety of yeasts and filamentous fungi including *Candida, Aspergillus, Cephalosporium, Fusarium,* and *Penicillium.* Before initiating therapy, determine the susceptibility of the infectious organism to drug in smears and cultures of corneal scrapings. Effectiveness of natamycin for use as single agent in fungal endophthalmitis not established.

Contraindications: Hypersensitivity to drug.

Precautions: Use with caution during lactation. Effectiveness as a single agent to treat fungal endophthalmitis has not been established. Safety and effectiveness have not been determined in children.

Route/Dosage
• **Ophthalmic Suspension (5%)**
   Fungal keratitis.
Initially, 1 gtt in conjunctival sac q 1–2 hr; can be reduced usually, after 3–4 days to 1 gtt 6–8 times/day. Continue therapy for 14–21 days, during which dosage can be reduced gradually at 4 to 7-day intervals.
   Fungal blepharitis/conjunctivitis.
1 gtt 4–6 times/day.
How Supplied: *Suspension:* 5%
Side Effects: Eye irritation, occasional allergies.

EMS CONSIDERATIONS

See also *Anti-Infectives.*

Nedocromil sodium
(neh-DAH-droh-mill)
Pregnancy Class: B
Tilade **(Rx)**
Classification: Antiasthmatic

Mechanism of Action: Inhibits the release of various mediators, such as histamine, leukotriene C_4, and prostaglandin D_2, from a variety of cell types associated with asthma. Has no intrinsic bronchodilator, antihistamine, or glucocorticoid activity.
Uses: Maintenance therapy in adults and children (age six and older) with mild to moderate bronchial asthma.
Contraindications: Use for the reversal of acute bronchospasms, especially status asthmaticus.
Precautions: Use with caution during lactation. Safety and efficacy have not been established in children less than 12 years of age. Has not been shown to be able to substitute for the total dose of corticosteroids.

Route/Dosage
• **Metered Dose Inhaler**
   Bronchial asthma.
Adults and children over 12 years of age: Two inhalations q.i.d. at regular intervals in order to provide 14 mg/day. If the patient is under good control on q.i.d. dosing (i.e., requir-

ing inhaled or oral beta agonist no more than twice a week or no worsening of symptoms occur with respiratory infections), a lower dose can be tried. In such instances, reduce the dose to 10.5 mg/day (i.e., used t.i.d.); then, after several weeks with good control, the dose can be reduced to 7 mg/day (i.e., used b.i.d.).
How Supplied: *Metered dose inhaler:* 1.75 mg/inh
Side Effects: *Respiratory:* Coughing, pharyngitis, rhinitis, URTI, increased sputum, bronchitis, dyspnea, **bronchospasm.** *GI tract:* N&V, dyspepsia, abdominal pain, dry mouth, diarrhea. *CNS:* Dizziness, dysphonia. *Skin:* Rash, sensation of warmth. *Body as a whole:* Headache, chest pain, fatigue, arthritis. *Miscellaneous:* Viral infection, unpleasant taste.

EMS CONSIDERATIONS
None.

Nefazodone hydrochloride
(nih-FAY-zoh-dohn)
Pregnancy Class: C
Serzone **(Rx)**
Classification: Antidepressant

Mechanism of Action: Exact antidepressant mechanism not known. Inhibits neuronal uptake of serotonin and norepinephrine and antagonizes central 5-HT$_2$ receptors and alpha-1-adrenergic receptors (which may cause postural hypotension). Produces none to slight anticholinergic effects, moderate sedation, and slight orthostatic hypotension.
Uses: Maintenance treatment of depression and for depression in hospitalized patients.
Contraindications: Use with terfenadine or astemizole; in combination with an MAO inhibitor or within 14 days of discontinuing MAO inhibitor therapy. Patients hypersensitive to nefazodone or other phenylpiperazine antidepressants.
Precautions: Use with caution in patients with a recent history of MI, unstable heart disease and taking di-

goxin, or a history of mania. Use with caution during lactation. Safety and efficacy have not been determined in individuals below 18 years of age. There is a possibility of a suicide attempt in depression that may persist until significant remission occurs.

Route/Dosage
• **Tablets**
Antidepressant.
Adults, initial: 200 mg/day given in two divided doses. Increase dose in increments of 100–200 mg/day at intervals of no less than 1 week. The effective dose range is 300–600 mg/day. The initial dose for elderly or debilitated patients is 100 mg/day given in two divided doses.
How Supplied: *Tablet:* 100 mg, 150 mg, 200 mg, 250 mg

Side Effects: *CNS:* Dizziness, insomnia, agitation, somnolence, lightheadedness, activation of mania or hypomania, confusion, memory impairment, paresthesia, abnormal dreams, decreased concentration, ataxia, incoordination, psychomotor retardation, tremor, hypertonia, decreased libido, vertigo, twitching, depersonalization, hallucinations, *suicide thoughts/attempt,* apathy, euphoria, hostility, abnormal gait, abnormal thinking, derealization, paranoid reaction, dysarthria, myoclonus, *neuroleptic malignant syndrome (rare).* *CV:* Postural hypotension, hypotension, sinus bradycardia, tachycardia, hypertension, syncope, ventricular extrasystoles, angina pectoris, *CVA (rare).* *GI:* Nausea, dry mouth, constipation, dyspepsia, diarrhea, increased appetite, vomiting, eructation, periodontal abscess, gingivitis, colitis, gastritis, mouth ulceration, stomatitis, esophagitis, peptic ulcer, rectal hemorrhage. *Dermatologic:* Pruritus, dry skin, acne, alopecia, urticaria, maculopapular rash, vesiculobullous rash, eczema. *Musculoskeletal:* Asthenia, arthralgia, arthritis, tenosynovitis, muscle stiffness, bursitis. *Respiratory:* Pharyngitis, increased cough, dyspnea, bronchitis, asthma, pneumonia, laryngitis, voice alteration, epistaxis, hiccups. *Hematologic:* Ecchymosis, anemia, leukopenia, lymphadenopathy. *Ophthalmologic:* Blurred vision, abnormal vision, visual field defect, dry eye, eye pain, abnormal accommodation, diplopia, conjunctivitis, mydriasis, keratoconjunctivitis, photophobia, night blindness. *Body as a whole:* Headache, infection, flu syndrome, chills, fever, neck rigidity, allergic reaction, malaise, photosensitivity, facial edema, hangover effect, enlarged abdomen, hernia, pelvic pain, halitosis, cellulitis, weight loss, gout, dehydration. *GU:* Urinary frequency, UTI, urinary retention, vaginitis, breast pain, cystitis, urinary urgency, metrorrhagia, amenorrhea, polyuria, vaginal hemorrhage, breast enlargement, menorrhagia, urinary incontinence, abnormal ejaculation, hematuria, nocturia, kidney calculus. *Miscellaneous:* Peripheral edema, thirst, abnormal LFTs, ear pain, hyperacusis, deafness, taste loss.

OD Overdose Management: *Symptoms:* N&V, somnolence, increased incidence of severity of any of the reported side effects. *Treatment:* Symptomatic and supportive in the cases of hypotension or excessive sedation. Gastric lavage may be used.

Drug Interactions
Alprazolam / ↑ Plasma levels of alprazolam
Astemizole / ↑ Plasma levels of astemizole resulting in QT prolongation and possible serious CV events, including death due to ventricular tachycardia of the torsades de pointes type
Cisapride / ↑ Risk of serious cardiac arrhythmias
Digoxin / ↑ Plasma levels of digoxin
MAO inhibitors / Serious and possibly fatal reactions including symptoms of hyperthermia, rigidity, myoclonus, autonomic instability with possible rigid fluctuations of VS, and mental status changes that may include extreme agitation progressing to delirium and coma

N

---

bold italic = life threatening side effect

Propranolol / ↓ Plasma levels of propranolol
Terfenadine / ↑ Plasma levels of terfenadine resulting in QT prolongation and possible serious CV events, including death due to ventricular tachycardia of the torsades de pointes type
Triazolam / ↑ Plasma levels of triazolam

EMS CONSIDERATIONS
None.

Nelfinavir mesylate
(nel-FIN-ah-veer)
Pregnancy Class: B
Viracept **(Rx)**
Classification: Antiviral, protease inhibitor

Mechanism of Action: HIV-1 protease inhibitor, resulting in prevention of cleavage of gagpol polyprotein resulting in production of immature, non-infectious viruses. Activity is increased when used with didanosine, lamivudine, stavudine, zalcitabine, or zidovudine.
Uses: Treat HIV infection when antiretroviral therapy is required.
Contraindications: Administration with astemizole, cisapride, midazolam, rifampin, terfenadine, or triazolam.
Precautions: Use with caution with hepatic impairment. Safety and efficacy have not been determined in children less than 2 years of age.

Route/Dosage
• **Powder, Tablets**
  HIV.
Adults: 750 mg (i.e., 3-250 mg tablets) t.i.d. in combination with nucleoside analogs. **Children, 2 to 13 years:** 20-30 mg/kg/dose t.i.d.
How Supplied: *Powder for Reconstitution:* 50 mg/1 g; *Suspension:* 50 mg/5 mL; *Tablets:* 250 mg
Side Effects: Side effects were determined when used in combination with other antiviral drugs. *GI:* N&V, diarrhea, flatulence, abdominal pain, anorexia, dyspepsia, epigastric pain,

GI bleeding, hepatitis, mouth ulcers, pancreatitis. *CNS:* Anxiety, depression, dizziness, emotional lability, hyperkinesia, insomnia, migraine, paresthesia, *seizures,* sleep disorder, somnolence, *suicide ideation. Hematologic:* Anemia, leukopenia, thrombocytopenia. *Respiratory:* Dyspnea, rhinitis, sinusitis, pharyngitis. *GU:* Kidney calculus, sexual dysfunction, urine abnormality. *Ophthalmic:* Eye disorder, acute iritis. *Musculoskeletal:* Arthralgia, arthritis, cramps, myalgia, myasthenia, myopathy. *Dermatologic:* Dermatitis, folliculitis, fungal dermatitis, maculopapular rash, pruritus, urticaria, sweating. *Miscellaneous:* Asthenia, dehydration, allergic reaction, back pain, fever, headache, malaise, pain, accidental injury.
OD **Overdose Management:** *Symptoms:* See side effects. *Treatment:* Emesis or gastric lavage, followed by activated charcoal.
Drug Interactions
Anticonvulsants / Possible ↓ plasma levels of nelfinavir
Astemizole / Potential for serious and life-threatening cardiac arrhythmias
Didanosine / ↓ Absorption of nelfinavir
Indinavir / Significant ↑ in nelfinavir levels
Oral contraceptives / ↓ Effect of oral contraceptives; use alternative contraceptive measures
Rifabutin / ↑ Levels of rifabutin; reduce dose of rifabutin by one-half
Rifampin / Significant ↓ in nelfinavir levels; do not coadminister
Terfenadine / Potential for serious and life-threatening cardiac arrhythmias

EMS CONSIDERATIONS
See also *Antiviral Drugs.*

Neomycin sulfate
(nee-oh-MY-sin)
Pregnancy Class: D
Mycifradin Sulfate, Myciguent, Neobiotic **(Rx)**
Classification: Antibiotic, aminoglycoside

Uses: PO: Hepatic coma, sterilization of gut prior to surgery, inhibition of ammonia-forming bacteria in GI tract in hepatic encephalopathy. Therapy of intestinal infections due to pathogenic strains of *Escherichia coli,* primarily in children. *Investigational:* Hypercholesterolemia.

Topical: Prophylaxis or treatment of infection in burns, minor cuts, wounds, and skin abrasions. As an aid to healing and for treating superficial skin infections.

Contraindications: Additional: Intestinal obstruction (PO). Use of topical products in or around the eyes.

Precautions: Safe use during pregnancy has not been determined. Due to the possibility of toxicity, some recommend not to use parenteral neomycin for any purpose. Use with caution in patients with extensive burns, trophic ulceration, or other conditions where significant systemic absorption is possible.

Route/Dosage ———————
• **Oral Solution**
   Preoperatively in colorectal surgery.
1 g each of neomycin and erythromycin base for a total of three doses: the first two doses 1 hr apart the afternoon before surgery and the third dose at bedtime the night before surgery.
   Hepatic coma, adjunct.
Adults, 4–12 g/day in divided doses for 5–6 days; **children:** 50–100 mg/kg/day in divided doses for 5–6 days.

• **Topical Cream, Ointment**
Neomycin alone or in combination with other antibiotics (bacitracin or gramicidin) and/or an anti-inflammatory agent (corticosteroid). Apply ointment (0.5%) or cream (0.5%) 1–3 times/day to affected area. If necessary, a bandage may be used to cover the area.

How Supplied: *Cream:* 5 mg/g; *Ointment:* 5 mg/g; *Solution:* 125 mg/5 mL; *Tablet:* 500 mg

Side Effects: Chronic use of topical neomycin to inflamed skin of those with contact dermatitis and chronic dermatosis increases the chance of hypersensitivity. Ototoxicity, nephrotoxicity. Sprue-like syndrome with steatorrhea, malabsorption, and electrolyte imbalance. Skin rashes after topical or parenteral administration. Chronic use in allergic contact dermatitis and chronic dermatoses increases the risk of sensitization.

Drug Interactions: Additional: *Digoxin/* ↓ Effect of digoxin due to ↓ absorption from GI tract. *Penicillin V/* ↓ Effect of penicillin due to ↓ absorption from GI tract. *Procainamide/* ↑ Muslce relaxation produced by neomycin.

EMS CONSIDERATIONS
None.

Neostigmine bromide
Neostigmine methylsulfate
(nee-oh-STIG-meen)
Pregnancy Class: C
Bromide (Prostigmin Bromide **(Rx)**)Methylsulfate (Prostigmin Injection **(Rx)** Bromide (Prostigmin Bromide **(Rx)**)
Classification: Indirectly acting cholinergic-acetylcholinesterase inhibitor

Mechanism of Action: Acetylcholinesterase inhibitor that causes an increase in the concentration of acetylcholine at the myoneural junction, thus facilitating transmission of impulses across the myoneural junction. In myasthenia gravis, muscle strength is increased. May also act on the autonomic ganglia of the CNS. Prevents or relieves postoperative distention by increasing gastric motility and tone and prevents or relieves urinary retention by increasing the tone of the detrusor muscle of the bladder. Shorter acting than ambenonium chloride and pyridostigmine. Atropine is often given concomitantly to control side effects.

N

---
bold italic = life threatening side effect

Onset of Action: PO: 45-75 min; **IM:** 20-30 min; **IV:** 4-8 min; **Time to peak effect, parenteral:** 20-30 min. **Duration of Action:** All routes, 2.5-4 hr.

Uses: Diagnosis and treatment of myasthenia gravis. Prophylaxis and treatment of postoperative distention or urinary retention. Antidote for tubocurarine and other nondepolarizing drugs.

Contraindications: Hypersensitivity, mechanical obstruction of GI or urinary tract, peritonitis, history of bromide sensitivity. Vesical neck obstruction of urinary bladder. Lactation.

Precautions: Safety and effectiveness in children have not been established. Use with caution in patients with bronchial asthma, bradycardia, vagotonia, epilepsy, hyperthyroidism, peptic ulcer, cardiac arrhythmias, or recent coronary occlusion. May cause uterine irritability and premature labor if given IV to pregnant women near term. In geriatric patients, the duration of action may be increased.

N

Route/Dosage
NEOSTIGMINE BROMIDE
• **Tablets**
Treat myasthenia gravis.
Adults: 15 mg q 3–4 hr; adjust dose and frequency as needed. **Usual maintenance:** 150 mg/day with dosing intervals determined by patient response. **Pediatric,** 2 mg/kg (60 mg/m²) daily in six to eight divided doses.

NEOSTIGMINE METHYLSULFATE
• **IM, IV, SC**
Diagnosis of myasthenia gravis.
Adults, IM, SC: 1.5 mg given with 0.6 mg atropine; **pediatric, IM:** 0.04 mg/kg (1 mg/m²); or, **IV:** 0.02 mg/kg (0.5 mg/m²).
Treat myasthenia gravis.
Adults, IM, SC: 0.5 mg. **Pediatric, IM, SC:** 0.01–0.04 mg/kg q 2–3 hr.
Antidote for tubocurarine.
Adults, IV: 0.5–2 mg slowly with 0.6–1.2 mg atropine sulfate. Can repeat if necessary up to total dose of 5 mg. **Pediatric, IV:** 0.04 mg/kg with 0.02 mg/kg atropine sulfate.

Prevention of postoperative GI distention or urinary retention.
Adults, IM, SC: 0.25 mg (1 mL of the 1:4,000 solution) immediately after surgery repeated q 4–6 hr for 2–3 days.
Treatment of postoperative GI distention.
Adults, IM, SC: 0.5 mg (1 mL of the 1:2,000 solution) as required.
Treatment of urinary retention.
Adults, IM, SC: 0.5 mg (1 mL of the 1:2,000 solution). If urination does not occur within 1 hr after 0.5 mg, the patient should be catheterized. After the bladder is emptied, 0.5 mg is given q 3 hr for at least five injections.

How Supplied: Neostigmine bromide: *Tablet:* 15 mg. Neostigmine methylsulfate: *Injection:* 0.5 mg/mL, 1 mg/mL

Side Effects: *GI:* N&V, diarrhea, abdominal cramps, involuntary defecation, salivation, dysphagia, flatulence, increased gastric and intestinal secretions. *CV:* Bradycardia, tachycardia, hypotension, ECG changes, nodal rhythm, *cardiac arrest,* syncope, *AV block,* substernal pain, thrombophlebitis after IV use. *CNS:* Headache, *seizures,* malaise, weakness, dysarthria, dizziness, drowsiness, loss of consciousness. *Respiratory:* Increased oral, pharyngeal, and bronchial secretions; *bronchospasms, skeletal muscle paralysis, laryngospasm, central respiratory paralysis, respiratory depression or arrest,* dyspnea. *Ophthalmologic:* Miosis, double vision, lacrimation, accommodation difficulties, hyperemia of conjunctiva, visual changes. *Musculoskeletal:* Muscle fasciculations or weakness, muscle cramps or spasms, arthralgia. *Other:* Skin rashes, urinary frequency and incontinence, sweating, flushing, allergic reactions, anaphylaxis, urticaria. These effects can usually be reversed by parenteral administration of 0.6 mg of atropine sulfate, which should be readily available.

Cholinergic crisis, due to overdosage, must be distinguished from myasthenic crisis (worsening of the disease), since cholinergic crisis involves removal of drug therapy, while myasthenic crisis involves an increase in anticholinesterase therapy.

OD Overdose Management: *Symptoms:* Abdominal cramps, vomiting, diarrhea, epigastric distress, excessive salivation, cold sweating, pallor, blurred vision, urinary urgency, fasciculation and *paralysis of voluntary muscles (including the tongue),* miosis, increased BP (may be accompanied by bradycardia), sensation of internal trembling, panic, severe anxiety. *Treatment:* Discontinue medication temporarily. Give atropine, 0.5–1 mg IV (up to 5–10 or more mg may be needed to get the HR to 80 beats/min). Supportive treatment including artificial respiration and oxygen.

Drug Interactions
Aminoglycosides / ↑ Neuromuscular blockade
Atropine / Atropine suppresses symptoms of excess GI stimulation caused by cholinergic drugs
Corticosteroids / ↓ Effect of neostigmine
Magnesium salts / Antagonize the effects of anticholinesterases
Mecamylamine / Intense hypotensive response
Organophosphate-type insecticides/pesticides / Added systemic effects with cholinesterase inhibitors
Succinylcholine / ↑ Neuromuscular blocking effects

EMS CONSIDERATIONS
None.

Nevirapine
(neh-VYE-rah-peen)
Pregnancy Class: C
Viramune **(Rx)**
Classification: Antiviral

Mechanism of Action: By binding tightly to reverse transcriptase, nevirapine prevents viral RNA from being converted into DNA. In combination with a nucleoside analogue, it reduces the amount of virus circulating in the body and increases CD4+ cell counts.

Uses: In combination with nucleoside analogues (e.g., AZT, lamivudine, didanosine, zalcitabine) or protease inhibitors (e.g., saquinavir, indinavir, ritonavir) for the treatment of HIV-1 infections in adults who have experienced clinical and immunologic deterioration. Always use in combination with at least one other antiretroviral agent, as resistant viruses emerge rapidly when nevirapine is used alone.

Contraindications: Lactation.

Precautions: The duration of benefit from therapy may be limited. Is not a cure for HIV infections; patients may continue to experience illnesses associated with HIV infections, including opportunistic infections. Has not been shown to reduce the risk of transmitting HIV to others through sexual contact or blood contamination. Use with caution in impaired renal or hepatic function.

Route/Dosage
• **Suspension, Tablets**
  HIV-1 infections.
Initial: 200 mg/day for 14 days.
Maintenance: 200 mg b.i.d. (e.g., 7:00 a.m. and 7:00 p.m.) in combination with a nucleoside analogue antiretroviral agent.

How Supplied: *Suspension:* 50 mg/5 mL; *Tablet:* 200 mg

Side Effects: *GI:* Nausea, abnormal LFTs, diarrhea, abdominal pain, ulcerative stomatitis, hepatitis. *CNS:* Headache, fatigue, paresthesia. *Hematologic:* Decreased hemoglobin, decreased platelets, decreased neutrophils. *Miscellaneous:* **Rash (may be severe and life-threatening),** fever, peripheral neuropathy, myalgia.

Drug Interactions
Oral contraceptives / ↓ Plasma levels of oral contraceptives → ↓ effect
Protease inhibitors / ↓ Plasma levels of protease inhibitors
Rifabutin / ↓ Nevirapine trough concentrations
Rifampin / Nevirapine trough concentrations

N

---

bold italic = life threatening side effect

EMS CONSIDERATIONS

See also *Antiviral Drugs,* and *Anti-Infectives,* .

Niacin (Nicotinic acid) Niacinamide

Niacin (Nicotinic acid): (NYE-ah-sin, nih-koh-TIN-ick AH-sid)Niacinamide: (nye-ah-SIN-ah-myd)
Pregnancy Class: C
Niacin (Nia-Bid, Niaspan, Nico-400, Nicobid, Nicolar, Nicotinex, Slo-Niacin, SpanNiacin, Tega-Span (Rx and OTC) Niacinamide (Rx; injection; OTC; tablets)
Classification: Vitamin B complex

Mechanism of Action: Niacin (nicotinic acid) and niacinamide are water-soluble, heat-resistant vitamins prepared synthetically. Niacin (after conversion to the active niacinamide) is a component of the coenzymes nicotinamide-adenine dinucleotide and nicotinamide-adenine dinucleotide phosphate, which are essential for oxidation-reduction reactions involved in lipid metabolism, glycogenolysis, and tissue respiration. Deficiency of niacin results in pellagra, the most common symptoms of which are dermatitis, diarrhea, and dementia. In high doses niacin also produces vasodilation. Reduces serum cholesterol and triglycerides in types II, III, IV, and V hyperlipoproteinemia (mechanism unknown).
Uses: Prophylaxis and treatment of pellagra; niacin deficiency. Treat hyperlipidemia in patients not responding to either diet or weight loss. Reduce the risk of recurrent nonfatal MI and promote regression of atherosclerosis when combined with bile-binding resins.
Contraindications: Severe hypotension, hemorrhage, arterial bleeding, liver dysfunction, active peptic ulcer. Use of the extended-release tablets and capsules in children.
Precautions: Extended-release niacin may be hepatotoxic. Use with caution in diabetics, gall bladder disease, in

those who consume a large amount of alcohol, and patients with gout.

Route/Dosage ————————
NIACIN
• **Extended-Release Capsules, Tablets, Extended-Release Tablets, Capsules, Elixir**
Vitamin.
Adults: Up to 500 mg/day; **pediatric:** Up to 300 mg/day.
Antihyperlipidemic.
Adults, initial: 1 g t.i.d.; **then:** increase dose in increments of 500 mg/day q 2–4 weeks as needed. **Maintenance:** 1–2 g t.i.d. (up to a maximum of 8 g/day). **Niaspan:** Week 1, 375 mg hs; week 2, 500 mg; week 3, 750 mg hs; then, dose may be increased by no more than 500 mg in any 4- week period; do not give doses greater than 2,000 mg/day.
• **IM, IV**
Pellagra.
Adults, IM: 50–100 mg 5 or more times/day. **IV, slow:** 25–100 mg 2 or more times/day. **Pediatric, IV slow:** Up to 300 mg/day.
NIACINAMIDE
• **Tablets**
Vitamin.
Adults: Up to 500 mg/day. **Pediatric:** Up to 300 mg/day. Capsules not recommended for use in children.
How Supplied: Niacin: *Capsule:* 100 mg; *Capsule, Extended Release:* 125 mg, 250 mg, 400 mg, 500 mg, 750 mg; *Elixir:* 50 mg/5 mL; *Tablet:* 50 mg, 100 mg, 250 mg, 500 mg; *Tablet, Extended Release:* 500 mg, 750 mg, 1,000 mg. Niacinamide: *Tablet:* 50 mg, 100 mg, 500 mg
Side Effects: *GI:* N&V, diarrhea, peptic ulcer activation, abdominal pain. *Dermatologic:* Flushing, warm feeling, skin rash, pruritus, dry skin, itching and tingling feeling, keratosis nigricans. *Other:* Hypotension, headache, macular cystoid edema, amblyopia. *NOTE:* Megadoses are accompanied by serious toxicity including the symptoms listed in the preceding as well as liver damage, hyperglycemia, hyperuricemia, arrhythmias, tachycardia, and dermatoses.

Drug Interactions

Chenodiol / ↓ Effect of chenodiol

Probenecid / Niacin may ↓ uricosuric effect of probenecid

Sulfinpyrazone / Niacin ↓ uricosuric effect of sulfinpyrazone

Sympathetic blocking agents / Additive vasodilating effects → postural hypotension

EMS CONSIDERATIONS

None.

Nicardipine hydrochloride

(nye-KAR-dih-peen)

Pregnancy Class: C

Cardene, Cardene IV, Cardene SR **(Rx)**

Classification: Calcium channel blocking agent (antianginal, antihypertensive)

Mechanism of Action: Moderately increases CO and significantly decreases peripheral vascular resistance.

Onset of Action: 20 min; **Maximum BP lowering effects, immediate release:** 1-2 hr; **maximum BP lowering effects, sustained release:** 2-6 hr.

Duration of Action: 8 hr.

Uses: Immediate release: Chronic stable angina (effort-associated angina) alone or in combination with beta-adrenergic blocking agents.

Immediate and sustained released: Hypertension alone or in combination with other antihypertensive drugs.

IV: Short-term treatment of hypertension when PO therapy is not desired or possible.

Investigational: CHF.

Contraindications: Use in advanced aortic stenosis due to the effect on reducing afterload. During lactation.

Precautions: Safety and efficacy in children less than 18 years of age have not been established. Use with caution in patients with CHF, especially in combination with a beta blocker due to the possibility of a negative inotropic effect. Use with caution in patients with impaired liver function, reduced hepatic blood flow, or impaired renal function. Initial increase in frequency, duration, or severity of angina.

Route/Dosage

• **Capsules, Immediate Release**

Angina, hypertension.

Initial, usual: 20 mg t.i.d. (range: 20–40 mg t.i.d.). Wait 3 days before increasing dose to ensure steady-state plasma levels.

• **Capsules, Sustained Release**

Hypertension.

Initial: 30 mg b.i.d. (range: 30–60 mg b.i.d.).

NOTE: Initial dose in renal impairment: 20 mg t.i.d. Initial dose in hepatic impairment: 20 mg b.i.d.

• **IV**

Hypertension.

Individualize dose. Initial: 5 mg/hr; the infusion rate may be increased to a maximum of 15 mg/hr (by 2.5-mg/hr increments q 15 min). For a more rapid reduction in BP, initiate at 5 mg/hr but increase the rate q 5 min in 2.5-mg/hr increments until a maximum of 15 mg/hr is reached.

Maintenance: 3 mg/hr. The IV infusion rate to produce an average plasma level similar to a particular PO dose is as follows: 20 mg q 8 hr is equivalent to 0.5 mg/hr; 30 mg q 8 hr is equivalent to 1.2 mg/hr; and 40 mg q 8 hr is equivalent to 2.2 mg/hr.

How Supplied: *Capsule:* 20 mg, 30 mg; *Capsule, Extended Release:* 30 mg, 45 mg, 60 mg; *Injection:* 2.5 mg/mL

Side Effects: *CV:* Pedal edema, flushing, increased angina, palpitations, tachycardia, other edema, abnormal ECG, hypotension, postural hypotension, syncope, *MI, AV block,* ventricular extrasystoles, peripheral vascular disease. *CNS:* Dizziness, headache, somnolence, malaise, nervousness, insomnia, abnormal dreams, vertigo, depression, confusion, amnesia, anx-

N

---

iety, weakness, psychoses, hallucinations, paranoia. *GI:* N&V, dyspepsia, dry mouth, constipation, sore throat. *Neuromuscular:* Asthenia, myalgia, paresthesia, hyperkinesia, arthralgia. *Miscellaneous:* Rash, dyspnea, SOB, nocturia, polyuria, allergic reactions, abnormal liver chemistries, hot flashes, impotence, rhinitis, sinusitis, nasal congestion, chest congestion, tinnitus, equilibrium disturbances, abnormal or blurred vision, infection, atypical chest pain.

OD **Overdose Management:** *Symptoms:* Marked hypotension, bradycardia, palpitations, flushing, drowsiness, confusion, and slurred speech following PO overdose. Lethal overdose may cause systemic hypotension, bradycardia (following initial tachycardia), and progressive AV block. *Treatment:*

• Treatment is supportive. Monitor cardiac and respiratory function.

• If patient is seen soon after ingestion, emetics or gastric lavage should be considered, followed by cathartics.

• *Hypotension:* IV calcium, dopamine, isoproterenol, metaraminol, or norepinephrine. Also, provide IV fluids. Place patient in Trendelenburg position.

• *Ventricular tachycardia:* IV procainamide or lidocaine; cardioversion may be necessary. Also, provide slow-drip IV fluids.

• *Bradycardia, asystole, AV block:* IV atropine sulfate (0.6–1 mg), calcium gluconate (10% solution), isoproterenol, norepinephrine; also, cardiac pacing may be indicated. Provide slow-drip IV fluids.

Drug Interactions
Cimetidine / ↑ Bioavailability of nicardipine → ↑ plasma levels
Cyclosporine / ↑ Plasma levels of cyclosporine possibly leading to renal toxicity
Ranitidine / ↑ Bioavailability of nicardipine

EMS CONSIDERATIONS

See also *Calcium Channel Blocking Agents*.

Nicotine polacrilex (Nicotine Resin Complex)
(NIK-oh-teen)
Pregnancy Class: X
Nicorette, Nicorette DS **(OTC)**
Classification: Smoking deterrent

Mechanism of Action: Following chewing, nicotine is released from an ion exchange resin in the gum product, providing blood nicotine levels approximating those produced by smoking cigarettes. The amount of nicotine released depends on the rate and duration of chewing.

Uses: Adjunct with behavioral modification in smokers wishing to give up the smoking habit. Is considered only as an initial aid, with the ultimate goal being abstention from all forms of nicotine. Most likely to benefit are individuals with the following characteristics:

a. smoke brands of cigarettes containing more than 0.9 mg nicotine;
b. smoke more than 15 cigarettes daily;
c. inhale cigarette smoke deeply and frequently;
d. smoke most frequently during the morning;
e. smoke the first cigarette of the day within 30 min of arising;
f. indicate cigarettes smoked in the morning are the most difficult to give up;
g. smoke even if the individual is ill and confined to bed;
h. find it necessary to smoke in places where smoking is not allowed. *NOTE:* Nicotine may be effective in improving the course of difficult-to-treat ulcerative colitis.

Contraindications: Pregnancy, lactation, nonsmokers, serious arrhythmias, angina, vasospastic disease, active temporomandibular joint disease. Use in individuals less than 18 years of age.

Precautions: Safety and effectiveness in children and adolescents who smoke have not been determined. Use with caution in hypertension, PUD, oral or pharyngeal inflammation, gastritis, stomatitis, hyperthyroidism, IDDM, and pheochromocytoma.

Route/Dosage
• **Gum**
Initial: One piece of gum chewed whenever the urge to smoke occurs; best results are obtained when the gum is chewed on a fixed schedule, at intervals of 1 to 2 hr, with at least 9 pieces chewed per day. **maintenance:** 9–12 pieces of gum daily during the first month, not to exceed 30 pieces daily of the 2-mg strength and 20 pieces daily of the 4-mg strength.

How Supplied: *Gum:* 2 mg, 4 mg

Side Effects: *CNS:* Dizziness, irritability, headache. *GI:* N&V, indigestion, GI upset, salivation, eructation. *Other:* Sore mouth or throat, hiccoughs, sore jaw muscles.

OD **Overdose Management:** *Symptoms: GI:* N&V, diarrhea, salivation, abdominal pain. *CNS:* Headache, dizziness, confusion, weakness, fainting, *seizures. Respiratory:* Labored breathing, *respiratory paralysis (cause of death).* Other: Cold sweat, disturbed hearing and vision, hypotension, and rapid, weak pulse. *Treatment:* Syrup of ipecac if vomiting has not occurred, saline laxative, gastric lavage followed by activated charcoal (if patient is unconscious), maintenance of respiration, maintenance of CV function.

Drug Interactions
Caffeine / Possibly ↓ blood levels of caffeine due to ↑ rate of breakdown by liver
Catecholamines / ↑ Levels of catecholamines
Cortisol / ↑ Levels of cortisol
Furosemide / Possible ↓ diuretic effect of furosemide
Glutethimide / Possible ↓ absorption of glutethimide
Imipramine / Possibly ↓ blood levels of imipramine due to ↑ rate of breakdown by liver
Pentazocine / Possibly ↓ blood levels of pentazocine due to ↑ rate of breakdown by liver

Theophylline / Possibly ↓ blood levels of theophylline due to ↑ rate of breakdown by liver

EMS CONSIDERATIONS
None.

Nicotine transdermal system

(NIK-oh-teen)
Pregnancy Class: D
Habitrol, Prostep **(Rx)**, Nicoderm CQ Step 1, 2, or Step 3, Nicotrol **(OTC)**
Classification: Smoking deterrent

Mechanism of Action: Nicotine transdermal system is a multilayered film that provides systemic delivery of varying amounts of nicotine over a 24-hr period after applying to the skin. Nicotine's reinforcing activity is due to stimulation of the cortex (via the locus ceruleus), producing increased alertness and cognitive performance and a "reward" effect due to an action in the limbic system. At low doses the stimulatory effects predominate, whereas at high doses the reward effects predominate. The nicotine transdermal system produces an initial (first day of use) increase in BP, an increase in HR (3%–7%), and a decrease in SV after 10 days.

Uses: As an aid to stopping smoking for the relief of nicotine withdrawal symptoms. Should be used in conjunction with a comprehensive behavioral smoking cessation program.

Contraindications: Hypersensitivity or allergy to nicotine or any components of the therapeutic system. Use in children and during pregnancy, labor, delivery, and lactation. Use in those with heart disease, hypertension, a recent MI, severe or worsening angina pectoris, those taking certain antidepressants or antiasthmatic drugs, or in severe renal impairment.

Precautions: Encourage pregnant smokers to try to stop smoking using educational and behavioral interventions before using the nicotine transdermal system. Use during pregnan-

N

cy only if the potential benefit outweighs the potential risk of nicotine to the fetus. The use of nicotine transdermal systems for longer than 3 months has not been studied. Before use, screen patients with coronary heart disease (history of MI and/or angina pectoris), serious cardiac arrhythmias, or vasospastic diseases (e.g., Buerger's disease, Prinzmetal's variant angina) carefully. Use with caution in patients with hyperthyroidism, pheochromocytoma, IDDM (nicotine causes the release of catecholamines), in active peptic ulcers, in accelerated hypertension, and during lactation.

Route/Dosage
• **Transdermal System**
HABITROL (Rx)
Healthy patients, initial: 21 mg/day for 4–8 weeks; **then,** 14 mg/day for 2–4 weeks and 7 mg/day for 2–4 weeks. **Light smokers, those who weigh less than 100 lb or who have CV disease:** 14 mg/day for 4–8 weeks; **then,** 7 mg/day for 2–4 weeks.
PROSTEP (Rx)
Patients weighing 100 lb or more: 22 mg/day for 4–8 weeks; **then,** 11 mg/day for 2–4 weeks. **Patients weighing less than 100 lb:** 11 mg/day for 4–8 weeks.
NICODERM CQ (OTC)
Light smokers (10 or less cigarettes/day): One 14-mg/24-hr patch for 16 or 24 hr/day for 6 weeks; **then,** one 7-mg/24-hr patch for 16 or 24 hr/day for 2 weeks. **Heavy smokers (> 10 cigarettes/day):** One 21-mg/24-hr patch for 16 or 24 hr/day for 6 weeks; **then,** one 14-mg/24-hr patch for 16 or 24 hr/day for 2 weeks, followed by one 7-mg/24-hr patch for 16 or 24 hr for 2 weeks.
NICOTROL (OTC)
Those who smoke > 10 cigarettes/day: 15 mg/day for 6 weeks. The patch is to be worn for 16 hr and removed at bedtime.
How Supplied: *Film, Extended Release:* 7 mg/24 hr, 14 mg/24 hr, 15 mg/16 hr, 21 mg/24 hr

Side Effects: *NOTE:* The incidence of side effects is complicated by the fact that patients manifest effects of nicotine withdrawal or by concurrent smoking.
Dermatologic: Erythema, pruritus, or burning at the site of application; cutaneous hypersensitivity, sweating, rash at application site. *Body as a whole:* Allergy, back pain. *GI:* Diarrhea, dyspepsia, dry mouth, abdominal pain, constipation, N&V. *Musculoskeletal:* Arthralgia, myalgia. *CNS:* Abnormal dreams, somnolence, dizziness, impaired concentration, headache, insomnia. *CV:* Tachycardia, hypertension. *Respiratory:* Increased cough, pharyngitis, sinusitis. *GU:* Dysmenorrhea.

OD **Overdose Management:** *Symptoms:* Pallor, cold sweat, N&V, abdominal pain, salivation, diarrhea, headache, dizziness, disturbed hearing and vision, mental confusion, weakness, tremor. Large overdoses may cause prostration, hypotension, *respiratory failure, seizures, and death. Treatment:* Remove the transdermal system immediately. The surface of the skin may be flushed with water and dried; soap should not be used as it may increase the absorption of nicotine. Diazepam or barbiturates may be used to treat seizures and atropine can be given for excessive bronchial secretions or diarrhea. Respiratory support for respiratory failure and fluid support for hypotension and CV collapse. If transdermal systems are ingested PO, activated charcoal should be given to prevent seizures. If the patient is unconscious, the charcoal should be administered by an NGT. A saline cathartic or sorbitol added to the first dose of activated charcoal may hasten GI passage of the system. Doses of activated charcoal should be repeated as long as the system remains in the GI tract as nicotine will continue to be released for many hours.

EMS CONSIDERATIONS
None.

Nifedipine

(nye-FED-ih-peen)
Pregnancy Class: C
Adalat, Adalat CC, Procardia, Procardia XL **(Rx)**
Classification: Calcium channel blocking agent (antianginal, antihypertensive)

Mechanism of Action: Variable effects on AV node effective and functional refractory periods. CO is moderately increased while peripheral vascular resistance is significantly decreased.
Onset of Action: 20 min.
Duration of Action: 4-8 hr (12 hr for extended-release).
Uses: Vasospastic (Prinzmetal's or variant) angina. Chronic stable angina without vasospasm, including angina due to increased effort (especially in patients who cannot take beta blockers or nitrates or who remain symptomatic following clinical doses of these drugs). Essential hypertension (sustained-release only). *Investigational:* PO, sublingually, or chewed in hypertensive emergencies. Also prophylaxis of migraine headaches, primary pulmonary hypertension, severe pregnancy-associated hypertension, esophageal diseases, Raynaud's phenomenon, CHF, asthma, premature labor, biliary and renal colic, and cardiomyopathy. To prevent strokes and to decrease the risk of CHF in geriatric hypertensives.
Contraindications: Hypersensitivity. Lactation.
Precautions: Use with caution in impaired hepatic or renal function and in elderly patients. Initial increase in frequency, duration, or severity of angina (may also be seen in patients being withdrawn from beta blockers and who begin taking nifedipine).

Route/Dosage
• **Capsules**
Individualized. Initial: 10 mg t.i.d. (range: 10–20 mg t.i.d.); **maintenance:** 10–30 mg t.i.d.–q.i.d. Patients with coronary artery spasm

may respond better to 20–30 mg t.i.d.–q.i.d. Doses greater than 120 mg/day are rarely needed while doses greater than 180 mg/day are not recommended.
• **Sustained-Release Tablets**
Initial: 30 or 60 mg once daily for Procardia XL and 30 mg once daily for Adalat CC. Titrate over a 7- to 14-day period. Dosage can be increased as required and as tolerated, to a maximum of 120 mg/day for Procardia XL and 90 mg/day for Adalat CC.
Investigational, hypertensive emergencies.
10–20 mg given PO (capsule is punctured several times and then chewed).
How Supplied: *Capsule:* 10 mg, 20 mg; *Tablet, Extended Release:* 30 mg, 60 mg, 90 mg
Side Effects: *CV:* Peripheral and pulmonary edema, MI, hypotension, palpitations, syncope, CHF (especially if used with a beta blocker), decreased platelet aggregation, arrhythmias, tachycardia. Increased frequency, length, and duration of angina when beginning nifedipine therapy. *GI:* Nausea, diarrhea, constipation, flatulence, abdominal cramps, dysgeusia, vomiting, dry mouth, eructation, gastroesophageal reflux, melena. *CNS:* Dizziness, lightheadedness, giddiness, nervousness, sleep disturbances, headache, weakness, depression, migraine, psychoses, hallucinations, disturbances in equilibrium, somnolence, insomnia, abnormal dreams, malaise, anxiety. *Dermatologic:* Rash, dermatitis, urticaria, pruritus, photosensitivity, erythema multiforme, *Stevens-Johnson syndrome.* *Respiratory:* Dyspnea, cough, wheezing, SOB, respiratory infection, throat, nasal, or chest congestion. *Musculoskeletal:* Muscle cramps or inflammation, joint pain or stiffness, arthritis, ataxia, myoclonic dystonia, hypertonia, asthenia. *Hematologic:* Thrombocytopenia, leukopenia, purpura, anemia. *Other:* Fever, chills, sweating, blurred vision, sexual difficulties, flushing, transient blindness,

N

---

bold italic = life threatening side effect

hyperglycemia, hypokalemia, gingival hyperplasia, allergic hepatitis, hepatitis, tinnitus, gynecomastia, polyuria, nocturia, erythromelalgia, weight gain, epistaxis, facial and periorbital edema, hypoesthesia, gout, abnormal lacrimation, breast pain, dysuria, hematuria.

EMS CONSIDERATIONS

See also *Calcium Channel Blocking Agents.*

Nilutamide
(nye-LOO-tah-myd)
Pregnancy Class: C
Nilanderon **(Rx)**
Classification: Antineoplastic, hormone

Mechanism of Action: Antiandrogen activity with no estrogen, progesterone, mineralocorticoid, or glucocorticoid effects. Binds to the androgen receptor, thus preventing the normal androgenic response.
Uses: In combination with surgical castration for the treatment of metastatic prostate cancer (stage D_2).
Contraindications: Severe hepatic impairment, severe respiratory insufficiency, hypersensitivity to nilutamide.
Precautions: Many patients experience a delay in adaptation to the dark ranging from seconds to a few minutes. Safety and efficacy have not been determined in children.

Route/Dosage ———————
• **Tablets**
   Metastatic prostate cancer.
300 mg (six 50-mg tablets) once daily for 30 days followed by 150 mg (three 50-mg tablets) once daily.
How Supplied: *Tablet:* 50 mg
Side Effects: *GI:* Nausea, constipation, dry mouth, diarrhea, hepatitis, GI disorder, *GI hemorrhage,* melena. *CNS:* Dizziness, paresthesia, nervousness. *CV:* Hypertension, *heart failure,* angina, syncope. *Respiratory:* Interstitial pneumonitis, dyspnea, lung disorder, increased cough, rhinitis. *Metabolic/nutritional:* Edema, weight loss, intolerance to alcohol. *Ophthalmic:* Cataract, photophobia, impaired adaptation to dark, abnormal vision. *Miscellaneous:* Leukopenia, hot flushes, UTI, malaise, pruritus, arthritis, aplastic anemia (rare).
Drug Interactions
Phenytoin / ↓ Metabolism of phenytoin → delayed elimination and ↑ risk of toxicity
Theophylline / Metabolism of theophylline delayed elimination and risk of toxicity
Vitamin K antagonists / Metabolism of vitamin K antagonists delayed elimination and risk of toxicity

EMS CONSIDERATIONS

None.

Nimodipine
(nye-MOH-dih-peen)
Pregnancy Class: C
Nimotop **(Rx)**
Classification: Calcium channel blocking agent

Mechanism of Action: Has a greater effect on cerebral arteries than arteries elsewhere in the body (probably due to its highly lipophilic properties). Mechanism to reduce neurologic deficits following subarachnoid hemorrhage not known.
Uses: Improvement of neurologic deficits due to spasm following subarachnoid hemorrhage from ruptured congenital intracranial aneurysms; patients should have Hunt and Hess grades of I–III. *Investigational:* Migraine headaches and cluster headaches.
Contraindications: Lactation.
Precautions: Safety and efficacy have not been established in children. Use with caution in patients with impaired hepatic function and reduced hepatic blood flow. The half-life may be increased in geriatric patients.

Route/Dosage ———————
• **Capsules**
Adults: 60 mg q 4 hr beginning within 96 hr after subarachnoid hemorrhage and continuing for 21 consecutive days. Reduce the dose to 30 mg q 4 hr in patients with hepatic impairment.

How Supplied: *Capsule:* 30 mg
Side Effects: *CV:* Hypotension, peripheral edema, CHF, ECG abnormalities, tachycardia, bradycardia, palpitations, rebound vasospasm, hypertension, hematoma, **DIC, DVT.** *GI:* Nausea, dyspepsia, diarrhea, abdominal discomfort, cramps, **GI hemorrhage,** vomiting. *CNS:* Headache, depression, lightheadedness, dizziness. *Hepatic:* Abnormal LFT, hepatitis, jaundice. *Hematologic:* Thrombocytopenia, anemia, purpura, ecchymosis. *Dermatologic:* Rash, dermatitis, pruritus, urticaria. *Miscellaneous:* Dyspnea, muscle pain or cramps, acne, itching, flushing, diaphoresis, wheezing, hyponatremia.

EMS CONSIDERATIONS

See also *Calcium Channel Blocking Agents.*

Nisoldipine
(NYE-sohl-dih-peen)
Pregnancy Class: C
Sular **(Rx)**
Classification: Calcium channel blocking drug

Mechanism of Action: Inhibits the transmembrane influx of calcium into vascular smooth muscle and cardiac muscle, resulting in dilation of arterioles. Has greater potency on vascular smooth muscle than on cardiac muscle. Chronic use results in a sustained decrease in vascular resistance and small increases in SI and LV ejection fraction. Weak diuretic effect and no clinically important chronotropic effects.
Uses: Treatment of hypertension alone or in combination with other antihypertensive drugs.
Contraindications: Use with grapefruit juice as it interferes with metabolism, resulting in a significant increase in plasma levels of the drug. Use in those with known hypersensitivity to dihydropyridine calcium channel blockers. Lactation.
Precautions: Geriatric patients may show a two- to threefold higher plasma concentration; use caution in

dosing. Use with caution and at lower doses in those with hepatic insufficiency. Use with caution in patients with CHF or compromised ventricular function, especially in combination with a beta blocker.

Route/Dosage
• **Tablets, Extended-Release**
Hypertension.
Dose must be adjusted to the needs of each person. **Initial:** 20 mg once daily; **then,** increase by 10 mg/week or longer intervals to reach adequate BP control. **Usual maintenance:** 20–40 mg once daily. Doses beyond 60 mg once daily are not recommended. **Initial dose, patients over 65 years and those with impaired renal function:** 10 mg once daily.
How Supplied: *Extended-Release Tablets:* 10 mg, 20 mg, 30 mg, 40 mg.
Side Effects: *CV:* Increased angina and/or MI in patients with CAD. Initially, excessive hypotension, especially in those taking other antihypertensive drugs. Vasodilation, palpitation, atrial fibrillation, **CVA, MI,** CHF, first-degree AV block, hypertension, hypotension, jugular venous distension, migraine, postural hypotension, ventricular extrasystoles, SVT, syncope, systolic ejection murmur, T-wave abnormalities on ECG, venous insufficiency. *Body as a whole:* Peripheral edema, cellulitis, chills, facial edema, fever, flu syndrome, malaise. *GI:* Anorexia, nausea, colitis, diarrhea, dry mouth, dyspepsia, dysphagia, flatulence, gastritis, **GI hemorrhage,** gingival hyperplasia, glossitis, hepatomegaly, increased appetite, melena, mouth ulceration. *CNS:* Headache, dizziness, abnormal dreams, abnormal thinking and confusion, amnesia, anxiety, ataxia, cerebral ischemia, decreased libido, depression, hypesthesia, hypertonia, insomnia, nervousness, paresthesia, somnolence, tremor, vertigo. *Musculoskeletal:* Arthralgia, arthritis, leg cramps, myalgia, myasthenia, myositis, tenosynovitis. *Hematologic:* Anemia, ecchymoses, leukopenia,

N

---
bold italic = life threatening side effect

petechiae. *Respiratory:* Pharyngitis, sinusitis, asthma, dyspnea, end-inspiratory wheeze and fine rales, epistaxis, increased cough, laryngitis, pleural effusion, rhinitis. *Dermatologic:* Acne, alopecia, dry skin, exfoliative dermatitis, fungal dermatitis, herpes simplex, herpes zoster, maculopapular rash, pruritus, pustular rash, skin discoloration, skin ulcer, sweating, urticaria. *GU:* Dysuria, hematuria, impotence, nocturia, urinary frequency, vaginal hemorrhage, vaginitis. *Metabolic:* Gout, hypokalemia, weight gain or loss. *Ophthalmic:* Abnormal vision, amblyopia, blepharitis, conjunctivitis, glaucoma, itchy eyes, keratoconjunctivitis, retinal detachment, temporary unilateral loss of vision, vitreous floater, watery eyes. *Miscellaneous:* Diabetes mellitus, thyroiditis, chest pain, ear pain, otitis media, tinnitus, taste disturbance.

OD **Overdose Management:** *Symptoms:* Pronounced hypotension. *Treatment:* Active CV support, including monitoring of CV and respiratory function, elevation of extremities, judicious use of calcium infusion, pressor agents, and fluids. Dialysis is not likely to be beneficial, although plasmapheresis may be helpful.

Drug Interactions: Cimetidine significantly ↑ the plasma levels of nislodipine.

EMS CONSIDERATIONS

See also *Calcium Channel Blocking Agents.*

Nitrofurantoin
Nitrofurantoin
macrocrystals
(nye-troh-fyour-AN-toyn)
Pregnancy Class: B
Nitrofurantoin (Furadantin **(Rx)**) Nitrofurantoin macrocrystals (Macrobid, Macrodantin **(Rx)**)
Classification: Urinary germicide

Mechanism of Action: Interferes with bacterial carbohydrate metabolism by inhibiting acetyl coenzyme A; also interferes with bacterial cell wall synthesis. Bacteriostatic at low concentrations and bactericidal at high concentrations.

Uses: UTIs due to susceptible strains of *Escherichia coli, Staphylococcus aureus* (not for treatment of pyelonephritis or perinephric abscesses), enterococci, and certain strains of *Enterobacter* and *Klebsiella.*

Contraindications: Anuria, oliguria, and patients with impaired renal function (C_{CR} below 40 mL/min); pregnant women, especially near term; infants less than 1 month of age; and lactation.

Precautions: Use with extreme caution in anemia, diabetes, electrolyte imbalance, avitaminosis B, or a debilitating disease. Safety during lactation has not been established.

Route/Dosage ———————
• **Capsules, Oral Suspension**
UTIs.
Adults: 50–100 mg q.i.d., not to exceed 600 mg/day. For cystitis, Macrobid is given in doses of 100 mg b.i.d. for 7 days. **Pediatric, 1 month of age and over:** 5–7 mg/kg/day in four equal doses.
Prophylaxis of UTIs.
Adults: 50–100 mg at bedtime. **Pediatric, 1 month of age and over:** 1 mg/kg/day at bedtime or in two divided doses daily.

How Supplied: *Capsule:* 25 mg, 50 mg, 100 mg; *Suspension:* 25 mg/5 mL (Nitrofurantoin)

Side Effects: Nitrofurantoin is a potentially toxic drug with many side effects. *GI:* N&V, anorexia, diarrhea, abdominal pain, parotitis, pancreatitis. *CNS:* Headache, dizziness, vertigo, drowsiness, nystagmus, confusion, depression, euphoria, psychotic reactions (rare). *Hematologic:* Leukopenia, thrombocytopenia, eosinophilia, megaloblastic anemia, *ag- ranulocytosis,* granulocytopenia, *he- molytic anemia (especially in patients with G6PD deficiency).* *Allergic:* Drug fever, skin rashes, pruritus, urticaria, angioedema, exfoliative dermatitis, erythema multiforme *(rarely, Stevens- Johnson syndrome), anaphylaxis,* arthralgia, myalgia, chills, sialadenitis, asthma symptoms in susceptible patients; maculopapular, erythematous, or eczematous eruption. *Pulmonary:* Sudden onset of dyspnea, cough, chest pain, fever and chills; pulmonary infiltration with consolidation or pleural effusion on x-ray, elevated ESR, eosinophilia. *After subacute or chronic use:* dyspnea, nonproductive cough, malaise, interstitial pneumonitis. Permanent impairment of pulmonary function with chronic therapy. A lupus-like syndrome associated with pulmonary reactions. *Hepatic:* Hepatitis, cholestatic jaundice, chronic active hepatitis, hepatic necrosis (rare). *CV:* Benign intracranial hypertension, changes in ECG, collapse, cyanosis. *Miscellaneous:* Peripheral neuropathy, asthenia, alopecia, superinfections of the GU tract, muscle pain.

OD **Overdose Management:** *Symptoms:* Vomiting (most common). *Treatment:* Induce emesis. High fluid intake to promote urinary excretion. The drug is dialyzable.

Drug Interactions

Acetazolamide / ↓ Effect of nitrofurantoin due to ↑ alkalinity of urine produced by acetazolamide

Antacids, oral / ↓ Effect of nitrofurantoin due to ↓ absorption from GI tract

Anticholinergic drugs / ↑ Effect of nitrofurantoin due to ↑ absorption from stomach

Magnesium trisilicate / ↓ Absorption of nitrofurantoin from GI tract

Nalidixic acid / Nitrofurantoin ↓ effect of nalidixic acid

Probenecid / High doses ↓ secretion of nitrofurantoin → toxicity

Sodium bicarbonate / ↓ Effect of nitrofurantoin due to ↑ alkalinity of urine produced by sodium bicarbonate

EMS CONSIDERATIONS

See also *Anit-Infectives.*

Nitroglycerin IV
(nye-troh-GLIH-sir-in)
Pregnancy Class: C

Nitro-Bid IV, Nitroglycerin in 5% Dextrose, Tridil **(Rx)**
Classification: Antianginal agent (coronary vasodilator)

Onset of Action: 1-2 min.
Duration of Action: 3-5 min (dose-dependent).

Uses: Hypertension associated with surgery (e.g., associated with ET intubation, skin incision, sternotomy, anesthesia, cardiac bypass, immediate postsurgical period). CHF associated with acute MI. Angina unresponsive to usual doses of organic nitrate or beta-adrenergic blocking agents. Cardiac-load reducing agent. Produce controlled hypotension during surgical procedures.

Precautions: Dosage has not been established in children.

Route/Dosage
- **IV Infusion Only**
Initial: 5 mcg/min delivered by precise infusion pump. May be increased by 5 mcg/min q 3–5 min until response is seen. If no response seen at 20 mcg/min, dose can be increased by 10–20 mcg/min until response noted. Monitor titration continuously until patient reaches desired level of response.
How Supplied: *Injection:* 5 mg/mL

EMS CONSIDERATIONS

See also *Antianginal Drugs, Nitrates/Nitrites.*

Administration/Storage
IV 1. Dilute with D5W USP or 0.9% NaCl injection. Not for direct IV use; must first be diluted.
2. Use glass IV bottle only and administration set provided by the manufacturer; is readily adsorbed onto many plastics. Avoid adding unnecessary plastic to IV system.
Assessment: Assess and rate pain, noting location, onset, duration, and any precipitating factors.
Interventions
1. Monitor VS and ECG. Note any evidence of hypotension, nausea, sweating, and/or vomiting.
- Elevate the legs to restore BP.

---

bold italic = life threatening side effect

• Reduce the rate of flow or administer additional IV fluids.
2. Assess for thrombophlebitis at the IV site; remove if reddened.
3. Wean from IV nitroglycerin by gradually decreasing doses to avoid posttherapy or CV distress.

Nitroglycerin sublingual
(nye-troh-GLIH-sir-in)
Pregnancy Class: C
Nitrostat **(Rx)**
Classification: Antianginal agent (coronary vasodilator)

Onset of Action: 1-3 min.
Duration of Action: 30-60 min.
Uses: Agents of choice for prophylaxis and treatment of angina pectoris.
Precautions: Dosage has not been established in children.

Route/Dosage
• **Sublingual Tablets**
150–600 mcg under the tongue or in the buccal pouch at first sign of attack; may be repeated in 5 min if necessary (no more than 3 tablets should be taken within 15 min). For prophylaxis, tablets may be taken 5–10 min prior to activities that may precipitate an attack.
How Supplied: *Tablet:* 0.3 mg, 0.4 mg, 0.6 mg

EMS CONSIDERATIONS

See also *Antianginal Drugs, Nitrates/Nitrites.*
Administration/Storage
1. Place sublingual tablets under the tongue and allow to dissolve; do not swallow.
2. Store in the original container at room temperature protected from moisture. Discard unused tablets if 6 months has elapsed since the original container was opened.

Nitroglycerin sustained-release capsules
Nitroglycerin sustained-release tablets
(nye-troh-GLIH-sir-in)
Pregnancy Class: C

Capsules (Nitroglyn **(Rx)**) Tablets (Nitrong **(Rx)**)
Classification: Antianginal agent (coronary vasodilator)

Onset of Action: 20-45 min.
Duration of Action: 3-8 hr.
Uses: To prevent anginal attacks. "Possibly effective" for the prophylaxis or treatment of anginal attacks.
Precautions: Dosage has not been established in children.

Route/Dosage
• **Sustained-Release Capsules**
2.5, 6.5, or 9 mg q 8–12 hr.
• **Sustained-Release Tablets**
1.3, 2.6, or 6.5 mg q 8–12 hr.
How Supplied: Nitroclycerin sustained-release capsules: *Capsule, Extended Release:* 2.5 mg, 6.5 mg, 9 mg. Nitroglycerin sustained-release tablets: *Tablet, Extended Release:* 2 mg

EMS CONSIDERATIONS

See also *Antianginal Drugs, Nitrates/Nitrites.*

Nitroglycerin topical ointment
(nye-troh-GLIH-sir-in)
Pregnancy Class: C
Nitro-Bid, Nitrol **(Rx)**
Classification: Antianginal agent (coronary vasodilator)

Onset of Action: 30-60 min.
Duration of Action: 2-12 hr (depending on amount used per unit of surface area).
Uses: Prophylaxis and treatment of angina pectoris due to CAD.
Precautions: Dosage has not been established in children.

Route/Dosage
• **Topical Ointment (2%)**
1–2 in. (15–30 mg) q 8 hr; up to 4–5 in. (60–75 mg) q 4 hr may be necessary. One inch equals approximately 15 mg nitroglycerin. Determine optimum dosage by starting with ½ in. q 8 hr and increasing by ½ in. with each successive dose until headache occurs; then, decrease to largest dose that does not cause headache.

When ending treatment, reduce both the dose and frequency of administration over 4–6 weeks to prevent sudden withdrawal reactions.
How Supplied: *Ointment:* 2%

EMS CONSIDERATIONS

See also *Antianginal Drugs, Nitrates/Nitriates.*

Nitroglycerin transdermal system

(nye-troh-GLIH-sir-in)
Pregnancy Class: C
Deponit 0.2 mg/hr and 0.4 mg/hr, Minitran 0.1 mg/hr, 0.2 mg/hr, 0.4 mg/hr, and 0.6 mg/hr, Nitrek 0.2 mg/hr, 0.3 mg/hr, and 0.4 mg/hr, Nitro-Dur 0.1 mg/hr, 0.2 mg/hr, 0.3 mg/hr, 0.4 mg/hr, 0.6 and 0.8 mg/hr, TransdermNitro 0.1 mg/hr, 0.2 mg/hr, 0.4 mg/hr, and 0.6 mg/hr **(Rx)**
Classification: Antianginal agent (coronary vasodilator)

Onset of Action: 30-60 min.
Duration of Action: 8-24 hr. The amount released each hour is indicated in the name.
Uses: Prophylaxis of angina pectoris due to CAD. *NOTE:* There is some evidence that nitroglycerin patches stop preterm labor.
Precautions: Dosage has not been established in children.

Route/Dosage —————
• **Topical Patch**
Initial: 0.2–0.4 mg/hr (initially the smallest available dose in the dosage series) applied each day to skin site free of hair and free of excessive movement (e.g., chest, upper arm).
Maintenance: Additional systems or strengths may be added depending on the clinical response.
How Supplied: *Film, Extended Release:* 0.1 mg/hr, 0.2 mg/hr, 0.3 mg/hr, 0.4 mg/hr, 0.6 mg/hr, 0.8 mg/hr

EMS CONSIDERATIONS

See also *Antianginal Drugs, Nitrates/Nitrites.*

Nitroglycerin translingual spray

(nye-troh-GLIH-sir-in)
Pregnancy Class: C
Nitrolingual **(Rx)**
Classification: Antianginal agent (coronary vasodilator)

Onset of Action: 2 min.
Duration of Action: 30-60 min.
Uses: Coronary artery disease to relieve an acute attack or used prophylactically 10–15 min before beginning activities that can cause an acute anginal attack.
Precautions: Dosage has not been established in children.

Route/Dosage —————
• **Spray**
Termination of acute attack.
One to two metered doses (400–800 mcg) on or under the tongue q 5 min as needed; no more than three metered doses should be administered within a 15-min period.
Prophylaxis.
One to two metered doses 5–10 min before beginning activities that might precipitate an acute attack.
How Supplied: *Spray:* 0.4 mg/Spray

EMS CONSIDERATIONS

See also *Antianginal Drugs, Nitrates/Nitrites.*

Nitroprusside sodium

(nye-troh-PRUS-eyed)
Pregnancy Class: C
Nitropress **(Rx)**
Classification: Antihypertensive, direct action on vascular smooth muscle

Mechanism of Action: Direct action on vascular smooth muscle, leading to peripheral vasodilation of arteries and veins. Acts on excitation-contraction coupling of vascular smooth muscle by interfering with both influx and intracellular activation of calcium. No effect on smooth muscle of the duodenum or uterus and is more active on veins than on arteries. May also improve CHF by decreasing systemic resistance, preload and afterload reduction, and improved CO. Reacts with hemoglobin to produce cyanmethemoglobin and cyanide ion. Caution must be exercised as nitroprusside injection can result in toxic levels of cyanide. However, when used briefly or at low infusion rates, the cyanide produced reacts with thiosulfate to produce thiocyanate, which is excreted in the urine.

Onset of Action: Drug must be given by IV infusion; 0.5-1 min; **peak effect:** 1-2 min.

Duration of Action: Up to 10 min after infusion stopped.

Uses: Hypertensive crisis to reduce BP immediately. To produce controlled hypotension during anesthesia to reduce bleeding. Acute CHF. *Investigational:* In combination with dopamine for acute MI. Left ventricular failure with coadministration of oxygen, morphine, and a loop diuretic.

Contraindications: Compensatory hypertension where the primary hemodynamic lesion is aortic coarctation or AV shunting. Use to produce controlled hypotension during surgery in patients with known inadequate cerebral circulation or in moribund patients. Patients with congenital optic atrophy or tobacco amblyopia (both of which are rare). Acute CHF associated with decreased peripheral vascular resistance (e.g., high-output heart failure that may be seen in endotoxic sepsis). Lactation.

Precautions: Use with caution in hypothyroidism, liver or kidney impairment, during lactation, and in the presence of increased ICP. Geriatric patients may be more sensitive to the hypotensive effects of nitroprusside; also, a decrease in dose may be necessary in these patients due to age-related decreases in renal function.

Route/Dosage ───────────
• **IV Infusion Only**
Hypertensive crisis.
Adults: average, 3 mcg/kg/min. **Range:** 0.3–10 mcg/kg/min. Smaller dose is required for patients receiving other antihypertensives. **Pediatric:**

1.4 mcg/kg/min adjusted slowly depending on the response.

Monitor BP and use as guide to regulate rate of administration to maintain desired antihypertensive effect. Do not exceed a rate of administration of 10 mcg/kg/min.

How Supplied: *Injection:* 25 mg/mL; *Powder for injection:* 50 mg

Side Effects: Excessive hypotension. *Large doses may lead to cyanide toxicity. Following rapid BP reduction:* Dizziness, nausea, restlessness, headache, sweating, muscle twitching, palpitations, abdominal pain, apprehension, retching, retrosternal discomfort. *Other side effects:* Bradycardia, tachycardia, ECG changes, venous streaking, rash, methemoglobinemia, decreased platelet aggregation, flushing, hypothyroidism, ileus, irritation at injection site, hypothyroidism. *Symptoms of thiocyanate toxicity:* Blurred vision, tinnitus, confusion, hyperreflexia, seizures. *CNS symptoms (transitory):* Restlessness, agitation, increased ICP, and muscle twitching. Vomiting or skin rash.

OD Overdose Management: *Symptoms:* Excessive hypotension, cyanide toxicity, thiocyanate toxicity. *Treatment:*
• Measure cyanide levels and blood gases to determine venous hyperoxemia or acidosis.
• To treat cyanide toxicity, discontinue nitroprusside and give sodium nitrite, 4–6 mg/kg (about 0.2 mL/kg) over 2–4 min (to convert hemoglobin into methemoglobin); follow by sodium thiosulfate, 150–200 mg/kg (about 50 mL of the 25% solution). This regimen can be given again, at half the original doses, after 2 hr.

Drug Interactions: Concomitant use of other antihypertensives, volatile liquid anesthetics, or certain depressants ↑ response to nitroprusside.

EMS CONSIDERATIONS

See also *Antihypertensive Agents.*
Administration/Storage
IV 1. Dissolve contents of the vial (50 mg) in 2–3 mL of D5W. This stock solution must be diluted further in 250–1,000 mL D5W.

2. Discard solutions that are any color but light brown.

3. Protect dilute solutions during administration by wrapping bag and tubing with opaque material such as aluminum foil or foil-lined bags.

Interventions: Monitor VS, and ECG. Monitor BP closely and titrate infusion.

Nizatidine
(nye-ZAY-tih-deen)
Pregnancy Class: C
name>Axid **(Rx)**, Axid AR **(OTC)**
Classification: Histamine H_2 receptor antagonist

Mechanism of Action: Decreases gastric acid secretion by blocking the effect of histamine on histamine H_2 receptors.

Onset of Action: 30 min; **time to peak effect:** 0.5-3 hr.

Duration of Action: Nocturnal: Up to 12 hr; **basal:** up to 8 hr.

Uses: Treatment of acute duodenal ulcer and maintenance following healing of a duodenal ulcer. GERD, including erosive and ulcerative esophagitis. Short-term treatment of benign gastric ulcer. OTC use to prevent meal-induced heartburn.

Contraindications: Hypersensitivity to H_2 receptor antagonists. Cirrhosis of the liver, impaired renal or hepatic function. Lactation.

Precautions: Safety and efficacy have not been determined in children.

Route/Dosage
AXID
• **Capsules**
   Active duodenal ulcer.
Adults: Either 300 mg once daily at bedtime or 150 mg b.i.d. If the C_{CR} is 20–50 mL/min: 150 mg/day; if C_{CR} is less than 20 mL/min: 150 mg every other day.
   Prophylaxis following healing of duodenal ulcer.
Adults: 150 mg/day at bedtime. If C_{CR} is 20–50 mL/min: 150 mg every other day; if C_{CR} is less than 20 mL/min: 150 mg every 3 days.
   Treatment of benign gastric ulcer.

Adults: 150 mg b.i.d. or 300 mg at bedtime
   GERD, including erosive and ulcerative esophagitis.
Adults: 150 mg b.i.d.
AXID AR
• **Tablets**
   Heartburn.
1 tablet b.i.d.
How Supplied: *Capsule:* 150 mg, 300 mg; *Tablet:* 75 mg

Side Effects: *CNS:* Headache, fatigue, somnolence, insomnia, dizziness, abnormal dreams, anxiety, nervousness, confusion (rare). *GI:* N&V, diarrhea, pancreatitis, constipation, abdominal discomfort, flatulence, dyspepsia, anorexia, dry mouth. *Dermatologic:* Exfoliative dermatitis, erythroderma, pruritus, urticaria, erythema multiforme. *CV:* Asymptomatic VT; *rarely, cardiac arrhythmias or arrest following rapid IV use.* *Respiratory:* Rhinitis, pharyngitis, sinusitis, cough. *Body as a whole:* Asthenia, back pain, chest pain, infection, fever, myalgia. *Miscellaneous:* Impotence, loss of libido, thrombocytopenia, sweating, gynecomastia, hyperuricemia, eosinophilia, gout, and cholestatic or hepatocellular effects (resulting in increased AST, ALT, or alkaline phosphatase).

Drug Interactions
Antacids containing Al and Mg hydroxides / ↓ Nizatidine absorption by about 10%
Aspirin, high doses / ↑ Salicylate serum levels
Simethicone / ↓ Nizatidine absorption by about 10%

EMS CONSIDERATIONS
See also *Histamine H_2* Antagonists.

Norfloxacin
(nor-FLOX-ah-sin)
Pregnancy Class: C
Chilbroxin Ophthalmic Solution, Noroxin **(Rx)**
Classification: Fluoroquinolone anti-infective

Mechanism of Action: Active against gram-positive and gram-neg-

---
bold italic = life threatening side effect

ative organisms by inhibiting bacterial DNA synthesis.

Uses: Systemic: Uncomplicated UTIs caused by *Escherichia coli, Klebsiella pneumoniae, Enterobacter cloacae, Proteus mirabilis, P. vulgaris, Pseudomonas aeruginosa, Citrobacter freundii, Staphylococcus aureus, S. epidermidis, Enterococcus faecalis, Enterobacter aerogenes, S. saprophyticus,* and *S. agalactiae.* Complicated UTIs caused by *Enterococcus faecalis, E. coli, K. pneumoniae, P. mirabilis, P. aeruginosa,* or *Serratia marcescens.* Urethral gonorrhea and endocervical gonococcal infections due to penicillinase- or non-penicillinase-producing *Neisseria gonorrhoeae.* Prostatitis due to *E. coli.*

Ophthalmic: Superficial ocular infections involving the cornea or conjunctiva due to *Staphylococcus, S. aureus, Streptococcus pneumoniae, E. coli, Haemophilus aegyptius, H. influenzae, Klebsiella pneumoniae, Neisseria gonorrhoeae, Proteus* species, *Enterobacter aerogenes, Serratia marcescens, Pseudomonas aeruginosa,* and *Vibrio* species.

Contraindications: Hypersensitivity to nalidixic acid, cinoxacin, or norfloxacin. Lactation, infants, and children. Ophthalmic use for dendritic keratitis, vaccinia, varicella, mycobacterial infections of the eye, fungal disease of the eye, and use with steroid combinations after uncomplicated removal of a corneal foreign body.

Precautions: Use with caution in patients with a history of seizures and in impaired renal function. Geriatric patients eliminate norfloxacin more slowly.

Route/Dosage ————————

• **Tablets**

Uncomplicated UTIs due to E. coli, K. pneumoniae, or P. mirabilis.
400 mg q 12 hr for 3 days.
Uncomplicated UTIs due to other organisms.
400 mg q 12 hr for 7–10 days.
Complicated UTIs.
400 mg q 12 hr for 10–21 days. Maximum dose for UTIs should not exceed 800 mg/day.

Uncomplicated gonorrhea.
800 mg as a single dose.
Impaired renal function, with C_{CR} *equal to or less than 30 mL/min/1.73 m².*
400 mg/day for 7–10 days.
Prostatis due to E. coli.
400 mg q 12 hr for 28 days.

• **Ophthalmic Solution**
Acute infections.
Initially, 1–2 gtt q 15–30 min; **then,** reduce frequency as infection is controlled.
Moderate infections.
1–2 gtt 4–6 times/day.
How Supplied: *Ophthalmic solution:* 0.3%; *Tablet:* 400 mg
Side Effects: See also *Side Effects* for *Fluoroquinolones.*

GI: N&V, diarrhea, abdominal pain or discomfort, dry/painful mouth, dyspepsia, flatulence, constipation, pseudomembranous colitis, stomatitis. *CNS:* Headache, dizziness, fatigue, malaise, drowsiness, depression, insomnia, confusion, psychoses. *Hematologic:* Decreased hematocrit, eosinophilia, leukopenia, neutropenia, either increased or decreased platelets. *Dermatologic:* Photosensitivity, rash, pruritus, exfoliative dermatitis, **toxic epidermal necrolysis,** erythema, erythema multiforme, **Stevens-Johnson syndrome.** *Other:* Paresthesia, hypersensitivity, fever, visual disturbances, hearing loss, crystalluria, cylindruria, candiduria, myoclonus (rare), hepatitis, pancreatitis, arthralgia.

Following ophthalmic use: Conjunctival hyperemia, photophobia, chemosis, bitter taste in mouth.
Drug Interactions: Additional: Nitrofurantoin ↓ antibacterial effect of norfloxacin.

EMS CONSIDERATIONS

None.

Nortriptyline hydrochloride
(nor-TRIP-tih-leen)
Pregnancy Class: C
Aventyl, Pamelor **(Rx)**
Classification: Antidepressant, tricyclic

Mechanism of Action: Manifests moderate anticholinergic and sedative effects but slight orthostatic hypotensive effects.

Uses: Treatment of symptoms of depression. Chronic, severe neurogenic pain. Dermatologic disorders including chronic urticaria, angioedema, and nocturnal pruritus in atopic eczema.

Contraindications: Use in children (safety and efficacy have not been determined).

Route/Dosage —————
• **Capsules, Oral Solution**
Depression.
Adults: 25 mg t.i.d.–q.i.d. Dose individualized; begin at a low dosage and increase as needed. **Doses above 150 mg/day are not recommended. Elderly patients:** 30–50 mg/day in divided doses.
Dermatologic disorders.
75 mg/day.
How Supplied: *Capsule:* 10 mg, 25 mg, 50 mg, 75 mg; *Solution:* 10 mg/5 mL

EMS CONSIDERATIONS

See also *Antidepressants, Tricyclic.*

Nystatin
(nye-STAT-in)
Pregnancy Class: C (A for vaginal use)
Tablets: Mycostatin, Nilstat; **Oral Suspension:** Mycostatin, Nilstat, Nystex; **Troches:** Mycostatin; **Topical:** Mycostatin, Nilstat, Nystex, Nystop; **Topical Powder:** Nystop **(Rx)**
Classification: Antibiotic, antifungal

Mechanism of Action: Derived from *Streptomyces noursei*; is both fungistatic and fungicidal against all species of *Candida*. Binds to fungal cell membranes (sterols), resulting in altered cellular permeability and leakage of potassium and other essential intracellular components.

Uses: *Candida* infections of the skin, mucous membranes, GI tract, vagina, and mouth (thrush). The drug is too toxic for systemic infections although it can be given PO for intestinal moniliasis infections, as it is not absorbed from the GI tract.

Contraindications: Use for systemic mycoses. Use of topical products in or around the eyes.

Precautions: Do not use occlusive dressings when treating candidiasis. Do not use lozenges in children less than 5 years of age.

Route/Dosage —————
• **Capsule, Lozenge, Oral Suspension, Tablets**
Intestinal candidiasis.
Tablets, 500,000–1,000,000 units t.i.d.; continue treatment for 48 hr after cure to prevent relapse.
Oral candidiasis.
Oral Suspension, adults and children: 400,000–600,000 units q.i.d. (1/2 dose in each side of mouth, held as long as possible before swallowing); **infants:** 200,000 units q.i.d. (same procedure as with adults); **premature or low birth weight infants:** 100,000 units q.i.d. **Lozenge, adults and children:** 200,000–400,000 units 4–5 times/day, up to 14 days. *NOTE:* Lozenges should not be chewed or swallowed.
• **Vaginal Tablets**
100,000 units (1 tablet) inserted in vagina once each day for 2 weeks.
• **Topical Cream, Ointment, Powder (100,000 units/g each)**
Apply to affected areas b.i.d.–t.i.d., or as indicated, until healing is complete.
How Supplied: *Capsule:* 500,000 U, 1 million U; *Cream:* 100,000 U/gm; *Lozenge/troche:* 200,000 U; *Ointment:* 100,000 U/gm; *Powder:* 100,000 U/gm; *Suspension:* 100,000 U/mL; *Tablet:* 100,000 U, 500,000 U

Side Effects: Nystatin has few toxic effects. *GI:* Epigastric distress, N&V, diarrhea. *Other:* Rarely, irritation.

EMS CONSIDERATIONS

See also *Anit-Infectives.*

Octreotide acetate
(ock-TREE-oh-tyd)
Pregnancy Class: B
Sandostatin **(Rx)**
Classification: Antineoplastic

Mechanism of Action: Similar to the natural hormone somatostatin. It suppresses secretions of serotonin and GI peptides including gastrin, insulin, glucagon, secretin, motilin, vasoactive intestinal peptide, and pancreatic polypeptide. Stimulates fluid and electrolyte absorption from the GI tract and inhibits growth hormone.
Uses: Metastatic carcinoid tumors; vasoactive intestinal tumors (VIPomas). The drug inhibits severe diarrhea in both situations and causes improvement in hypokalemia in VIPomas. Acromegaly. *Investigational:* GI fistula, variceral bleeding, pancreatic fistula, irritable bowel syndrome, and dumping syndrome. Also, treatment of diarrhea due to AIDS, short bowel syndrome, diabetes, pancreatic cholera syndrome, chemotherapy or radiation therapy in cancer patients, and idiopathic secretory diarrhea. Other potential uses include enteric fistula, pancreatitis, pancreatic surgery, glucagonoma, insulinoma, Zollinger-Ellison syndrome, intestinal obstruction, local radiotherapy, chronic pain management, antineoplastic therapy, to decrease insulin requirements in diabetes mellitus, in thyrotropin- and TSH-secreting tumors.
Precautions: Use with caution in diabetics, in patients with gallbladder disease, in patients with severe renal failure requiring dialysis, and during lactation.

Route/Dosage
• **SC (Recommended), IV Bolus (Emergencies)**
Metastatic carcinoid tumors.
Initial, SC: 50 mcg 1–2 times/day.
Then, 100–600 mcg/day in two to four divided doses for the first 2 weeks; **maintenance, usual:** 450 mcg/day (range: 50–1,500 mcg/day).
VIPomas.
Initial, SC: 200–300 mcg/day in two to four divided doses during the initial 2 weeks of therapy (range: 150–750 mcg/day). Doses may then be adjusted but the daily dose usually does not exceed 450 mcg.
Acromegaly.
Initial: 50 mcg t.i.d.; **then,** 100–500 mcg t.i.d. The goal is to achieve growth hormone levels less than 5 ng/mL or IGF-1 levels less than 1.9 U/mL in males and less than 2.2 U/mL in females.
GI fistula.
50–200 mcg q 8 hr.
Variceal bleeding.
25–50 mcg/hr via continuous IV infusion for 18 hr to 5 days.
AIDS-related diarrhea.
100–500 mcg SC t.i.d.
Idiopathic secretory diarrhea, short-bowel syndrome.
Either 25 mcg/hr by IV infusion or 50 mcg SC b.i.d.
Diabetes, pancreatic cholera syndrome, diarrhea due to chemotherapy or radiation therapy in cancer patients.
50–100 mcg SC t.i.d. for 3 days.
Pancreatic fistula.
50–200 mcg q 8 hr.
Irritable bowel syndrome.
100 mcg as a single dose to 125 mcg SC b.i.d.
Dumping syndrome.
50–150 mcg/day.
How Supplied: *Injection:* 50 mcg/mL, 100 mcg/mL, 200 mcg/mL, 500 mcg/mL, 1000 mcg/mL
Side Effects: *GI:* Nausea, diarrhea or loose stools, abdominal pain or distention, malabsorption of fat, vomiting; less commonly, constipation, pancreatitis, anorexia, flatulence, abdominal distention, abnormal stools, hepatitis, jaundice, appendicitis, GI bleeding, hemorrhoids. *CNS:* Headache, dizziness, lightheadedness, fa-

tigue; less commonly, anxiety, seizures, depression, vertigo, decrease in libido, syncope, tremor, Bell's palsy, paranoia, pituitary apoplexy. *CV:* Sinus bradycardia in acromegalics, hypertension, thrombophlebitis, SOB, CHF, ischemia, palpitations, orthostatic hypotension, conduction abnormalities, hypertensive reaction, tachycardia, arrhythmias, chest pain. *Endocrine:* Hyperglycemia or hypoglycemia in acromegalics, biochemical hypothyroidism in acromegalics. Galactorrhea, hypoadrenalism, diabetes insipidus, gynecomastia, amenorrhea, polymenorrhea, vaginitis. *Musculoskeletal:* Backache, joint pain, arthritis, joint effusion, muscle pain, Raynaud's phenomenon. *Dermatologic:* Pain, wheal, or erythema at injection site; flushing, edema, pruritus, hair loss, rash, cellulitis, petechiae, urticaria. *GU:* Pollakiuria, UTI, nephrolithiasis, hematuria. *Hematologic:* Hematoma at injection site, bruise, iron deficiency anemia, epistaxis. *Other:* Gallbladder abnormalities, especially stones or biliary sludge; flu symptoms, malabsorption of fat, blurred vision, otitis, allergic reaction, visual disturbances, ***anaphylactoid reactions, including anaphylactic shock.***

OD Overdose Management: *Symptoms:* Hyperglycemia and hypoglycemia manifested by dizziness, drowsiness, loss of sensory or motor function, incoordination, disturbed consciousness, and visual blurring. *Treatment:* Withdraw drug temporarily and treat symptomatically.

Drug Interactions: Octreotide may interfere with drugs such as diazoxide, insulin, beta-adrenergic blocking agents, or sulfonylureas. Close monitoring is necessary.

EMS CONSIDERATIONS

None.

Ofloxacin
(oh-FLOS-ah-zeen)
Pregnancy Class: C

Floxin, Floxin Otic, Ocuflox **(Rx)**
Classification: Antibacterial, fluoroquinolone

Mechanism of Action: Effective against a wide range of gram-positive and gram-negative aerobic and anaerobic bacteria. Penicillinase has no effect on the activity of ofloxacin.

Uses: Systemic: Pneumonia or acute bacterial exacerbations of chronic bronchitis or community-acquired pneumonia due to *Haemophilus influenzae* or *Streptococcus pneumoniae.* Not a drug of first choice in the treatment of presumed or confirmed pneumococcal pneumonia. Not effective for syphilis.

Acute, uncomplicated urethral and cervical gonorrhea due to *Neisseria gonorrhoeae;* nongonococcal urethritis, and cervicitis due to *Chlamydia trachomatis.* Mixed infections of the urethra and cervix due to *N. gonorrhoeae* and *C. trachomatis.*

Mild to moderate skin and skin structure infections due to *Staphylococcus aureus, Streptococcus pyogenes,* or *Proteus mirabilis.*

Uncomplicated cystitis due to *Citrobacter diversus, Enterobacter aerogenes, E. coli, Klebsiella pneumoniae, Proteus mirabilis,* or *Pseudomonas aeruginosa.* Complicated UTIs due to *Escherichia coli, K. pneumoniae, P. mirabilis, C. diversus,* or *P. aeruginosa.* Prostatitis due to *E. coli.* Monotherapy for PID.

Ophthalmic: Treatment of conjunctivitis caused by *S. aureus, Staphylococcus epidermidis, S. pneumoniae, Enterobacter cloacae, H. influenzae, P. mirabilis,* and *P. aeruginosa.* Corneal ulcers caused by susceptible organisms.

Otic: Otitis externa due to *S. aureus* and *P. aeruginosa* in patients one year of age and older. Acute otitis media with tympanostomy tubes due to *S. aureus, S. pneumoniae, H. influenzae, Moraxella catarrhalis,* and *P. aeruginosa* (from age one to twelve). Chronic suppurative otitis media due to *S. aureus, P. mirabilis,* and *P. aeruginosa* in those twelve years and older who have perforated tympanic membranes.

Contraindications: Hypersensitivity to quinolone antibacterial agents. Use during lactation. Use for syphilis (ineffective). Ophthalmic use in dendritic keratitis, vaccinia, varicella, mycobacterial infections of the eye, fungal diseases of the eye, and with steroid combinations after uncomplicated removal of a corneal foreign body.

Precautions: Safety and effectiveness of the systemic forms have not been established in children, adolescents under the age of 18 years, pregnant women, and lactating women. Safety and effectiveness of the ophthalmic form have not been established in children less than 1 year of age. Use with caution in patients with known or suspected CNS disorders such as severe cerebral atherosclerosis, epilepsy, or factors that predispose to seizures.

Route/Dosage ───────────

• **Tablets**

Pneumonia, exacerbation of chronic bronchitis.

400 mg q 12 hr for 10 days.

Acute uncomplicated gonorrhea.

One 400-mg dose. The Centers for Disease Control also recommend adding doxycycline.

Cervicitis/urethritis due to C. trachomatis or N. gonorrhoeae.

300 mg q 12 hr for 7 days.

Mild to moderate skin and skin structure infections.

400 mg q 12 hr for 10 days.

Cystitis due to E. coli or K. pneumoniae.

200 mg q 12 hr for 3 days.

Cystitis due to other organisms.

200 mg q 12 hr for 7 days.

Complicated UTIs.

200 mg q 12 hr for 10 days.

Prostatitis.

300 mg q 12 hr for 6 weeks.

Chlamydia.

300 mg PO b.i.d. for 7 days.

Epididymitis.

300 mg PO b.i.d. for 10 days.

PID, outpatient.

400 mg PO b.i.d. for 14 days.

NOTE: The dose should be adjusted in patients with a C_{CR} of 50 mL/min or less. If the C_{CR} is 10–50 mL/min, the dosage interval should be q 24 hr, and if C_{CR} is less than 10 mL/min, the dose should be half the recommended dose given q 24 hr.

• **Ophthalmic Solution (0.3%)**

Conjunctivitis.

Initial: 1–2 gtt in the affected eye(s) q 2–4 hr for the first 2 days; **then,** 1–2 gtt q.i.d. for five additional days.

• **Otic Solution (0.3%)**

Otitis externa, otitis media.

Apply b.i.d.

How Supplied: *Ophthalmic solution:* 0.3%; *Otic Solution:* 0.3%; *Tablet:* 200 mg, 300 mg, 400 mg

Side Effects: See also *Side Effects* for *Fluroquinolones.*

GI: Nausea, diarrhea, vomiting, abdominal pain or discomfort, dry or painful mouth, dyspepsia, flatulence, constipation, pseudomembranous colitis, dysgeusia, decreased appetite. *CNS:* Headache, dizziness, fatigue, malaise, somnolence, depression, insomnia, seizures, sleep disorders, nervousness, anxiety, cognitive change, dream abnormality, euphoria, hallucinations, vertigo. *CV:* Chest pain, edema, hypertension, palpitations, vasodilation. *Hypersensitivity reactions:* Dyspnea, **anaphylaxis.** *GU:* External genital pruritus in women, vaginitis, vaginal discharge; burning, irritation, pain, and rash of the female genitalia; glucosuria, proteinuria, hematuria, pyuria, dysmenorrhea, menorrhagia, metrorrhagia, urinary frequency or pain. *Respiratory:* Cough, rhinorrhea. *Dermatologic:* Diaphoresis, vasculitis, photosensitivity, rash, pruritus. *Hematologic:* Leukocytosis, lymphocytopenia, eosinophilia. *Musculoskeletal:* Asthenia, extremity pain, arthralgia, myalgia, possibility of osteochondrosis. *Miscellaneous:* Chills, malaise, syncope, hyperglycemia or hypoglycemia, whole body pain, thirst, weight loss, photophobia, trunk pain, paresthesia, visual disturbances, hypersensitivity, hearing loss, fever.

After ophthalmic use: Transient ocular burning or discomfort, stinging, redness, itching, photophobia, tearing, and dryness.

After otic use: Pruritus, application site reaction, dizziness, earache, vertigo, taste perversion, paresthesia, rash.

EMS CONSIDERATIONS

See also *Anti-Infectives.*

Olanzapine

(oh-LAN-zah-peen)
Pregnancy Class: C
Zyprexa **(Rx)**
Classification: Antipsychotic agent, miscellaneous

Mechanism of Action: A thienbenzodiazepine antipsychotic believed to act by antagonizing dopamine D_{1-4} and serotonin ($5HT_2$) receptors. Also binds to muscarinic, histamine H_1 and alpha-1 adrenergic receptors, which can explain many of the side effects.

Uses: Management of psychotic disorders. *Investigational:* Treatment of mania.

Contraindications: Lactation.

Precautions: Use with caution in geriatric patients, as the drug may be excreted more slowly in this population. Use with caution in impaired hepatic function and in those where there is a chance of increased core body temperature (e.g., strenuous exercise, exposure to extreme heat, concomitant anticholinergic drug administration, dehydration). Due to anticholinergic side effects, use with caution in patients with significant prostatic hypertrophy, narrow-angle glaucoma, or a history of paralytic ileus. Safety and efficacy have not been determined in children less than 18 years of age.

Route/Dosage

• **Tablets**
Psychoses.
Adults, initial: 5–10 mg once daily without regard to meals. Goal is 10 mg daily; increments to reach 10 mg can be in 5-mg amounts but at an interval

of 1 week. Doses higher than 10 mg daily are recommended only after clinical assessment and should not be greater than 20 mg/day. The recommended initial dose is 5 mg in those who are debilitated, who have a predisposition to hypotensive reactions, who may have factors that cause a slower metabolism of olanzapine (e.g., nonsmoking female patients over 65 years of age), or who may be more sensitive to the drug. It is recommended that patients who respond to the drug be continued on it at the lowest possible dose to maintain remission with periodic evaluation to determine continued need for the drug.

Mania.
5–20 mg daily.

How Supplied: *Tablet:* 2.5 mg, 5 mg, 7.5 mg, 10 mg

Side Effects: *Neuroleptic malignant syndrome:* Hyperpyrexia, muscle rigidity, altered mental status, irregular pulse or BP, tachycardia, diaphoresis, cardiac dysrhythmia, rhabdomyolysis, *acute renal failure, death. GI:* Dysphagia, constipation, dry mouth, increased appetite, increased salivation, N&V, thirst, aphthous stomatitis, eructation, esophagitis, rectal incontinence, flatulence, gastritis, gastroenteritis, gingivitis, glossitis, hepatitis, melena, mouth ulceration, oral moniliasis, periodontal abscess, *rectal hemorrhage,* tongue edema. *CNS:* Tardive dyskinesia, seizures, somnolence, agitation, insomnia, nervousness, hostility, dizziness, anxiety, personality disorder, akathisia, hypertonia, tremor, amnesia, impaired articulation, euphoria, stuttering, *suicide,* abnormal gait, alcohol misuse, antisocial reaction, ataxia, CNS stimulation, coma, delirium, depersonalization, hypesthesia, hypotonia, incoordination, decreased libido, obsessive-compulsive symptoms, phobias, somatization, stimulant misuse, stupor, vertigo, withdrawal syndrome. *CV:* Tachycardia, orthostatic/postural hypotension, hypotension, *CVA, hemorrhage, heart arrest,* migraine,

---

bold italic = life threatening side effect

palpitation, vasodilation, ventricular extrasystoles. *Body as a whole:* Headache, fever, abdominal pain, chest pain, neck rigidity, intentional injury, flu syndrome, chills, facial edema, hangover effect, malaise, moniliasis, neck pain, pelvic pain, photosensitivity. *Respiratory:* Rhinitis, increased cough, pharyngitis, dyspnea, apnea, asthma, epistaxis, hemoptysis, hyperventilation, voice alteration. *GU:* Premenstrual syndrome, hematuria, metrorrhagia, urinary incontinence, UTI, abnormal ejaculation, amenorrhea, breast pain, cystitis, decreased or increased menstruation, dysuria, female lactation, impotence, menorrhagia, polyuria, pyuria, urinary retention, urinary frequency, impaired urination, enlarged uterine fibroids. *Hematologic:* Leukocytosis, lymphadenopathy, thrombocytopenia. *Metabolic/nutritional:* Weight gain or loss, peripheral edema, lower extremity edema, dehydration, hyperglycemia, hyperkalemia, hyperuricemia, hypoglycemia, hypokalemia, hyponatremia, ketosis, water intoxication. *Musculoskeletal:* Joint pain, extremity pain, twitching, arthritis, back and hip pain, bursitis, leg cramps, myasthenia, rheumatoid arthritis. *Dermatologic:* Vesiculobullous rash, alopecia, contact dermatitis, dry skin, eczema, hirsutism, seborrhea, skin ulcer, urticaria. *Ophthalmic:* Amblyopia, blepharitis, corneal lesion, cataract, diplopia, dry eyes, eye hemorrhage, eye inflammation, eye pain, ocular muscle abnormality. *Otic:* Deafness, ear pain, tinnitus. *Miscellaneous:* Diabetes mellitus, goiter, cyanosis, taste perversion.

OD Overdose Management: *Symptoms:* Drowsiness, slurred speech. Possible obtundation, seizures, dystonic reaction of the head and neck. CV symptoms, arrhythmias. *Treatment:* Establish and maintain an airway and ensure adequate oxygenation and ventilation. Gastric lavage followed by activated charcoal and a laxative can be considered, although dystonic reaction may cause aspiration with induced emesis. Begin CV monitoring immediately with continuous ECG monitoring to detect possible arrhythmias. Hypotension and circulatory collapse are treated with IV fluids or sympathomimetic agents. Do not use epinephrine, dopamine, or other sympathomimetics with beta-agonist activity, as beta stimulation may worsen hypotension.

Drug Interactions
Antihypertensive agents / ↑ Effect of antihypertensive agents
Carbamazepine / ↑ Clearance of olanzepine due to ↑ rate of metabolism
CNS depressants / ↑ Effect of CNS depressants
Levodopa and Dopamine agonists / Olanzapine may antagonize the effects of levodopa and dopamine agonists

EMS CONSIDERATIONS
None.

Olopatadine hydrochloride
(oh-loh-pah-TIH-deen)
Pregnancy Class: C
Patanol **(Rx)**
Classification: Antihistamine, ophthalmic

Mechanism of Action: Selective histamine H-1 receptor antagonist. Little is absorbed into the systemic circulation.
Uses: Prevention of itching in allergic conjunctivitis.
Contraindications: Not to be injected. Not to be instilled while the patient is wearing contact lenses.
Precautions: Use with caution during lactation. Safety and efficacy have not been determined for children less than 3 years of age.

Route/Dosage
• **Solution (0.1%)**
  Allergic conjunctivitis.
Adults and children over 3 years of age: 1–2 drops in each affected eye b.i.d. at an interval of 6–8 hr.
How Supplied: *Solution:* 1%
Side Effects: *Ophthalmic:* Burning or stinging, dry eye, foreign body

sensation, hyperemia, keratitis, lid edema, pruritus. Nose/throat: Pharyngitis, rhinitis, sinusitis. *Miscellaneous:* Headache, asthenia, cold syndrome, taste perversion.

EMS CONSIDERATIONS
See also *Antihistamines.*

Olsalazine sodium
(ohl-SAL-ah-zeen)
Pregnancy Class: C
Dipentum **(Rx)**
Classification: Anti-inflammatory drug

Mechanism of Action: A salicylate that is converted by bacteria in the colon to 5-PAS (5-para-aminosalicylate), which exerts an anti-inflammatory effect for the treatment of ulcerative colitis. 5-PAS is slowly absorbed resulting in a high concentration of drug in the colon. The anti-inflammatory activity is likely due to inhibition of synthesis of prostaglandins in the colon.
Uses: To maintain remission of ulcerative colitis in patients who cannot take sulfasalazine.
Contraindications: Hypersensitivity to salicylates.
Precautions: Use with caution during lactation. Safety and efficacy have not been established in children. May cause worsening of symptoms of colitis.

Route/Dosage
• **Capsules**
Adults: Total of 1 g/day in two divided doses.
How Supplied: *Capsule:* 250 mg
Side Effects: *GI:* Diarrhea (common), pain or cramps, nausea, dyspepsia, bloating, anorexia, vomiting, stomatitis. *CNS:* Headache, drowsiness, lethargy, fatigue, dizziness, vertigo. *Miscellaneous:* Arthralgia, rash, itching, upper respiratory tract infection. *NOTE:* The following symptoms have been reported on withdrawal of therapy: diarrhea, nausea, abdominal pain, rash, itching, headache,

heartburn, insomnia, anorexia, dizziness, lightheadedness, rectal bleeding, depression.
OD Overdose Management: *Symptoms:* Diarrhea, decreased motor activity. *Treatment:* Treat symptoms.

EMS CONSIDERATIONS
None.

Omeprazole
(oh-MEH-prah-zohl)
Pregnancy Class: C
Prilosec **(Rx)**
Classification: Agent to suppress gastric acid secretion

Mechanism of Action: Thought to be a gastric pump inhibitor in that it blocks the final step of acid production by inhibiting the H^+-K^+ ATPase system at the secretory surface of the gastric parietal cell. Both basal and stimulated acid secretions are inhibited. Serum gastrin levels are increased during the first 1 or 2 weeks of therapy and are maintained at such levels during the course of therapy. Because omeprazole is acid-labile, the product contains an enteric-coated granule formulation; however, absorption is rapid.
Onset of Action: Within 1 hr.
Duration of Action: Up to 72 hr.
Uses: Short-term (4 to 8-week) treatment of active duodenal ulcer, active benign gastric ulcer, erosive esophagitis (all grades), and heartburn and other symptoms associated with GERD. In combination with clarithromycin for eradication of *Helicobacter pylori* and treatment of active duodenal ulcer. In combination with clarithromycin and amoxicillin for eradication of *H. pylori* and treatment of active duodenal ulcer. Long-term maintenance therapy for healed erosive esophagitis. Long-term treatment of pathologic hypersecretory conditions such as Zollinger-Ellison syndrome, multiple endocrine adenomas, and systemic mastocytosis. *Investigational:* Posterior laryngitis,

enhanced efficacy of pancreatin for treating steatorrhea in cystic fibrosis. **Contraindications:** Lactation. Use as maintenance therapy for duodenal ulcer disease.

Precautions: Bioavailability may be increased in geriatric patients. Use with caution during lactation. Symptomatic effects with omeprazole do not preclude gastric malignancy. Safety and effectiveness have not been determined in children.

Route/Dosage ─────────────
* **Capsules, Enteric-Coated**
  Active duodenal ulcer.
Adults, 20 mg/day for 4–8 weeks.
  Erosive esophagitis, heartburn, symptoms associated with GERD.
Adults: 20 mg/day for 4–8 weeks.
Maintenance of healing erosive esophagitis: 20 mg daily.
  Treatment of H. pylori, reduction of risk of duodenal ulcer recurrence.
Days 1–14: Omeprazole, 40 mg daily in the morning, plus clarithromycin, 500 mg t.i.d. **Days 15–28:** Omeprazole, 20 mg daily. Or, omeprazole, 20 mg b.i.d.; clarithromycin, 500 mg b.i.d.; and amoxicillin, 1 g b.i.d. for 10 days. If an ulcer is present, continue omeprazole, 20 mg once daily, for an additional 18 days.
  Pathologic hypersecretory conditions.
Adults, initial: 60 mg/day; then, dose individualized although doses up to 120 mg t.i.d. have been used. Daily doses greater than 80 mg should be divided.
  Gastric ulcers.
Adults: 40 mg once daily for 4–8 weeks.
How Supplied: *Enteric Coated Capsule:* 10 mg, 20 mg, 40 mg
Side Effects: *CNS:* Headache, dizziness. Possibly, anxiety disorders, abnormal dreams, vertigo, insomnia, nervousness, apathy, paresthesia, somnolence, depression, aggression, hallucinations, hemifacial dysesthesia, tremors, confusion. *GI:* Diarrhea, N&V, abdominal pain, abdominal swellling, constipation, flatulence, anorexia, fecal discoloration, esophageal candidiasis, mucosal atrophy

of the tongue, dry mouth, irritable colon, gastric fundic gland polyps, gastroduodenal carcinoids. *Hepatic: **Pancreatitis.*** Overt liver disease, including hepatocellular, cholestatic, or mixed hepatitis; *liver **necrosis, hepatic failure,*** hepatic encephalopathy. *CV:* Angina, chest pain, tachycardia, bradycardia, palpitation, peripheral edema, elevated BP. *Respiratory:* URI, pharyngeal pain, bronchospasms, cough, epistaxis. *Dermatologic:* Rash, severe generalized skin reaction including ***toxic epidermal necrolysis, Stevens-Johnson syndrome;*** erythema multiforme, skin inflammation, urticaria, pruritus, alopecia, dry skin, hyperhidrosis. *GU:* UTI, acute interstitial nephritis, urinary frequency, hematuria, proteinuria, glycosuria, testicular pain, microscopic pyuria, gynecomastia. *Hematologic:* Pancytopenia, thrombocytopenia, anemia, leukocytosis, neutropenia, hemolytic anemia, ***agranulocytosis.*** *Musculoskeletal:* Asthenia, back pain, myalgia, joint pain, muscle cramps, muscle weakness, leg pain. *Miscellaneous:* Rash, angioedema, fever, pain, gout, fatigue, malaise, weight gain, tinnitus, alteration in taste.

When used with clarithromycin the following *additional* side effects were noted: Tongue discoloration, rhinitis, pharyngitis, and flu syndrome.

NOTE: Data are lacking on the effect of long-term hypochlorhydria and hypergastrinemia on the risk of developing tumors.

OD Overdose Management: *Symptoms:* Confusion, drowsiness, blurred vision, tachycardia, nausea, diaphoresis, flushing, headache, dry mouth. *Treatment:* Symptomatic and supportive. Omeprazole is not readily dialyzable.

Drug Interactions
Ampicillin (esters) / Possible ↓ absorption of ampicillin esters due to ↑ pH of stomach
Clarithromycin / Possible ↑ plasma levels of both drugs
Diazepam / ↑ Plasma levels of diazepam due to ↓ rate of metabolism by the liver

Iron salts / Possible ↓ absorption of iron salts due to ↑ pH of stomach
Ketoconazole / Possible ↓ absorption of ketoconazole due to ↑ pH of stomach
Phenytoin / ↑ Plasma levels of phenytoin due to ↓ rate of metabolism of the liver
Sucralfate / ↓ Absorption of omeprazole; take 30 min before sucralfate
Warfarin / Prolonged rate of elimination of warfarin due to ↓ rate of metabolism by the liver

EMS CONSIDERATIONS
None.

Ondansetron hydrochloride
(on-DAN-sih-tron)
Pregnancy Class: B
Zofran **(Rx)**
Classification: Antiemetic

Mechanism of Action: Cytotoxic chemotherapy is thought to release serotonin from enterochromoffin cells of the small intestine. The released serotonin may stimulate the vagal afferent nerves through the 5-HT$_3$ receptors, thus stimulating the vomiting reflex. Ondansetron, a 5-HT$_3$ antagonist, blocks this effect of serotonin. Whether the drug acts centrally and/or peripherally to antagonize the effect of serotonin is not known. **Uses: Parenteral:** Prevent N&V resulting from initial and repeated courses of cancer chemotherapy, including high-dose cisplatin. Prophylaxis and treatment of selected cases of postoperative N&V, especially situations where there is multiple retching and long periods of N&V. **Oral:** Prevention of N&V due to initial and repeated courses of cancer chemotherapy. Prevenion of N&V associated with radiotherapy in patients receiving either total body irradiation, single high-dose fraction, or daily fractions to the abdomen. Prevention of postoperative N&V.
Precautions: Use with caution during lactation. Safety and effectiveness in children 3 years of age and younger are not known.

Route/Dosage
• **IM, IV**
Prevention of N&V due to chemotherapy.
Adults and children, 4–18 years: Three doses of 0.15 mg/kg each. The first dose is infused over 15 min starting 30 min before the start of chemotherapy; the second and third doses are given 4 hr and 8 hr, respectively, after the first dose. Alternatively, a single 32-mg dose may be given over 15 min beginning 30 min before the start of chemotherapy.
N&V postoperatively.
Adults: 4 mg over 2–5 min immediately before induction of anesthesia or postoperatively as needed. **Children, 2 to 12 years weighing 40 kg or less:** 0.1 mg/kg over 2–5 min. **Children, 2 to 12 years weighing over 40 kg:** 4 mg over 2–5 min.
• **Tablets**
In patients receiving moderately emetogenic chemotherapy agents.
Adults and children over 12 years of age: 8 mg 30 min before treatment followed by a second 8-mg dose 8 hr after the first dose; **then,** 8 mg b.i.d. for 1–2 days after chemotherapy. **Children, 4–12 years:** 4 mg t.i.d. The first dose is given 30 min before chemotherapy with subsequent doses 4 and 8 hr after the first dose. **Then,** 4 mg q 8 hr for 1–2 days after completion of chemotherapy.
Prevention of N&V due to total body irradiation.
8 mg 1–2 hr before each fraction of radiotherapy administered each day.
Prevention of N&V in single high-dose fraction radiotherapy to the abdomen.
8 mg 1–2 hr before radiotherapy with subsequent doses 8 hr after the first dose for 1–2 days after completion of radiotherapy.
Prevention of N&V due to daily fractionated radiotherapy to the abdomen.

8 mg 1–2 hr before radiotherapy, with subsequent doses 8 hr after the first dose for each day radiotherapy is given.

Prevention of postoperative N&V.
Adults: 16 mg given as a single dose 1 hr before induction of anesthesia. –
How Supplied: *Injection:* 2 mg/mL, 32 mg/50 mL; *Oral Solution:* 4 mg/5 mL; *Tablet:* 4 mg, 8 mg
Side Effects: *GI:* Diarrhea (most common), constipation, xerostomia, abdominal pain. *CNS:* Headache, dizziness, drowsiness, sedation, malaise, fatigue, anxiety, agitation, extrapyramidal syndrome, **clonic-tonic seizures.** *CV:* Tachycardia, chest pain, hypotension, ECG alterations, angina, bradycardia, syncope, vascular occlusive events. *Dermatologic:* Pain, redness, and burning at injection site; cold sensation, pruritus, paresthesia. *Hypersensitivity (rare):* **Anaphylaxis, bronchospasm, shock,** SOB, hypotension, angioedema, urticaria. *Miscellaneous:* Rash, **bronchospasm,** transient blurred vision, hypokalemia, weakness, fever, musculoskeletal pain, shivers, dysuria, postoperative carbon dioxide-related pain, akathisia, acute dystonic reactions, gynecologic disorder, urinary retention, wound problem.

EMS CONSIDERATIONS

See also *Antiemetics.*

Oprelvekin (Interleukin 11)

(oh-PREL-veh-kin)
Pregnancy Class: C
Neumega **(Rx)**
Classification: Recombinant human interleukin

Mechanism of Action: Produced by DNA recombinant technology. Interleukin 11 is a thrombopoietic growth factor that directly stimulates proliferation of hematopoietic stem cells and megakaryocyte progenitor cells and induces megakaryocyte maturation. This results in increased platelet production.

Uses: Prevention of thrombocytopenia following myelosuppressive chemotherapy in patients with nonmyeloid malignancies who are at high risk of severe thrombocytopenia.
Contraindications: Use following myeloablative chemotherapy. Lactation.
Precautions: Use with caution in CHF or those who may be susceptible to developing CHF, and in those with history of heart failure who are well compensated and receiving appropriate medical therapy. Use with caution in those with history of atrial arrhythmia, in preexisting papilledema or with tumors involving CNS. Safety and efficacy have not been determined in children.

Route/Dosage
• **SC Injection**
Prevent thrombocytopenia.
Adults: 50 mcg/kg once daily SC either in the abdomen, thigh, or hip. Dose of 75–100 mcg/kg in children will produce plasma levels consistent with a 50 mcg/kg dose in adults.
How Supplied: *Powder for injection, lyophilized:* 5 mg
Side Effects: *Body as a whole:* Edema, neutropenic fever, headache, fever, rash, conjunctival infection, asthenia, chills, pain, infection, flu-like symptoms. *GI:* N&V, mucositis, diarrhea, oral moniliasis, abdominal pain, constipation, dyspepsia. *CV:* Tachycardia, vasodilation, palpitations, syncope, atrial fibrillation or flutter, thrombocytosis, thrombotic events. *CNS:* Dizziness, insomnia, nervousness. *Respiratory:* Dyspnea, rhinitis, increased cough, pharyngitis, pleural effusion. *Miscellaneous:* Anorexia, ecchymosis, myalgia, bone pain, alopecia, mild visual blurring (transient).

In cancer patients: Also, amblyopia, dehydration, exfoliative dermatitis, eye hemorrhage, paresthesia, skin discoloration.
OD Overdose Management: *Symptoms:* Increased incidence of cardiovascular events if doses greater than 50 mcg/kg are given. *Treatment:* Dis-

continue drug and observe for signs
of toxicity.

EMS CONSIDERATIONS
None.

Oseltamivir phosphate
(oh-sell-TAM-ih-vir)
Pregnancy Class: C
Tamiflu **(Rx)**
Classification: Antiviral drug

Mechanism of Action: Hydrolyzed
by hepatic esterases to the active
oseltamivir carboxylate. May act by inhibiting the flu virus neuraminidase
with possible alteration of virus particle aggregation and release. Drug
resistance to influenza A virus is
possible.
Uses: Treatment of uncomplicated
acute influenza A or B infection in
adults who have been symptomatic
for 2 days or less.
Precautions: Use during lactation
only if potential benefits outweigh
the potential risk to the infant. Efficacy in patients who begin treatment after 40 hr of symptoms, for prophylactic use to prevent influenza, or for
repeated treatment courses have not
been determined. Safety and efficacy
have not been determined in children less than 18 years of age.

Route/Dosage
• **Capsules**
  Influenza A or B infection.
75 mg b.i.d. for 5 days. Begin treatment within 2 days of onset of flu
symptoms.
How Supplied: *Capsules:* 75 mg
Side Effects: *GI:* N&V, diarrhea, abdominal pain. *CNS:* Dizziness, headache, insomnia, vertigo. *Miscellaneous:* Bronchitis, cough, fatigue.

EMS CONSIDERATIONS
None.

Oxacillin sodium
(ox-ah-SILL-in)
Pregnancy Class: B

Bactocill **(Rx)**
Classification: Antibiotic, penicillin

Mechanism of Action: Penicillinase-
resistant, acid-stable drug used for resistant staphylococcal infections.
Uses: Infections caused by penicillinase-producing staphylococci; may
be used to initiate therapy when a
staphylococcal infection is suspected.

Route/Dosage
• **Capsules, Oral Solution**
  *Mild to moderate infections of the
  upper respiratory tract, skin, soft tissue.*
Adults and children (over 20 kg):
500 mg q 4–6 hr for at least 5 days.
Children less than 20 kg: 50 mg/
kg/day in equally divided doses q 6
hr for at least 5 days.
  Septicemia, deep-seated infections.
Parenteral therapy (see below) followed by PO therapy. **Adults:** 1 g q
4–6 hr; **children:** 100 mg/kg/day in
equally divided doses q 4–6 hr.
• **IM, IV**
  Mild to moderate infections.
Adults and children over 40 kg:
250–500 mg q 4–6 hr. **Children less
than 40 kg:** 50 mg/kg/day in equally divided doses q 6 hr.
  *Severe infections of the lower respir-
  atory tract or disseminated infections.*
Adults and children over 40 kg: 1
g q 4–6 hr. **Children less than 40 kg:**
100 mg/kg/day in equally divided
doses q 4–6 hr. **Neonates and premature infants, less than 2,000 g:**
50 mg/kg/day divided q 12 hr if less
than 7 days of age and 100 mg/
kg/day divided q 8 hr if more than 7
days of age. **Neonates and premature infants, more than 2,000 g:**
75 mg/kg/day divided q 8 hr if less
than 7 days of age and 150 mg/
kg/day divided q 6 hr if more than
7 days of age. Maximum daily dose:
Adults, 12 g; **children,** 100–300
mg/kg.
How Supplied: *Capsule:* 250 mg,
500 mg; *Injection:* 1 g/50 mL, 2 g/50
mL; *Powder for injection:* 500 mg, 1 g,

2 g, 10 g; *Powder for reconstitution:* 250 mg/5 mL

EMS CONSIDERATIONS

See also *Anti-Infectives* and *Penicillins.*

Oxaprozin
(ox-ah-PROH-zin)
Pregnancy Class: C
Daypro **(Rx)**
Classification: Nonsteroidal anti-inflammatory drug

Uses: Acute and chronic management of rheumatoid arthritis and osteoarthritis.

Route/Dosage
• **Tablets**
Rheumatoid arthritis.
Adults: 1,200 mg once daily. Lower and higher doses may be required in certain patients.
Osteoarthritis.
Adults: 1,200 mg once daily. For patients with a lower body weight or with a milder disease, 600 mg/day may be appropriate.
Maximum daily dose for either rheumatoid arthritis or osteoarthritis: 1,800 mg (or 26 mg/kg, whichever is lower) given in divided doses.
How Supplied: *Tablet:* 600 mg

EMS CONSIDERATIONS

None.

Oxazepam
(ox-AY-zeh-pam)
Pregnancy Class: D
Serax **(C-IV) (Rx)**
Classification: Antianxiety agent, benzodiazepine

Mechanism of Action: Absorbed more slowly than most benzodiazepines.
Uses: Anxiety, tension, anxiety with depression. Adjunct in acute alcohol withdrawal.
Precautions: Dosage has not been established in children less than 12 years of age; use is not recommended in children less than 6 years of age.

Route/Dosage
• **Capsules, Tablets**
Anxiety, mild to moderate.
Adults: 10–30 mg t.i.d.–q.i.d.
Anxiety, tension, irritability, agitation.
Geriatric and debilitated patients: 10 mg t.i.d.; can be increased to 15 mg t.i.d.–q.i.d.
Alcohol withdrawal.
Adults: 15–30 mg t.i.d.–q.i.d.
How Supplied: *Capsule:* 10 mg, 15 mg, 30 mg; *Tablet:* 15 mg
Side Effects: Additional: Paradoxical reactions characterized by sleep disorders and hyperexcitability during first weeks of therapy. Hypotension after parenteral administration.

EMS CONSIDERATIONS

None.

Oxiconazole nitrate
(ox-ee-KON-ah-zohl)
Pregnancy Class: B
Oxistat **(Rx)**
Classification: Antifungal agent, topical

Mechanism of Action: Acts by inhibiting ergosterol synthesis, which is required for cytoplasmic membrane integrity of fungi. Active against a broad range of organisms including many strains of *Trichophyton rubrum* and *T. mentagrophytes.*
Uses: Topical treatment of tinea pedis (athlete's foot), tinea cruris (jock itch), tinea versicolor, and tinea corporis (ringworm) due to *Trichophyton rubrum, T. mentagrophytes,* and *Epidermophyton floccosum.* Cream only to treat tinea versicolor due to *Malassezia furfur* in adults and children.
Contraindications: Ophthalmic or vaginal use.
Precautions: Use with caution during lactation.

Route/Dosage
• **Cream (1%), Lotion (1%)**
Adults and childen: Apply 1% cream or lotion to cover affected areas and immediately surrounding areas once or twice daily for tinea

pedis, tinea corporis, and tinea cruris. Apply cream only to affected areas once daily for tinea versicolor. To prevent recurrence, continue treatment for 2 weeks for tinea corporis, tinea versicolor, and tinea cruris and for 1 month for tinea pedis.

How Supplied: *Cream:* 1%; *Lotion:* 1%

Side Effects: *Dermatologic:* Pruritus, burning, stinging, irritation, erythema, fissuring, maceration, contact dermatitis, scaling, tingling, pain, dyshidrotic eczema, folliculitis, papules, rash, nodules.

EMS CONSIDERATIONS

See also *Anti-Infectives*.

Oxybutynin chloride

(ox-ee-BYOU-tih-nin)
Pregnancy Class: B
Ditropan **(Rx)**
Classification: Antispasmodic

Mechanism of Action: Causes increased vesicle capacity, decreases frequency of uninhibited contractions of the detrusor muscle, and delays initial urgency to void by exerting a direct antispasmodic effect. Has no effect at either the neuromuscular junction or autonomic ganglia. Has 4–10 times the antispasmodic effect of atropine but only one-fifth the anticholinergic activity.

Onset of Action: 30-60 min; **Time to peak effect:** 3-6 hr.

Duration of Action: 6-10 hr.

Uses: Neurogenic bladder disease characterized by urinary retention, urinary overflow, incontinence, nocturia, urinary frequency or urgency, reflex neurogenic bladder.

Contraindications: Glaucoma (angle closure), untreated narrow anterior chamber angles, GI obstruction, paralytic ileus, intestinal atony (in elderly or debilitated), megacolon, toxic megacolon complicating ulcerative colitis, severe colitis, myasthenia gravis, obstructive uropathy, unstable CV status in acute hemorrhage.

Precautions: *Use with caution when increased cholinergic effect is undesirable and in the elderly.* Safe use in children less than 5 years of age has not been determined. Use with caution in geriatric patients; during lactation; in patients with autonomic neuropathy, renal, or hepatic disease; and in patients with hiatal hernia with reflex esophagitis. Heat stroke and fever (due to decreased sweating) may occur if given at high environmental temperatures.

Route/Dosage ———————
• **Syrup, Tablets**

Adults: 5 mg b.i.d.–t.i.d. Maximum dose: 5 mg q.i.d. **Children, over 5 years:** 5 mg b.i.d. Maximum dose: 5 mg t.i.d.

How Supplied: *Syrup:* 5 mg/5 mL; *Tablet:* 5 mg

Side Effects: *GI:* N&V, constipation, bloated feeling, decreased GI motility. *CNS:* Drowsiness, insomnia, weakness, dizziness, restlessness, hallucinations. *EENT:* Dry mouth, decreased lacrimation, mydriasis, amblyopia, cycloplegia. *CV:* Tachycardia, palpitations, vasodilation. *Miscellaneous:* Decreased sweating, urinary hesitancy and retention, impotence, suppression of lactation, *severe allergic reactions,* drug idiosyncrasies, urticaria, and other dermal manifestations. *NOTE:* The drug may aggravate symptoms of prostatic hypertrophy, hypertension, coronary heart disease, CHF, hyperthyroidism, cardiac arrhythmias, and tachycardia.

OD **Overdose Management:** *Symptoms:* Intense CNS disturbances (restlessness, psychoses), circulatory changes (flushing, hypotension) and failure, respiratory failure, paralysis, coma. *Treatment:* Stomach lavage, physostigmine (0.5–2 mg IV; repeat as necessary up to maximum of 5 mg). Supportive therapy, if necessary. Counteract excitement with sodium thiopental (2%) or chloral hydrate (100–200 mL of 2% solution) rectally. Artificial respiration may be necessary if respiratory muscles become paralyzed.

---

bold italic = life threatening side effect

Drug Interactions: See *Cholinergic Blocking Agents.*

EMS CONSIDERATIONS

See also *Cholinergic Blocking Agents.*

————COMBINATION DRUG————

Oxycodone and acetaminophen

(ox-ee-KOH-dohn, ah-SEAT-ah-MIN-oh-fen)
Pregnancy Class: C
Endocet, Percocet, Roxicet **(C-II) (Rx)**
Classification: Analgesic

Uses: Relief of moderate to moderately severe pain.

Contraindications: Hypersensitivity to either oxycodone or acetaminophen.

Precautions: Can produce drug dependence and has abuse potential. The respiratory depressant effects of oxycodone can be exaggerated in patients with head injury, other intracranial lesions, or a preexisting increase in intracranial pressure. Use with caution in patients who are elderly, are debilitated, have severely impaired hepatic or renal function, are hyperthyroid, have Addison's disease, have prostatic hypertrophy, or have urethral stricture. Use for acute abdominal conditions may obscure the diagnosis or clinical course. Use with caution during lactation. Safety and efficacy in children have not been established.

Route/Dosage
- **Oral Solution, Tablets**
  Analgesic.
Adults: 5 mL of the oral solution q 6 hr or 1 tablet q 6 hr as needed for pain.

How Supplied: Endocet and Roxicet Tablets: *Narcotic analgesic:* Oxycodone hydrochloride, 5 mg. *Analgesic:* Acetaminophen, 325 mg.
Roxicet Oral Solution: *Narcotic analgesic:* Oxycodone hydrochloride, 5 mg/5 mL. *Analgesic:* Acetaminophen, 325 mg/5 mL.

Side Effects: Commonly, dizziness, lightheadedness, N&V, and sedation; these effects are more common in ambulatory patients than nonambulatory patients. Other side effects include euphoria, dysphoria, constipation, skin rash, and pruritus. See also individual components.

Drug Interactions
Anticholinergic drugs / Production of paralytic ileus
Antidepressants, tricyclic / ↑ Effect of either the tricyclic antidepressant or oxycodone
CNS depressants (including other narcotic analgesics, phenothiazines, antianxiety drugs, sedative-hypnotics, anesthetics, alcohol) / Additive CNS depression
MAO inhibitors / ↑ Effect of either the MAO inhibitor or oxycodone

EMS CONSIDERATIONS

See also *Acetaminophen* and *Narcotic Analgesics.*

Oxycodone hydrochloride

(ox-ee-KOH-dohn)
Pregnancy Class: C
OxyContin, Percolone CII, Roxicodone, Roxicodone Intensol **(C-II) (Rx)**
Classification: Narcotic analgesic, morphine type

Mechanism of Action: Semisynthetic opiate causing mild sedation and little or no antitussive effect. Most effective in relieving acute pain. Dependence liability is moderate.
Onset of Action: 15-30 min; **Peak effect:** 60 min.
Duration of Action: 4-6 hr.

Uses: Moderate to severe pain. The extended-release product (OxyContin) is indicated for moderate to severe pain, including that due to cancer, injuries, arthritis, lower back problems, and other musculoskeletal conditions that require treatment for more than a few days.

Contraindications: Additional: Use in children.

Precautions: OxyContin 80 mg controlled release is indicated only for opiate-tolerant patients.

Route/Dosage
• **Capsule, Oral Solution, Concentrated Solution, Tablet, Extended Release Tablet**
Analgesia.
Adults: 5 mg q 6 hr.
• **Extended Release Tablet**
Analgesia.
Adults, opioid-naive: 10 mg q 12 hr. **Adults, with prior narcotic therapy:** 10–30 mg b.i.d.
How Supplied: *Capsule:* 5 mg; *Concentrate:* 20 mg/mL; *Solution:* 5 mg/5 mL; *Tablet:* 5 mg; *Tablet, Extended Release:* 10 mg, 20 mg, 40 mg, 80 mg
Drug Interactions: Additional: Cients with gastric distress, such as colitis or gastric or duodenal ulcer, and patients who have glaucoma should not receive Percodan, which also contains aspirin.

EMS CONSIDERATIONS
See also *Narcotic Analgesics.*

Oxymorphone hydrochloride
(ox-ee-MOR-fohn)
Pregnancy Class: C
Numorphan **(C-I) (Rx)**
Classification: Narcotic analgesic, morphine type

Mechanism of Action: On a weight basis, is 2–10 times more potent as an analgesic than morphine, although potency depends on the route of administration. Produces mild depression of the cough reflex and significant respiratory depression and emesis.
Onset of Action: 5-10 min; **Peak effect:** 30-60 min.
Duration of Action: 3-6 hr.
Uses: Moderate to severe pain. **Parenteral:** Preoperative analgesia, to support anesthesia, obstetrics, relief of anxiety in patients with dyspnea associated with acute LV failure and pulmonary edema.

Route/Dosage
• **SC, IM**

Analgesia.
Adults, initial: 1–1.5 mg q 4–6 hr; dose can be increased carefully until analgesic response obtained.
Analgesia during labor.
Adults: 0.5–1.0 mg IM.
• **IV**
Analgesia.
Adults, initial: 0.5 mg.
• **Suppositories**
Analgesia.
Adults: 5 mg q 4–6 hr. **Not recommended for children under 12 years of age.**
How Supplied: *Injection:* 1 mg/mL, 1.5 mg/mL; *Suppository:* 5 mg

EMS CONSIDERATIONS
See also *Narcotic Analgesics.*

Oxytocin, parenteral
(ox-eh-TOE-sin)
Pregnancy Class: X
Pitocin **(Rx)**
Classification: Oxytocic agent

Mechanism of Action: Synthetic compound identical to the natural hormone isolated from the posterior pituitary. Has uterine stimulant, vasopressor, and weak antidiuretic properties. May act on uterine myofibril activity to increase the number of contracting myofibrils. Uterine sensitivity to oxytocin, as well as amplitude and duration of uterine contractions, increases gradually during gestation and just before parturition increases rapidly. Facilitates ejection of milk from the breasts by stimulating smooth muscle.
Onset of Action: IV: immediate; **IM:** 3-5 min; **Peak effects:** 40 min.
Duration of Action: IV: 20 min after infusion is stopped; **IM:** 2-3 hr.
Uses: *Antepartum:* Induction or stimulation of labor at term. To overcome true primary or secondary uterine inertia. Induction of labor with oxytocin is indicated only under certain *specific* conditions and is not usual because serious toxic effects can occur.
Oxytocin is indicated:
1. For uterine inertia.

2. For induction of labor in cases of erythroblastosis fetalis, maternal diabetes mellitus, preeclampsia, and eclampsia.

3. For induction of labor after premature rupture of membranes in last month of pregnancy when labor fails to develop spontaneously within 12 hr.

4. For routine control of postpartum hemorrhage and uterine atony.

5. To hasten uterine involution.

6. To complete inevitable abortions after the 20th week of pregnancy.

7. Intranasally for initial letdown of milk.

Investigational: Breast engorgement, oxytocin challenge test for determining antepartum fetal HR.

Contraindications: Hypersensitivity to drug. Significant cephalopelvic disproportion; unfavorable fetal positions or presentations that are undeliverable without conversion prior to delivery. In obstetric emergencies where the benefit-to-risk ratio for either the mother or fetus favors surgical intervention. Fetal distress where delivery is not imminent, prolonged use in uterine inertia or severe toxemia, hypertonic or hyperactive uterine patterns, when adequate uterine activity does not achieve satisfactory progress. Induction of augmentation of labor where vaginal delivery is contraindicated, including invasive cervical cancer, cord presentation or prolapse, total placenta previa and vasa previa, active herpes genitalis. Use of oxytocin citrate in severe toxemia, CV or renal disease. Use of intranasal oxytocin during pregnancy.

Also, predisposition to thromboplastin and amniotic fluid embolism (dead fetus, abruptio placentae), history of previous traumatic deliveries, or women with four or more deliveries. Never give oxytocin IV undiluted or in high concentrations.

Route/Dosage
• **IV Infusion, IM**
Induction or stimulation of labor.
Dilute 10 units (1 mL) to 1,000 mL isotonic saline or 5% dextrose for IV infusion. **Initial:** 0.001–0.002 unit/min (0.1–0.2 mL/min); dose can be gradually increased at 15- to 30-min intervals by 0.001 unit/min (0.1 mL/min) to maximum of 0.02 unit/min (2 mL/min).

Reduction of postpartum bleeding. Dilute 10–40 units (1–4 mL) to 1,000 mL with isotonic saline or 5% dextrose for IV infusion. Administer at a rate to control uterine atony, usually at a rate of 0.02–0.1 unit/min.

Incomplete or therapeutic abortion.
10 units at a rate of 0.02–0.04 unit/min by IV infusion or 10 units IM after placental delivery.

How Supplied: *Injection:* 10 U/mL.
Side Effects: *Mother:* Tetanic uterine contractions, *anaphylaxis,* cardiac arrhythmia, *fatal afibrinogenemia,* N&V, PVCs, increased blood loss, pelvic hematoma, hypertension, tachycardia, and ECG changes. Also, rarely, anxiety, dyspnea, precordial pain, edema, cyanosis or reddening of the skin, and CV spasm. Water intoxication from prolonged IV infusion, *death due to hypertensive episodes, SAH, postpartum hemorrhage, or uterine rupture.* Excessive dosage may cause uterine hypertonicity, spasm, tetanic contraction, or uterine rupture.

Fetus: *Death,* PVCs, bradycardia, tachycardia, arrhythmias, hypoxia, *intracranial hemorrhage due to overstimulation of the uterus during labor leads to uterine tetany with marked impairment of uteroplacental blood flow.*

NOTE: Hypersensitivity reactions occur rarely. When they do, they occur most often with natural oxytocin administered IM or in concentrated IV doses and least frequently after IV infusion or diluted doses. Accidental swallowing of buccal tablets is not harmful.

OD **Overdose Management:** *Symptoms: Hyperstimulation of the uterus resulting in hypertonic or tetanic contractions. Or, a resting tone of 15–20 cm water between contractions can result in uterine rupture, cervical and vaginal lacerations, tumultuous labor, uteroplacental* *hypoperfusion, postpartum hemorrhage, and a variable deceleration of fetal heart rate, fetal hypoxia, hypercapnia, or death. Water intoxication with seizures can occur if large doses (40–50 mL/min) of the drug are infused for long periods of time.* Treatment: Discontinue the drug and restrict fluid intake. Start diuresis and give a hypertonic saline solution IV. Correct electrolyte imbalance and control seizures with a barbiturate. If the patient is comatose, provide special nursing care.

Drug Interactions
Cyclopropane / Hypotension; also, maternal sinus bradycardia with abnormal AV rhythms

Sympathomimetic amines / Severe hypertension and possible stroke

EMS CONSIDERATIONS
Administration/Storage
IV 1. Use Y-tubing system, with one bottle containing IV solution and oxytocin, and the other containing only the IV solution. This allows for the discontinuation of the drug while maintaining the patency of the vein when it is decided to change to the drug-free infusion bottle.
2. Have magnesium sulfate immediately available to relax the uterus in case of tetanic uterine contractions.
Interventions: Monitor VS until stable.

Pancrelipase
(Lipancreatin)
(pan-kree-LY-payz)
Pregnancy Class: C
Cotazym, Cotazym-S, Creon 5, 10, or 20, Ilozyme, Ku-Zyme HP, Pancrease, Pancrease MT 4, 10, 16, or 20, Protilase, Viokase, Ultrase MT12, 20 or 24, Zymase **(Rx)**
Classification: Digestant

Mechanism of Action: Enzyme concentrate from hog pancreas, which contains lipase, amylase, and protease, enzymes that replace or supplement naturally occurring enzymes.
Uses: Pancreatic deficiency diseases such as chronic pancreatitis, cystic fibrosis of the pancreas, pancreatectomy, ductal obstructions caused by cancer of the pancreas or common bile duct, steatorrhea of malabsorption syndrome or postgastrectomy or postgastrointestinal surgery. Presumptive test for pancreatic function, especially in insufficiency due to chronic pancreatitis.
Contraindications: Hog protein sensitivity. Acute pancreatitis, acute exacerbation of chronic pancreatic disease.

Precautions: Safety for use during lactation and in children less than 6 months of age not established. Methacrylic acid copolymer, which is found in the enteric coating of certain products, may cause fibrosing colonopathy.

Route/Dosage
• **Capsules; Enteric-Coated Microspheres, Microtablets, Spheres, Pellets; Powder; Tablets**
Pancreatic insufficiency.
Adults and children over 12 years of age: 4,000–48,000 units of lipase with each meal and with snacks.
Children, 7–12 years: 4,000–12,000 units of lipase with each meal and snacks; **1–6 years:** 4,000–8,000 units of lipase with each meal and 4,000 units lipase with snacks. **6–12 months:** 2,000 units lipase with each meal. Dosage has not been established in children less than 6 months of age. Severe deficiencies may require up to 64,000–88,000 units of lipase with meals (or the frequency of administration can be increased if side effects are not manifested).

Pancreatectomy or obstruction of pancreatic ducts.
Adults: 8,000–16,000 units of lipase at 2 hr intervals or as directed by a physician.
Cystic fibrosis.
Use 0.7 g of the powder with meals.
How Supplied: *Capsule; Enteric Coated capsule; Enteric Coated tablet; Powder; Tablet*
Side Effects: *GI:* Nausea, diarrhea, abdominal cramps following high doses. *Other:* Inhalation of the powder is irritating to the skin and mucous membranes and may result in an asthma attack. High doses cause hyperuricemia and hyperuricosuria.
OD Overdose Management: *Symptoms:* Diarrhea, intestinal upset.
Drug Interactions
Calcium carbonate / ↓ Effect of pancreatic enzymes
Iron / Response to oral iron may ↓ if given with pancreatic enzymes
Magnesium hydroxide / ↓ Effect of pancreatic enzymes

EMS CONSIDERATIONS

None.

Pancuronium bromide
(pan-kyou-ROH-nee-um)
Pregnancy Class: C
Pavulon **(Rx)**
Classification: Neuromuscular blocking agent, nondepolarizing

Mechanism of Action: Anticholinesterase agents will reverse effects. Possesses vagolytic activity although it is not likely to cause histamine release.
Onset of Action: Within 45 sec;
Time to peak effect: 3-4.5 min (depending on the dose).
Duration of Action: 35-45 min (increased with multiple doses).
Uses: Adjunct to anesthesia to produce relaxation of skeletal muscle. Facilitate ET intubation. Facilitate management of patients undergoing mechanical ventilation.
Precautions: Children up to 1 month of age may be more sensitive to the effects of atracurium. Patients

with myasthenia gravis or Eaton-Lambert syndrome may have profound effects from small doses.

Route/Dosage
• **IV Only**
Muscle relaxation during anesthesia.
Adults and children over 1 month of age, initial: 0.04–0.1 mg/kg. Additional doses of 0.01 mg/kg may be administered as required (usually q 20–60 min). **Neonates:** Administer a test dose of 0.02 mg/kg first to determine responsiveness.
ET intubation.
0.06–0.1 mg/kg as a bolus dose. Can undertake intubation in 2 to 3 min.
How Supplied: *Injection:* 1 mg/mL, 2 mg/mL
Side Effects: Additional: *Respiratory:***Apnea, respiratory insufficiency.** *CV:* Increased HR and MAP. *Miscellaneous:* Salivation, akin rashes, **hypersensitivity reactions (e.g., bronchospasm,** flushing, hypotension, redness, tachycardia).

Drug Interactions: Additional: *Azathioprine* / Reverses effects of pancuronium. *Bacitracin* / Additive muscle relaxation. *Enflurane/* ↑ Muscle relaxation. *Isoflurane* / ↑ Muscle relaxation. *Metocurine* / ↑ Muscle relaxation, but duration is not prolonged. *Quinine* / ↑ Effect of pancuronium. *Sodium colistimethate* / ↑ Muslce relaxation. *Succinylcholine* / ↑ Intensity and duration of action of pancuronium. *Tetracyclines* / Additive muscle relaxation. *Theophyllines* / ↓ Effects of pancuronium; also, possible cardiac arrhythmias. *Tricyclic antidepressants with halothane* / Administration of pancuronium may cause severe arrhythmias. *Tubocurarine* / ↑ Muscle relaxation but duration is not prolonged.

EMS CONSIDERATIONS

See also *Neuromuscular Blocking Agents.*
Administration/Storage
IV 1. May be mixed with D5W, RL, and 0.9% NSS.
2. Administer in a continuously monitored environment.

3. Have appropriate anticholineste-rase agents available to reverse drug effects; pyridostigmine bromide, neostigmine, or edrophonium and are usually administered with atropine or glycopyrrolate.

Interventions

1. Provide ventilatory support.

2. Monitor and record VS, ECG. Drug can cause vagal stimulation resulting in bradycardia, hypotension, and cardiac arrhythmias.

3. Consciousness is not affected by pancuronium. Explain all procedures and provide emotional support. Do not conduct any discussions that should not be overheard.

4. With short-term therapy, reassure that they will be able to talk and move once the drug effects are reversed.

5. Assess airway at frequent intervals. Have a suction machine at the bedside.

6. *Never* leave patient unmonitored.

7. Determine patient need and administer medications for anxiety, pain, and/or sedation regularly.

Papaverine
(pah-PAV-er-een)
Pregnancy Class: C
Pavabid Plateau Caps, Pavagen TD
(Rx)
Classification: Peripheral vasodilator

Mechanism of Action: Direct spasmolytic effect on smooth muscle, possibly by inhibiting cyclic nucleotide phosphodiesterase, thus increasing levels of cyclic AMP. This effect is seen in the vascular system, bronchial muscle, and in the GI, biliary, and urinary tracts. Large doses produce CNS sedation and sleepiness. May also directly relax cerebral vessels as it increases cerebral blood flow and decreases cerebral vascular resistance. Depresses cardiac conduction and irritability and prolongs the myocardial refractory period.

Uses: Relief of cerebral and peripheral ischemia associated with arterial spasm and myocardial ischemia complicated by arrhythmias.

Contraindications: Complete AV block.

Precautions: Safe use during lactation or for children not established. Use with extreme caution in coronary insufficiency and glaucoma.

Route/Dosage ———————
• **Capsules, Timed-Release**
Ischemia.
150 mg q 12 hr. May be increased to 150 mg q 8 hr or 300 mg q 12 hr in difficult cases.

How Supplied: *Capsule, Extended Release:* 150 mg; *Injection:* 30 mg/mL

Side Effects: *CV:* Flushing of face, hypertension, increase in HR and depth of respiration. Large doses can depress AV and intraventricular conduction, causing serious arrhythmias. *GI:* Nausea, anorexia, abdominal distress, constipation or diarrhea, dry mouth and throat. *CNS:* Headache, drowsiness, sedation, vertigo. *Miscellaneous:* Sweating, malaise, pruritus, skin rashes, chronic hepatitis, hepatic hypersensitivity, jaundice, eosinophilia, altered LFTs.

OD Overdose Management: *NOTE:* Both acute and chronic poisoning may result from use of papaverine. Symptoms are extensions of side effects.

Symptoms (Acute Poisoning): Nystagmus, diplopia, drowsiness, weakness, lassitude, incoordination, coma, cyanosis, *respiratory depression. Treatment (Acute Poisoning):* Delay absorption by giving tap water, milk, or activated charcoal followed by gastric lavage or induction of vomiting and then a cathartic. Maintin BP and take measures to treat respiratory depression and coma. Hemodialysis is effective.

Symptoms (Chronic Poisoning): Ataxia, blurred vision, drowsiness, anxiety, headache, GI upset, depression, urticaria, erythematous macular eruptions, blood dyscrasias, hypotension. *Treatment (Chronic Poisoning):* Discontinue medication.

P

---

bold italic = life threatening side effect

Monitor and treat blood dyscrasias. Provide symptomatic treatment. Treat hypotension by IV fluids, elevation of legs, and a vasopressor with inotropic effects.

Drug Interactions
Diazoxide IV / Additive hypotensive effect
Levodopa / Papaverine ↓ effect of levodopa by blocking dopamine receptors

EMS CONSIDERATIONS
None.

Paregoric (Camphorated opium tincture)
(pair-eh-GOR-ick)
Pregnancy Class: C
(C-III) (Rx)
Classification: Antidiarrheal agent, systemic

Mechanism of Action: The active principle of the mixture is opium (0.04% of morphine). The preparation also contains benzoic acid, camphor, and anise oil. Morphine increases the muscular tone of the intestinal tract, decreases digestive secretions, and inhibits normal peristalsis. The slowed passage of the feces through the intestines promotes desiccation, which is a function of the time the feces spend in the intestine.
Duration of Action: 4-5 hr.
Uses: Acute diarrhea.
Contraindications: See *Morphine Sulfate.* Use in patients with diarrhea caused by poisoning until toxic substance has been eliminated. Treatment of pseudomembranous colitis due to lincomycin, penicillins, and cephalosporins. Rubbing paregoric on the gums of a teething child. Use to treat neonatal opioid dependence.

Route/Dosage
• **Liquid**
Adult: 5–10 mL 1–4 times/day (5 mL contains 2 mg of morphine). **Pediatric:** 0.25–0.5 mL/kg 1–4 times/day.
How Supplied: *Oral Liquid*: 2 mg/5 mL

Side Effects: See *Narcotic Analgesics.*
Drug Interactions: See *Narcotic Analgesics.*

EMS CONSIDERATIONS
See also *Narcotic Analgesics.*

Paricalcitol
(pair-ee-KAL-sih-tohl)
Pregnancy Class: C
Zemplar **(Rx)**
Classification: Drug for hyperparathyroidism

Mechanism of Action: Synthetic vitamin D analog that reduces parathyroid hormone levels in chronic renal failure with no significant changes in the incidence of hypercalcemia or hyperphosphatemia. Serum phosphorous, calcium, and calcium x phosphorous product may increase.
Uses: Prevention and treatment of secondary hyperparathyroidism associated with chronic renal failure.
Contraindications: Evidence of vitamin D toxicity, hypercalemia, or hypersensitivity to any part of the product. Use of phosphate or vitamin D-related compounds concomitantly with paricalcitol.
Precautions: Use with caution during lactation or if given with digitalis compounds. Safety and efficacy have not been determined in children.

Route/Dosage
• **Injection**
Treat hyperparathyroidism associated with chronic renal failure.
Initial: 0.04–0.1 mcg/kg (2.8 to 7 mcg) as a bolus dose no more frequently than every other day at any time during dialysis. Doses as high as 0.24 mcg/kg (16.8 mcg) have been used safely. If a satisfactory response is not seen, the dose may be increased by 2 to 4 mcg at 2– 4–week intervals. During any dosage adjustment period, monitor serum calcum and phosphorous levels more frequently. If an elevated calcium level or Ca x P product greater than 75 is noted, immediately reduce or stop

the drug until parameters are normal. Then, restart at a lower dose. Doses may need to be decreased as the parathyroid levels decrease in response to therapy.

How Supplied: *Injection:* 5 mcg/mL

Side Effects: *GI:* N&V, GI bleeding, dry mouth. *CV:* Palpitation. *CNS:* Lightheadedness. *Respiratory:* Pneumonia. *Miscellaneous:* Edema, chills, fever, flu, sepsis, not feeling well.

OD **Overdose Management:** *Symptoms:* Hypercalcemia. Early symptoms include weakness, headache, somnolence, nausea, vomiting, dry mouth, constipation, muscle pain, bone pain, and metallic taste. Late symptoms include anorexia, weight loss, conjunctivitis, pancreatitis, photophobia, rhinorrhea, pruritus, hyperthermia, decreased libido, elevated BUN, hypercholesterolemia, elevated AST and ALT, ectopic calcification, hypertension, cardiac arrhythmias, somnolence, overt psychosis, death (rarely). *Treatment:* Immediately reduce or discontinue therapy. Institute a low calcium diet and withdraw calcium supplements. Mobilize patient, give attention to fluid and electrolyte imbalances, assess ECG abnormalities (especially if also taking digitalis), and undertake hemodialysis or peritoneal dialysis against a calcium-free dialysate. Monitor serum calcium levels frequentlly until normal values are obtained.

Drug Interactions: Digitalis toxicity is potentiated by hypercalcemia.

EMS CONSIDERATIONS
None.

Paromomycin sulfate
(pair-oh-moh-MY-sin)
Humatin **(Rx)**
Classification: Antibiotic, aminoglycoside

Mechanism of Action: Obtained from *Streptomyces rimosus forma paromomycina.*

Uses: Inhibition of ammonia-forming bacteria in GI tract in hepatic encephalopathy, intestinal amebiasis, preoperative suppression of intestinal flora. Hepatic coma. *Investigational:* Anthelmintic, to treat *Dientamoeba fragilis, Diphyllobothrium latum, Taenia saginata, T. solium, Dipylidium caninum,* and *Hymenolepis nana.*

Contraindications: Intestinal obstruction.

Precautions: Use during pregnancy only if benefits outweigh risks. Use with caution in the presence of GI ulceration because of possible systemic absorption.

Route/Dosage
• **Capsules**
  Hepatic coma.
Adults: 4 g/day in divided doses for 5–6 days.
  Intestinal amebiasis.
Adults and children: 25–35 mg/kg/day administered in three doses with meals for 5–10 days.
  D. fragilis infections.
25–30 mg/kg/day in three divided doses for 1 week.
  H. nana infections.
45 mg/kg/day for 5–7 days.
  D. latum, T. saginata, T. solium, D. caninum infections.
Adults: 1 g/ q 15 min for a total of four doses; **pediatric:** 11 mg/kg/15 min for four doses.

How Supplied: *Capsule:* 250 mg

Side Effects: Additional: Diarrhea or loose stools. Heartburn, emesis, and pruritus ani. Superinfections, especially by monilia.

Drug Interactions: Penicillin is inhibited by paromomycin.

EMS CONSIDERATIONS
None.

Paroxetine hydrochloride
(pah-ROX-eh-teen)
Pregnancy Class: B
Paxil **(Rx)**
Classification: Antidepressant

Mechanism of Action: Inhibits neuronal reuptake of serotonin in the CNS resulting in potentiation of serotonergic activity in the CNS. Weak effects on neuronal uptake of norepinephrine and dopamine. Does not cause anticholinergic effects or orthostatic hypotension; slight sedative effects.

Uses: Treatment of major depressive episodes, panic disorder with or without agoraphobia (as defined in DSM-IV), and obsessive-compulsive disorders (as defined in DSM-III-R). *Investigational:* Headaches, diabetic neuropathy, premature ejaculation.

Contraindications: Use of alcohol and in patients taking MAO inhibitors.

Precautions: Use with caution and initially at reduced dosage in elderly patients as well as in those with impaired hepatic or renal function, with a history of mania, with a history of seizures, in patients with diseases or conditions that could affect metabolism or hemodynamic responses, and during lactation. Concurrent administration of paroxetine with lithium or digoxin should be undertaken with caution. Safety and efficacy have not been determined in children.

Route/Dosage
• **Tablets**
Depression.
Adults: 20 mg/day, usually given as a single dose in the morning. Some patients not responding to the 20-mg dose may benefit from increasing the dose in 10-mg/day increments, up to a maximum of 50 mg/day. Make dose changes at intervals of at least 1 week.
Panic disorders.
Adults, initial: 10 mg/day usually given in the morning; **then,** increase by 10-mg increments each week until a dose of 40 mg/day is reached. Maximum daily dose: 60 mg.
Obsessive-compulsive disorders.
Adults, initial: 20 mg/kg; **then,** increase by 10-mg increments a day in intervals of at least 1 week until a dose of 40 mg/kg is reached. Maximum daily dose: 60 mg.
Headaches.
10–50 mg/day.
Diabetic neuropathy.
10–60 mg/day.
Premature ejaculation in men.
20 mg/day.
NOTE: Geriatric or debilitated patients, those with severe hepatic or renal impairment, **initial:** 10 mg/day, up to a maximum of 40 mg/day for all uses.

How Supplied: *Suspension:* 10 mg/5 mL; *Tablet:* 10 mg, 20 mg, 30 mg, 40 mg

Side Effects: The side effects listed were observed with a frequency up to 1 in 1,000 patients.

CNS: Headache, somnolence, insomnia, agitation, *seizures,* tremor, anxiety, activation of mania or hypomania, dizziness, nervousness, paresthesia, drugged feeling, myoclonus, CNS stimulation, confusion, amnesia, impaired concentration, depression, emotional lability, vertigo, abnormal thinking, akinesia, alcohol abuse, ataxia, *convulsions, possibility of a suicide attempt* depersonalization, hallucinations, hyperkinesia, hypertonia, incoordination, lack of emotion, manic reaction, paranoid reaction. *GI:* Nausea, abdominal pain, diarrhea, dry mouth, vomiting, constipation, decreased appetite, flatulence, oropharynx disorder ("lump" in throat, tightness in throat), dyspepsia, increased appetite, bruxism, dysphagia, eructation, gastritis, glossitis, increased salivation, mouth ulceration, *rectal hemorrhage,* abnormal LFTs. *Hematologic:* Anemia, leukopenia, lymphadenopathy, purpura. *CV:* Palpitation, vasodilation, postural hypotension, hypertension, syncope, tachycardia, bradycardia, conduction abnormalities, abnormal ECG, hypotension, migraine, peripheral vascular disorder. *Dermatologic:* Sweating, rash, pruritus, acne, alopecia, dry skin, ecchymosis, eczema, furunculosis, urticaria. *Metabolic/Nutritional:* Edema, weight gain, weight loss, hyperglycemia, peripheral edema, thirst. *Respiratory:* Respiratory disorder (cold symptoms or URI), pharyngitis, yawn, increased cough, rhinitis, asthma, bronchitis, dyspnea, epistaxis, hyperventilation, pneumonia, respiratory flu, sinusitis. *GU:* Abnormal ejaculation (usually delay), erectile difficulties, sexual dysfunction, impotence, urinary frequency, urinary difficulty or hesitancy, decreased libido, anorgasmia in women, difficulty in reaching climax/orgasm in women, abortion, amenorrhea, breast pain, cystitis, dysmenorrhea, dysuria, menorrhagia, nocturia, polyuria, urethritis, urinary incontinence, urinary retention, vaginitis. *Musculoskeletal:* Asthenia, back pain, myopathy, myalgia, myasthenia, neck pain, arthralgia, arthritis. *Ophthalmologic:* Blurred vision, abnormality of accommodation, eye pain, mydriasis. *Otic:* Ear pain, otitis media, tinnitus. *Miscellaneous:* Fever, chest pain, trauma, taste perversion or loss, chills, malaise, allergic reaction, **carcinoma,** face edema, moniliasis, anorexia.

NOTE: Over 4- to 6-week period, there was evidence of adaptation to side effects such as nausea and dizziness but less adaptation to dry mouth, somnolence, and asthenia.

OD Overdose Management: *Symptoms:* N&V, drowsiness, sinus tachycardia, dilated pupils. *Treatment:*
• Establish and maintain an airway.
• Ensure adequate oxygenation and ventilation.
• Induction of emesis, lavage, or both; following evacuation, 20–30 g activated charcoal may be given q 4–6 hr during the first 24–48 hr after ingestion.
• Take an ECG and monitor cardiac function if there is any evidence of abnormality.
• Provide supportive care with monitoring of VS.

Drug Interactions
Antiarrhythmics, Type IC / Possible ↑ effect due to ↓ liver breakdown
Cimetidine / ↑ Effect of paroxetine due to ↓ breakdown by the liver
Digoxin / Possible ↓ plasma levels
MAO inhibitors / Possibility of serious, and sometimes fatal, reactions including hyperthermia, rigidity, myoclonus, autonomic instability with possible rapid fluctuations in VS, and mental status changes in-

cluding extreme agitation progressing to delirium and coma
Phenobarbital / Possible ↓ effect of paroxetine due to ↑ breakdown by the liver
Phenytoin / Possible ↓ effect of paroxetine due to ↑ breakdown by the liver; also, paroxetine ↓ levels of phenytoin
Procyclidine / ↓ Dose of procyclidine as significant anticholinergic effects are seen
Theophylline / ↑ Theophylline levels
Tryptophan / Possibility of headache, nausea, sweating, and dizziness when taken together
Warfarin / Possibility of ↑ bleeding tendencies

EMS CONSIDERATIONS
None.

Pediazole
(PEE-dee-ah-zohl)
Pregnancy Class: C
(Rx)
Classification: Antibacterial

Uses: Acute otitis media in children caused by *Haemophilus influenzae.*
Contraindications: Pregnancy at term and in children less than 2 months of age. Use with caution during other times of pregnancy.

Route/Dosage
• **Oral Suspension**
Usual: Equivalent of 50 mg/kg/day of erythromycin and 150 mg/kg/day of sulfisoxazole, up to a maximum of 6 g/day. **Over 45 kg:** 10 mL q 6 hr; **24 kg:** 7.5 mL q 6 hr; **16 kg:** 5 mL q 6 hr; **8 kg:** 2.5 mL q 6 hr; **less than 8 kg:** Calculate dose according to body weight.
How Supplied: This product is available as granules that, when reconstituted, provide an oral suspension.

Antibacterial, antibiotic: Erythromycin ethylsuccinate, 200 mg/5 mL erythromycin activity. *Antibacterial, sulfonamide:* Sulfisoxazole, 600 mg/5 mL. See also information on individual components.

EMS CONSIDERATIONS

See also *All Anti-Infectives* and *Sulfonamides*.

Pemirolast potassium ophthalmic solution

(peh-MEER-oh-last)
Pregnancy Class: C
Alamast **(Rx)**
Classification: Mast cell stabilizier, ophthalmic drug

Mechanism of Action: Inhibits the antigen-induced release of inflammatory mediators such as histamine and leukotriene C_4, D_4, and E_4, from human mast cells. Also inhibits the chemotaxis of eosinophils into ocular tissue and blocks the release of mediators from human eosinophils. Probably acts by preventing calcium influx into mast cells upon antigen stimulation.

Uses: Prevent itching of the eye due to allergic conjunctivitis.

Contraindications: Use by injection or PO.

Precautions: Use with caution during lactation. Safety and efficacy have not been determined in children less than 3 years of age.

Route/Dosage
• **Ophthalmic Solution**
   Allergic conjunctivitis.
1–2 gtt in each affected eye q.i.d. Effect may be evident within a few days but frequently requires up to four weeks.

How Supplied: *Ophthalmic Solution:* 0.1%

Side Effects: *Ophthalmic:* Burning, dry eye, foreign body sensation, ocular discomfort. *Respiratory:* Rhinitis, cold/flu symptoms, bronchitis, cough, sinusitis, sneezing/nasal congestion. *Miscellaneous:* Headache, allergy, back pain, dysmenorrhea, fever.

EMS CONSIDERATIONS

None.

Pemoline

(PEM-oh-leen)
Pregnancy Class: Pregnancy Class: B
Cylert, Cylert Chewable **(C-IV) (Rx)**
Classification: CNS stimulant

Mechanism of Action: Believed to act by dopaminergic mechanisms. Causes a decrease in hyperactivity and a prolonged attention span in children.

Duration of Action: Up to 8 hr.

Uses: Attention-deficit disorders. Due to possible life-threatening hepatic failure, not usually first-line therapy. *Investigational:* Narcolepsy.

Contraindications: Hypersensitivity to drug. Tourette's syndrome. Children under 6 years of age.

Precautions: Safe use during lactation has not been established. Use with caution in impaired renal or kidney function. Chronic use in children may cause growth suppression.

Route/Dosage
• **Tablets, Chewable Tablets**
   Attention-deficit disorders.
Children, 6 years and older, initial: 37.5 mg/day as a single dose in the morning; increase at 1-week intervals by 18.75 mg until desired response is attained up to maximum of 112.5 mg/day. **Usual maintenance:** 56.25–75 mg/day.
   Narcolepsy.
Adults: 50–200 mg/day in two divided doses.

How Supplied: *Chew Tablet:* 37.5 mg; *Tablet:* 18.75 mg, 37.5 mg, 75 mg

Side Effects: *CNS:* Insomnia (most common). Dyskinesia of the face, tongue, lips, and extremities; precipitation of Tourette's syndrome. Mild depression, headache, nystagmus, dizziness, hallucinations, irritability, **seizures.** Exacerbation of behavior disturbances and thought disorders in psychotic children. *GI:* Transient weight loss, gastric upset, nausea. *Miscellaneous:* Skin rash, **hepatic failure.**

OD Overdose Management: *Symptoms:* Symptoms of CNS stimulation and sympathomimetic effects including agitation, confusion, delirium, euphoria, headache, muscle twitching, mydriasis, vomiting, hallucinations, flushing, sweating, tachycardia, hyperreflexia, tremors, ***hyperpyrexia,*** hypertension, ***seizures (may be followed by coma).*** *Treatment:* Reduce external stimuli. If symptoms are not severe, induce vomiting or undertake gastric lavage. Chlorpromazine can be used to decrease the CNS stimulation and sympathomimetic effects.

EMS CONSIDERATIONS
None.

Penbutolol sulfate
(pen-BYOU-toe-lohl)
Pregnancy Class: C
Levatol **(Rx)**
Classification: Beta-adrenergic blocking agent

Mechanism of Action: Has both beta-1- and beta-2-receptor blocking activity. It has no membrane-stabilizing activity but does possess minimal intrinsic sympathomimetic activity.
Uses: Mild to moderate arterial hypertension.
Contraindications: Bronchial asthma or bronchospasms, including severe COPD.
Precautions: Dosage has not been established in children. Geriatric patients may manifest increased or decreased sensitivity to the usual adult dose.

Route/Dosage ————————
• **Tablets**
  Hypertension.
Initial: 20 mg/day either alone or with other antihypertensive agents.
Maintenance: Same as initial dose. Doses greater than 40 mg/day do not result in a greater antihypertensive effect.
How Supplied: *Tablet:* 20 mg

EMS CONSIDERATIONS
See also *Beta-Adrenergic Blocking Agents, and Antihypertensive Agents.*

Penciclovir
(pen-SIGH-kloh-veer)
Pregnancy Class: B
Denavir **(Rx)**
Classification: Antiviral drug

Mechanism of Action: Active against herpes simplex viruses (HSVs), including HSV-1 and HSV-2. In infected cells, viral thymidine kinase phosphorylates penciclovir to a monophosphate form which then is converted to penciclovir triphosphate by cellular kinases. Penciclovir triphosphate inhibits HSV polymerase competitively with deoxyguanosine triphosphate which inhibits herpes viral DNA synthesis and replication.
Uses: Treatment of recurrent herpes labialis (cold sores) in adults.
Contraindications: Lactation. Application of the drug to mucous membranes.
Precautions: Use with caution if applied around the eyes due to the possibility of irritation. The effect of the drug in immunocompromised patients has not been determined. Safety and efficacy have not been determined in children.

Route/Dosage ————————
• **Cream (10 mg/g)**
  Cold sores.
Apply q 2 hr while awake for 4 days.
How Supplied: *Cream:* 10 mg/g.
Side Effects: *Dermatologic:* Reaction at the site of application, hypesthesia, local anesthesia, erythematous rash, mild erythema. *Miscellaneous:* Headache, taste perversion.

EMS CONSIDERATIONS
See also *Antiviral Drugs.*

Penicillamine
(pen-ih-SILL-ah-meen)
Pregnancy Class: D
Cuprimine, Depen **(Rx)**
Classification: Antirheumatic, heavy metal antagonist, to treat cystinuria

Mechanism of Action: A chelating agent for mercury, lead, iron, and

P

copper; forms soluble complexes, thus decreasing toxic levels of the metal (e.g., copper in Wilson's disease). Anti-inflammatory activity may be due to its ability to inhibit T-lymphocyte function and therefore decrease cell-mediated immune response. May also protect lymphocytes from hydrogen peroxide generated at the site of inflammation by inhibiting release of lysosomal enzymes and oxygen radicals. Beneficial effects may not be seen for 2 to 3 months when used for rheumatoid arthritis. In cystinuria, is able to reduce excess cystine excretion, probably by disulfide interchange between penicillamine and cystine. This results in penicillamine-cysteine disulfide, which is a complex that is more soluble than cystine and is thus readily excreted.

Uses: Wilson's disease, cystinuria, and rheumatoid arthritis (severe active disease unresponsive to conventional therapy). Heavy metal antagonist. *Investigational:* Primary biliary cirrhosis. Scleroderma.

Contraindications: Pregnancy, lactation, penicillinase-related aplastic anemia or agranulocytosis, hypersensitivity to drug. Patients allergic to penicillin may cross-react with penicillamine. Renal insufficiency or history thereof.

Precautions: Use for juvenile rheumatoid arthritis has not been established. Patients older than 65 years may be at greater risk of developing hematologic side effects.

Route/Dosage ─────────
• **Capsules, Tablets**
   Rheumatoid arthritis.
Adults, individualized, initial: 125–250 mg/day. Dosage may be increased at 1- to 3-month intervals by 125- to 250-mg increments until adequate response is attained. **Maximum:** 500–750 mg/day. Up to 500 mg/day can be given as a single dose; higher dosages should be divided. **Maintenance, individualized. Range:** 500–750 mg/day. If the patient is in remission for 6 or more months, a gradual stepwise decrease in dose

of 125 or 250 mg/day at about 3-month intervals can be attempted.
Wilson's disease.
Dosage is usually calculated on the basis of the urinary excretion of copper. One gram of penicillamine promotes excretion of 2 mg of copper. **Adults and adolescents, usual, initial:** 250 mg q.i.d. Dosage may have to be increased to 2 g/day. A further increase does not produce additional excretion. **Pediatric, 6 months—young children:** 250 mg as a single dose given in fruit juice.
Antidote for heavy metals.
Adults: 0.5–1.5 g/day for 1–2 months; **pediatric:** 30–40 mg/kg/day (600–750 mg/m²/day) for 1–6 months.
Cystinuria.
Individualized and based on excretion rate of cystine (100–200 mg/day in patients with no history of stones, below 100 mg with patients with history of stones or pain). Initiate at low dosage (250 mg/day) and increase gradually to minimum effective dosage. **Adult, usual:** 2 g/day (range: 1–4 g/day); **pediatric:** 7.5 mg/kg q.i.d. If divided in fewer than four doses, give larger dose at night.
Primary biliary cirrhosis.
Adults: 600–900 mg/day.
How Supplied: *Capsule:* 125 mg, 250 mg; *Tablet:* 250 mg

Side Effects: This drug manifests a large number of potentially serious side effects. Patients should be carefully monitored. *GI:* Altered taste perception (common), N&V, diarrhea, anorexia, GI pain, stomatitis, oral ulcerations, reactivation of peptic ulcer, glossitis, cheilosis, colitis, gingivostomatitis (rare). *CNS:* Tinnitus, myasthenia gravis, peripheral sensory and motor neuropathies (with or without muscle weakness), reversible optic neuritis, polyradiculopathy (rare). *Hematologic:* Thrombocytopenia, leukopenia, *agranulocytosis, aplastic anemia,* eosinophilia, monocytosis, red cell aplasia, thrombocytopenia, *hemolytic anemia,* leukocytosis, thrombocytosis. *Renal:* Proteinuria, hematuria, nephrotic syndrome, *Goodpasture's syndrome* (a severe and ultimately fatal glomerulonephritis). *Aller-*

gic: Rashes (common), lupus-like syndrome, drug fever, pruritus, pemphigoid-type symptoms (e.g., bullous lesions), arthralgia, lymphadenopathy, dermatoses, urticaria, thyroiditis, hypoglycemia, migratory polyarthralgia, polymyositis, allergic alveolitis. *Respiratory:* Obliterative bronchiolitis, pulmonary fibrosis, pneumonitis, bronchial asthma, interstitial pneumonitis. *Dermatologic:* Increased skin friability, excessive skin wrinkling, development of small white papules at venipuncture and surgical sites, alopecia or falling hair, lichen planus, dermatomyositis, nail disorders, ***toxic epidermal necrolysis,*** cutaneous macular atrophy. *Hepatic:* Pancreatitis, hepatic dysfunction, intrahepatic cholestasis, toxic hepatitis (rare). *Other:* Thrombophlebitis, hyperpyrexia, polymyositis, mammary hyperplasia, renal vasculitis (may be fatal), hot flashes, lupus erythematosus–like syndrome.

Drug Interactions
Antacids / ↓ Effect of penicillamine due to ↓ absorption from GI tract
Antimalarial drugs / ↑ Risk of blood dyscrasias and adverse renal effects
Cytotoxic drugs / ↑ Risk of blood dyscrasias and adverse renal effects
Digoxin / Penicillamine ↓ effect of digoxin
Gold therapy / ↑ Risk of blood dyscrasias and adverse renal effects
Iron salts / ↓ Effect of penicillamine due to ↓ absorption from GI tract

EMS CONSIDERATIONS
None.

Penicillin G benzathine and Procaine combined, intramuscular
(pen-ih-SILL-in, BEN-zah-theen, PROH-kain)
Pregnancy Class: B
Bicillin C-R, Bicillin C-R 900/300 **(Rx)**
Classification: Antibiotic, penicillin

Uses: Streptococcal infections (A, C, G, H, L, and M) without bacteremia, of the upper respiratory tract, skin, and soft tissues. Scarlet fever, erysipelas, pneumococcal infections, and otitis media. *Note:* For severe pneumonia, empyema, bacteremia, pericarditis, meningitis, peritonitis, and arthritis of pneumococcal etiology, use aqueous penicillin G during the acute stage.
Contraindications: Use to treat syphilis, gonorrhea, yaws, bejel, and pinta.

Route/Dosage
- **IM Only**
  Streptococcal infections.
Adults and children over 27 kg: 2,400,000 units, given at a single session using multiple injection sites or, alternatively, in divided doses on days 1 and 3; **children 13.5–27 kg:** 900,000–1,200,000 units; **infants and children under 13.5 kg:** 600,000 units.
  Pneumococcal infections, except meningitis.
Adults: 1,200,000 units; **pediatric:** 600,000 units. Give q 2–3 days until temperature is normal for 48 hr.
How Supplied: The injection contains the following: *300,000 units/dose:* 150,000 units each of penicillin G benzathine and penicillin G procaine. *600,000 units/dose:* 300,000 units each of penicillin G benzathine and penicillin G procaine. *1,200,000 units/dose:* 600,000 units each of penicillin G benzathine and penicillin G procaine. *2,400,000 units/dose:* 1,200,000 units each of penicillin G benzathine and penicillin G procaine. *Injection, 900/300 per dose.* 900,000 units of penicillin G benzathine and 300,000 units of penicillin G procaine.
Drug Interactions: Additional: Aspirin, ethacrynic acid, furosemide, indomethacin, sulfonamides, or thiazide diuretics may compete with penicillin G for renal tubular secretion → prolongation of serum t½ of penicillin.

P

---

bold italic = life threatening side effect

EMS CONSIDERATIONS

See also *Anti-Infectives* and *Penicillins*.

Penicillin G benathine, intramuscular

(pen-ih-SILL-in, BEN-zah-theen)
Pregnancy Class: B
Bicillin L-A, Permapen **(Rx)**
Classification: Antibiotic, penicillin

Mechanism of Action: Penicillin G is neither penicillinase resistant nor acid stable. The product is a long-acting (repository) form of penicillin in an aqueous vehicle; it is administered as a sterile suspension.

Uses: Infections due to penicillin G sensitive microorganisms susceptible to low and prolonged serum levels. Mild to moderate URTI due to susceptible streptococci. Syphilis, yaws, bejel, and pinta. Prophylaxis of rheumatic fever or chorea. Follow-up prophylactic therapy for rheumatic heart disease and acute glomerulonephritis.

Contraindications: IV use.

Route/Dosage

• **Parenteral Suspension (IM Only)**

URTI due to Group A streptococcus.
Adults: 1,200,000 units as a single dose; **older children:** 900,000 units as a single dose; **children under 27 kg:** 300,000–600,000 units as a single dose; **neonates:** 50,000 units/kg as a single dose.

Early syphilis (primary, secondary, or latent).
Adults: 2,400,000 units as a single dose. **Children:** 50,000 units/kg, up to the adult dose.

Gummas and cardiovascular syphilis.
Adults: 2,400,000 units q 7 days for 3 weeks. **Children:** 50,000 units/kg, up to adult dose.

Neurosyphilis.
Adults: Aqueous penicillin G, 18,000,000–24,000,000 units IV/day for 10–14 days followed by penicillin G benzathine, 2,400,000 units IM q week for 3 weeks.

Yaws, bejel, pinta.
1,200,000 units in a single dose.

Prophylaxis of rheumatic fever and glomerulonephritis.
Following an acute attack, 1,200,000 units once a month or 600,000 units q 2 weeks.

How Supplied: *Injection:* 300,000 U/mL, 600,000 U/mL

Drug Interactions: Additional: Aspirin, ethacrynic acid, furosemide, indomethacin, sulfonamides, or thiazide diuretics may compete with penicillin G for renal tubular secretion → prolongation of serum t½ of penicillin.

EMS CONSIDERATIONS

See also *Anti-Infectives* and *Penicillins*.

Penicillin G potassium for injection
Penicillin G (Aqueous) sodium for injection

(pen-ih-SILL-in)
Pregnancy Class: B
Potassium (Pfizerpen **(Rx)**) Sodium **(Rx)**
Classification: Antibiotic, penicillin

Mechanism of Action: The first choice for treatment of many infections due to low cost. Rapid onset makes it especially suitable for fulminating infections.

Uses: Streptococci of groups A, C, G, H, L, and M are sensitive to penicillin G. High serum levels are effective against streptococci of the D group.

Route/Dosage

• **Penicillin G Potassium and Sodium Injections (IM, Continuous IV Infusion)**

Serious streptococcal infections (empyema, endocarditis, meningitis, pericarditis, pneumonia).
Adults: 5–24 million units/day in divided doses q 4 to 6 hr. **Pediatric:** 150,000 units/kg/day given in equal doses q 4 to 6 hr. **Infants over 7 days of age:** 75,000 units/kg/day in

divided doses q 8 hr. **Infants less than 7 days of age:** 50,000 units/kg/day given in divided doses q 12 hr. For group B streptococcus, give 100,000 units/kg/day.

Meningococcal meningitis/septicemia.

Adults: 1–2 million units IM q 2 hr or 20–30 million units/day continuous IV drip for 14 days or until afebrile for 7 days. Or, 200,000–300,000 units/kg/day q 2–4 hr in divided doses for a total of 24 doses.

Meningitis due to susceptible strains of Pneumococcus or Meningococcus.

Children: 250,000 units/kg/day divided in equal doses q 4 to 6 hr for 7 to 14 days (maximum daily dose: 12–20 million units). **Infants over 7 days of age:** 200,000–300,0000 units/kg/day divided into equal doses given q 6 hr. **Infants less than 7 days of age:** 100,000–150,000 units/kg/day.

Anthrax.

Adults: A minimum of 5 million units/day (up to 12–20 million units have been used).

Clostridial infections.

Adults: 20 million units/day used with an antitoxin.

Actinomycosis.

Adults: *Cervicofacial:* 1–6 million units/day. *Thoracic and abdominal disease:* **initial,** 10–20 million units/day divided into equal doses given q 6 hr IV for 6 weeks followed by penicillin V, PO, 500 mg q.i.d. for 2–3 months.

Rat-bite fever, Haverhill fever.

Adults: 12–20 million units/day q 4 to 6 hr for 3–4 weeks. **Children:** 150,000–250,000 units/kg/day in equal doses q 4 hr for 4 weeks.

Endocarditis due to Listeria.

Adults: 15–20 million units/day q 4 to 6 hr for 4 weeks.

Endocarditis due to Erysipelothrix rhusiopathiae.

Adults: 12–20 million units/day q 4 to 6 hr for 4–6 weeks.

Meningitis due to Listeria.

Adults: 15–20 million units/day q 4 to 6 hr for 2 weeks.

Pasteurella infections causing bacteremia and meningitis.

Adults: 4–6 million units/day q 4 to 6 hr for 2 weeks.

Severe fusospirochetal infections of the oropharynx, lower respiratory tract, and genital area.

Adults: 5–10 million units/day q 4 to 6 hr.

Pneumococcal infections causing empyema.

Adults: 5–24 million units/day in divided doses q 4–6 hr.

Pneumococcal infections causing meningitis.

Adults: 20–24 million units/day for 14 days.

Pneumococcal infections causing endocarditis, pericarditis, peritonitis, suppurative arthritis, osteomyelitis, mastoiditis.

Adults: 12–20 million units/day for 2–4 weeks.

Adjunct with antitoxin to prevent diphtheria.

Adults: 2–3 million units/day in divided doses q 4 to 6 hr for 10–12 days.

Children: 150,000–250,000 units/kg/day in equal doses q 6 hr for 10 days.

Neurosyphilis.

Adults: 18–24 million units/day (3–4 million units q 4 hr) for 10–14 days (can be followed by benzathine penicillin G, 2.4 million units IM weekly for 3 weeks).

Disseminated gonococcal infections.

Adults: 10 million units/day q 4 to 6 hr (for meningococcal meningitis/septicemia, give q 3 hr). **Children, less than 45 kg:** Arthritis, 100,000 units/kg/day in 4 equally divided doses for 7 to 10 days. Endocarditis: 250,000 units/kg/day in equal doses q 4 hr for 4 weeks. Meningitis: 250,000 units/kg/day in equal doses q 4 hr for 10 to 14 days. **Children, over 45 kg:** Arthritis, endocarditis, meningitis: 10 million units/day in 4 equally divided doses (duration depends on type of infection).

P

Congenital syphilis after the new-born period.
50,000 units/kg IV q 4–6 hr for 10–14 days.

Symptomatic or asymptomatic congenital syphilis in infants.
Infants: 50,000 units/kg IV q 12 hr the first 7 days; then, q 8 hr for a total of 10 days. **Children:** 50,000 units/kg q 4 to 6 hr for 10 days.

How Supplied: Penicillin G potassium for injection: *Injection:* 1 million U/50 mL, 2 million U/50 mL, 3 million U/50 mL; *Powder for injection:* 1 million U, 5 million U, 10 million U, 20 million U Penicillin G (Aqueous) sodium for injection: *Powder for injection:* 5 million U

Side Effects: Additional: Rapid IV administration may cause hyperkalemia and cardiac arrhythmias. Renal damage occurs rarely.

Drug Interactions: Additional: Aspirin, ethacrynic acid, furosemide, indomethacin, sulfonamides, or thiazide diuretics may compete with penicillin G for renal tubular secretion → prolongation of serum t½ of penicillin.

EMS CONSIDERATIONS

See also *Anti-Infectives* and *Penicillins*.

Penicillin G procaine, intramuscular

(pen-ih-SILL-in, PROH-caine)
Pregnancy Class: B
Wycillin **(Rx)**
Classification: Antibiotic, penicillin

Mechanism of Action: Long-acting (repository) form in aqueous or oily vehicle. Because of slow onset, a soluble penicillin is often administered concomitantly for fulminating infections.

Uses: Penicillin-sensitive staphylococci, pneumococci, streptococci, and bacterial endocarditis (for *Streptococcus viridans* and *S. bovis* infections). Gonorrhea, all stages of syphilis. *Prophylaxis:* Rheumatic fever, pre- and postsurgery. Diphtheria, anthrax, fusospirochetosis (Vincent's

infection), erysipeloid, rat-bite fever. *Note:* Severe pneumonia, empyema, bacteremia, pericarditis, meningitis, peritonitis, and purulent or septic arthritis due to pneumococcus are better treated with aqueous penicillin G during the acute phase.

Contraindications: Use in newborns due to possible sterile abcesses and procaine toxicity.

Route/Dosage

• **IM Only**

Pneumococccal, staphylococcal, streptococcal infections; erysipeloid, rat-bite fever, anthrax, fusospirochetosis.
Adults, usual: 600,000–1 million units/day for 10–14 days. **Children, less than 27.2 kg:** 300,000 units/day.

Bacterial endocarditis (only very sensitive S. viridans or S. bovis infections).
Adults: 600,000–1 million units/day.

Diphtheria carrier state.
300,000 units/day for 10 days.

Diphtheria, adjunct with antitoxin.
300,000–600,000 units/day.

Anthrax (cutaneous), erysipeloid, rate-bite fever.
600,000 to 1 million units/day.

Fusospirochetosis: Vincent's gingivitis, pharyngitis.
600,000 to 1 million units/day. Obtain necessary dental care.

Gonococcal infections.
4.8 million units divided into at least two doses at one visit and given with 1 g PO probenecid (given 30 min before the injections).

Neurosyphilis.
2.4 million units/day for 10 to 14 days (given at two sites) with probenecid 500 mg PO q.i.d.; **then,** benzathine penicillin G, 2.4 million units/week for 3 weeks. *Note:* For yaws, bejel, and pinta, treat the same as syphilis in corresponding stage of disease.

Congenital syphilis in infants, symptomatic and asymptomatic.
50,000 units/kg/day for 10 days.

Syphilis: primary, secondary, latent with negative spinal fluid.

Adults and children over 12 years: 600,000 units/day for 8 days (total of 4.8 million units).

Syphilis: tertiary, neurosyphilis, latent with positive spinal-fluid.
Adults: 600,000 units/day for 10 to 15 days (total of 6 to 9 million units).

How Supplied: *Injection:* 600,000 U/mL

Drug Interactions: Additional: Aspirin, ethacrynic acid, furosemide, indomethacin, sulfonamides, or thiazide diuretics may compete with penicillin G for renal tubular secretion → prolongation of serum t½ of penicillin.

EMS CONSIDERATIONS

See also *Anti-Infectives* and *Penicillins.*

Penicillin V potassium (Phenoxymethyl-penicillin potassium)

(pen-ih-SILL-in)

Pregnancy Class: B
Beepen-VK, Penicillin VK, Pen-Vee K, Veetids `250' **(Rx)**
Classification: Antibiotic, penicillin

Mechanism of Action: Related closely to penicillin G.

Uses: Mild to moderate upper respiratory tract streptococcal infections, including scarlet fever and erysipelas. Mild to moderate upper respiratory tract pneumococcal infections, including otitis media. Mild staphylococcal infections of the skin and soft tissue. Mild to moderate fusospirochetosis (Vincent's infection) of the oropharynx. Prophylaxis of recurrence following rheumatic fever or chorea. *Investigational:* Prophylactially to reduce *S. pneumoniae* septicemia in children with sickle cell anemia, mild to moderate anaerobic infections, Lyme disease.

Contraindications: PO penicillin V to treat severe pneumonia, empyema, bacteremia, pericarditis, meningitis, and arthritis during the acute stage. Prophylactic uses for GU instrumentation or surgery, sigmoidoscopy, or childbirth.

Precautions: More and more strains of staphylococci are resistant to penicillin V, necessitating culture and sensitivity studies.

Route/Dosage

• **Oral Solution, Tablets**
Streptococcal infections, including scarlet fever and mild erysipelas.
Adults and children over 12 years: 125–250 mg q 6–8 hr for 10 days. **Children, usual:** 500 mg q 8 hr for pharyngitis.
Staphylococcal infections (including skin and soft tissue), fusospirochetosis of oropharynx.
Adults and children over 12 years: 250 mg q 6–8 hr.
Pneumococcal infections, including otitis media.
Adults and children over 12 years: 250 mg q 6 hr until afebrile for at least 2 days.
Prophylaxis of recurrence of rheumatic fever/chorea.
Adults and children over 12 years: 125–250 mg b.i.d., on a continuing basis.
Prophylaxis of septicemia caused by Staphylococcus pneumoniae *in children with sickle cell anemia.*
125 mg b.i.d.
Anaerobic infections.
250 mg q.i.d. See also *Penicillin G, Procaine, Aqueous, Sterile.*
Lyme disease.
250–500 mg q.i.d. for 10–20 days (for children less than 2 years of age, 50 mg/kg/day in four divided doses for 10–20 days).
NOTE: 250 mg penicillin V is equivalent to 400,000 units.

How Supplied: *Powder for reconstitution:* 125 mg/5 mL, 250 mg/5 mL; *Tablet:* 250 mg, 500 mg

Drug Interactions: Additional: *Contraceptives, oral /* ↓ Effectiveness of oral contraceptives.*Neomycin, oral /* ↓ Absorption of penicillin V.

EMS CONSIDERATIONS

See also *Anti-Infectives* and *Penicillins.*

P

---

bold italic = life threatening side effect

Pentamidine isethionate

(pen-TAM-ih-deen)
Pregnancy Class: C
NebuPent, Pentam **(Rx)**
Classification: Antibiotic, miscellaneous (antiprotozoal)

Mechanism of Action: Inhibits synthesis of DNA, RNA, phospholipids, and proteins, thereby interfering with cell metabolism. May interfere also with folate transformation.

Uses: Parenteral: Pneumonia caused by *Pneumocystis carinii*. **Inhalation:** Prophylaxis of *P. carinii* in high-risk HIV-infected patients defined by one or both of the following: (a) a history of one or more cases of pneumonia caused by *P. carinii* and/or (b) a peripheral CD4+ lymphocyte count less than 200/mm^3. *Investigational:* Trypanosomiasis, visceral leishmaniasis.

Contraindications: Anaphylaxis to inhaled or parenteral pentamidine.

Precautions: Use with caution in patients with hepatic or kidney disease, hypertension or hypotension, hyperglycemia or hypoglycemia, hypocalcemia, leukopenia, thrombocytopenia, anemia, ventricular tachycardia, pancreatitis, Stevens-Johnson syndrome.

Route/Dosage
• **IV, Deep IM**
Adults and children: 4 mg/kg/day for 14 days. Dosage should be reduced in renal disease.
• **Aerosol**
Prevention of P. carinii pneumonia.
300 mg q 4 weeks given via the Respirgard II nebulizer.

How Supplied: *Powder for injection,* 300 mg; *Powder for inhalation,* 300 mg

Side Effects: Parenteral. *CV:* Hypotension, *ventricular tachycardia,* phlebitis. *GI:* Nausea, anorexia, bad taste in mouth. *Hematologic:* Leukopenia, thrombocytopenia, anemia. *Electrolytes/glucose:* Hypoglycemia, hypocalcemia, hyperkalemia. *CNS:* Dizziness without hypotension, confusion, hallucinations. *Miscellaneous:* Acute renal failure, *Stevens-*

Johnson syndrome, elevated serum creatinine, elevated LFTs, pain or induration at IM injection site, sterile abscess at injection site, rash, neuralgia.

Inhalation. Most frequent include the following. *GI:* Decreased appetite, N&V, metallic taste, diarrhea, abdominal pain. *CNS:* Fatigue, dizziness, headache. *Respiratory:* SOB, cough, pharyngitis, chest pain, chest congestion, *bronchospasm,* pneumothorax. *Miscellaneous:* Rash, night sweats, chills, myalgia, headache, anemia, edema.

EMS CONSIDERATIONS

See also *Anti-Infectives.*

---COMBINATION DRUG---

Pentazocine hydrochloride with Naloxone hydrochloride Pentazocine lactate

(pen-TAZ-oh-seen, nah-LOX-ohn)
Pregnancy Class: C
Pentazocine hydrochloride with Naloxone hydrochloride (Talwin NX **(C-IV) (Rx)**) Pentazocine lactate (Talwin **(C-IV) (Rx)**)
Classification: Narcotic agonist/antagonist

Mechanism of Action: Manifests both narcotic agonist and antagonist properties. Agonist effects are due to combination with kappa and sigma opioid receptors; antagonistic effect is due to an action on mu opioid receptors. Also elevates systemic and pulmonary arterial pressure, systemic vascular resistance, and LV end-diastolic pressure, which results in an increased cardiac workload. One-third as potent as morphine as an analgesic.

To reduce the possibility of abuse, the PO dosage form of pentazocine has been combined with naloxone (Talwin NX), which will prevent the effects of IV administered pentazocine but will not affect the efficacy of pentazocine when taken PO. If pentazocine with naloxone is used IV, fatal reactions may occur, which include vascular occlusion, pulmonary emboli, ulceration, and abscesses, and withdrawal in narcotic-dependent individuals.

Onset of Action: IM: 15-20 min; **PO:** 15-30 min; **IV:** 2-3 min. **Peak effect: IM,** 15-60 min; **PO,** 60-180 min. **Duration of Action: All routes:** 3 hr. However, onset, duration, and degree of relief depend on both dose and severity of pain.

Uses: PO: Moderate to severe pain. **Parenteral:** Preoperative or preanesthetic medication, obstetrics, supplement to surgical anesthesia. Moderate to severe pain.

Contraindications: Additional: Increased ICP or head injury. Use in children under 12 years of age. Use of methadone or other narcotics for pentazocine withdrawal.

Precautions: Use with caution in impaired renal or hepatic function, as well as after MI, when N&V are present. Use with caution in women delivering premature infants and in patients with respiratory depression. Safety and efficacy in children less than 12 years of age have not been determined.

Route/Dosage

PENTAZOCINE HYDROCHLORIDE WITH NALOXONE

• **Tablets**
  Analgesia.
Adults: 50 mg q 3–4 hr, up to 100 mg. Daily dose should not exceed 600 mg.

PENTAZOCINE LACTATE

• **IM, IV, SC**
  Analgesia.
Adults: 30 mg q 3–4 hr; doses exceeding 30 mg IV or 60 mg IM not recommended. Do not exceed a total daily dosage of 360 mg.
  Obstetric analgesia.
Adults: 30 mg IM given once; or, 20 mg IV q 2–3 hr for two or three doses.

How Supplied: Each tablet of pentazocine HCl with naloxone HCl contains: pentazocine HCl, 50 mg, and naloxone HCl, 0.5 mg.

Side Effects: Additional: *CNS:* Syncope, dysphoria, nightmares, hallu-cinations, disorientation, paresthesias, confusion, *seizures, Miscellaneous:* Dedcreased WBCs, edema of the face, chills. Both psychologic and physical dependence are possible, although the addiction liability is thought to be no greater than for codeine. Multiple parenteral doses may cause severe sclerosis of the skin, SC tissues, and underlying muscle.

EMS CONSIDERATIONS

See also *Narcotic Analgesics.*

Pentobarbital
Pentobarbital sodium
(pen-toe-BAR-bih-tal)
Pregnancy Class: D
Pentobarbital (Nembutal **(C-II) (Rx)**)
Pentobarbital sodium (Nembutal Sodium **(C-II) (Rx)**)
Classification: Sedative-hypnotic, barbiturate type

Mechanism of Action: Short-acting.
Uses: PO: Sedative. Short-term treatment of insomnia (no more than 2 weeks). Preanesthetic. **Rectal:** Sedation, short-term treatment of insomnia (no more than 2 weeks). **Parenteral:** Short-term treatment of insomnia (no more than 2 weeks). Preanesthetic. Anticonvulsant in anesthetic doses for emergency treatment of acute convulsive states (e.g., status epilepticus, eclampsia, meningitis, tetanus, and toxic reactions to strychnine or local anesthetics). *Investigational:* Parenterally to induce coma to protect the brain from ischemia and increased ICP following stroke and head trauma.
Precautions: Reduce dose in geriatric and debilitated patients and in impaired hepatic or renal function.

Route/Dosage
• **Capsules**
  Sedation.
Adults: 20 mg t.i.d.–q.i.d. **Pediatric:** 2–6 mg/kg/day, depending on age,

P

weight, and degree of sedation desired.

Preoperative sedation.
Adults: 100 mg. **Pediatric:** 2–6 mg/kg/day (maximum of 100 mg), depending on age, weight, and degree of sedation desired.

Hypnotic.
Adults: 100 mg at bedtime.

* **Suppositories, Rectal**
Hypnotic.
Adults: 120–200 mg at bedtime; **infants, 2–12 months (4.5–9 kg):** 30 mg; **1–4 years (9–18.2 kg):** 30 or 60 mg; **5–12 years (18.2–36.4 kg):** 60 mg; **12–14 years (36.4–50 kg):** 60 or 120 mg.

* **IM**
Hypnotic/preoperative sedation.
Adults: 150–200 mg; **pediatric:** 2–6 mg/kg (not to exceed 100 mg).

Anticonvulsant.
Pediatric, initially: 50 mg; **then,** after 1 min, additional small doses may be given, if needed, until the desired effect is achieved.

* **IV**
Sedative/hypnotic.
Adults: 100 mg followed in 1 min by additional small doses, if required, up to a total of 500 mg.

Anticonvulsant.
Adults, initial: 100 mg; **then,** after 1 min, additional small doses may be given, if needed, up to a total of 500 mg. **Pediatric, initially:** 50 mg; **then,** after 1 min, additional small doses may be given, if needed, until the desired effect is achieved.

How Supplied: Pentobarbital: *Elixir:* 18.2 mg/5 mL. Pentobarbital sodium: *Capsule:* 50 mg, 100 mg; *Injection:* 50 mg/mL; *Suppository:* 30 mg, 60 mg, 120 mg, 200 mg

EMS CONSIDERATIONS

See also *Barbiturates.*

Pentosan polysulfate sodium
(PEN-toh-san)
Pregnancy Class: B
Elmiron **(Rx)**
Classification: Urinary analgesic

Mechanism of Action: Mechanism for urinary analgesic activity is not known. It appears to adhere to the bladder wall mucosal membrane and may act as a buffer to control cell permeability, thus preventing irritating solutes in the urine from reaching the cells.

Uses: Relief of bladder pain or discomfort associated with interstitial cystitis.

Contraindications: Hypersensitivity to pentosan polysulfate sodium or related compounds.

Precautions: Use with caution during lactation, in those with hepatic insufficiency or spleen disorders, and in those who have a history of heparin-induced thrombocytopenia. Safety and efficacy have not been determined in children less than 16 years of age.

Route/Dosage ————————

* **Capsules**
Interstitial cystitis.
100 mg t.i.d.

How Supplied: *Capsule:* 100 mg

Side Effects: *GI:* Diarrhea, N&V, abdominal pain, dyspepsia, anorexia, colitis, constipation, esophagitis, flatulence, gastritis, mouth ulcer. *CNS:* Headache, severe emotional lability or depression, hyperkinesia, dizziness, insomnia. *CV:* Bleeding complications, including ecchymosis, epistaxis, gum hemorrhage. *Hematologic:* Anemia, leukopenia, thrombocytopenia. *Respiratory:* Dyspnea, pharyngitis, rhinitis. *Dermatologic:* Alopecia, rash, pruritus, urticaria, increased sweating. *Ophthalmic:* Amblyopia, conjunctivitis, optic neuritis, retinal hemorrhage. *Miscellaneous:* Hepatic toxicity, liver function abnormalities, allergic reactions, tinnitus, photosensitivity.

EMS CONSIDERATIONS

None.

Pentoxifylline
(pen-tox-EYE-fih-leen)
Pregnancy Class: C

Trental **(Rx)**
Classification: Agent affecting blood viscosity

Mechanism of Action: Drug and active metabolites decrease the viscosity of blood and improve erythrocyte flexibility. Results in increased blood flow to the microcirculation and an increase in tissue oxygen levels. Mechanism may include (1) decreased synthesis of thromboxane A_2, thus decreasing platelet aggregation, (2) increased blood fibrinolytic activity (decreasing fibrinogen levels), and (3) decreased RBC aggregation and local hyperviscosity by increasing cellular ATP.

Uses: Intermittent claudication; not intended to replace surgery. *Investigational:* To improve circulation in patients with cerebrovascular insufficiency, TIAs, sickle cell thalassemia, diabetic angiopathies and neuropathies, high-altitude sickness, strokes, acute and chronic hearing disorders, circulation disorders of the eye, severe recurrent aphthous stomatitis, leg ulcers, asthenozoospermia, and Raynaud's phenomenon.

Contraindications: Intolerance to pentoxifylline, caffeine, theophylline, or theobromine. Recent cerebral or retinal hemorrhage.

Precautions: Use with caution in impaired renal function and during lactation. Safety and efficacy in children less than 18 years of age not established. Geriatric patients may be at greater risk for manifesting side effects.

Route/Dosage
- **Extended-Release Tablets**
  Intermittent claudication.
  Adults: 400 mg t.i.d. with meals for at least 8 weeks. If side effects occur, reduce dose to 400 mg b.i.d.
  Severe idiopathic recurrent aphthous stomatitis.
  400 mg t.i.d. for 1 month.
How Supplied: *Tablet, Extended Release:* 400 mg

Side Effects: *CV:* Angina, chest pain, hypotension, edema. *GI:* Abdominal pain, flatus/bloating, dyspepsia, salivation, bad taste in mouth, N&V, anorexia, constipation, dry mouth and thirst, cholecystitis. *CNS:* Dizziness, headache, tremor, malaise, anxiety, confusion, depression, *seizures.* *Ophthalmologic:* Blurred vision, conjunctivitis, scotomata. *Dermatologic:* Pruritus, rash, urticaria, brittle fingernails, angioedema. *Respiratory:* Dyspnea, laryngitis, nasal congestion, epistaxis. *Miscellaneous:* Flu-like symptoms, leukopenia, sore throat, swollen neck glands, change in weight, earache, malaise.

OD Overdose Management: *Symptoms:* Agitation, fever, flushing, hypotension, nervousness, *seizures,* somnolence, tremors, loss of consciousness. *Treatment:* Gastric lavage followed by activated charcoal. Monitor BP and ECG. Support respiration, control seizures, and treat arrhythmias.

Drug Interactions
Antihypertensives / Small ↓ in BP; dose of antihypertensive may need to be ↑
Theophylline / ↑ Theophylline levels → ↑ risk of toxicitiy
Warfarin / Prolonged PT

EMS CONSIDERATIONS
None.

Percocet
(PER-koh-set)
Pregnancy Class: C
(C-II) (Rx)
Classification: Analgesic

Uses: Moderate to moderately severe pain.

Precautions: Use with caution during lactation. Safety and effectiveness have not been determined in children. Dependence to oxycodone can occur.

Route/Dosage
- **Tablets**
Adults, usual: 1 tablet q 6 hr as required for pain.
How Supplied: Each tablet contains: *Nonnarcotic analgesic:* Ace-

---

bold italic = life threatening side effect

taminophen, 325 mg. *Narcotic analgesic:* Oxycodone HCl, 5 mg. Also see information on individual components.

EMS CONSIDERATIONS

See also *Acetaminophen* and *Narcotic Analgesics.*

Pergolide mesylate
(PER-go-lyd)
Pregnancy Class: B
Permax **(Rx)**
Classification: Antiparkinson agent

Mechanism of Action: Potent dopamine receptor (both D_1 and D_2) agonist. May act by directly stimulating postsynaptic dopamine receptors in the nigrostriatal system, thus relieving symptoms of parkinsonism. Also inhibits prolactin secretion; causes a transient rise in serum levels of growth hormone and a decrease in serum levels of LH.

Uses: Adjunct with levodopa/carbidopa in Parkinson's disease.

Precautions: Use with caution during lactation and in patients prone to cardiac dysrhythmias, preexisting dyskinesia, and preexisting states of confusion or hallucinations. Safety and efficacy have not been determined in children.

Route/Dosage
• **Tablets**
    Parkinsonism.

Adults, initial: 0.05 mg/day for the first 2 days; **then,** increase dose gradually by 0.1 or 0.15 mg/day every third day over the next 12 days. The dosage may then be increased by 0.25 mg/day every third day until the therapeutic dosage level is reached. The mean therapeutic daily dosage is 3 mg used concurrently with levodopa/carbidopa (expressed as levodopa) at a dose of 650 mg/day. The effectiveness of doses of pergolide greater than 5 mg/day has not been evaluated.

How Supplied: *Tablet:* 0.05 mg, 0.25 mg, 1 mg

Side Effects: The most common side effects are listed. *CV:* Postural hypotension, palpitation, vasodilation, syncope, hypotension, hypertension, **arrhythmias, MI.** *GI:* Nausea (common), vomiting, diarrhea, constipation, dyspepsia, anorexia, dry mouth. *CNS:* Dyskinesia (common), dizziness, dystonia, hallucinations, confusion, insomnia, somnolence, anxiety, tremor, depression, abnormal dreams, psychosis, personality disorder, extrapyramidal syndrome, akathisia, paresthesia, incoordination, akinesia, neuralgia, hypertonia, speech disorders. *Musculoskeletal:* Arthralgia, bursitis, twitching, myalgia. *Respiratory:* Rhinitis, dyspnea, hiccup, epistaxis. *Dermatologic:* Sweating, rash. *Ophthalmologic:* Abnormal vision, double vision, eye disorders. *GU:* UTI, urinary frequency, hematuria. *Whole body:* Pain in chest, abdomen, neck, or back; headache, asthenia, flu syndrome, chills, facial edema, infection. *Miscellaneous:* Taste alteration, peripheral edema, anemia, weight gain.

OD Overdose Management: *Symptoms:* Include agitation, hypotension, N&V, hallucinations, involuntary movements, palpitations, tingling of arms and legs. *Treatment:* Activated charcoal (usually recommended instead of or in addition to gastric lavage or induction of vomiting). Maintain BP. An antiarrhythmic drug may be helpful. A phenothiazine or butyrophenone may help any CNS stimulation. Support ventilation.

Drug Interactions
Butyrophenones / ↓ Effect of pergolide due to dopamine antagonist effect
Metoclopramide / ↓ Effect of pergolide due to dopamine antagonist effect
Phenothiazines / ↓ Effect of pergolide due to dopamine antagonist effect
Thioxanthines / ↓ Effect of pergolide due to dopamine antagonist effect

EMS CONSIDERATIONS

None.

Perindopril erbumine

(per-IN-doh-pril)
Pregnancy Class: C (first trimester), D (second and third trimesters)
Aceon **(Rx)**
Classification: Antihypertensive, ACE Inhibitor

Uses: Treatment of essential hypertension, either alone or combined with other antihypertensive classes, especially thiazide diuretics.

Contraindications: Use in those with a history of angioedema related to previous ACE inhibitor therapy.

Precautions: Safety and efficacy have not been determined in patients with a C_{CR} less than 30 mL/min. There is a higher incidence of angioedema in blacks compared to nonblacks. Use with caution during lactation. Safety and efficacy have not been determined in children.

Route/Dosage

• **Tablets**

Uncomplicated essential hypertension.

Adults, initial: 4 mg once daily (may also be given in 2 divided doses). May increase dose until BP, when measured just before the next dose, is controlled. **Usual maintenance:** 4–8 mg, up to a maximum of 16 mg/day. For elderly patients, give doses greater than 8 mg/day cautiously.

Use with a diuretic for essential hypertension.

If possible, discontinue the diuretic 2–3 days before beginning perindopril therapy. If BP is not controlled with perindopril, resume the diuretic. When using both drugs, use an initial dose of 2–4 mg of perindopril daily in 1 or 2 divided doses. Carefully supervise until BP has stabilized.

In patients with a C_{CR} greater than 30 mL/min, give an initial dose of 2 mg/day. Daily dose should not exceed 8 mg.

How Supplied: *Tablets:* 2 mg, 4 mg, 8 mg

Side Effects: *GI:* Diarrhea, abdominal pain, N&V, dyspepsia, flatulence, dry mouth, dry mucous membrane, increased appetite, gastroenteritis, *hepatic necrosis/failure*. *CNS:* Headache, dizziness, sleep disorder, paresthesia, depression, migraine, amnesia, vertigo, anxiety, psychosexual disorder. *CV:* Palpitation, abnormal ECG, *CVA, MI,* orthostatic symptoms, hypotension, ventricular extrasystole, vasodilation, syncope, abnormal conduction, heart murmur. *Respiratory:* Cough, sinusitis, URTI, rhinitis, pharyngitis, posterior nasal drip, bronchitis, rhinorrhea, throat disorder, dyspnea, sneezing, epistaxis, hoarseness, pulmonary fibrosis. *Body as a whole:* Asthenia, viral infection, fever, edema, rash, seasonal allergy, malaise, pain, cold/hot sensation, chills, fluid retention, angioedema, *anaphylaxis*. *Musculoskeletal:* Back pain, upper extremity pain, lower extremity pain, chest pain, neck pain, myalgia, arthralgia, arthritis. *GU:* UTI, male sexual dysfunction, menstrual disorder, vaginitis, kidney stone, flank pain, urinary frequency, urinary retention. *Dermatologic:* Sweating, skin infection, tinea, pruritus, dry skin, erythema, fever blisters, purpura, hematoma. *Miscellaneous:* Hypertonia, ear infection, injury, tinnitus, facial edema, gout, ecchymosis.

Drug Interactions: Concomitant use of diuretics may cause an excessive ↓ BP.

EMS CONSIDERATIONS

None.

Perphenazine

(per-FEN-aah-zeen)
Pregnancy Class: C
Trilafon **(Rx)**
Classification: Antipsychotic, antiemetic, piperazine-type phenothiazine

Mechanism of Action: Resembles chlorpromazine. High incidence of extrapyramidal effects; strong antiemetic effects; moderate anticholinergic effects; and a low incidence of

P

orthostatic hypotension and sedation.

Onset of Action: IM: 10 min; **Maximum effect IM:** 1-2 hr.

Duration of Action: IM: 6 hr (up to 24 hr).

Uses: Psychotic disorders. IV to treat severe N&V and intractable hiccoughs.

Precautions: Use during pregnancy only if benefits clearly outweigh risks. Dosage has not been established in children less than 12 years of age. Geriatric, emaciated, or debilitated patients usually require a lower initial dose.

Route/Dosage ————————

- **Concentrate, Tablets**
  Psychoses.

Nonhospitalized patients: 4–8 mg t.i.d. **Hospitalized patients:** 8–16 mg b.i.d.–q.i.d. Avoid doses greater than 64 mg/day.

- **IM**
  Psychotic disorders.

Adults and adolescents, nonhospitalized: 5 mg q 6 hr, not to exceed 15 mg/day. **Hospitalized patients: initial,** 5–10 mg; total daily dose should not exceed 30 mg.

- **IV**
  Severe N&V.

Adults: Up to 5 mg diluted to 0.5 mg/mL with 0.9% sodium chloride injection. Give in divided doses of not more than 1 mg q 1–3 hr. Can also be given as an infusion at a rate not to exceed 1 mg/min. Restrict use to hospitalized recumbent adults. Do not exceed a single dose of 5 mg.

How Supplied: *Concentrate:* 16 mg/5 mL; *Injection:* 5 mg/mL; *Tablet:* 2 mg, 4 mg, 8 mg, 16 mg

EMS CONSIDERATIONS

See also *Antipsychotic Agents, Phenothiazines.*

Phenazopyridine hydrochloride (Phenylazodiamino-pyridine HCl)

(fen-AY-zoh-PEER-ih-deen)

Pregnancy Class: B
Azo-Standard, Baridium, Prodium, Pyridiate, Pyridiate No. 2, Pyridium, Urogesic **(OTC) (Rx)**
Classification: Urinary analgesic

Mechanism of Action: An azo dye with local analgesic and anesthetic effects on the urinary tract.

Uses: Relief of pain, urgency or frequency, and burning in chronic UTIs or irritation, including cystitis, urethritis and pyelitis, trauma, surgery, or urinary tract instrumentation. As an adjunct to antibacterial therapy. Determine the underlying cause of the irritation.

Contraindications: Renal insufficiency. Use in children less than 12 years of age. Chronic use to treat undiagnosed pain of the urinary tract.

Route/Dosage ————————

- **Tablets**

Adults: 200 mg t.i.d. with or after meals for not more than 2 days when used together with an antibacterial agent for UTI. **Pediatric, 6–12 years:** 4 mg/kg t.i.d. with food for 2 days.

How Supplied: *Tablet:* 95 mg, 97.2 mg, 100 mg, 200 mg

Side Effects: *GI:* Nausea. *Hematologic:* Methemoglobinemia, **hemolytic anemia** (especially in patients with G6PD deficiency). *Dermatologic:* Yellowish tinge of the skin or sclerae may indicate accumulation of drug due to renal insufficiency, pruritus, rash. *Miscellaneous:* Renal and hepatic toxicity, headache, anaphylactoid reaction, staining of contact lenses.

OD Overdose Management: *Symptoms:* Methemoglobinemia following massive overdoses. Hemolysis due to G6PD deficiency. *Treatment:* Methylene blue, 1–2 mg/kg IV or 100–200 mg PO of ascorbic acid to treat methemoglobinemia.

EMS CONSIDERATIONS

None.

Phendimetrazine tartrate

(fen-dye-ME-trah-zeen)
Pregnancy Class: C
Adipost, Bontril PDM and Slow-Release, Dital, Dyrexan-OD, Melflat-

105 Unicelles, Plegine, Prelu-2, Rexigen Forte **(Rx)**
Classification: Anorexiant

Uses: Short-term (8–12 weeks) treatment of exogenous obesity in conjunction with a weight reduction program including exercise, reduced caloric intake, and behavior modification.

Route/Dosage
• **Capsules, Tablets**
Adults: 35 mg 2–3 times/day 1 hr before meals. **Maximum daily dose:** 70 mg t.i.d.
• **Extended-Release Capsules, Extended-Release Tablets**
Adults: 105 mg/day 30–60 min before the morning meal.
How Supplied: *Capsule:* 35 mg; *Capsule, Extended Release:* 105 mg; *Tablet:* 35 mg

EMS CONSIDERATIONS

See also *Amphetamines and Derivatives*.

Phenelzine sulfate

(FEN-ell-zeen)
Pregnancy Class: C
Nardil **(Rx)**
Classification: Antidepressant, monoamine oxidase inhibitor

Mechanism of Action: MAO inhibitor that prevents MAO from metabolizing biogenic amines. Antidepressant effect due to accumulation of biogenic amines in presynaptic granules, increasing the concentration of neurotransmitter released upon nerve stimulation. Slight anticholinergic, sedative, and orthostatic hypotensive effects.
Onset of Action: Few days to several months. Beneficial effects at doses of 60 mg/day may not be seen for at least 4 weeks. Clinical effects of the drug may be observed for up to 2 weeks after termination of therapy.
Uses: Depression characterized as atypical, nonendogenous, or neurotic; most often used in those patients who have mixed anxiety and depression and phobic or hypochon-

driacal symptoms. Not usually first-line therapy; reserve for those who have failed to respond to drugs more commonly used. *Investigational:* Alone or as an adjunct to treat bulimia nervosa, agoraphobia with panic attcks, globus hystericus syndrome, and chronic headache. Also for orthostatic hypotension, refractory migraine headaches, narcolepsy, obsessive-compulsive disorder, panic attacks, posttraumatic stress disorder, and social phobia.
Contraindications: Pheochromocytoma, CHF, history of liver disease, abnormal LFTs. Use with other sympathomimetic drugs due to the possibility of hypertensive crisis. Contraindicated with the use of many other drugs (see *Drug Interactions*). Use in children under the age of 16 years.
Precautions: Use with caution in combination with antihypertensive drugs, including thiazide diuretics and β-blockers, due to the possibility of severe hypotensive effects. The safe use during pregnancy or lactation has not been determined. Use with caution in geriatric patients.

Route/Dosage
• **Tablets**
Treatment of depression.
Adults, initial: 15 mg t.i.d.; **then,** increase the dose to 60 mg/day at a fairly rapid pace (some may require 90 mg/day). **Maintenance:** After the maximum beneficial effect has been observed, the dose should be reduced slowly over several weeks to a range of 15 mg/day or every other day to as high as 45 mg/day or every other day. **Geriatric, initial:** 0.8–1 mg/kg daily in divided doses; **then,** increase s needed to a maximum of 60 mg/day.
How Supplied: *Tablets:* 15 mg.
Side Effects: *CNS:* Dizziness, headache, drowsiness, sleep disturbances (insomnia, hypersomnia), fatigue, weakness, tremors, twitching, myoclonic movements, hyperreflexia, jitteriness, palilalia, euphoria, nystagmus, paresthesias, ataxia, ***shock-like***

P

---

bold italic = life threatening side effect

coma, toxic delirium, manic reaction, *convulsions,* acute anxiety reaction, precipitation of schizophrenia. *GI:* Constipation, dry mouth, GI disturbances, reversible jaundice. Rarely, *fatal necrotizing hepatocellular damage. CV:* Postural hypotension, edema. *GU:* Anorgasmia, ejaculatory disturbances, urinary retention. *Metabolic:* Weight gain, hypernatremia, hypermetabolic syndrome. *Dermatologic:* Skin rash, sweating. *Ophthalmic:* Blurred vision, glaucoma. *Miscellaneous:* Leukopenia, edema of the glottis, fever associated with increased muscle tone.

OD Overdose Management: *Symptoms:* Drowsiness, dizziness, fainting, irritability, hyperactivity, agitation, severe headache, hallucinations, trismus, opisthotonus, rigidity, convulsions, coma, rapid and irregular pulse, hypertension, hypotension, cardiovascular collapse, precordial pain, respiratory depression, respiratory failure, hyperpyrexia, diaphoresis, cold and clammy skin, death. Symptoms of overdose may be absent or minimal during the initial 12-hr period after ingestion but then slowly increase, reaching a maximum effect within 24 to 48 hr. *Treatment:* If detected early, induction of emesis or gastric lavage followed by a charcoal slurry. Use of IV diazepam for CNS symptoms. For hypotension and CV collapse, IV fluids and, if necessary, BP titration with an IV infusion of a dilute pressor drug. Respirations should be supported by use of supplemental oxygen and mechanical ventilation. Fluid and electrolyte balance must be maintained. Do **not** use phenothiazine derivatives or CNS stimulants.

Drug Interactions

Alcohol / Possibility of excitation, seizures, delirium, hyperpyrexia, circulatory collapse, coma, death

Anesthetics, general / ↑ Hypotensive effect; use together with caution. Discontinue phenelzine at least 10 days before elective surgery

Anticholinergic drugs, atropine / MAO inhibitors ↑ effect of anticholinergic drugs

Antidepressants, tricyclic / Comcomitant use may result in excitation, sweating, tachycardia, tachypnea, hyperpyrexia, disseminated intravascular coagulation, delirium, tremors, convulsions, death. At least 7-10 days should elapse between discontinuing a MAO inhibitor and initiating a new drug. However, such combinations have been used together successfully

Antidiabetic drugs / Potentiatioin of hypoglycemic response and delayed recovery from hypoglycemia

Antihypertensive drugs / Exaggerated hypotensive effects

Beta-adrenergic blocking drugs / Exaggerated hypotensive effects; development of bradycardia

Bupropion / Concomitant use contraindicated; allow at least 10 days between discontinuing phenelzine and starting bupropion

Buspirone / Elevated BP

Carbamazepine / Possible hypertensive crisis, severe seizures, coma, or circulatory collapse; do not use together

Dextromethorphan / Possible hyperpyrexia, abnormal muscle movement, psychosis, bizarre behavior, hypotension, coma, and death; do not use together

Fluoxetine / Possibility of hyperthermia, rigidity, myoclonic movements, death. At least 10 days should elapse between discontinuation of phenelzine and initiation of fluoxetine; and, at least 5 weeks should elapse between discontinuing fluoxetine and beginning phenelzine

Guanethidine / Inhibition of the hypotensive effect of guanethidine

Levodopa / Possible hypertensive reactions

Meperidine / Possibility of agitation, excitation, seizures, diaphoresis, delirium, hyperpyrexia, apnea, coma, death; do not use together

Methyldopa / Loss of BP control or signs of central stimulation

Metrizamide / Possible ↓ of seizure threshold

Narcotics / Use with caution with phenelzine

Phenothiazines / ↑ Effect of phenothizines due to ↓ breakdown by the liver; also, ↑ chance of severe extrapyramidal effects and hypertensive crisis

Succinylcholine / ↑ Effect of succinylcholine due to ↓ breakdown in the plasma by pseudocholinesterase

Sulfonamides / Either sulfonamide or phenelzine toxicity

Sumatriptan / ↑ Risk of sumatriptan toxicity

Sympathomimetic drugs—amphetamine, cocaine, dopa, ephedrine, epinephrine, metaraminol, methyldopa, methylphenidate, norepinephrine, phenylephrine, phenylpropanolamine. Many OTC cold products, hay fever medications, and nasal decongestants contain one or more of these drugs / All peripheral, metabolic, cardiac, and central effects are potentiated for up to 2 weeks after termination of MAO inhibitor therapy. Symptoms include acute hypertensive crisis with possible intracranial hemorrhage, hyperthermia, coma, and possibly death

Thiazide diuretics / Exaggerated hypotensive effects

Tryptophan / Possibility of behavioral and neurologic effects, including disorientation, confusion, amnesia, delirium, agitation, hypomania, ataxia, myoclonus, hyperreflexia, shivering, ocular oscillation,and Babinski signs

Tyramine-rich foods—beer, broad beans, certain cheeses (Brie, cheddar, Camembert, Stilton), Chianti wine, chicken livers, caffeine, cola beverages, figs, licorice, liver, pickled or kippered herring, dry sausage (Genoa salami, hard salami, pepperoni, Lebanon bologna), tea, cream, yogurt, yeast extract, and chocolate / Possible precipitation of hypertensive crisis, including severe headache, **hyperension, intracranial hemorrhage, death**

EMS CONSIDERATIONS
None.

Phenobarbital
Phenobarbital sodium
(fee-no-BAR-bih-tal)

Pregnancy Class: D
Phenobarbital (Solfoton **(C-IV) (Rx)**)
Phenobarbital sodium (Luminal Sodium **(C-IC) (Rx)**)
Classification: Sedative, anticonvulsant, barbiturate type

Mechanism of Action: Long-acting. **Onset of Action:** 30 to more than 60 min; **Time for peak effect, after IV:** up to 15 min.

Duration of Action: 10-16 hr.

Uses: PO: Sedative, hypnotic (short-term), anticonvulsant (partial and generalized tonic-clonic or cortical focal seizures); emergency control of acute seizure disorders such as status epilepticus, meningitis, tetanus, eclampsia, toxicity of local anesthetics. **Parenteral:** Sedative, hypnotic (short-term), preanesthetic, anticonvulsant, emergency control of acute seizure disorders.

Precautions: Reduce the dose in geriatric and debilitated patients,as well as those with impaired hepatic or renal function.

Route/Dosage
PHENOBARBITAL, PHENOBARBITAL SODIUM

• **Capsules, Elixir, Tablets**
  Sedation.

Adults: 30–120 mg/day in two to three divided doses. **Pediatric:** 2 mg/kg (60 mg/m²) t.i.d.
  Hypnotic.

Adults: 100–200 mg at bedtime. **Pediatric:** Dose should be determined by provider, based on age and weight.
  Anticonvulsant.

Adults: 60–200 mg/day in single or divided doses. **Pediatric:** 3–6 mg/kg/day in single or divided doses.

• **IM, IV**
  Sedation.

Adults: 30–120 mg/day in two to three divided doses.
  Preoperative sedation.

Adults: 100–200 mg IM only, 60–90 min before surgery. **Pediatric:** 1–3

P

mg/kg IM or IV 60–90 min prior to surgery.
Hypnotic.
Adults: 100–320 mg IM or IV.
Acute convulsions.
Adults: 200–320 mg IM or IV; may be repeated in 6 hr if needed. **Pediatric:** 4–6 mg/kg/day for 7–10 days to achieve a blood level of 10–15 mcg/mL (or 15 mg/kg/day, IV or IM).
Status epilepticus.
Adults: 15–20 mg/kg IV (given over 10–15 min); may be repeated if needed. **Pediatric:** 15–20 mg/kg given over a 10- to 15-min period.
How Supplied: Phenobarbital: *Elixir:* 20 mg/5 mL; *Tablet:* 15 mg, 16.2 mg, 30 mg, 60 mg, 100 mg. Phenobarbital sodium: *Injection:* 30 mg/mL, 60 mg/mL, 65 mg/mL, 130 mg/mL
Side Effects: Additional: Chronic use may result in headache, fever, and magaloblastic anemia.

EMS CONSIDERATIONS

See also *Barbiturates.*
Administration/Storage
1. When used as an anticonvulsant in infants and children, a loading dose of 15–20 mg/kg achieves blood levels of about 20 mcg/mL shortly after administration. To achieve therapeutic blood levels of 10–20 mcg/mL, higher doses per kilogram may be needed compared with adults.
IV 2. For IV administration, inject slowly at a rate of 50 mg/min.
3. Avoid extravasation as tissue damage and necrosis may result.
Assessment: Assess liver and renal function studies. Reduce dose with impairment and in debilitated/elderly patients.

Phensuximide
(fen-SUCKS-ih-myd)
Milontin **(Rx)**
Classification: Anticonvulsant, succinimide type

Mechanism of Action: Less effective and less toxic than other succinimides. May color the urine pink, red, or red-brown.
Onset of Action: Peak effect: 1-4 hr.

Uses: Absence seizures.
Precautions: Use with caution in patients with intermittent porphyria.

Route/Dosage
• **Capsules**
Absence seizures.
Adults and children, initial: 0.5 g b.i.d.; **then,** dose can be increased by 0.5 g/day at 1-week intervals until seizures are controlled or the daily dosage reaches 3 g. May be used with other anticonvulsants in the presence of multiple types of epilepsy.
How Supplied: *Capsule:* 0.5 g
Side Effects: Additional: Kidney damage, hematuria, urinary frequency.

EMS CONSIDERATIONS

See also *Anticonvulsants* and *Succinimides.*

Phentolamine mesylate
(fen-TOLL-ah-meen)
Pregnancy Class: C
Regitine, Vasomax **(Rx)**
Classification: Alpha-adrenergic blocking agent

Mechanism of Action: Phentolamine competitively blocks both presynaptic (alpha-2) and postsynaptic (alpha-1) adrenergic receptors producing vasodilation and a decrease in peripheral resistance. The drug has little effect on BP. In CHF, phentolamine reduces afterload and pulmonary arterial pressure as well as increases CO.
Onset of Action: Parenteral: Immediate.
Duration of Action: Short.
Uses: Dermal necrosis and sloughing following IV use or extravasation of norepinephrine. *Investigational:* Hypertensive crisis secondary to MAO inhibitor/sympathomimetic amine interactions, as well as rebound hypertension due to withdrawal of clonidine, propranolol, or other antihypertensive drugs. In combination with papaverine as an intracavernous injection for impotence. PO to treat erectile dysfunction.

Contraindications: CAD including angina, MI, or coronary insufficiency.
Precautions: Use during pregnancy and lactation only if benefits clearly outweigh risks. Geriatric patients may have a greater risk of developing hypothermia. Use with great caution in the presence of gastritis, ulcers, and patients with a history thereof. Defer use of cardiac glycosides until cardiac rhythm returns to normal.

Route/Dosage ───────────────

Dermal necrosis/sloughing following IV or extravasation of norepinephrine.
Prevention: 10 mg/1,000 mL norepinephrine solution; *treatment:* 5–10 mg/10 mL saline injected into area of extravasation within 12 hr. **Pediatric:** 0.1–0.2 mg/kg to a maximum of 10 mg.
CHF.
Adults, IV infusion: 0.17–0.4 mg/min.

• **Intracavernosal**
  Impotence.
Adults: Papaverine, 30 mg, and 0.5–1 mg phentolamine; adjust dose according to response.
How Supplied: *Powder for injection:* 5 mg
Side Effects: *CV:* Acute and prolonged hypotension, tachycardia, *MI, cerebrovascular spasm, cerebrovascular occlusion,* and arrhythmias, especially after parenteral administration. Orthostatic hypotension, flushing. *GI:* N&V, diarrhea. *Other:* Dizziness, weakness, nasal stuffiness.

OD **Overdose Management:** *Symptoms: Hypotension, shock. Treatment:* Maintain BP by giving IV norepinephrine (DO NOT USE EPINEPHRINE).
Drug Interactions
Ephedrine / Phentolamine antagonizes vasoconstrictor and hypertensive effect
Epinephrine / Phentolamine antagonizes vasoconstrictor and hypertensive effect
Norepinephrine / Suitable antagonist to treat overdosage induced by phentolamine

Propranolol / Concomitant use during surgery for pheochromocytoma is indicated

EMS CONSIDERATIONS
None.

Phenylephrine hydrochloride
(fen-ill-EF-rin)
Pregnancy Class: C
Nasal: Alconefrin 12, 25, and 50, Children's Nostril, Doktors,.Duration, Neo-Synephrine Solution, Nostril, Rhinall, Vicks Sinex. **Ophthalmic:** Ak-Dilate, Mydfrin 2.5%, Neo-Sunephrine, Neo-Synephrine Viscous, Phenoptic, Prefrin Liquifilm, Relief. **Parenteral:** Neo-synephrine. (Rx: Parenteral and Ophthalmic Solutions 2.5% or greater; OTC: Nasal products and ophthalmic solutions 0.12% or less)
Classification: Alpha-adrenergic agent (sympathomimetic)

Mechanism of Action: Stimulates alpha-adrenergic receptors, producing pronounced vasoconstriction and hence an increase in both SBP and DBP; reflex bradycardia results from increased vagal activity. Also acts on alpha receptors producing vasoconstriction in the skin, mucous membranes, and the mucosa as well as mydriasis by contracting the dilator muscle of the pupil. Resembles epinephrine, but it has more prolonged action and few cardiac effects.
Onset of Action: IV: immediate; **IM, SC:** 10-15 min; *Nasal decongestion (topical):* 15-20 min; *Ophthalmic:* **Time to peak effect for mydriasis:** 15-60 min for 2.5% solution and 10-90 min for 10% solution.
Duration of Action: IV: 15-20 min; **IM:** 0.5-2 hr; **SC:** 50-60 min; *Nasal decongestion (topical):* 30 min-4hr; *Ophthalmic:* 0.5-1.5 hr for 0.12%, 3 hr for 2.5%, and 5-7 hr with 10% (when used for mydriasis).
Uses: Systemic: Vascular failure in shock, shock-like states, drug-induced hypotension or hypersensitivity. To maintain BP during spinal and inhala-

P

tion anesthesia; to prolong spinal anesthesia. As a vasoconstrictor in regional analgesia. Paroxysmal SVT. **Nasal:** Nasal congestion due to allergies, sinusitis, common cold, or hay fever. **Ophthalmologic: 0.12%:** Temporary relief of redness of the eye associated with colds, hay fever, wind, dust, sun, smog, smoke, contact lens. **2.5% and 10%:** Decongestant and vasoconstrictor, treatment of uveitis with posterior synechiae, open-angle glaucoma, refraction without cycloplegia, ophthalmoscopic examination, funduscopy, prior to surgery.

Contraindications: Severe hypertension, VT.

Precautions: Use with extreme caution in geriatric patients, severe arteriosclerosis, bradycardia, partial heart block, myocardial disease, hyperthyroidism and during pregnancy and lactation. Systemic absorption with nasal or ophthalmic use. Use of the 2.5% or 10% ophthalmic solutions in children may cause hypertension and irregular heart beat. In geriatric patients, chronic use of the 2.5% or 10% ophthalmic solutions may cause rebound miosis and a decreased mydriatic effect.

Route/Dosage

• **IM, IV, SC**

Vasopressor, mild to moderate hypotension.

Adults: 2–5 mg (range: 1–10 mg), not to exceed an initial dose of 5 mg IM or SC repeated no more often than q 10–15 min; or, 0.2 mg (range: 0.1–0.5 mg), not to exceed an initial dose of 0.5 mg IV repeated no more often than q 10–15 min. **Pediatric:** 0.1 mg/kg (3 mg/m²) IM or SC repeated in 1–2 hr if needed.

Vasopressor, severe hypotension and shock.

Adults: 10 mg by continuous IV infusion using 250–500 mL D5W or 0.9% NaCl injection given at a rate of 0.1–0.18 mg/min initial; **then,** give at a rate of 0.04–0.06 mg/min.

Prophylaxis of hypotension during spinal anesthesia.

Adults: 2–3 mg IM or SC 3–4 min before anesthetic given; subsequent

doses should not exceed the previous dose by more than 0.1–0.2 mg. No more than 0.5 mg should be given in a single dose. **Pediatric:** 0.044–0.088 mg/kg IM or SC.

Hypotensive emergencies during spinal anesthesia.

Adults, initial: 0.2 mg IV; dose can be increased by no more than 0.2 mg for each subsequent dose not to exceed 0.5 mg/dose.

Prolongation of spinal anesthesia. 2–5 mg added to the anesthetic solution increases the duration of action up to 50% without increasing side effects or complications.

Vasoconstrictor for regional anesthesia.

Add 1 mg to every 20 mL of local anesthetic solution. If more than 2 mg phenylephrine is used, pressor reactions can be expected.

Paroxysmal SVT.

Initial: 0.5 mg (maximum) given by rapid IV injection (over 20–30 seconds). Subsequent doses are determined by BP and should not exceed the previous dose by more than 0.1–0.2 mg and should never be more than 1 mg.

• **Nasal Solution, Nasal Spray**

Adults and children over 12 years of age: 2–3 gtt of the 0.25% or 0.5% solution into each nostril q 3–4 hr as needed. In resistant cases, the 1% solution can be used but no more often than q 4 hr. **Children, 6–12 years of age:** 2–3 gtt of the 0.25% solution q 3–4 hr as needed. **Infants, greater than 6 months of age:** 1–2 gtt of the 0.16% solution into each nostril q 3–4 hr.

• **Ophthalmic Solution, 0.12%, 2.5%, 10%**

Vasoconstriction, pupillary dilation.

1 gtt of the 2.5% or 10% solution on the upper limbus a few minutes following 1 gtt of topical anesthetic (prevents stinging and dilution of solution by lacrimation). An additional drop may be needed after 1 hr.

Uveitis.

1 gtt of the 2.5% or 10% solution with atropine. To free recently formed posterior synechiae, 1 gtt of

the 2.5% or 10% solution to the upper surface of the cornea. Continue treatment the following day, if needed. In the interim, apply hot compresses for 5–10 min t.i.d. using 1 gtt of 1% or 2% atropine sulfate before and after each series of compresses.

Glaucoma.

1 gtt of 10% solution on the upper surface of the cornea as needed. Both the 2.5% and 10% solutions may be used with miotics in patients with open-angle glaucoma.

Surgery.

2.5% or 10% solution 30–60 min before surgery for wide dilation of the pupil.

Refraction.

Adults: 1 gtt of a cycloplegic (homatropine HBr, atropine sulfate, cyclopentolate, tropicamide HCl, or a combination of homatropine and cocaine HCl) in each eye followed in 5 min with 1 gtt of 2.5% phenylephrine solution and in 10 min with another drop of cycloplegic. The eyes are ready for refraction in 50–60 min. **Children:** 1 gtt of atropine sulfate, 1%, in each eye followed in 10–15 min with 1 gtt of phenylephrine solution, 2.5%, and in 5–10 min with a second drop of atropine sulfate, 1%. The eyes are ready for refraction in 1–2 hr.

Ophthalmoscopic examination.

1 gtt of 2.5% solution in each eye. The eyes are ready for examination in 15– 30 min and the effect lasts for 1–3 hr.

Minor eye irritations.

1–2 gtt of the 0.12% solution in the eye(s) up to q.i.d. as needed.

How Supplied: *Injection:* 10 mg/mL; *Liquid:* 5 mg/5 mL; *Nasal Solution:* 0.125%, 0.25%, 0.5%, 1%; *Ophthalmic Solution:* 0.12%, 2.5%, 10%; *Nasal Spray:* 0.25%, 0.5%, 1%

Side Effects: *CV:* Reflex bradycardia, arrhythmias (rare). *CNS:* Headache, excitability, restlessness. *Ophthalmologic:* Rebound miosis and decreased mydriatic response in geriatric patients, blurred vision.

OD **Overdose Management:** *Symptoms:* Ventricular extrasystoles, short paroxysms of ventricular tachycardia, sensation of fullness in the head, tingling of extremities. *Treatment:* Administer an alpha-adrenergic blocking agent (e.g., phentolamine).

Drug Interactions: Additional: *Anesthetics, halogenated hydrocarbon /* May sensitize myocardium → serious arrhythmias. *Bretylium /* ↑ Effect of phenylephrine → possible arrhythmias.

EMS CONSIDERATIONS

See also *Sympathomimetic Drugs.*
Administration/Storage
IV 1. For IV administration, dilute each 1 mg with 9 mL of sterile water and administer over 1 min. Further dilution of 10 mg in 500 mL of dextrose, Ringer's, or saline solution may be titrated to patient response.
2. When used parenterally, monitor infusion site closely to avoid extravasation. If evident, administer SC phentolamine locally to prevent tissue necrosis.
3. Do not use solution if it changes color, becomes cloudy, or contains a precipitate.
Assessment: During IV administration monitor cardiac rhythm and BP continuously until stabilized, noting any evidence of bradycardia or arrhythmias.

Phenylpropanolamine hydrochloride

(fen-ill-proh-pah-NOHL-ah-meen)
Pregnancy Class: Pregnancy Class: C
Acutrim 16 Hour, Acutrim Late Day, Acutrim II Maximum Strength, Control, Dexatrim, Dexatrim Maximum Strength and Maximum Strength Caplets, Dexatrim Maximum Strength Pre-Meal Caplets, Efed II Yellow, Malgret-50, Phenyldrine, Propagest, Unitrol (OTC except Malgret-50 and Rhindecon)
Classification: Sympathomimetic decongestant, appetite suppressant

Mechanism of Action: Thought to stimulate both alpha and beta receptors as well as to act indirectly through release of norepinephrine from storage sites. Increases in BP are due mainly to increased CO rather than to vasoconstriction; has minimal CNS effects. Acts on alpha-adrenergic receptors to produce a decongestant effect in the nasal mucosa.

Onset of Action: Decongestant: 15-30 min.

Duration of Action: Capsules and tablets: 3 hr; **extended-release tablets:** 12-16 hr.

Uses: Nasal congestion due to colds, hay fever, allergies. Short-term (8–12 weeks) treatment of exogenous obesity in conjunction with a weight reduction program including reduced caloric intake, exercise, and behavior modification. *Investigational:* Mild to moderate stress incontinence in women.

Contraindications: Arteriosclerosis, depression, glaucoma, hypertension, diabetes, kidney disease, hyperthyroidism, during or within 14 days of use of MAO inhibitors, hypersensitivity to sympathomimetics. Use as an anorexiant for children less than 12 years of age. Sustained-release forms during lactation and in children less than 12 years of age.

Precautions: Safety and efficacy during pregnancy and lactation and for children not established. Children less than 6 years of age may be at greater risk for developing psychiatric disorders when using phenylpropanolamine. Individualize the anorexiant dose for children 12–18 years of age.

Route/Dosage
• **Capsules, Tablets**
    Decongestant.
Adults: 25 mg q 4 hr or 50 mg q 6–8 hr (not to exceed 150 mg/day); **Children, 2–6 years:** 6.25 mg q 4 hr, not to exceed 37.5 mg in 24 hr; **6–12 years:** 12.5 mg q 4 hr, not to exceed 75 mg in 24 hr.
    Anorexiant.

Adults: 25 mg t.i.d. 30 min before meals, not to exceed 75 mg in 24 hr.
• **Extended-Release   Capsules, Extended-Release Tablets**
    Decongestant.
Adults: 75 mg q 12 hr.
    Anorexiant.
Adults: 75 mg once daily in the morning.

How Supplied: *Capsule:* 37.5 mg; *Capsule, Extended Release:* 75 mg; *Tablet:* 25 mg, 37.5 mg, 50 mg; *Tablet, Extended Release:* 75 mg

Side Effects: *CNS:* Dizziness, headache, insomnia, restlessness, bizarre behavior. Serious effects due to abuse include: agitation, tremor, increased motor activity, hallucinations, *seizures, stroke, and death.* *CV:* Palpitations, *hypertension (may be severe and lead to crisis),* tachycardia. *Miscellaneous:* Dry mouth, dysuria, renal failure, nausea, nasal dryness.

Drug Interactions: Additional: *Bromocriptine /* Worsening of side effects of bromocriptine; possibility of ventricular tachycardia and cardiac dysfunction.*Caffeine /* ↑ Serum caffeine levels, ↑ risk of pharmacologic and toxic effects.*Indomethacin /* Possibility of severe hypertensive episode.

EMS CONSIDERATIONS

Phenytoin (Diphenylhydantoin)
Phenytoin sodium, extended
Phenytoin sodium, parenteral
Phenytoin sodium prompt
(FEN-ih-toyn)

Pregnancy Class: C
Phenytoin (Diphenylhydantoin): Dilantin Infatab, Dilantin-125 **(Rx)** Phenytoin sodium, extended (Dilantin Kapseals **(Rx)**))Phenytoin sodium, parenteral (Dilantin Sodium **(Rx)**) Phenytoin sodium prompt (Diphenylan Sodium **(Rx)**)
Classification: Anticonvulsant, hydantoin type; antiarrhythmic (type I)

Mechanism of Action: Acts in the motor cortex of the brain to reduce the spread of electrical discharges from the rapidly firing epileptic foci in this area. This is accomplished by stabilizing hyperexcitable cells possibly by affecting sodium efflux. Also, phenytoin decreases activity of centers in the brain stem responsible for the tonic phase of grand mal seizures. Has few sedative effects.

Phenytoin extended is designed for once-a-day dosage. Since the rate and extent of absorption depend on the particular preparation, the same product should be used for a particular patient.

As an antiarrhythmic, phenytoin increases the electrical stimulation threshold of heart muscle, although it is less effective than quinidine, procainamide, or lidocaine.

Onset of Action: 30-60 min.

Duration of Action: 24 hr or more.

Uses: Chronic epilepsy, especially of the tonic-clonic, psychomotor type. Not effective against absence seizures and may even increase the frequency of seizures in this disorder. Parenteral phenytoin is sometimes used to treat status epilepticus and to control seizures during neurosurgery.

PO for certain PVCs and IV for PVCs and tachycardia. Particularly useful for arrhythmias produced by digitalis overdosage.

Investigational: Paroxysmal choreoathetosis; to treat blistering and erosions in patients with recessive dystrophic epidermolysis bullosa; episodic dyscontrol; trigeminal neuralgia; as a muscle relaxant in neuromyotonia, myotonia congenita, or myotonic muscular dystrophy; to treat cardiac symptoms in overdosage of tricyclic antidepressants. Severe preeclampsia.

Contraindications: Hypersensitivity to hydantoins, exfoliative dermatitis, sinus bradycardia, second- and third-degree AV block, patients with Adams-Stokes syndrome, SA block. Lactation.

Precautions: Use with caution in acute, intermittent porphyria. Administer with extreme caution to patients with a history of asthma or other allergies, impaired renal or hepatic function, and heart disease (hypotension, severe myocardial insufficiency). Abrupt withdrawal may cause status epilepticus. Combined drug therapy is required if petit mal seizures are also present.

Route/Dosage

• **Oral Suspension, Chewable Tablets**

Seizures.

Adults, initial: 100 mg (125 mg of the suspension) t.i.d.; adjust dosage at 7- to 10-day intervals until seizures are controlled; **usual, maintenance:** 300–400 mg/day, although 600 mg/day (625 mg of the suspension) may be required in some. **Pediatric, initial:** 5 mg/kg/day in two to three divided doses; **maintenance,** 4–8 mg/kg (up to maximum of 300 mg/day). Children over 6 years may require up to 300 mg/day. **Geriatric:** 3 mg/kg initially in divided doses; **then,** adjust dosage according to serum levels and response. Once dosage level has been established, the extended capsules may be used for once-a-day dosage.

• **Capsules, Extended-Release Capsules**

Seizures.

Adults, initial: 100 mg t.i.d.; adjust dose at 7- to 10-day intervals until control is achieved. An initial loading dose of 12–15 mg/kg divided into two to three doses over 6 hr followed by 100 mg t.i.d. on subsequent days may be preferred if seizures are frequent. **Pediatric:** See dose for Oral Suspension and Chewable Tablets.

Arrhythmias.

Adults: 200–400 mg/day.

• **IV**

Status epilepticus.

Adults, loading dose: 10–15 mg/kg at a rate not to exceed 50 mg/min; **then,** 100 mg PO or IV q 6–8 hr. **Pe-**

P

diatric, loading dose: 15–20 mg/kg in divided doses of 5–10 mg/kg given at a rate of 1–3 mg/kg/min.

Arrhythmias.
Adults: 100 mg q 5 min up to maximum of 1 g.

• **IM**
Dose should be 50% greater than the PO dose.

Neurosurgery.
100–200 mg q 4 hr during and after surgery (during first 24 hr, administer no more than 1,000 mg; after first day, give maintenance dosage).

How Supplied: Phenytoin: *Chew Tablet:* 50 mg; *Suspension:* 100 mg/4 mL, 125 mg/5 mL; Phenytoin sodium, extended: *Capsule, Extended Release:* 30 mg, 100 mg; Phenytoin sodium, parenteral: *Injection:* 50 mg/mL; Phenytoin sodium prompt: *Capsule:* 100 mg

Side Effects: *CNS:* Most commonly, drowsiness, ataxia, dysarthria, confusion, insomnia, nervousness, irritability, depression, tremor, numbness, headache, psychoses, *increased seizures.* Choreoathetosis following IV use. *GI:* Gingival hyperplasia, N&V, either diarrhea or constipation. *Dermatologic:* Various dermatoses including a measles-like rash (common), scarlatiniform, maculopapular, and urticarial rashes. Rarely, drug-induced lupus erythematosus, *Stevens-Johnson syndrome,* exfoliative or purpuric dermatitis, and *toxic epidermal necrolysis.* Alopecia, hirsutism. Skin reactions may necessitate withdrawal of therapy. *Hematopoietic:* Leukopenia, granulocytopenia, thrombocytopenia, pancytopenia, *agranulocytosis,* macrocytosis, megaloblastic anemia, leukocytosis, monocytosis, eosinophilia, simple anemia, *aplastic anemia, hemolytic anemia.* *Hepatic:* Liver damage, toxic hepatitis, hypersensitivity reactions involving the liver including hepatocellular degeneration and *fatal hepatocellular necrosis.* *Ophthalmic:* Diplopia, nystagmus, conjunctivitis. *Miscellaneous:* Hyperglycemia, chest pain, edema, fever, photophobia, weight gain, *pulmonary fibrosis,* lymph node hyperplasia, gynecomastia, periarteritis nodosa,

depression of IgA, soft tissue injury at injection site, coarsening of facial features, Peyronie's disease, enlarged lips.

Rapid parenteral administration may cause serious CV effects, including hypotension, arrhythmias, CV collapse, and heart block, as well as CNS depression.

Many patients have a partial deficiency in the ability of the liver to degrade phenytoin, and as a result, toxicity may develop after a small PO dose. Liver and kidney function tests and hematopoietic studies are indicated prior to and periodically during drug therapy.

OD Overdose Management: *Symptoms:* Initially, ataxia, dysarthria, and nystagmus followed by unresponsive pupils, hypotension, and *coma.* Plasma levels greater than 40 mcg/mL result in significant decreases in mental capacity. *Treatment:* Treat symptoms. Hemodialysis may be effective. In children, total-exchange transfusion has been used.

Drug Interactions
Acetaminophen / ↓ Effect of acetaminophen due to ↑ breakdown by liver; however, hepatotoxicity may be ↑
Alcohol, ethyl / In alcoholics, ↓ effect of phenytoin due to ↑ breakdown by liver
Allopurinol / ↑ Effect of phenytoin due to ↓ breakdown in liver
Amiodarone / ↑ Effect of phenytoin or amiodarone due to ↓ breakdown by liver
Antacids / ↓ Effect of phenytoin due to ↓ GI absorption
Anticoagulants, oral / ↑ Effect of phenytoin due to ↓ breakdown by liver. Also, possible ↑ anticoagulant effect due to ↓ plasma protein binding
Antidepressants, tricyclic / May ↑ incidence of epileptic seizures or ↑ effect of phenytoin by ↓ plasma protein binding
Barbiturates / Effect of phenytoin may be ↑, ↓, or not changed; possible ↑ effect of barbiturates
Benzodiazepines / ↑ Effect of phenytoin due to ↓ breakdown by liver

Carbamazepine / ↓ Effect of phenytoin or carbamazepine due to ↑ breakdown by liver

Charcoal / ↓ Effect of phenytoin due to ↓ absorption from GI tract

Chloramphenicol / ↑ Effect of phenytoin due to ↓ breakdown by liver

Chlorpheniramine / ↑ Effect of phenytoin

Cimetidine / ↑ Effect of phenytoin due to ↓ breakdown by liver

Clonazepam / ↓ Plasma levels of clonazepam or phenytoin; or, ↑ risk of phenytoin toxicity

Contraceptives, oral / Estrogen-induced fluid retention may precipitate seizures; also, ↓ effect of contraceptives due to ↑ breakdown by liver

Corticosteroids / Effect of corticosteroids ↓ due to ↑ breakdown by liver; also, corticosteroids may mask hypersensitivity reactions due to phenytoin

Cyclosporine / ↓ Effect of cyclosporine due to ↑ breakdown by liver

Diazoxide / ↓ Effect of phenytoin due to ↑ breakdown by liver

Dicumarol / Phenytoin ↓ effect of dicumarol due to ↑ breakdown by liver

Digitalis glycosides / ↓ Effect of digitalis glycosides due to ↑ breakdown by liver

Disopyrimide / ↓ Effect of disopyramide due to ↑ breakdown by liver

Disulfiram / ↑ Effect of phenytoin due to ↓ breakdown by liver

Dopamine / IV phenytoin results in hypotension and bradycardia; also, ↓ effect of dopamine

Doxycycline / ↓ Effect of doxycycline due to ↑ breakdown by liver

Estrogens / See *Contraceptives, oral*

Fluconazole / ↑ Effect of phenytoin due to ↓ breakdown by liver

Folic acid / ↓ Effect of phenytoin

Furosemide / ↓ Effect of furosemide due to ↓ absorption

Haloperidol / ↓ Effect of haloperidol due to ↑ breakdown by liver

Ibuprofen / ↑ Effect of phenytoin

Isoniazid / ↑ Effect of phenytoin due to ↓ breakdown by liver

Levodopa / Phenytoin ↓ effect of levodopa

Levonorgestrel / ↓ Effect of norgestrel

Lithium / ↑ Risk of lithium toxicity

Loxapine / ↓ Effect of phenytoin

Mebendazole / ↓ Effect of mebendazole

Meperidine / ↓ Effect of meperidine due to ↑ breakdown by liver; toxic effects of meperidine may ↑ due to accumulation of active metabolite (normeperidine)

Methadone / ↓ Effect of methadone due to ↑ breakdown by liver

Metronidazole / ↑ Effect of phenytoin due to ↓ breakdown by liver

Metyrapone / ↓ Effect of metyrapone due to ↑ breakdown by liver

Mexiletine / ↓ Effect of mexiletine due to ↑ breakdown by liver

Miconazole / ↑ Effect of phenytoin due to ↓ breakdown by liver

Nitrofurantoin / ↓ Effect of phenytoin

Omeprazole / ↑ Effect of phenytoin due to ↓ breakdown by liver

Phenacemide / ↑ Effect of phenytoin due to ↓ breakdown by liver

Phenothiazines / ↑ Effect of phenytoin due to ↓ breakdown by liver

Phenylbutazone / ↑ Effect of phenytoin due to ↓ breakdown by liver and ↓ plasma protein binding

Primidone / Possible ↑ effect of primidone

Pyridoxine / ↓ Effect of phenytoin

Quinidine / ↓ Effect of quinidine due to ↑ breakdown by liver

Rifampin / ↓ Effect of phenytoin due to ↑ breakdown by liver

Salicylates / ↑ Effect of phenytoin by ↓ plasma protein binding

Sucralfate / ↓ Effect of phenytoin due to ↓ absorption from GI tract

Sulfonamides / ↑ Effect of phenytoin due to ↓ breakdown in liver

Sulfonylureas / ↓ Effect of sulfonylureas

Theophylline / ↓ Effect of both drugs due to ↑ breakdown by liver

Trimethoprim / ↑ Effect of phenytoin due to ↓ breakdown by liver

P

---

bold italic = life threatening side effect

Valproic acid / ↑ Effect of phenytoin due to ↓ breakdown by liver and ↓ plasma protein binding; phenytoin may also ↓ effect of valproic acid due to ↑ breakdown by liver

EMS CONSIDERATIONS

See also *Anticonvulsants* and *Antiarrhythmic Agents*.

Administration/Storage

IV 1. For parenteral preparations:
• Use only a clear solution.
• Dilute with special diluent supplied by manufacturer.
• Shake the vials until the solution is clear. It may take about 10 min for the drug to dissolve.
2. If IV infusion is used, a rate of 50 mg/min should not be exceeded in adults.
3. For treatment of status epilepticus, inject IV slowly at a rate not to exceed 50 mg/min. May repeat the dose 30 min after the initial administration if needed.
Assessment: Monitor ECG.
Interventions: During IV administration, monitor for hypotension.

Phosphorated carbohydrate solution

(FOS-for-ay-ted kar-boh-HIGH-drayt)

Emetrol, Nausea Relief, Nausetrol **(OTC)**

Classification: Antiemetic

Mechanism of Action: A hyperosmolar carbohydrate solution containing fructose, dextrose, and orthophosphoric acid with controlled hydrogen ion concentration. It relieves N&V due to a direct action on the wall of the GI tract that decreases smooth muscle contraction and delays gastric emptying time; the effect is directly related to the amount used.

Uses: Symptomatic relief of nausea due to upset stomach from intestinal flu, stomach flu, and food or drink. *Investigational:* Morning or motion sickness, regurgitation in infants, N&V due to drug therapy or inhaled anesthetics.

Contraindications: Diabetic patients due to the presence of carbohydrates. Individuals with hereditary fructose intolerance.

Precautions: Since nausea may be a symptom of a serious condition, a physician should be consulted if symptoms are not relieved or recur often.

Route/Dosage
• **Oral Solution**
Nausea.
Adults: 15–30 mL at 15-min intervals until vomiting ceases; if the first dose is rejected, the same dosage should be given in 5 min. Should not be taken for more than five doses (1 hr). **Children, 2 to 12 years:** 5–10 mL at 15-min intervals in the same manner as adults.
Regurgitation in infants.
5 or 10 mL, 10–15 min before each feeding; in refractory cases, 10 or 15 mL, 30 min before feeding.
Morning sickness.
15–30 mL on arising; repeat q 3 hr or when nausea threatens.
N&V due to drug therapy or inhalation anesthesia, motion sickness.
Adults and older children: 15 mL; **young children:** 5 mL.
How Supplied: *Solution:* Liquid
Side Effects: *GI:* Abdominal pain and diarrhea due to large doses of fructose.

EMS CONSIDERATIONS

See also *Antiemetics*.

Physostigmine salicylate
Physostigmine sulfate

(fye-zoh-STIG-meen)

Pregnancy Class: C

Salicylate (Antilirium **(Rx)**) Sulfate (Eserine Sulfate **(Rx)**)

Classification: Indirectly acting cholinergic-acetylcholinesterase inhibitor

Mechanism of Action: Reversible acetylcholinesterase inhibitor causing an increased concentration of acetylcholine at nerve endings; antagonizes anticholinergic drugs. Produces miosis, increased accommodation, and a decrease in intraocular pressure with decreased resistance to outflow of aqueous humor. When used for chronic open-angle glaucoma, ciliary muscle contraction may open the intertrabecular spaces, facilitating aqueous humor outflow.

Onset of Action: IV: 3-5 min; **miosis:** 20-30 min; **Reduction of IOP, peak:** 2-6 hr.

Duration of Action: IV: 1-2 hr; **miosis:** 12-36 hr; **Reduction of IOP:** 12-36 hr.

Uses: Overdosage due to cholinergic blocking drugs (e.g., atropine) and tricyclic antidepressant overdosage. Reduce intraocular pressure in open-angle glaucoma. Friedreich's and other inherited ataxias (FDA has granted orphan status for this use). *Investigational:* Angle-closure glaucoma during or after iridectomy, secondary glaucoma if no inflammation present. Treat delirium tremens (DTs) and Alzheimer's disease. May also antagonize the CNS depressant effect of diazepam.

Contraindications: Active uveal inflammation, any inflammatory disease of the iris or ciliary body, glaucoma associated with iridocyclitis. Asthma, gangrene, diabetes, CV disease, GI or GU tract obstruction, any vagotonic state, in those receiving choline esters or depolarizing neuromuscular blocking drugs.

Precautions: Use with caution during lactation, in patients with chronic angle-closure glaucoma, or in patients with narrow angles. Safety and efficacy have not been established for ophthalmic use in children. Reserve systemic use in children for life-threatening situations only. Benzyl alcohol, found in the parenteral product, may cause a fatal "gasping syndrome" in premature infants. The parenteral form also contains sulfites that may cause allergic reactions.

Route/Dosage
• **IM, IV**
  Anticholinergic drug overdose.

Adults, IM, IV: 0.5–2 mg at a rate of 1 mg/min; may be repeated if necessary. **Pediatric, IV:** 0.02 mg/kg IM or by slow IV injection (0.5 mg given over a period of at least 1 min). Dose may be repeated at 5–10 min if needed to a maximum of 2 mg if no toxic effects are manifested.
  Postanesthesia.
0.5–1 mg given IM or by slow IV (less than 1 mg/min). May be repeated at 10- to 30-min intervals to attain desired response.
• **Ophthalmic Ointment**
  Glaucoma.

Adults and children: 1 cm of the 0.25% sulfate ointment applied to the lower fornix up to t.i.d.

How Supplied: Physostigmine salicylate: *Injection:* 1 mg/mL. Physostigmine sulfate: *Ophthalmic Ointment:* 0.25%

Side Effects: Additional: If IV administration is too rapid, bradycardia, hypersalivation, breathing difficulties, and *seizures* may occur. Conjunctivitis when used for glaucoma.

OD Overdose Management: *Symptoms:* Cholinergic crisis. *Treatment:* IV atropine sulfate: **Adults:** 0.4–0.6 mg; **infants and children up to 12 years of age:** 0.01 mg/kg q 2 hr as needed (maximum single dose should not exceed 0.4 mg). A short-acting barbiturate may be used for seizures not relieved by atropine.

Drug Interactions
Anticholinesterases, systemic / Additive effects → toxicity
Succinylcholine / ↑ Risk of respiratory and CV collapse

EMS CONSIDERATIONS

IV Administration/Storage: May administer IV undiluted: 1 mg/min; 0.5 mg/min for children.

Assessment: Determine type of overdosage (drug or plant ingestion), amount and time ingested.

Interventions: During IV administration, monitor ECG and VS; report any bradycardia, hypersalivation, respiratory difficulty, or seizure activity.

---

bold italic = life threatening side effect

Phytonadione (Vitamin K₁)

(fye-toe-nah-DYE-ohn)
Pregnancy Class: C
Aqua-Mephyton, Mephyton **(Rx)**
Classification: Fat-soluble vitamin

Mechanism of Action: Vitamin K is essential for the hepatic synthesis of factors II, VII, IX, and X, all of which are essential for blood clotting. Vitamin K deficiency causes an increase in bleeding tendency, demonstrated by ecchymoses, epistaxis, hematuria, GI bleeding, and postoperative and intracranial hemorrhage. Phytonadione is similar to natural vitamin K.

Onset of Action: IM: 1-2 hr. *Control of bleeding:* Parenteral, 3-6 hr; **PO:** 6-12 hr.

Uses: Primary and drug-induced hypoprothrombinemia, especially that caused by anticoagulants of the coumarin and phenindione type. Vitamin K cannot reverse the anticoagulant activity of heparin.

Parenteral use for vitamin K malabsorption syndromes. Adjunct during whole blood transfusions. Preoperatively to prevent the danger of hemorrhages in surgical patients who may require anticoagulant therapy.

Certain forms of liver disease. Hemorrhagic states associated with obstructive jaundice, celiac disease, ulcerative colitis, sprue, biliary fistula, cystic fibrosis of the pancreas, regional enteritis, resection of intestine. Prophylaxis of hemorrhagic disease of the newborn.

Contraindications: Severe liver disease.

Precautions: Use with caution in patients with sulfite sensitivity and during lactation as phytonadione is excreted in breast milk. Safety and efficacy have not been determined in children. Benzyl alcohol, contained in some preparations, may cause toxicity in newborns.

Route/Dosage

• **Tablets**

Hypoprothrombinemia, drug-induced.

Adults: 2.5–10 mg (up to 25 mg); dose may be repeated after 12–48 hr if needed.

Vitamin supplement, prothrombogenic, drug-induced hypoprothrombinemia.

Pediatric: 5–10 mg.

• **IM, SC**

Vitamin supplement, prothrombogenic, drug-induced hypoprothrombinemia.

Adults: 2.5–10 mg (up to 25 mg) which may be repeated after 6–8 hr if needed. **Infants:** 1–2 mg; **children:** 5–10 mg.

Prophylaxis of hypoprothrombinemia during prolonged TPN.

Adults, IM: 5–10 mg once weekly; **pediatric:** 2–5 mg IM once weekly.

Infants receiving milk substitutes or who are breastfed.

1 mg/month if vitamin K in diet is less than 0.1 mg/L.

Prevention of hemorrhagic disease in the newborn.

0.5–1 mg IM within 1 hr after delivery. The dose may be repeated in 2–3 weeks if the mother took anticoagulant, anticonvulsant, antituberculosis, or recent antibiotic therapy during pregnancy. Alternatively, 1–5 mg given to the mother 12–24 hr before delivery.

Treatment of hemorrhagic disease in the newborn.

1 mg SC or IM (higher doses may be needed if the mother has been taking oral anticoagulants).

How Supplied: *Injection:* 1 mg/0.5 mL, 10 mg /mL; *Tablet:* 0.1 mg, 5 mg

Side Effects: May be transient flushing of the face, sweating, a sense of constriction of the chest, and weakness. Cramp-like pain, weak and rapid pulse, convulsive movements, chills and fever, hypotension, cyanosis, or hemoglobinuria has been reported occasionally. ***Shock and cardiac and respiratory failure*** may be observed. *Allergic:* Rash, urticaria, ***anaphylaxis.*** *After PO use:* N&V, stomach upset, headache. *After parenteral use:* Flushing, alteration of taste, sweating, hypotension, dizziness, rapid and weak pulse, dyspnea, cyanosis, delayed skin reactions. Pain, swelling, and tenderness at injection site. *IV administration may cause severe reactions (e.g., shock, cardiac or respiratory arrest, anaphylaxis) leading to death.* These effects may occur when receiving vitamin K for the first time. *Newborns: Fatal kernicterus,* hemolysis, jaundice, hyperbilirubinemia (especially in premature infants).

Drug Interactions

Antibiotics / May inhibit the body's production of vitamin K and may lead to bleeding. Vitamin K supplements should be given

Anticoagulants, oral / Vitamin K antagonizes anticoagulant effect

Cholestyramine / ↓ Effect of phytonadione due to ↓ absorption from GI tract

Colestipol / ↓ Effect of phytonadione due to ↓ absorption from GI tract

Hemolytics / ↑ Potential for toxicity

Mineral oil / ↓ Effect of phytonadione due to ↓ absorption from GI tract

Quinidine, Quinine / ↑ Requirement for vitamin K

Salicylates / High doses of salicylates → ↑ requirements for vitamin K

Sulfonamides / ↑ Requirements for vitamin K

Sucralfate / ↓ Effect of phytonadione due to ↓ absorption from GI tract

EMS CONSIDERATIONS

None.

Pilocarpine hydrochloride
Pilocarpine ocular therapeutic system

(pie-low-CAR-peen)

Pregnancy Class: C

Hydrochloride (Adsorbocarpine, Akarpine, Isopto Carpine, Pilocar, Pilopine HS, Piloptic-1/2-1, -2, -3, -4, and -6, Pilopto-Carpine, Pilostat, Salagen **(Rx)**) Ocular therapeutic system (Ocusert Pilo-20 and -40 **(Rx)**)

Classification: Direct-acting cholinergic agent (miotic)

Mechanism of Action: *Nitrate:* The ocular therapeutic system is placed in the cul-de-sac of the eye for release of pilocarpine. The drug is released from the ocular therapeutic system three times faster during the first few hours and then decreases (within 6 hr) to a rate of 20 or 40 mcg/hr for 1 week. When used to treat dry mouth due to radiotherapy in head and neck cancer patients, pilocarpine stimulates residual functioning salivary gland tissue to increase saliva production.

Onset of Action: *Hydrochloride Gel:* 60 min; **peak effect:** 3-12 hr; *Ocular system:* 60 min; **peak effect:** 1.5-2 hr.

Duration of Action: *Hydrochloride Gel:* 18-24 hr; *Ocular system:* 7 days.

Uses: HCl: Chronic simple glaucoma (especially open-angle). Chronic angle-closure glaucoma, including after iridectomy. Acute angle-closure glaucoma (alone or with other miotics, epinephrine, beta-adrenergic blocking agents, carbonic anhydrase inhibitors, or hyperosmotic agents). To reverse mydriasis (i.e., after cycloplegic and mydriatic drugs). Pre- and postoperative intraocular tension. The nitrate product is also used for emergency miosis. Salagen (Pilocarpine HCl) has been approved for treatment of radiation-induced dry mouth in head and neck cancer patients, as well as in Sjogren's syndrome. **Ocular Therapeutic System:** Glaucoma alone or with other ophthalmic medications. *Investigational:* Hydrochloride used to treat xerostomia in patients with malfunctioning salivary glands.

Contraindications: Lactation.

Precautions: Use with caution during lactation, in those with narrow angles (angle closure may result), in those with known or suspected cholelithiasis or biliary tract disease, and in patients with controlled asthma, chronic bronchitis, or COPD. Safety and efficacy have not been established in children.

Route/Dosage

PILOCARPINE HYDROCHLORIDE
• **Ophthalmic Gel, 4%**

bold italic = life threatening side effect

Glaucoma.
Adults and adolescents: 1/2-in. ribbon in the lower conjunctival sac of the affected eye(s) once daily at bedtime.
• **Ophthalmic Solution,** 1/4%, 1/2%, 1%, 2%, 3%, 4%, 5%, 6%, 8%
Doses listed are all for adults and adolescents.
Chronic glaucoma.
1 gtt of a 0.5%–4% solution q.i.d.
Acute angle-closure glaucoma.
1 gtt of a 1% or 2% solution q 5–10 min for three to six doses; then, 1 gtt q 1–3 hr until pressure is decreased.
Miotic, to counteract sympathomimetics.
1 gtt of a 1% solution.
Miosis, prior to surgery.
1 gtt of a 2% solution q 4–6 hr for one or two doses before surgery.
Miosis before iridectomy.
1 gtt of a 2% solution for four doses immediately before surgery.
• **Ocular System**
Insert and remove as directed on package insert or by physician. Ocusert Pilo-20 is approximately equal to the 0.5% or 1% drops, while Ocusert Pilo-40 is approximately equal to the 2% or 3% solution.
• **Tablets (Salagen)**
Treat radiation-induced dry mouth in head and neck cancer patients.
Initial: 5 mg t.i.d.; **then,** up to 10 mg t.i.d., if needed.
How Supplied: Pilocarpine hydrochloride: *Device:* 20 mcg/hr, 40 mcg/hr; *Ophthalmic gel:* 4%; *Ophthalmic Solution:* 0.25%, 0.5%, 1%, 2%, 3%, 4%, 5%, 6%, 8%; *Tablet:* 5 mg. Pilocarpine ocular therapeutic system: *Device:* 20 mcg/hr, 40 mcg/hr
Side Effects: Additional: The following side effects have been attributed to the pilocarpine ocular system. *Ophthalmic:* Conjunctival irritation, including mild erythema with or without a slight increase in mucous secretion upon initial use.
OD Overdose Management: *Treatment:* Titrate with atropine (0.5–1 mg SC or IM) and supportive measures to maintain circulation and respiration. If there is severe cardiovascular depression or bronchoconstriction, epinephrine (0.3–1 mg SC or IV) may be used.

EMS CONSIDERATIONS

None.

Pindolol
(PIN-doh-lohl)
Pregnancy Class: B
Visken **(Rx)**
Classification: Beta-adrenergic blocking agent

Mechanism of Action: Manifests both beta-1 and beta-2 adrenergic blocking activity. Also has significant intrinsic sympathomimetic effects and minimal membrane-stabilizing activity.
Uses: Hypertension (alone or in combination with other antihypertensive agents as thiazide diuretics). *Investigational:* Ventricular arrhythmias and tachycardias, antipsychotic-induced akathisia, situational anxiety.
Contraindications: Bronchial asthma or bronchospasm, including severe COPD.
Precautions: Dosage has not been established in children.

Route/Dosage
• **Tablets**
Hypertension.
Initial: 5 mg b.i.d. (alone or with other antihypertensive drugs). If no response in 3–4 weeks, increase by 10 mg/day q 3–4 weeks to a maximum of 60 mg/day.
Antipsychotic-induced akathisia.
5 mg/day.
How Supplied: *Tablet:* 5 mg, 10 mg

EMS CONSIDERATIONS

See also *Beta-Adrenergic Blocking Agents.*

Pioglitazone hydrochloride
(pie-oh-GLIT-ah-zohn)
Pregnancy Class: C
Actos **(Rx)**
Classification: Oral hypoglycemic agent

Mechanism of Action: Depends on the presence of insulin to act. Decreases insulin resistance in the periphery and liver resulting in increased insulin-dependent glucose disposal and decreased hepatic glucose output. It is not an insulin secretagogue. Is an agonist for peroxisome proliferator-activated receptor (PPAR) gamma, which is found in adipose tissue, skeletal muscle, and liver. Activation of these receptors modulates the transcription of a number of insulin responsive genes that control glucose and lipid metabolism.

Uses: Adjunct to diet and exercise in type 2 diabetes. Used either as monotherapy or in combination with a sulfonylurea, metformin, or insulin when diet and exercise plus the single drug does not adequately control blood glucose.

Contraindications: In type I diabetes, diabetic ketoacidosis, active liver disease, with ALT levels that exceed 2.5 times ULN, in patients with NYHA Class II or IV cardiac status, or during lactation.

Precautions: Treatment may result in resumption of ovulation in premenopausal anovulatory patients with insulin resistance. Use with caution in patients with edema. Safety and efficacy have not been determined in children.

Route/Dosage ⸻
- **Tablets**
  Type II diabetes as monotherapy.
Adults: 15 mg or 30 mg once daily in patients not adequately controlled with diet and exercise. Initial dose can be increased up to 45 mg once daily for those who respond inadequately.
  Type II diabetes as combination therapy.
If combined with a sulfonylurea, initiate pioglitazone at 15 or 30 mg once daily. The current sulfonylurea dose can be continued unless hypoglycemia occurs; then, reduce the sulfonylurea dose. If combined with metformin, initiate pioglitazone at 15 or 30 mg once daily. The current metformin dose can be continued; it

is unlikely the metformin dose will have to be adjusted due to hypoglycemia. If combined with insulin, initiate pioglitazone at 15 or 30 mg once daily. The current insulin dose can be continued unless hypoglycemia occurs or plasma glucose levels decrease to less than 100 mg/dL; then, decrease the insulin dose by 10% to 25%. Individualize further dosage adjustments based on glucose-lowering response.

Daily dose should not exceed 45 mg.

How Supplied: *Tablets:* 15 mg, 30 mg, 45 mg

Side Effects: *Metabolic:* Hypoglycemia, aggravation of diabetes mellitus. *Respiratory:* URTI, sinusitis, pharyngitis. *Miscellaneous:* Headache, myalgia, tooth disorder, anemia, edema.

Drug Interactions

Ketoconazole / Significant inhibition of pioglitazone metabolism

Oral contraceptives (containing ethinyl estradiol/norethindrone / ↓ Plasma levels of both hormones; possible loss of contraception

EMS CONSIDERATIONS

None.

⸻

P

Piperacillin sodium
(pie-PER-ah-sill-in)
Pregnancy Class: B
Pipracil **(Rx)**
Classification: Antibiotic, penicillin

Mechanism of Action: Semisynthetic, broad-spectrum penicillin for parenteral use.

Uses: (1) Intra-abdominal infections (including hepatobiliary and surgical infections) due to *Escherichia coli, Pseudomonas aeruginosa, Clostridium* sp., enterococci, anaerobic cocci, *Bacteroides* sp., including *B. fragilis.* (2) URIs due to *E. coli, P. aeruginosa, Proteus* sp. (including *P. mirabilis* and enterococci), *Klebsiella* sp. (3) Gynecologic infections (including endometritis, PID, pelvic cellulitis) due to *Bacteroides* sp. (including *B. fragilis)*, anaerobic cocci, enterococci (*Streptococcus faecalis*), *Neisseria gonorrhoeae*. (4) Septicemia (including bacteremia) due to *E. coli*, *P. mirabilis*, *S. pneumoniae*, *P. aeruginosa*, *Klebsiella* sp., *Enterobacter* sp., *Serratia* sp., *Bacteroides* sp., anaerobic cocci. (5) Lower respiratory tract infections due to *E. coli*, *P. aeruginosa*, *Haemophilus influenzae*, *Klebsiella* sp., *Enterobacter* sp., *Serratia* sp., *Bacteroides* sp., anaerobic cocci. (6) Skin and skin structure infections due to *E. coli*, *Klebsiella* sp., *Serratia* sp., *Acinetobacter* sp., *Enterobacter* sp., *P. aeruginosa*, *P. mirabilis*, indole-positive *Proteus* sp., *Bacteroides* sp. (including *B. fragilis*), anaeroabic cocci, enterococci. (7) Bone and joint infections due to *P. aeruginosa*, *Bacteroides* sp., enterococci, anaerobic cocci. (8) Uncomplicated gonococcal urethritis. (9) Infections due to streptococcus species, including Group A β–hemolytic streptococcus and *S. pneumoniae*. (10) Prophylaxis in surgery, including GI and biliary procedures, vaginal and abdominal hysterectomy, and cesarean section.

Route/Dosage

• **IM, IV**

Serious infections, including septicemia, nosocomial pneumonia, intra-abdominal infections, aerobic and anaerobic gyn infections, and skin and soft tissue infections.

Adults, IV: 3–4 g q 4–6 hr (12–18 g/day, not to exceed 24 g/day) as a 20- to 30-min infusion. Average duration is 7 to 10 days (3 to 10 days for gynecologic infections and at least 10 days for group A β–hemolytic streptococcal infections). If C_{CR} is 20–40 mL/min, give 12 g/day (4 g q 8 hr); if C_{CR} is less than 20 mL/min, give 8 g/day (4 g q 12 hr). Dosage has not been determined for children less than 12 years of age. However, use the following guidelines: **Neonates, less than 36 weeks old:** 75 mg/kg IV q 12 hr during the first week of life; **then,** q 8 hr during the second week. **Full-term:** 75 mg/kg IV q 8 hr during the first week of life; **then,** q 6 hr thereafter. **Children, other conditions:** 200–300 mg/kg/day, up to a maximum of 24 g/day divided q 4 to 6 hr.

Complicated UTIs.

Adults, IV: 8–16 g/day (125–200 mg/kg/day) in divided doses q 6–8 hr. If C_{CR} is 20–40 mL/min, give 9 g/day (3 g q 8 hr); if C_{CR} is less than 20 mL/min, give 6 g/day (3 g q 12 hr).

Uncomplicated UTIs and most community-acquired pneumonias.

Adults, IM, IV: 6–8 g/day (100–125 mg/kg/day) in divided doses q 6–12 hr. If C_{CR} is less than 20 mL/min, give 6 g/day (3 g q 12 hr).

Uncomplicated gonorrhea infections.

2 g **IM** with 1 g probenecid **PO** 30 min before injection (both given as single dose).

Prophylaxis in surgery.

Intra-abdominal surgery: 2 g IV just prior to anesthesia, 2 g during surgery, and 2 g q 6 hr post surgery for no more than 24 hr. *Vaginal hysterectomy:* 2 g IV just prior to anesthesia, 2 g 6 hr after initial dose, and 2 g 12 hr after first dose. *Cesarean section:* 2 g IV after cord is clamped, 2 g 4 hr after initial dose, and 2 g 8 hr after first dose. *Abdominal hysterectomy:* 2 g IV just prior to anesthesia, 2 g on return to recovery room, and 2 g after 6 hr.

For cystic fibrosis.

350–500 mg/kg/day divided q 4–6 hr.

How Supplied: *Powder for injection:* 2g, 3g, 4g, 40g

Side Effects: Additional: Rarely, prolonged muscle relaxation.

Drug Interactions: Additional: Pipercillin may prolong the neuromuscular blockade of vecuronium.

EMS CONSIDERATIONS

See also *Penicillins*.

───────COMBINATION DRUG───────

Piperacillin sodium and Tazobactam sodium

(pie-PER-ah-sill-in, tay-zoh-BAC-tam)

Pregnancy Class: B

Zosyn **(Rx)**

Classification: Antibiotic, penicillin

Mechanism of Action: A combination of piperacillin sodium and tazobactam sodium, a beta-lactamase inhibitor. Tazobactam inhibits beta-lactamases, thus ensuring activity of piperacillin against beta-lactamase-producing microorganisms. Thus, tazobactam broadens the antibiotic spectrum of piperacillin to those bacteria normally resistant to it.

Uses: (1) Appendicitis complicated by rupture or abscess and peritonitis caused by piperacillin-resistant, beta-lactamase-producing strains of *Escherichia coli, Bacteroides fragilis, B. ovatus, B. thetaiotaomicron,* or *B. vulgatus.* (2) Uncomplicated and complicated skin and skin structure infections (including cellulitis, cutaneous abscesses, and ischemic/diabetic foot infections) caused by piperacillin-resistant, beta-lactamase-producing strains of *Staphylococcus aureus.* (3) Postpartum endometritis or PID caused by piperacillin-resistant, beta-lactamase-producing strains of *E. coli.* (4) Community-acquired pneumonia of moderate severity caused by piperacillin-resistant, beta-lactamase-producing strains of *Haemophilus influenzae.* (5) Moderate to severe nosocomial pneumonia caused by piperacillin-resistant, beta-lactamase-producing strains of *S. aureus.* (6) Infections caused by piperacillin-susceptible organisms for which piperacillin is effective may also be treated with this combination. The treatment of mixed infections caused by piperacillin-susceptible organisms and piperacillin-resistant, beta-lactamase-producing organisms susceptible to this combination does not require addition of another antibiotic.

Contraindications: Hypersensitivity to penicillins, cephalosporins, or beta-lactamase inhibitors.

Precautions: Use with caution during lactation. Safety and efficacy have not been determined in children less than 12 years of age.

Route/Dosage ———————
- **IV Infusion**
  Susceptible infections.

Adults: 12 g/day piperacillin and 1.5 g/day tazobactam, given as 3.375 g (i.e., 3 g piperacillin and 0.375 g tazobactam) q 6 hr for 7–10 days. In patients with renal insufficiency, the IV dose is adjusted depending on the extent of impaired function. If C_{CR} is 20–40 mL/min, the dose is 8 g/day piperacillin and 1 g/day tazobactam in divided doses of 2.25 g q 6 hr. If the C_{CR} is less than 20 mL/min, the dose is 6 g/day piperacillin and 0.75 g/day tazobactam in divided doses of 2.25 g q 8 hr.

Moderate to severe nosocomial pneumonia due to piperacillin-resistant, beta-lacatamase-producing S. aureus.

Adults: 3.375 g q 4 hr with an aminoglycoside for 7 to 14 days.

How Supplied: *Injection:* 40 mg-5 mg/mL, 60 mg-7.5 mg/mL, 4 g-0.5 g/100 mL; *Powder for Injection:* 2 g-0.25 g, 3 g-0.375 g, 4 g-0.5 g, 36 g-4.5g

Side Effects: See *Penicillins(/italic>. The highest incidence of side effects include the following.* GI: *Diarrhea, constipation, N&V, dyspepsia, stool changes, abdominal pain.* CNS: *Headache, insomnia, fever, agitation, dizziness, anxiety.* Dermatologic: *Rash, including maculopapular, bullous, urticarial, and eczematoid; pruritus.* Hematologic: *Thrombocytopenia, eosinophilia, leukopenia, neutropenia. Miscellaneous:* Pain, moniliasis, hypertension, chest pain, edema, rhinitis, dyspnea.

Drug Interactions
Heparin / Possible ↑ effect of heparin
Oral anticoagulants / Possible ↑ effect of oral anticoagulants
Tobramycin / ↓ Area under the curve, renal clearance, and urinary recovery of tobramycin
Vecuronium / Prolongation of the neuromuscular blockade of vecuronium

EMS CONSIDERATIONS

See also *Piperacillin sodium* and *Penicillins.*

---

bold italic = life threatening side effect

Piperazine citrate
(pie-PER-ah-zeen)
Pregnancy Class: B
(Rx)
Classification: Anthelmintic

Mechanism of Action: Acts to paralyze the muscles of parasites; this dislodges the parasites and promotes their elimination by peristalsis. Has little effect on larvae in tissues.
Uses: Pinworm (oxyuriasis) and roundworm (ascariasis) infestations. Particularly recommended for pediatric use.
Contraindications: Impaired liver or kidney function, seizure disorders, hypersensitivity. Lactation.
Precautions: Safe use during pregnancy has not been established. Due to neurotoxicity, avoid prolonged, repeated, or excessive use in children.

Route/Dosage —————————
* **Syrup, Tablets**
    Pinworms.
Adults and children: 65 mg/kg/day as a single dose for 7 days up to a maximum daily dose of 2.5 g.
    Roundworms.
Adults: One dose of 3.5 g/day for 2 consecutive days; **pediatric:** One dose of 75 mg/kg/day for 2 consecutive days, not to exceed 3.5 g/day. For severe infections, repeat therapy after 1 week.
How Supplied: *Tablet:* 250 mg
Side Effects: Piperazine has low toxicity. *GI:* N&V, diarrhea, cramps. *CNS:* Tremors, headache, vertigo, decreased reflexes, paresthesias, *seizures,* ataxia, chorea, memory decrement. *Ophthalmologic:* Nystagmus, blurred vision, cataracts, strabismus. *Allergic:* Urticaria, fever, skin reactions, purpura, lacrimation, rhinorrhea, arthralgia, *bronchospasm,* cough. *Miscellaneous:* Muscle weakness.
Drug Interactions: Concomitant administration of piperazine and phenothiazines may result in an increase in extrapyramidal effects (including violent convulsions) caused by phenothiazines.

EMS CONSIDERATIONS
None.

Pipobroman
(pip-oh-BROH-man)
Pregnancy Class: D
Classification: Antineoplastic, alkylating agent.

Uses: Polycythemia vera; chronic granulocytic leukemia in patients refractory to busulfan.
Contraindications: Additionl: Children under 15 years of age. Lactation. Bone marrow depression due to chemotherapy or X rays.
Precautions: Bone marrow depression may not occur for 4 or more weeks after therapy is started.

Route/Dosage —————————
* **Tablets**
    Polycythemia vera.
1 mg/kg/day. Up to 1.5–3 mg/kg/day may be required in patients refractory to other treatment; do not use such doses until a dose of 1 mg/kg/day has been given for at least 30 days with no improvement. When hematocrit has been reduced to 50%–55%, **maintenance dosage** of 100–200 mcg/kg is instituted.
    Chronic granulocytic leukemia.
Initial: 1.5–2.5 mg/kg/day; **maintenance:** 7–175 mg/day, to be instituted when leukocyte count approaches 10,000/mm³.
How Supplied: *Tablet:* 25 mg
Side Effects: *Hematologic:* Leukopenia, anemia, thrombocytopenia. *GI:* N&V, diarrhea, abdominal cramps. *Dermatologic:* Skin rashes.
OD Overdose Management: *Symptoms:* Hematologic toxicity, especially with chronic overdosage. *Treatment:* Monitor hematologic status; if necessary, begin vigorous supportive treatment.

EMS CONSIDERATIONS
None.

Pirbuterol acetate
(peer-BYOU-ter-ohl)
Pregnancy Class: C

Maxair Autohaler (Rx)
Classification: Sympathomimetic, bronchodilator

Mechanism of Action: Causes bronchodilation by stimulating beta-2-adrenergic receptors. Has minimal effects on beta-1 receptors. Also inhibits histamine release from mast cells, causes vasodilation, and increases ciliary motility.
Onset of Action: Inhalation: Approximately 5 min; **time to peak effect:** 30-60 min.
Duration of Action: 5 hr.
Uses: Alone or with theophylline or steroids for prophylaxis and treatment of bronchospasm in asthma and other conditions with reversible bronchospasms, including bronchitis, emphysema, bronchiectasis, obstructive pulmonary disease.
Contraindications: Cardiac arrhythmias due to tachycardia; tachycardia caused by digitalis toxicity.
Precautions: Safety and efficacy have not been determined in children less than 12 years of age.

Route/Dosage ───────────
• **Inhalation Aerosol**
Adults and children over 12 years: 0.2–0.4 mg (1–2 inhalations) q 4–6 hr, not to exceed 12 inhalations (2.4 mg) daily.
How Supplied: *Aerosol Solid w/Adapter:* 0.2 mg/inh
Side Effects: Additional: *CV:* PVCs, hypotension. *CNS:* Hyperactivity, hyperkinesia, anxiety, confusion, depression, fatigue, syncope. *GI:* Diarrhea, dry mouth, anorexia, loss of appetite, bad taste or taste change, abdominal pain, abdominal cramps, stomatitis, glossitis. *Dermatologic:* Rash, edema, pruritus, alopecia. *Miscellaneous:* Flushing, numbness in extremities, weight gain.

EMS CONSIDERATIONS

See also *Sympathomimetic Drugs*.

Piroxicam
(peer-OX-ih-kam)

Feldene (Rx)
Classification: Nonsteroidal anti-inflammatory drug

Mechanism of Action: May inhibit prostaglandin synthesis. Effect is comparable to that of aspirin, but with fewer GI side effects and less tinnitus.
Onset of Action: Analgesia: 1 hr; **Anti-inflammatory activity:** 7-12 days.
Duration of Action: Analgesia: 2-3 days; **Anti-inflammatory activity:** 2-3 weeks.
Uses: Acute and chronic treatment of rheumatoid arthritis and osteoarthritis. *Investigational:* Juvenile rheumatoid arthritis, primary dysmenorrhea, sunburn.
Contraindications: Safe use during pregnancy has not been determined. Use in children less than 14 years old. Lactation.
Precautions: Safety and efficacy have not been established in children. Increased plasma levels and elimination half-life may be observed in geriatric patients (especially women).

Route/Dosage ───────────
• **Capsules**
  Anti-inflammatory, antirheumatic.
Adults: 20 mg/day in one or more divided doses. Do not assess the effect of therapy for 2 weeks.
How Supplied: *Capsule:* 10 mg, 20 mg

EMS CONSIDERATIONS

None.

Podofilox
(poh-DAHF-ih-lox)
Pregnancy Class: C
Condylox (Rx)
Classification: Keratolytic

Mechanism of Action: An antimitotic agent that causes necrosis of visible wart tissue when applied topically.

P

---

bold italic = life threatening side effect

Uses: Topical treatment of external genital warts and perianal warts (gel only). *Investigational:* Systemically for treatment of cancer.

Contraindications: Use of solution or gel for mucous membrane warts or solution for perianal warts. Lactation.

Precautions: Genital warts must be distinguished from squamous cell carcinoma prior to initiation of treatment. Safety and effectiveness have not been demonstrated in children. Avoid contact with the eyes.

Route/Dosage

• **Topical Solution, Topical Gel**
External genital warts, perianal warts (gel only).

Adults, initial: Apply b.i.d. in the morning and evening (i.e., q 12 hr) for 3 consecutive days; **then,** withhold use for 4 consecutive days. The 1-week cycle of treatment may be repeated up to 4 times until there is no visible sign of wart tissue. Consider alternative treatment if the response is incomplete after four treatments.

How Supplied: *Solution:* 0.5%, *Gel:* 0.5%

Side Effects: Solution. D*ermatologic:* Commonly, burning, pain, inflammation, erosion, and itching. Also, tenderness, chafing, scarring, vesicle formation, dryness and peeling, tingling, bleeding, ulceration, malodor, crusting edema, foreskin irretraction. *Miscellaneous:* Pain with intercourse, insomnia, dizziness, hematuria, vomiting.

Gel. *Dermatologic:* Commonly, burning, pain, inflammation, erosion, itching, and bleeding. Also, stinging, erythema, desquamation, scabbing, discoloration, tenderness, dryness, crusting, fissures, soreness, ulceration, swelling/edema, tingling, rash, blisters.

Systemic Use. G*I:* N&V, diarrhea, oral ulcers. *Hematologic:* Bone marrow depression, leukocytosis, pancytosis. *CNS:* Altered mental status, lethargy, *coma, seizures. Miscellaneous:* Peripheral neuropathy, fever, tachypnea, *respiratory failure,* hematuria, renal failure.

OD Overdose Management: *Symptoms:* N&V, diarrhea, fever, altered mental status, hematologic toxicity, peripheral neuropathy, lethargy, tachypnea, *respiratory failure,* hematuria, leukocytosis, pancytosis, renal failure, *seizures, coma. Treatment:* Wash the skin free of any remaining drug. General supportive therapy to treat symptoms.

EMS CONSIDERATIONS

None.

Polymyxin B sulfate, parenteral
Polymyxin B sulfate, sterile ophthalmic
(pol-ee-MIX-in)

Pregnancy Class: C
Parenteral (Aerosporin **(Rx)**) Ophthalmic **(Rx)**
Classification: Antibiotic, polymyxin

Mechanism of Action: Derived from the spore-forming soil bacterium *Bacillus polymyxa.* Bactericidal against most gram-negative organisms; rapidly inactivated by alkali, strong acid, and certain metal ions. Increases the permeability of the plasma cell membrane of the bacterium (i.e., similar to detergents), causing leakage of essential metabolites and ultimately inactivation.

Uses: Systemic: Acute infections of the urinary tract and meninges, septicemia caused by *Pseudomonas aeruginosa.* Meningeal infections caused by *Haemophilus influenzae,* UTIs caused by *Escherichia coli,* bacteremia caused by *Enterobacter aerogenes* or *Klebsiella pneumoniae.* Combined with neomycin for irrigation of the urinary bladder to prevent bacteriuria and bacteremia from indwelling catheters.

Ophthalmic: Conjunctival and corneal infections (e.g., conjunctivitis, keratitis, keratoconjunctivitis, corneal ulcers, blepharitis, blepharoconjunctivitis, acute meibomianitis, dacryocystitis) due to *E. coli, H. influenzae, H. parainfluenzae, K. pneumoniae, E.*

aerogenes, and *P. aeruginosa.* Used alone or in combination for ear infections.

Contraindications: Hypersensitivity. A potentially toxic drug to be reserved for the treatment of severe, resistant infections in hospitalized patients. Not indicated for patients with severely impaired renal function or nitrogen retention. Ophthalmic use in dendritic keratitis, vaccinia, varicella, mycobacterial infections of the eye, fungal diseases of the eye, use with steroid combinations after uncomplicated removal of a foreign body from the cornea. Ophthalmic use in deep-seated ophthalmic infections or in those likely to become systemic infections.

Precautions: Safe use during pregnancy has not been established.

Route/Dosage ───────────

• **IV**
   Infections.
Adults and children: 15,000 25,000 units/kg/day (maximum) in divided doses q 12 hr. **Infants,** up to 40,000 units/kg/day.

• **IM**
Not usually recommended due to pain at injection site.
   Infections.
Adults and children: 25,000–30,000 units/kg/day in divided doses q 4–6 hr. **Infants,** up to 40,000 units/kg/day.
Both IV and IM doses should be reduced in renal impairment.

• **Intrathecal**
   Meningitis.
Adults and children over 2 years: 50,000 units/day for 3–4 days; **then,** 50,000 units every other day until 2 weeks after cultures are negative; **children under 2 years,** 20,000 units/day for 3–4 days or 25,000 units once every other day; dosage of 25,000 units should be continued every other day for 2 weeks after cultures are negative.

• **Ophthalmic Solution**
1–2 gtt 2–6 times/day, depending on the infection. Treatment may be necessary for 1–2 months or longer.

How Supplied: *Powder for injection:* 500,000 U

Side Effects: *Nephrotoxic:* Albuminuria, cylindruria, azotemia, hematuria, proteinuria, leukocyturia, electrolyte loss. *Neurologic:* Dizziness, flushing of face, mental confusion, irritability, nystagmus, muscle weakness, drowsiness, paresthesias, blurred vision, slurred speech, ataxia, ***coma, seizures. Neuromuscular blockade may lead to respiratory paralysis.*** *GI:* N&V, diarrhea, abdominal cramps. *Miscellaneous:* Fever, urticaria, skin exanthemata, eosinophilia, ***anaphylaxis.***

Following intrathecal use: Meningeal irritation with fever, stiff neck, headache, increase in leukocytes and protein in the CSF. Nerve-root irritation may result in neuritic pain and urine retention. *Following IM use:* Irritation, severe pain. *Following IV use:* Thrombophlebitis. *Following ophthalmic use:* Burning, stinging, irritation, inflammation, angioneurotic edema, itching, urticaria, vesicular and maculopapular dermatitis.

Drug Interactions
Aminoglycoside antibiotics / Additive nephrotoxic effects
Cephalosporins / ↑ Risk of renal toxicity
Phenothiazines / ↑ Risk of respiratory depression
Skeletal muscle relaxants (surgical) / Additive muscle relaxation

EMS CONSIDERATIONS
See also *Anti-Infectives.*

Potassium Salts:
Potassium acetate, parenteral
Potassium acetate, bicarbonate, and citrate, (Trikates)
Potassium bicarbonate

P

Potassium bicarbonate and Citric acid
Potassium bicarbonate and Potassium chloride
Potassium bicarbonate and Potassium citrate
Potassium chloride
Potassium chloride, Potassium bicarbonate, and Potassium citrate
Potassium gluconate
Potassium gluconate and Potassium chloride
Potassium gluconate and Potassium citrate

Pregnancy Class: C
Potassium Salts Potassium acetate, parenteral **(Rx)** Potassium acetate, Potassium bicarbonate, and Potassium citrate (Trikates): **Oral solution:** Tri-K **(Rx)** Potassium bicarbonate: K + Care ET **(Rx)** Potassium bicarbonate and Citric acid: **Effervescent Tablets:** K+ Care ET Potassium bicarbonate and Potassium chloride: **Effervescent Granules (Rx); Effervescent Tablets:** Klorvess, K-Lyte/Cl, K-Lyte/Cl 50 **(Rx)** Potassium bicarbonate and Potassium citrate: **Effervescent Tablets:** Effer-K, Effervescent Potassium, K-Lyte **(Rx)** Potassium chloride: **Extended-Release Capsules:** K-Lease, K-Norm, Micro-K Extencaps, Micro-K 10 Extencaps **(Rx). Injection:** Potassium Chloride for Injection Concentrate **(Rx). Oral Solution:** Cena-K 10% and 20%, Kaochlor 10% Liquid, Potasalan, Rum-K **(Rx). Powder for Oral Solution:** Gen-K, Kay Ciel, K+ Care, K-Lor, Klor-Con Powder, Micro-K LS **(Rx). Extended-Release Tablets:** K+ 10, Kaon-Cl, Kaon-Cl-10, K-Dur 10 and 20, Klor-Con 8 and 10, Klotrix, K-Tab, Slow-K, Ten-K **(Rx)** Potassium Chloride, Potassium bicarbonate, and Potassium citrate: **Effervescent Granules:** Klorvess Effervescent Granules **(Rx)** Potassium gluconate: **Elixir:** Kaon, Kaylixir, K-G Elixir **(Rx)** Potassium gluconate and Potassium chloride: **Oral Solution and Powder for Oral Solution:** Kolyum **(Rx)**

Potassium gluconate and Potassium citrate: **Oral Solution:** Twin-K **(Rx)**
Classification: Electrolyte

Mechanism of Action
Though a number of salts can be used to supply the potassium cation, potassium chloride is the agent of choice since hypochloremia frequently accompanies potassium deficiency. Dietary measures can often prevent and even correct potassium deficiencies. Potassium-rich foods include most meats (beef, chicken, ham, turkey, veal), fish, beans, broccoli, brussels sprouts, lentils, spinach, potatoes, milk, bananas, dates, prunes, raisins, avocados, watermelon, cantaloupe, apricots, and molasses.

Uses: PO: Treat hypokalemia due to digitalis intoxication, diabetic acidosis, diarrhea and vomiting, familial periodic paralysis, certain cases of uremia, hyperadrenalism, starvation and debilitation, and corticosteroid or diuretic therapy. Also, hypokalemia with or without metabolic acidosis and following surgical conditions accompanied by nitrogen loss, vomiting and diarrhea, suction drainage, and increased urinary excretion of potassium. Prophylaxis of potassium depletion when dietary intake is not adequate in the following conditions: patients on digitalis and diuretics for CHF, hepatic cirrhosis with ascites, excess aldosterone with normal renal function, significant cardiac arrhythmias, potassium-losing nephropathy, and certain states accompanied by diarrhea. *Investigational:* Mild hypertension.

NOTE: Use potassium chloride when hypokalemia is associated with alkalosis; potassium bicarbonate, citrate, acetate, or gluconate should be used when hypokalemia is associated with acidosis.

IV: Prophylaxis and treatment of moderate to severe potassium loss when PO therapy is not feasible. Potassium acetate is used as an additive for preparing specific IV formulas when patient needs cannot be met by usual nutrient or electrolyte preparations. Potassium acetate is also used in the following conditions: marked loss of GI secretions due to vomiting, diarrhea, GI intubation, or fistulas; prolonged parenteral use of potassium-free fluids (e.g., dextrose or NSS); diabetic acidosis, especially during treatment with insulin and dextrose infusions; prolonged diuresis; metabolic alkalosis; hyperadrenocorticism; primary aldosteronism; overdose of adrenocortical steroids, testosterone, or corticotropin; attacks of hereditary or familial periodic paralysis; during the healing phase of burns or scalds; and cardiac arrhythmias, especially due to digitalis glycosides.

Contraindications: Severe renal function impairment with azotemia or oliguria, postoperatively before urine flow has been reestablished. Crush syndrome, Addison's disease, hyperkalemia from any cause, anuria, heat cramps, acute dehydration, severe hemolytic reactions, adynamia episodica hereditaria, patients receiving potassium-sparing diuretics or aldosterone-inhibiting drugs. Solid dosage forms in patients in whom there is a reason for delay or arrest in passage of tablets through the GI tract.

Precautions: Safety during lactation and in children has not been established. Geriatric patients are at greater risk of developing hyperkalemia due to age-related changes in renal function. Administer with caution in the presence of cardiac and renal disease. Potassium loss is often accompanied by an obligatory loss of chloride resulting in hypochloremic metabolic alkalosis; thus, the underlying cause of the potassium loss should be treated.

Route/Dosage —————

Highly individualized. Oral administration is preferred because the slow absorption from the GI tract prevents sudden, large increases in plasma potassium levels. Dosage is usually expressed as mEq/L of potassium. The bicarbonate, chloride,

citrate, and gluconate salts are usually administered PO. The chloride, acetate, and phosphate may be administered by **slow IV** infusion.

• **IV Infusion**
  Serum K less than 2.0 mEq/L.
400 mEq/day at a rate not to exceed 40 mEq/hr. Use a maximum concentration of 80 mEq/L.
  Serum K more than 2.5 mEq/L.
200 mEq/day at a rate not to exceed 20 mEq/hr. Use a maximum concentration of 40 mEq/L.
  Pediatric: Up to 3 mEq potassium/kg (or 40 mEq/m^2) daily. Adjust the volume administered depending on the body size.

• **Effervescent Granules, Effervescent Tablets, Elixir, Extended-Release Capsules, Extended Release Granules, Extended-Release Tablets, Oral Solution, Powder for Oral Solution, Tablets**
  Prophylaxis of hypokalemia.
16–24 mEq/day.
  Potassium depletion.
40–100 mEq/day.
  NOTE: Usual dietary intake of potassium is 40–250 mEq/day.

For patients with accompanying metabolic acidosis, use an alkalizing potassium salt (potassium bicarbonate, potassium citrate, or potassium acetate).

How Supplied: Potassium acetate, parenteral: *Injection:* 2 mEq/mL, 4 mEq/mL; Potassium acetate, potassium bicarbonate, and potassium citrate: *Liquid:* 45 mEq/15 mL; Potassium bicarbonate: *Tablet, effervescent:* 25 mEq, 650 mg; Potassium bicarbonate and potassium citrate: *Tablet, effervescent:* 25 mEq; Potassium bicarbonate and potassium chloride: *Granule for reconstitution:* 20 mEq; *Tablet, effervescent:* 25 mEq, 50 mEq; Potassium chloride: *Capsule, extended release:* 8 mEq, 10 mEq; *Injection:* 1.5 mEq/mL, 2 mEq/mL, 10 mEq/50 mL, 10 mEq/100 mL, 20 mEq/50 mL, 20 mEq/100 mL, 30 mEq/100 mL, 40 mEq/100 mL, 100 mEq/L, 200 mEq/L; *Liquid:* 20 mEq/15 mL, 30 mEq/15 mL, 40 mEq/15 mL; *Powder*

P

for reconstitution: 20 mEq, 25 mEq, 200 mEq; *Tablet:* 180 mg; *Tablet, extended release:* 8 mEq, 10 mEq, 20 mEq; Potassium gluconate: *Elixir:* 20 mEq/15 mL; *Tablet:* 486 mg, 500 mg, 550 mg, 595 mg, 610 mg, 620 mg; *Tablet, extended release:* 595 mg; Potassium gluconate and potassium citrate: *Liquid:* 20 mEq/15 mL

Side Effects: Hypokalemia. *CNS:* Dizziness, mental confusion. *CV:* Arrhythmias; weak, irregular pulse; hypotension, *heart block,* ECG abnormalities, *cardiac arrest.* *GI:* Abdominal distention, anorexia, N&V, *Neuromuscular:* Weakness, paresthesia of extremities, flaccid paralysis, areflexia, muscle or *respiratory paralysis,* weakness and heaviness of legs. *Other:* Malaise.

Hyperkalemia. *CV:* Bradycardia, then tachycardia, *cardiac arrest.* *GI:* N&V, diarrhea, abdominal cramps, GI bleeding or obstruction. Ulceration or perforation of the small bowel from enteric-coated potassium chloride tablets. *GU:* Oliguria, anuria. *Neuromuscular:* Weakness, tingling, paralysis. *Other:* Skin rashes, hyperkalemia.

Effects due to solution or IV technique used. Fever, infection at injection site, venous thrombosis, phlebitis extending from injection site, extravasation, venospasm, hypervolemia, hyperkalemia.

OD **Overdose Management:** *Symptoms:* Mild (5.5–6.5 mEq/L) to moderate (6.5–8 mEq/L) hyperkalemia (may be asymptomatic except for ECG changes). ECG changes include progression in height and peak of T waves, lowering of the R wave, decreased amplitude and eventually disappearance of P waves, prolonged PR interval and QRS complex, shortening of the QT interval, *ventricular fibrillation, death. Muscle weakness that may progress to flaccid quadriplegia and respiratory failure,* although dangerous cardiac arrhythmias usually occur before onset of complete paralysis. *Treatment (plasma potassium levels greater than 6.5 mEq/L):* All measures must be monitored by ECG. Measures consist of actions taken to shift potassium ions from plasma into cells by:

• **Sodium bicarbonate:** IV infusion of 50–100 mEq over period of 5 min. May be repeated after 10–15 minutes if ECG abnormalities persist.
• **Glucose and insulin:** IV infusion of 3 g glucose to 1 unit regular insulin to shift potassium into cells.
• **Calcium gluconate—or other calcium salt** (only for patients not on digitalis or other cardiotonic glycosides): IV infusion of 0.5–1 g (5–10 mL of a 10% solution) over period of 2 min. Dosage may be repeated after 1–2 min if ECG remains abnormal. When ECG is approximately normal, the excess potassium should be removed from the body by administration of polystyrene sulfonate, hemodialysis or peritoneal dialysis (patients with renal insufficiency), or other means.
• **Sodium polystyrene sulfonate, hemodialysis, peritoneal dialysis:** To remove potassium from the body.

Drug Interactions
ACE inhibitors / May cause potassium retention → hyperkalemia
Digitalis glycosides / Cardiac arrhythmias
Potassium-sparing diuretics / Severe hyperkalemia with possibility of cardiac arrhythmias or arrest

EMS CONSIDERATIONS
Administration/Storage
IV 1. Do not administer potassium IV undiluted. Usual method is to administer by slow IV infusion in dextrose solution at a concentration of 40–80 mEq/L and at a rate not to exceed 10–20 mEq/hr.
2. Check site of administration frequently for pain and redness because drug is extremely irritating.
Interventions
1. Complaints of weakness, fatigue, or the presence of cardiac arrhythmias may be symptoms of hypokalemia indicating a low *intracellular* potassium level, although the level may appear to be within normal limits.
2. Report complaints of weakness or heaviness of the legs, the presence of a gray pallor, cold skin, listlessness, mental confusion, flaccid

paralysis, hypotension, or cardiac arrhythmias (S&S of hyperkalemia).

Pramipexole
(prah-mih-PEX-ohl)
Pregnancy Class: C
Mirapex **(Rx)**
Classification: Antiparkinson drug

Mechanism of Action: Thought to act by stimulating dopamine (especially D₃) receptors in striatum.

D_3

Uses: Idiopathic Parkinson's disease.
Contraindications: Lactation.
Precautions: Safety and efficacy have not been determined in children.

Route/Dosage
• **Tablets**
  Parkinsonism.
Initial: Start with 0.125 mg t.i.d.; **then,** increase dose by 0.125 mg t.i.d. weekly for seven weeks (i.e., dose at week seven is 1.5 mg t.i.d.). **Maintenance:** 1.5–4.5 mg/day in equally divided doses t.i.d. with or without comcomitant levodopa (about 800 mg/day). Impaired renal function, C_{CR}, over 60 mL/min: Start with 0.125 mg t.i.d., up to maximum of 1.5 mg t.i.d. C_{CR}, 25–59 mL/min: Start with 0.125 mg b.i.d., up to maximum of 1.5 mg b.i.d. C_{CR}, 15–24 mL/min: Start with 0.125 mg once daily, up to maximum of 1.5 mg once daily.
How Supplied: *Tablets:* 0.125 mg, 0.25 mg, 0.5 mg, 1 mg, 1.5 mg
Side Effects: *CNS:* Hallucinations (especially in elderly), dizziness, somnolence, insomnia, confusion, amnesia, hypesthesia, dystonia, akathisia, abnormal thinking, decreased libido, myoclonus. *CV:* Orthostatic hypotension. *Body as a whole:* Asthenia, general edema, malaise, fever. *GI:* Nausea, constipation, anorexia, dysphagia. *Miscellaneous:* Vision abnormalities, impotence, peripheral edema, decreased weight.
Drug Interactions
Butyrophenones / Possible ↓ effect of pramipexole

Cimetidine / ↑ Levodopa levels and half-life
CNS Depressants / Additive CNS depression
Levodopa / ↑ Levodopa levels; also, may cause or worsen pre-existing dyskinesia
Metoclopramide / Possible ↓ effect of pramipexole
Phenothiazines / Possible ↓ effect of pramipexole
Thioxanthines / Possible ↓ effect of pramipexole

EMS CONSIDERATIONS
None.

Pravastatin sodium
(prah-vah-STAH-tin)
Pregnancy Class: X
Pravachol **(Rx)**
Classification: Antihyperlipidemic agent

Mechanism of Action: Competitively inhibits HMG-CoA reductase, the enzyme catalyzing the conversion of HMG-CoA to mevalonate in the biosynthesis of cholesterol. This results in an increased number of LDL receptors on cell surfaces and enhanced receptor-mediated catabolism and clearance of circulating LDL. Also inhibits LDL production by inhibiting hepatic synthesis of VLDL, the precursor of LDL. Elevated levels of total cholesterol, dLDL cholesterol, and apolipoprotein B (a membrane transport complex for LDL) promote development of atherosclerosis and are lowered by pravastatin. Drug increases survival in heart transplant recipients.
Uses: Adjunct to diet for reducing elevated total and LDL cholesterol levels in patients with primary hypercholesterolemia (type IIa and IIb) and mixed dyslipidemia when the response to a diet with restricted saturated fat and cholesterol has not been effective. Reduce the risk of heart attack with and without established CHD and slow progression of coronary atherosclerosis in those

P

with hypercholesterolemia and heart disease. To reduce the risk of stroke or TIA. *Investigational:* To lower cholesterol levels in those with heterozygous familial hypercholesterolemia, familial combined hyperlipidemia, diabetic dyslipidemia in non-insulin-dependent diabetics, hypercholesterolemia secondary to nephrotic syndrome, homozygous familial hypercholesterolemia in those not completely devoid of LDL receptors but who have a decreased level of LDL receptor activity.

Contraindications: To treat hypercholesterolemia due to hyperalphaproteinemia. Active liver disease; unexplained, persistent elevations in LFTs. Use during pregnancy and lactation and in children less than 18 years of age.

Precautions: Use with caution in patients with a history of liver disease, renal insufficiency, or heavy alcohol use.

Route/Dosage
• **Tablets**
Initial: 10–20 mg once daily at bedtime (geriatric patients should take 10 mg once daily at bedtime). **Maintenance dose:** 10–40 mg once daily at bedtime (maximum dose for geriatric patients is 20 mg/day). Use a starting dose of 10 mg/day at bedtime in renal/hepatic dysfunction and in the elderly.

How Supplied: *Tablet:* 10 mg, 20 mg, 40 mg

Side Effects: *Musculoskeletal:* Rhabdomyolysis with renal dysfunction secondary to myoglobinuria, myalgia, myopathy, arthralgias, localized pain, muscle cramps, leg cramps, bursitis, tenosynovitis, myasthenia, tendinous contracture, myositis. *CNS:* CNS vascular lesions characterized by **perivascular hemorrhage,** edema, and mononuclear cell infiltration of perivascular spaces; headache, dizziness, psychic disturbances. Dizziness, vertigo, memory loss, anxiety, insomnia, somnolence, abnormal dreams, emotional lability, incoordination, hyperkinesia, torticollis, psychic disturbances. *GI:* N&V, diarrhea, abdominal pain, cramps, constipation, flatulence, heartburn, anorexia, gastroenteritis, dry mouth, rectal hemorrhage, esophagitis, eructation, glossitis, mouth ulceration, increased appetite, stomatitis, cheilitis, duodenal ulcer, dysphagia, enteritis, melena, gum hemorrhage, stomach ulcer, tenesmus, ulcerative stomach. *CV:* Palpitation, vasodilation, syncope, migraine, postural hypotension, phlebitis, arrhythmia. *Hepatic:* Hepatitis (including chronic active hepatitis), fatty change in liver, cirrhosis, **fulminant hepatic necrosis, hepatoma,** pancreatitis, cholestatic jaundice, biliary pain. *GU:* Gynecomastia, erectile dysfunction, loss of libido, cystitis, hematuria, impotence, dysuria, kidney calculus, nocturia, epididymitis, fibrocystic breast, albuminuria, breast enlargement, nephritis, urinary frequency, incontinence, retention and urgency, abnormal ejaculation, vaginal or uterine hemorrhage, metrorrhagia, UTI. *Ophthalmic:* Progression of cataracts, lens opacities, ophthalmoplegia. *Hypersensitivity reaction:* Vasculitis, purpura, polymyalgia rheumatica, **angioedema,** lupus erythematosus–like syndrome, thrombocytopenia, **hemolytic anemia,** leukopenia, positive ANA, arthritis, arthralgia, urticaria, asthenia, ESR increase, fever, chills, photosensitivity, malaise, dyspnea, **toxic epidermal necrolysis, Stevens-Johnson syndrome.** *Dermatologic:* Alopecia, pruritus, rash, skin nodules, discoloration of skin, dryness of skin and mucous membranes, changes in hair and nails, contact dermatitis, sweating, acne, urticaria, eczema, seborrhea, skin ulcer. *Neurologic:* Dysfunction of certain cranial nerves resulting in alteration of taste, impairment of extraocular movement, and facial paresis; paresthesia, peripheral neuropathy, tremor, vertigo, memory loss peripheral nerve palsy. *Respiratory:* Common cold, rhinitis, cough. *Hematologic:* Anemia, transient asymptomatic eosinophilia, thrombocytopenia, leukopenia, ecchymosis, lymphadenopathy, petechiae. *Miscellaneous:* Cardiac chest pain, fatigue, influenza.

Drug Interactions
Bile acid sequestrants / ↓ Bioavailability of pravastatin
Clofibrate / ↑ Risk of myopathy
Cyclosporine / ↑ Risk of myopathy or rhabdomyolysis
Erythromycin / ↑ Risk of myopathy or rhabdomyolysis
Gemfibrozil / ↑ Risk of myopathy or rhabdomyolysis
Niacin / ↑ Risk of myopathy or rhabdomyolysis
Warfarin / ↑ Anticoagulant effect of warfarin

EMS CONSIDERATIONS
None.

Praziquantel
(pray-zih-KWON-tell)
Pregnancy Class: B
Biltricide **(Rx)**
Classification: Anthelmintic

Mechanism of Action: Causes increased cell permeability in the helminth, resulting in a loss of intracellular calcium with massive contractions, and paralysis of musculature with breakdown of the integrity of the organism. Also causes vacuolization and disintegration of phagocytes to the parasite, resulting in death.
Uses: Schistosomal infections due to *Schistosoma japonicum, S. mansoni, S. mekongi,* and *S. hematobium.* Liver flukes (*Clonorchis sinensis, Opisthorchis viverrini*). *Investigational:* Neurocysticercosis, other tissue flukes, and intestinal cestodes. Low doses of oxamniquine and praziquantel as a single-dose treatment of schistosomiasis.
Contraindications: Ocular cysticercosis. Lactation.
Precautions: Safety in children less than 4 years of age not established.

Route/Dosage
• **Tablets**
Schistosomiasis.
Three doses of 20 mg/kg as a 1-day treatment with an interval between doses not less than 4 hr or more than 6 hr.

Chonorchiasis and opisthorchiasis.
Three doses of 25 mg/kg as a 1-day treatment with an interval between doses not less than 4 hr or more than 6 hr.
How Supplied: *Tablet:* 600 mg
Side Effects: *GI:* Nausea, abdominal discomfort. *CNS:* Malaise, headache, dizziness, drowsiness. *Miscellaneous:* Fever, urticaria (rare). *NOTE:* These side effects may also be due to the helminth infection itself.
OD Overdose Management: *Symptoms:* Extension of side effects. *Treatment:* Administer a fast-acting laxative.
Drug Interactions: Hydantoins may decrease serum praziquantel levels, resulting in ineffective treatment.

EMS CONSIDERATIONS
None.

Prazossin hydrochloride
(PRAY-zoh-sin)
Pregnancy Class: C
Minipress **(Rx)**
Classification: Antihypertensive, alpha-1-adrenergic blocking agent

Mechanism of Action: Produces selective blockade of postsynaptic alpha-1-adrenergic receptors. Dilates arterioles and veins, thereby decreasing total peripheral resistance and decreasing DBP more than SBP. CO, HR, and renal blood flow are not affected. Can be used to initiate antihypertensive therapy; most effective when used with other agents (e.g., diuretics, beta-adrenergic blocking agents).
Onset of Action: 2 hr; **Maximum effect:** 2-3 hr.
Duration of Action: 6-12 hr. Full therapeutic effect: 4-6 weeks.
Uses: Mild to moderate hypertension alone or in combination with other antihypertensive drugs. *Investigational:* CHF refractory to other treatment. Raynaud's disease, BPH.
Precautions: Safe use in children has not been established. Use with caution during lactation. Geriatric

bold italic = life threatening side effect

patients may be more sensitive to the hypotensive and hypothermic effects; may be necessary to decrease the dose in these patients due to age-related decreases in renal function.

Route/Dosage ————————
• **Capsules**
  Hypertension.
Individualized: Initial, 1 mg b.i.d.–t.i.d.; **maintenance:** if necessary, increase gradually to 6–15 mg/day in two to three divided doses. Do not exceed 20 mg/day, although some patients have benefitted from doses of 40 mg daily. If used with diuretics or other antihypertensives, reduce dose to 1–2 mg t.i.d. **Pediatric, less than 7 years of age, initial:** 0.25 mg b.i.d.–t.i.d. adjusted according to response. **Pediatric, 7–12 years of age, initial:** 0.5 mg b.i.d.–t.i.d. adjusted according to response.
How Supplied: *Capsule:* 1 mg, 2 mg, 5 mg

Side Effects: First-dose effect: *Marked hypotension* and syncope 30–90 min after administration of initial dose (usually 2 or more mg), increase of dosage, or addition of other antihypertensive agent. *CNS:* Dizziness, drowsiness, headache, fatigue, paresthesias, depression, vertigo, nervousness, hallucinations. *CV:* Palpitations, syncope, tachycardia, orthostatic hypotension, aggravation of angina. *GI:* N&V, diarrhea or constipation, dry mouth, abdominal pain, pancreatitis. *GU:* Urinary frequency or incontinence, impotence, priapism. *Respiratory:* Dyspnea, nasal congestion, epistaxis. *Dermatologic:* Pruritus, rash, sweating, alopecia, lichen planus. *Miscellaneous:* Asthenia, edema, symptoms of lupus erythematosus, blurred vision, tinnitus, arthralgia, myalgia, reddening of sclera, eye pain, conjunctivitis, edema, fever.
OD Overdose Management: *Symptoms:* Hypotension, **shock.** *Treatment:* Keep patient supine to restore BP and HR. If shock is manifested, use volume expanders and vasopressors; maintain renal function.

Drug Interactions
Antihypertensives (other) / ↑ Antihypertensive effect
Beta-adrenergic blocking agents / Enhanced acute postural hypotension following the first dose of prazosin
Clonidine / ↓ Antihypertensive effect of clonidine
Diuretics / ↑ Antihypertensive effect
Indomethacin / ↓ Effect of prazosin
Nifedipine / ↑ Hypotensive effect
Propranolol / Especially pronounced additive hypotensive effect
Verapamil / ↑ Hypotensive effect; ↑ sensitivity to prazosin-induced postural hypotension

EMS CONSIDERATIONS

See also *Alpha-1-Adrenergic Blocking Agents* and *Antihypertensive Agents.*

Prednisolone
Prednisolone acetate
Prednisolone acetate and Prednisolone sodium phosphate
Prednisolone sodium phosphate
Prednisolone tebutate
(pred-NISS-oh-lohn)
Pregnancy Class: C
Prednisolone: **Syrup:** Prelone, **Tablets:** Delta-Cortef **(Rx)** Prednisolone acetate: **Parenteral:** Articulose-50, Key-Pred 25 and 50, Predalone 50, **Ophthalmic Suspension:** Econopred, Econopred Plus, Pred Forte Ophthalmic, Pred Mild Ophthalmic **(Rx)** Prednisolone acetate and Prednisolone sodium phosphate: **(Rx)** Prednisolone sodium phosphate: **Oral Solution:** Prediapred **(Rx)**, **Ophthalmic Solution:** AK-Pred Ophthalmic, Inflamase Forte Ophthalmic, Inflamase Mild Ophthalmic **(Rx)**. **Parenteral:** Hydeltrasol, Key-Pred-SP **(Rx)** Prednisolone tebutate: Hydeltra-T.B.A., Prednisol TPA **(Rx)** **Classification:** Corticosteroid, synthetic

Mechanism of Action: Intermediate-acting. Is five times more potent than hydrocortisone and cortisone. Minimal side effects except for GI distress. Moderate mineralocorticoid activity.

Contraindications: Lactation.

Precautions: Use with particular caution in diabetes.

Route/Dosage ───────────

PREDNISOLONE

• **Tablets, Syrup**

Most uses.

5–60 mg/day, depending on disease being treated.

Multiple sclerosis (exacerbation).

200 mg/day for 1 week; **then,** 80 mg on alternate days for 1 month.

Pleurisy of tuberculosis.

0.75 mg/kg/day (then taper) given concurrently with antituberculosis therapy.

PREDNISOLONE ACETATE

• **IM**

4–60 mg/day. **Not for IV use.**

Multiple sclerosis (exacerbation).

See *Prednisolone.*

• **Intralesional, Intra-articular, Soft Tissue Injection**

4–100 mg (larger doses for large joints).

• **Ophthalmic Suspension (0.12%, 0.125%, 1%)**

Instill 1–2 gtt into the conjunctival sac b.i.d.–q.i.d. During the first 24 to 48 hr, the frequency of dosing may be increased if necessary.

PREDNISOLONE ACETATE AND PREDNISOLONE SODIUM PHOSPHATE

• **IM Only**

20–80 mg acetate and 5–20 mg sodium phosphate every few days for 3–4 weeks.

• **Intra-articular, Intrasynovial**

20–40 mg prednisolone acetate and 5–10 mg prednisolone sodium phosphate.

PREDNISOLONE SODIUM PHOSPHATE

• **PO Solution**

Most uses.

5–60 mg/day in single or divided doses.

Adrenocortical insufficiency.

Pediatric: 0.14 mg/kg (4 mg/m²) daily in three to four divided doses.

Other pediatric uses.

0.5–2 mg/kg (15–60 mg/m²) daily in three to four divided doses.

• **IM, IV**

4–60 mg/day.

Multiple sclerosis (exacerbation).

See *Prednisolone.*

• **Intralesional, Intra-articular, Soft Tissue Injection**

2–30 mg, depending on site and severity of disease.

• **Ophthalmic Solution (0.125%, 1%)**

1–2 gtt into the conjunctival sac q hr during the day and q 2 hr during the night; **then,** after response obtained, decrease dose to 1 gtt/ q 4 hr and then later 1 gtt t.i.d.–q.i.d.

PREDNISOLONE TEBUTATE

• **Intra-articular, Intralesional, Soft Tissue Injection**

4–30 mg, depending on site and severity of disease. Doses higher than 40 mg are not recommended.

How Supplied: Prednisolone: *Syrup:* 5 mg/5 mL, 15 mg/5 mL; *Tablet:* 5 mg. Prednisolone acetate: *Injection:* 25 mg/mL, 50 mg/mL; *Ophthalmic Suspension:* 0.12%, 0.125%, 1%. Prednisolone sodium phosphate: *Liquid:* 5 mg/5 mL; *Ophthalmic Solution:* 0.125%, 1%. Prednisolone tebutate: *Injection:* 20 mg/mL.

EMS CONSIDERATIONS

See also *Corticosteroids.*

Prednisone
(PRED-nih-sohn)

Pregnancy Class: C

Oral Solution: Prednisone Intensol Concentrate **(Rx). Syrup:** Liquid Pred **(Rx). Tablets:** Deltasone, Meticorten, Orasone 1, 5, 10, 20, and 50, Panasol-S, Sterapred DS **(Rx)**

Classification: Corticosteroid, synthetic

Mechanism of Action: Three to five times as potent as cortisone or hydrocortisone. May cause moderate fluid retention.

─────────────────────────

bold italic = life threatening side effect

Precautions: Dose must be highly individualized.

Route/Dosage ————————
• **Oral Concentrate, Syrup, Tablets**
   Acute, severe conditions.
Initial: 5–60 mg/day in four equally divided doses after meals and at bedtime. Decrease gradually by 5–10 mg q 4–5 days to establish minimum maintenance dosage (5–10 mg) or discontinue altogether until symptoms recur.
   Replacement.
Pediatric: 0.1–0.15 mg/kg/day.
   COPD.
30–60 mg/day for 1–2 weeks; then taper.
   Ophthalmopathy due to Graves' disease.
60 mg/day; **then,** taper to 20 mg/day.
   Duchenne's muscular dystrophy.
0.75–1.5 mg/kg/day (used to improve strength).
How Supplied: *Concentrate:* 5 mg/mL; *Solution:* 5 mg/5 mL; *Syrup:* 5 mg/5 mL; *Tablet:* 1 mg, 2.5 mg, 5 mg, 10 mg, 20 mg, 50 mg

EMS CONSIDERATIONS

See also *Corticosteroids.*

Primaquine phosphate
(PRIM-ah-kwin)
Pregnancy Class: C
(Rx)
Classification: 8-Aminoquinoline, antimalarial

Mechanism of Action: Mechanism of action not known, but the drug binds to and may alter the properties of DNA leading to decreased protein synthesis. Both the gametocyte and exoerythrocyte forms are inhibited. Some gametocytes are destroyed while others cannot undergo maturation division in the gut of the mosquito.

Uses: Only for the radical cure of *Plasmodium vivax* malaria, the prophylaxis of relapse in *P. vivax* malaria, or following the termination of chloroquine phosphate suppressive

therapy in areas where *P. vivax* is endemic.

Contraindications: Concomitant use with quinacrine. In patients with rheumatoid arthritis or lupus erythematosus who are acutely ill or who have a tendency to develop granulocytopenia. Concomitant use with other bone marrow depressants or hemolytic drugs.

Precautions: Use during pregnancy only when benefits outweigh risks.

Route/Dosage ————————
• **Tablets**
   Acute attack of vivax malaria, patients with parasitized RBCs.
15 mg (base) daily for 14 days together with chloroquine phosphate (to destroy erythrocytic parasites).
   Suppression of malaria.
Adults: 26.3 mg (15 mg base) daily for 14 days or 78.9 mg once a week for 8 weeks; **children:** 0.5 mg/kg/day (0.3 mg/kg base) for 14 days.
How Supplied: *Tablet:* 26.3 mg

Side Effects: *GI:* Abdominal cramps, epigastric distress, N&V. *Hematologic:* Leukopenia. Methemoglobinemia in NADH methemoglobin reductase deficient individuals. Blacks and members of certain Mediterranean ethnic groups (Sardinians, Sephardic Jews, Greeks, Iranians) manifest a high incidence of G6PD deficiency and as a result have a low tolerance for primaquine. These individuals manifest *marked hemolytic anemia* following primaquine administration. *Miscellaneous:* Headache, pruritus, interference with visual accommodation, *cardiac arrhythmias,* hypertension.

OD **Overdose Management:** *Symptoms:* Abdominal cramps, vomiting, burning and epigastric distress, cyanosis, methemoglobinemia, anemia, moderate leukocytosis or leukopenia, CNS and CV disturbances. Granulocytopenia and *acute hemolytic anemia* in sensitive patients. *Treatment:* Treat symptoms.

Drug Interactions
Bone marrow depressants, hemolytic drugs / Additive side effects
Quinacrine / Quinacrine interferes with metabolic degradation of prim-

aquine and thus enhances its toxic side reactions. **Do not give primaquine** to patients who are receiving or have received quinacrine within the past 3 months.

EMS CONSIDERATIONS
None.

Primidone
(PRIH-mih-dohn)
Mysoline **(Rx)**
Classification: Anticonvulsant, miscellaneous

Mechanism of Action: Closely related to the barbiturates; however, the anticonvulsant mechanism is unknown. Produces a greater sedative effect than barbiturates when used for seizure treatment. Side effects usually subside with use.
Uses: Alone or with other anticonvulsants to treat psychomotor seizures, focal seizures, or tonic-clonic seizures (including those refractory to barbiturate-hydantoin regimens). *Investigational:* Benign familial tremor.
Contraindications: Porphyria. Hypersensitivity to phenobarbital. Lactation.
Precautions: Safe use during pregnancy has not been determined. Use during lactation may result in drowsiness in the neonate. Children and geriatric patients may react to primidone with restlessness and excitement. Due to differences in bioavailability, brand interchange is not recommended.

Route/Dosage
• **Oral Suspension, Tablets**
Seizures, in patients on no other anticonvulsant medication.
Adults and children over 8 years, initial: Days 1–3, 100–125 mg at bedtime; days 4–6, 100–125 mg b.i.d.; days 7–9, 100–125 mg t.i.d.; **maintenance:** 250 mg t.i.d.–q.i.d. (may be increased to 250 mg 5–6 times/day; not to exceed 500 mg

q.i.d.). **Children under 8 years, initial:** days 1–3, 50 mg at bedtime; days 4–6, 50 mg b.i.d.; days 7–9, 100 mg b.i.d.; **maintenance:** 125 mg b.i.d.–250 mg t.i.d. (10–25 mg/kg in divided doses).
Seizures, in patients receiving other anticonvulsants.
Initial: 100–125 mg at bedtime; **then,** increase to maintenance levels as other drug is slowly withdrawn (transition should take at least 2 weeks).
Benign familial tremor.
750 mg/day.
How Supplied: *Suspension:* 250 mg/5 mL; *Tablet:* 50 mg, 250 mg
Side Effects: *CNS:* Drowsiness, ataxia, vertigo, fatigue, hyperirritability, emotional disturbances, personality disturbances with mood changes and paranoia. *GI:* N&V, anorexia, painful gums. *Hematologic:* Megaloblastic anemia, thrombocytopenia. *Ophthalmologic:* Diplopia, nystagmus. *Miscellaneous:* Impotence, morbilliform and maculopapular skin rashes. Occasionally has caused hyperexcitability, especially in children. ***Postpartum hemorrhage and hemorrhagic disease of the newborn.*** Symptoms of SLE.
Drug Interactions: See also *Barbiturates.*
Acetazolamide / ↓ Effect of primidone due to ↓ levels
Carbamazepine / ↓ Plasma levels of primidone and phenobarbital and ↑ plasma levels of carbamazepine
Hydantoins / ↑ Plasma levels of primidone, phenobarbital, and PEMA
Isoniazid / ↑ Effect of primidone due to ↓ breakdown by liver
Nicotinamide / ↑ Effect of primidone due to ↓ rate of clearance from body
Succinimides / ↓ Plasma levels of primidone and phenobarbital

EMS CONSIDERATIONS
None.

Probenecid
(proh-BEN-ih-sid)
Pregnancy Class: B
Benemid **(Rx)**
Classification: Antigout agent, uricosuric agent

Mechanism of Action: A uricosuric agent that increases the excretion of uric acid by inhibiting the tubular reabsorption of uric acid; this results in a decreased serum level of uric acid. Also inhibits the renal secretion of penicillins and cephalosporins; this effect is often taken advantage of in the treatment of infections because concomitant administration of probenecid will increase plasma levels of antibiotics.
Onset of Action: Time to peak effect, uricosuric: 0.5 hr; **for suppression of penicillin excretion:** 2 hr.
Duration of Action: For inhibition of pencicillin excretion: 8 hr.
Uses: Hyperuricemia in chronic gout and gouty arthritis. Adjunct in therapy with penicillins or cephalosporins to elevate and prolong plasma antibiotic levels.
Contraindications: Hypersensitivity to drug, blood dyscrasias, uric acid, and kidney stones. Use for hyperuricemia in neoplastic disease or its treatment. Use in children less than 2 years of age. Concomitant use of salicylates or use with penicillin in renal impairment.
Precautions: Use with caution in renal disease, porphyria, G6PD deficiency, history of allergy to sulfa drugs, and peptic ulcer.

Route/Dosage ———————————
• **Tablets**
  Gout.
Adults, initial: 250 mg b.i.d. for 1 week. **Maintenance:** 500 mg b.i.d. Dosage may have to be increased further (by 500 mg/day q 4 weeks to maximum of 2 g) until urate excretion is less than 700 mg in 24 hr. Colbenemid, a combination tablet containing colchicine (0.5 mg) and probenecid (500 mg), is available.
  Adjunct to penicillin or cephalosporin therapy.

Adults: 500 mg q.i.d. Dosage is decreased for elderly patients with renal damage. **Pediatric, 2–14 years, initial:** 25 mg/kg (or 700 mg/m^2); **maintenance,** 10 mg/kg q.i.d. (or 300 mg/m^2 q.i.d.). **For children 50 kg or more:** give adult dosage.
  Gonorrhea, uncomplicated.
Adults: 1 g (as a single dose) 30 min before 4.8 million units of penicillin G procaine aqueous; **pediatric, less than 45 kg:** 25 mg/kg (up to a maximum of 1 g) with appropriate antibiotic therapy.
  Neurosyphilis.
Adults: 0.5 g q.i.d. with penicillin G procaine aqueous, 2.4 million units/day IM, both for 10–14 days.
  Pelvic inflammatory disease.
Adults: 1 g (as a single dose) plus cefoxitin, 2 g IM given concurrently.
How Supplied: *Tablet:* 500 mg
Side Effects: *CNS:* Headaches, dizziness. *GI:* Anorexia, N&V, diarrhea, constipation, and abdominal discomfort. *Allergic:* Skin rash, dermatitis, pruritus, drug fever, and rarely **anaphylaxis.** *GU:* Nephrotic syndrome, uric acid stones with or without hematuria, urinary frequency, renal colic or costovertebral pain. *Miscellaneous:* Flushing, **hemolytic anemia (possibly related to G6PD deficiency),** anemia, sore gums, **hepatic necrosis, aplastic anemia.**
  Initially, the drug may increase frequency of acute gout attacks due to mobilization of uric acid.
Drug Interactions
Acyclovir / Probenecid ↓ renal excretion of acyclovir
Allopurinol / Additive effects to ↓ uric acid serum levels
AZT / ↑ Bioavailability of AZT; possible malaise, myalgia, fever
Benzodiazepines / More rapid onset and longer duration of the effects of benzodiazepines
Cephalosporins / ↑ Effect of cephalosporins due to ↓ excretion by kidney
Ciprofloxacin / 50% ↑ in systemic levels of ciprofloxacin
Clofibrate / ↑ Levels of clofibric acid (active) → ↑ effects
Dapsone / ↑ Effect of dapsone

Dyphylline / ↑ Effect of dyphylline due to ↓ excretion by kidney

Methotrexate / ↑ Effect and toxicity of methotrexate due to ↓ excretion by kidney

NSAIDs / ↑ Effect of NSAIDs due to ↓ excretion by kidney

Pantothenic acid / ↑ Effects of pantothenic acid

Penicillamine / ↓ Effect of penicillamine

Penicillins / ↑ Effect of penicillins due to ↓ excretion by kidney

Pyrazinamide / Probenecid inhibits hyperuricemia produced by pyrazinamide

Rifampin / ↑ Effect of rifampin due to ↓ excretion by kidney

Salicylates / Salicylates inhibit uricosuric activity of probenecid

Sulfinpyrazone / ↑ Effect of sulfinpyrazone due to ↓ excretion by kidney

Sulfonamides / ↑ Effect of sulfonamides due to ↓ plasma protein binding

Sulfonylureas, oral / ↑ Action of sulfonylureas → hypoglycemia

Thiopental / ↑ Effect of thiopental

EMS CONSIDERATIONS
None.

Procainamide hydrochloride
(proh-KAYN-ah-myd)
Pregnancy Class: C
Procanbid, Pronestyl, Pronestyl-SR
(Rx)
Classification: Antiarrhythmic, class IA

Mechanism of Action: Produces a direct cardiac effect to prolong the refractory period of the atria and to a lesser extent the bundle of His-Purkinje system and ventricles. Large doses may cause AV block. Some anticholinergic and local anesthetic effects. **Onset of Action: PO:** 30 min; **IV:** 1-5 min; **Time to peak effect, PO:** 90-120 min; **IM:** 15-60 min; **IV:** immediate.

Duration of Action: 3 hr; **t½:** 2.5-4.7 hr.

Uses: Documented ventricular arrhythmias (e.g., sustained ventricular tachycardia) that may be life threatening in patients where benefits of treatment clearly outweigh risks. Antiarrhythmic drugs have not been shown to improve survival in patients with ventricular arrhythmias.

Contraindications: Hypersensitivity to drug, complete AV heart block, lupus erythematosus, torsades de pointes, asymptomatic ventricular premature contractions. Lactation.

Precautions: There is an increased risk of death in those with non-life-threatening arrhythmias. Although used in children, safety and efficacy have not been established. Use with extreme caution in patients for whom a sudden drop in BP could be detrimental, in CHF, acute ischemic heart disease, or cardiomyopathy. Also, use with caution in patients with liver or kidney dysfunction, preexisting bone marrow failure or cytopenia of any type, development of first-degree heart block while on procainamide, myasthenia gravis, and those with bronchial asthma or other respiratory disorders. May cause more hypotension in geriatric patients; also, in this population, the dose may have to be decreased due to age-related decreases in renal function.

Route/Dosage
• **Capsules, Extended-Release Tablets, Tablets**
Adults, initial: 50 mg/kg/day in divided doses q 3 hr. **Usual, 40–50 kg:** 250 mg q 3 hr of standard formulation or 500 mg q 6 hr of sustained-release; **60–70 kg:** 375 mg q 3 hr of standard formulation or 750 mg q 6 hr of sustained-release; **80–90 kg:** 500 mg q 3 hr of standard formulation or 1 g q 6 hr of sustained-release; **over 100 kg:** 625 mg q 3 hr of standard formulation or 1.25 g q 6 hr of sustained-release. **Pediatric:** 15–50 mg/

P

---

bold italic = life threatening side effect

kg/day divided q 3–6 hr (up to a maximum of 4 g/day).

- **Procanbid   Extended-Release Tablets**

Life-threatening arrhythmias.
500 or 1,000 mg b.i.d.

- **IM**

Ventricular arrhythmias.

Adults, initial: 50 mg/kg/day divided into fractional doses of $\frac{1}{8}$–$\frac{1}{4}$ given q 3–6 hr until PO therapy is possible. **Pediatric:** 20–30 mg/kg/day divided q 4–6 hr (up to a maximum of 4 g/day).

Arrhythmias associated with surgery or anesthesia.

Adults: 100–500 mg.

- **IV**

Initial loading infusion: 20 mg/min (for up to 25–30 min). **Maintenance infusion:** 2–6 mg/min. **Pediatric, initial loading dose:** 3–5 mg/kg/dose over 5 min (maximum of 100 mg); **maintenance:** 20–80 mcg/kg/min continuous infusion (maximum of 2 g/day).

How Supplied: *Capsule:* 250 mg, 375 mg, 500 mg; *Injection:* 100 mg/mL, 500 mg/mL; *Tablet:* 250 mg, 375 mg, 500 mg; *Tablet, extended release:* 250 mg, 500 mg, 750 mg, 1000 mg

Side Effects: *Body as a whole:* Lupus erythematosus–like syndrome especially in those on maintenance therapy and who are slow acetylators. Symptoms include arthralgia, pleural or abdominal pain, arthritis, pleural effusion, pericarditis, fever, chills, myalgia, skin lesions, hematologic changes. *CV:* Following IV use: Hypotension, ***ventricular asystole or fibrillation, partial or complete heart block.*** Rarely, second-degree heart block after PO use. *GI:* N&V, diarrhea, anorexia, bitter taste, abdominal pain. *Hematologic:* Thrombocytopenia, ***agranulocytosis,*** neutropenia. ***Rarely, hemolytic anemia.*** *Dermatologic:* Urticaria, pruritus, angioneurotic edema, flushing, maculopapular rash. *CNS:* Depression, dizziness, weakness, giddiness, psychoses, hallucinations. *Other:* Granulomatous hepatitis, weakness, fever, chills.

OD **Overdose Management:** *Symptoms:* Plasma levels of 10–15 mcg/mL are associated with toxic symptoms. Progressive widening of the QRS complex, prolonged QT or PR intervals, lowering of R and T waves, increased AV block, increased ventricular extrasystoles, ***ventricular tachycardia or fibrillation. IV overdose may result in hypotension, CNS depression, tremor, respiratory depression.*** *Treatment:*

- Induce emesis or perform gastric lavage followed by administration of activated charcoal.
- To treat hypotension, give IV fluids and/or a vasopressor (dopamine, phenylephrine, or norepinephrine).
- Infusion of $\frac{1}{6}$ molar sodium lactate IV reduces the cardiotoxic effects.
- Hemodialysis (but not peritoneal dialysis) is effective in reducing serum levels.
- Renal clearance can be enhanced by acidification of the urine and with high flow rates.
- A ventricular pacing electrode can be inserted as a precaution in the event AV block develops.

Drug Interactions

Acetazolamide / ↑ Effect of procainamide due to ↓ excretion by kidney

Anticholinergic agents, atropine / Additive anticholinergic effects

Antihypertensive agents / Additive hypotensive effect

Cholinergic agents / Anticholinergic activity of procainamide antagonizes effect of cholinergic drugs

Cimetidine / ↑ Effect of procainamide due to ↑ bioavailability

Disopyramide / ↑ Risk of enhanced prolongation of conduction or depression of contractility and hypotension

Ethanol / Effect of procainamide may be altered, but because the main metabolite is active as an antiarrhythmic, specific outcome not clear

Kanamycin / Procainamide ↑ muscle relaxation produced by kanamycin

Lidocaine / Additive cardiodepressant effects

Magnesium salts / Procainamide ↑ muscle relaxation produced by magnesium salts

Neomycin / Procainamide ↑ muscle relaxation produced by neomycin

Propranolol / ↑ Serum procainamide levels

Quinidine / ↑ Risk of enhanced prolongation of conduction or depression of contractility and hypotension

Ranitidine / ↑ Effect of procainamide due to ↑ bioavailability

Sodium bicarbonate / ↑ Effect of procainamide due to ↓ excretion by the kidney

Succinylcholine / Procainamide ↑ muscle relaxation produced by succinylcholine

Trimethoprim / ↑ Effect of procainamide due to ↑ serum levels

EMS CONSIDERATIONS

See also *Antiarrhythmic Agents*.
Administration/Storage
IV 1. Reserve IV use for emergency situations.
2. For IV initial therapy, dilute the drug with D5W; give a maximum of 1 g slowly to minimize side effects by one of the following methods:
• Direct injection into a vein or into tubing of an established infusion line at a rate not to exceed 50 mg/min. Dilute either the 100- or 500-mg/mL vials prior to injection to facilitate control of the dosage rate. Doses of 100 mg may be given q 5 min until arrhythmia is suppressed or until 500 mg has been given (then wait 10 or more min before resuming administration).
• Loading infusion containing 20 mg/mL (1 g diluted with 50 mL of D5W) given at a constant rate of 1 mL/min for 25–30 min to deliver 500–600 mg.
3. For IV maintenance infusion, the dose is usually 2–6 mg/min.
4. Discard solutions that are darker than light amber or otherwise colored. Solutions that have turned slightly yellow on standing may be used.

Assessment: Monitor ECG.
Interventions: Place in a supine position during IV infusion and monitor BP. Discontinue if SBP falls 15 mm Hg or more during administration or if increased SA or AV block is noted.

Procarbazine hydrochloride (MIH, N-Methylhydrazine)
(pro-KAR-bah-zeen)
Pregnancy Class: D
Matulane (Abbreviation: PCB) **(Rx)**
Classification: Antineoplastic, miscellaneous

Mechanism of Action: May inhibit synthesis of protein, RNA, and DNA and inhibit transmethylation of methyl groups of methionine into t-RNA. Absences of t-RNA could result in cessation of protein synthesis and subsequently DNA and RNA synthesis. Also, hydrogen peroxide formed during auto-oxidation of the drug may attack protein sulfhydryl groups found in residual protein that is tightly bound to DNA.
Uses: As an adjunct in the treatment of Hodgkin's disease (stage III and stage IV) as part of MOPP (nitrogen mustard, vincristine, procarbazine, prednisone) or ChIVPP (chlorambucil, vinblastine, procarbazine, prednisone) therapies. *Investigational:* Non-Hodgkin's lymphomas, malignant melanoma, primary brain tumors, lung cancer, multiple myeloma, polycythemia vera.
Contraindications: Inadequate bone marrow reserve as shown by bone marrow aspiration (i.e., in patients with leukopenia, thrombocytopenia, or anemia). Lactation. Hypersensitivity to drug.
Precautions: Use with caution in impaired kidney or liver function. Due to the possibility of tremors, convulsions, and coma, close monitoring is necessary when used in children.

P

---

bold italic = life threatening side effect

Route/Dosage
• **Capsules**
When used alone.
Adults: 2–4 mg/kg/day for first week; **then,** 4–6 mg/kg/day until leukocyte count falls below 4,000/mm³ or platelet count falls below 100,000/mm³. If toxic symptoms appear, discontinue drug and resume treatment at rate of 1–2 mg/kg/day; **maintenance:** 1–2 mg/kg/day.
Children, highly individualized: 50 mg/m²/day for first week; then 100 mg/m² (to nearest 50 mg) until maximum response obtained or until leukopenia or thrombocytopenia occurs. When maximum response is reached, maintain the dose at 50 mg/m²/day.
When used in combination with other antineoplastic drugs (e.g., MOPP or ChIVPP therapies).
100 mg/m² for 14 days.
How Supplied: *Capsule:* 50 mg
Side Effects: *GI:* N&V, anorexia, stomatitis, dry mouth, dysphagia, abdominal pain, hematemesis, melena, diarrhea, constipation. *CNS:* Paresthesias, neuropathies, headache, dizziness, depression, apprehension, nervousness, insomnia, nightmares, hallucinations, falling, weakness, fatigue, lethargy, drowsiness, unsteadiness, ataxia, foot drop, decreased reflexes, tremors, confusion, *coma, convulsions. CV:* Hypotension, tachycardia, syncope. *Respiratory:* Pleural effusion, pneumonitis, cough. *Hematologic:* Leukopenia, anemia, thrombocytopenia, pancytopenia, eosinophilia, *hemolytic anemia,* petechiae, purpura, epistaxis, hemoptysis. *GU:* Hematuria, urinary frequency, nocturia. *Dermatologic:* Dermatitis, pruritus, rash, urticaria, herpes, hyperpigmentation, flushing, alopecia. *Ophthalmic:* Retinal hemorrhage, nystagmus, photophobia, diplopia, inability to focus, papilledema. *Hepatic:* Jaundice, hepatic dysfunction. *Miscellaneous:* Gynecomastia in prepubertal and early pubertal boys, pain, myalgia and arthralgia, pyrexia, diaphoresis, chills, intercurrent infections, edema, hoarseness, generalized allergic reactions, hearing loss, slurred speech, second nonlymphoid malignancies (including acute myelocytic leukemia, malignant myelosclerosis) and azoospermia in those treated with procarbazine combined with other chemotherapy or radiation.

OD Overdose Management: *Symptoms:* N&V, diarrhea, enteritis, hypotension, tremors, seizures, coma, hematologic and hepatic toxicity. *Treatment:* Induce vomiting or undertake gastric lavage. IV fluids. Perform trequent blood counts and LFTs.

Drug Interactions
Alcohol / Antabuse-like reaction
Antihistamines / Additive CNS depression
Antihypertensive drugs / Additive CNS depression
Barbiturates / Additive CNS depression
Chemotherapy / Depressed bone marrow activity
Digoxin / ↓ Digoxin plasma levels
Guanethidine / Excitation and hypertension
Hypoglycemic agents, oral / ↑ Hypoglycemic effect
Insulin / ↑ Hypoglycemic effect
Levodopa / Flushing and hypertension within 1 hr of levodopa administration
MAO inhibitors / Possibility of hypertensive crisis
Methyldopa / Excitation and hypertension
Narcotics / Significant CNS depression → possible deep coma and death
Phenothiazines / Additive CNS depression; also, possibility of hypertensive crisis
Reserpine / Excitation and hypertension
Sympathomimetics, indirectly acting / Possibility of hypertensive crisis
Tricyclic antidepressants / Possible toxic and fatal reactions, including excitability, fluctuations in BP, seizures, and coma
Tyramine-containing foods / Possibility of hypertensive crisis

EMS CONSIDERATIONS

None.

Prochlorperazine
Prochlorperazine edisylate
Prochlorperazine maleate

(proh-klor-PAIR-ah-zeen)

Compazine **(Rx)**

Classification: Antipsychotic, antiemetic, piperazine-type phenothiazine

Mechanism of Action: Prochlorperazine causes a high incidence of extrapyramidal and antiemetic effects, moderate sedative effects, and a low incidence of anticholinergic effects and orthostatic hypotension. It also possesses significant antiemetic effects.

Uses: Psychotic disorders. Short-term treatment of generalized nonpsychotic anxiety (not drug of choice). Postoperative N&V, radiation sickness, vomiting due to toxins. Severe N&V. *Investigational:* Acute headache.

Contraindications: Use in patients who weigh less than 44 kg or who are under 2 years of age.

Precautions: Safe use during pregnancy has not been established. Geriatric, emaciated, and debilitated patients usually require a lower initial dose.

Route/Dosage

• **Edisylate Syrup, Maleate Extended-Release Capsules, Tablets**

Psychotic disorders.

Adults and adolescents: 5 or 10 mg t.i.d. or q.i.d. for mild conditions. For severe conditions, for hospitalized, or adequately supervised patients: 10 mg t.i.d. or q.i.d. Dose can be increased gradually q 2–3 days as needed and tolerated. For extended-release capsules, up to 100–150 mg/day can be given. **Pediatric, 2–12 years:** 2.5 mg b.i.d.–t.i.d. Do not give more than 10 mg on the first day.

N&V.

Adults and adolescents: 5–10 mg t.i.d.–q.i.d. (up to 40 mg/day). For extended-release capsules, the dose is 15–30 mg once daily in the morning (or 10 mg q 12 hr, up to 40 mg/day). **Pediatric, 18–39 kg:** 2.5 mg (base) t.i.d. (or 5 mg b.i.d.), not to exceed 15 mg/day; **14–17 kg:** 2.5 mg (base) b.i.d.–t.i.d., not to exceed 10 mg/day; **9–13 kg:** 2.5 mg (base) 1–2 times/day, not to exceed 7.5 mg/day. The total daily dose for children should not exceed 10 mg the first day; on subsequent days, the total daily dose should not exceed 20 mg for children 2–5 years of age or 25 mg for children 6–12 years of age.

Anxiety.

Adults and adolescents: 5 mg t.i.d.–q.i.d. on arising. Or, 15 mg sustained release on arising or 10 mg sustained release q 12 hr. Do not give more than 20 mg/day for more than 12 weeks.

• **IM, Edisylate Injection**

Psychotic disorders, for immediate control of severely disturbed patients.

Adults and adolescents, initial: 10–20 mg; dose can be repeated q 2–4 hr as needed (usually up to three or four doses). If prolonged therapy is needed: 10–20 mg q 4–6 hr. **Children, less than 12 years of age:** 0.03 mg/kg by deep IM injection. After control is achieved (usually after 1 injection), switch to PO at same dosage level or higher.

N&V.

Adults and adolescents: 5–10 mg; repeat the dose q 3–4 hr as needed. **Pediatric, 2–12 years:** 0.132 mg/kg.

N&V during surgery.

Adults and adolescents: 5–10 mg (base) given as a slow injection or infusion 15–30 min before induction of anesthesia; to control symptoms during or after surgery the dose can be repeated once. The rate of infusion should not exceed 5 mg/mL/min.

• **Rectal Suppositories**

Pediatric, 2–12 years: 2.5 mg b.i.d.–t.i.d. with no more than 10 mg given on the first day. No more than 20 mg/day for children 2–5 years of age and 25 mg/day for children 6–12 years of age.

P

How Supplied: Prochlorperazine: *Suppository:* 2.5 mg, 5 mg, 25 mg; Prochlorperazine Edisylate: *Injection:* 5 mg/mL; *Syrup:* 5 mg/5 mL; Prochlorperazine maleate: *Capsule, extended release:* 10 mg, 15 mg; *Tablet:* 5 mg, 10 mg

EMS CONSIDERATIONS
None.

Progesterone gel
(pro-JES-ter-ohn)
Crinone 4%, Crinone 8% **(Rx)**
Classification: Progesterone product

Uses: Progesterone supplementation or replacement as part of assisted reproductive technology treatment for infertile women with progesterone deficiency. Secondary amenorrhea.
Contraindications: Undiagnosed vaginal bleeding, liver disease or dysfunction, known or suspected malignancy of breast or genital organs, missed abortion, active thrombophlebitis or thromboembolic disease (or history of such). Concurrent use with other local intravaginal therapy.
Precautions: Safety and efficacy have not been determined in children.

Route/Dosage
• **Vaginal gel: Crinone 8%**
Assisted reproductive technology.
90 mg once daily for women who require progesterone supplementation. Administer 90 mg b.i.d. in women with partial or complete ovarian failure who require progesterone replacement. If pregnancy occurs, treatment may be continued until placental autonomy has been achieved (up to 10–12 weeks).
• **Vaginal gel: Crinone 4%**
Secondary amenorrhea.
45 mg every other day up to total of 6 doses. For women who fail to respond, Crinone 8% (90 mg) may be given every other day up to total of 6 doses.
How Supplied: *Vaginal applicator:* 90 mg/1.125 g (Crinone 8%), 45 mg 1.125 g (Crinone 4%)

Side Effects: See Progesterone and Progestins.

EMS CONSIDERATIONS
None.

Promazine hydrochloride
(PROH-mah-zeen)
Pregnancy Class: C
Sparine **(Rx)**
Classification: Antipsychotic, dimethylaminopropyl-type phenothiazine

Mechanism of Action: Significant anticholinergic, sedative, and hypotensive effects; moderate antiemetic effect; and weak extrapyramidal effects. Ineffective in reducing destructive behavior in acutely agitated psychotic patients.
Uses: Psychotic disorders.
Precautions: Safe use during pregnancy has not been established. Dosage has not been established in children less than 12 years of age. Geriatric, emaciated, and debilitated patients may require a lower initial dosage.

Route/Dosage
• **Tablets**
Psychotic disorders.
Adults: 10–200 mg q 4–6 hr; adjust dose as needed and tolerated. Total daily dose should not exceed 1,000 mg. **Pediatric, 12 years and older:** 10–25 mg q 4–6 hr; adjust dose as needed and tolerated.
• **IM**
Psychotic disorders, severe and moderate agitation.
Adults, initial: 50–150 mg; if desired calming effect is not seen after 30 min, give additional doses up to a total of 300 mg. **Maintenance:** 10–200 mg q 4–6 hr as needed and tolerated. Switch to PO therapy as soon as possible. **Pediatric over 12 years:** 10–25 mg q 4–6 hr for chronic psychotic disorders (maximum dose: 1 g/day).
How Supplied: *Injection:* 25 mg/mL, 50 mg/mL; *Tablet:* 50 mg

EMS CONSIDERATIONS

See also *Antipsychotic Agents, Phenothiazines.*

Promethazine hydrochloride

(proh-METH-ah-zeen)
Pregnancy Class: C
Parenteral: Anergan 50, Phenergan,
Suppositories: Phenergan, **Syrup:**
Phenergan Fortis, Phenergan Plain,
Tablets: Phernergan **(Rx)**
Classification: Antihistamine, phenothiazine-type

Mechanism of Action: Antiemetic effects are likely due to inhibition of the CTZ. Effective in vertigo by its central anticholinergic effect which inhibits the vestibular apparatus and the integrative vomiting center as well as the CTZ. May cause severe drowsiness.
Onset of Action: PO, IM, PR: 20 min; **IV:** 3-5 min.
Duration of Action: Antihistaminic: 6-12 hr; **sedative:** 2-8 hr.
Uses: PO and PR for prophylaxis and treatment of motion sickness. Prophylaxis of N&V due to anesthesia or surgery (also postoperatively). Pre- or postoperative sedative, obstetric sedative. Hypersensitivity reactions, including perennial and seasonal allergic rhinitis, vasomotor rhinitis, allergic conjunctivitis, urticaria, angioedema, allergic reactions to blood or plasma, dermographism. Adjunct in the treatment of anaphylaxis or anaphylactoid reactions. Adjunct to analgesics for postoperative pain. IV with meperidine or other narcotics in special surgical procedures as bronchoscopy, ophthalmic surgery, or in poor-risk patients.
Contraindications: Lactation. Comatose patients. CNS depression due to drugs, previous phenothiazine idiosyncrasy, acutely ill or dehydrated children (due to greater susceptibility to dystonias). Children up to 2 years of age. SC or intra-arterial use due to tissue necrosis and gangrene.

Precautions: Safe use during pregnancy has not been established. Use in children may cause paradoxical hyperexcitability and nightmares. Geriatric patients are more likely to experience confusion, dizziness, hypotension, and sedation.

Route/Dosage
- **Suppositories, Syrup, Tablets**
Hypersensitivity reactions.
Adults: 12.5 mg q.i.d. before meals and at bedtime (or 25 mg at bedtime if needed). **Pediatric over 2 years:** 0.125 mg/kg (3.75 mg/m²) q 4–6 hr; 0.5 mg/kg (15 mg/m²) at bedtime if needed; or, 6.25–12. mg t.i.d. (or 25 mg at bedtime if needed).
Antiemetic.
Adults: 25 mg (usual); 12.5–25 mg q 4–6 hr as needed. **Pediatric, over 2 years:** 0.25–0.5 mg/kg (7.5–15 mg/m²) q 4–6 hr as needed (or 12.5–25 mg q 4–6 hr).
Sedation.
Adults: 25–50 mg at bedtime; **pediatric, over 2 years:** 0.5–1 mg/kg (15–30 mg/m²) or 12.5–25 mg at bedtime.
Motion sickness.
Adults: 25 mg b.i.d. **Pediatric, over 2 years:** 12.5–25 mg b.i.d.
Analgesia adjunct.
Adults: 50 mg with an equal amount of meperidine and an appropriate dose of an atropine-like agent. **Pediatric, over 2 years:** 1.2 mg/kg with an equal amount of meperidine and an atropine-like agent.
- **IM, IV**
Hypersensitivity reactions.
Adults: 25 mg repeated in 2 hr if needed; **pediatric, 2–12 years:** 12.5 mg or less, not to exceed half the adult dose. Resume PO therapy as soon as possible.
Antiemetic.
Adults: 12.5–25 mg q 4 hr if needed. If used postoperatively, reduce doses of concomitant hypnotics, analgesics, or barbiturates. **Pediatric, 2–12 years:** Do not exceed half the adult dose. Do not use when the cause of vomiting is unknown.

P

---

bold italic = life threatening side effect

Sedation.

Adults: 25–50 mg at bedtime. May be combined with hypnotics for pre- and postoperative sedation. **Pediatric, 2–12 years:** Do not exceed half the adult dose.

Sedation during labor.

Adults: 50 mg during early stages of labor, not to exceed 100 mg/24 hr.

Analgesia adjunct.

Adults: 25–50 mg in combination with reduced doses of analgesics and hypnotics; give atropine-like drugs as needed. **Pediatric, 2–12 years:** 1.2 mg/kg in combination with an equal dose of analgesic or barbiturate and an appropriate dose of an atropine-like drug.

How Supplied: *Injection:* 25 mg/mL, 50 mg/mL; *Suppository:* 12.5 mg, 25 mg, 50 mg; *Syrup:* 6.25 mg/5 mL, 25 mg/5 mL; *Tablet:* 12.5 mg, 25 mg, 50 mg

Side Effects: Additional: Leukipenia and ***agranulocytosis (especially if used with cytotoxic agents).***

EMS CONSIDERATIONS

See also *Antihistamines* and *Antiemetics.*

P

Propafenone hydrochloride

(proh-pah-FEN-ohn)
Pregnancy Class: C
Rythmol **(Rx)**
Classification: Antiarrhythmic, class IC

Mechanism of Action: Manifests local anesthetic effects and a direct stabilizing action on the myocardium. Reduces upstroke velocity (Phase O) of the monophasic action potential, reduces the fast inward current carried by sodium ions in the Purkinje fibers, increases diastolic excitability threshold, and prolongs the effective refractory period. Also, spontaneous activity is decreased. Slows AV conduction and causes first-degree heart block. Has slight beta-adrenergic blocking activity.

Uses: Documented life-threatening ventricular arrhythmias, such as sustained ventricular tachycardia where the benefits outweigh the risks. Paroxysmal atrial fibrillation or flutter and paroxysmal supraventricular tachycardia associated with disabling symptoms. Do not use in less severe ventricular arrhythmias even if the patient is symptomatic. Antiarrhythmic drugs have not been shown to improve survival in patients with ventricular arrhythmias. *Investigational:* Arrhythmias associated with Wolff-Parkinson-White syndrome.

Contraindications: Uncontrolled CHF, cardiogenic shock, sick sinus node syndrome or AV block in the absence of an artificial pacemaker, bradycardia, marked hypotension, bronchospastic disorders, electrolyte disorders, hypersensitivity to the drug. MI more than 6 days but less than 2 years previously. Lactation.

Precautions: There is an increased risk of death in those with non-life-threatening arrhythmias. Use with caution during labor and delivery. Safety and effectiveness have not been determined in children. Use with caution in patients with impaired hepatic or renal function. Geriatric patients may require lower dosage.

Route/Dosage
• **Tablets**

Adults, initial: 150 mg q 8 hr; dose may be increased at a minimum of q 3–4 days to 225 mg q 8 hr and, if necessary, to 300 mg q 8 hr.

How Supplied: *Tablet:* 150 mg, 225 mg, 300 mg

Side Effects: *CV: **New or worsened arrhythmias.*** First-degree AV block, intraventricular conduction delay, palpitations, PVCs, proarrhythmia, bradycardia, atrial fibrillation, angina, syncope, CHF, ***ventricular tachycardia, second-degree AV block,*** increased QRS duration, chest pain, hypotension, bundle branch block. Less commonly, atrial flutter, AV dissociation, flushing, hot flashes, sick sinus syndrome, sinus pause or arrest, SVT, ***cardiac arrest.*** *CNS:* Dizziness, headache, anxiety, drowsiness, fatigue, loss of balance, ataxia, insomnia. Less commonly, abnormal speech, abnormal dreams, abnormal vision, confusion, depression, memory loss, **apnea,** psychosis/mania, vertigo, **seizures, coma,** numbness, paresthesias. *GI:* Unusual taste, constipation, nausea and/or vomiting, dry mouth, anorexia, flatulence, abdominal pain, cramps, diarrhea, dyspepsia. Less commonly, gastroenteritis and liver abnormalities (cholestasis, hepatitis, elevated enzymes, hepatitis). *Hematologic:* **Agranulocytosis,** increased bleeding time, anemia, granulocytopenia, bruising, leukopenia, purpura, anemia, thrombocytopenia. *Miscellaneous:* Blurred vision, dyspnea, weakness, rash, edema, tremors, diaphoresis, joint pain, possible decrease in spermatogenesis. Less commonly, tinnitus, unusual smell sensation, alopecia, eye irritation, hyponatremia, inappropriate ADH secretion, impotence, increased glucose, kidney failure, lupus erythematosus, muscle cramps or weakness, nephrotic syndrome, pain, pruritus.

OD **Overdose Management:** *Symptoms:* Bradycardia, hypotension, IA and intraventricular conduction disturbances, somnolence. **Rarely, high-grade ventricular arrhythmias and seizures.** *Treatment:* To control BP and cardiac rhythm, defibrillation and infusion of dopamine or isoproterenol. If seizures occur, diazepam, IV, can be given. External cardiac massage and mechanical respiratory assistance may be required.

Drug Interactions
Beta-adrenergic blockers / ↑ Plasma levels of beta blockers metabolized by the liver
Cimetidine / ↓ Plasma levels of propafenone
Cyclosporine / ↑ Blood trough levels of cyclosporine; ↓ renal function
Digoxin / ↑ Plasma levels of digoxin necessitating a ↓ in the dose of digoxin

Local anesthetics / May ↑ risk of CNS side effects
Quinidine / ↑ Serum levels of propafenone in rapid metabolizers → possible ↑ effect
Rifampin / ↓ Effect of propafenone due to ↑ clearance
Warfarin / May ↑ plasma levels of warfarin necessitating ↓ dose of warfarin

EMS CONSIDERATIONS
See also *Antiarrhythmic Agents.*

Propantheline bromide
(proh-PAN-thih-leen)
Pregnancy Class: C
Norpanth, Pro-Banthine **(Rx)**
Classification: Anticholinergic, antispasmodic (quaternary ammonium compound)

Uses: Adjunct in peptic ulcer therapy. Spastic and inflammatory disease of GI and urinary tracts. Control of salivation and enuresis. Duodenography. Second-line therapy for urinary incontinence.
Precautions: Safety and effectiveness for use in children with peptic ulcer have not been established.

Route/Dosage
• **Tablets**
  GI problems.
Adults: 15 mg 30 min before meals and 30 mg at bedtime. Reduce dose to 7.5 mg t.i.d. for mild symptoms, geriatric patients, or patients of small stature. **Pediatric:** 0.375 mg/kg (10 mg/m^2) q.i.d. with dose being adjusted as needed.
  Urinary incontinence.
Adults: 7.5–30 mg 3–5 times/day; in some, doses as high as 15–60 mg q.i.d. may be needed.
How Supplied: *Tablet:* 7.5 mg, 15 mg

EMS CONSIDERATIONS
See also *Cholinergic Blocking Agents.*

P

---

bold italic = life threatening side effect

Propoxyphene hydrochloride
Propoxyphene napsylate
(proh-POX-ih-feen)
Pregnancy Class: C
Hydrochloride: Darvon, Dolene, Doloxene, Doraphen, Doxaphene, Profene, Progesic, Pro Pox, Propoxycon **(C-IV) (Rx)** Napsylate: Darvon-N **(C-IV) (Rx)**
Classification: Analgesic, narcotic, miscellaneous

Mechanism of Action: Resembles narcotics with respect to its mechanism and analgesic effect; it is one-half to one-third as potent as codeine. Is devoid of antitussive, anti-inflammatory, or antipyretic activity. When taken in excessive doses for long periods, psychologic dependence and occasionally physical dependence and tolerance will be manifested.

Onset of Action: Analgesic: 30-60 min; **peak analgesic effect:** 2-2.5 hr. **Duration of Action:** 4-6 hr.

Uses: Relief of mild to moderate pain. Napsylate has been used experimentally to suppress the withdrawal syndrome from narcotics.

Contraindications: Hypersensitivity to drug. Use in children.

Precautions: Safe use during pregnancy has not been established. Use with caution during lactation.

Route/Dosage
- **Capsules (Hydrochloride)**
  Analgesia.
Adults: 65 mg q 4 hr, not to exceed 390 mg/day.
- **Tablets (Napsylate)**
  Analgesia.
Adults: 100 mg q 4 hr, not to exceed 600 mg/day. Reduce the dose of propoxyphene in renal or hepatic impairment.

How Supplied: Propoxyphene hydrochloride: *Capsule:* 65 mg; Propoxyphene napsylate: *Tablet:* 100 mg
Side Effects: *GI:* N&V, constipation, abdominal pain. *CNS:* Sedation, dizziness, lightheadedness, headache, weakness, euphoria, dysphoria. *Other:* Skin rashes, visual disturbances. Propoxyphene can produce psycho-logic dependence, as well as physical dependence and tolerance.

OD Overdose Management: *Symptoms:* Stupor, respiratory depression, *apnea,* hypotension, pulmonary edema, *circulatory collapse, cardiac arrhythmias,* conduction abnormalities, *coma, seizures,* respiratory-metabolic acidosis. *Treatment:* Maintain an adequate airway, artificial respiration, and naloxone, 0.4–2 mg IV (repeat at 2- to 3-min intervals) to combat respiratory depression. Gastric lavage or administration of activated charcoal may be helpful. Correct acidosis and electrolyte imbalance. Acidosis due to lactic acid may require IV sodium bicarbonate.

Drug Interactions
Alcohol, antianxiety drugs, antipsychotic agents, narcotics, sedative-hypnotics / Concomitant use may lead to drowsiness, lethargy, stupor, respiratory, depression, and coma
Carbamazepine / ↑ Effect of carbamazepine due to ↓ breakdown by liver
CNS depressants / Additive CNS depression
Orphenadrine / Concomitant use may lead to confusion, anxiety, and tremors
Phenobarbital / ↑ Effect of phenobarbital due to ↓ breakdown by liver
Skeletal muscle relaxants / Additive respiratory depression
Warfarin / ↑ Hypoprothrombinemic effects of warfarin

EMS CONSIDERATIONS
None.

————COMBINATION DRUG————
Propranolol hydrochloride and Hydrochlorothiazide
(proh-PRAN-oh-lohl, hy-droh-klor-oh-THIGH-ah-zyd)
Pregnancy Class: C
Inderide 40/25, Inderide 80/25, Inderide LA 80/50, Inderide LA 120/50, Inderide LA 160/50 **(Rx)**
Classification: Antihypertensive

Uses: Hypertension (not indicated for initial therapy).

Precautions: Use with caution during lactation. Safety and effectiveness have not been established in children. The risk of hypothermia is increased in geriatric patients.

Route/Dosage
• **Inderide Tablets**
Individualized: 1–2 tablets b.i.d., up to 320 mg propranolol HCl daily.
• **Inderide LA Capsules**
1 capsule once daily.
How Supplied: *Antihypertensive/diuretic:* Hydrochlorothiazide, 25 mg (Inderide) or 50 mg (Inderide LA).*Beta-adrenergic blocking agent:* Propranolol HCl, 40 or 80 mg (Inderide) or 80, 120, or 160 mg (Inderide LA).

EMS CONSIDERATIONS

See also *Antihypertensive Agents.*

Propranolol hydrochloride
(proh-PRAN-oh-lohl)
Pregnancy Class: C
Inderal, Inderal 10, 20, 40, 60, 80, and 90, Inderal LA, Propranolol Intensol
(Rx)
Classification: Beta-adrenergic blocking agent; antiarrhythmic (type II)

Mechanism of Action: Manifests both beta-1- and beta-2-adrenergic blocking activity. Antiarrhythmic action is due to both beta-adrenergic receptor blockade and a direct membrane-stabilizing action on the cardiac cell. Has no intrinsic sympathomimetic activity.
Onset of Action: PO: 30 min; **IV:** immediate; **maximum effect:** 1-1.5 hr.
Duration of Action: 3-5 hr.
Uses: Hypertension (alone or in combination with other antihypertensive agents). Angina pectoris, hypertrophic subaortic stenosis, prophylaxis of MI, pheochromocytoma, prophylaxis of migraine, essential tremor. Cardiac arrhythmias including ventricular tachycardias and ar-

rhythmias, tachycardias due to digitalis intoxication, supraventricular arrhythmias, PVCs, resistant tachyarrhythmias due to anesthesia/catecholamines.
Investigational: Schizophrenia, tremors due to parkinsonism, aggressive behavior, antipsychotic-induced akathisia, rebleeding due to esophageal varices, situational anxiety, acute panic attacks, gastric bleeding in portal hypertension, vaginal contraceptive, anxiety, alcohol withdrawal syndrome, winter depression.
Contraindications: Bronchial asthma, bronchospasms including severe COPD.
Precautions: It is dangerous to use propranolol for pheochromocytoma unless an alpha-adrenergic blocking agent is already in use.

Route/Dosage
• **Tablets, Sustained-Release Capsules, Oral Solution, Concentrate**
Hypertension.
Initial: 40 mg b.i.d. or 80 mg of sustained-release/day; **then,** increase dose to maintenance level of 120–240 mg/day given in two to three divided doses or 120–160 mg of sustained-release medication once daily. Do not exceed 640 mg/day. **Pediatric, initial:** 0.5 mg/kg b.i.d.; dose may be increased at 3- to 5-day intervals to a maximum of 1 mg/kg b.i.d. Calculate the dosage range by weight and not by body surface area.
Angina.
Initial: 80–320 mg b.i.d., t.i.d., or q.i.d.; or, 80 mg of sustained-release once daily; **then,** increase dose gradually to maintenance level of 160 mg/day of sustained-release capsule. Do not exceed 320 mg/day.
Arrhythmias.
10–30 mg t.i.d.–q.i.d. given after meals and at bedtime.
Hypertrophic subaortic stenosis.
20–40 mg t.i.d.–q.i.d. before meals and at bedtime or 80–160 mg of sus-

P

---

bold italic = life threatening side effect

tained-release medication given once daily.

MI prophylaxis.
180–240 mg/day given in three to four divided doses. Do not exceed 240 mg/day.

Pheochromocytoma, preoperatively.
60 mg/day for 3 days before surgery, given concomitantly with an alpha-adrenergic blocking agent.

Inoperable tumors.
30 mg/day in divided doses.

Migraine.
Initial: 80 mg sustained-release medication given once daily; **then,** increase dose gradually to maintenance of 160–240 mg/day in divided doses. If a satisfactory response has not been observed after 4–6 weeks, discontinue the drug and withdraw gradually.

Essential tremor.
Initial: 40 mg b.i.d.; **then,** 120 mg/day up to a maximum of 320 mg/day.

Aggressive behavior.
80–300 mg/day.

Antipsychotic-induced akathisia.
20–80 mg/day.

Tremors associated with Parkinson's disease.
160 mg/day.

Rebleeding from esophageal varices.
20–180 mg b.i.d.

Schizophrenia.
300–5,000 mg/day.

Acute panic symptoms.
40–320 mg/day.

Anxiety.
80–320 mg/day.

Intermittent explosive disorder.
50–1,600 mg/day.

Nonvariceal gastric bleeding in portal hypertension.
24–480 mg/day.

• **IV**
Life-threatening arrhythmias or those occurring under anesthesia.
1–3 mg not to exceed 1 mg/min; a second dose may be given after 2 min, with subsequent doses q 4 hr. Begin PO therapy as soon as possible. Although use in pediatrics is not recommended, investigational doses of 0.01–0.1 mg/kg/dose, up to a max-

imum of 1 mg/dose (by slow push), have been used for arrhythmias.

How Supplied: *Capsule, extended release:* 60 mg, 80 mg, 120 mg, 160 mg; *Concentrate:* 80 mg/mL; *Injection:* 1 mg/mL; *Solution:* 20 mg/5 mL, 40 mg/5 mL; *Tablet:* 10 mg, 20 mg, 40 mg, 60 mg, 80 mg

Side Effects: Additional: Psoriasis-like eruptions, skin necrosis, SLE (rare).

Drug Interactions: Additional:
Haloperidol / Severe hypotension. *Hydralazine /* ↑ Effect of both agents. *Methimazole /* May ↑ effects of propranolol. *Phenobarbital /* ↓ Effect of propranolol dur to ↑ breakdown by liver. *Propylthiouracil /* May ↑ the effects of propranolol. *Rifampin /* ↓ Effect of propranolol due to ↑ breakdown by liver. *Smoking /* ↓ Serum levels and ↑ clearance of propranolol.

EMS CONSIDERATIONS

See also *Beta-Adrenergic Blocking Agents.*

Administration/Storage

IV 1. For IV use, dilute 1 mg in 10 mL of D5W and administer IV over at least 1 min. May be further reconstituted in 50 mL of dextrose or saline solution and infused IVPB over 10–15 min.

2. After IV administration, have emergency drugs and equipment available to combat hypotension or circulatory collapse.

Assessment

1. Note ECG, VS, and cardiopulmonary assessment.

2. Monitor VS. Observe for S&S of CHF (e.g., SOB, rales, edema, and weight gain).

Propylthiouracil
(proh-pill-thigh-oh-YOUR-ah-sill)
Pregnancy Class: D
(Rx)
Classification: Antithyroid preparation

Mechanism of Action: May be preferred for treatment of thyroid storm, as it inhibits peripheral conversion of thyroxine to triiodothyronine.

Onset of Action: 10-20 days; **Time to peak effect:** 2-10 weeks.
Duration of Action: 2-3 hr.
Precautions: Incidence of vasculitis is increased.

Route/Dosage —————————
• **Tablets**
  Hyperthyroidism.
Adults, initial: 300 mg/day (up to 900 mg/day may be required in some patients with severe hyperthyroidism) given as one to four divided doses; **maintenance, usual:** 100–150 mg/day. **Pediatric, 6–10 years, initial:** 50–150 mg/day in one to four divided doses; **over 10 years, initial:** 150–300 mg/day in one to four divided doses. Maintenance for all pediatric use is based on response. **Alternative dose for children, initial:** 5–7 mg/kg/day (150–200 mg/m²/day) in divided doses q 8 hr; **maintenance:** ⅓–⅔ the initial dose when the patient is euthyroid.
  Thyrotoxic crisis.
Adults: 200–400 mg q 4 hr during the first day as an adjunct to other treatments.
  Neonatal thyrotoxicosis.
10 mg/kg daily in divided doses.
How Supplied: *Tablet:* 50 mg
Drug Interactions: Propylthiouracil may produce hypoprothrombinemia, adding to the effect of anticoagulants.

—————————————————————
EMS CONSIDERATIONS
None.

—————————————————————
Protamine sulfate
(PROH-tah-meen)
Pregnancy Class: C
(Rx)
Classification: Heparin antagonist

Mechanism of Action: A strong basic polypeptide that complexes with strongly acidic heparin to form an inactive stable salt. The complex has no anticoagulant activity. Heparin is neutralized within 5 min after IV protamine. The t½ of protamine is shorter than heparin; thus, repeated doses may be required. Upon metabolism, the complex may liberate heparin (heparin rebound).
Duration of Action: 2 hr (but depends on body temperature).
Uses: Only for treatment of heparin overdose.
Contraindications: Previous intolerance to protamine. Use to treat spontaneous hemorrhage, postpartum hemorrhage, menorrhagia, or uterine bleeding. Administration of over 50 mg over a short period.
Precautions: Use with caution during lactation. Safety and efficacy have not been determined in children. Rapid administration may cause severe hypotension and anaphylaxis.

Route/Dosage —————————
• **Slow IV**
Give no more than 50 mg of protamine sulfate in any 10-min period. One mg of protamine sulfate can neutralize about 90 USP units of heparin derived from lung tissue or about 115 USP units of heparin derived from intestinal mucosa. *NOTE:* The dose of protamine sulfate depends on the amount of time that has elapsed since IV heparin administration. For example, if 30 min has elapsed, one-half the usual dose of protamine sulfate may be sufficient because heparin is cleared rapidly from the circulation.
How Supplied: *Injection:* 10 mg/mL
Side Effects: *CV:* Sudden fall in BP, bradycardia, transitory flushing, warm feeling, *acute pulmonary hypertension, circulatory collapse (possibly irreversible) with myocardial failure* and decreased CO. Pulmonary edema in patients on cardiopulmonary bypass undergoing CV surgery. *Anaphylaxis:* Severe respiratory distress, capillary leak, and noncardiogenic pulmonary edema. *GI:* N&V. *CNS:* Lassitude. *Other:* Dyspnea, back pain in conscious patients undergoing cardiac catheterization, hypersensitivity reactions.
OD Overdose Management: *Symptoms:* Bleeding. Rapid administration may cause dyspnea, bradycardia,

flushing, warm feeling, severe hypotension, hypertension. In assessing overdose, there may be the possibility of multiple drug overdoses leading to drug interactions and unusual pharmacokinetics. *Treatment:* Replace blood loss with blood transfusions or fresh frozen plasma. Fluids, epinephrine, dobutamine, or dopamine to treat hypotension.

EMS CONSIDERATIONS

None.

Pseudoephedrine hydrochloride
Pseudoephedrine sulfate

(soo-doh-eh-FED-rin)

Pregnancy Class: B

Hydrochloride: Allermed, Cenafed, Children's Congestion Relief, Children's Sudafed Liquid, Congestion Relief, Decofed Syrup, DeFed-60, Dorcol Children's Decongestant Liquid, Efidac/24, Genaphed, Halofed, PediaCare Infants' Oral Decongestant Drops, Pseudo, Pseudo-Gest, Seudotabs, Sinustop Pro, Sudafed, Sudafed 12 Hour **(OTC)** Sulfate: Afrin Extended-Release Tablets, Drixoral Non-Drowsy Formula **(OTC)**

Classification: Direct- and indirect-acting sympathomimetic, nasal decongestant

Mechanism of Action: Produces direct stimulation of both alpha- (pronounced) and beta-adrenergic receptors, as well as indirect stimulation through release of norepinephrine from storage sites. Results in decongestant effect on the nasal mucosa. Systemic administration eliminates possible damage to the nasal mucosa. **Onset of Action:** 15-30 min; **Time to peak effect:** 30-60 min.
Duration of Action: 3-4 hr; **Extended-release:** 8-12 hr.
Uses: Nasal congestion associated with sinus conditions, otitis, allergies. Relief of eustachian tube congestion.
Contraindications: Additional: Lactation. Use of sustained-release products in children less than 12 years of age.

Precautions: Use with caution in newborn and premature infants due to a higher risk of side effects. Geriatric patients may be more prone to age-related prostatic hypertrophy.

Route/Dosage

HYDROCHLORIDE
• **Oral Solution, Syrup, Tablets**
Decongestant.
Adults: 60 mg q 4–6 hr, not to exceed 240 mg in 24 hr. **Pediatric, 6–12 years:** 30 mg using the oral solution or syrup q 4–6 hr, not to exceed 120 mg in 24 hr; **2–6 years:** 15 mg using the oral solution or syrup q 4–6 hr, not to exceed 60 mg in 24 hr. Individualize the dose for children less than 2 years of age.
• **Extended-Release   Capsules, Tablets**
Decongestant.
Adults and children over 12 years: 120 mg q 12 hr or 240 mg q 24 hr. Use is not recommended for children less than 12 years of age.
SULFATE
• **Extended-Release Tablets**
Decongestant.
Adults and children over 12 years: 120 mg q 12 hr. Use is not recommended for children less than 12 years of age.
How Supplied: Pseudoephedrine hydrochloride: *Liquid:* 7.5 mg/0.8 mL, 30 mg/5 mL; *Syrup:* 15 mg/5 mL, 30 mg/5 mL; *Tablet:* 30 mg, 60 mg; *Tablet, extended release:* 120 mg, 240 mg. Pseudoephedrine sulfate: *Tablet:* 60 mg

EMS CONSIDERATIONS

See also *Sympathomimetic Drugs.*

Psyllium hydrophilic muciloid

(SILL-ee-um hi-droh-FILL-ik)

Effer-syllium, Fiberall Natural Flavor, Fiberall Orange Flavor, Fiberall Wafers, Hydrocil Instant, Konsyl, Konsyl-D, Metamucil, Metamucil Lemon-Lime Flavor, Metamucil Orange Flavor, Metamucil Sugar Free, Metamucil Sugar Free Orange Flavor, Modane Bulk, Natural Vegeta-

bale, Perdiem Fiber, Reguloid Natural, Reguloid Orange, Reguloid Sugar Free Orange, Reguloid Sugar Free Regular, Serutan, Siblin, Syllact, V-Lax **(OTC)**
Classification: Laxative, bulk-forming

Mechanism of Action: Obtained from the fruit of various species of plantago. The powder forms a gelatinous mass with water, which adds bulk to the stools and stimulates peristalsis. Also has a demulcent effect on an inflamed intestinal mucosa. Products may also contain dextrose, sodium bicarbonate, monobasic potassium phosphate, citric acid, and benzyl benzoate. Laxative effects usually occur in 12–24 hr. The full effect may take 2–3 days. Dependence may occur.
Uses: Prophylaxis of constipation in patients who should not strain during defecation. Short-term treatment of constipation; useful in geriatric patients with diminished colonic motor response and during pregnancy and postpartum to reestablish normal bowel function. To soften feces during fecal impaction.
Contraindications: Severe abdominal pain or intestinal obstruction.

Route/Dosage —————————
Dose depends on the product. General information on adult dosage follows.
• **Granules/Flakes**
Adults: 1–2 teaspoons 1–3 times/day spread on food or with a glass of water.
• **Powder**
Adults: 1 rounded teaspoon in 8 oz of liquid 1–3 times/day.
• **Effervescent Powder**
Adults: 1 packet in water 1–3 times/day.
• **Chewable Pieces**
Adults: 2 pieces followed by a glass of water 1–3 times/day.
How Supplied: *Capsule*; *Granule*; *Granule for reconstitution*; *Powder for reconstitution:* 3.4 g/15 mL; *Wafer*
Side Effects: Obstruction of the esophagus, stomach, small intestine, and rectum.

Drug Interactions: Do not use concomitantly with salicylates, nitrofurantoin, or cardiac glycosides (e.g., digitalis).

EMS CONSIDERATIONS
See also *Laxatives.*

Pyrantel pamoate
(pie-RAN-tell)
Pregnancy Class: C
Antiminth, Pin-Rid, Pin-X, Reese's Pinworm **(OTC)**
Classification: Anthelmintic

Mechanism of Action: Has neuromuscular blocking effect which paralyzes the helminth, allowing it to be expelled through the feces. Also inhibits cholinesterases.
Uses: Pinworm (enterobiasis) and roundworm (ascariasis) infestations. Multiple helminth infections, as it is also effective against roundworm and hookworm.
Contraindications: Pregnancy. Hepatic disease.
Precautions: Use with caution in presence of liver dysfunction. Safe use in children less than 2 years of age has not been established.

Route/Dosage —————————
• **Liquid Oral Suspension, Tablets**
Adults and children: One dose of 11 mg/kg (maximum). **Maximum total dose:** 1.0 g.
How Supplied: *Suspension:* 144 mg/30 mL, 720 mg/5 mL; *Tablet:* 180 mg
Side Effects: *GI* (most frequent): Anorexia, N&V, abdominal cramps, diarrhea. *Hepatic:* Transient elevation of AST. *CNS:* Headache, dizziness, drowsiness, insomnia. *Miscellaneous:* Skin rashes.
Drug Interactions: Use with piperazine for ascariasis results in antagonism of the effect of both drugs.

EMS CONSIDERATIONS
None.

P

Pyridostigmine bromide

(peer-id-oh-STIG-meen)
Pregnancy Class: C
Mestinon, Regonol **(Rx)**
Classification: Indirectly acting cholinergic-acetylcholinesterase inhibitor

Mechanism of Action: Has a slower onset, longer duration of action, and fewer side effects than neostigmine.

Onset of Action: PO: 30-45 min for syrup and tablets and 30-60 min for extended-release tablets; **IM:** 15 min; **IV:** 2-5 min.

Duration of Action: PO: 3-6 hr for syrup and tablets and 6-12 hr for extended-release tablets; **IM, IV:** 2-4 hr.

Uses: Myasthenia gravis. Antidote for nondepolarizing muscle relaxants (e.g., tubocurarine).

Contraindications: Additional: Sensitivity to bromides.

Precautions: Safe use during pregnancy and during lactation has not been established. May cause uterine irritability and premature labor if given IV to pregnant women near term. Duration of action may be increased in the elderly.

Route/Dosage
• **Syrup, Tablets**
  Myasthenia gravis.
Adults: 60–120 mg q 3–4 hr with dosage adjusted to patient response. **Maintenance:** 600 mg/day (range: 60 mg–1.5 g). **Pediatric:** 7 mg/kg (200 mg/m²) daily in five to six divided doses.
• **Sustained-Release Tablets**
  Myasthenia gravis.
Adults: 180–540 mg 1–2 times/day with at least 6 hr between doses. Sustained-release tablets not recommended for use in children.
• **IM, IV**
  Myasthenia gravis.
Adults, IM, IV: 2 mg (about 1/30 the adult dose) q 2–3 hr.
  Neonates of myasthenic mothers.
IM: 0.05–0.15 mg/kg q 4–6 hr.
  Antidote for nondepolarizing drugs.

Adults, IV: 10–20 mg with 0.6–1.2 mg atropine sulfate given IV.

How Supplied: *Injection:* 5 mg/mL; *Syrup:* 60 mg/5 mL; *Tablet:* 60 mg; *Tablet, extended release:* 180 mg

Side Effects: Additional: Skin rash. Thrombophlebitis after IV use.

OD Overdose Management: *Symptoms:* Abdominal cramps, vomiting, diarrhea, epigastric distress, excessive salivation, cold sweating, pallor, blurred vision, urinary urgency, fasciculation and *paralysis of voluntary muscles* (including the tongue), miosis, increased BP (may be accompanied by bradycardia), sensation of internal trembling, panic, severe anxiety. *Treatment:* Discontinue medication temporarily. Give atropine, 0.5–1 mg IV (up to 5–10 mg or more may be needed to get HR to 80 beats/min). Supportive treatment including artificial respiration and oxygen.

EMS CONSIDERATIONS

None.

Pyridoxine hydrochloride (Vitamin B₆)

(peer-ih-DOX-een)
Pregnancy Class: A
Nestrex (Rx: Injection; OTC: Tablets)
Classification: Vitamin B complex

Mechanism of Action: A water-soluble, heat-resistant vitamin that is destroyed by light. Acts as a coenzyme in the metabolism of protein, carbohydrates, and fat. As the amount of protein increases in the diet, the pyridoxine requirement increases. However, pyridoxine deficiency alone is rare.

Uses: Pyridoxine deficiency including poor diet, drug-induced (e.g., oral contraceptives, isoniazid), and inborn errors of metabolism. *Investigational:* Hydrazine poisoning, PMS, high urine oxalate levels, N&V due to pregnancy.

Precautions: Safety and effectiveness have not been established in children.

Route/Dosage

• **Capsules, Enteric-Coated Tablets, Extended-Release Tablets, Tablets**

Dietary supplement.

Adults: 10–20 mg/day for 2 weeks; **then,** 2–5 mg/day as part of a multivitamin preparation for several weeks. **Pediatric,** 2.5–10 mg/day for 3 weeks; **then,** 2–5 mg/day as part of a multivitamin preparation for several weeks.

Pyridoxine dependency syndrome.

Adults and children, initial: 30–600 mg/day; **maintenance,** 30 mg/day for life. **Infants, maintenance:** 2–10 mg/day for life.

Drug-induced deficiency.

Adults, prophylaxis: 10–50 mg/day for penicillamine or 100–300 mg/day for cycloserine, hydralazine, or isoniazid. **Adults, treatment:** 50–200 mg/day for 3 weeks followed by 25–100 mg/day to prevent relapse. **Adults, alcoholism:** 50 mg/day for 2–4 weeks; if anemia responds, continue pyridoxine indefinitely.

Hereditary sideroblastic anemia.

Adults: 200–600 mg/day for 1–2 months; **then,** 30–50 mg/day for life.

• **IM, IV**

Pyridoxine dependency syndrome.

Adults: 30–600 mg/day. **Pediatric:** 10–100 mg initially.

Drug-induced deficiency.

Adults: 50–200 mg/day for 3 weeks followed by 25–100 mg/day as needed.

Cycloserine poisoning.

Adults: 300 mg/day.

Isoniazid poisoning.

Adults: 1 g for each gram of isoniazid taken.

How Supplied: *Capsule:* 150 mg, 500 mg; *Enteric coated tablet:* 20 mg;

Injection: 100 mg/mL; *Tablet:* 10 mg, 25 mg, 32.5 mg, 50 mg, 100 mg, 200 mg, 250 mg, 500 mg; *Tablet, extended release:* 200 mg

Side Effects: *CNS:* Unstable gait; decreased sensation to touch, temperature, and vibration; paresthesia, sleepiness; numbness of feet; awkwardness of hands; perioral numbness. *NOTE:* Abuse and dependence have been noted in adults administered 200 mg/day.

OD Overdose Management: *Symptoms:* Ataxia, severe sensory neuropathy. *Treatment:* Discontinue pyridoxine; allow up to 6 months for CNS sensation to return.

Drug Interactions

Chloramphenicol / ↑ Pyridoxine requirements

Contraceptives, oral / ↑ Pyridoxine requirements

Cycloserine / ↑ Pyridoxine requirements

Ethionamide / ↑ Pyridoxine requirements

Hydralazine / ↑ Pyridoxine requirements

Immunosuppressants / ↑ Pyridoxine requirements

Isoniazid / ↑ Pyridoxine requirements

Levodopa / Daily doses exceeding 5 mg pyridoxine antagonize the therapeutic effect of levodopa

Penicillamine / ↑ Pyridoxine requirements

Phenobarbital / Pyridoxine ↓ serum levels of phenobarbital

Phenytoin / Pyridoxine ↓ serum levels of phenytoin

EMS CONSIDERATIONS

None.

Q

Quetiapine fumarate
(kweh-TYE-ah-peen)
Pregnancy Class: C
Seroquel **(Rx)**
Classification: Antipsychotic drug

Mechanism of Action: Mechanism unknown but may act as an antagonist at dopamine D_2 and serotonin $5HT_2$ receptors. Side effects may be due to antagonism of other receptors (e.g., histamine H_1, dopamine D_1, adrenergic alpha-1 and alpha-2, serotonin $5HT_{1A}$).
Uses: Management of psychoses.
Contraindications: Lactation.
Precautions: Use with caution in liver disease, in those at risk for aspiration pneumonia, and in those with history of seizures or conditions that lower seizure threshold (e.g., Alzheimer's). Safety and efficacy have not been determined in children.

Route/Dosage
• **Tablets**
  Psychoses.
Initial: 25 mg b.i.d., with increases of 25 to 50 mg b.i.d. or t.i.d. on second and third day, as tolerated. Target dose range, by fourth day, is 300 to 400 mg daily. Further dosage adjustments can occur at intervals of two or more days. The antipsychotic dose range is 150 to 750 mg/day.
How Supplied: *Tablets:* 25 mg, 100 mg, 200 mg
Side Effects: Side effects with incidence of 1% or more are listed. *Body as a whole:* Asthenia, rash, fever, weight gain, back pain, flu syndrome. *CNS:* Headache, somnolence, dizziness, hypertonia, dysarthria. *GI:* Constipation, dry mouth, dyspepsia, anorexia, abdominal pain. *CV:* Orthostatic hypotension, syncope, tachycardia, palpitation. *Respiratory:* Pharyngitis, rhinitis, increased cough, dyspnea. *Miscellaneous:* Peripheral edema, sweating, leukopenia, ear pain. *Note: **Neuroleptic malignant syndrome** and **seizures,** although rare, may occur.*

OD Overdose Management: *Symptoms:* Drowsiness, sedation, tachycardia, hypotension, dystonic reaction of the head and neck, seizures, obtundation. *Treatment:* Cardiovascular monitoring for arrhythmias. If antiarrhythmic therapy is used, disopyramide, procainamide, and quinidine increase risk of prolongation of QT. Treat hypotension and circulatory shock with IV fluids or sympathomimetic drugs (do not use epinephrine or dopamine as they may worsen hypotension). Use anticholinergic drugs to treat severe extrapyramidal symptoms.
Drug Interactions
Barbiturates / ↓ Effect of quetiapine due to ↑ breakdown by liver
Carbamazepine / ↓ Effect of quetiapine due to ↑ breakdown by liver
Dopamine agonists / Quetiapine antagonizes effect
Glucocorticoids / ↓ Effect of quetiapine due to ↑ breakdown by liver
Levodopa / Quetiapine antagonizes effect
Phenytoin / ↓ Effect of quetiapine due to ↑ breakdown by liver
Rifampin / ↓ Effect of quetiapine due to ↑ breakdown by liver
Thioridazine / ↑ Clearance of quetiapine

EMS CONSIDERATIONS
None.

Quinapril hydrochloride
(KWIN-ah-prill)
Pregnancy Class: D
Accupril **(Rx)**
Classification: Angiotensin-converting enzyme inhibitor

Onset of Action: 1 hr.
Duration of Action: 18-24 hr.
Uses: Alone or in combination with a thiazide diuretic for the treatment of hypertension. Adjunct with a diuret-

ic or digitalis to treat CHF in those not responding adequately to diuretics or digitalis.

Precautions: Use with caution during lactation. Safety and effectiveness have not been determined in children. Geriatric patients may be more sensitive to the effects of quinapril and manifest higher peak quinaprilat blood levels.

Route/Dosage

• **Tablets**
  Hypertension.
  Initial: 10 or 20 mg once daily; **then,** adjust dosage based on BP response at peak (2–6 hr) and trough (predose) blood levels. The dose should be adjusted at 2-week intervals. **Maintenance:** 20, 40, or 80 mg daily as a single dose or in two equally divided doses. With impaired renal function, the initial dose should be 10 mg if the C_{CR} is greater than 60 mL/min, 5 mg if the C_{CR} is between 30 and 60 mL/min, and 2.5 mg if the C_{CR} is between 10 and 30 mL/min. If the initial dose is well tolerated, the drug may be given the following day as a b.i.d. regimen.
  CHF.
  Initial: 5 mg b.i.d. If this dose is well tolerated, titrate patients at weekly intervals until an effective dose, usually 20–40 mg daily in two equally divided doses, is attained. Undesirable hypotension, orthostasis, or azotemia may prevent this dosage level from being reached.

How Supplied: *Tablet:* 5 mg, 10 mg, 20 mg, 40 mg

Side Effects: *CV:* Vasodilation, tachycardia, ***heart failure,*** palpitations, chest pain, hypotension, ***MI, CVA, hypertensive crisis,*** angina pectoris, orthostatic hypotension, ***cardiac rhythm disturbances, cardiogenic shock.*** *GI:* Dry mouth or throat, constipation, diarrhea, N&V, abdominal pain, hepatitis, pancreatitis, ***GI hemorrhage.*** *CNS:* Somnolence, vertigo, insomnia, sleep disturbances, paresthesias, nervousness, depression, headache, dizziness, fatigue. *Hematologic:* ***Agranu-***

locytosis, bone marrow depression, thrombocytopenia. *Dermatologic:* ***Angioedema of the lips, tongue, glottis, and larynx;*** sweating, pruritus, exfoliative dermatitis, photosensitivity, dermatopolymyositis, flushing, rash. *Body as a whole:* Malaise, back pain. *GU:* Oliguria and/or progressive azotemia and rarely ***acute renal failure and/or death in severe heart failure.*** Impotence. Worsening renal failure. *Respiratory:* Pharyngitis, cough, asthma, bronchospasm, dyspnea. *Miscellaneous:* Oligohydramnios in fetuses exposed to the drug in utero. Abnormal liver function tests, syncope, hyperkalemia, amblyopia, syncope, malagia, viral infections.

OD **Overdose Management:** *Symptoms:* Commonly, hypotension. *Treatment:* IV infusion of normal saline to restore blood pressure.

Drug Interactions
Potassium-containing salt substitutes / ↑ Risk of hyperkalemia
Potassium-sparing diuretics / ↑ Risk of hyperkalemia
Potassium supplements / ↑ Risk of hyperkalemia
Tetracyclines / ↓ Absorption of tetracycline due to high magnesium content of quinapril tablets

EMS CONSIDERATIONS
None.

Quinidine bisulfate
Quinidine gluconate
Quinidine polygalacturonate
Quinidine sulfate
(KWIN-ih-deen)

Pregnancy Class: bisulfate: D; gluconate, polygalacturonate, sulfate: C.
Bisulfate: **(Rx)** Gluconate: Quinaglute Dura-Tabs, Quinalan **(Rx)** Polygalacturonate: Cardioquin **(Rx)** Sulfate: Quinidex Extentabs, Quinora **(Rx)**
Classification: Antiarrhythmic, class IA

Mechanism of Action: Reduces the excitability of the heart and depresses conduction velocity and contractility. Prolongs the refractory period and increases conduction time. It also decreases CO and possesses anticholinergic, antimalarial, antipyretic, and oxytocic properties.

Onset of Action: PO: 0.5-3 hr; **IM:** 1 hr; **Maximum effects, after IM:** 30-90 min.

Duration of Action: 6-8 hr for tablets/capsules and 12 hr for extended-release tablets.

Uses: Premature atrial, AV junctional, and ventricular contractions. Treatment and control of atrial flutter, established atrial fibrillation, paroxysmal atrial tachycardia, paroxysmal AV junctional rhythm, paroxysmal and chronic atrial fibrillation, paroxysmal ventricular tachycardia not associated with complete heart block, maintenance therapy after electrical conversion of atrial flutter or fibrillation. The parenteral route is indicated when PO therapy is not feasible or immediate effects are required. *Investigational:* Gluconate salt for life-threatening *Plasmodium falciparum* malaria.

Contraindications: Hypersensitivity to drug or other cinchona drugs. Myasthenia gravis, history of thrombocytopenic purpura associated with quinidine use, digitalis intoxication evidenced by arrhythmias or AV conduction disorders. Also, complete heart block, left bundle branch block, or other intraventricular conduction defects manifested by marked QRS widening or bizarre complexes. Complete AV block with an AV nodal or idioventricular pacemaker, aberrant ectopic impulses and abnormal rhythms due to escape mechanisms. History of drug-induced torsades de pointes or long QT syndrome.

Precautions: Safety in children and during lactation has not been established. Use with extreme caution in patients in whom a sudden change in BP might be detrimental or in those suffering from extensive myocardial damage, subacute endocarditis, bradycardia, coronary occlusion, distur-

bances in impulse conduction, chronic valvular disease, considerable cardiac enlargement, frank CHF, and renal or hepatic disease. Use with caution in acute infections, hyperthyroidism, muscular weakness, respiratory distress, and bronchial asthma. The dose in geriatric patients may have to be reduced due to age-related changes in renal function.

Route/Dosage ——————
• **Quinidine Bisulfate Sustained-Release Tablets**
Antiarrhythmic.
Initial: Test dose of 200 mg in the morning (to ascertain hypersensitivity). In the evening, administer 500 mg. **Then,** beginning the next day, 500–750 mg/12 hr. **Maintenance:** 0.5–1.25 g morning and evening.
• **Quinidine Polygalacturonate Tablets, Quinidine Sulfate Tablets**
Premature atrial and ventricular contractions.
Adults: 200–300 mg t.i.d.–q.i.d.
Paroxysmal SVTs.
Adults: 400–600 mg q 2–3 hr until the paroxysm is terminated.
Conversion of atrial flutter.
Adults: 200 mg q 2–3 hr for five to eight doses; daily doses can be increased until rhythm is restored or toxic effects occur.
Conversion of atrial flutter, maintenance therapy.
Adults: 200–300 mg t.i.d.–q.i.d. Large doses or more frequent administration may be required in some patients.
• **Quinidine Gluconate Extended-Release Tablets, Quinidine Sulfate Extended-Release Tablets**
All uses.
Adults: 300–600 mg q 8–12 hr.
• **Quinidine Gluconate Injection (IM or IV)**
Acute tachycardia.
Adults, initial: 600 mg IM; **then,** 400 mg IM repeated as often as q 2 hr.
Arrhythmias.
Adults: 330 mg IM or less IV (as much as 500–750 mg may be required).
P. falciparum malaria.

Two regimens may be used. (1) *Loading dose:* 15 mg/kg in 250 mL NSS given over 4 hr; **then,** 24 hr after beginning the loading dose, institute 7.5 mg/kg infused over 4 hr and given q 8 hr for 7 days or until PO therapy can be started. (2) *Loading dose:* 10 mg/kg in 250 mL NSS infused over 1–2 hr followed immediately by 0.02 mg/kg/min for up to 72 hr or until parasitemia decreases to less than 1% or PO therapy can be started.

How Supplied: Quinidine bisulfate: *Sustained-release tablet:* 250 mg. Quinidine gluconate: *Injection:* 80 mg/mL; *Tablet, extended release:* 324 mg. Quinidine polygalacturonate: *Tablet:* 275 mg. Quinidine sulfate: *Tablet:* 200 mg, 300 mg; *Tablet, extended release:* 300 mg

Side Effects: *CV:* Widening of QRS complex, hypotension, *cardiac asystole,* ectopic ventricular beats, *ventricular tachycardia or fibrillation, torsades de pointes,* paradoxical tachycardia, *arterial embolism,* ventricular extrasystoles (one or more every 6 beats), prolonged QT interval, *complete AV block, ventricular flutter.* *GI:* N&V, abdominal pain, anorexia, diarrhea, urge to defecate as well as urinate, esophagitis (rare). *CNS:* Syncope, headache, confusion, excitement, vertigo, apprehension, delirium, dementia, ataxia, depression. *Dermatologic:* Rash, urticaria, exfoliative dermatitis, photosensitivity, flushing with intense pruritus, eczema, psoriasis, pigmentation abnormalities. *Allergic:* Acute asthma, angioneurotic edema, *respiratory arrest,* dyspnea, fever, *vascular collapse,* purpura, vasculitis, hepatic dysfunction (including granulomatous hepatitis), *hepatic toxicity.* *Hematologic:* Hypoprothrombinemia, *acute hemolytic anemia,* thrombocytopenic purpura, *agranulocytosis,* thrombocytopenia, leukocytosis, neutropenia, shift to left in WBC differential. *Ophthalmologic:* Blurred vision, mydriasis, alterations in color perception, decreased field of vision, double vision, photophobia, optic neuritis, night blindness, scotomata. *Other:* Liver toxicity including hepatitis, lupus nephritis, tinnitus, decreased hearing acuity, arthritis, myalgia, increase in serum skeletal muscle CPK, lupus erythematosus.

OD Overdose Management: *Symptoms:* *CNS:* Lethargy, confusion, *coma, seizures, respiratory depression or arrest,* headache, paresthesia, vertigo. CNS symptoms may be seen after onset of CV toxicity. *GI:* Vomiting, diarrhea, abdominal pain, hypokalemia, nausea. *CV:* Sinus tachycardia, *ventricular tachycardia or fibrillation, torsades de pointes, depressed automaticity and conduction* (including bundle branch block, sinus bradycardia, SA block, prolongation of QRS and QTc, sinus arrest, AV block, ST depression, T inversion), syncope, *heart failure.* Hypotension due to decreased conduction and CO and vasodilation. *Miscellaneous:* Cinchonism, visual and auditory disturbances, hypokalemia, tinnitus, acidosis. *Treatment:*
• Perform gastric lavage, induce vomiting, and administer activated charcoal if ingestion is recent.
• Monitor ECG, blood gases, serum electrolytes, and BP.
• Institute cardiac pacing, if necessary.
• Acidify the urine.
• Use artificial respiration and other supportive measures.
• Infusions of 1/6 molar sodium lactate IV may decrease the cardiotoxic effects.
• Treat hypotension with metaraminol or norepinephrine after fluid volume replacement.
• Use phenytoin or lidocaine to treat tachydysrhythmias.
• Hemodialysis is effective but not often required.

Drug Interactions
Acetazolamide, Antacids / ↑ Effect of quinidine due to ↓ renal excretion
Amiodarone / ↑ Quinidine levels with possible fatal cardiac dysrhythmias
Anticholinergic agents, Atropine / Additive effect on blockade of vagus nerve action

Anticoagulants, oral / Additive hypoprothrombinemia with possible hemorrhage

Barbiturates / ↓ Effect of quinidine due to ↑ breakdown by liver

Cholinergic agents / Quinidine antagonizes effect of cholinergic drugs

Cimetidine / ↑ Effect of quinidine due to ↓ breakdown by liver

Digoxin, Digitoxin / ↑ Symptoms of digoxin or digitoxin toxicity

Disopyramide / Either ↑ disopyramide levels or ↓ quinidine levels

Guanethidine / Additive hypotensive effect

Methyldopa / Additive hypotensive effect

Metoprolol / ↑ Effect of propranolol in fast metabolizers

Neuromuscular blocking agents / ↑ Respiratory depression

Nifedipine / ↓ Effect of quinidine

Phenobarbital, Phenytoin / ↓ Effect of quinidine by ↑ rate of metabolism in liver

Potassium / ↑ Effect of quinidine

Procainamide / ↑ Effects of procainamide with possible toxicity

Propafenone / ↑ Serum propafenone levels in rapid metabolizers

Propranolol / ↑ Effect of propranolol in fast metabolizers

Reserpine / Additive cardiac depressant effects

Rifampin / ↓ Effect of quinidine due to ↑ breakdown by liver

Skeletal muscle relaxants / ↑ Skeletal muscle relaxation

Sodium bicarbonate / ↑ Effect of quinidine due to ↓ renal excretion

Sucralfate / ↓ Serum levels of quinidine → ↓ effect

Thiazide diuretics / ↑ Effect of quinidine due to ↓ renal excretion

Tricyclic antidepressants / ↑ Effect of antidepressant due to ↓ clearance

Verapamil / ↓ Clearance of verapamil → ↑ hypotension, bradycardia, AV block, ventricular tachycardia, and pulmonary edema

---

EMS CONSIDERATIONS

See also *Antiarrhythmic Agents.*

Quinine sulfate

(KWYE-nine)
Pregnancy Class: X
Formula Q, Legatrim, M-KYA, Quinamm **(Rx)**
Classification: Antimalarial

Mechanism of Action: Natural alkaloid having antimalarial, antipyretic, analgesic, and oxytocic properties. Use in treating malaria is important due to emergence of resistant forms of vivax and falciparum; no resistant forms of the parasite have been found for quinine. Antimalarial mechanism not known precisely; quinine does affect DNA replication and may raise intracellular pH. Eradicates the erythrocytic stages of plasmodia. Increases the refractory period of skeletal muscle, decreases the excitability of the motor end-plate region, and affects the distribution of calcium within the muscle fiber, thus making it useful for nocturnal leg cramps. Is oxytocic and may cause congenital malformations.

Uses: Alone or in combination with pyrimethamine and a sulfonamide or a tetracycline for resistant forms of *Plasmodium falciparum.* As alternative therapy for chloroquine, sensitive stains of *P. falciparum, P. malariae, P. ovale,* and *P. vivax.* Mefloquine and clindamycin may also be used with quinine, depending on where the malaria was acquired. *Investigational:* Prevention and treatment of nocturnal recumbency leg cramps.

Contraindications: Use with tinnitus, G6PD deficiency, optic neuritis, history of blackwater fever, and thrombocytopenia purpura associated with previous use of quinine.

Precautions: Use with caution in patients with cardiac arrhythmias and during lactation. Hemolysis, with a potential for hemolytic anemia, may occur in patients with G6PD deficiency.

Route/Dosage ————————

• **Capsules, Tablets**
  Chloroquine-resistant malaria.
Adults: 650 mg q 8 hr for at least 3 days (7 days in Southeast Asia)

along with pyrimethamine, 25 mg b.i.d. for the first 3 days and sulfadiazine, 2 g/day for the first 5 days. There are two alternative regimens: (1) quinine, 650 mg q 8 hr for at least 3 days (7 days in Southeast Asia) along with a tetracycline, 250 mg q 6 hr for 10 days or (2) quinine, 650 mg q 8 hr for 3 days with sulfadoxine, 1.5 g and pyrimethamine, 75 mg as a single dose.

Chloroquine-sensitive malaria.
Adults: 600 mg q 8 hr for 5–7 days.
Pediatric: 10 mg/kg q 8 hr for 5–7 days.

Nocturnal leg cramps.
Adults: 260–300 mg at bedtime.
How Supplied: *Capsule:* 180 mg, 200 mg, 324 mg, 325 mg; *Tablet:* 260 mg

Side Effects: Use of quinine may result in a syndrome referred to as *cinchonism.* Mild cinchonism is characterized by tinnitus, headache, nausea, slight visual disturbances. Larger doses, however, may cause severe CNS, CV, GI, or dermatologic effects.

Allergic: Flushing, cutaneous rashes (papular, scarlatinal, urticarial), fever, facial edema, pruritus, dyspnea, tinnitus, sweating, asthmatic symptoms, visual impairment, gastric upset. *GI:* N&V, epigastric pain, hepatitis. *Ophthalmologic:* Blurred vision with scotomata, photophobia, diplopia, night blindness, decreased visual fields, impaired color vision and perception, amblyopia, mydriasis, optic atrophy. *CNS:* Headache, confusion, restlessness, vertigo, syncope, fever, apprehension, excitement, delirium, hypothermia, dizziness, **convulsions.** *Otic:* Tinnitus, deafness. *Hematologic:* Acute hemolysis, hemolytic anemia, thrombocytopenic purpura, agranulocytosis, hypoprothrombinemia. *CV:* Symptoms of angina, ventricular tachycardia, conduction disturbances, vasculitis. *Miscellaneous:* Sweating, hypoglycemia, lichenoid photosensitivity.

OD Overdose Management: *Symptoms:* Dizziness, intestinal cramping, skin rash, tinnitus. With higher doses, symptoms include apprehension, confusion, fever, headache, vomiting, and seizures. *Treatment:*
• Induce vomiting or undertake gastric lavage.
• Maintain BP and renal function.
• If necessary, provide artificial respiration.
• Sedatives, oxygen, and other supportive measures may be required.
• Give IV fluids to maintain fluid and electrolyte balance.
• Treat angioedema or asthma with epinephrine, corticosteroids, and antihistamines.
• Urinary acidification will hasten excretion; however, in the presence of hemoglobinuria, acidification of the urine will increase renal blockade.

Drug Interactions
Acetazolamide / ↑ Blood levels (and therefore potential for toxicity) of quinine due to ↓ rate of elimination
Aluminum-containing antacids / Absorption of quinine ↓ or delayed
Anticoagulants, oral / Additive hypoprothrombinemia due to ↓ synthesis of vitamin K–dependent clotting factors
Cimetidine / ↑ Effect of quinine due to ↓ rate of excretion
Digoxin / ↑ Serum levels of digoxin
Heparin / Effect ↓ by quinine
Mefloquine / ↑ Risk of ECG abnormalities or cardiac arrest; also, ↑ risk of convulsions. Do **not** use together; delay mefloquine administration at least 12 hr after the last dose of quinine
Neuromuscular blocking agents (depolarizing and nondepolarizing) / ↑ Respiratory depression and apnea
Rifabutin, Rifampin / ↑ Hepatic clearance of quinine; can persist for several days following discontinuation of the rifampin
Sodium bicarbonate / ↑ Blood levels (and therefore potential for toxicity) of quinine due to ↓ rate of elimination

EMS CONSIDERATIONS
See also *Anti-Infectives.*

R

Rabeprazole sodium
(rah-BEP-rah-zohl)
Pregnancy Class: B
Aciphex **(Rx)**
Classification: GI drug

Mechanism of Action: Suppresses gastric secretion by inhibiting gastric H+,K+ATPase at the secretory surface of parietal cells, i.e., is a gastric proton-pump inhibitor. Blocks the final step of gastric acid secretion.

Uses: Short-term (4–8 weeks) treatment in the healing and symptomatic relief of erosive or ulcerative gastroesophageal reflux disease (GERD). Maintenance of healing and reduction in relapse rates of heartburn symptoms in patients with erosive or ulcerative GERD. Short-term (up to 4 weeks) treatment in healing and symptomatic relief of duodenal ulcers. Long-term treatment of pathological hypersecretory symptoms, including Zollinger-Ellison syndrome.

Contraindications: Known sensitivity to rabeprazole or substituted benzimidazoles. Lactation.

Precautions: Safety and efficacy have not been determined in children. Greater sensitivity in some geriatric patients is possible. Symptomatic response to therapy does not preclude presence of gastric malignancy. Use with caution in severe hepatic impairment.

Route/Dosage
• **Tablet, Enteric-Coated**
Healing of erosive or ulcerative GERD.
Adults: 20 mg once daily for 4–8 weeks. An additional 8 weeks of therapy may be considered for those who have not healed.
Maintenance of healing of erosive or ulcerative GERD.
Adults: 20 mg once daily.
Healing of duodenal ulcers.
Adults: 20 mg once daily after the morning meal for up to 4 weeks. A few patients may require additional time to heal.

Treatment of pathological hypersecretory conditions.
Adults, initial: 60 mg once a day. Adjust dosage to individual patient needs (doses up to 100 mg/day and 60 mg b.i.d. have been used). Continue as long as clinically needed.

How Supplied: *Tablet, Enteric-Coated:* 20 mg

Side Effects: *GI:* Diarrhea, N&V, abdominal pain, dyspepsia, flatulence, constipation, dry mouth, eructation, gastroenteritis, rectal hemorrhage, melena, anorexia, cholelithiasis, mouth ulceration, stomatitis, dysphagia, gingivitis, cholecystitis, increased appetite, abnormal stools, colitis, esophagitis, glossitis, pancreatitis, proctitis. *CNS:* Insomnia, anxiety, dizziness, depression, nervousness, somnolence, hypertonia, neuralgia, vertigo, convulsions, abnormal dreams, decreased libido, neuropathy, paresthesia, tremor, coma, disorientation, delirium. *CV:* Hypertension, *MI* , abnormal EEG, migraine, syncope, angina pectoris, bundle branch block, palpitation, sinus bradycardia, tachycardia. *Musculoskeletal:* Myalgia, arthritis, leg cramps, bone pain, arthrosis, bursitis, neck rigidity, rhabdomyolysis. *Respiratory:* Dyspnea, asthma, epistaxis, laryngitis, hiccough, hyperventilation, interstitial pneumonia. *Dermatologic:* Rash, pruritus, sweating, urticaria, alopecia, jaundice, bullous and other skin eruptions. *GU:* Cystitis, urinary frequency, dysmenorrhea, dysuria, kidney calculus, metorrhagia, polyuria. *Endocrine:* Hyperthyroidism, hypothyroidism. *Hematologic:* Anemia, ecchymosis, lymphadenopathy, hypochromic anemia, agranulocytosis, hemolytic anemia, leukopenia, pancytopenia, thrombocytopenia. *Metabolic:* Peripheral edema, edema, weight gain, gout, dehydration, weight loss. *Body as a whole:* Asthenia, fever, allergic reaction, chills, malaise, substernal chest pain, photosensitivity reaction, **sudden death**. *Ophthalmic:* Cataract, amblyopia, glaucoma, dry eyes, abnormal vision. *Otic:* Tinnitus, otitis media.

Drug Interactions

Digoxin / ↑ Plama levels of digoxin R/T changes in gastric pH

Ketoconazole / ↓ Plasma levels of ketoconazole R/T changes in gastric pH

EMS CONSIDERATIONS

None.

Raloxifene hydrochloride

(ral-OX-ih-feen)

Pregnancy Class: X

Evista **(Rx)**

Classification: Estrogen receptor modulator

Mechanism of Action: Selective estrogen receptor modulator that reduces bone resorption and decreases overall bone turnover. Considered an estrogen antagonist that acts by combining with estrogen receptors. Has not been associated with endometrial proliferation, breast enlargement, breast pain, or increased risk of breast cancer. Also decreases total and LDL cholesterol levels.

Uses: Prevention of osteoporosis in postmenopausal women. Not effective in reducing hot flashes or flushes associated with estrogen deficiency. *Investigational:* Reduce risk of breast cancer in postmenopausal women.

Contraindications: In women who are or who might become pregnant, active or history of venous thromboembolic events (e.g., DVT, pulmonary embolism, retinal vein thrombosis). Use in premenopausal women, during lactation, or in pediatric patients. Concurrent use with systemic estrogen or hormone replacement therapy.

Precautions: Use with caution with highly protein-bound drugs, including clofibrate, diazepam, diazoxide, ibuprofen, indomethacin, and naproxen. Effect on bone mass density beyond 2 years of treatment is not known.

Route/Dosage

• **Tablets**

Prevention of osteoporosis in postmenopausal women.

Adults: 60 mg once daily.

How Supplied: *Tablets:* 60 mg

Side Effects: *CV:* Hot flashes, migraine. *Body as a whole:* Infection, flu syndrome, chest pain, fever, weight gain, peripheral edema. *CNS:* Depression, insomnia. *GI:* Nausea, dyspepsia, vomiting, flatulence, GI disorder, gastroenteritis. *GU:* Vaginitis, UTI, cystitis, leukorrhea, endometrial disorder. *Respiratory:* Sinusitis, pharyngitis, increased cough, pneumonia, laryngitis. *Musculoskeletal:* Arthralgia, myalgia, leg cramps, arthritis. *Dermatologic:* Rash, sweating.

Drug Interactions

Cholestryamine / ↓ Absorption of raloxifene

Warfarin / ↓ Prothrombin time

EMS CONSIDERATIONS

None.

Ramipril

(RAM-ih-prill)

Pregnancy Class: D

Altace **(Rx)**

Classification: Angiotensin-converting enzyme inhibitor

Onset of Action: 1-2 hr; **Peak effect:** 3-6 hr.

Duration of Action: 24 hr.

Uses: Alone or in combination with other antihypertensive agents (especially thiazide diuretics) for the treatment of hypertension. Treatment of CHF following MI to decrease risk of CV death and decrease the risk of failure-related hospitalization and progression to severe or resistant heart failure.

Contraindications: Lactation.

Precautions: Geriatric patients may manifest higher peak blood levels of ramiprilat.

R

Route/Dosage
- **Capsules**

Hypertension.
Initial: 2.5 mg once daily in patients not taking a diuretic; **maintenance:** 2.5–20 mg/day as a single dose or two equally divided doses. *Patients taking diuretics or who have a C_{CR} less than 40 mL/min/1.73 m²: initially 1.25 mg/day; dose may then be increased to a maximum of 5 mg/day.*

CHF following MI.
Initial: 2.5 mg b.i.d. Patients intolerant of this dose may be started on 1.25 mg b.i.d. The target maintenance dose is 5 mg b.i.d.

How Supplied: *Capsule:* 1.25 mg, 2.5 mg, 5 mg, 10 mg

Side Effects: *CV:* Hypotension, chest pain, palpitations, angina pectoris, orthostatic hypotension, *MI, CVA, arrhythmias.* *GI:* N&V, abdominal pain, diarrhea, dysgeusia, anorexia, constipation, dry mouth, dyspepsia, enzyme changes suggesting pancreatitis, dysphagia, gastroenteritis, increased salivation. *CNS:* Headache, dizziness, fatigue, insomnia, sleep disturbances, somnolence, depression, nervousness, malaise, vertigo, anxiety, amnesia, *convulsions,* tremor. *Respiratory:* Cough, dyspnea, URI, asthma, *bronchospasm.* *Hematologic:* Leukopenia, anemia, eosinophilia. Rarely, decreases in hemoglobin or hematocrit. *Dermatologic:* Diaphoresis, photosensitivity, pruritus, rash, dermatitis, purpura, alopecia, erythema multiforme, urticaria. *Body as a whole:* Paresthesias, angioedema, asthenia, syncope, fever, muscle cramps, myalgia, arthralgia, arthritis, neuralgia, neuropathy, influenza, edema. *Miscellaneous:* Impotence, tinnitus, hearing loss, vision disturbances, epistaxis, weight gain, proteinuria, angioneurotic edema, edema, flu syndrome.

EMS CONSIDERATIONS
None.

Ranitidine bismuth citrate
(rah-NIH-tih-deen BIS-muth)

Pregnancy Class: C, when used with clarithromycin.
Tritec **(Rx)**
Classification: Histamine H_2 antagonist/treatment for H. pylori

Mechanism of Action: A complex of ranitidine and bismuth citrate which is freely soluble in water; solubility decreases as pH is decreased. The complex is more soluble than either ranitidine or bismuth citrate given separately. Is believed the greater solubility of the complex facilitates penetration of the drug into the mucous layer that protects the epithelial cells in the GI mucosa.

Uses: In combination with clarithromycin for treatment of active duodenal ulcers associated with *Helicobacter pylori* infections. *NOTE:* Ranitidine bismuth citrate should not be prescribed alone for the treatment of active duodenal ulcer.

Contraindications: Hypersensitivity to the complex or any of its ingredients. Hangover. Use in those with a history of acute porphyria or in those with a C_{CR} less than 25 mL/min.

Precautions: Use with caution during lactation. Safety and efficacy of ranitidine bismuth citrate plus clarithromycin in pediatric patients have not been determined.

Route/Dosage
- **Tablets**

Eradication of H. pylori *infection.*
Ranitidine bismuth citrate: 400 mg b.i.d. for 4 weeks. *Clarithromycin:* 500 mg t.i.d. for the first 2 weeks of therapy.

How Supplied: *Tablet:* 400 mg

Side Effects: See also side effects for *Ranitidine.* *GI:* N&V, diarrhea, constipation, abdominal discomfort, gastric pain. *CNS:* Headache, dizziness, sleep disorder, tremors (rare). *Hypersensitivity:* Rash, anaphylaxis (rare). *Miscellaneous:* Pruritus, gynecologic problems, taste disturbance, chest symptoms, transient changes in liver enzymes.

Drug Interactions
Antacids / Possible ↓ plasma levels of ranitidine and bismuth

Clarithromycin / ↑ Plasma levels of ranitidine and bismuth

EMS CONSIDERATIONS
None.

Ranitidine hydrochloride
(rah-NIH-tih-deen)

Pregnancy Class: B
Zantac, Zantac Efferdose, Zantac GELdose Capsules **(Rx)** Zantac 75 **(OTC)**

Classification: H_2 receptor antagonist

Mechanism of Action: Competitively inhibits gastric acid secretion by blocking the effect of histamine on histamine H_2 receptors. Both daytime and nocturnal basal gastric acid secretion, as well as food- and pentagastrin-stimulated gastric acid are inhibited.

Onset of Action: Peak effect: PO: 1–3 hr; **IM, IV:** 15 min.

Duration of Action: Nocturnal: 13 hr; **basal:** 4hr.

Uses: Short-term (4–8 weeks) and maintenance treatment of duodenal ulcer. Pathologic hypersecretory conditions such as Zollinger-Ellison syndrome and systemic mastocytosis. Short-term treatment of active, benign gastric ulcers. Maintenance of healing of gastric ulcers. Gastroesophageal reflux disease, including erosive esophagitis. Maintenance of healing of erosive esophagitis. *Investigational:* Prophylaxis of pulmonary aspiration of acid during anesthesia, prevent gastric damage from NSAIDs, prevent stress ulcers, prevent acute upper GI bleeding, as part of multidrug regimen to eradicate Helicobacter pylori.

Contraindications: Cirrhosis of the liver, impaired renal or hepatic function.

Precautions: Use with caution during lactation and in patients with decreased hepatic or renal function. Safety and efficacy not established in children.

Route/Dosage ――――――――
• **Capsules (Soft Gelatin), Effer-**

vescent Tablets and Granules, Syrup, Tablets

Duodenal ulcer, short-term.
Adults: 150 mg b.i.d. or 300 mg at bedtime to heal ulcer, although 100 mg b.i.d. will inhibit acid secretion and may be as effective as the higher dose. **Maintenance:** 150 mg at bedtime.

Pathologic hypersecretory conditions.
Adults: 150 mg b.i.d. (up to 6 g/day has been used in severe cases).

Benign gastric ulcer.
Adults: 150 mg b.i.d. for active ulcer.
Maintenance: 150 mg at bedtime

Gastroesophageal reflux disease.
Adults: 150 mg b.i.d.

Erosive esophagitis.
Adults: 150 mg q.i.d.

Maintenenace of healing of erosive esophagitis.
Adults: 150 mg b.i.d.

• **IM, IV**

Treatment and maintenance for duodenal ulcer, hypersecretory conditions, gastroesophageal reflux.
Adults, IM: 50 mg q 6–8 hr. **Intermittent IV injection or infusion:** 50 mg q 6–8 hr, not to exceed 400 mg/day. **Continuous IV infusion:** 6.25 mg/hr.

Zollinger-Ellison patients.
Continuous IV infusion: Dilute ranitidine in D5W to a concentration no greater than 2.5 mg/mL with an initial infusion rate of 1 mg/kg/hr. If after 4 hr the patient shows a gastric acid output of greater than 10 mEq/hr or if symptoms appear, increase the dose by 0.5-mg/kg/hr increments and measure the acid output. Doses up to 2.5 mg/kg/hr may be necessary.

How Supplied: *Capsule:* 150 mg, 300 mg; *Granule for reconstitution:* 150 mg; *Injection:* 1 mg/mL, 25 mg/mL; *Syrup:* 15 mg/mL; *Tablet:* 75 mg, 150 mg, 300 mg; *Tablet, effervescent:* 150 mg

Side Effects: *GI:* Constipation, N&V, diarrhea, abdominal pain, pancreatitis (rare). *CNS:* Headache, dizziness, malaise, insomnia, vertigo, confusion, anxiety, agitation, depres-

R

---

bold italic = life threatening side effect

sion, fatigue, somnolence, hallucinations. *CV:* Bradycardia or tachycardia, premature ventricular beats following rapid IV use (especially in patients predisposed to cardiac rhythm disturbances), *cardiac arrest.* *Hematologic:* Thrombocytopenia, granulocytopenia, leukopenia, pancytopenia (sometimes with marrow hypoplasia), *agranulocytosis, autoimmune hemolytic or aplastic anemia.* *Hepatic:* Hepatotoxicity, jaundice, hepatitis, increase in ALT. *Dermatologic:* Erythema multiforme, rash, alopecia. *Allergic:* *Bronchospasm, anaphylaxis,* angioneurotic edema (rare), rashes, fever, eosinophilia. *Other:* Arthralgia, gynecomastia, impotence, loss of libido, blurred vision, pain at injection site, local burning or itching following IV use.

Drug Interactions
Antacids / Antacids may ↓ the absorption of ranitidine
Diazepam / ↓ Effect of diazepam due to ↓ absorption from GI tract
Glipizide / Ranitidine ↑ effect of glipizide
Procainamide / Ranitidine ↓ excretion of procainamide → possible ↑ effect
Theophylline / Possible ↑ pharmacologic and toxicologic effects of theophylline
Warfarin / Ranitidine may ↑ hypoprothrombinemic effects of warfarin

EMS CONSIDERATIONS
See also *Histamine H_2 Antagonists.*

Rapacuronium bromide
(rap-ah-kyou-ROH-nee-um)
Pregnancy Class: C
Raplon **(Rx)**
Classification: Neuromuscular Blocking Agent

Mechanism of Action: Rapid onset (about 90 sec); dose-dependent duration (about 15 min using a dose of 1.5 mg/kg). The mean clinical duration (time from injection to return to 25% of control T_1) in adults was 24 min. Dose-related increases in HR and decreases in mean arterial pressure are seen in both adults and children.

Uses: Adjunct to general anesthesia to facilitate tracheal intubation; provide skeletal muscle relaxation during surgery.
Precautions: Use with caution during lactation. Safety in children less than 1 month of age has not been determined. Dosage has not been established for adolescents, aged 13–17 years.

Route/Dosage
• **IV only**
   Tracheal intubation.
Adults/elderly: 1.5 mg/kg for short surgical procedures.
   Intubation with cesarean section.
2.5 mg/kg with thiopental induction.
   Repeat dosing (bolus) in adults.
Following an intubating dose of 1.5 mg/kg, up to 3 maintenance doses of 0.5 mg/kg given at 25% recovery of control T_1 provided a mean clinical duration of 12–16 min under opioid/nitrous oxide/oxygen anesthesia. Duration of blockade increases with each additional dose.
   Children, under halothane anesthesia.
Ages, 1 month –12 years, initial: 2 mg/kg. Acceptable intubating conditions reached within 60 sec with maximum block at 90 seconds; duration was about 15 min. For patients, 13–17 years of age, consider physical maturity, height, and weight in determining the dose. The adult (1.5 mg/kg), pediatric (2 mg/kg), and cesarean section (2.5 mg/kg) doses may serve as a general guideline.
How Supplied: *Injection:* 100 mg, 200 mg
Side Effects: Listed are side effects with an incidence of 0.1% or greater. *CV:* Hypertension, tachycardia, bradycardia, extrasystoles, abnormal ECG, arrhythmia, cerebrovascular disorder, *ventricular fibrillation,* atrial fibrillation, ventricular tachycardia. *CNS:* Hypoestheisa, hemiparesis, hypertonia, prolonged neuromuscular blockade, prolonged emergence from anesthesia. *GI:* N&V, ileus, increased saliva. *Respiratory:* Hypoxia, increased airway pressure, hypoventilation, laryngismus, coughing, ap-

nea, respiratory depression, upper airway obstruction, **neonatal respiratory distress syndrome,** pneumothorax, pulmonary edema, respiratory insufficiency, stridor. *Dermatologic:* Erythematous rash, injection site reaction or pain, rash, urticaria, pruritus, increased sweating. *Hematologic:* Thrombosis, postoperative bleeding. *Musculoskeletal:* Myalgia. *GU:* Urinary retention, oliguria. *Miscellaneous:* Fever, rigors, back pain, hypothermia, chest pain, peripheral edema, pain.

EMS CONSIDERATIONS

See also *Neuromuscular Blocking Agents.*
Administration/Storage
IV 1. Compatible in solution with 0.9% NaCl, D5W, 5% dextrose in saline, sterile water for injection, lactated Ringer's, and bacteriostatic water for injection.
2. May store prepared solutions at room temperature; use within 24 hr of mixing.
3. Rapacuronium is physically incompatible when mixed with cefuroxime, danaparoid sodium, diazaepam, nitroglycerin, and thiopental.
4. Do not mix reconstituted rapacuronium, which has a pH of 4, with alkaline solutions (e.g., barbiturate solutions) in the same syringe or through the same IV infusion needle.
5. Do not use bacteriostatic water for injection in newborns as it contains benzyl alcohol.
6. Discard unused portion; single use only.
7. For obese patients, base the initial dose on actual body weight.

Repaglinide
(re-PAY-glin-eyed)
Pregnancy Class: C
Prandin **(Rx)**
Classification: Oral antidiabetic

Mechanism of Action: Lowers blood glucose by stimulating release of insulin from pancreas. Action depends on functioning beta cells in pancreatic islets. Drug closes ATP-dependent potassium channels in beta-cell membrane due to binding at sites. Blockade of potassium channel depolarizes beta cell which leads to opening of calcium channels. This causes calcium influx which induces insulin secretion.

Uses: Adjunct to diet and exercise in type 2 diabetes mellitus. In combination with metformin to lower blood glucose where hyperglycemia can not be controlled by exercise, diet, or either drug alone.

Contraindications: Lactation. Diabetic ketoacidosis, with or without coma. Type 1 diabetes.
Precautions: Use with caution in impaired hepatic function. Safety and efficacy have not been determined in children.

Route/Dosage
• **Tablets**
Type 2 diabetes mellitus.
Individualize dosage. **Initial:** In those not previously treated or whose HbA1-C is less than 8%, give 0.5 mg. For those previously treated or whose HbA1-C is 8% or more, give 1 or 2 mg before each meal. **Dose range:** 0.5–4 mg taken with meals. **Maximum daily dose:** 16 mg.
How Supplied: *Tablets:* 0.5 mg, 1 mg, 2 mg
Side Effects: *CV:* Chest pain, angina, ischemia. *GI:* Nausea, diarrhea, constipation, vomiting, dyspepsia. *Respiratory:* URI, sinusitis, rhinitis, bronchitis. *Musculoskeletal:* Arthralgia, back pain. *Miscellaneous:* Hypoglycemia, headache, paresthesia, chest pain, UTI, tooth disorder, allergy.
OD Overdose Management: *Symptoms:* Hypoglycemia. *Treatment:* Oral glucose. Also adjust drug dosage or meal patterns.
Drug Interactions: See *Antidiabetic Agents, Hypoglycemic Agents.*

EMS CONSIDERATIONS

See also *Antidiabetic Agents, Hypoglycemic Agents.*

R

---

bold italic = life threatening side effect

Respiratory Syncytial Virus Immune Globulin Intravenous (Human) (RSV-IGIV)

Pregnancy Class: C
(Rx)
Classification: Immunosuppressant

Mechanism of Action: Is an IgG containing neutralizing antibody to RSV. The immunoglobulin is obtained and purified from pooled adult human plasma that has been selected for high titers of neutralizing antibody against RSV. Each milliliter contains 50 mg of immunoglobulin, primarily IgG with trace amounts of IgA and IgM.

Uses: Prevention of serious lower respiratory tract infection caused by RSV in children less than 24 months old with bronchopulmonary dysplasia or a history of premature birth (less than 35 weeks gestation).

Contraindications: History of a severe prior reaction associated with administration of RSV-IGIV or other human immunoglobulin products. Patients with selective IgA deficiency who have the potential for developing antibodies to IgA and which could cause anaphylaxis or allergic reactions to blood products that contain IgA.

Route/Dosage
• **IV Injection**
Prevention of RSV infections.
1.5 mL/kg/hr for 15 min. If the clinical condition of the patient allows, the rate can be increased to 3 mL/kg/hr for the next 15-min period and, finally, increased to a maximum rate of 6 mL/kg/hr from 30 min to the end of the infusion. *Do not exceed these rates of infusion.*

How Supplied: *Injection:* 2,500 mg RSV Immunoglobulin.

Side Effects: Infusion of RSV-IGIV may cause fluid overload, especially in children with bronchopulmonary dysplasia. Aseptic meningitis syndrome has been reported within several hours to 2 days following RSV-IGIV treatment. Symptoms include severe headache, drowsiness, fever, photophobia, painful eye movements, muscle rigidity, nausea, and vomiting. The CSF shows pleocytosis, predominately granulocytic, as well as elevated protein levels.

Allergic: Hypotension, **anaphylaxis, angioneurotic edema,** respiratory distress. *CNS:* Fever, pyrexia, sleepiness. *Respiratory:* Respiratory distress, wheezing, rales, tachypnea, cough. *GI:* Vomiting, diarrhea, gagging, gastroenteritis. *CV:* Tachycardia, increased pulse rate, hypertension, hypotension, heart murmur. *Dermatologic:* Rash, pallor, cyanosis, eczema, cold and clammy skin. *Miscellaneous:* Hypoxia, hypoxemia, inflammation at injection site, edema, rhinorrhea, conjunctival hemorrhage.

Reactions similar to other immunoglobulins may occur as follows. *Body as a whole:* Dizziness, flushing, **immediate allergic, anaphylactic, or hypersensitivity reactions.** *CV:* Blood pressure changes, palpitations, chest tightness. *Miscellaneous:* Anxiety, dyspnea, abdominal cramps, pruritus, myalgia, arthralgia.

OD **Overdose Management:** *Symptoms:* Symptoms due to fluid volume overload. *Treatment:* Administration of diuretics and modification of the infusion rate.

Drug Interactions: Antibodies found in immunoglobulin products may interfere with the immune response to live virus vaccines, including those for mumps, rubella, and measles. Also, the antibody response to diphtheria, tetanus, pertussis, and *Haemophilus influenzae b* may be lower in RSV-IGIV recipients.

EMS CONSIDERATIONS
Administration/Storage
IV 1. Enter the single-use vial only once. Initiate infusion within 6 hr and complete within 12 hr of removal from the vial.
2. Do not use if the solution is turbid.
3. Give separately from other drugs or medications.
4. Give through an IV line (preferably

a separate line) using a constant infusion pump. Administration may be "piggy-backed" into an existing line if that line contains one of the following dextrose solutions (with or without NaCl): 2.5%, 5%, 10%, or 20% dextrose in water. If a preexisting line must be used, do not dilute RSV-IGIV more than 1:2 with one of the above solutions. Do not predilute RSV-IGIV before infusion.

5. Although use of filters is not necessary, an in-line filter with a pore size greater than 15 µm may be used.

6. Store the injection at 2°C–8°C (35.6°F–46.4°F). Do not freeze or shake (to prevent foaming).

Assessment

1. Document indications for therapy, any previous experiences with this drug and the outcome.

2. Note any IgA deficiency.

3. Assess VS, I&O, and cardiopulmonary status prior to infusion, before each rate increase, and thereafter at 30-min intervals until 30 min following infusion completion. Observe for fluid overload (increased HR, increased respiratory rate, rales, retractions), especially in infants with bronchopulmonary dysplasia. A loop diuretic (e.g., furosemide or bumetanide) should be available for management of fluid overload.

Reteplase recombinant
(REE-teh-place)
Pregnancy Class: C
Retavase **(Rx)**
Classification: Inhibitor of platelet aggregation

Mechanism of Action: Plasminogen activator that catalyzes the cleavage of endogenous plasminogen to generate plasmin. Plasmin, in turn, degrades the matrix of the thrombus, causing a thrombolytic effect. **t^1/$_2$:** 13 to 16 min.

Uses: In adults for the management of acute MI for improvement of ventricular function, reduction of the incidence of CHF, and reduction of mortality.

Contraindications: Active internal bleeding; history of CVA; recent intracranial or intraspinal surgery or trauma; intracranial neoplasm, arteriovenous malformation, or aneurysm; known bleeding diathesis; severe uncontrolled hypertension.

Precautions: Use with caution during lactation. Safety and efficacy have not been determined in children.

Route/Dosage ———————
• **IV only**
   Acute MI.
Adults: 10 + 10 unit double-bolus. Each bolus is given over 2 min, with the second bolus given 30 min after initiation of the first bolus injection.

How Supplied: *Kit:* 10.8 mg

Side Effects: *Bleeding disorders:* From internal bleeding sites, including intracranial, retroperitoneal, GI, GU, or respiratory. ***Hemorrhage may occur.*** From superficial bleeding sites, including venous cutdowns, arterial punctures, sites of recent surgery. *CV:* ***Cholesterol embolism,*** coronary thrombolysis resulting in arrhythmias associated with perfusion (no different from those seen in the ordinary course of acute MI), cardiogenic shock, sinus bradycardia, accelerated idioventricular rhythm, ventricular premature depolarizations, SVT, ventricular tachycardia, ***ventricular fibrillation,*** AV block, pulmonary edema, ***heart failure, cardiac arrest, recurrent ischemia, myocardial rupture, cardiac tamponade, venous thrombosis or embolism, electromechanical dissociation, mitral regurgitation, pericardial effusion, pericarditis.*** *Hypersensitivity:* Serious allergic reactions. *NOTE:* Many of the CV side effects listed are frequent sequelae of MI and may or may not be attributable to reteplase recombinant.

Drug Interactions: Use with abciximab, aspirin, dipyridamole, heparin, or vitamin K antagonists may increase the risk of bleeding.

EMS CONSIDERATIONS
See also *Alteplase.*

R

---

bold italic = life threatening side effect

Administration/Storage

IV 1. Initiate treatment as soon as possible after symptom onset.

2. Have available antiarrhythmic therapy for bradycardia and/or ventricular irritability.

3. Reconstitution is performed using the diluent, syringe, needle, and dispensing pin provided with the drug as follows:

• Remove the flip-cap from one vial of sterile water (preservative free), and, with the syringe provided, withdraw 10 mL of the sterile water.

• Open the package containing the dispensing pin. Remove the needle from the syringe and discard. Remove the protective cap from the spike end of the dispensing pin and connect the syringe to the dispensing pin. Remove the protective flip-cap from one vial of reteplase.

• Remove the protective cap from the spike end of the dispensing pin, and insert the spike into the vial of reteplase. Transfer the 10 mL of sterile water through the dispensing pin into the vial

• With the dispensing pin and syringe still attached to the vial, gently swirl the vial to dissolve the reteplase. *Do not shake.*

• Withdraw the 10 mL of reconstituted reteplase back into the syringe (a small amount will remain due to overfill).

• Detach the syringe from the dispensing pin, and attach the sterile 20-gauge needle provided. The solution is ready to administer.

Assessment: Note cardiopulmonary assessments and ECG.

Interventions

1. During administration, continuously monitor cardiac rhythm. Have medications available for management of arrhythmias.

2. Record VS every 15 min during infusion and for 2 hr following.

3. Administer first dose over 2 min and the second dose 30 min later if no serious bleeding is observed. In the event of any uncontrolled bleeding, terminate the heparin infusion and withhold the second dose.

4. Observe all puncture sites and areas for evidence of bleeding.

5. Assess for reperfusion reactions such as:

• Arrhythmias usually of short duration, which may include bradycardia or ventricular tachycardia

• Reduction of chest pain

• Return of elevated ST segment and smaller Q waves

Ribavirin and Interferon alfa-2b recombinant

(rye-bah-VYE-rin/in-ter-FEER-on)
Pregnancy Class: X
Rebetron **(Rx)**
Classification: Drug for chronic hepatitis C

Mechanism of Action: The mechanism of action of the combination in inhibiting the hepatitis C virus is not known.

Uses: Treatment of chronic hepatitis C in patients with compensated liver disease who have relapsed following alpha interferon therapy.

Contraindications: Pregnancy and in those who may become pregnant. Lactation. Hypersensitivity or history thereof to alpha interferons and/or ribavirin. Use in patients with autoimmune hepatitis.

Precautions: Use with extreme caution in those with pre-existing psychiatric disorders who report a history of severe depression. Use with caution if C_{CR} is less than 50 mL/min or in pre-existing cardiac disease. Safety and efficacy have not been determined in children less than 18 years of age.

Route/Dosage

• **Capsules (Rebetol), SC (Intron A)**

Chronic hepatitis C.

Adults, 75 kg or less: Rebetol: 2 x 200 mg capsules in the a.m. and 3 x 200 mg capsules in the p.m. Intron A: 3 million I.U. 3 times weekly SC. **Adults, more than 75 kg:** Rebetol: 3 x 200 mg capsules in the a.m. and 3 x 200 mg capsules in the p.m. Intron A: 3 million I.U. three times a week SC. Reduce the dose of Rebetol by 600 mg daily and Intron A by 1.5 million I.U. three times a week if the hemoglobin is less than 10 g/dL.

How Supplied: Combination packages containing ribavirin (Rebetol) capsules, 200 mg, and interferon alfa-2b recombinant (Introl A) injectable.

Side Effects: See individual drugs; selected treatment-emergent side effects follow. *Hematologic:* Anemia. *GI:* N&V, anorexia, dyspepsia. *CNS:* Depression, suicidal behavior, dizziness, insomnia, irritability, emotional lability, impaired concentration, nervousness. *Respiratory:* Dyspnea, pulmonary infiltrates, pneumonitis, pneumonia, sinusitis. *Musculoskeletal:* Myalgia, arthralgia, musculoskeletal pain. *Dermatologic:* Alopecia, rash, pruritus. *Body as a whole:* Headache, fatigue, rigors, fever, flu-like symptoms, asthenia, chest pain. *Miscellaneous:* Taste perversion, injection site inflammation or reaction.

Drug Interactions: See individual drugs.

EMS CONSIDERATIONS

None.

Rifabutin

(rif-ah-BYOU-tin)
Pregnancy Class: B
Mycobutin **(Rx)**
Classification: Antitubercular drug

Mechanism of Action: Inhibits DNA-dependent RNA polymerase in susceptible strains of *Escherichia coli* and *Bacillus subtilis*.

Uses: Prevention of disseminated *Mycobacterium avium* complex (MAC) disease in patients with advanced HIV infection.

Contraindications: Hypersensitivity to rifabutin or other rifamycins (e.g., rifampin). Use in active tuberculosis. Lactation.

Precautions: Safety and efficacy have not been determined in children, although the drug has been used in HIV-positive children.

Route/Dosage
• **Capsules**
Prophylaxis of MAC disease in patients with advanced HIV infection.
Adults: 300 mg/day.
How Supplied: *Capsule:* 150 mg
Side Effects: *GI:* Anorexia, abdominal pain, diarrhea, dyspepsia, eructation, flatulence, N&V, taste perversion. *Respiratory:* Chest pain, chest pressure or pain with dyspnea. *CNS:* Insomnia, *seizures*, paresthesia, aphasia, confusion. *Musculoskeletal:* Asthenia, myalgia, arthralgia, myositis. *Body as a whole:* Fever, headache, generalized pain, flu-like syndrome. *Dermatologic:* Rash, skin discoloration. *Hematologic:* Neutropenia, leukopenia, anemia, eosinophilia, thrombocytopenia. *Miscellaneous:* Discolored urine, nonspecific T wave changes on ECG, hepatitis, hemolysis, uveitis.

OD **Overdose Management:** *Symptoms:* Worsening of side effects. *Treatment:* Gastric lavage followed by instillation into the stomach of an activated charcoal slurry.

Drug Interactions: Rifabutin has liver enzyme-inducing properties and may be expected to have similar interactions as does rifampin. However, rifabutin is a less potent enzyme inducer than rifampin.
AZT / ↓ Steady-state plasma levels of AZT after repeated rifabutin dosing
Oral contraceptives / Rifabutin may ↓ the effectiveness of oral contraceptives

EMS CONSIDERATIONS

See also *Anti-Infectives*.

Rifampin

(rih-FAM-pin)
Pregnancy Class: C
Rifadin, Rimactane **(Rx)**
Classification: Primary antitubercular agent

Mechanism of Action: Semisynthetic antibiotic derived from *Streptomyces mediterranei*. Suppresses RNA

R

synthesis by binding to the beta subunit of DNA-dependent RNA polymerase. This prevents attachment of the enzyme to DNA and blockade of RNA transcription. Both bacteriostatic and bactericidal; most active against rapidly replicating organisms.

Uses: All types of tuberculosis. Must be used in conjunction with at least one other tuberculostatic drug (such as isoniazid, ethambutol, pyrazinamide) but is the drug of choice for retreatment. Also for treatment of asymptomatic meningococcal carriers to eliminate *Neisseria meningitidis. Investigational:* Used in combination for infections due to *Staphylococcus aureus* and *S. epidermidis* (endocarditis, osteomyelitis, prostatitis); Legionnaire's disease; in combination with dapsone for leprosy; prophylaxis of meningitis due to *Haemophilus influenzae* and gram-negative bacteremia in infants.

Contraindications: Hypersensitivity; not recommended for intermittent therapy.

Precautions: Safe use during lactation has not been established. Safety and effectiveness not determined in children less than 5 years of age. Use with extreme caution in patients with hepatic dysfunction.

Route/Dosage ⸻
• **Capsules, IV**
  Pulmonary tuberculosis.
  Adults: Single dose of 600 mg/day; **children over 5 years:** 10–20 mg/kg/day, not to exceed 600 mg/day.
  Meningococcal carriers.
  Adults: 600 mg b.i.d. for 2 days; **children:** 10–20 mg/kg q 12 hr for four doses, not to exceed 600 mg/day.

How Supplied: *Capsule:* 150 mg, 300 mg; *Powder for injection:* 600 mg

Side Effects: *GI:* N&V, diarrhea, anorexia, gas, pseudomembranous colitis, pancreatitis, sore mouth and tongue, cramps, heartburn, flatulence. *CNS:* Headache, drowsiness, fatigue, ataxia, dizziness, confusion, generalized numbness, fever, diffi-culty in concentrating. *Hepatic:* Jaundice, hepatitis. Increases in AST, ALT, bilirubin, alkaline phosphatase. *Hematologic:* Thrombocytopenia, eosinophilia, hemolysis, leukopenia, **hemolytic anemia.** *Allergic:* Flu-like symptoms, dyspnea, wheezing, SOB, purpura, pruritus, urticaria, skin rashes, sore mouth and tongue, conjunctivitis. *Renal:* Hematuria, hemoglobinuria, renal insufficiency, acute renal failure. *Miscellaneous:* Visual disturbances, muscle weakness or pain, arthralgia, decreased BP, osteomalacia, menstrual disturbances, edema of face and extremities, adrenocortical insufficiency, increases in BUN and serum uric acid. *NOTE:* Body fluids and feces may be red-orange.

OD **Overdose Management:** *Symptoms:* Shortly after ingestion, N&V, and lethargy will occur. Followed by severe hepatic involvement (liver enlargement with tenderness, increased direct and total bilirubin, change in hepatic enzymes) with unconsciousness. Also, brownish red or orange discoloration of urine, saliva, tears, sweat, skin, and feces. *Treatment:* Gastric lavage followed by activated charcoal slurry introduced into the stomach. Antiemetics to control N&V. Forced diuresis to enhance excretion. If hepatic function is seriously impaired, bile drainage may be required. Extracorporeal hemodialysis may be necessary.

Drug Interactions
Acetaminophen / ↓ Effect of acetaminophen due to ↑ breakdown by liver
Aminophylline / ↓ Effect of aminophylline due to ↑ breakdown by liver
Anticoagulants, oral / ↓ Effect of anticoagulants due to ↑ breakdown by liver
Antidiabetics, oral / ↓ Effect of oral antidiabetic due to ↑ breakdown by liver
Barbiturates / ↓ Effect of barbiturates due to ↑ breakdown by liver
Benzodiazepines / ↓ Effect of benzodiazepines due to ↑ breakdown by liver

Beta-adrenergic blocking agents / ↓ Effect of beta-blocking agents due to ↑ breakdown by liver

Chloramphenicol / ↓ Effect of chloramphenicol due to ↑ breakdown by liver

Clofibrate / ↓ Effect of clofibrate due to ↑ breakdown by liver

Contraceptives, oral / ↓ Effect of oral contraceptives due to ↑ breakdown by liver

Corticosteroids / ↓ Effect of corticosteroids due to ↑ breakdown by liver

Cyclosporine / ↓ Effect of cyclosporine due to ↑ breakdown by liver

Digitoxin / ↓ Effect of digitoxin due to ↑ breakdown by liver

Digoxin / ↓ Serum levels of digoxin

Disopyramide / ↓ Effect of disopyramide due to ↑ breakdown by liver

Estrogens / ↓ Effect of estrogens due to ↑ breakdown by liver

Halothane / ↑ Risk of hepatotoxicity and hepatic encephalopathy

Hydantoins / ↓ Effect of hydantoins due to ↑ breakdown by liver

Isoniazid / ↑ Risk of hepatotoxicity

Ketoconazole / ↓ Effect of either ketoconazole or rifampin

Methadone / ↓ Effect of methadone due to ↑ breakdown by liver

Mexiletine / ↓ Effect of mexiletine due to ↑ breakdown by liver

Quinidine / ↓ Effect of quinidine due to ↑ breakdown by liver

Sulfones / ↓ Effect of sulfones due to ↑ breakdown by liver

Theophylline / ↓ Effect of theophylline due to ↑ breakdown by liver

Tocainide / ↓ Effect of tocainide due to ↑ breakdown by liver

Verapamil / ↓ Effect of verapamil due to ↑ breakdown by liver

EMS CONSIDERATIONS
See also *Anti-Infectives*.

———COMBINATION DRUG———
Rifampin and Isoniazid
(rih-FAM-pin/eye-sNYE-ah-zid)
Pregnancy Class: C
Rifamate, Rimactane/INH Dual Pack
(Rx)

Classification: Antitubercular drug combination

Uses: Pulmonary tuberculosis following completion of initial therapy. Concomitant treatment with pyridoxine is recommended in malnourished patients, in those predisposed to neuropathy (e.g., alcoholics, diabetics), and in adolescents.

Contraindications: To treat meningococcal infections or asymptomatic carriers of *Neisseria meningitidis* to eliminate meningococci from the nasopharynx. In those who have previous isoniazid-induced hepatic injury or who have had severe side effects to isoniazid.

Precautions: Use with caution in impaired liver function, as rifampin and isoniazid can cause liver dysfunction and fatal hepatitis, respectively. Use with caution, if at all, during lactation.

Route/Dosage
• **Capsules**
  Pulmonary tuberculosis.
Adults: Two capsules once daily.
How Supplied: Each capsule contains the following antituberculosis drugs: rifampin, 300 mg, and isoniazid, 150 mg.
Side Effects: See individual entries for *Rifampin* and *Isoniazid*.

EMS CONSIDERATIONS
None.

———COMBINATION DRUG———
Rifampin, Isoniazid, and Pyrazinamide
(rih-FAM-pin/eye-soh-NYE-ah-zid/pie-rah-ZIN-ah-myd)
Pregnancy Class: C
Rifater **(Rx)**
Classification: Antitubercular drug combination

Uses: Initial phase of the short-course (2-month) treatment of pulmonary tuberculosis. Either streptomycin or ethambutol may be added unless the likelihood of resistance to isoniazid or rifampin is low. Concomitant treatment with pyridoxine

R

---
bold italic = life threatening side effect

is recommended in malnourished patient's, in those predisposed to neuropathy (e.g., alcoholics, diabetics), and in adolescents. The 2-month treatment with Rifater is followed by a 4-month course of therapy with rifampin and isoniazid (Rifamate).

Contraindications: Hypersensitivity to any of the components. Severe hepatic damage, acute gout. Lactation.

Precautions: Use with caution in impaired liver function, as rifampin and isoniazid can cause liver dysfunction and fatal hepatitis, respectively. Use with caution in diabetes mellitus. Safety and efficacy have not been determined in children less than 15 years of age.

Route/Dosage
* **Tablets**
  Short-course treatment of pulmonary tuberculosis.
Patients weighing less than 44 kg: 4 tablets/day given at the same time. **Patients weighing 45–54 kg:** 5 tablets/day given at the same time. **Patients weighing more than 55 kg:** 6 tablets/day given at the same time.

How Supplied: Each tablet contains the following antituberculosis drugs: rifampin, 120 mg; isoniazid, 50 mg; and pyrazinamide, 300 mg.

Side Effects: For side effects caused by isoniazid or rifampin, consult those drug entries. The side effects due to pyrazinamide follow. *Hepatic:* Hepatotoxicity, porphyria. *GI:* N&V, anorexia. *Hematologic:* Thrombocytopenia, sideroblastic anemia with erythroid hyperplasia, vacuolation of erythrocytes, and increased serum concentration. *Hypersensitivity:* Rashes, urticaria, pruritus. *Miscellaneous:* Hyperuricemia, gout, mild arthralgia and myalgia, fever, acne, photosensitivity, dysuria, interstitial nephritis.

EMS CONSIDERATIONS
None.

Rifapentine
(rih-fah-PEN-teen)

Pregnancy Class: C
Priftin **(Rx)**
Classification: Antituberculosis drug

Mechanism of Action: Similar activity to rifampin. Inhibits DNA–dependent RNA polymerase in susceptible strains of *Mycobacterium tuberculosis*, but not in mammalian cells. Is bactericidal against both intracellular and extracellular organisms.

Uses: Treatment of pulmonary tuberculosis. Must be used with at least one other antituberculosis drug.

Contraindications: Hypersensitivity to other rifamycins (e.g., rifampin or rifabutin). Lactation.

Precautions: Experience is limited in HIV-infected patients. Organisms resistant to other rifamycins are likely to be resistant to rifapentine. Use with caution in patients with abnormal liver tests or liver disease. Safety and efficacy have not been determined in children less than 12 years of age.

Route/Dosage
* **Tablets**
  Tuberculosis, intensive phase.
600 mg (four 150 mg tablets) twice weekly with an interval of 72 hr or more between doses continued for 2 months.
  Tuberculosis, continuation phase
Continue rifapentine therapy once weekly for 4 months in combination with isoniazid or another antituberculosis drug. If the patient is still sputum-smear- or culture-positive, if resistant organisms are present, or if the patient is HIV-positive, follow ATS/CDC treatment guidelines.

How Supplied: *Tablets:* 150 mg

Side Effects: Side effects listed occurred in 1% or more of patients and were seen when rifapentine was used in combination with other antituberculosis drugs (e.g., isoniazid, pyrazinamide, ethambutol). *GI:* N&V, dyspepsia, diarrhea, hemoptysis. *CNS:* Anorexia, headache, dizziness. *GU:* Pyuria, proteinuria, hematuria, urinary casts. *Dermatologic:* Rash, acne, maculopapular rash. *Hematologic:* Neutropenia, lymphopenia, anemia, leukopenia, thrombocytosis. *Miscellaneous:* Hyperuricemia (probably due to pyrizinamide), hypertension, pruritus, arthralgia, pain, red coloration of body tissues and fluids.

Drug Interactions

Cytochrome P450 / Rifapentine is an inducer of certain cytochromes P450 → reduced activity of a number of drugs (See *Rifampin*). Dosage adjustment may be required

Indinavir / Three-fold ↑ in clearance of indinavir.

EMS CONSIDERATIONS
None.

Riluzole
(RIL-you-zohl)
Pregnancy Class: C
Rilutek **(Rx)**
Classification: Drug for amyotrophic lateral sclerosis

Mechanism of Action: Mechanism not known. Possible effects include (a) inhibition of glutamate release, (b) inactivation of voltage-dependent sodium channels, and (c) interference with intracellular events that follow transmitter binding at excitatory amino acid receptors.

Uses: Treatment of patients with ALS; the drug extends both survival and time to tracheostomy.

Contraindications: Lactation.

Precautions: Use with caution in hepatic and renal impairment due to decreased excretion and higher plasma levels. Use with caution in the elderly, as age-related changes in renal and hepatic function may cause a decreased clearance. Clearance of riluzole in Japanese patients is 50% lower compared with Caucasians; clearance may also be lower in women. Safety and efficacy have not been determined in children.

Route/Dosage
• **Tablets**
Treatment of ALS.
50 mg q 12 hr. Higher daily doses will not increase the beneficial effect but

will increase the incidence of side effects.

How Supplied: *Tablets:* 50 mg.

Side Effects: Side effects listed occurred at a frequency of 0.1% or more. *GI:* N&V, diarrhea, anorexia, abdominal pain, dyspepsia, flatulence, dry mouth, stomatitis, tooth disorder, oral moniliasis, dysphagia, constipation, increased appetite, intestinal obstruction, fecal impaction, *GI hemorrhage,* GI ulceration, gastritis, fecal incontinence, jaundice, hepatitis, glossitis, gum hemorrhage, pancreatitis, tenesmus, esophageal stenosis. *Body as a whole:* Asthenia, malaise, weight loss or gain, peripheral edema, flu syndrome, hostility, abscess, *sepsis,* photosensitivity reaction, cellulitis, facial edema, hernia, peritonitis, reaction at injection site, chills, *attempted suicide,* enlarged abdomen, neoplasm. *CNS:* Dizziness (more common in women), vertigo, somnolence, circumoral paresthesia, headache, aggravation reaction, hypertonia, depression, insomnia, agitation, tremor, hallucination, personality disorders, abnormal thinking, coma, paranoid reaction, manic reaction, ataxia, extrapyramidal syndrome, hypokinesis, emotional lability, delusions, apathy, hypesthesia, incoordination, confusion, *convulsion,* amnesia, increased libido, stupor subdural hematoma, abnormal gait, delirium, depersonalization, facial paralysis, hemiplegia, decreased libido. *CV:* Hypertension, tachycardia, phlebitis, palpitation, postural hypotension, *heart arrest, heart failure,* syncope, hypotension, migraine, peripheral vascular disease, angina pectoris, *MI,* ventricular extrasystoles, *cerebral hemorrhage,* atrial fibrillation, bundle branch block, CHF, pericarditis, lower extremity embolus, *myocardial ischemia, shock.* *Hematologic:* Neutropenia, anemia, leukocytosis, leukopenia, ecchymosis. *Respiratory:* Decreased lung function, pneumonia, rhinitis, increased cough, sinusitis, apnea, bronchitis, dyspnea, respiratory dis-

R

bold italic = life threatening side effect

order, increased sputum, hiccup, pleural disorder, asthma, epistaxis, hemoptysis, yawn, hyperventilation, lung edema, hypoventilation, *lung carcinoma,* hypoxia, laryngitis, pleural effusion, pneumothorax, respiratory moniliasis, stridor. *Musculoskeletal:* Arthralgia, back pain, leg cramps, dysarthria, myoclonus, arthrosis, myasthenia, *bone neoplasm. GU:* Urinary retention, urinary urgency, urine abnormality, urinary incontinence, kidney calculus, hematuria, impotence, *prostate carcinoma,* kidney pain, metrorrhagia, priapism. *Dermatologic:* Pruritus, eczema, alopecia, exfoliative dermatitis, skin ulceration, urticaria, psoriasis, seborrhea, skin disorder, fungal dermatitis. *Metabolic:* Gout, respiratory acidosis, edema, thirst, hypokalemia, hyponatremia. *Miscellaneous:* Accidental or intentional injury, *death,* diabetes mellitus, thyroid neoplasia, amblyopia, ophthalmitis.

Drug Interactions

Amitriptyline / ↓ Elimination of riluzole → higher plasma levels

Caffeine / ↓ Elimination of riluzole → higher plasma levels

Charcoal-broiled foods / ↑ Elimination of riluzole → lower plasma levels

Omeprazole / ↑ Elimination of riluzole → lower plasma levels

Quinolones / ↓ Elimination of riluzole → higher plasma levels

Rifampin / ↑ Elimination of riluzole → lower plasma levels

Smoking (cigarettes) / ↑ Elimination of riluzole → lower plasma levels

Theophyllines / ↓ Elimination of riluzole → higher plasma levels

EMS CONSIDERATIONS

None.

Rimanatadine hydrochloride

(rih-MAN-tih-deen)

Pregnancy Class: C

Flumadine **(Rx)**

Classification: Antiviral agent

Mechanism of Action: May act early in the viral replication cycle, possibly by inhibiting the uncoating of the virus. A virus protein specified by the virion M_2 gene may play an important role in the inhibition of the influenza A virus by rimantadine. Has little or no activity against influenza B virus.

Uses: In adults for prophylaxis and treatment of illness caused by strains of influenza A virus. In children for prophylaxis against influenza A virus.

Contraindications: Hypersensitivity to amantadine, rimantadine, or other drugs in the adamantine class. Lactation.

Precautions: Use with caution in patients with renal or hepatic insufficiency. An increased incidence of seizures is possible in patients with a history of epilepsy who have received amantadine. Influenza A virus strains resistant to rimantadine can emerge during treatment and be transmitted, causing symptoms of influenza. Safety and efficacy of rimantadine in the treatment of symptomatic influenza infections in children have not been established. Safety and efficacy for prophylaxis of infections have not been determined in children less than 1 year of age. The incidence of side effects in geriatric patients is higher than in other patients.

Route/Dosage

• **Syrup, Tablets**

Prophylaxis.

Adults and children over 10 years of age: 100 mg b.i.d. In patients with severe hepatic dysfunction (C_{CR} < 10 mL/min) and in elderly nursing home patients, reduce the dose to 100 mg/day. **Children, less than 10 years of age:** 5 mg/kg once daily, not to exceed a total dose of 150 mg/day.

Treatment.

Adults: 100 mg b.i.d. In patients with severe hepatic dysfunction and in elderly nursing home patients, reduce the dose to 100 mg/day.

How Supplied: *Syrup:* 50 mg/5 mL; *Tablet:* 100 mg

Side Effects: GI and CNS side effects are the most common. *GI:* N&V, anorexia, dry mouth, abdominal pain, diarrhea, dyspepsia, constipation, dysphagia, stomatitis. *CNS:* Insomnia, dizziness, headache, nervousness, fatigue, asthenia, impairment of concentration, ataxia, somnolence, agitation, depression, gait abnormality, euphoria, hyperkinesia, tremor, hallucinations, confusion, ***convulsions,*** agitation, diaphoresis, hypesthesia. *Respiratory:* Dyspnea, ***bronchospasm,*** cough. *CV:* Pallor, palpitation, hypertension, ***cerebrovascular disorder, cardiac failure,*** pedal edema, heart block, tachycardia, syncope. *Miscellaneous:* Tinnitus, taste loss or change, parosmia, eye pain, rash, nonpuerperal lactation, increased lacrimation, increased frequency of micturition, fever, rigors.

OD Overdose Management: *Symptoms:* Extensions of side effects including the possibility of agitation, hallucinations, ***cardiac arrhythmias, and death.*** *Treatment:* Supportive therapy. IV physostigmine at doses of 1–2 mg IV in adults and 0.5 mg in children, not to exceed 2 mg/hr, has been reported to be beneficial in treating overdose for amantadine (a related drug).

Drug Interactions
Acetaminophen / ↓ Peak concentration and area under the curve for rimantadine
Aspirin / ↓ Peak plasma levels and area under the curve for rimantadine
Cimetidine / ↓ Clearance of rimantadine

EMS CONSIDERATIONS
See also *Antiviral Drugs.*

Rimexolone
(rih-MEX-ah-lohn)
Pregnancy Class: C
Vexol **(Rx)**
Classification: Corticosteroid, ophthalmic

Uses: Treatment of postoperative inflammation following ocular surgery. Treatment of anterior uveitis.

Contraindications: Use in epithelial herpes simplex keratitis; vaccinia, varicella, and most other viral infections of the cornea or conjunctiva; mycobacterial infections of the eye; fungal infections of the eye; any acute, untreated eye infection.

Precautions: Acute purulent ocular infections may be masked if used in bacterial, fungal, or viral eye infections. Safety and efficacy have not been determined in children.

Route/Dosage ————————
• **Ophthalmic Suspension**
Postoperative inflammation following ocular surgery.
Adults: 1–2 gtt in the conjunctival sac(s) q.i.d. beginning 24 hr after surgery and continuing for 2 weeks.
Anterior uveitis.
Adults: 1–2 gtt in the conjunctival sac(s) q hr during waking hours during the first week and 1 gtt q 2 hr during the second week; then, taper the dose until uveitis is resolved.

How Supplied: *Ophthalmic Suspension:* 1%

Side Effects: *Ophthalmic:* Elevated IOP, blurred vision, discharge, discomfort, ocular pain, foreign body sensation, hyperemia, pruritus, sticky sensation, increased fibrin, dry eye, conjunctival edema, corneal staining, keratitis, tearing, photophobia, edema, irritation, corneal ulcer, browache, lid margin crusting, corneal edema, infiltrate, corneal erosion. *Respiratory:* Pharyngitis, rhinitis. *Miscellaneous:* Headache, taste perversion. *Prolonged use:* Ocular hypertension, glaucoma, optic nerve damage, defects in visual acuity and visual fields, posterior subcapsular formation, secondary ocular infections, perforation of the globe where there is thinning of the cornea or sclera.

EMS CONSIDERATIONS
None.

R

Risedronate sodium
(rih-SEH-droh-nayt)
Pregnancy Class: C
Actonel **(Rx)**
Classification: Biphosphonate for Paget's disease

Mechanism of Action: Inhibits osteoclasts, thus leading to decreased bone resorption.

Uses: Treatment of Paget's disease in those who (1) have a serum alkaline phosphatase level at least two times the upper limit of normal, (2) are symptomatic, or (3) are at risk for future complications from the disease.

Contraindications: Use in those with C_{CR} less than 30 mL/min. Hypocalcemia. Lactation.

Precautions: May cause upper GI disorders, including dysphagia, esophagitis, esophageal ulcer, or gastric ulcer. Use with caution in those with a history of UGI disorders. Safety and efficacy have not been determined in children.

Route/Dosage
• **Tablets**
   Treat Paget's disease.
Adults: 30 mg once daily for 2 months.

How Supplied: *Tablets:* 30 mg

Side Effects: *GI:* Diarrhea, abdominal pain, nausea, constipation, belching, colitis. *CNS:* Headache, dizziness. *Body as a whole:* Flu syndrome, chest pain, asthenia, neoplasm. *Musculoskeletal:* Arthralgia, bone pain, leg cramps, myasthenia. *Respiratory:* Sinusitis, bronchitis. *Ophthalmic:* Amblyopia, dry eye. *Miscellaneous:* Peripheral edema, skin rash, tinnitus.

OD Overdose Management: *Symptoms:* Hypocalemia. *Treatment:* Gastric lavage to remove unabsorbed drug. Milk or antacids to bind risedronate. IV calcium.

Drug Interactions
Antacids, calcium-containing / ↓ Absorption of risedronate
Bone imaging agents / Risedronate interferes with these agents
Calcium / ↓ Absorption of risedronate

NSAIDs / Possible additive GI side effects

EMS CONSIDERATIONS
None.

Risperidone
(ris-PAIR-ih-dohn)
Pregnancy Class: C
Risperdal **(Rx)**
Classification: Antipsychotic

Mechanism of Action: Mechanism may be due to a combination of antagonism of dopamine (D_2) and serotonin (5-HT_2) receptors. Also has high affinity for the alpha-1, alpha-2, and histamine-1 receptors.

Uses: Treatment of psychotic disorders.

Contraindications: Lactation.

Precautions: Use with caution in patients with known CV disease (including history of MI or ischemia, heart failure, conduction abnormalities), cerebrovascular disease, and conditions that predispose the patient to hypotension (e.g., dehydration, hypovolemia, use of antihypertensive drugs). Use with caution in patients who will be exposed to extreme heat or when taken with other CNS drugs or alcohol. The effectiveness of risperidone for more than 6–8 weeks has not been studied. Safety and effectiveness have not been established for children.

Route/Dosage
• **Oral Solution, Tablets**
   Antipsychotic.
Adults, initial: 1 mg b.i.d. Once daily dosing can also be used. Can be increased by 1 mg b.i.d. on the second and third days, as tolerated, to reach a dose of 3 mg b.i.d. by the third day. Further increases in dose should occur at intervals of about 1 week. **Maximal effect:** 4–6 mg/day. Doses greater than 6 mg/day were not shown to be more effective and were associated with greater incidence of side effects. Safety of doses greater than 16 mg/day have not been studied. **Maintenance:** Use lowest dose that will maintain remis-

sion. The initial dose is 0.5 mg b.i.d. for patients who are elderly or debilitated, those with severe renal or hepatic impairment, and those predisposed to hypotension or in whom hypotension would pose a risk. Dosage increases in these patients should be in increments of 0.5 mg b.i.d. Dosage increases above 1.5 mg b.i.d. should occur at intervals of about 1 week.

How Supplied: *Solution:* 1 mg/mL; *Tablet:* 1 mg, 2 mg, 3 mg, 4 mg

Side Effects: *Neuroleptic malignant syndrome:* Hyperpyrexia, muscle rigidity, altered mental status, autonomic instability (i.e., irregular pulse or BP, tachycardia, diaphoresis, cardiac dysrhythmia), elevated CPK, rhabdomyolysis, *acute renal failure, death. CNS:* Tardive dyskinesia (especially in geriatric patients), somnolence, insomnia, agitation, anxiety, aggressive reaction, extrapyramidal symptoms, headache, dizziness, increased dream activity, decreased sexual desire, nervousness, impaired concentration, depression, apathy, catatonia, euphoria, increased libido, amnesia, increased duration of sleep, dysarthria, vertigo, stupor, paresthesia, confusion. *GI:* Constipation, nausea, dyspepsia, vomiting, abdominal pain, increased or decreased salivation, toothache, anorexia, flatulence, diarrhea, increased appetite, stomatitis, melena, dysphagia, hemorrhoids, gastritis. *CV:* Prolongation of the QT interval that might lead to *torsades de pointes,*. Orthostatic hypotension, tachycardia, palpitation, hypertension or hypotension, *AV block, MI. Respiratory:* Rhinitis, coughing, URI, sinusitis, pharyngitis, dyspnea. *Body as a whole:* Arthralgia, back pain, chest pain, fever, fatigue, rigors, malaise, edema, flu-like symptoms, increase or decrease in weight. *Hematologic:* Purpura, anemia, hypochromic anemia. *GU:* Polyuria, polydipsia, urinary incontinence, hematuria, dysuria, menorrhagia, orgasmic dysfunction, dry vagina, erectile dysfunction, nonpuerperal lactation, amenorrhea, female breast pain, leukorrhea, mastitis, dysmenorrhea, female perineal pain, intermenstrual bleeding, *vaginal hemorrhage,* failure to ejaculate. *Dermatologic:* Rash, dry skin, seborrhea, increased pigmentation, increased or decreased sweating, acne, alopecia, hyperkeratosis, pruritus, skin exfoliation. *Ophthalmic:* Abnormal vision, abnormal accommodation, xerophthalmia. *Miscellaneous:* Increased prolactin, photosensitivity, diabetes mellitus, thirst, myalgia, epistaxis.

OD Overdose Management: *Symptoms:* Exaggeration of known effects, especially drowsiness, sedation, tachycardia, hypotension, and extrapyramidal symptoms. *Treatment:* Establish and secure airway, and ensure adequate oxygenation and ventilation. Follow gastric lavage with activated charcoal and a laxative. Monitor CV system, including continuous ECG readings. Provide general supportive measures. Treat hypotension and circulatory collapse with IV fluids or sympathomimetic drugs; however, do not use epinephrine and dopamine, as beta stimulation may worsen hypotension due to risperidone-induced alpha blockade. Anticholinergic drugs can be given for severe extrapyramidal symptoms.

Drug Interactions

Carbamazepine / ↑ Clearance of risperidone following chronic use of carbamazepine

Clozapine / ↓ Clearance of risperidone following chronic use of clozapine

Levodopa / Risperidone antagonizes the effects of levodopa and dopamine agonists

EMS CONSIDERATIONS

See also *Antipsychotic Drugs.*

Ritodrine hydrochloride
(RYE-toe-dreen)
Pregnancy Class: B

R

Ritodrine HCl in 5% Dextrose, Yutopar
(Rx)
Classification: Uterine relaxant

Mechanism of Action: Stimulates beta-2 receptors of smooth muscle of the uterus, which results in inhibition of uterine contractility. May also directly inhibit the actin-myosin interaction.

Onset of Action: IV: 5 min.

Uses: Management of preterm labor in selected patients after week 20 of gestation. When indicated, initiate therapy as early as possible after diagnosis. However, decision to use ritodrine should include determination of fetal maturity.

Contraindications: Before week 20 of pregnancy and when continuation of pregnancy is hazardous to mother (e.g., eclampsia, severe preeclampsia, intrauterine fetal death, antepartum hemorrhage, pulmonary hypertension, chorioamnionitis, and maternal hyperthyroidism, cardiac disease or uncontrolled diabetes mellitus). Also, medical conditions (e.g., uncontrolled hypertension, pheochromocytoma, bronchial asthma, hypovolemia, cardiac arrhythmias due to tachycardia or digitalis toxicity) that would be aggravated by beta-adrenergic agonists. Use in diabetics.

Precautions: Maternal pulmonary edema has been noted in women treated with ritodrine. The use in advanced labor (i.e., greater than 4 cm cervical dilation or effacement greater than 80%) has not been established.

Route/Dosage ────────────

• **IV**

  Preterm labor.

Initial: 0.05 mg/min (10 gtt/min using microdrip chamber); **then,** depending on response, increase by 0.05 mg/min (10 microdrops/min) q 10 min until desired response occurs. **Effective dose range:** 0.15–0.35 mg/min (30–70 gtt/min). Continue infusion antepartum for a minimum of 12 hr after contractions cease.

How Supplied: *Injection:* 10 mg/mL, 15 mg/mL

Side Effects: All effects are related to the stimulation of beta receptors by the drug. **IV.** *CV:* Increase in maternal and fetal HR, increase in maternal systolic and marked decrease in diastolic BP (widening of pulse pressure), persistent tachycardia (may indicate pulmonary edema), palpitations, **arrhythmias including VT,** chest pain or tightness, angina, heart murmur, **myocardial ischemia.** Sinus bradycardia following drug withdrawal. *GI:* N&V, bloating, ileus, epigastric distress, diarrhea or constipation. *CNS:* Headache, migraine headache, tremors, malaise, nervousness, jitteriness, restlessness, anxiety, emotional changes, drowsiness, weakness. *Metabolic:* Transient increases in insulin and blood glucose, increases in cyclic AMP and free fatty acids, decrease in potassium, glycosuria, lactic acidosis. *Respiratory:* Dyspnea, **maternal pulmonary edema,** hyperventilation. *Hematologic:* Leukopenia or agranulocytosis after 2–3 weeks of IV therapy (leukocyte count returned to normal after cessation of drug). *Other:* Erythema, **anaphylactic shock,** rash, intrauterine growth retardation, hemolytic icterus, sweating, chills, impaired liver function. *NOTE:* Neonatal effects are infrequent but may include hypoglycemia and ileus; also, hypocalcemia and hypotension in neonates whose mothers were treated with other betamimetic drugs.

OD Overdose Management: *Symptoms:* Excessive beta-adrenergic stimulation, including tachycardia (in both the mother and fetus), palpitations, **cardiac arrhythmias,** hypotension, dyspnea, tremor, dyspnea, nervousness, N&V. *Treatment:* Supportive measures. A beta-adrenergic blocking agent can be used as an antidote. The drug is dialyzable.

Drug Interactions

Anesthetics, general / Additive hypotension or cardiac arrhythmias
Atropine / ↑ Systemic hypertension
Beta-adrenergic blocking agents / Inhibition of the effect of ritodrine
Corticosteroids / ↑ Risk of pulmonary edema

Diazoxide / Additive hypotension or cardiac arrhythmias

Magnesium sulfate / Additive hypotension or cardiac arrhythmias

Meperidine / Additive hypotension or cardiac arrhythmias

Sympathomimetics / Additive or potentiated effects of sympathomimetics

EMS CONSIDERATIONS
None.

Ritonavir
(rih-TOH-nah-veer)

Pregnancy Class: B

Norvir **(Rx)**

Classification: Antiviral drug, protease inhibitor

Mechanism of Action: A peptidomimetic inhibitor of both the HIV-1 and HIV-2 proteases. Inhibition of HIV protease results in the enzyme incapable of processing the "gag-pool" polyprotein precursor that leads to production of noninfectious immature HIV particles.

Uses: Alone or in combination with nucleoside analogues (ddC or AZT) for the treatment of HIV infection. Use of ritonavir may result in a reduction in both mortality and AIDS-defining clinical events. Clinical benefit has not been determined for periods longer than 6 months.

Precautions: Not considered a cure for HIV infection; patients may continue to manifest illnesses associated with advanced HIV infection, including opportunistic infections. Also, therapy with ritonavir has not been shown to decrease the risk of transmitting HIV to others through sexual contact or blood contamination. Use with caution in those with impaired hepatic function and during lactation. Hemophiliacs treated with protease inhibitors may manifest spontaneous bleeding episodes. Safety and efficacy have not been determined in children less than 12 years of age.

Route/Dosage
• **Capsules, Oral Solution**

Treatment of HIV infection.
600 mg b.i.d. If nausea is experienced upon initiation of therapy, dose escalation may be tried as follows: 300 mg b.i.d. for 1 day, 400 mg b.i.d. for 2 days, 500 mg b.i.d. for 1 day, and then 600 mg b.i.d. thereafter.

How Supplied: *Capsules:* 100 mg; *Oral Solution:* 600 mg/7.5 mL.

Side Effects: Side effects listed are those with a frequency of 2% or greater. *GI:* N&V, diarrhea, taste perversion, anorexia, flatulence, constipation, abdominal pain, dyspepsia, local throat irritation. *Nervous:* Circumoral paresthesia, peripheral paresthesia, dizziness, insomnia, paresthesia, somnolence, abnormal thinking. *Body as a whole:* Asthenia, headache, malaise, fever. *Dermatologic:* Sweating, rash. *Miscellaneous:* Vasodilation, hyperlipidemia, myalgia, pharyngitis.

OD **Overdose Management:** *Symptoms:* Extension of side effects. *Treatment:* General supportive measures, including monitoring of VS and observing the clinical status. Elimination of unabsorbed drug may be assisted by emesis or gastric lavage, with attention given to maintaining a patent airway. Activated charcoal may also help in removing any unabsorbed drug. Dialysis is not likely to be of benefit in removing the drug from the body.

Drug Interactions: Ritonavir is expected to produce large increases in the plasma levels of a number of drugs, including amiodarone, astemizole, bepridil, bupropion, cisapride, clozapine, encainide, erythromycin, flecainide, meperidine, methylphenidate, pentoxifylline, phenothiazines, piroxicam, propafenone, propoxyphene, quinidine, rifabutin, tefenadine, and warfarin. This may lead to an increased risk of arrhythmias, hematologic complications, seizures, or other serious adverse effects.

Ritonavir may produce a decrease in the plasma levels of the following drugs: atovaquone, clofibrate, daunorubicin, diphenoxylate, metoclopramide, and sedative/hypnotics.

Coadministration of ritonavir with

R

the following drugs may cause extreme sedation and respiratory depression and thus should not be combined: alprazolam, clorazepate, diazepam, estazolam, flurazepam, midazolam, triazolam, and zolpidem.

Clarithromycin / ↑ Clarithromycin levels; reduce clarithromycin dose

Desipramine / Significant ↑ desipramine levels; reduce desipramine dose

Ethinyl estradiol / ↓ Ethyinyl estradiol levels; use alternative contraceptive

Propulsid / ↑ Risk of serious cardiac arrhythmias

Saquinavir / Significant ↑ in saquinavir blood levels

Theophylline / ↓ Theophylline levels

EMS CONSIDERATIONS
See also *Antiviral Drugs.*

Rizatriptan benzoate
(rise-ah-TRIP-tan)
Pregnancy Class: C
Maxalt, Maxalt-MLT **(Rx)**
Classification: Antimigraine drug

Mechanism of Action: Binds to 5-HT$_{1B/1D}$ receptors, resulting in cranial vessel vasocontriction, inhibition of neuropeptide release, and reduced transmission in trigeminal pain pathways.

Uses: Acute treatment of migraine attacks in adults with or without aura.

Contraindications: Use in children less than 18 years of age, as prophylactic therapy of migraine, or use in the management of hemiplegic or basilar migraine. Use in those with ischemic heart disease or vasospastic coronary artery disease, uncontrolled hypertension, within 24 hr of treatment with another 5-HT$_1$ agonist or an ergotamine-containing or ergot-type medication (e.g., dihydroergotamine, methysergide). Use concurrently with MAO inhibitors or use of rizatriptan within 2 weeks of discontinuing a MAO inhibitor. Strongly recommended the drug not be given in unrecognized coronary artery disease (CAD) predicted by the presence of risk factors, including hypertension, hypercholesterolemia, smoking, obesity, diabetes, strong family history of CAD, female with surgical or physiological menopause, or males over 40, unless a CV evaluation reveals the patient is free from CAD or ischemic myocardial disease.

Precautions: Safety and efficacy have not been determined for use in cluster headache or in children. Use with caution during lactation, with diseases that may alter the absorption, metabolism, or excretion of drugs; in dialysis patients, and in moderate hepatic insufficiency. Maxalt-MLT tablets contain phenylalanine; may be of concern to phenylketonurics.

Route/Dosage ───────
• **Oral Disintegrating Tablets, Tablets**
Acute treatment of migraine.
Adults: Single dose of 5 mg or 10 mg of Maxalt or Maxalt-MLT. Doses should be separated by at least 2 hr, with no more than 30 mg taken in any 24-hr period.

How Supplied: *Orally Disintegrating Tablets:* 5 mg, 10 mg; *Tablets:* 5 mg, 10 mg.

Side Effects: *CV: **Acute MI, coronary artery vasospasm, life-threatening disturbances in cardiac rhythm (VT, ventricular fibrillation), death, cerebral hemorrhage, subarachnoid hemorrhage, stroke, hypertensive crisis.** Also, transient myocardial ischemia, peripheral vascular ischemia, colonic ischemia with abdominal pain and bloody diarrhea, palpitation, tachycardia, cold extremities, hypertension, arrhythmia, bradycardia. GI:* Nausea, dry mouth, abdominal distention, vomiting, dyspepsia, thirst, acid regurgitation, dysphagia, constipation, flatulence, tongue edema. *CNS:* Somnolence, headache, dizziness, paresthesias, hypesthesia, decreased mental acuity, euphoria, tremor, nervousness, vertigo, insomnia, anxiety, depression, disorientation, ataxia, dysarthria, confusion, dream abnormality, abnormal gait, irritability, impaired memory, agitation, hyperesthesia. *Pain and pressure sensations:* Chest tightness/pressure and/or heaviness; pain/tightness/pressure in the precordium, neck, throat, jaw; regional pain, tightness, pressure, or heaviness; or unspecified pain. *Musculoskeletal:* Muscle weakness, stiffness, myalgia, muscle cramps, musculoskeletal pain, arthralgia, muscle spasm. *Respiratory:* Dyspnea, pharyngitis, nasal irritation, nasal congestion, dry throat, URI, yawning, dry nose, epistaxis, sinus disorder. *GU:* Urinary frequency, polyuria, menstrual disorder. *Dermatologic:* Flushing, sweating, pruritus, rash, urticaria. *Body as a whole:* Asthenia, fatigue, chills, heat sensitivity, hangover effect, warm/cold sensations, dehydration, hot flashes. *Ophthalmic:* Blurred vision, dry eyes, burning eye, eye pain, eye irritation, tearing. *Miscellaneous:* Facial edema, tinnitus, ear pain.

Drug Interactions
Dihydroergotamine / Additive vasospastic reactions; do not use within 24 hr of each other
MAO Inhibitors / ↑ Plasma levels of rizatriptan; do not use together
Methysergide / Additive vasospastic reactions; do not use within 24 hr of each other
Propranolol / ↑ Plasma levels of rizatriptan

EMS CONSIDERATIONS
None.

Rofecoxib
(roh-feh-KOX-ib)
Pregnancy Class: C
Vioxx **(Rx)**
Classification: NSAID, COX-2 inhibitor

Mechanism of Action: NSAID that acts by inhibiting prostaglandin synthesis via inhibition of cyclooxygenase-2 (COX-2).
Uses: Relieve signs and symptoms of osteoarthritis, acute pain in

adults, and treatment of dysmenorrhea.
Contraindications: Advanced renal disease. Use in patients who manifested asthma, urticaria, or allergic-type reactions after taking aspirin or other NSAIDs. Use in late pregnancy due to premature closure of the ductus arteriosus. Lactation.
Precautions: Use with extreme caution in those with a prior history of ulcer disease or GI bleeding. Use with caution in fluid retention, hypertension, or heart failure. Most fatal GI events are in elderly or debilitated patients. Safety and efficacy have not been determined in children less than 18 years of age.

Route/Dosage
• **Oral Suspension, Tablets**
Osteoarthritis.
Adults, initial: 12.5 mg once daily, up to a maximum of 25 mg once daily.
Acute pain, primary dysmenorrhea.
Adults, initial: 50 mg once daily; **then,** 50 mg once daily as needed.
How Supplied: *Oral Suspension:* 12.5 mg/5 mL, 25 mg/mL; *Tablets:* 12.5 mg, 25 mg
Side Effects: Side effects listed occurred in at least 2% of patients. *GI:* Diarrhea, nausea, constipation, heartburn, epigastric discomfort, dyspepsia, abdominal pain. *CNS:* Headache. *Respiratory:* Bronchitis, upper respiratory tract infection. *CV:* Hypertension. *GU:* UTI. *Body as a whole:* Lower extremity edema, asthenia, fatigue, dizziness, flu-like disease, fever. *Miscellaneous:* Back pain, sinusitis, post-dental extraction alveolitis.
Drug Interactions
ACE inhibitors / ↓ ACE inhibitor effect
Antacids (Mg-Al containing, Calcium carbonate) / ↓ Absorption of rofecoxib
Aspirin / ↑ Risk of GI ulceration and other complications
Furosemide / ↓ Natriuretic effect of furosemide
Lithium / ↑ Risk of lithium toxicity

R

Methotrexate / ↑ Risk of methotrexate toxicity
Rifampin / ↓ Plasma levels of rifampin R/T ↑ liver metabolism
Thiazide diuretics / ↓ Natriuretic effect of thiazides
Warfarin / ↑ PT

EMS CONSIDERATIONS
None.

Ropinirole hydrochloride
(roh-PIN-ih-roll)
Pregnancy Class: C
Requip **(Rx)**
Classification: Antiparkinson agent

Mechanism of Action: Mechanism is not known but believed to involve stimulation of postsynaptic D_2 dopamine receptors in caudate-putamen in brain. Causes decreases in both systolic and diastolic BP at doses above 0.25 mg.
Uses: Treat signs and symptoms of idiopathic Parkinson's disease.
Contraindications: Lactation.
Precautions: Safety and efficacy have not been determined in children.

Route/Dosage
• **Tablets**
Parkinson's disease.
Week 1: 0.25 mg t.i.d. **Week 2:** 0.5 mg t.i.d. **Week 3:** 0.75 mg t.i.d. **Week 4:** 1 mg t.i.d. After week 4, daily dose, if necessary, may be increased by 1.5 mg/day on weekly basis up to dose of 9 mg/day. This may be followed by increase of up to 3 mg/day weekly to total dose of 24 mg/day.
How Supplied: *Tablets:* 0.25 mg, 0.5 mg, 1 mg, 2 mg, 5 mg.
Side Effects: *CNS:* Hallucinations, cause and/or exacerbate pre-existing dyskinesia. *CV:* Syncope (sometimes with bradycardia), postural hypotension.
OD Overdose Management: *Symptoms:* Agitation, increased dyskinesia, grogginess, sedation, orthostatic hypotension, chest pain, confusion, N&V. *Treatment:* General suppportive measures. Maintain vital signs. Gastric lavage.

Drug Interactions
Ciprofloxacin / Significant ↑ in ropinirole plasma levels
Estrogens / ↓ Oral clearance of ropinirole

EMS CONSIDERATIONS
None.
Administration/Storage
1. If taken with l-dopa, decrease dose of l-dopa gradually, as tolerated.
2. When discontinued, do so gradually over 7-day period. Reduce frequency of administration to twice daily for 4 days. For remaining 3 days, reduce frequency to once daily prior to complete withdrawal.

Rosiglitazone maleate
(roh-sih-GLIH-tah-zohn)
Pregnancy Class: C
Avelox, Avandia **(Rx)**
Classification: Oral hypoglycemic agent.

Mechanism of Action: Improves blood glucose levels by improving insulin sensitivity in type II diabetes insulin resistance. Active only in the presence of insulin. A highly selective and potent agonist for the peroxisome proliferator-activated receptor (PPAR)-gamma which is found in adipose tissue, skeletal muscle, and liver. Activation of these receptors regulates the transcription of insulin-responsive genes involved in the control of glucose production, transport, and use. The genes also participate in regulation of fatty acid metabolism.
Uses: As an adjunct to diet and exercise to improve glycemic control in type II diabetes. Used either as monotherapy or in combination witih metformin when diet, exercise, and rosiglitazone alone do not control blood glucose.
Contraindications: Type I diabetes, diabetic ketoacidosis, active liver disease, if serum ALT levels are 2.5 times ULN, in patients with NYHA Class III and IV cardiac status (unless the expected benefit outweighs the potential risk), and during lactation.

Precautions: Treatment may result in resumption of ovulation in premenopausal anovulatory patients with insulin resistance. Use with caution in patients with edema. Safety and efficacy have not been determined in patients less than 18 years of age.

Route/Dosage
• **Tablets**
Type II diabetes, monotherapy.
Adults, initial: 4 mg once daily or in divided doses b.i.d. If the response is inadequate after 12 weeks, the dose can be increased to 8 mg as a single dose once daily or in divided doses b.i.d. A dose of 4 mg b.i.d. resulted in the greatest decrease in fasting blood glucose and HbA1c.

Type II diabetes, combination therapy with metformin.
Adults, initial: 4 mg once daily or in divided doses b.i.d. If the response is inadequate after 12 weeks, the dose can be increased to 8 mg as a single dose once daily or in divided doses b.i.d.
How Supplied: *Tablets:* 2 mg, 4 mg, 8 mg
Side Effects: *Respiratory:* URTI, sinusitis. *Metabolic:* Hyperglycemia, hypoglycemia. *Miscellaneous:* Injury, headache, back ache, fatigue, diarrhea, anemia, edema.

EMS CONSIDERATIONS
None.

S

Sacrosidase
(sac-roh-SIGH-dace)
Pregnancy Class: C
Sucraid **(Rx)**
Classification: Enzyme

Mechanism of Action: Enzyme replacement for those with genetic sucrase deficiency. In the absence of sucrase, sucrose is not metabolized and is thus not absorbed from the intestine. This results in osmotic water retention, loose stools, excessive gas, bloating, abdominal cramps, nausea, and vomiting. Chronic malabsorption of disaccharides may result in malnutrition.
Uses: Oral replacement therapy for sucrase deficiency, which is part of congenital sucrase-isomaltase deficiency. Safe and effective for use in children.
Contraindications: Hypersensitivity to yeast, yeast products, or glycerin.

Route/Dosage
• **Solution**
Treat sucrase deficiency.
Patients 15 kg or less: 1 mL (8500 IU)—1 full measuring scoop or 22 drops per meal or snack. **Patients over 15 kg:** 2 mL (17,000 IU)—2 full measuring scoops or 44 drops per meal or snack. Dosage may be measured with the 1 mL measuring scoop provided or by drop count method using the guide of 1 mL equals 22 drops from the sacrosidase container tip.
How Supplied: *Solution:* 8500 IU/mL
Side Effects: *GI:* Abdominal pain, N&V, diarrhea, constipation. *CNS:* Insomnia, headache, nervousness. *Miscellaneous:* Hypersensitivity reactions, dehydration.

EMS CONSIDERATIONS
None.

Salmeterol xinafoate
(sal-MET-er-ole)
Pregnancy Class: C
Serevent **(Rx)**
Classification: Beta-2 adrenergic agonist

Mechanism of Action: Selective for beta-2 adrenergic receptors, located in the bronchi and heart. Acts by

---

bold italic = life threatening side effect

stimulating intracellular adenyl cyclase, the enzyme that converts ATP to cyclic AMP. Increased AMP levels cause relaxation of bronchial smooth muscle and inhibition of release of mediators of immediate hypersensitivity, especially from mast cells.

Uses: Long-term maintenance treatment of asthma or bronchospasm associated with COPD. Prevention of bronchospasms in patients over 12 years of age with reversible obstructive airway disease, including nocturnal asthma. Prevention of exercise-induced bronchospasms. Inhalation powder for long-term maintenance treatment of asthma in patients aged 12 years or older.

Contraindications: Use in patients who can be controlled by short-acting, inhaled beta-2 agonists. Use to treat acute symptoms of asthma or in those who have worsening or deteriorating asthma. Lactation.

Precautions: Not a substitute for PO or inhaled corticosteroids. The safety and efficacy of using salmeterol with a spacer or other devices has not been studied adequately. Use with caution in impaired hepatic function; with cardiovascular disorders, including coronary insufficiency, cardiac arrhythmias, and hypertension; with convulsive disorders or thyrotoxicosis; and in patients who respond unusually to sympathomimetic amines. Because of the potential of the drug interfering with uterine contractility, use of salmeterol during labor should be restricted to those in whom benefits clearly outweigh risks. Safety and efficacy have not been determined in children less than 12 years of age.

Route/Dosage ───────────

• **Metered Dose Inhaler**
Maintenance of bronchodilation, prevention of symptoms of asthma, including nocturnal asthma.
Adults and children over 12 years of age: Two inhalations (42 mcg) b.i.d. (morning and evening, approximately 12 hr apart).
Prevention of exercise-induced bronchospasms.

Adults and children over 12 years of age: Two inhalations (42 mcg) at least 30–60 min before exercise. Additional doses should not be used for 12 hr.
• **Inhalation Powder (Diskus)**
Maintenance treatment of asthma or bronchospasm associated with COPD.
Adults and children over 12 years of age: 50 mcg (one inhalation) b.i.d. in the morning and evening. *NOTE:* Even though the metered dose inhaler and the inhalation powder are used for the same conditions, they are not interchangeable.

How Supplied: *Metered dose inhaler:* 21 mcg/inh; *Powder for Inhalation:* 46 mcg/inh

Side Effects: *Respiratory:* Paradoxical bronchospasms, upper or lower respiratory tract infection, nasopharyngitis, disease of nasal cavity/sinus, cough, pharyngitis, allergic rhinitis, laryngitis, tracheitis, bronchitis. *Allergic: **Immediate hypersensitivity reactions,** including urticaria, rash, and **bronchospasm.** CV:* Palpitations, chest pain, increased BP, tachycardia. *CNS:* Headache, sinus headache, tremors, nervousness, malaise, fatigue, dizziness, giddiness. *GI:* Stomachache. *Musculoskeletal:* Joint pain, back pain, muscle cramps, muscle contractions, myalgia, myositis, muscle soreness. *Miscellaneous:* Flu, dental pain, rash, skin eruption, dysmenorrhea.

OD **Overdose Management:** *Symptoms:* Tachycardia, arrhythmia, tremors, headache, muscle cramps, hypokalemia, hyperglycemia. *Treatment:* Supportive therapy. Consider judicious use of a beta-adrenergic blocking agent, although these drugs can cause bronchospasms. Cardiac monitoring is necessary. Dialysis is not an appropriate treatment of overdosage.

Drug Interactions
MAO Inhibitors / Potentiation of the effect of salmeterol
Tricyclic antidepressants / Potentiation of the effect of salmeterol

───────────

EMS CONSIDERATIONS

See also *Sympathomimetic Drugs.*

Saquinavir mesylate

(sah-KWIN-ah-veer)
Pregnancy Class: B
Fortovase, Invirase **(Rx)**
Classification: Antiviral drug, protease inhibitor

Mechanism of Action: HIV protease cleaves viral polyprotein precursors to form functional proteins in HIV-infected cells. Cleavage of viral polyprotein precursors is required for maturation of the infectious virus. Saquinavir inhibits the activity of HIV protease and prevents the cleavage of viral polyproteins.

Uses: Combined with AZT or zalcitabine (ddC) for treatment of advanced HIV infection in selected patients. No data are available regarding the benefit of combination therapy of saquinavir with AZT or ddC on HIV disease progression or survival.

Contraindications: Lactation. Use with astemizole, cisapride, ergot derivatives, midazolam, terfenadine, triazolam.

Precautions: Photoallergy or phototoxicity may occur; take protective measures against exposure to ultraviolet or sunlight until tolerance is assessed. Use with caution in those with hepatic insufficiency. Hemophiliacs treated with protease inhibitors for HIV infections may manifest spontaneous bleeding episodes. Safety and efficacy have not been determined in HIV-infected children or adolescents less than 16 years of age.

Route/Dosage
- **Fortovase Capsules**
  HIV infections in combination with AZT or ddC.
  Six 200-mg capsules (i.e., 1,200 mg) taken t.i.d. with meals or up to 2 hr after meals.
- **Invirase Capsules**
  HIV infections in combination with AZT or ddC.
  Three 200-mg capsules of saquinavir t.i.d. taken within 2 hr of a full meal. The recommended doses of AZT or ddC as part of combination therapy are: AZT, 200 mg t.i.d., or ddC, 0.75

mg t.i.d. However, base dosage adjustments of AZT or ddC on the known toxicity profile of the individual drug. This form of the drug will be phased out.

How Supplied: *Capsules:* 200 mg.

Side Effects: Side effects listed are for saquinavir combined with either AZT or ddC. *GI:* Diarrhea, abdominal discomfort, nausea, dyspepsia, abdominal pain, ulceration of buccal mucosa, cheilitis, constipation, dysphagia, eructation, blood-stained or discolored feces, gastralgia, gastritis, GI inflammation, gingivitis, glossitis, *rectal hemorrhage,* hemorrhoids, hepatomegaly, hepatosplenomegaly, melena, pain, painful defecation, pancreatitis, parotid disorder, pelvic salivary glands disorder, stomatitis, tooth disorder, vomiting, frequent bowel movements, dry mouth, alteration in taste. *CNS:* Headache, paresthesia, numbness of extremity, dizziness, peripheral neuropathy, ataxia, confusion, *convulsions,* dysarthria, dysesthesia, hyperesthesia, hyperreflexia, hyporeflexia, face numbness, facial pain, paresis, poliomyelitis, progressive multifocal leukoencephalopathy, spasms, tremor, agitation, amnesia, anxiety, depression, excessive dreaming, euphoria, hallucinations, insomnia, reduced intellectual ability, irritability, lethargy, libido disorder, overdose effect, psychic disorder, somnolence, speech disorder. *Musculoskeletal:* Musculoskeletal pain, myalgia, arthralgia, arthritis, back pain, muscle cramps, musculoskeletal disorder, stiffness, tissue changes, trauma. *Body as a whole:* Allergic reaction, chest pain, edema, fever, intoxication, external parasites, retrosternal pain, shivering, wasting syndrome, weight decrease, abscess, angina tonsillaris, candidiasis, hepatitis, herpes simplex, herpes zoster, infections (bacterial, mycotic, staphylococcal), influenza, lymphadenopathy, tumor. *CV:* Cyanosis, heart murmur, heart valve disorder, hypertension, hypotension, syncope, distended vein, HR disorder. *Metabolic:* Dehydration, hyperglycemia, weight

S

decrease, worsening of existing diabetes mellitus. *Hematologic:* Anemia, microhemorrhages, pancytopenia, splenomegaly, thrombocytopenia. *Respiratory:* Bronchitis, cough, dyspnea, epistaxis, hemoptysis, laryngitis, pharyngitis, pneumonia, respiratory disorder rhinitis, sinusitis, URTI. *GU:* Enlarged prostate, vaginal discharge, micturition disorder, UTI. *Dermatologic:* Acne, dermatitis, seborrheic dermatitis, eczema, erythema, folliculitis, furunculosis, hair changes, hot flushes, photosensitivity reaction, changes in skin pigment, maculopapular rash, skin disorder, skin nodules, skin ulceration, increased sweating, urticaria, verruca, xeroderma. *Ophthalmic:* Dry eye syndrome, xerophthalmia, blepharitis, eye irritation, visual disturbance. *Otic:* Earache, ear pressure, decreased hearing, otitis, tinnitus.

Drug Interactions

Astemizole / Possibility of serious or life-threatening cardiac arrhythmias or prolonged sedation

Carbamazepine / ↓ Blood levels of saquinavir

Cisapride / Possibility of serious or life-threatening cardiac arrhythmias or prolonged sedation

Clarithromycin / ↑ Blood levels of both drugs

Dexamethasone / ↓ Blood levels of saquinavir

Ergot derivatives / Possibility of serious or life-threatening cardiac arrhythmias or prolonged sedation

Ketconazole / ↑ Blood levels of saquinavir

Midazolam / Possibility of serious or life-threatening cardiac arrhythmias or prolonged sedation

Phenobarbital / ↓ Blood levels of saquinavir

Phenytoin / ↓ Blood levels of saquinavir

Rifampin / ↓ Blood levels of saquinavir

Ritonavir / ↑ Blood levels of saquinavir

Terfenadine / Possibility of serious or life-threatening cardiac arrhythmias or prolonged sedation

Triazolam / Possibility of serious or life-threatening cardiac arrhythmias or prolonged sedation

EMS CONSIDERATIONS

See also *Antiviral Drugs.*

Sargramostim
(sar-GRAM-oh-stim)
Pregnancy Class: C
Leukine **(Rx)**
Classification: Colony-stimulating factor

Mechanism of Action: A granulocyte-macrophage colony-stimulating factor (rhu GM-CSF) produced by recombinant DNA technology in a yeast expression system. GM-CSF stimulates the proliferation and differentiation of hematopoietic progenitor cells. It stimulates partially committed progenitor cells to divide and differentiate in the granulocyte-macrophage pathways. Division, maturation, and activation are induced through GM-CSF binding to specific receptors located on the surface of target cells. Also activates mature granulocytes and macrophages. Increases the cytotoxicity of monocytes toward certain neoplastic cell lines as well as activates polymorphonuclear neutrophils, thus inhibiting the growth of tumor cells.

Onset of Action: Peak levels: 2-3 hr, depending on the dose.

Uses: Increased myeloid recovery in patients with non-Hodgkin's lymphoma, ALL, and Hodgkin's disease undergoing autologous bone marrow transplantation. Bone marrow transplantation failure or engraftment delay. To shorten recovery time to neutrophil recovery and to decrease the incidence of severe and life-threatening infections in older adult patients with acute myelogenous leukemia. To mobilize hematopoietic progenitor cells into peripheral blood collection by leukapheresis. For acceleration of myeloid recovery in allogenic bone marrow transplantation from human lymphocyte antigen-matched related donors. *Investigational:* To increase WBC counts in patients with myelodysplastic syndrome and in AIDS patients taking AZT; to correct neutropenia in patients with aplastic anemia; to decrease the nadir of leukopenia secondary to myelosuppressive chemotherapy and to decrease myelosuppression in preleukemic patients; and to decrease organ system damage following transplantation, especially in the liver and kidney.

Contraindications: More than 10% leukemic myeloid blasts in the bone marrow or peripheral blood. Known hypersensitivity to GM-CSF, yeast-derived products, or any component of the product. Simultaneous use with cytotoxic chemotherapy or radiotherapy or use within 24 hr preceding or following chemotherapy or radiotherapy.

Precautions: Use with caution in patients with preexisting cardiac disease and hypoxia and during lactation. Safety and effectiveness have not been determined in children although it appears the drug is no more toxic in children than in adults. May aggravate fluid retention in patients with preexisting peripheral edema, or pleural or pericardial effusion. Insufficient data on effectiveness of sargramostim in increasing myeloid recovery after peripheral blood stem cell transplantation. It is possible that sargramostim can act as a growth factor for any tumor type, especially myeloid malignancies; thus, use with caution in any malignancy with myeloid characteristics.

Route/Dosage
• **IV Infusion, SC**

Myeloid reconstitution after autologous or allogenic bone marrow transplantation.

250 mcg/m²/day for 21 days as a 2-hr infusion beginning 2–4 hr after the autologous bone marrow infusion and greater than 24 hr after the last dose of chemotherapy and 12 hr after the last dose of radiotherapy. Do not give drug until the postmarrow infusion absolute neutrophil count is less than 500 cells/mm³.

Bone marrow transplantation failure or engraftment delay.

250 mcg/m²/day for 14 days as a 2-hr IV infusion. If engraftment has not occurred, therapy may be repeated after 7 days off therapy. A third course of 250 mcg/m²/day may be undertaken after another 7 days off therapy. However, if no response occurs after three courses, it is unlikely the drug will be beneficial.

Neutrophil recovery following chemotherapy in acute myelogenous leukemia.

250 mcg/m²/day given over a 4-hr period staring at about day 11 or 4 days following completion of induction chemotherapy. Use if the day 10 bone marrow is hypoplastic with less than 5% blasts. If a second cycle of therapy is needed, give about 4 days after the completion of chemotherapy if the bone marrow is hypoplastic with less than 5% blasts. Continue therapy until an absolute neutrophil count greater than 1,500/mm³ is noted for 3 consecutive days or a maximum of 42 days. If a severe adverse reaction occurs, decrease the dose by 50% or discontinue temporarily until the drug reaction is reduced.

Mobilization of peripheral blood progenitor cells (PBPCs).

250 mcg/m²/day IV over 24 hr or SC once daily. Use this dose throughout the PBPC collection period. If the WBC count is greater than 50,000 cells/mm³, reduce the dose by 50%. If sufficient numbers of progenitor cells are not collected, use other mobilization therapy.

Postperipheral blood progenitor cell transplantation.

250 mcg/m²/day IV over 24 hr or SC once daily beginning immediately after infusion of progenitor cells and continuing until an absolute neutrophil count greater than 1,500 is reached for 3 consecutive days.

How Supplied: *Injection:* 500 mcg/mL; *Powder for injection:* 250 mcg, 500 mcg

Side Effects: *First-dose effects (rare):* Respiratory distress, hypoxia, flush-

S

ing, hypotension, syncope, tachycardia. *CV:* Hypertension, **hemorrhage,** edema, hypotension, peripheral edema, cardiac event, tachycardia, pericardial effusion, pleural effusion, capillary leak syndrome. *GI:* N&V, diarrhea, abdominal pain, GI disorder, stomatitis, dyspepsia, anorexia, hematemesis, dysphagia, **GI hemorrhage,** constipation, abdominal distension, liver damage. *CNS:* Neuroclinical, neuromotor, neuropsychiatric, and neurosensory side effects. Paresthesia, headache, CNS disorder, insomnia, anxiety. *Respiratory:* Pulmonary event, pharyngitis, lung disorder, epistaxis, dyspnea, rhinitis. *Hematologic:* Blood dyscrasias, thrombocytopenia, leukopenia, petechia, agranulocytosis, coagulation disorders. *Musculoskeletal:* Bone pain, arthralgia, asthenia. *Dermatologic:* Rash, alopecia, pruritus. *GU:* Urinary tract disorder, hematuria, abnormal kidney function. *Miscellaneous:* Fever, infection, malaise, weight loss, chills, pain, chest pain, allergy, **sepsis,** eye hemorrhage, back pain, weight gain, sweating.

OD **Overdose Management:** *Symptoms:* Dyspnea, malaise, nausea, fever, rash, sinus tachycardia, chills, headache. *Treatment:* Discontinue therapy. Monitor for increases in WBCs and for respiratory symptoms.

Drug Interactions: Drugs such as corticosteroids and lithium may ↑ the myeloproliferative effects of sargramostim. The effect of sargramostim may be limited in those who have received alkylating agents, anthracycline antibiotics, or antimetabolites.

EMS CONSIDERATIONS

None.

Scopolamine hydrobromide
Scopolamine transdermal therapeutic system
(scoh-POLL-ah-meen)
Pregnancy Class: C
Hydrobromide: Hyoscine Hydrobromide, Isopto Hyoscine Ophthalmic,

Scopace **(Rx)** Transdermal therapeutic system: Transderm-Scop **(Rx)**
Classification: Anticholinergic, antiemetic

Mechanism of Action: Anticholinergic with CNS depressant effects; produces amnesia when given with morphine or meperidine. In the presence of pain, delirium may be produced. Causes pupillary dilation and paralyzes the muscle required to accommodate for close vision (cycloplegia). This enables the physician to examine the inner structure of the eye, including the retina, as well as to examine refractive errors of the lens without automatic accommodation by the patient. Tolerance may develop if scopolamine is used alone. Recovery time can be reduced by using 1–2 gtt pilocarpine (1% or 2%). To reduce absorption, apply pressure over the nasolacrimal sac for 2–3 min.

The transdermal therapeutic system contains 1.5 mg scopolamine, which is slowly released from a mineral oil–polyisobutylene matrix. Approximately 0.5 mg is released from the system per day.

Onset of Action: When used for refraction: **peak for mydriasis,** 20-30 min; **peak for cycloplegia,** 30-60 min.
Duration of Action: 24 hr (residual cycloplegia and mydriasis may last for 3-7 days).
Uses: Ophthalmic: For cycloplegia and mydriasis in diagnostic procedures. Preoperatively and postoperatively in the treatment of iridocyclitis. Dilate the pupil in treatment of uveitis or posterior synechiae. *Investigational:* Prophylaxis of synechiae, treatment of iridocyclitis. **Parenteral:** Antiemetic, antivertigo. Preanesthetic sedation and obstetric amnesia. Antiarrhythmic during anesthesia and surgery. **Oral:** Prevention of motion sickness. **Transdermal:** Antiemetic, antivertigo. Prevention of motion sickness.
Contraindications: Additional: Use of the transdermal system in children or lactating women. Ophthalmic use in glaucome or infants less than 3 months of age. Use for prophylaxis of

excess secretions in children less than 4 months of age.

Precautions: Use with caution in children, infants, geriatric patients, diabetes, hypo- or hyperthyroidism, narrow anterior chamber angle.

Route/Dosage
• **Ophthalmic Solution**
Cycloplegia/mydriasis.
Adults: 1–2 gtt of the 0.25% solution in the conjunctiva 1 hr prior to refraction; **children:** 1 gtt of the 0.25% solution b.i.d. for 2 days prior to refraction.

Uveitis.
Adults and children: 1 gtt of the 0.25% solution in the conjunctiva 1–4 times/day, depending on the severity of the condition.

Treatment of posterior synechiae.
Adults and children: 1 gtt of the 0.25% solution q min for 5 min. (1 gtt of either a 2.5% or 10% solution of phenylephrine instilled q min for 3 min will enhance the effect of scopolamine.)

Postoperative mydriasis.
Adults: 1 gtt of the 0.25% solution once daily. For dark brown irides, administration 2 or 3 times/day may be required.

Pre- or Postoperative iridocyclitis.
Adults and children: 1 gtt of the 0.25% solution 1–4 times/day as required. Individualize the pediatric dose based on age, weight, and severity of the inflammation.
• **Injection (IM, IV, SC)**
Anticholinergic, antiemetic.
Adults: 0.3–0.6 mg (single dose).
Pediatric: 0.006 mg/kg (0.2 mg/m²) as a single dose.

Prophylaxis of excessive salivation and respiratory tract secretions in anesthesia.
Adults: 0.2–0.6 mg 30–60 min before induction of anesthesia. **Pediatric (given IM): 8–12 years:** 0.3 mg; **3–8 years:** 0.2 mg; **7 months–3 years:** 0.15 mg; **4–7 months:** 0.1 mg. Not recommended for children less than 4 months of age.

Adjunct to anesthesia, sedative-hypnotic.

Adults: 0.6 mg t.i.d–q.i.d.
Adjunct to anesthesia, amnesia.
Adults: 0.32–0.65 mg.
• **Tablets**
Prevent motion sickness.
0.4–0.8 mg taken 1 hr before travel.
• **Transdermal System**
Antiemetic, antivertigo.
Adults: 1 transdermal system placed on the postauricular skin to deliver either 1 mg or 0.33 mg over 3 days (apply at least 4 hr before antiemetic effect is required). The Canadian product should be applied about 12 hr before the antiemetic effect is desired.

How Supplied: Scopolamine hydrobromide: *Injection:* 0.4 mg/mL, 1 mg/mL; *Ophthalmic Solution:* 0.25%; *Tablet:* 0.4 mg. Scopolamine transdermal therapeutic system: *Film, extended release:* 0.33 mg/24 hr, 0.5 mg/24 hr

Side Effects: Additional: Disorientation, delirium, increased HR, decreased respiratory rate. *Ophthalmologic:* Blurred vision, stinging, increased intraocular pressure. Long-term use may cause irritation, photophobia, conjunctivitis, hyperemia, or edema.

EMS CONSIDERATIONS

See also *Cholinergic Blocking Agents.*

Secobarbital sodium
(see-koh-BAR-bih-tal)
Pregnancy Class: D
Seconal Sodium **(C-II) (Rx)**
Classification: Barbiturate sedative-hypnotic

S

Mechanism of Action: Short-acting.
Onset of Action: 10-15 min.
Duration of Action: 3-4 hr.
Uses: Short-term treatment of insomnia (2 weeks or less).
Precautions: Elderly or debilitated patients may be more sensitive to the drug and require reduced dosage.

Route/Dosage
• **Capsule**
Hypnotic.
Adults: 100 mg at bedtime.

---

bold italic = life threatening side effect

How Supplied: *Capsule:* 100 mg

EMS CONSIDERATIONS
See also *Barbiturates*.

Sertraline hydrochloride
(SIR-trah-leen)
Pregnancy Class: B
Zoloft **(Rx)**
Classification: Antidepressant

Mechanism of Action: Believed to act by inhibiting CNS neuronal uptake of serotonin. No significant affinity for adrenergic, cholinergic, dopaminergic, histaminergic, serotonergic, GABA, or benzodiazepine receptors. **Uses:** Treatment of depression with reduced psychomotor agitation, anxiety, and insomnia. Obsessive-compulsive disorders in adults and children as defined in DSM-III-R. Treatment of panic disorder, with or without agoraphobia.

Contraindications: Use in combination with a MAO inhibitor or within 14 days of discontinuing treatment with a MAO inhibitor.

Precautions: Use with caution in hepatic or renal dysfunction, with seizure disorders, during lactation, and in diseases or conditions that may affect hemodynamic responses or metabolism. Safety and efficacy have not been determined in children. The plasma clearance may be lower in elderly patients. The possibility of a suicide attempt is possible in depression and may persist until significant remission occurs.

Route/Dosage
• **Tablets**
   Depression.
Adults, initial: 50 mg once daily either in the morning or evening. Patients not responding to a 50-mg dose may benefit from doses up to a maximum of 200 mg/day.
   Obsessive-compulsive disorder.
Adults: 50–200 mg/day. **Children, 6 to 12 years:** 25 mg once a day; **adolescents, 13 to 17 years:** 50 mg once a day.
   Panic attacks.

Adults, initial: 25 mg/day for the first week; **then,** dosage ranges from 50–200 mg/day, based on response and tolerance.

How Supplied: *Tablet:* 25 mg, 50 mg, 100 mg

Side Effects: A large number of side effects is possible; listed are those side effects with a frequency of 0.1% or greater. *GI:* Nausea and diarrhea (common), dry mouth, constipation, dyspepsia, vomiting, flatulence, anorexia, abdominal pain, thirst, increased salivation, increased appetite, gastroenteritis, teeth-grinding, dysphagia, eructation, taste perversion or change. *CV:* Palpitations, hot flushes, edema, hypertension, hypotension, peripheral ischemia, postural hypotension or dizziness, syncope, tachycardia. *CNS:* Headache (common), insomnia (common), somnolence, agitation, nervousness, anxiety, dizziness, tremor, fatigue, impaired concentration, yawning, paresthesia, hypoesthesia, twitching, hypertonia, confusion, ataxia or abnormal coordination, abnormal gait, hyperesthesia, hyperkinesia, abnormal dreams, aggressive reaction, amnesia, apathy, delusion, depersonalization, depression, aggravated depression, emotional lability, euphoria, hallucinations, neurosis, paranoid reaction, *suicide ideation or attempt,* abnormal thinking, hypokinesia, migraine, nystagmus, vertigo. *Dermatologic:* Rash, acne, excessive sweating, alopecia, pruritus, cold and clammy skin, facial edema, erythematous rash, maculopapular rash, dry skin. *Musculoskeletal:* Myalgia, arthralgia, arthrosis, dystonia, muscle cramps or weakness. *GU:* Urinary frequency, micturition disorders, menstrual disorders, dysmenorrhea, dysuria, painful menstruation, intermenstrual bleeding, sexual dysfunction and decreased libido, nocturia, polyuria, dysuria, urinary incontinence. *Respiratory:* Rhinitis, pharyngitis, yawning, bronchospasm, coughing, dyspnea, epistaxis. *Ophthalmologic:* Blurred vision, abnormal vision, abnormal accommodation, conjunctivitis, diplopia, eye pain, xerophthalmia. *Otic:* Tinnitus, earache. *Body as a whole:* Asthenia, fever, chest pain, chills, back pain, weight loss or weight gain, generalized edema, malaise, flushing, hot flashes, rigors, lymphadenopathy, purpura.

OD Overdose Management: *Symptoms:* Intensification of side effects. *Treatment:*

• Establish and maintain an airway, ensuring adequate oxygenation and ventilation.

• Activated charcoal, with or without sorbitol, may be as or more effective than emesis or lavage.

• Cardiac and VS should be monitored.

• Provide general supportive measures and symptomatic treatment.

• Since sertraline has a large volume of distribution, it is unlikely that dialysis, forced diuresis, hemoperfusion, or exchange transfusion will be beneficial.

Drug Interactions: Because sertraline is highly bound to plasma proteins, its use with other drugs that are also highly protein bound may lead to displacement, resulting in higher plasma levels of the drug and possibly increased side effects.

Alcohol / Concurrent use is not recommended in depressed patients

Benzodiazepines / ↓ Clearance of benzodiazepines metabolized by hepatic oxidation

Cimetidine / ↑ Half-life and blood levels of sertraline

Diazepam / ↑ Plasma levels of desmethyldiazepam (significance not known)

MAO inhibitors / Serious and possibly fatal reactions including hyperthermia, rigidity, autonomic instability with possible rapid fluctuation of VS, myoclonus, changes in mental status (e.g., extreme agitation, delirium, coma)

Warfarin / ↑ PT and delayed normalization of PT

EMS CONSIDERATIONS
None.

Sevelamer hydrochloride
(seh-VEL-ah-mer)
Pregnancy Class: C
Renagel **(Rx)**
Classification: Urinary tract product for end-stage renal disease (ESRD)

Mechanism of Action: A polymeric phosphate binder that decreases intestinal phosphate absorption. A decrease in serum phosphate decreases ectopic calcification and osteitis fibrosa. Also lowers LDL and total serum cholesterol.

Uses: To reduce serum phosphorous in ESRD in patients on hemodialysis.

Contraindications: Hypophosphatemia, bowel obstruction.

Precautions: No well controlled studies in lactating mothers. Use with caution in dysphagia, swallowing disorders, severe GI motility disorders, or major GI tract surgery. Safety and efficacy have not been determined in children.

Route/Dosage
• **Capsules**
Hyperphosphatemia in ESRD
Adults, initial: 2–4 capsules with each meal, based on the following serum phosphorus levels: **Greater than 6 but less than 7.5 mg/dL:** 2 capsules t.i.d.; **7.5 mg/dL or more but less than 9 mg/dL:** 3 capsules t.i.d.; **9 mg/dL or more:** 4 capsules t.i.d. Adjust dosage to lower serum phosphorus to 6 mg/dL or less. Increase or decrease the dose by 1 capsule/meal as needed.

How Supplied: *Capsules:* 340 mg

Side Effects: *GI:* Diarrhea, dyspepsia, vomiting. *CV:* Hypotension or hypertension, *thrombosis*. *Body as a whole:* Infection, pain, headache. *Respiratory:* Increased cough.

Drug Interactions: Sevelamer may bind antiarrhythmic or anticonvulsant drugs → ↓ absorption.

EMS CONSIDERATIONS
None.

S

Sibutramine hydrochloride monohydrate
(sih-BYOU-trah-meen)
Pregnancy Class: C
Meridia **(C-IV) (Rx)**
Classification: Anti-obesity drug

Mechanism of Action: Main effect is likely due to primary and secondary amine metabolites of sibutramine. Inhibits reuptake of norepinephrine (NE) and serotonin (5HT), resulting in enhanced NE and 5HT activity and reduced food intake.

Uses: Management of obesity, including weight loss and maintenance of weight loss. Recommended for obese patients with initial body mass index of 30 kg/m² or more or 27 kg/m² in presence of hypertension, diabetes, or dyslipidemia. Use in conjunction with reduced calorie diet. Safety and efficacy have not been determined for more than 1 year.

Contraindications: Lactation. Use in patients receiving MAO inhibitors, who have anorexia nervosa, those taking centrally-acting appetite suppressant drugs, those with history of coronary artery disease, CHF, arrhythmias, or stroke. Use in severe renal impairment or hepatic dysfunction. Use with serotonergic drugs, such as fluoxetine, fluvoxamine, paroxetine, sertraline, venlafaxine, sumatriptan, and dihydroergotamine; also, use with dextromethorphan, meperidine, pentazocine, fentanyl, lithium, or tryptophan.

Precautions: Use with caution in geriatric patients. Safety and efficacy have not been determined in children less than 16 years of age. Use with caution in narrow angle glaucoma, history of seizures, or with drugs that may raise BP (e.g., phenylpropanolamine, ephedrine, pseudoephedrine). Exclude organic causes (e.g., untreated hypothyroidism) before use.

Route/Dosage
• **Capsules**
  Obesity.

Adults, initial: 10 mg once daily (usually in morning) with or without food. If there is inadequate weight loss, dose may be titrated after 4 weeks to total of 15 mg once daily. Do not exceed 15 mg daily.

How Supplied: *Capsules:* 5 mg, 10 mg, 15 mg

Side Effects: *Body as a whole:* Headache, back pain, flu syndrome, injury/accident, asthenia, chest pain, neck pain, allergic reaction. *GI:* Dry mouth, anorexia, abdominal pain, constipation, N&V, rectal disorder, increased appetite, dyspepsia, gastritis. *CNS:* Insomnia, dizziness, paresthesia, nervousness, anxiety, depression, somnolence, CNS stimulation, emotional lability. *CV:* Increased blood pressure, tachycardia, vasodilation, migraine, palpitation. *Dermatologic:* Sweating, rash, herpes simplex, acne. *Musculoskeletal:* Arthralgia, myalgia, tenosynovitis, joint disorder. *Respiratory:* Rhinitis, pharyngitis, sinusitis, increase cough, laryngitis. *GU:* Dysmenorrhea, UTI, vaginal monilia, metrorrhagia. *Otic:* Ear disorder, ear pain. *Miscellaneous:* Thirst, generalized edema, taste perversion.

Drug Interactions: [0]

EMS CONSIDERATIONS
None.

Sildenafil citrate
(sill-DEN-ah-fill)
Pregnancy Class: C
Viagra **(Rx)**
Classification: Drug for erectile dysfunction

Mechanism of Action: Nitric oxide activates the enzyme guanylate cyclase, which causes increased levels of guanosine monophosphate (cGMP) and subsequently smooth muscle relaxation in the corpus cavernosum and allowing inflow of blood. Sildenafil enhances effect of nitric oxide by inhibiting phosphodiesterase type 5 which is responsible for degradation of cGMP in the corpus cavernosum. When sexual stimulation causes local release of nitric oxide, inhibition of phosphodiesterse type 5 by sildenafil causes increased levels of cGMP in the corpus cavernosum and thus smooth muscle relaxation and inflow of blood resulting in an erection. Drug has no effect in absence of sexual stimulation.

Uses: Treatment of erectile dysfunction.

Contraindications: Concomitant use with organic nitrates in any form or with other treatments for erectile dysfunction. Use in newborns, children, or women.

Precautions: Use with caution in patients with anatomical deformation of penis, in those with predisposition to priapism (e.g., sickle cell anemia, multiple myeloma, leukemia), in bleeding disorders or active peptic ulceration, and in those with genetic disorders of retinal phosphodiesterases.

Route/Dosage
• **Tablets**
Treat erectile dysfunction.
For most patients, 50 mg no more than once daily, as needed, about 1 hr before sexual activity. Take anywhere from 0.5 hr to 4 hr before sexual activity. Depending on tolerance and effectiveness, dose may be increased to maximum of 100 mg or decreased to 25 mg. Consider a starting dose of 25 mg in those with hepatic or renal impairment or if taken with erythromycin, itraconzole, or ketoconazole.

How Supplied: *Tablets:* 25 mg, 50 mg, 100 mg

Side Effects: Listed are side effects with incidence of 2% or greater. *CNS:* Headache, dizziness. *GI:* Dyspepsia, diarrhea. *Dermatologic:* Flushing, rash. *Ophthalmic:* Mild and transient predominantly color tinge to vision, increased sensitivity to light, blurred vision. *Respiratory:* Nasal congestion, respiratory tract infection. *Miscellaneous:* UTI, back pain, flu syndrome, arthralgia. *Note:* Death has occurred in some patients following use of the drug.

OD Overdose Management: *Symptoms:* Extension of side effects. *Treatment:* Standard supportive measures.

Drug Interactions
Cimetadine / ↑ Plasma levels of sildenafil
Erythromycin / ↑ Plasma levels of sildenafil
Itraconazole / ↑ Plasma levels of sildenafil
Ketoconazole / ↑ Plasma levels of sildenafil
Mibefradil / ↑ Plasma levels of sildenafil
Rifampin / ↓ Plasma levels of sildenafil

EMS CONSIDERATIONS
None.

Simvastatin
(sim-vah-STAH-tin)
Pregnancy Class: X
Zocor **(Rx)**
Classification: Antihyperlipidemic

Mechanism of Action: Inhibits HMG-CoA reductase, an enzyme that is necessary to convert HMG-CoA to mevalonate (an early step in the biosynthesis of cholesterol). Levels of VLDL and LDL cholesterol and plasma triglycerides are reduced while the plasma concentration of HDL cholesterol is increased.

Onset of Action: Peak therapeutic resonse: 4-6 weeks.

Uses: Adjunct to diet for the reduction of elevated total and LDL cholesterol levels in types IIa and IIb hypercholesterolemia when the response to diet and other approaches has been inadequate. In coronary heart disease and hypercholesterolemia to reduce risk of total mortality by reducing coronary death; to reduce the risk of non-fatal MI; to reduce the risk for undergoing myocardial revascularization procedures; to reduce the risk of stroke or TIAs. *Investigational:* Heterozygous familial hypercholesterolemia, familial combined hyperlipidemia, diabetic dyslipidemia in non-insulin-dependent diabetes, hyperlipidemia secondary to the nephrotic syndrome, and homozygous familial hypercholesterolemia in patients with defective LDL receptors.

Contraindications: Active liver disease or unexplained persistent increases in LFTs. Use in pregnancy, during lactation, or in children.

Precautions: Use with caution in patients who have a history of liver disease/consume large quantities of alcohol or with drugs that affect steroid levels or activity. Higher plasma levels may be observed in patients with hepatic and severe renal insufficiency. Safety and efficacy have not been determined in children less than 18 years of age.

Route/Dosage
• **Tablets**
Adults, initially: 20 mg once daily in the evening; **maintenance:** 5–80 mg/day as a single dose in the evening. Consider a starting dose of 5 mg/day for patients on immunosuppressives or those with LDL less than 190 mg/dL and 10 mg/day for patients with LDL greater than 190 mg/dL. For geriatric patients, the starting dose should be 5 mg/day with maximum LDL reductions seen with 20 mg or less daily.

How Supplied: *Tablet:* 5 mg, 10 mg, 20 mg, 40 mg, 80 mg

Side Effects: *Musculoskeletal:* Rhabdomyolysis with renal dysfunction secondary to myoglobinuria, myopathy, arthralgias. *GI:* N&V, diarrhea, abdominal pain, constipation, flatulence, dyspepsia, pancreatitis, anorexia, stomatitis. *Hepatic:* Hepatitis (including chronic active hepatitis), cholestatic jaundice, cirrhosis, fatty change in liver, *fulminant hepatic necrosis, hepatoma. Neurologic:* Dysfunction of certain cranial nerves resulting in alteration of taste, impairment of extraocular movement, and facial paresis. Paresthesia, peripheral neuropathy, peripheral nerve palsy. *CNS:* Headache, tremor, vertigo, memory loss, anxiety, insomnia, depression. *Hypersensitivity Reactions:* Although rare, the following symptoms have been noted. *Angioedema,*

anaphylaxis, lupus erythematous–like syndrome, vasculitis, purpura, thrombocytopenia, leukopenia, *hemolytic anemia,* polymyalgia rheumatica, positive ANA, ESR increase, arthritis, arthralgia, asthenia, urticaria, photosensitivity, chills, fever, flushing, malaise, dyspnea, *toxic epidermal necrolysis, erythema multiforme (including Stevens-Johnson syndrome). GU:* Gynecomastia, loss of libido, erectile dysfunction. *Ophthalmologic:* Lens opacities, ophthalmoplegia. *Hematologic:* Transient asymptomatic eosinophilia, anemia, thrombocytopenia, leukopenia. *Miscellaneous:* URI, asthenia, alopecia, edema.

Drug Interactions: Additional: *Gemfibrozil /* Possible severe myopathy or rhabdomyolysis. *Warfarin /* ↑ Anticoagulant effect of warfarin.

EMS CONSIDERATIONS
None.

Sirolimus
(sir-oh-LIH-mus)
Pregnancy Class: C
Rapamune **(Rx)**
Classification: Immunosuppressive drug

Mechanism of Action: Inhibits both T-lymphocyte activation and proliferation that occurs in response to antigenic and interleukin IL-2, IL-4, and IL-15 stimulation. Also inhibits antibody production. Rapidly absorbed after PO use.

Uses: Prevent organ rejection in renal transplants. *Investigational:* Treatment of psoriasis.

Contraindications: Hypersensitivity to sirolimus, its derivatives, or any component of the drug product. Lactation.

Precautions: Use with caution in those with impaired renal function or when using with drugs that impair renal function (e.g., aminoglycosides, amphotericin B). Safety and efficacy have not been determined in combination with other immunosuppressant drugs or in pediatric patients less than 13 years of age.

Route/Dosage

• **Oral Solution**

Prophylaxis of rejection following kidney transplantation.

Loading dose, initial: 2 mg; **maintenance dose:** 2 mg/day. Or, **Loading dose, initial:** 15 mg; **maintenance:** 5 mg/day. **Patients, 13 years and older weighing <40 kg:** Adjust the initial dose based on body surface area to 1 mg/m²/day. The loading dose should be 3 mg/m². Reduce the maintenance dose by about 33% in patients with impaired hepatic function; it is not necessary to reduce the initial loading dose.

How Supplied: *Oral Solution:* 1 mg/mL

Side Effects: *GI:* Diarrhea, nausea, constipation, vomiting, dyspepsia, anorexia, dysphagia, eructation, esophagitis, flatulence, gastritis, gastroenteritis, gingivitis, gum hyperplasia, ileus, mouth ulceration, oral moniliasis, stomatitis. *CNS:* Tremor, insomnia, anxiety, confusion, depression, dizziness, emotional lability, hypertonia, hypesthesia, hypotonia, insomnia, neuropathy, paresthesia, somnolence. *CV:* Hypertension, atrial fibrillation, CHF, ***hemorrhage,*** hypervolemia, hypotension, palpitation, peripheral vascular disorder, postural hypotension, syncope, tachycardia, thrombophlebitis, thrombosis, vasodilation. *Dermatologic:* Acne, rash, fungal dermatitis, hirsutism, pruritus, skin hypertrophy, skin ulcer, sweating. *Respiratory:* Dyspnea, URTI, pharyngitis, asthma, atelectasis, bronchitis, increased cough, epistaxis, hypoxia, lung edema, pleural effusion, pneumonia, rhinitis, sinusitis. *Hematologic:* Anemia, thrombocytopenia, leukopenia, leukocytosis, lymphadenopathy, polycythemia, thrombotic thrombocytopenic purpura (hemolytic uremic syndrome). *GU:* UTI, bladder pain, dysuria, hematuria, hydronephrosis, impotence, kidney pain, kidney tubular necrosis, nocturia, oliguria, pyuria, scrotal edema, testis disorder, toxic nephrotoxicity, increased urinary frequency, urinary incontinence, urinary retention. *Musculoskeletal:* Arthralgia, arthrosis, bone necrosis, leg cramps, myalgia, osteoporosis, tetany. *Endocrine:* Cushing's syndrome, diabetes mellitus, glycosuria. *Ophthalmic:* Abnormal vision, cataract, conjunctivitis. *Otic:* Deafness, ear pain, otitis media, tinnitus. *Miscellaneous:* Abdominal pain, asthenia, back pain, chest pain, fever, headache, pain, arthralgia, ecchymosis, dehydration, abnormal healing, weight loss, enlarged abdomen, abscess, ascites, cellulitis, chills, facial edema, flu syndrome, generalized edema, hernia, infection, lymphocele, malaise, pelvic pain, peritonitis, ***sepsis***, increased susceptibility to infection and possible development of lymphoma.

Drug Interactions

Bromocriptine / ↑ Sirolimus blood levels R/T ↓ metabolism
Carbamazepine / ↓ Sirolimus blood levels R/T ↑ metabolism
Cimetidine / ↑ Sirolimus blood levels R/T ↓ metabolism
Cisapride / ↑ Sirolimus blood levels R/T ↓ metabolism
Clarithromycin / ↑ Sirolimus blood levels R/T ↓ metabolism
Clotrimazole / ↑ Sirolimus blood levels R/T ↓ metabolism
Cyclosporine / ↑ Sirolimus plasma levels
Danazol / ↑ Sirolimus blood levels R/T ↓ metabolism
Diltiazem / ↑ Sirolimus plasma levels
Erythromycin / ↑ Sirolimus blood levels R/T ↓ metabolism
Fluconazole / ↑ Sirolimus blood levels R/T ↓ metabolism
HIV-protease inhibitors / ↑ Sirolimus blood levels R/T ↓ metabolism
Itraconazole / ↑ Sirolimus blood levels R/T ↓ metabolism
Ketoconazole Significant ↑ sirolimus plasma levels; do not use together
Metoclopramide / ↑ Sirolimus blood levels R/T ↓ metabolism
Nicardipine / ↑ Sirolimus blood levels R/T ↓ metabolism

S

Phenobarbital / ↓ Sirolimus blood levels R/T ↑ metabolism
Phenytoin / ↓ Sirolimus blood levels R/T ↑ metabolism
Rifabutin / ↓ Sirolimus blood levels R/T ↑ metabolism
Rifampin / ↓ Sirolimus plasma levels R/T ↑ metabolism
Rifapentine/ ↓ Sirolimus blood levels R/T ↑ metabolism
Troleandomycin / ↑ Sirolimus blood levels R/T ↓ metabolism
Vaccines / Vaccines may be less effective
Verapamil / ↑ Sirolimus blood levels R/T ↓ metabolism

EMS CONSIDERATIONS
None.

Sodium bicarbonate
(SO-dee-um bye-KAR-bon-ayt)
Pregnancy Class: C
Arm and Hammer Pure Baking Soda, Bell/ans, Citrocarbonate, Neut, Soda Mint (Rx and OTC)
Classification: Alkalinizing agent, antacid, electrolyte

Mechanism of Action: The antacid action is due to neutralization of hydrochloric acid by forming sodium chloride and carbon dioxide (1 g of sodium bicarbonate neutralizes 12 mEq of acid). Provides temporary relief of peptic ulcer pain and of discomfort associated with indigestion. Although widely used by the public, sodium bicarbonate is rarely prescribed as an antacid because of its high sodium content, short duration of action, and ability to cause alkalosis (sometimes desired). Is also a systemic and urinary alkalinizer by increasing plasma and urinary bicarbonate, respectively.
Uses: Treatment of hyperacidity, severe diarrhea (where there is loss of bicarbonate). Alkalization of the urine to treat drug toxicity (e.g., due to barbiturates, salicylates, methanol). Treatment of acute mild to moderate metabolic acidosis due to shock, severe dehydration, anoxia, uncontrolled diabetes, renal disease, cardiac arrest, extracorporeal circulation of blood, severe primary lactic acidosis. Prophylaxis of renal calculi in gout. During sulfonamide therapy to prevent renal calculi and nephrotoxicity. Neutralizing additive solution to decrease chemical phlebitis and patient discomfort due to vein irritation at or near the site of infusion of IV acid solutions. *Investigational:* Sickle cell anemia.
Contraindications: Chloride loss due to vomiting or from continuous GI suction. With diuretics known to produce a hypochloremic alkalosis. Metabolic and respiratory alkalosis. Hypocalcemia in which alkalosis may cause tetany. Hypertension, convulsions, CHF, and other situations where administration of sodium can be dangerous. As a systemic alkalizer when used as a neutralizing additive solution. As an antidote for strong mineral acids because carbon dioxide is formed, which may cause discomfort and even perforation.
Precautions: Use with caution in impaired renal function, toxemia of pregnancy, with oliguria or anuria, during lactation, in edema, CHF, liver cirrhosis, with low-salt diets, and in geriatric or postoperative patients with renal or CV insufficiency with or without CHF.

Route/Dosage
• **Effervescent Powder**
   Antacid.
Adults: 3.9–10 g in a glass of cold water after meals. **Geriatric and pediatric, 6–12 years:** 1.9–3.9 g after meals.
• **Oral Powder**
   Antacid.
Adults: ½ teaspoon in a glass of water q 2 hr; adjust dosage as required.
   Urinary alkalinizer.
Adults: 1 teaspoon in a glass of water q 4 hr; adjust dosage as required. Dosage not established for this form for children.
• **Tablets**
   Antacid.
Adults: 0.325–2 g 1–4 times/day; pediatric, 6–12 years: 520 mg; may be repeated once after 30 min.

Urinary alkalinizer.
Adults, initial: 4 g; **then,** 1–2 g q 4 hr. **Pediatric:** 23–230 mg/kg/day; adjust dosage as needed.
• **IV**
Cardiac arrest.
Adults: 200–300 mEq given rapidly as a 7.5% or 8.4% solution. In emergencies, 300–500 mL of a 5% solution given as rapidly as possible without overalkalinizing the patient. **Infants, less than 2 years of age, initial:** 1–2 mEq/kg/min given over 1–2 min; **then,** 1 mEq/kg q 10 min of arrest. Do not exceed 8 mEq/kg/day.
Severe metabolic acidosis.
90–180 mEq/L (about 7.5–15 g) at a rate of 1–1.5 L during the first hour. Adjust to needs of patient.
Less severe metabolic acidosis.
Add to other IV fluids. **Adults and older children:** 2–5 mEq/kg given over a 4- to 8-hr period.
Neutralizing additive solution.
One vial of neutralizing additive solution added to 1 L of commonly used parenteral solutions, including dextrose, NaCl, and Ringer's.
How Supplied: *Granule, effervescent*; *Injection:* 4%, 4.2%, 5%, 7.5%, 8.4%; *Powder*; *Tablet:* 325 mg, 520 mg, 648 mg, 650 mg
Side Effects: *GI:* Acid rebound, gastric distention. *Milk-alkali syndrome:* Hypercalcemia, metabolic alkalosis (dizziness, cramps, thirst, anorexia, N&V, hyperexcitability, tetany, diminished breathing, *seizures*), renal dysfunction. *Miscellaneous:* Systemic alkalosis after prolonged use. *Following rapid infusion:* Hypernatremia, alkalosis, hyperirritability, tetany, fluid or solute overload. Extravasation following IV use may manifest ulceration, sloughing, cellulitis, or tissue necrosis at the site of injection.
OD Overdose Management: *Symptoms:* Severe alkalosis that may be accompanied by tetany or hyperirritability. *Treatment:* Discontinue sodium bicarbonate. Reverse symptoms of alkalosis by rebreathing expired air from a paper bag or using a rebreathing mask. Use an IV infusion of ammo-

nium chloride solution, 2.14%, to control severe cases. Treat hypokalemia by IV sodium chloride or potassium chloride. Calcium gluconate will control tetany.
Drug Interactions
Amphetamines / ↑ Effect of amphetamines by ↑ renal tubular reabsorption
Antidepressants, tricyclic / ↑ Effect of tricyclics by ↑ renal tubular reabsorption
Benzodiazepines / ↓ Effect due to ↑ alkalinity of urine
Chlorpropamide / ↑ Rate of excretion due to alkalinization of the urine
Ephedrine / ↑ Effect of ephedrine by ↑ renal tubular reabsorption
Erythromycin / ↑ Effect of erythromycin in urine due to ↑ alkalinity of urine
Flecainide / ↑ Effect due to ↑ alkalinity of urine
Iron products / ↓ Effect due to ↑ alkalinity of urine
Ketoconazole / ↓ Effect due to ↑ alkalinity of urine
Lithium carbonate / Excretion of lithium is proportional to amount of sodium ingested. If patient on sodium-free diet, may develop lithium toxicity because less lithium is excreted
Mecamylamine / ↓ Excretion due to alkalinization of the urine
Methenamine compounds / ↓ Effect of methenamine due to ↑ alkalinity of urine
Methotrexate / ↑ Renal excretion due to alkalinization of the urine
Nitrofurantoin / ↓ Effect of nitrofurantoin due to ↑ alkalinity of urine
Procainamide / ↑ Effect of procainamide due to ↓ excretion by kidney
Pseudoephedrine / ↑ Effect of pseudoephedrine due to ↑ tubular reabsorption
Quinidine / ↑ Effect of quinidine by ↑ renal tubular reabsorption
Salicylates / ↑ Rate of excretion due to alkalinization of the urine

S

Sulfonylureas / ↓ Effect due to ↑ alkalinity of urine

Sympathomimetics / ↓ Renal excretion due to alkalinization of the urine

Tetracyclines / ↓ Effect of tetracyclines due to ↑ excretion by kidney

EMS CONSIDERATIONS
Administration/Storage
IV 1. Avoid extravasation as tissue irritation or cellulitis may result.

2. May be given IV push in an arrest situation.

3. Administer isotonic solutions slowly; too-rapid administration may result in death due to cellular acidity.

4. If only the 7.5% or 8.4% solution is available, dilute 1:1 with D5W when used in infants for cardiac arrest.

5. Do not exceed a rate of administration of 8 mEq/kg/day in infants with cardiac arrest to guard against hypernatremia, induction of intracranial hemorrhage, and decreasing CSF pressure.

6. In the event of severe alkalosis or tetany, have available a parenteral solution of calcium gluconate and 2.14% ammonium chloride .

7. Norepinephrine and dobutamine are incompatible with $NaHCO_3$.

Sodium chloride
(SO-dee-um KLOR-eyed)
Pregnancy Class: C
Topical: Ayr Saline, HuMist Saline Nasal, NaSal Salaine Nasal, Ocean Mist, Salinex Nasal Mist; **Ophthalmic:** Adsorbonac Ophthalmic, AK-NaCl, Hypersal 5%, Muro-128 Ophthalmic, Muroptic-5; **Parenteral:** Sodium Chloride IV Infusions (0.45%, 0.9%, 3%, 5%), Sodium Chloride Injection for Admixtures (50, 100, 625 mEq/vial), Sodium Chloride Diluent (0.9%), concentrated Sodium Chloride Injection (14.6%, 23.4%) (parenteral is Rx; topical and ophthalmic are OTC)
Classification: Electrolyte

Mechanism of Action: Sodium is the major cation of the body's extracellular fluid. It plays a crucial role in maintaining the fluid and electrolyte balance. Excess retention of sodium results in overhydration (edema, hypervolemia), which is often treated with diuretics. Abnormally low levels of sodium result in dehydration. The average daily requirement of salt is approximately 5 g.

Uses: PO: Prophylaxis of heat prostration or muscle cramps, chloride deficiency due to diuresis or salt restriction, prevention or treatment of extracellular volume depletion.

Parenteral:

0.9% (Isotonic) NaCl. To restore sodium and chloride losses; to dilute or dissolve drugs for IV, IM, or SC use; flushing of IV catheters; extracellular fluid replacement; priming solution for hemodialysis; initiate and terminate blood transfusions so RBCs will not hemolyze; metabolic alkalosis when there is fluid loss and mild sodium depletion.

0.45% (Hypotonic) NaCl. Fluid replacement when fluid loss exceeds depletion of electrolytes; hyperosmolar diabetes when dextrose should not be used (need for large volume of fluid but without excess sodium ions).

3% or 5% (Hypertonic) NaCl. Hyponatremia and hypochloremia due to electrolyte losses; to dilute body water significantly following excessive fluid intake; emergency treatment of severe salt depletion.

Concentrated NaCl. Additive in parenteral therapy for patients with special needs for sodium intake.

Bacteriostatic NaCl. Used only to dilute or dissolve drugs for IM, IV, or SC injection.

Topical: Relief of inflamed, dry, or crusted nasal membranes; irrigating solution. **Ophthalmic:** Use hypertonic solutions to decrease corneal edema due to bullous keratitis; as an aid to facilitate ophthalmoscopic examination in gonioscopy, biomicroscopy, and funduscopy.

Contraindications: Congestive heart failure, severely impaired renal function, hypernatremia, fluid retention. Use of the 3% or 5% solutions in elevated, normal, or only slightly depressed levels of plasma sodium and chloride. Use of bacteriostatic NaCl injection in newborns.

Precautions: Use with caution in CV, cirrhotic, or renal disease; in presence of hyperproteinemia, hypervolemia, urinary tract obstruction, and CHF; in those with concurrent edema and sodium retention and in patients receiving corticosteroids or corticotropin; and during lactation. Use with caution in geriatric or postoperative patients with renal or CV insufficiency with or without CHF.

Route/Dosage

• **Tablets (Including Extended-Release and Enteric-Coated)**
Heat cramps/dehydration.
0.5–1 g with 8 oz water up to 10 times/day; total daily dose should not exceed 4.8 g.

• **IV**
Individualized. Daily requirements of sodium and chloride can be met by administering 1 L of 0.9% NaCl.
To calculate sodium deficit.
Amount of sodium to be given to raise serum sodium to the desired level:

Total body water (TBW): sodium deficit (mEq) = TBW × (desired plasma Na − observed plasma Na).

• **Ophthalmic Solution 2% or 5%**
1–2 gtt in eye q 3–4 hr.

• **Ophthalmic Ointment 5%**
A small amount (approximately ¼ in.) to the inside of the affected eye(s) (i.e., by pulling down the lower eyelid) q 3–4 hr.

How Supplied: *Dressing; Injection:* 0.45%, 0.9%, 2.5%, 3%, 5%, 14.6%, 23.4%; *Inhalation solution:* 0.45%, 0.9%, 3%, 10%; *Irrigation solution:* 0.45%, 0.9%; *Nasal solution:* 0.4%, 0.75%; *Ophthalmic ointment:* 5%; *Ophthalmic solution:* 0.44%, 2%, 5%; *Powder for reconstitution; Tablet:* 250 mg, 1 g

Side Effects: Hypernatremia. Excessive NaCl may lead to hypopotassemia and acidosis. Fluid and solute overload leading to dilution of serum electrolyte levels, CHF, overhydration, *acute pulmonary edema* (especially in patients with CV disease or in those receiving corticosteroids or other drugs that cause sodium retention). Too rapid administration may cause local pain and venous irritation.

Postoperative intolerance of NaCl: Cellular dehydration, weakness, asthenia, disorientation, anorexia, nausea, oliguria, increased BUN levels, distention, deep respiration.

Symptoms due to solution or administration technique: Fever, abscess, tissue necrosis, infection at injection site, venous thrombosis or phlebitis extending from injection site, local tenderness, extravasation, hypervolemia.

Inadvertent administration of concentrated NaCl (i.e., without dilution) will cause sudden hypernatremia with the possibility of CV shock, extensive hemolysis, CNS problems, necrosis of the cortex of the kidneys, local tissue necrosis (if given extravascularly).

OD **Overdose Management:** *Symptoms:* Irritation of GI mucosa, N&V, abdominal cramps, diarrhea, edema. Hypernatremia symptoms include: irritability, restlessness, *weakness, seizures,* coma, tachycardia, hypertension, fluid accumulation, *pulmonary edema, respiratory arrest. Treatment:* Supportive measures, including gastric lavage, induction of vomiting, provide adequate airway and ventilation, maintain vascular volume and tissue perfusion. Magnesium sulfate given as a cathartic.

EMS CONSIDERATIONS
None.

Sodium polystyrene sulfonate
(SO-dee-um pol-ee-STY-reen SUL-fon-ayt)
Pregnancy Class: C
Kayexalate, Kionex, SPS **(Rx)**
Classification: Potassium ion exchange resin

Mechanism of Action: Resin that exchanges sodium ions for potassium ions primarily in the large intestine. Thus, excess amounts of potassium (as well as calcium and magnesium) may be removed.

Onset of Action: PO: 2-12 hr.

Uses: Hyperkalemia.

Precautions: Use with caution in geriatric patients because they are more likely to develop fecal impaction. Use with caution in patients sensitive to sodium overload (e.g., in CV disease) or for those receiving digitalis preparations because the action of these agents is potentiated by hypokalemia. Effective decreases in potassium may take several hours to accomplish; other treatment (e.g., IV calcium or sodium bicarbonate or glucose and insulin) may be considered in states of severe hyperkalemia (e.g., burns, renal failure).

Route/Dosage

• **Powder for Suspension, Suspension**

Hyperkalemia.

Adults: 15 g resin suspended in 20–100 mL water or syrup (to increase palatability) 1–4 times/day. Up to 40 g/day has been used. **Pediatric:** To calculate dose, use an exchange ratio of 1 mEq potassium/g resin (usually, 1 g/kg dose).

• **Enema**

Hyperkalemia.

Adults: 30–50 g suspended in 100 mL sorbitol or 20% dextrose in water q 6 hr.

How Supplied: *Powder for reconstitution*; *Suspension:* 15 g/60 mL, 50 g/200 mL

Side Effects: *GI:* N&V, constipation, anorexia, gastric irritation, diarrhea (rarely). Fecal impaction in geriatric patients. *Electrolyte:* Sodium retention, hypokalemia, hypocalcemia, hypomagnesemia. *Other:* Overhydration, ***pulmonary edema.***

Drug Interactions

Aluminum hydroxide / ↑ Risk of intestinal obstruction

Calcium- or magnesium-containing antacids or laxatives / ↑ Risk of metabolic alkalosis

EMS CONSIDERATIONS

None.

Somatrem
Somatropin

Somatrem: (SO-mah-trem)Somatropin: (so-mah-TROH-pin)

Pregnancy Class: C, (Serostim is B)

Somatrem: Protropin **(Rx)** Somatropin: Genotropin, Humatrope, Norditropin, Nutropin, Nutropin AQ, Saizen, Serostim **(Rx)**

Classification: Growth hormone

Mechanism of Action: Both somatrem and somatropin are derived from recombinant DNA technology. Somatrem contains the same sequence of amino acids (191) as human growth hormone derived from the pituitary gland plus one additional amino acid (methionine). Somatropin has the identical sequence of amino acids as does human growth hormone of pituitary origin. These agents stimulate linear growth by increasing somatomedin-C serum levels, which, in turn, increases the incorporation of sulfate into proteoglycans, thereby stimulating skeletal growth. They also increase the number and size of muscle cells, increase synthesis of collagen, increase protein synthesis, and increase internal organ size. Serum insulin levels increase (indicative of insulin resistance), and there is acute mobilization of lipid.

Uses: Treat growth failure associated with chronic renal insufficiency up to the time of renal transplantation. Except for Serostim to stimulate linear growth of children who suffer from lack of adequate levels of endogenous growth hormone. Humatrope and Genotropin have been approved for the treatment of somatropin deficiency syndrome in adults. In adults, Humatrope produces increased lean muscle mass and exercise capacity, decreased body fat, and normalized high-density lipoprotein cholesterol levels. Humatrope, Nutropin, and Nutropin AQ for long-term treatment of short stature associated with Turner's syndrome. Serostim is approved for the treatment of AIDS wasting (i.e., cachexia). *Investigational:* Short children due to intrauterine growth retardation.

Contraindications: In patients in whom epiphyses have closed. Active intracranial lesions, sensitivity to benzyl alcohol (somatrem); sensitivity to m-cresol or glycerin (diluent in Humatrope). Use of Genotropin to treat acute catabolism in critically ill patients. *NOTE:* Hypothyroidism (which may be induced by the drug) decreases the response to somatrem.

Precautions: Use with caution during lactation. Concomitant use of glucocorticoids may decrease the response to growth hormone.

Route/Dosage
SOMATREM (PROTROPIN)
• **IM, SC**
Individualized. Usual: Up to 0.1 mg/kg (0.26 IU/kg) 3 times/week, not to exceed a weekly dosage of 0.30 mg/kg (about 0.90 IU/kg). The incidence of side effects increases if the dose is greater than 0.1 mg/kg.
SOMATROPIN (GENOTROPIN)
• **SC**
0.16–0.24 mg/kg/week divided into 6 or 7 SC injections.
SOMATROPIN (HUMATROPE)
• **IM, SC**
Adults: Individualized. Initial: 0.006 mg/kg/day (0.018 IU/kg/day) or less SC. May be increased, depending on need, to a maximum of 0.0125 mg/kg/day (0.0375 IU/kg/day). **Pediatric:** 0.18 mg/kg/week (0.54 IU/kg/week) SC or IM divided into equal doses given either on 3 alternate days or 6 times a week. Maximum weekly dose is 0.3 mg/kg (0.9 IU/kg) divided into equal doses and given on 3 alternate days.
SOMATRIPIN (NORDITROPIN)
• **SC**
0.024–0.034 mg/kg 6 to 7 times a week.
SOMATROPIN (NUTROPIN, NUTROPIN AQ)
• **SC**
Growth hormone deficiency.
Individualized. Usual: Give a weekly dose of 0.3 mg/kg (about 0.9 IU/kg).

Chronic renal insufficiency.
Individualized. Usual: Give a weekly dose of 0.35 mg/kg (about 1.05 IU/kg). This dose can be given up to the time of renal transplantation.
Turner Syndrome.
Give a weekly dose of 0.375 (or less) mg/kg (about 1.125 IU/kg) divided into equal doses 3 to 7 times/week.
SOMATROPIN (SAIZEN)
• **IM, SC**
0.06 mg/kg (about 0.18 IU/kg) 3 times weekly. Discontinue when epiphyses fuse.
SOMATROPIN (SEROSTIM)
• **SC**
Weight > 55 kg: 6 mg daily; **45–55 kg:** 5 mg daily; **35–45 kg:** 4 mg daily; **less than 35 kg:** 0.1 mg/kg. Give daily dose at bedtime.
How Supplied: Somatrem:*Powder for injection:* 5 mg, 10 mg; Somatropin: *Injection:* 5 mg/mL; *Powder for injection:* 1.5 mg, 5 mg, 5.8 mg, 6 mg, 10 mg

Side Effects: Development of persistent antibodies to growth hormone (30%–40% taking somatrem and 2% taking somatropin). Development of insulin resistance; hypothyroidism. Sodium retention and mild edema (especially in adults). Slipped capital femoral epiphysis or avascular necrosis of the femoral head in children with advanced renal osteodystrophy. Intracranial hypertension manifested by papilledema, visual changes, headache, N&V. *In adults:* Hyperglycemia, glucosuria; mild, transient edema; headache, weakness, muscle pain. *In children:* Injection site pain, leukemia.

Nutropin AQ: CTS, increased growth of preexisting nevi, gynecomastia, peripheral edema (rare), pancreatitis (rare). *Somatropin:* In adults, headache, localized muscle pain, weakness, mild hyperglycemia, glucosuria, mild transient edema during early treatment.

OD Overdose Management: *Symptons:* In acute overdose, hypoglycemia followed by hyperglycemia. Long-term overdose can result in S&S of acromegaly or gigantism.

Drug Interactions: Glucocorticoids inhibit the effect of somatrem on growth.

EMS CONSIDERATIONS

None.

Sotalol hydrochloride
(SOH-tah-lol)
Pregnancy Class: B
Betapace **(Rx)**
Classification: Beta-adrenergic blocking agent

Mechanism of Action: Blocks both beta-1- and beta-2-adrenergic receptors; has no membrane-stabilizing activity or intrinsic sympathomimetic activity. Has both Group II and Group III antiarrhythmic properties (dose dependent). Significantly increases the refractory period of the atria, His-Purkinje fibers, and ventricles. Also prolongs the QTc and JT intervals.

Uses: Treatment of documented ventricular arrhythmias such as life-threatening sustained VT.

Contraindications: Use in asymptomatic PVCs or supraventricular arrhythmias due to the proarrhythmic effects of sotalol. Congenital or acquired long QT syndromes. Use in patients with hypokalemia or hypomagnesemia until the imbalance is corrected, as these conditions aggravate the degree of QT prolongation and increase the risk for torsades de pointes.

Precautions: Patients with sustained ventricular tachycardia and a history of CHF appear to be at the highest risk for serious proarrhythmia. Dose, presence of sustained ventricular tachycardia, females, excessive prolongation of the QTc interval, and history of cardiomegaly or CHF are risk factors for torsades de pointes. Use with caution in patients with chronic bronchitis or emphysema and in asthma if an IV agent is required. Use with extreme caution in patients with sick sinus syndrome associated with symptomatic arrhythmias due to the increased risk of sinus bradycardia, sinus pauses, or sinus arrest. Reduce dosage in impaired renal function. Safety and efficacy in children have not been established.

Route/Dosage
• **Tablets**
  Ventricular arrhythmias.
Adults, initial: 80 mg b.i.d. The dose may be increased to 240 or 320 mg/day after appropriate evaluation. **Usual:** 160–320 mg/day given in two or three divided doses. Patients with life-threatening refractory ventricular arrhythmias may require doses ranging from 480 to 640 mg/day (due to potential proarrhythmias, use these doses only if the potential benefit outweighs the increased risk of side effects).

How Supplied: *Tablet:* 80 mg, 120 mg, 160 mg, 240 mg

Side Effects: Additional: *CV:New or worsened ventriclular arrhythmias, including sustained VT or ventricular fibrillation that might be fatal. Torsades de pointes.*

EMS CONSIDERATIONS

See also *Beta-Adrenergic Blocking Agents.*

Sparfloxacin
(spar-FLOX-ah-sin)
Pregnancy Class: C
Zagam **(Rx)**
Classification: Fluoroquinolone antibiotic

Uses: Community acquired pneumonia due to *Chlamydia pneumoniae, Haemophilus influenzae, Haemophilus parainfluenzae, Moraxella catarrhalis, Mycoplasma pneumoniae,* or *Streptococcus pneumoniae.* Acute bacterial exacerbations of chronic bronchitis caused by *C. pneumoniae, Enterobacter cloacae, H. influenzae, H. parainfluenzae, Klebsiella pneumoniae, M. catarrhalis, Staphylococcus aureus,* or *S. pneumoniae.*

Precautions: Safety and efficacy have not been determined in children less than 18 years of age.

Route/Dosage
- **Tablets**

Community-acquired pneumonia, acute bacterial exacerbations of chronic bronchitis.

Adults over 18 years of age: Two - 200 mg tablets taken on the first day as a loading dose. Then, one - 200 mg tablet q 24 hr for a total of 10 days of therapy (i.e., a total of 11 tablets). For patients with a C_{CR} less than 50 mL/min, the loading dose is two - 200 mg tablets taken on the first day. Then, one - 200 mg tablet q 48 hr for a total of 9 days (i.e., a total of 6 tablets).

How Supplied: *Tablets:* 200 mg.

EMS CONSIDERATIONS

None.

Spectinomycin hydrochloride
(speck-tin-oh-MY-sin)
Pregnancy Class: B
Trobicin **(Rx)**
Classification: Antibiotic, miscellaneous

Mechanism of Action: Produced by *Streptomyces spectabilis*. It inhibits bacterial protein synthesis by binding to ribosomes (30S subunit), thereby interfering with transmission of genetic information crucial to life of microorganism. Mainly bacteriostatic.

Uses: Acute gonorrheal proctitis and urethritis in males and acute gonorrheal cervicitis and proctitis in females due to susceptible strains of *Neisseria gonorrhoeae*. For pharyngeal infections, use only in those intolerant to cephalosporins or quinolones. It is ineffective against pharyngeal infections and against syphilis; is a poor drug to choose when mixed infections are present.

Contraindications: Sensitivity to drug.

Precautions: Safe use during pregnancy, in infants, and in children has not been established. Benzyl alcohol in the product may cause a fatal gasping syndrome in infants.

Route/Dosage
- **IM Only**

Gonorrheal urethritis in males, proctitis, and cervicitis.

2 g. In geographic areas where antibiotic resistance is known to be prevalent, give 4 g divided between two gluteal injection sites.

Alternative regimen for urethral, endocervical, or rectal gonococcal infections in patients who cannot take ceftriaxone.

Adults and children weighing more than 45 kg: Spectinomycin, 2 g, as a single dose followed by doxycycline. **Children weighing less than 45 kg:** 40 mg/kg given IM once.

Gonococcal infections in pregnancy where patient is allergic to beta-lactams.

2 g followed by erythromycin.

Disseminated gonococcal infection where patient is allergic to beta-lactams.

2 g q 12 hr.

How Supplied: *Powder for injection:* 2 g

Side Effects: A single dose of spectinomycin has caused soreness at the site of injection, urticaria, dizziness, nausea, chills, fever, and insomnia. Multiple doses have caused a decrease in H&H and C_{CR} and an increase in alkaline phosphatase, BUN, and ALT. In single or multiple doses, decrease in urine output.

EMS CONSIDERATIONS

See also *Anti-Infectives*.

Spironolactone
(speer-no-LAK-tohn)
Pregnancy Class: D
Aldactone **(Rx)**
Classification: Diuretic, potassium-sparing

S

---

bold italic = life threatening side effect

Mechanism of Action: Mild diuretic that acts on the distal tubule to inhibit sodium exchange for potassium, resulting in increased secretion of sodium and water and conservation of potassium. An aldosterone antagonist.

Onset of Action: Urine output increases over 1-2 days; **Peak:** 2-3 days.

Duration of Action: 2-3 days, and declines thereafter.

Uses: Primary hyperaldosteronism, including diagnosis, short-term preoperative treatment, long-term maintenance therapy for those who are poor surgical risks and those with bilateral micronodular or macronodular adrenal hyperplasia. To treat edema when other approaches are inadequate or ineffective (e.g., CHF, cirrhosis of the liver, nephrotic syndrome). Essential hypertension (usually in combination with other drugs). Prophylaxis of hypokalemia in patients taking digitalis. *Investigational:* Hirsutism, treat symptoms of PMS, with testolactone to treat familial male precocious puberty (short-term treatment), acne vulgaris.

Contraindications: Acute renal insufficiency, progressive renal failure, hyperkalemia, and anuria. Patients receiving potassium supplements, amiloride, or triamterene.

Precautions: Use during pregnancy only if benefits clearly outweigh risks. Use with caution in impaired renal function. Geriatric patients may be more sensitive to the usual adult dose.

S

Route/Dosage ————————
• **Tablets**
  Edema.

Adults, initial: 100 mg/day (range: 25–200 mg/day) in two to four divided doses for at least 5 days; **maintenance:** 75–400 mg/day in two to four divided doses. **Pediatric:** 3.3 mg/kg/day as a single dose or as two to four divided doses.
  Antihypertensive.

Adults, initial: 50–100 mg/day as a single dose or as two to four divided doses—give for at least 2 weeks;

maintenance: adjust to individual response. **Pediatric:** 1–2 mg/kg in a single dose or in two to four divided doses.
  Hypokalemia.

Adults: 25–100 mg/day as a single dose or two to four divided doses.
  Diagnosis of primary hyperaldosteronism.

Adults: 400 mg/day for either 4 days (short-test) or 3–4 weeks (long-test).
  Hyperaldosteronism, prior to surgery.

Adults: 100–400 mg/day in two to four doses prior to surgery.
  Hyperaldosteronism, chronic-therapy.

Use lowest possible dose.
  Hirsutim.

50–200 mg/day.
  Symptoms of PMS.

25 mg q.i.d. beginning on day 14 of the menstrual cycle.
  Familial male precocious puberty, short-term.

Spironolactone, 2 mg/kg/day, and testolactone, 20–40 mg/kg/day, for at least 6 months.
  Acne vulgaris.

100 mg/day.

How Supplied: *Tablet:* 25 mg, 50 mg, 100 mg

Side Effects: *Electrolyte:* Hyperkalemia, hyponatremia (characterized by lethargy, dry mouth, thirst, tiredness). *GI:* Diarrhea, cramps, ulcers, gastritis, gastric bleeding, vomiting. *CNS:* Drowsiness, ataxia, lethargy, mental confusion, headache. *Endocrine:* Gynecomastia, menstrual irregularities, impotence, bleeding in postmenopausal women, deepening of voice, hirsutism. *Dermatologic:* Maculopapular or erythematous cutaneous eruptions, urticaria. *Miscellaneous:* Drug fever, breast carcinoma, gynecomastia, hyperchloremic metabolic acidosis in hepatic cirrhosis (decompensated), ***agranulocytosis.*** *NOTE:* Spironolactone has been shown to be tumorigenic in chronic rodent studies.

Drug Interactions
Anesthetics, general / Additive hypotension

ACE inhibitors / Significant hyperkalemia

Anticoagulants, oral / Inhibited by spironolactone

Antihypertensives / Potentiation of hypotensive effect of both agents. Reduce dosage, especially of ganglionic blockers, by one-half

Captopril / ↑ Risk of significant hyperkalemia

Digitalis / ↑ Half-life of digoxin → ↓ clearance. Spironolactone may ↓ inotropic effect of digoxin. Spironolactone both ↑ and ↓ elimination t½ of digitoxin

Diuretics, others / Often administered concurrently because of potassium-sparing effect of spironolactone. Severe hyponatremia may occur. Monitor closely

Lithium / ↑ Chance of lithium toxicity due to ↓ renal clearance

Norepinephrine / ↓ Responsiveness to norepinephrine

Potassium salts / Since spironolactone conserves potassium excessively, hyperkalemia may result. Rarely used together

Salicylates / Large doses may ↓ effects of spironolactone

Triamterene / Hazardous hyperkalemia may result from combination

EMS CONSIDERATIONS

See also *Diuretics, Thiazides.*

————COMBINATION DRUG————
Spironolactone and Hydrochlorothiazide
(speer-oh-no-LAK-tohn)(hy-droh-klor-oh-THIGH-ah-zyd)
Pregnancy Class: D
Aldactazide **(Rx)**
Classification: Antihypertensive, diuretic

Mechanism of Action: This drug is a combination of a thiazide and potassium-sparing diuretic.

Uses: Congestive heart failure, essential hypertension, nephrotic syndrome. Edema and/or ascites in cirrhosis of the liver.

Contraindications: Use in pregnancy only if benefits outweigh risks.

Route/Dosage —————
• **Tablets**
Edema.
Adults, usual: 100 mg of each drug daily (range: 25–200 mg), given as single or divided doses. **Pediatric, usual:** equivalent to 1.65–3.3 mg/kg spironolactone.

Essential hypertension.
Adults, usual: 50–100 mg of each drug daily in single or divided doses.
How Supplied: Spironolactone - Hydrochlorothiazide: *Tablets:* 25 mg - 25 mg, 50 mg - 50 mg

EMS CONSIDERATIONS
None.

Stavudine
(STAH-vyou-deen)
Pregnancy Class: C
Zerit
Classification: Antiviral agent

Mechanism of Action: Inhibits replication of HIV due to phosphorylation by cellular kinases to stavudine triphosphate, which has antiviral activity. The mechanism for the antiviral activity includes inhibition of HIV reverse transcriptase by competing with the natural substrate deoxythymidine triphosphate and by causing DNA chain termination, thereby inhibiting viral DNA synthesis.

Uses: Treatment of adults with advanced HIV infection who cannot tolerate approved therapies or who have experienced significant clinical or immunologic deterioration while receiving such therapies (or for whom such therapies are contraindicated).

Contraindications: Lactation.

Precautions: The effect of stavudine on the clinical progression of HIV infection, such as incidence of opportunistic infections or survival, has not been determined.

S

Route/Dosage

• **Capsules**

Advanced HIV infections.

Adults, initial: 40 mg b.i.d. for patients weighing 60 or more kg and 30 mg b.i.d. for patients weighing less than 60 kg. In patients developing peripheral neuropathy, the following dosage schedule may be used if symptoms of neuropathy resolve completely: 20 mg b.i.d. for patients weighing 60 or more kg and 15 mg b.i.d. for patients weighing less than 60 kg.

The following dosage schedule is recommended for patients with impaired renal function: (a) C_{CR} greater than 50 mL/min: 40 mg q 12 hr for patients weighing 60 or more kg and 30 mg q 12 hr for patients weighing less than 60 kg; (b) C_{CR} 26–50 mL/min: 20 mg q 12 hr for patients weighing 60 or more kg and 15 mg q 12 hr for patients weighing less than 60 kg; (c) C_{CR} 10–25 mL/min: 20 mg q 24 hr for patients weighing 60 or more kg and 15 mg q 24 hr for patients weighing less than 60 kg. Insufficient data are available to recommend doses for a C_{CR} less than 10 mL/min or for patients undergoing dialysis.

How Supplied: *Capsule:* 15 mg, 20 mg, 30 mg, 40 mg; *Powder for Injection:* 1 mg/mL

Side Effects: *Neurologic:* Peripheral neuropathy (common), including numbness, tingling, or pain in feet or hands. *CNS:* Insomnia, anxiety, depression, nervousness, dizziness, confusion, migraine, somnolence, tremor, neuralgia, dementia. *GI:* Diarrhea, N&V, anorexia, dyspepsia, constipation, ulcerative stomatitis, aphthous stomatitis, pancreatitis. *Body as a whole:* Headache, chills, fever, asthenia, abdominal pain, back pain, malaise, weight loss, allergic reactions, flu syndrome, lymphadenopathy, pelvic pain, neoplasms, death. *CV:* Chest pain, vasodilation, hypertension, peripheral vascular disorder, syncope. *GU:* Dysuria, genital pain, dysmenorrhea, vaginitis, urinary frequency, hematuria, impotence, urogenital neoplasm.

Respiratory: Dyspnea, pneumonia, asthma. *Dermatologic:* Rash, sweating, pruritus, maculopapular rash, benign skin neoplasm, urticaria, exfoliative dermatitis. *Ophthalmic:* Conjunctivitis, abnormal vision.

EMS CONSIDERATIONS

See also *Antiviral Agents.*

Streptokinase

(strep-toe-KYE-nayz)

Pregnancy Class: C

Kabikinase, Streptase **(Rx)**

Classification: Thrombolytic agent

Mechanism of Action: Most patients have a natural resistance to streptokinase that must be overcome with the loading dose before the drug becomes effective. Streptokinase acts with plasminogen to produce an "activator complex," which enhances the conversion of plasminogen to plasmin. Plasmin then breaks down fibrinogen, fibrin clots, and other plasma proteins, promoting the dissolution (lysis) of the insoluble fibrin trapped in intravascular emboli and thrombi. Also, inhibitors of streptokinase, such as alpha-2-macroglobulin, are rapidly inactivated by streptokinase.

Onset of Action: Rapid.

Duration of Action: 12 hr.

Uses: DVT; arterial thrombosis and embolism; acute evolving transmural MI; pulmonary embolism. Also, clearing of occluded arteriovenous and IV cannulae.

Contraindications: Any condition presenting a risk of hemorrhage, such as recent surgery or biopsies, delivery within 10 days, ulcerative disease. Arterial emboli originating from the left side of the heart. Also, hepatic or renal insufficiency, tuberculosis, recent cerebral embolism, thrombosis, hemorrhage, SBE, rheumatic valvular disease, thrombocytopenia. Streptokinase resistance in excess of 1 million IU.

Precautions: The use of streptokinase in septic thrombophlebitis may be hazardous. History of significant allergic response. Safety in children has not been established. Geriatric patients have an increased risk of bleeding during therapy.

Route/Dosage ————————
• **IV Infusion**
DVT, pulmonary embolism, arterial thrombosis or embolism.
Loading dose: 250,000 IU over 30 min (use the 1,500,000 IU vial diluted to 90 mL); **maintenance:** 100,000 IU/hr for 24–72 hr for arterial thrombosis or embolism, 72 hr for deep vein thrombosis, and 24 hr (72 hr if deep vein thrombosis is suspected) for pulmonary embolism.
Acute evolving transmural MI.
1,500,000 IU within 60 min (use the 1,500,000 IU vial diluted to a total of 45 mL).
Arteriovenous cannula occlusion.
250,000 IU in 2-mL IV solution into each occluded limb of cannula and clamp off; **then,** after 2 hr aspirate cannula limbs, flush with saline, and reconnect cannula.
• **Intracoronary Infusion**
Acute evolving transmural MI.
20,000 IU by bolus; **then,** 2,000 IU/min for 60 min (total dose of 140,000 IU). Use the 250,000 IU vial diluted to 125 mL.
How Supplied: *Powder for injection:* 250,000 IU, 750,000 IU, 1.5 million IU

Side Effects: *CV:* Superficial bleeding, **severe internal bleeding.** *Allergic:* Nausea, headache, breathing difficulties, **bronchospasm, angioneurotic edema,** urticaria, flushing, musculoskeletal pain, vasculitis, interstitial nephritis, periorbital swelling. *Other:* Fever, possible development of Guillain-Barre syndrome, development of antistreptokinase antibody (i.e., streptokinase may be ineffective if administered between 5 days and 6 months following prior use of streptokinase or following streptococcal infections).

Drug Interactions: The following drugs increase the chance of bleeding when given concomitantly with streptokinase: anticoagulants, aspirin, heparin, indomethacin, and phenylbutazone.

EMS CONSIDERATIONS
See also *Alteplase, Recombinant.*
Administration/Storage
IV 1. NaCl injection USP or D5W is the preferred diluent for IV use.
2. Reconstitute gently, as directed by manufacturer, without shaking vial.
3. Note any redness and/or pain at the site of infusion; may need to further dilute solution to prevent phlebitis.
4. Have emergency drugs and equipment available.
Assessment: Drug may not be effective if administered within 5 days to 6 months of a strep infection.
Interventions
1. Observe in a closely monitored environment; document rhythm strips and VS q 15–30 min initially.
2. Check access sites for evidence of bleeding.
3. If excessive bleeding develops from an invasive procedure, discontinue therapy.
4. Following recanalization of an occluded coronary artery, patients may develop reperfusion reactions; these may include:
• Reperfusion arrhythmias (accelerated idioventricular rhythm, sinus bradycardia) usually of short duration.
• Reduction of chest pain
• Return of elevated ST segment to near baseline levels

Strontium-89 Chloride
(STRON-shee-um)
Pregnancy Class: D
Metastron **(Rx)**
Classification: Antineoplastic, radiopharmaceutical

Mechanism of Action: Taken up preferentially in sites of active osteogenesis leading to significant accumulation in primary bone tumors and areas of metastatic involvement. As a beta emitter, it selectively irradi-

---

ates primary metastatic bone involvement with minimal irradiation of soft tissues distant from bone lesions. Retained in metastatic areas significantly longer than in normal bone.

Uses: Relief of bone pain in patients with painful skeletal metastases.

Contraindications: Use in patients with seriously compromised bone marrow from previous therapy or disease without an assessment of benefit vs. risk. Lactation.

Precautions: Potential carcinogen. Use with caution in patients with platelet counts below 60,000 and WBC counts less than 2,400. Safety and efficacy in children less than 18 years of age have not been determined.

Route/Dosage
• **Slow IV Injection**
  Pain from bone metastases.
148 MBq, 4 mCi, given by slow IV injection over 1–2 min. An alternative dose is 1.5–2.2 MBq/kg, 40–60 mcCi/kg.

How Supplied: *Injection:* 1 mCi/mL
Side Effects: Calcium-like flushing following rapid (< 30 sec) administration. Increase in bone pain between 36 and 72 hr following injection. Bone marrow depression.

EMS CONSIDERATIONS

None.

Succinylcholine chloride
(suck-sin-ill-KOH-leen)
Pregnancy Class: C
Anectine, Anectine Flo-Pack, Quelicin, Succinylcholine Chloride Min-I-Mix **(Rx)**
Classification: Depolarizing neuromuscular blocking agent

Mechanism of Action: Initially excites skeletal muscle by combining with cholinergic receptors preferentially to acetylcholine. Subsequently, it prevents the muscle from contracting by prolonging the time during which the receptors at the neuromuscular junction cannot respond to acetylcholine. The order of paralysis

is levator muscles of the eyelid, mastication muscles, limb muscles, abdominal muscles, glottis muscles, the intercostals, the diaphragm, and all other skeletal muscles. Prolonged use may change from a depolarizing neuromuscular block (phase I block) to a block that resembles a nondepolarizing block (phase II block). This may be associated with prolonged respiratory depression and apnea. No effect on pain threshold, cerebration, or consciousness; use with sufficient anesthesia. Effects are not blocked by anticholinesterase drugs and may even be enhanced by them. May cause a change in myocardial rhythm due to vagal stimulation due to surgical procedures (especially in children) and from potassium-mediated alterations in electrical conductivity (enhanced by cyclopropane and halogenated anesthetics).

Onset of Action: IV: 30-60 sec; **IM:** 2-3 min.

Duration of Action: IV: 4-6 min; **recovery:** 8-10 min; **IM:** 10-30 min.

Uses: Adjunct to general anesthesia to facilitate ET intubation and to induce relaxation of skeletal muscle during surgery or mechanical ventilation. *Investigational:* Reduce intensity of electrically induced seizures or seizures due to drugs.

Contraindications: Use in genetically determined disorders of plasma pseudocholinesterase. Personal or family history of malignant hyperthermia. Myopathies associated with elevated CPK values. Acute narrow-angle glaucoma or penetrating eye injuries. Use of IV infusion in children due to the risk of malignant hyperpyrexia.

Precautions: Use with caution during lactation. Pediatric patients may be especially prone to myoglobinemia, myoglobinuria, and cardiac effects. Use with caution in patients with severe liver disease, severe anemia, malnutrition, impaired cholinesterase activity, fractures. Also, use with caution in CV, pulmonary, renal, or metabolic diseases. Use with great caution in those with severe burns, electrolyte imbalance, hyperkalemia, those receiving quinidine, and those who are digitalized or recovering from severe trauma, as serious cardiac arrhythmias or cardiac arrest may result. Patients with myasthenia gravis may show resistance to succinylcholine. Those with fractures or muscle spasms may manifest additional trauma due to succinylcholine-induced muscle fasciculations.

Route/Dosage

• **IM, IV**

Short or prolonged surgical procedures.

Adults, IV, initial: 0.3–1.1 mg/kg (average: 0.6 mg/kg); **then,** repeated doses can be given based on patient response. **Adults, IM:** 3–4 mg/kg, not to exceed a total dose of 150 mg.

• **IV Infusion (Preferred)**

Prolonged surgical procedures.

Adults: Average rate ranges from 2.5 to 4.3 mg/min. Most commonly used are 0.1%–0.2% solutions in 5% dextrose, sodium chloride injection, or other diluent given at a rate of 0.5–10 mg/min depending on patient response and degree of relaxation desired, for up to 1 hr.

• **Intermittent IV**

Prolonged muscle relaxation.

Initial: 0.3–1.1 mg/kg; **then,** 0.04–0.07 mg/kg at appropriate intervals to maintain required level of relaxation.

• **IM, IV**

Electroshock therapy.

Adults, IV: 10–30 mg given 1 min prior to the shock (individualize dosage). **IM:** Up to 2.5 mg/kg, not to exceed a total dose of 150 mg.

ET intubation.

Pediatric, IV: 1–2 mg/kg; if necessary, dose can be repeated. **IM:** 3–4 mg/kg, not to exceed a total dose of 150 mg.

How Supplied: *Injection:* 20 mg/mL, 50 mg/mL, 100 mg/mL; *Powder for injection:* 500 mg, 1 g

Side Effects: *Skeletal muscle:* May cause *severe, persistent respiratory depression or apnea.* Muscle fascicula-

tions, postoperative muscle pain. *CV:* Bradycardia or tachycardia, hypertension, hypotension, *arrhythmias, cardiac arrest. Respiratory:* **Apnea, respiratory depression.** *Other:* Fever, salivation, hyperkalemia, postoperative muscle pain, *anaphylaxis,* myoglobinemia, myoglobinuria, skin rashes, increased intraocular pressure, muscle fasciculation, myalgia, jaw rigidity, perioperative dreams in children, rhabdomyolysis with possible myoglobinuric acute renal failure. Repeated doses may cause tachyphylaxis.

Malignant hyperthermia: Muscle rigidity (especially of the jaw), tachycardia, tachypnea unresponsive to increased depth of anesthesia, increased oxygen requirement and carbon dioxide production, increased body temperature, metabolic acidosis.

OD Overdose Management: *Symptoms:* Skeletal muscle weakness, decreased respiratory reserve, low tidal volume, apnea. *Treatment:* Maintain a patent airway and respiratory support until normal respiration is ensured.

Drug Interactions

Aminoglycoside antibiotics / Additive skeletal muscle blockade

Amphotericin B / ↑ Effect of succinylcholine due to induced electrolyte imbalance

Antibiotics, nonpenicillin / Additive skeletal muscle blockade

Beta-adrenergic blocking agents / Additive skeletal muscle blockade

Chloroquine / Additive skeletal muscle blockade

Cimetidine / Cimetidine inhibits pseudocholinesterase

Clindamycin / Additive skeletal muscle blockade

Cyclophosphamide / ↑ Effect of succinylcholine by ↓ breakdown of drug in plasma by pseudocholinesterase

Cyclopropane / ↑ Risk of bradycardia, arrhythmias, sinus arrest, apnea, and malignant hyperthermia

Diazepam / ↓ Effect of succinylcholine

S

---

bold italic = life threatening side effect

Digitalis glycosides / ↑ Chance of cardiac arrhythmias, including ventricular fibrillation

Echothiophate iodide / ↑ Effect of succinylcholine by ↓ breakdown of drug in plasma by pseudocholinesterase

Furosemide / ↑ Skeletal muscle blockade

Halothane / ↑ Risk of bradycardia, arrhythmias, sinus arrest, apnea, and malignant hyperthermia

Isoflurane / Additive skeletal muscle blockade

Lidocaine / Additive skeletal muscle blockade

Lincomycin / Additive skeletal muscle blockade

Lithium carbonate / ↑ Skeletal muscle blockade

Magnesium salts / Additive skeletal muscle blockade

Narcotics / ↑ Risk of bradycardia and sinus arrest

Nitrous oxide / ↑ Risk of bradycardia, arrhythmias, sinus arrest, apnea, and malignant hyperthermia

Oxytocin / ↑ Effect of succinylcholine

Phenelzine / ↑ Effect of succinylcholine

Phenothiazines / ↑ Effect of succinylcholine

Polymyxin / Additive skeletal muscle blockade

Procainamide / ↑ Effect of succinylcholine

Procaine / ↑ Effect of succinylcholine by inhibiting plasma pseudocholinesterase activity

Promazine / ↑ Effect of succinylcholine

Quinidine / Additive skeletal muscle blockade

Quinine / Additive skeletal muscle blockade

Tacrine / ↑ Effect of succinylcholine

Thiazide diuretics / ↑ Effect of succinylcholine due to induced electrolyte imbalance

Thiotepa / ↑ Effect of succinylcholine by ↓ breakdown of drug in plasma by pseudocholinesterase

Trimethaphan / ↑ Effect of succinylcholine by inhibiting plasma pseudocholinesterase activity

EMS CONSIDERATIONS

See also *Neuromuscular Blocking Agents.*

IV **Administration/Storage:** For IV infusion, use 1 or 2 mg/mL solution of drug in D5W, 0.9% NaCl, or other suitable IV solution; drug is not compatible with alkaline solutions.

Interventions

1. Monitor VS and ECG; can cause vagal stimulation resulting in bradycardia, hypotension, and cardiac arrhythmias, especially in children.

2. Monitor for evidence of malignant hyperthermia, unresponsive tachycardia, jaw spasm, or lack of laryngeal relaxation.

3. Patient fully conscious and aware of surroundings/conversations.

4. Drug does not affect pain or anxiety; administer analgesics and antianxiety agents as indicated.

Sucralfate

(sue-KRAL-fayt)
Pregnancy Class: B
Carafate **(Rx)**
Classification: Antiulcer drug

Mechanism of Action: Thought to form an ulcer-adherent complex with albumin and fibrinogen at the site of the ulcer, protecting it from further damage by gastric acid. May also form a viscous, adhesive barrier on the surface of the gastric mucosa and duodenum. It adsorbs pepsin, thus inhibiting its activity. May be used in conjunction with antacids.

Duration of Action: 5 hr.

Uses: Short-term treatment (up to 8 weeks) of active duodenal ulcers. Maintenance for duodenal ulcer at decreased dosage after healing of acute ulcers. *Investigational:* Hasten healing of gastric ulcers, chronic treatment of gastric ulcers. Treatment of reflux and peptic esophagitis. Treatment of aspirin- and NSAID-induced GI symptoms; prevention of stress ulcers and GI bleeding in critically ill patients. The suspension has been used to treat oral and esophageal ulcers due to chemotherapy, radiation, or sclerotherapy.

Note: Even though healing of ulcers may result, the frequency or severity of subsequent attacks is not altered.

Precautions: Safety for use in children and during lactation has not been fully established. A successful course resulting in healing of ulcers will not alter posthealing frequency or severity of duodenal ulceration.

Route/Dosage
• **Suspension, Tablets**
Adults: usual: 1 g q.i.d. (10 mL of the suspension) 1 hr before meals and at bedtime (it may also be taken 2 hr after meals). Take for 4–8 weeks unless X-ray films or endoscopy have indicated significant healing. **Maintenance (tablets only):** 1 g b.i.d.

How Supplied: *Suspension:* 1 g/10 mL; *Tablet:* 1 g

Side Effects: *GI:* Constipation (most common); also, N&V, diarrhea, indigestion, flatulence, dry mouth, gastric discomfort. *Hypersensitivity:* Urticaria, **angioedema, respiratory difficulty,** rhinitis. *Miscellaneous:* Back pain, dizziness, sleepiness, vertigo, rash, pruritus, facial swelling, **laryngospasm.**

Drug Interactions
Antacids containing aluminum / ↑ Total body burden of aluminum
Anticoagulants / ↓ Hypoprothrombinemic effect of warfarin
Cimetidine / ↓ Absorption of cimetidine due to binding to sucralfate
Ciprofloxacin / ↓ Absorption of ciprofloxacin due to binding to sucralfate
Digoxin / ↓ Absorption of digoxin due to binding to sucralfate
Ketoconazole / ↓ Bioavailability of ketoconazole
Norfloxacin / ↓ Absorption of norfloxacin due to binding to sucralfate
Phenytoin / ↓ Absorption of phenytoin due to binding to sucralfate

Quinidine / ↓ Quinidine levels → ↓ effect
Ranitidine / ↓ Absorption of ranitidine due to binding to sucralfate
Tetracycline / ↓ Absorption of tetracycline due to binding to sucralfate
Theophylline / ↓ Absorption of theophylline due to binding to sucralfate

EMS CONSIDERATIONS
None.

Sulfacetamide sodium
(sul-fah-SEAT-ah-myd)
Bleph-10, Cetamide, Isopto-Cetamide, I-Sulfacet, Ocu-Sul-10, Ocu-Sul-15, Ocu-Sul-30, Ocusulf-10, Ophthacet, Sebizon, Sodium Sulamyd, Spectro-Sulf, Steri-Units Sulfacetamide, Sulf-10, Sulfair, Sulfair 10, Sulfair 15, Sulfair Forte, Sulfamide, Sulten-10 **(Rx)**
Classification: Sulfonamide, topical

Uses: Topically for conjunctivitis, corneal ulcer, and other superficial ocular infections. As an adjunct to systemic sulfonamides to treat trachoma.

Contraindications: In infants less than 2 months of age. Use in the presence of epithelial herpes simplex keratitis, vaccinia, varicella, and other viral diseases of the cornea and conjunctiva. Mycobacterial or fungal infections of the ocular structures. After uncomplicated removal of a corneal foreign body.

Precautions: Safe use during pregnancy and lactation or in children less than 12 years of age has not been established. Use with caution in patients with dry eye syndrome. Ophthalmic ointments may retard corneal wound healing.

Route/Dosage
• **Ophthalmic Solution, 10%, 15%, 20%**
Conjunctivitis or other superficial ocular infections.
1–2 gtt in the conjunctival sac q 1–4 hr. Doses may be tapered by in-

S

---

bold italic = life threatening side effect

creasing the time interval between doses as the condition improves.

Trachoma.

2 gtt q 2 hr with concomitant systemic sulfonamide therapy.

• **Ophthalmic Ointment (10%)**

Apply approximately ¼ in. into the lower conjunctival sac 3–4 times/day and at bedtime. Alternatively, 0.5–1 in. is placed in the conjunctival sac at bedtime along with use of drops during the day.

For cutaneous infections.

Apply locally (10%) to affected area b.i.d.–q.i.d.

• **Lotion**

Seborrheic dermatitis.

Apply 1–2 times/day (for mild cases, apply overnight).

Cutaneous bacterial infections.

Apply b.i.d.–q.i.d. until infection clears.

How Supplied: *Lotion:* 10%; *Ophthalmic Ointment:* 10%; *Ophthalmic Solution:* 10%, 15%, 30%

Side Effects: *When used topically:* Itching, local irritation, periorbital edema, burning and transient stinging, headache, bacterial or fungal corneal ulcers. *NOTE:* Sulfonamides may cause serious systemic side effects, including severe hypersensitivity reactions. Symptoms include fever, skin rash, GI disturbances, bone marrow depression, ***Stevens-Johnson syndrome, toxic epidermal necrolysis,*** exfoliative dermatitis, photosensitivity. Fatalities have occurred.

Drug Interactions: Preparations containing silver are incompatible with sulfacetamide sodium.

EMS CONSIDERATIONS

See also *Anti-Infectives* and *Sulfonamides.*

Sulfadiazine
Sulfadiazine sodium

(sul-fah-DYE-ah-zeen)

Pregnancy Class: C

Sulfadiazine: Microsulfon **(Rx)** Sulfadiazine sodium: **(Rx)**

Classification: Sulfonamide

Mechanism of Action: Short-acting; often combined with other anti-infectives.

Uses: UTIs caused by *Escherichia coli, Klebsiella, Enterobacter, Staphylococcus aureus, Proteus mirabilis, and Proteus vulgaris.* Chancroid, inclusion conjunctivitis, adjunct in treating chloroquine-resistant strains of *Plasmodium falciparum,* meningitis caused by *Haemophilus influenzae,* meningococcal meningitis for sulfonamide-sensitive group A strains, nocardiosis, with penicillin to treat acute otitis media caused by *H. influenzae,* rheumatic fever prophylaxis, adjunct with pyrimethamine for toxoplasmosis in selected immunocompromised patients (e.g., those with AIDS, neoplastic disease, or congenital immune compromise), trachoma.

Contraindications: Use in infants less than 2 months of age unless combined with pyrimethamine to treat congenital toxoplasmosis.

Precautions: Safe use during pregnancy has not been established.

Route/Dosage ——————

• **Tablets**

General use.

Adults, loading dose: 2–4 g; **maintenance:** 2–4 g/day in 3 to 6 divided doses; **infants over 2 months, loading dose:** 75 mg/kg/day (2 g/m²); **maintenance:** 150 mg/kg/day (4 g/m²/day) in 4 to 6 divided doses, not to exceed 6 g/day.

Rheumatic fever prophylaxis.

Under 30 kg: 0.5 g/day; **over 30 kg:** 1 g/day.

As adjunct with pyrimethamine in congenital toxoplasmosis.

Infants less than 2 months: 25 mg/kg q.i.d. for 3 to 4 weeks. **Children greater than 2 months:** 25–50 mg/kg q.i.d. for 3 to 4 weeks. **How Supplied:** *Tablet:* 500 mg

EMS CONSIDERATIONS

See also *Anti-Infectives* and for *Sulfonamides.*

S

Sulfamethoxazole

(sul-fah-meth-OX-ah-zohl)
Pregnancy Class: C
Gantanol **(Rx)**
Classification: Sulfonamide, intermediate-acting

Uses: UTIs caused by *Escherichia coli, Klebsiella, Enterobacter, Staphylococcus aureus, Proteus mirabilis,* and *Proteus vulgaris.* Chancroid, inclusion conjunctivitis, adjunct in treating chloroquine-resistant strains of *Plasmodium falciparum,* meningococcal meningitis for sulfonamide-sensitive group A strains, nocardiosis, with penicillin to treat acute otitis media caused by *H. influenzae,* adjunct with pyrimethamine for toxoplasmosis in selected immunocompromised patients (e.g., those with AIDS, neoplastic disease, or congenital immune compromise), trachoma.
Precautions: May be an increased risk of severe side effects in elderly patients.

Route/Dosage ——————
• **Tablets**
Mild to moderate infections.
Adults, initially: 2 g; **then,** 1 g in morning and evening.
Severe infections.
Adults, initially: 2 g; **then,** 1 g t.i.d. **Infants over 2 months, initial:** 50–60 mg/kg; **then,** 25–30 mg/kg in morning and evening, not to exceed 75 mg/kg/day. Alternative dosing: 50–60 mg/kg/day divided q 12 hr, not to exceed 3 g/24 hr.
How Supplied: *Tablet:* 500 mg

EMS CONSIDERATIONS

See also *All Anti-Infectives*

Sulfasalazine

(sul-fah-SAL-ah-zeen)
Pregnancy Class: B
Azulfidine, Azulfidine EN-Tabs, **(Rx)**
Classification: Sulfonamide

Uses: Ulcerative colitis. Azulfidine EN-tabs are also used to treat rheumatoid arthritis in patients who do not respond well to NSAIDs. *Investiga-*

tional: Ankylosing spondylitis, collagenous colitis, Crohn's disease, psoriasis, juvenile chronic arthritis, psoriatic arthritis.
Contraindications: Additional: Children below 2 years. In persons with marked sulfonamide, salicylate, or related drug hypersensitivity. Intestinal or urinary obstruction.
Precautions: Use with caution during lactation.

Route/Dosage ——————
• **Enteric-Coated Tablets, Tablets**
Ulcerative colitis.
Adults, initial: 3–4 g/day in divided doses (1–2 g/day may decrease side effects); **maintenance:** 500 mg q.i.d.
Pediatric, over 2 years of age, initial: 40–60 mg/kg/day in 3 to 6 equally divided doses; **maintenance:** 30 mg/kg/day in 4 divided doses.
For desensitization to sulfasalazine.
Reinstitute at level of 50–250 mg/day; **then,** give double dose q 4–7 days until desired therapeutic level reached. Do not attempt in those with a history of agranulocytosis or who have experienced anaphylaxis previously with sulfasalazine.
Collagenous colitis.
2–3 g/day.
Psoriasis.
3–4 g/day.
Juvenile chronic arthritis.
50 mg/kg.
Psoriatic arthritis.
2 g/day.
How Supplied: *Enteric Coated Tablet:* 500 mg; *Tablet:* 500 mg
Side Effects: Most common include anorexia, headache, N&V, gastric distress, reversible oligospermia. Less frequently, pruritus, urticaria, fever, Heinz body anemia, hemolytic anemia, cyanosis.
Drug Interactions
Digoxin / ↓ Absorption of digoxin
Folic acid / ↓ Absorption of folic acid

EMS CONSIDERATIONS

See also *Anti-Infectives* and for *Sulfonamides.*

S

Sulfinpyrazone
(sul-fin-PEER-ah-zohn)
Classification: Antigout agent, uricosuric

Uses: Chronic and intermittent gouty arthritis. Not effective during acute attacks of gout and may even increase the frequency of acute episodes during the initiation of therapy. However, do not discontinue during acute attacks. Concomitant administration of colchicine during initiation of therapy is recommended. *Investigational:* To decrease sudden death during first year after MI.
Contraindications: Active peptic ulcer or symptoms of GI inflammation or ulceration. Blood dyscrasias. Sensitivity to phenylbutazone or other pyrazoles. Use to control hyperuricemia secondary to treatment of malignancies.
Precautions: Use with caution in pregnant women. Dosage has not been established in children. Use with extreme caution in patients with impaired renal function and in those with a history of peptic ulcers.

Route/Dosage ———————
• **Capsules, Tablets**
Gout.
Adults, initial: 200–400 mg/day in two divided doses with meals or milk. Patients who are transferred from other uricosuric agents can receive full dose at once. **Maintenance:** 100–400 mg b.i.d. Maintain full dosage without interruption even during acute attacks of gout.
Following MI.
Adults: 300 mg q.i.d. or 400 mg b.i.d.
How Supplied: *Capsule:* 200 mg; *Tablet:* 100 mg
Side Effects: *GI:* N&V, abdominal discomfort. May reactivate peptic ulcer. *Hematologic:* Leukopenia, **agranulocytosis,** anemia, thrombocytopenia, **aplastic anemia.** *Miscellaneous:* Skin rash (which usually disappears with usage), **bronchoconstriction in aspirin-induced asthma.** Acute attacks of gout may become more frequent during initial therapy. Give concomitantly with colchicine at this time.
OD **Overdose Management:** *Symptoms:* N&V, diarrhea, epigastric pain, labored respiration, ataxia, seizures, coma. *Treatment:* Supportive measures.
Drug Interactions
Acetaminophen / ↑ Risk of acetaminophen hepatotoxicity; ↓ effect of acetaminophen
Anticoagulants / ↑ Effect of anticoagulants due to ↓ plasma protein binding
Niacin / ↓ Uricosuric effect of sulfinpyrazone
Salicylates / Inhibit uricosuric effect of sulfinpyrazone
Theophylline / ↓ Effect of theophylline due to ↑ plasma clearance
Tolbutamide / ↑ Risk of hypoglycemia
Verapamil / ↓ Effect of verapamil due to ↑ plasma clearance

EMS CONSIDERATIONS
None.

Sulfisoxazole
Sulfisoxazole diolamine
(sul-fih-SOX-ah-zohl)
Pregnancy Class: C
(Rx) for both.
Classification: Sulfonamide, short-acting

Uses: UTIs caused by *Escherichia coli, Klebsiella, Enterobacter, Staphylococcus aureus, Proteus mirabilis,* and *Proteus vulgaris.* Chancroid, inclusion conjunctivitis, adjunct in treating chloroquine-resistant strains of *Plasmodium falciparum,* meningitis caused by *Haemophilus influenzae,* meningococcal meningitis for sulfonamide-sensitive group A strains, nocardiosis, with penicillin to treat acute otitis media caused by *H. influenzae,* adjunct with pyrimethamine for toxoplasmosis in selected immunocompromised patients (e.g., those with AIDS, neoplastic disease, or congenital immune compromise). Ophthalmically as an adjunct with systemic sulfonamides to treat trachoma.

Contraindications: Additional: Use in infants less than 2 months of age except as adjunct with pyrimethamine to treat congenital toxoplasmosis. Use in the presence of epithelial herpes simplex keratitis, vaccinia, varicella, and other viral diseases of the cornea and conjuctiva. Mycobacterial or fungal infections of the ocular structures. After uncomplicated removal of a corneal foreign body.

Precautions: Safety and efficacy of the ophthalmic products have not been established in children. Use with caution in patients with severe dry eye.

Route/Dosage ————
• **Tablets**
Adults, loading dose: 2–4 g; **maintenance:** 4–8 g/day in 4 to 6 divided doses, depending on severity of the infection. **Infants over 2 months, initial:** 75 mg/kg/day; **maintenance:** 150 mg/kg/day (4 g/m²/day) in 4 to 6 divided doses, not to exceed 6 g/day.
• **Ophthalmic Solution (4%)**
Conjunctivitis or corneal ulcer.
1–2 gtt into conjunctival sac q 1–4 hr, depending on the severity of the infection. Dose may be tapered by increasing the time interval between doses as the condition improves.
Trachoma.
2 qtt q 2 hr with concomitant systemic therapy.

How Supplied: Sulfisoxazole: *Tablet:* 500 mg. Sulfisoxazole acetyl: *Suspension:* 500 mg/5 mL Sulfisoxazole diolamine: *Ophthalmic Solution:* 4%

EMS CONSIDERATIONS

See also *Anti-Infectives* and *Sulfonamides.*

Sulindac
(su-IN-dak)
Clinoril, **(Rx)**
Classification: Nonsteroidal anti-inflammatory drug

Onset of Action: Anti-Inflammatory effect: within 1 week.
Duration of Action: Anti-Inflammatory effect: 1-2 weeks.
Uses: Acute and chronic treatment of rheumatoid arthritis, osteoarthritis, ankylosing spondylitis, acute gouty arthritis; acute, painful shoulder; tendinitis, bursitis. *Investigational:* Juvenile rheumatoid arthritis, sunburn.
Contraindications: Use with active GI lesions or a history of recurrent GI lesions.
Precautions: Safety and efficacy have not been established for children. Safe use during pregnancy has not been established. Use with caution during lactation.

Route/Dosage ————
• **Tablets**
Osteoarthritis, rheumatoid arthritis, ankylosing spondylitis.
Adults: 150 mg b.i.d.
Acute painful shoulder, acute gouty arthritis.
Adults: 200 mg b.i.d. for 7–14 days.
Antigout.
Adults: 200 mg b.i.d. for 7 days.
How Supplied: *Tablet:* 150 mg, 200 mg
Side Effects: Additional: Hypersensitivity, pancreatitis, GI pain (common), maculopapular rash. Stupor, ***coma***, hypotension, and diminished urine output.
Drug Interactions: Additional: Sulindac ↑ effect of warfarin due to ↓ plasma protein binding.

EMS CONSIDERATIONS

See also *Nonsteroidal Anti-Inflammatory Drugs.*

Sumatriptan succinate
(soo-mah-TRIP-tan)
Pregnancy Class: C
Imitrex, **(Rx)**
Classification: Antimigraine drug

Mechanism of Action: Selective agonist for a vascular 5-HT₁ receptor subtype (probably 5-HT_{1D}) located on cranial arteries, on the basilar artery, and the vasculature of the dura mater. Activates the 5-HT$_1$ receptor, causing vasoconstriction and therefore relief of migraine. Transient increases in BP may be observed. No significant activity at 5-HT$_2$ or 5-HT$_3$ receptor subtypes; alpha-1-, alpha-2-, or beta-adrenergic receptors; dopamine-1 or dopamine-2 receptors; muscarinic receptors; or benzodiazepine receptors. **Onset of Action: Time to peak effect after SC:** 12 min after a 6-mg dose.

Uses: Treatment of acute migraine attacks with or without aura. Photophobia, phonophobia, N&V associated with migraine attacks are also relieved. Intended to relieve migraine, but not to prevent or reduce the number of attacks experienced. Acute treatment of cluster headaches (injection only).

Contraindications: Hypersensitivity to sumatriptan. IV use due to the possibility of coronary vasospasm. SC use in patients with ischemic heart disease, history of MI, documented silent ischemia, Prinzmetal's angina, or uncontrolled hypertension. Concomitant use with ergotamine-containing products or MAO inhibitor therapy (or within 2 weeks of discontinuing an MAO inhibitor). Use in patients with hemiplegic or basilar migraine. Use in women who are pregnant, think they may be pregnant, or are trying to get pregnant.

Precautions: Use with caution during lactation, in patients with impaired hepatic or renal function, and in patients with heart conditions. Patients with risk factors for CAD (e.g., men over 40, smokers, postmenopausal women, hypertension, obesity, diabetes, hypercholesterolemia, family history of heart disease) should be screened before initiating treatment. Safety and efficacy have not been determined for use in children.

Route/Dosage
• **SC**
Migraine headaches.
Adults: 6 mg. A second injection may be given if symptoms of mi-

graine come back but no more than two injections (6 mg each) should be taken in a 24-hr period and at least 1 hr should elapse between doses.
• **Tablets**
Adults: 25 mg with fluids as soon as symptoms of migraine appear. A second dose may be taken if symptoms return but not sooner than 2 hr following the first dose. **Maximum recommended dose:** 100 mg, with no more than 300 mg taken in a 24-hr period.
• **Nasal Spray**
A single dose of 5, 10, or 20 mg given in one nostril. The 20 mg dose increases the risk of side effects. The 10-mg dose may be given as a single 5-mg dose in each nostril. If the headache returns, repeat the dose once after 2 hr; not to exceed a total daily dose of 40 mg. The safety of treating an average of more than 4 headaches in a 30-day period has not been studied.

How Supplied: *Injection:* 6 mg/0.5 mL; *Kit:* 6 mg/0.5 mL; *Nasal spray:* 5 mg, 20 mg; *Tablet:* 25 mg, 50 mg

Side Effects: Side effects listed are for either SC or PO use of the drug. *CV:* Coronary vasospasm in patients with a history of CAD. ***Serious and/or life-threatening arrhythmias, including atrial fibrillation, ventricular fibrillation, ventricular tachycardia, MI, marked ischemic ST elevations,*** chest and arm discomfort representing angina pectoris. Flushing, hypertension, hypotension, bradycardia, tachycardia, palpitations, pulsating sensations, ECG changes (including nonspecific ST- or T-wave changes, prolongation of PR or QTc intervals, sinus arrhythmia, nonsustained ventricular premature beats, isolated junctional ectopic beats, atrial ectopic beats, and delayed activation of the right ventricle), syncope, pallor, abnormal pulse, vasodilatation, atherosclerosis, bradycardia, cerebral ischemia, CV lesion, heart block, peripheral cyanosis, thrombosis, transient myocardial ischemia, vasodilation, Raynaud's syndrome. *At injection site:* Pain, redness. *Atypical sensa-*

tions: Sensation of warmth, cold, tingling, or paresthesia. Localized or generalized feeling of pressure, burning, numbness, and tightness. Feeling of heaviness, feeling strange, tight feeling in head. *CNS:* Fatigue, dizziness, drowsiness, vertigo, sedation, headache, anxiety, malaise, confusion, euphoria, agitation, relaxation, chills, tremor, shivering, prickling or stinging sensations, phonophobia, depression, euphoria, facial pain, heat sensitivity, incoordination, monoplegia, sleep disturbances, shivering. *EENT:* Throat discomfort, discomfort in nasal cavity or sinuses. Vision alterations, eye irritation, photophobia, lacrimation, otalgia, feeling of fullness in ear, disorders of sclera, mydriasis. *GI:* Abdominal discomfort, dysphagia, discomfort of mouth and tongue, gastroesophageal reflux, diarrhea, peptic ulcer, retching, flatulence, eructation, gallstones, taste disturbances, GI bleeding, hematemesis, melena. *Respiratory:* Dyspnea, diseases of the lower respiratory tract, hiccoughs, influenza, asthma. *Dermatologic:* Erythema, pruritus, skin rashes, skin eruptions, skin tenderness, dry or scaly skin, tightness or wrinkling of skin. *GU:* Dysuria, dysmenorrhea, urinary frequency, renal calculus, breast tenderness, increased urination, intermenstrual bleeding, nipple discharge, abortion, hematuria. *Musculoskeletal:* Weakness, neck pain or stiffness, myalgia, muscle cramps, joint disturbances (pain, stiffness, swelling, ache), muscle stiffness, need to flex calf muscles, backache, muscle tiredness, swelling of the extremities, tetany. *Endocrine:* Elevated TSH levels, galactorrhea, hyperglycemia, hypoglycemia, hypothyroidism, weight gain or loss. *Miscellaneous:* Chest, jaw, or neck tightness. Sweating, thirst, polydipsia, chills, fever, dehydration.

OD Overdose Management: *Symptoms*: Tremor, ***convulsions,*** inactivity erythema of extremities, reduced respiratory rate, cyanosis, ataxia, mydriasis, injection site reactions (desquamation, hair loss, scab formation), paralysis. *Treatment:* Continuous monitoring of patient for at least 10 hr and especially when signs and symptoms persist.

Drug Interactions
Ergot drugs / Prolonged vasospastic reactions
Monoamine oxidase A inhibitors / ↑ t½ of sumatriptan
Selective Serotonin Reuptake Inhibitors (SSRIs) / Rarely, weakness, hyperreflexia, and incoordination

EMS CONSIDERATIONS
None.

T

Tacrine hydrochloride (THA, Tetrahydroaminoacridine)
(TAH-krin)
Pregnancy Class: C
Cognex **(Rx)**
Classification: Psychotherapeutic drug for Alzheimer's disease

Mechanism of Action: During early stages of Alzheimer's disease, cholinergic neuronal pathways that project from the basal forebrain to the cerebral cortex and hippocampus may be affected. Symptoms of dementia may be due to a deficiency of acetylcholine. As a reversible CNS cholinesterase inhibitor, tacrine elevates acetylcholine levels in the cerebral cortex. There is no evidence tacrine alters progression of dementia. **Uses:** Treatment of mild to moderate dementia of the Alzheimer's type. **Contraindications:** Hypersensitivity to tacrine or acridine derivatives. Use in patients previously treated

T

---

bold italic = life threatening side effect

with tacrine who developed jaundice (elevated total bilirubin > 3 mg/dL).

Precautions: May cause bradycardia—important in sick sinus syndrome. Use with caution in patients at risk for developing ulcers as the drug increases gastric acid secretion. Use with caution in patients with a history of abnormal liver function as indicated by abnormalities in serum ALT, AST, bilirubin, and GGT levels. Use with caution in patients with a history of asthma. There may be worsening of cognitive function following abrupt discontinuation of the drug. Safety and efficacy have not been determined in children with dementing illness.

Route/Dosage

• Capsules

Alzheimer's disease.

Initial: 10 mg q.i.d. for at least 6 weeks; **then,** after 6 weeks, increase the dose to 20 mg q.i.d., providing there are no significant transaminase elevations and the patient tolerates the treatment. Based on the degree of tolerance, the dose may be titrated, at 6-week intervals, to 30 or 40 mg q.i.d.

If transaminase elevations occur, modify the dose as follows:

• If transaminase levels are less than or equal to 2 × ULN, continue treatment according to recommended titration and monitoring schedule.

• If transaminse levels are greater than 2 but equal to or less than 3 × ULN, treatment is continued according to recommended titraiton but levels are monitored weekly until they return to normal levels.

• If transaminase levels are more than 3 but equal to or less than 5 × ULN, the daily dose is reduced by 40 mg/day. Monitor ALT/SGPT levels weekly. Dose titration is resumed and every other week monitoring is undertaken when levels return to within normal limits.

• If transaminase levels are greater than 5 × ULN, stop treatment. Monitor closely for signs and symptoms associated with hepatitis; monitor levels until they are within normal limits.

Patients who are required to stop treatment due to elevated transami-

nase levels may be rechallenged once levels return to within normal range. Weekly monitoring of serum ALT/SGPT levels should be undertaken after rechallenging occurs. If rechallenged, the initial dose is 10 mg t.i.d. with levels monitored weekly. After 6 weeks on this dose, the patient may begin dose titration if transaminase levels are acceptable.

How Supplied: *Capsule:* 10 mg, 20 mg, 30 mg, 40 mg

Side Effects: *Hepatic:* Increased transaminase levels (most common reason for stopping the drug during treatment). *GI:* N&V, diarrhea, dyspepsia, anorexia, abdominal pain, flatulence, constipation, glossitis, gingivitis, dry mouth or throat, stomatitis, increased salivation, dysphagia, esophagitis, gastritis, gastroenteritis, **GI hemorrhage,** stomach ulcer, hiatal hernia, hemorrhoids, bloody stools, diverticulitis, fecal impaction, fecal incontinence, **rectal hemorrhage,** cholelithiasis, cholecystitis, increased appetite. *Musculoskeletal:* Myalgia, fracture, arthralgia, arthritis, hypertonia, osteoporosis, tendinitis, bursitis, gout, myopathy. *CNS:* **Precipitation of seizures** (may also be due to Alzheimer's), dizziness, confusion, ataxia, insomnia, somnolence, tremor, agitation, depression, abnormal thinking, anxiety, hallucinations, hostility, migraine, **convulsions,** vertigo, syncope, hyperkinesia, paresthesia, abnormal dreams, dysarthria, aphasia, amnesia, twitching, hypesthesia, delirium, paralysis, bradykinesia, movement disorders, cogwheel rigidity, paresis, neuritis, hemiplegia, Parkinson's disease, neuropathy, extrapyramidal syndrome, decreased or absent reflexes, tardive dyskinesia, dysesthesia, dystonia, encephalitis, **coma,** apraxia, oculogyric crisis, akathisia, oral facial dyskinesia, Bell's palsy, nervousness, apathy, increased libido, paranoia, neurosis, **suicidal episodes,** psychosis, hysteria. *Respiratory:* Rhinitis, URI, coughing, pharyngitis, sinusitis, bronchitis, pneumonia, dyspnea, epistaxis, chest congestion, asthma, hyperventilation, lower respiratory infection, hemoptysis, lung

edema, *lung cancer, acute epiglottitis.*
CV: Hypotension, hypertension, *heart failure, MI, CVA,* angina pectoris, TIA, phlebitis, venous insufficiency, abdominal aortic aneurysm, atrial fibrillation or flutter, palpitation, tachycardia, bradycardia, *pulmonary embolus, heart arrest,* premature atrial contractions, *AV block,* bundle branch block. *Dermatologic:* Rash, facial and skin flushing, increased sweating, acne, alopecia, dermatitis, eczema, dry skin, herpes zoster, psoriasis, cellulitis, cyst, furunculosis, herpes simplex, hyperkeratosis, basal cell carcinoma, skin cancer, desquamation, seborrhea, squamous cell carcinoma, skin ulcer, skin necrosis, *melanoma. GU:* Bladder outflow obstruction, urinary frequency, urinary incontinence, UTI, hematuria, renal stone, kidney infection, glycosuria, dysuria, polyuria, nocturia, pyuria, cystitis, urinary retention, urinary urgency, *vaginal hemorrhage,* genital pruritus, breast pain, urinary obstruction, impotence, *prostate cancer, bladder tumor, renal tumor, renal failure, breast cancer, ovarian carcinoma,* epididymitis. *Body as a whole:* Headache, fatigue, chest pain, weight decrease, back pain, asthenia, chill, fever, malaise, peripheral edema, facial edema, dehydration, weight increase, cachexia, lipoma, heat exhaustion, sepsis, *cholinergic crisis, death. Hematologic:* Anemia, lymphadenopathy, leukopenia, thrombocytopenia, hemolysis, pancytopenia. *Ophthalmologic:* Conjunctivitis, cataract, dry eyes, eye pain, visual field defect, diplopia, amblyopia, glaucoma, hordeolum, vision loss, ptosis, blepharitis. *Otic:* Deafness, earache, tinnitus, inner ear infection, otitis media, labyrinthitis, inner ear disturbance. *Miscellaneous:* Purpura, hypercholesterolemia, diabetes mellitus, hypothyroid, hyperthyroid, unusual taste.

OD Overdose Management: *Symptoms:* Cholinergic crisis characterized by severe N&V, sweating, bradycardia, salivation, hypotension, *collapse,*

seizures, and increased muscle weakness (may paralyze respiratory muscles leading to death). Treatment: General supportive measures. IV atropine sulfate, titrated to effect, may be given in an initial dose of 1–2 mg IV with subsequent doses based on the response.

Drug Interactions
Anticholinergic drugs / Tacrine interferes with the action of these drugs
Bethanechol / Tacrine → synergistic effect with bethanechol
Cholinesterase inhibitors / Tacrine → synergistic effect with cholinesterase inhibitors
Cimetidine / Cimetidine ↑ maximum levels of tacrine
Succinylcholine / Tacrine ↑ muscle relaxation due to succinylcholine
Theophylline / Tacrine ↑ plasma levels of theophylline; ↓ theophylline dose recommended.

EMS CONSIDERATIONS
None.

Tacrolimus (FK506)
(tah-KROH-lih-mus)
Pregnancy Class: C
Prograf, (Rx)
Classification: Immunosuppressive drug

Mechanism of Action: Produced by *Streptomyces tsukubaensis.* Mechanism of action is not known but it inhibits T-lymphocyte formation leading to immunosuppression.
Uses: Prophylaxis of organ rejection in allogeneic liver transplants and kidney transplants; usually used with corticosteroids. *Investigational:* Transplants of bone marrow, heart, pancreas, pancreatic island cells, and small bowel. Treatment of autoimmune disease and severe recalcitrant psoriasis.
Contraindications: Hypersensitivity to tacrolimus or HCO-60 polyoxyl 60 hydrogenated castor oil (vehicle used for the injection). Lactation. Concomitant use with cyclosporine.

T

Precautions: Increased risk of developing lymphomas and other malignancies (especially of the skin).

Route/Dosage
• IV Infusion Only
Immunosuppression.
Initial: 0.05–0.1 mg/kg/day as a continuous IV infusion. Early in the period following transplantation, concomitant adrenal corticosteroid use is recommended.
• Capsules
Immunosuppression.
Initial: 0.15–0.3 mg/kg/day administered in two divided doses q 12 hr.
Maintenance: Titrate dose based on clinical assessment of rejection and tolerability. Lower doses may suffice for maintenance therapy.
How Supplied: *Capsule:* 1 mg, 5 mg; *Injection:* 5 mg/ml
Side Effects: *CNS:* Headache, tremor, insomnia, paresthesia, *seizures, coma,* delirium, abnormal dreams, anxiety, agitation, confusion, depression, dizziness, emotional lability, hallucinations, hypertonia, incoordination, myoclonus nervousness, psychosis, somnolence, abnormal thinking. *Neurotoxicity:* Changes in motor function, mental status, and sensory function; tremor, headache. *GI:* Diarrhea, nausea, constipation, abnormal LFT, anorexia, vomiting, dyspepsia, dysphasia, flatulence, *GI hemorrhage, GI perforation,* ileus, increased appetite, oral moniliasis. *Hepatic:* Hepatitis, cholangitis, cholestatic jaundice, jaundice, liver damage. *CV:* Hypertension, chest pain, abnormal ECG, *hemorrhage,* hypotension, tachycardia. *Hematologic:* Anemia, thrombocytopenia, leukocytosis, coagulation disorder, ecchymosis, hypochromic anemia, leukopenia, decreased prothrombin. *GU:* Abnormal kidney function, nephrotoxicity, UTI, oliguria, hematuria, *kidney failure. Metabolic:* Hyperkalemia, hypokalemia, hyperglycemia, hypomagnesemia, acidosis, alkalosis, hyperlipemia, hyperphosphatemia, hyperuricemia, hypocalcemia, hypophosphatemia, hyponatremia, hypoproteinemia, bilirubinemia. *Respiratory:* Pleural effusion, atelectasis, dyspnea, asthma, bronchitis, increased cough, pulmonary edema, pharyngitis, pneumonia, lung disorder, respiratory disorder, rhinitis, sinusitis, alteration in voice. *Musculoskeletal:* Arthralgia, leg cramps, myalgia, myasthenia, osteoporosis, generalized spasm. *Dermatologic:* Pruritus, rash, alopecia, herpes simplex, sweating, skin disorder, herpes simplex. *Miscellaneous:* Hypersensitivity reactions (including *anaphylaxis*), increased incidence of malignancies, lymphoma, diabetes mellitus, pain, fever, asthenia, back pain, ascites, peripheral edema, abdominal pain, enlarged abdomen, abscess, chills, hernia, photosensitivity, peritonitis, abnormal healing.

Drug Interactions
Aminoglycosides / Additive or synergistic impairment of renal function
Amphotericin B / Additive or synergistic impairment of renal function
Antifungal drugs / ↑ Tacrolimus blood levels
Bromocriptine / ↑ Tacrolimus blood levels
Calcium channel blocking drugs / ↑ Tacrolimus blood levels
Carbamazepine / ↓ Tacrolimus blood levels
Cimetidine / ↑ Tacrolimus blood levels
Cisplatin / Additive or synergistic impairment of renal function
Clarithromycin / ↑ Tacrolimus blood levels
Cyclosporine / Additive or synergistic nephrotoxicity; also, ↑ tacrolimus blood levels
Danazol / ↑ Tacrolimus blood levels
Diltiazem / ↑ Tacrolimus blood levels
Erythromycin / ↑ Tacrolimus blood levels
Methylprednisolone / ↑ Tacrolimus blood levels
Metoclopramide / ↑ Tacrolimus blood levels
Phenobarbital / ↓ Tacrolimus blood levels
Phenytoin / ↓ Tacrolimus blood levels

Rifamycin / ↓ Tacrolimus blood levels
Vaccines / ↓ Effectiveness of vaccines

EMS CONSIDERATIONS
None.

Tamoxifen
(tah-MOX-ih-fen)
Pregnancy Class: C
Nolvadex, **(Rx)**
Classification: Antiestrogen

Mechanism of Action: Antiestrogen believed to compete with estrogen for estrogen-binding sites in target tissue (breast); also blocks uptake of estradiol.

Uses: Adjuvant treatment of axillary node-negative or node-positive breast cancer in women following total or segmental mastectomy, axillary dissection, and breast irradiation. Metastatic breast cancer in premenopausal women as an alternative to oophorectomy or ovarian irradiation (especially in women with estrogen-positive tumors). Advanced metastatic breast cancer in men. Prophylaxis of breast cancer in high-risk women. *Investigational:* Mastalgia, gynecomastia (to treat pain and size), pancreatic carcinoma, advanced or recurrent endometrial and hepatocellular carcinoma.

Contraindications: Lactation.

Precautions: Use with caution in patients with leukopenia or thrombocytopenia. Women should not become pregnant while taking tamoxifen. Although the risk of breast cancer is significantly lowered, this benefit must be weighed against an increased risk of endometrial cancer, pulmonary embolism, and DVT.

Route/Dosage
• **Tablets**
Breast cancer.
10–20 mg b.i.d. (morning and evening) or 20 mg daily. Doses of 10 mg b.i.d.–t.i.d. for 2 years and 10 mg b.i.d. for 5 years have been used.

There is no evidence that doses greater than 20 mg daily are more effective.
Mastalgia.
10 mg/day for 4 months.

How Supplied: *Tablet:* 10 mg, 20 mg

Side Effects: *GI:* N&V, distaste for food, anorexia, diarrhea, abdominal cramps. *CV:* Peripheral edema, superficial phlebitis, DVT, ***pulmonary embolism, thromboembolic disorders (especially when tamoxifen is combined with other cytotoxic agents).*** *CNS:* Depression, dizziness, lightheadedness, headache, fatigue. *Hepatic:* Rarely, fatty liver, cholestasis, hepatitis, ***hepatic necrosis.*** *GU:* Hot flashes, vaginal bleeding and discharge, menstrual irregularities, pruritus vulvae, ovarian cysts, hyperplasia of the uterus, polyps, uterine carcinoma. *Other:* Skin rash, skin changes, hypercalcemia, musculoskeletal pain, hyperlipidemias, weight gain or loss, increased bone and tumor pain, mild to moderate thrombocytopenia and leukopenia, retinopathy, hair thinning or partial loss, fluid retention, coughing. In men, may be loss of libido and impotency. Impotence and loss of libido in males after discontinuing therapy.

Drug Interactions
Anticoagulants / ↑ Hypoprothrombinemic effect
Bromocriptine / ↑ Serum levels of tamoxifen and N-desmethyl tamoxifen

EMS CONSIDERATIONS
None.

Tamsulosin hydrochloride
(tam-SOO-loh-sin)
Pregnancy Class: B
Flomax, **(Rx)**
Classification: Alpha-1 adrenergic blocking agent

Mechanism of Action: Blockade of alpha-1 receptors (probably alpha$_{1A}$) in prostate results in relaxation of smooth muscles in bladder neck and

---

bold italic = life threatening side effect

prostate; thus, urine flow rate is improved and there is a decrease in symptoms of BPH.

Uses: Treatment of signs and symptoms of BPH. Rule out prostatic carcinoma before using tamsulosin.

Contraindications: Use to treat hypertension, with other alpha-adrenergic blocking agents, or in women or children.

Precautions: Use with caution with concurrent administration of warfarin.

Route/Dosage
• **Capsules**
  Benign prostatic hypertrophy.

Adult males: 0.4 mg daily given about 30 min after same meal each day. If, after 2 to 4 weeks, patients have not responded, dose can be increased to 0.8 mg daily.

How Supplied: *Capsules:* 0.4 mg

Side Effects: *Body as a whole:* Headache, infection, asthenia, back pain, chest pain. *CV:* Postural hypotension, syncope. *GI:* Diarrhea, nausea, tooth disorder. *CNS:* Dizziness, vertigo, somnolence, insomnia, decreased libido. *Respiratory:* Rhinitis, pharyngitis, increased cough, sinusitis. *GU:* Abnormal ejaculation. *Miscellaneous:* Amblyopia.

OD **Overdose Management:** *Symptoms:* Hypotension. *Treatment:* Keep patient in supine position to restore BP and normalize HR. If this is inadequate, consider IV fluids. Vasopressors may also be used; monitor renal function.

Drug Interactions: Cimetidine causes significant ↓ in clearance of tamsulosin.

EMS CONSIDERATIONS
None.

Tazarotene (Tazorac)
taz-AR-oh-teen
Pregnancy Class: X
Tazorac **(Rx)**
Classification: Antipsoriasis topical drug

Mechanism of Action: A retinoid prodrug converted by deesterification to active cognate carboxylic acid of tazarotene. Mechanism not known. Little systemic absorption.

t½, after topical use: About 18 hr. Parent drug and metabolite are further metabolized and excreted through urine and feces.

Uses: Stable plaque psoriasis. Mild to moderate facial acne vulgaris.

Contraindications: Pregnancy. Use on eczematous skin. Use of cosmetics or skin medications that have strong drying effect.

Route/Dosage
• **Gel**
  Acne vulgaris, Psoriasis.

After skin is dry following cleaning, apply thin film (2 mg/cm²) on lesions once daily in evening. Cover entire affected area. For psoriasis, do not apply to more than 20% of body surface area.

How Supplied: *Gel:* 0.05%, 0.1%

Side Effects: *Dermatologic:* Pruritus, photosensitivity, burning/stinging, erythema, worsening of psoriasis, skin pain, irritation, rash, desquamation, contact dermatitis, skin inflammation, fissuring, bleeding, dry skin, localized edema, skin discoloration.

OD **Overdose Management:** *Symptoms:* Marked redness, peeling, discomfort. *Treatment:* Decrease or discontinue dose.

Drug Interactions: ↑ Risk of photosensitivity when used with fluoroquinolones, phenothiazines, sulfonamides, tetracyclines, thiazides.

EMS CONSIDERATIONS
Administration/Storage: Avoid application to unaffected skin due to increased susceptibility to irritation.
Assessment
1. Document condition requiring treatment; may photograph to assess response.
2. Determine if pregnant and begin therapy during menstrual cycle.

Telmisartan (Micardis)
tell-mih-SAR-tan
Pregnancy Class: C (first trimester), D (second and third trimesters)
Micardis **(Rx)**
Classification: Antihypertensive, angiotensin II receptor antagonist

Mechanism of Action: Angiotensin II receptor (AT$_1$) antagonist that blocks the vasoconstrictor and al-dosterone-secreting effects of angiotensin II by blocking binding of angiotensin II to the AT$_1$ receptors. Over 99.5% bound to plasma protein. **t½, terminal:** About 24 hr. Excreted mainly in the feces by way of the bile.

Uses: Alone or in combination to treat hypertension.

Contraindications: Lactation.

Route/Dosage ─────────────

• **Tablets**

Antihypertensive.

Adults, initial: 40 mg/day. **Maintenance:** 20–80 mg/day. If additional BP reduction is desired beyond that achieved with 80 mg/day, add a diuretic.

How Supplied: *Tablets:* 40 mg, 80 mg

Side Effects: *GI:* Diarrhea, dyspepsia, heartburn, N&V, abdominal pain. *CNS:* Dizziness, headache, fatigue, anxiety, nervousness. *Musculoskeletal:* Pain, including back and neck pain; myalgia. *Respiratory:* URI, sinusitis, cough, pharyngitis, influenza. *Miscellaneous:* Chest pain, UTI, peripheral edema, hypertension.

OD Overdose Management: *Symptoms:* Hypotension, dizziness, tachycardia or bradycardia. *Treatment:* Supportive for hypotension.

Drug Interactions: ↑ Digoxin peak plasma and trough levels.

EMS CONSIDERATIONS

Administration/Storage: May be taken with or without food.

Assessment

1. Note onset and duration of disease, other agents trialed and the outcome.

2. Symptomatic hypotension may occur in patients who are volume- or salt-depleted. Correct prior to using telmisartan, use a lower starting dose and monitor closely.

3. With renal dialysis may develop orthostatic hypotension; monitor BP closely.

4. Monitor ECG, labs, and VS. With hepatic dysfunction, use cautiously.

─────────────────────

Temazepam
(teh-MAZ-eh-pam)
Pregnancy Class: X
Restoril **(C-IV) (Rx)**
Classification: Benzodiazepine hypnotic

Mechanism of Action: Benzodiazepine derivative. Disturbed nocturnal sleep may occur the first one or two nights following discontinuance of the drug. Prolonged administration is not recommended because physical dependence and tolerance may develop. See also *Flurazepam.*

Uses: Insomnia in patients unable to fall asleep, with frequent awakenings during the night and/or early morning awakenings.

Contraindications: Pregnancy.

Precautions: Use with caution in severely depressed patients. Use during lactation may cause sedation and feeding problems in the infant. Geriatric patients may be more sensitive to the effects of temazepam.

Route/Dosage ─────────────

• **Capsules**

Adults, usual: 15–30 mg at bedtime. **In elderly or debilitated patients, initial:** 15 mg; **then,** adjust dosage to response.

How Supplied: *Capsule:* 7.5 mg, 15 mg, 30 mg

Side Effects: *CNS:* Drowsiness (after daytime use) and dizziness are common. Lethargy, confusion, euphoria, weakness, ataxia, lack of concentration, hallucinations. In some patients, paradoxical excitement (less than 0.5%), including stimulation and hyperactivity, occurs. *GI:* Anorexia, diarrhea. *Other:* Tremors, horizontal nystagmus, falling, palpitations. Rarely, blood dyscrasias.

EMS CONSIDERATIONS

See also *Tranquilizers, Antimanic Drugs, and Hypnotics.*

T

---

bold italic = life threatening side effect

Temozolomide
tem-oh-ZOHL-oh-myd
Pregnancy Class: D
Temodar **(Rx)**
Classification: Antineoplastic, miscellaneous

Mechanism of Action: Temozolomide is a prodrug that is hydrolyzed, nonenzymatically, at physiologic pH to the reactive 3-methyl-(triazen-1-yl)imidazole-4-carboxamide (MTIC). MTIC methylates specific guanine-rich areas of DNA that initiate transcription, leading to cytotoxicity and antiproliferative effects.

Uses: Treat adults with refractory anaplastic astrocytoma, i.e., those at first relapse whose disease has progressed on a drug regimen containing a nitrosourea and procarbazine.

Contraindications: Hypersensitivity to dacarbazine (DTIC) because it is also metabolized to MTIC. Lactation.

Precautions: Use with caution in the elderly and in those with severe renal or hepatic impairment. Safety and efficacy have not been determined in pediatric patients.

Route/Dosage
• **Capsules**
Anaplastic astrocytoma.
Adults, initial: 150 mg/m^2 once daily for 5 consecutive days per 28-day treatment cycle. If both the nadir and day of dosing (day 29, day 1 of next cycle) ANC are equal to or greater than 1.5 x 10^9 (1500/mcL), the dose may be increased to 200 mg/m^2 for 5 consecutive days per 28-day treatment cycle.

During treatment, obtain a CBC on day 22 (21 days after the first dose) or within 48 hr of that day, and weekly until the ANC is greater than 1.5 x 10^9/L (1500/mcL) and the platelet count exceeds 100 x 10^9 (100,000/mcL). Do not start the next cycle until the ANC and platelet count exceed these levels. If the ANC falls to less than 1 x 10^9/L (1000/mcL) or the platelet count is less than 50 x 10^9/L (50,000/mcL) during any cycle, reduce the next cycle by 50 mg/m^2, but not less than 100 mg/m^2 (the lowest recommended dose).

How Supplied: *Capsules:* 5 mg, 20 mg, 100 mg, 250 mg

Side Effects: *Most common:* N&V, headache, fatigue. *Myelosuppression:* Thrombocytopenia, neutropenia. *CNS:* Convulsions, hemiparesis, dizziness, abnormal coordination, amnesia, insomnia, paresthesia, somnolence, paresis, ataxia, anxiety, dysphasia, depression, abnormal gait, confusion. *GI:* N&V, constipation, diarrhea, abdominal pain, anorexia. *Dermatologic:* Rash, pruritus. *Respiratory:* URTI, pharyngitis, sinusitis, coughing. *GU:* Urinary incontinence, UTI, increased frequency of micturition. *Ophthalmic:* Diplopia, blurred vision, visual deficit, vision changes, vision troubles. *Body as a whole:* Fatigue, asthenia, fever, viral infection, weight increase, myalgia. *Miscellaneous:* Headache, peripheral edema, back pain, adrenal hypercorticism, female breast pain.

OD Overdose Management: Hematologic evaluation. Supportive measures, as necessary.

EMS CONSIDERATIONS
None.

Terazosin
(ter-AY-zoh-sin)
Pregnancy Class: C
Hytrin **(Rx)**
Classification: Antihypertensive, alpha-1-adrenergic receptor blocking agent

Mechanism of Action: Blocks postsynaptic alpha-1-adrenergic receptors, leading to a dilation of both arterioles and veins, and ultimately, a reduction in BP. Both standing and supine BPs are lowered with no reflex tachycardia. Also relaxes smooth muscle of the prostate and bladder neck. Usefulness in BPH is due to alpha-1 receptor blockade, which relaxes the smooth muscle of the prostate and bladder neck and relieves pressure on the urethra.

Onset of Action: 15 min.
Duration of Action: 24 hr.

Uses: Alone or in combination with diuretics or beta-adrenergic blocking agents to treat hypertension. Treat symptoms of benign prostatic hyperplasia.

Precautions: Use with caution during lactation. Safety and efficacy have not been determined in children. Geriatric patients may be more sensitive to the hypotensive and hypothermic effects of terazosin.

Route/Dosage
* **Capsules**
  Hypertension.

Individualized, initial: 1 mg at bedtime (this dose is not to be exceeded); **then,** increase dose slowly to obtain desired response. **Range:** 1–5 mg/day; doses as high as 20 mg may be required in some patients. Doses greater than 20 mg daily do not provide further BP control.

Benign prostatic hyperplasia.

Initial: 1 mg/day; dose should be increased to 2 mg, 5 mg, and then 10 mg once daily to improve symptoms and/or urinary flow rates. Doses greater than 20 mg daily have not been studied.

How Supplied: *Capsule:* 1 mg, 2 mg, 5 mg, 10 mg

Side Effects: *First-dose effect:* Marked postural hypotension and syncope. *CV:* Palpitations, tachycardia, postural hypotension, syncope, ***arrhythmias,*** chest pain, vasodilation. *CNS:* Dizziness, headache, somnolence, drowsiness, nervousness, paresthesia, depression, anxiety, insomnia, vertigo. *Respiratory:* Nasal congestion, dyspnea, sinusitis, epistaxis, bronchitis, ***bronchospasm,*** cold or flu symptoms, increased cough, pharyngitis, rhinitis. *GI:* Nausea, constipation, diarrhea, dyspepsia, dry mouth, vomiting, flatulence, abdominal discomfort or pain. *Musculoskeletal:* Asthenia, arthritis, arthralgia, myalgia, joint disorders, back pain, pain in extremities, neck and shoulder pain, muscle cramps. *Miscellaneous:* Peripheral edema, weight gain, blurred vision, impotence, chest pain, fever, gout, pruritus, rash, sweating, urinary frequency, UTI, tinnitus, conjunctivitis, abnormal vision, edema, facial edema.

OD **Overdose Management:** *Symptoms:* Hypotension, drowsiness, shock. *Treatment:* Restore BP and HR. Patient should be kept supine; vasopressors may be indicated. Volume expanders can be used to treat shock.

EMS CONSIDERATIONS

See also *Antihypertensive Agents.*

Terbinafine hydrochloride
(ter-BIN-ah-feen)
Pregnancy Class: B
Lamisil **(Rx)**
Classification: Antifungal agent

Mechanism of Action: Inhibits squalene epoxidase, a key enzyme in the sterol biosynthesis in fungi. Results in ergosterol deficiency and a corresponding accumulation of squalene leading to fungal cell death.

Uses: Topical use: Interdigital tinea pedis (athletes' foot), tinea cruris (jock itch), or tinea corporis (ringworm) due to *Epidermophyton floccosum, Trichophyton mentagrophytes,* or *T. rubrum.* Plantar tinea pedis. Tinea versicolor due to *Malassezia furfur. Investigational:* Cutaneous candidiasis and tinea versicolor. **Oral use:** Onychomycosis of the toenail or fingernail due to dermatophytes.

Contraindications: Ophthalmic or intravaginal use. PO use in preexisting liver disease or renal impairment (C_{CR} less than 50 mL/min). Lactation.

Precautions: Safety and efficacy have not been determined in children less than 12 years of age.

Route/Dosage
* **Cream**
  Interdigital tinea pedis.

Apply to cover the affected and immediately surrounding areas b.i.d. until symptoms are significantly improved. Maintain therapy for a minimum of 1 week and not more than 4 weeks.

T

---

bold italic = life threatening side effect

Tinea cruris or tinea corporis.
Apply to cover the affected and immediately surrounding areas 1–2 times/day until symptoms are significantly improved. Maintain therapy for a minimum of 1 week and not more than 4 weeks.

- **Spray**
  Tinea pedis, Tinea versicolor.
  Spray b.i.d. for one week.
  Tinea corporis, Tinea cruris.
  Spray once daily for one week.
- **Tablets**
  Onychomycosis.
  250 mg/day for 6 weeks if fingernails are affected and 250 mg/day for 12 weeks if toenails are affected. Alternatively, intermittent dosing may be used: 500 mg daily for 1 week each month (use 2 months for fingernails and 4 months for toenails). The optimal clinical effect is observed several months after mycologic cure and cessation of treatment due to slow period for outgrowth of healthy nails.

How Supplied: *Cream:* 1%; *Spray:* 1%; *Tablet:* 250 mg

Side Effects: *Following topical use. Dermatologic:* Irritation, burning, itching, dryness.

Following oral use. GI: Diarrhea, dyspepsia, abdominal pain, nausea, flatulence. *Dermatologic:* Rash, pruritus, urticaria. *Other:* Headache, taste or visual disturbances. Rarely, symptomatic idiosyncratic hepatobiliary dysfunction (including cholestatic hepatitis), serious skin reactions, severe neutropenia, allergic reactions (including **anaphylaxis**).

Drug Interactions
Cimetidine / Terbinafine clearance is ↓ by one-third
Cyclosporine / ↑ Clearance of cyclosporine
Rifampin / ↑ Clearance (100%) of terbinafine
Terfenadine / ↓ Clearance of terbinafine

EMS CONSIDERATIONS
None.

Terbutaline sulfate
(ter-BYOU-tah-leen)
Pregnancy Class: B
Brethaire, Brethine, Bricanyl, **(Rx)**
Classification: Sympathomimetic, direct-acting; bronchodilator

Mechanism of Action: Specific beta-2 receptor stimulant, resulting in bronchodilation and relaxation of peripheral vasculature. Minimum beta-1 activity. Action resembles that of isoproterenol.

Onset of Action: PO: 30 min; **maximum effect:** 2-3 hr; **SC:** 5-15 min; **maximum effect:** 30 min - 1 hr; **Inhalation:** 5-30 min; **time to peak effect:** 1-2 hr.

Duration of Action: PO: 4-8 hr; **SC:** 1.5-4hr; **Inhalation:** 3-6 hr.

Uses: Bronchodilator in asthma, bronchitis, emphysema, bronchiectasis, pulmonary obstructive disease, and other conditions associated with reversible bronchospasms. Relief of reversible bronchospasms in patients age six and up who suffer from obstructive airway diseases. *Investigational:* Inhibit premature labor.

Contraindications: Lactation.

Precautions: Safe use in children less than 12 years of age not established.

Route/Dosage
- **Tablets**
  Bronchodilation.
  Adults and children over 15 years: 5 mg t.i.d. q 6 hr during waking hours, not to exceed 15 mg q 24 hr. If disturbing side effects are observed, dose can be reduced to 2.5 mg t.i.d. without loss of beneficial effects. Anticipate use of other therapeutic measures if patient fails to respond after second dose. **Children 12–15 years:** 2.5 mg t.i.d., not to exceed 7.5 mg q 24 hr.
  Premature labor.
  2.5 mg q 4–6 hr until term.
- **SC**
  Bronchodilation.
  Adults: 0.25 mg. May be repeated 1 time after 15–30 min if no significant

clinical improvement is noted. If patient does not respond to the second dose, undertake other measures. Do not exceed a dose of 0.5 mg over 4 hr.

- **IV Infusion**
  Premature labor.

10 mcg/min initially; **then,** increase rate by 0.005 mg/min q 10 min until contractions cease or a maximum dose of 80 mcg/min is reached. Continue the minimum effective dose for 4–8 hr after contractions cease. Terbutaline may also be given SC for preterm labor.

- **Metered Dose Inhaler**
  Bronchodilation.

Adults and children over 12 years: 0.2–0.5 mg (1–2 inhalations) q 4–6 hr. Inhalations should be separated by 60-sec intervals. Dosage may be repeated q 4–6 hr.

How Supplied: *Metered dose inhaler:* 0.2 mg/inh; *Injection:* 1 mg/mL; *Tablet:* 2.5 mg, 5 mg

Side Effects: Additional: *CV:* PVCs, ECG changes (e.g., atrial premature beats, AV block, sinus pause, ST-T wave depression, T-wave inversion, sinus bradycardia, atrial escape beat with aberrant conduction), tachycardia. *Respiratory:* Wheezing, *Micellaneous:* Hypersensitivity reactions (including vasculitis), flushing, sweating, bad taste or taste change, muscle cramps, CNS stimulation, pain at injection site.

EMS CONSIDERATIONS

See also *Sympathomimetic Drugs.*

Terconazole nitrate
(ter-KON-ah-zohl)
Pregnancy Class: C
Terazol 3, Terazol 7, **(Rx)**
Classification: Antifungal, vaginal

Mechanism of Action: May exert its antifungal activity by disrupting cell membrane permeability leading to loss of essential intracellular materials. Also inhibits synthesis of triglycerides and phospholipids as well as inhibiting oxidative and peroxida-tive enzyme activity. When used for *Candida,* terconazole inhibits transformation of blastospores into the invasive mycelial form.

Uses: Vulvovaginitis caused by *Candida.* Ineffective in infections due to *Trichomonas* or *Haemophilus vaginalis.*

Precautions: During lactation, consider discontinuing nursing or the drug. Safety and efficacy have not been established in children.

Route/Dosage —————

- **Vaginal Cream (0.4%, 0.8%)**
One applicator full (5 g) intravaginally, once daily at bedtime for 7 consecutive days for the 0.4% cream and for 3 consecutive days for the 0.8% cream.
- **Vaginal Suppository**
One 80-mg suppository once daily at bedtime for 3 consecutive days.

How Supplied: *Vaginal cream:* 0.4%, 0.8%; *Vaginal suppository:* 80 mg

Side Effects: *GU:* Vulvovaginal burning, irritation, or itching; dysmenorrhea, pain of the female genitalia. *Miscellaneous:* Headache (most common), body pain, photosensitivity, abdominal pain, chills, fever.

EMS CONSIDERATIONS
None.

Testolactone
(tes-toe-LACK-tohn)
Pregnancy Class: C
Teslac **(C-III) (Rx)**
Classification: Antineoplastic, androgen

Mechanism of Action: Synthetic steroid related to testosterone. May act to reduce synthesis of estrone from adrenal androstenedione by inhibiting steroid aromatase activity.

Uses: Palliative treatment of advanced disseminated mammary cancer in postmenopausal women or in premenopausal ovariectomized patients. Is effective in only 15% of patients.

Contraindications: Breast cancer in men. Lactation. Premenopausal women with intact ovaries.

Precautions: Safety and efficacy have not been determined in children.

Route/Dosage
- **Tablets**

250 mg q.i.d. Continue therapy for 3 months unless there is active progression of the disease.

How Supplied: *Tablet:* 50 mg

Drug Interactions: Testolactone may ↑ effect of oral anticoagulants.

EMS CONSIDERATIONS

See also *Testosterone*.

Testosterone aqueous suspension
Testosterone cypionate (in oil)
Testosterone enanthate (in oil)
Testosterone propionate (in oil)
Testosterone transdermal system

(tess-TOSS-ter-ohn)

Pregnancy Class: X

Testosterone aqueous suspension: Histerone 100, Tesamone 100, Testandro, **(Rx) (C-III)** Testosterone cypionate (in oil): depAndro 100 and 200, Depotest 100 and 200, Depo-Testosterone, Duratest-100 and -200, Scheinpharm, **(Rx) (C-III)** Testosterone enanthate (in oil): Andro L.A. 200, Andropository-200, Delatestryl, Durathate-200, Everone 200, **(Rx) (C-III)** Testosterone propionate (in oil): **(Rx) (C-III)** Testosterone transdermal system: Androderm, Testoderm, Testoderm TTS, Testoderm with Adhesive, **(Rx) (C-III)**

Classification: Androgen, natural hormone and salts of natural hormone

---

Mechanism of Action: Treatment with testosterone and its congeners is complicated by the fact that the exogenous supply of the hormone may depress secretion of the natural hormone through inhibitory effects on the pituitary. Too large a dose may cause permanent damage. Treatment is usually associated with a feeling of well-being.

Uses: Parenteral products: Replacement therapy in males for congenital or acquired primary hypogonadism or for congenital or acquired hypogonadotropic hypogonadism. Delayed puberty. In postmenopausal women to treat inoperable metastatic breast carcinoma or in premenopausal women following oophorectomy. Postpartum breast engorgement (evidence for effectiveness is lacking). *Investigational:* Male contraceptive (testosterone enanthate).

Transdermal products: Replacement therapy for acquired or congenital primary hypogonadism or for acquired or congenital secondary hypogonadotropic hypogonadism.

Contraindications: Serious renal, hepatic, or cardiac disease due to edema formation. Prostatic or breast (males) carcinoma. Use in pregnancy (masculinization of female fetus) and lactation. Discontinue if hypercalcemia occurs.

Precautions: Use with caution in young males who have not completed their growth (because of premature epiphyseal closure). Androgens may also cause virilization in females or precocious sexual development in males. Geriatric patients may manifest an increased risk of prostatic hypertrophy or prostatic carcinoma. Androgen therapy occasionally seems to accelerate metastatic breast carcinoma in women.

Route/Dosage

Testosterone aqueous suspension and Testosterone propionate in oil
- **IM Only**

    Replacement therapy.

25–50 mg 2–3 times/week.

    Breast cancer.

50–100 mg 3 times/week.

    Growth stimulation in Turner's syndrome or constitutional delay of puberty.

40–50 mg/m²/dose given monthly for 6 months.

Male hypogonadism, initiation of pubertal growth.

40–50 mg/m²/month until growth rate falls to prepubertal levels (about 5 cm/year).

Male hypogonadism, during terminal growth phase.

100 mg/m²/month until growth ceases.

Male hypogonadism, maintain virilization.

100 mg/m² twice monthly or 50–400 mg/dose q 2–4 weeks.

Postpartum breast engorgement.

25–50 mg of testostrone propionate for 3–4 days.

Testosterone enanthate and cypionate

• **IM Only**

Hypogonadism, replacement therapy.

50–400 mg q 2–4 weeks.

Delayed puberty.

50–200 mg q 2–4 weeks for no more than 4–6 months.

Palliation of inoperable breast cancer in women.

200–400 mg q 2–4 weeks.

• **Transdermal System**

Replacement therapy (congenital or acquired primary hypogonadism, congenital or acquired hypogonadotropic hypogonadism).

Testoderm: One 6-mg patch applied daily on clean, dry scrotal skin that has been dry-shaved to remove hair. Patients with a smaller scrotum can use a 4-mg patch. The patch should be worn for 22–24 hr/day for 6–8 weeks. *Testoderm TTS:* One 5-mg patch applied to the arm, back, or upper buttocks each day. The patch can be removed and reapplied if the patient wants to swim, bathe, or vigorously exercise.

Androderm: **Initial dose, usual:** Two systems applied nightly for 24 hr providing a total dose of 5 mg/day. The systems are applied to a clean, dry area of the skin on the back, abdomen, upper arms, or thighs.

How Supplied: Testosterone aqueous suspension: *Injection:* 50 mg/mL, 100 mg/mL. Testosterone cypionate: *Injection:* 200 mg/mL. Testosterone enanthate: *Injection:* 100 mg/mL, 200 mg/mL. Testosterone propionate: *Injection:* 100 mg/mL. Testosterone transdermal system: *Film, extended release:* 2.5 mg/24 hr, 4 mg/24 hr, 5 mg/24 hr, 6 mg/24 hr

Side Effects: *Hepatic:* Liver toxicity is the most serious side effect. Jaundice, cholestasis, alterations in BSP retention, AST, and ALT. Rarely, ***hepatic necrosis, hepatocellular neoplasms,*** peliosis hepatis, acute intermittent porphyria in patients with this disease. *GI:* N&V, diarrhea, anorexia, symptoms of peptic ulcer. *CNS:* Headache, anxiety, increased or decreased libido, insomnia, excitation, paresthesias, sleep apnea syndrome, ***CNS hemorrhage,*** chills, choreiform movements, habituation, confusion (toxic doses). *GU:* Testicular atrophy with inhibition of testicular function (e.g., oligospermia), impotence, epididymitis, irritable bladder, prepubertal phallic enlargement, gynecomastia. *Electrolyte:* Retention of sodium, chloride, calcium, potassium, phosphates. Edema. *Miscellaneous:* Acne, flushing, suppression of clotting factors (II, V, VII, X), polycythemia, leukopenia, rashes, dermatitis, ***anaphylaxis (rare),*** muscle cramps, hypercholesterolemia, male-pattern baldness, acne, seborrhea, hirsutism. Hypercalcemia, especially in immobilized patients or those with metastatic breast carcinoma. Virilization in women.

In females, menstrual irregularities (including amenorrhea), virilization, clitoral enlargement, hirsutism, increased libido, baldness (male pattern), virilization of external genitalia of female fetus.

In males, decreased ejaculatory volume, oligospermia (high doses), gynecomastia, increased frequency and duration of penile erections.

In children, disturbances of growth, premature closure of epiphyses, precocious sexual development.

---

bold italic = life threatening side effect

Inflammation and pain at site of IM or SC injection.

NOTE: Side effects of the cypionate and enanthate products are not readily reversible due to the long duration of action of these dosage forms.

The patch may cause itching, irritation, erythema, or discomfort of the scrotum (Testoderm) or on skin areas where applied (Androderm). Potentially, small amounts of testosterone may be transferred to a sex partner.

Drug Interactions

Anticoagulants, oral / Anabolic steroids ↑ effect of anticoagulants
Antidiabetic agents / Additive hypoglycemia
Barbiturates / ↓ Effect of androgens due to ↑ breakdown by liver
Corticosteroids / ↑ Chance of edema
Phenylbutazone / Certain androgens ↑ effect of phenylbutazone

EMS CONSIDERATIONS

None.

Tetracycline hydrochloride
(teh-trah-SYE-kleen)

Pregnancy Class: D
Achromycin Ophthalmic Ointment, Achromycin Ophthalmic Suspension, Actisite Periodontal Fiber, Nor-Tet, Panmycin, Robicaps, Sumycin 250 and 500, Sumycin Syrup, Tetracap, Topicycline Topical Solution, **(Rx)**
Classification: Antibiotic, tetracycline

Uses: Additional Use: Ophthalmic: Superficial ophthalmic infections due to *Staphylococcus aureus, Streptococcus, Streptococcus pneumoniae, Escherichia coli, Neisseria,* and *Bacteroides.* Prophylaxis of *Neisseria gonorrhoeae* in newborns. With oral therapy for treatment of *Chlamydia trachomatis.* **Topical:** Acne vulgaris, prophylaxis or treatment of infection following skin abrasions, minor cuts, wounds, or burns. **Tetracycline fiber:** Adult periodontitis. *Investigational:* Pleural sclerosing agent in malignant pleural effusions (administered by chest tube); in combination with gentamicin for *Vibrio vulnificus* infections due to wound ifection after trauma or by eating contaminated seafood. Mouthwash (use suspension) to treat nonspecific mouth ulcerations, canker sores, aphthous ulcers. Possible drug of choice for stage I Lyme disease.

Contraindications: Use of the topical ointment in or around the eyes. Ophthalmic products to treat fungal diseases of the eye, dendritic keratitis, vaccinia, varicella, mycobacterial eye infections, or following removal of a corneal foreign body.

Precautions: Use tetracycline fiber with caution in patients with a history of oral candidiasis. Use of the fiber in chronic abscesses has not been evaluated. Safety and efficacy of the fiber have not been determined in children.

Route/Dosage
• **Capsules, Syrup, Tablets**
  Mild to moderate infections.
Adults, usual: 500 mg b.i.d. or 250 mg q.i.d.
  Severe infections.
Adult: 500 mg q.i.d. **Children over 8 years:** 25–50 mg/kg/day in four equal doses.
  Brucellosis.
500 mg q.i.d. for 3 weeks with 1 g streptomycin IM b.i.d. for first week and once daily the second week.
  Syphilis.
Total of 30–40 g over 10–15 days.
  Gonorrhea.
Initially, 1.5 g; **then,** 500 mg q 6 hr until 9 g has been given.
  Gonorrhea sensitive to penicillin.
Initially, 1.5 g; **then,** 500 mg q 6 hr for 4 days (total: 9 g).
  GU or rectal Chlamydia trachomatis infections.
500 mg q.i.d. for minimum of 7 days.
  Severe acne.
Initially, 1 g/day; **then,** 125500 mg/day (long-term).
NOTE: The CDC have established treatment schedules for STDs.

Initially, 1 g/day; **then,** 125–500 mg/day (long-term).
* **Topical**
  Acne.
Apply topical solution to affected areas in the morning and at night, making sure that skin is completely wet after each application.
  Infections.
Apply OTC ointment (3%) to affected areas 1–4 times/day. A sterile bandage may be used.
* **Tetracycline Fiber**
  Adult periodontitis.
Place the fiber into the periodontal pocket until the pocket is filled (amount of fiber will vary with pocket depth and contour) ensuring that the fiber is in contact with the base of the pocket. Retain the fiber in place for 10 days, after which it is to be removed. The effectiveness of subsequent therapy with the fiber has not been assessed.

How Supplied: Tetracycline: *Syrup:* 125 mg/5 mL; Tetracycline hydrochloride: *Capsule:* 100 mg, 250 mg, 500 mg; *Ointment:* 3%; *Tablet:* 250 mg, 500 mg

Side Effects: Additional: Temporary blurring of vision or stinging following administration. Dermatitis and photosensitivity following ophthalmic use. *Use of the tetracycline fiber:* Oral candidiasis, glossitis, staining of the tongue, severe gingival hyperplasia, minor throat irritation, pain following placement in an abscessed area, throbbing pain, hypersensitivity reactions.

EMS CONSIDERATIONS

See also *Tetracyclines* and *Anti-Infectives.*

Thalidomide
(thah-LID-ah-myd)
Pregnancy Class: X
Thalomid, **(Rx)**
Classification: Dermatologic drug

Mechanism of Action: Immunomodulatory drug; mechanism of action not known. Drug may suppress excessive tumor necrosis factor–alpha (TNF–α) production and down–modulation of selected cell surface adhesion molecules involved in leukocyte migration.

Uses: Acute treatment of moderate to severe erythema nodosum leprosum (ENL). Maintenance therapy for prevention and suppression of the cutaneous symptoms of erythema nodosum leprosum recurrence.

Contraindications: Never to be used in pregnancy or in those who could become pregnant while taking the drug (even a single 50 mg dose can cause severe birth defects). Use in males unless the patient meets several conditions (see package insert). Use as monotherapy for ENL in the presence of moderate to severe neuritis. Lactation.

Precautions: Due to possible birth defects, thalidomide is marketed only under a special restricted distribution program called the "System for Thalidomide Education and Prescribing Safety (STEPS). Under this program only prescribers and pharmacists registered with the program are allowed to prescribe and dispense the drug. Safety and efficacy have not been determined in children less than 12 years of age.

Route/Dosage
* **Capsules**
  Cutaneous ENL, initial therapy.
Adults, initial: 100–300 mg once daily with water, preferably at bedtime and at least 1 hr after the evening meal. Patients weighing less then 50 kg should be started at the low end of the dose range. In those with severe cutaneous ENL or who have required higher doses previously, dosing may be started at doses up to 400 mg once daily at bedtime or in divided doses with water 1 hr after meals. Continue initial dosing until signs and symptoms of active reaction have been eliminated (usually at least 2 weeks). Following this, taper patients off medication in 50 mg decrements q 2 to 4 weeks.

T

Maintenance therapy for prevention and suppression of ENL recurrence.

Maintain on the minimum dose (see initial therapy) necessary to control the reaction. Attempt tapering of medication q 3 to 6 months, in decrements of 50 mg q 2 to 4 weeks.

How Supplied: *Capsules:* 50 mg

Side Effects: *Note:* Only the most common side effects are listed. **Human teratogenicity.** *GI:* Constipation, diarrhea, nausea, oral moniliasis, tooth pain, abdominal pain. *CNS:* Drowsiness, somnolence, dizziness, tremor, vertigo, headache. *Neurologic:* Peripheral neuropathy. *CV:* Orthostatic hypotension, bradycardia. *Respiratory:* Pharyngitis, rhinitis, sinusitis. *Hematologic:* Neutropenia. *Hypersensitivity:* Erythematous macular rash, fever, tachycardia, hypotension. *Dermatologic:* Photosensitivity, rash, dermatitis, fungal nail disorder, pruritus. *Musculoskeletal:* Back pain, neck pain, neck rigidity. *Miscellaneous:* HIV viral load increase, impotence, peripheral edema, accidental injury, asthenia, chills, facial edema, malaise, pain.

Drug Interactions

Alcohol / Enhanced sedative effects
Barbiturates / Enhanced sedative effects
Chlorpromazine / Enhanced sedative effects
Reserpine / Enhanced sedative effects

EMS CONSIDERATIONS

None.

Theophylline
(thee-OFF-ih-lin)

Pregnancy Class: C

Immediate-release Capsules, Tablets, **Liquid Products:** Accurbron, Aquaphyllin, Asmalix, Bronkadyl, Elixomin, Elixophyllin, Lanophyllin, Lixolin, Quibron-T Dividose, Slo-Phyllin, Solu-Phyllin, Somophyllin-T, Theo, Theoclear-80, Theolair, Theomar, Truxophyllin. **Timed-release Capsules and Tablets:** Aerolate III, Aerolate Jr., Aerolate Sr., Quibron-T/SR Dividose, Respid, SloBid Gyrocaps, Slo-Phyllin Gyrocaps, Somophyllin-CRT, Sustaire, Theo-24, Theo 260 Cenules, Theocot, Theochron, Theolair-SR, Theospan-SR, Theo-Time, Theophylline SR, Theo-Time, Theovent Long-Acting, Uni-Dur, Uniphyl, **(Rx)**

Classification: Antiasthmatic, bronchodilator

Onset of Action: Time to peak serum levels, oral solution: 1 hr; **uncoated tablets:** 2hrs; **chewable tablets:** 1-1.5 hr; **enteric-coated tablets:** 5 hr; **extended-release capsules and tablets:** 4-7 hr.

Uses: Additional Use: Oral liquid: Neonatal apnea as a respiratory stimulant. Theophylline and dextrose injection. Respiratory stimulant in neonatal apnea and Cheyne-Stokes respiration.

Route/Dosage ————————

• **Capsules, Tablets, Elixir, Oral Solution, Syrup**

See *Dosage* for *Oral Solution, Tablets,* under *Aminophylline.*

• **Extended-Release Capsules, Extended-Release Tablets**

See *Dosage* for *Extended-Release Tablets,* under *Aminophylline.*

• **Elixir, Oral Solution, Oral Suspension, Syrup**

Bronchodilator, chronic therapy.
9–12 years: 20 mg/kg/day; **6–9 years:** 24 mg/kg/day.

Neonatal apnea.
Loading dose: Using the equivalent of anhydrous theophylline administered by NGT, 5 mg/kg; **maintenance:** 2 mg/kg/day in two to three divided doses given by NGT.

How Supplied: *Capsule, extended release:* 50 mg, 65 mg, 75 mg, 100 mg, 125 mg, 130 mg, 200 mg, 260 mg, 300 mg, 400 mg; *Elixir:* 80 mg/15 mL; *Solution:* 80 mg/15 mL; *Syrup:* 80 mg/15 mL; *Tablet:* 100 mg, 125 mg, 200 mg, 250 mg, 300 mg; *Tablet, extended release:* 100 mg, 200 mg, 250 mg, 300 mg, 400 mg, 450 mg, 500 mg, 600 mg

---

EMS CONSIDERATIONS

See also *Theophylline Derivatives.*

Thiabendazole

(thigh-ah-BEN-dah-zohl)
Pregnancy Class: C
Mintezol **(Rx)**
Classification: Anthelmintic

Mechanism of Action: Interferes with the enzyme fumarate reductase, which is specific to several helminths.

Uses: Primarily for threadworm infections, cutaneous larva migrans, visceral larva migrans when these infections occur alone or if pinworm is also present. Use in the following infections only if specific therapy is not available or cannot be used or if a second drug is desirable: hookworm, whipworm, large roundworm. To reduce symptoms of trichinosis during the invasive phase.

Contraindications: Lactation. Use in mixed infections with ascaris as it may cause worms to migrate.

Precautions: Safety and efficacy not established in children less than 13.6 kg. Use with caution in patients with hepatic disease or impaired hepatic function.

Route/Dosage
• **Oral Suspension, Chewable Tablets**
Over 68 kg: 1.5 g/dose; **less than 68 kg:** 22 mg/kg/dose.

How Supplied: *Chew Tablet:* 500 mg; *Suspension:* 500 mg/5 mL

Side Effects: *GI:* N&V, anorexia, diarrhea, epigastric distress. *CNS:* Dizziness, drowsiness, headache, irritability, weariness, giddiness, numbness, psychic disturbances, collapse, *seizures. Allergic:* Pruritus, *angioedema,* flushing of face, chills, fever, skin rashes, ***Stevens-Johnson syndrome, anaphylaxis,*** lymphadenopathy, conjunctival injection, erythema multiforme. *Hepatic:* Jaundice, cholestasis, parenchymal liver damage. *GU:* Crystalluria, hematuria, enuresis, foul odor of urine. *Ophthalmic:* Blurred vision, abnormal sensation in the eyes, yellow appearance of objects, drying of mucous membranes. *Miscellaneous:* Tinnitus, hypotension, hyperglycemia, transient leukopenia, perianal rash, appearance of live *Ascaris* in nose and mouth.

OD **Overdose Management:** *Symptoms:* Psychic changes, transient vision changes. *Treatment:* Induce vomiting or perform gastric lavage. Treat symptoms.

Drug Interactions: ↑ Serum levels of xanthines to potentially toxic levels due to ↓ breakdown by liver.

EMS CONSIDERATIONS
None.

Thiamine hydrochloride (Vitamin B₁)

(THIGH-ah-min)
Pregnancy Class: A (parenteral use)
Thiamilate (Rx: Injection; OTC: Tablets)

Mechanism of Action: Water-soluble vitamin. Required for the synthesis of thiamine pyrophosphate, a coenzyme required in carbohydrate metabolism. The maximum amount absorbed PO is 8–15 mg/day although absorption may be increased by giving in divided doses with food.

Uses: Prophylaxis and treatment of thiamine deficiency states and associated neurologic and CV symptoms. Prophylaxis and treatment of beriberi. Alcoholic neuritis, neuritis of pellagra, and neuritis of pregnancy. To correct anorexia due to thiamine insufficiency. *Investigational:* Treatment of subacute necrotizing encephalomyelopathy, maple syrup urine disease, pyruvate carboxylase deficiency, hyperalaninemia.

Precautions: Use with caution during lactation.

Route/Dosage
• **Tablets, Enteric-Coated Tablets**
Mild beriberi or maintenance following severe beriberi.
Adults: 5–10 mg/day (as part of a multivitamin product); **infants:** 10 mg/day.
Treatment of deficiency.

---

bold italic = life threatening side effect

Adults: 5–10 mg/day; **pediatric:** 10–50 mg/day.
Alcohol-induced deficiency.
Adults: 40 mg/day.
Dietary supplement.
Adults: 1–2 mg/day; **pediatric:** 0.3–0.5 mg/day for infants and 0.5 mg/day for children.
Genetic enzyme deficiency disease.
10–20 mg/day (up to 4 g/day has been used in some patients).
• **Slow IV**
Wet beriberi with myocardial failure.
Adults: 10–30 mg t.i.d.
• **IM**
Beriberi.
10–20 mg t.i.d. for 2 weeks. Give a PO multivitamin product containing 5–10 mg/day thiamine for 1 month to cause body saturation.
Recommended dietary allowance.
Adult males: 1.2–1.5 mg; **adult females:** 1.1 mg.
How Supplied: *Enteric Coated Tablet:* 20 mg; *Injection:* 100 mg/mL; *Tablet:* 25 mg, 50 mg, 100 mg, 250 mg, 500 mg

Side Effects: *Serious hypersensitivity reactions;* thus, intradermal testing is recommended if sensitivity is suspected. *Dermatologic:* Pruritus, urticaria, sweating, feeling of warmth. *CNS:* Weakness, restlessness. *Other:* Nausea, tightness in throat, *angioneurotic edema,* cyanosis, *hemorrhage into the GI tract, pulmonary edema, CV collapse. Death has been reported. Following IM use:* Induration, tenderness.

Drug Interactions: Because vitamin B_1 is unstable in neutral or alkaline solutions, the vitamin should not be used with substances that yield alkaline solutions, such as citrates, barbiturates, carbonates, or erythromycin lactobionate IV.

EMS CONSIDERATIONS
None.

Thioguanine
(thigh-oh-GWON-een)

Pregnancy Class: D
TG, 6-Thioguanine (Abbreviation: 6-TG) **(Rx)**
Classification: Antimetabolite, purine analog

Mechanism of Action: Purine antagonist that is cell-cycle specific for the S phase of cell division. Converted to 6-thioguanylic acid, which in turn interferes with the synthesis of guanine nucleotides by competing with hypoxanthine and xanthine for the enzyme phosphoribosyltransferase (HGPRTase). Ultimately the synthesis of RNA and DNA is inhibited. Resistance to the drug may result from increased breakdown of 6-thioguanylic acid or loss of HGPRTase activity.

Uses: Acute and nonlymphocytic leukemias (usually in combination with other drugs such as cyclophosphamide, cytarabine, prednisone, vincristine). Chronic myelogenous leukemia (not first-line therapy).

Contraindications: Resistance to mercaptopurine or thioguanine. Lactation.

Route/Dosage ─────────
• **Tablets**
Individualized and determined by hematopoietic response.
Adults and pediatric, initial: 2 mg/kg/day (or 75–100 mg/m²) given at one time. From 2 to 4 weeks may elapse before beneficial results become apparent. Compute dose to nearest multiple of 20 mg. If no response, dosage may be increased to 3 mg/kg/day. **Usual maintenance dose (even during remissions):** 2–3 mg/kg/day (or 100 mg/m²). Dosage of thioguanine does not have to be decreased during administration of allopurinol (to inhibit uric acid production).

How Supplied: *Tablet:* 40 mg
Side Effects: Additional: Loss of vibration sense, unsteadiness of gait. *Hepatotoxicity,* myelosuppression (common), hyperuricemia. Adults tend to show a more rapid fall in WBC count than children.

OD Overdose Management: *Symptoms:* N&V, hypertension, malaise, and diaphoresis may be seen immediately, which may be followed by myelosuppression and azotemia. ***Severe hematologic toxicity.*** *Treatment:* Induce vomiting if patient is seen immediately after an acute overdosage. Treat symptoms. Hematologic toxicity may be treated by platelet transfusions (for bleeding) and granulocyte transfusions. Antibiotics are indicated for sepsis.

EMS CONSIDERATIONS
None.

Thioridazine hydrochloride
(thigh-oh-RID-ah-zeen)
Pregnancy Class: C
Mellaril, Mellaril-S, Thioridazine HCl Intensol Oral **(Rx)**
Classification: Antipsychotic, piperidine-type phenothiazine

Mechanism of Action: High incidence of hypotension; moderate incidence of sedative and anticholinergic effects and weak antiemetic and extrapyramidal effects. May be used in patients intolerant of other phenothiazines.

Uses: Management of psychotic disorders. Short-term treatment of moderate to marked depression with variable levels of anxiety in adults. Treat psychoneurotic symptoms in geriatric patients, including agitation, anxiety, depressed mood, tension, sleep disturbances, and fears. **In children:** Treat severe behavioral problems marked by combativeness or explosive hyperexcitable behavior. Short-term treatment of hyperactive children showing excessive motor activity with accompanying impulsivity, short attention span, aggressivity, mood lability, and poor frustration tolerance.

Precautions: Safe use during pregnancy has not been established. Dosage has not been Sestablished in children less than 2 years of age. Geriatric, emaciated, or debilitated patients usually require a lower initial dose.

Route/Dosage ————
• **Oral Suspension, Oral Solution, Tablets**
Psychotic disorders.
Adults, initial: 50–100 mg t.i.d. Increase gradually to a maximum of 800 mg/day, if needed to control symptoms. Then, reduce gradually to the minimum maintainence dose. Dose range: 200–800 mg/day divided into two to four doses.
Psychoneurotic symptoms.
Initial: 25 mg t.i.d. Dose range: 10 mg b.i.d.–q.i.d. in milder cases to 50 mg t.i.d. or q.i.d. Dose range: 20–200 mg/day.
Behavioral disorders in children.
Ages 2 to 12: 0.5 mg/kg/day to a maximum of 3 mg/kg/day. For moderate disorders, initially use 10 mg b.i.d.–t.i.d. For hospitalized, severely disturbed or psychotic children: 25 mg b.i.d.–t.i.d.
How Supplied: *Oral Concentrate:* 30 mg/mL, 100 mg/mL; *Tablet:* 10 mg, 15 mg, 25 mg, 50 mg, 100 mg, 150 mg, 200 mg
Side Effects: Additional: More likely to cause pigmentary retinopathy than other phenothiazines.

EMS CONSIDERATIONS
See also *Antipsychotic Agents, Phenothiazines.*

Thiothixene (Navane)
thigh-oh-THICKS-een
Pregnancy Class: C
Navane, Thiothixene HCl Intensol **(Rx)**
Classification: Antipsychotic, miscellaneous

Mechanism of Action: Mechanism of action may be due to blockade of postsynaptic dopamine receptors in the brain, especially at subcortical levels in the reticular formation, hypothalamus, and limbic system. Also causes cholinergic and alpha-adrenergic blocking effects, adrenergic

T

---

bold italic = life threatening side effect

potentiating effects, antiserotonin effects, and prevention of uptake of biogenic amines. This results in significant extrapyramidal symptoms and antiemetic effects and minimal sedation, orthostatic hypotension, and anticholinergic symptoms. The margin between a therapeutically effective dose and one that causes extrapyramidal symptoms is narrow. Well absorbed from the GI tract. **Peak plasma levels, PO:** 1–3 hr. **t½:** 34 hr. A therapeutic response may occur within 1 to 6 hr following IM use and within a few days to several weeks following PO use. Metabolized in the liver and excreted in the feces as both unchanged drug and metabolites.

Uses: Symptomatic treatment of psychotic disorders, including withdrawn, apathetic schizophrenia, delusions, and hallucinations.

Contraindications: Use in patients with circulatory collapse, comatose states, CNS depression due to any cause, and blood dyscrasias. Hypersensitivity to thiothixene and possibly phenothiazine derivatives. Use in children less than 12 years of age.

Route/Dosage ────────────
• **Capsules, Concentrate**
   Mild to moderate psychoses.
Adults, initial: 2 mg t.i.d., increased to 15 mg/day if necessary.
   Severe psychoses.
Adults, initial: 5 mg b.i.d., increased to 60 mg/day if necessary. The usual optimum dose is 20–30 mg/day. Doses greater than 60 mg/day rarely increase the therapeutic effect.
How Supplied: *Capsules:* 1 mg, 2 mg, 5 mg, 10 mg, 20 mg; *Concentrate:* 5 mg/mL

Side Effects: Since thiothixene has pharmacologic properties similar to phenothiazines, the side effects associated with phenothiazines should also be consulted. *CNS:* Drowsiness, extrapyramidal symptoms (especially akathisia and dystonia), persistent tardive dyskinesia (especially in female geriatric patients), lethargy, dizziness, restlessness, lightheaded-ness, agitation, insomnia, hyperpyrexia, weakness, fatigue. Rarely, seizures and paradoxical exacerbation of psychoses. *GI:* Dry mouth, constipation, increased salivation, adynamic ileus, anorexia, N&V, diarrhea, increase in appetite and weight, cholestatic jaundice. *CV:* Orthostatic hypotension, tachycardia, syncope, ECG changes. *Ophthalmic:* Blurred vision, miosis, mydriasis. *Hypersensitivity:* Rash, pruritus, urticaria, photosensitivity, ***anaphylaxis (rare).*** *GU:* Impotence, lactation, moderate breast enlargement in women, amenorrhea. *Hematologic:* Leukopenia, leukocytosis. *Miscellaneous:* **Neuroleptic malignant syndrome.** Increased sweating, nasal congestion, impotence, leg cramps, polydypsia, peripheral edema, fine lenticular pigmentation.

OD **Overdose Management:** *Symptoms:* Muscle twitching, drowsiness, dizziness. In severe cases, symptoms include rigidity, weakness, torticollis, tremor, salivation, dysphagia, disturbance of gait, CNS depression, coma. *Treatment:* General supportive measures, including maintaining an adequate airway and oxygenation. Gastric lavage, if overdose found early. Hypotension and circulatory collapse may be treated with IV fluids and/or vasopressor agents (epinephrine is not to be used). Antiparkinson drugs may be used to treat extrapyramidal symptoms. Do *not* use analeptic drugs.

Drug Interactions
Anticholinergic drugs / Additive or potentiation of anticholinergic effect
CNS depressants / Additive or potentiation of depressant effect
Hypotensive drugs / Additive or potentiation of hypotensive effect

EMS CONSIDERATIONS

See also *Nursing Considerations* for *Antipsychotics.*
Administration/Storage: For maintenance therapy, a single daily dose may be adequate.
Assessment
1. Document onset, duration, and characteristics of symptoms. List other agents trialed and the outcome.

2. Assess baseline mental status, noting mood, behavior, and any evidence of depression.

3. List drugs currently prescribed to ensure none interact.

4. Avoid drug with CNS depression, circulatory collapse, coma, blood dyscrasias, or uncontrolled seizure disorder.

5. Monitor CBC, LFTs, and ECG.

Tiagabine hydrochloride (Gabatril)

tye-AG-ah-been
Pregnancy Class: C
Gabatril **(Rx)**
Classification: Anticonvulsant, miscellaneous

Mechanism of Action: Mechanism not known but activity of GABA, an inhibitory neurotransmitter, may be enhanced. Drug may block uptake of GABA into presynaptic neurons allowing more GABA to bind to post-synaptic cells. This prevents propagation of neural impulses that contribute to seizures due to GABA-ergic action. **Peak plasma levels:** About 45 min when fasting. High fat meals decrease rate but not extent of absorption. Metabolized in liver; excreted in urine and feces. **t½, elimination:** 7–9 hr. Diurnal effect occurs with levels being lower in evening compared with morning.

Uses: Adjunctive therapy for partial seizures.

Contraindications: Lactation.

Route/Dosage
• **Tablets**
Partial seizures.
Adults and children over 18 years, initial: 4 mg once daily. Total daily dose may be increased by 4 to 8 mg at weekly intervals until clinical effect is observed or daily dose is 56 mg/day. **Children, 12 to 18 years, initial:** 4 mg once daily. Total daily dose may be increased by 4 mg at beginning of week 2. Thereafter, dose may be increased by 4 to 8 mg at weekly intervals until clinical effect is

seen or dose is 32 mg/day. For all ages, give total daily dose in 2 to 4 divided doses.

How Supplied: *Tablets:* 4 mg, 12 mg, 16 mg, 20 mg

Side Effects: *CNS:* Dizziness, asthenia, somnolence, nervousness, tremor, insomnia, difficulty with concentration or attention, ataxia, confusion, speech disorder, difficulty with memory, paresthesia, depression, emotional lability, abnormal gait, hostility, nystagmus, problems with language, agitation. *GI:* N&V, diarrhea, increased appetite, mouth ulceration. *Respiratory:* Pharyngitis, increased cough. *Dermatologic:* Rash, pruritus. *Miscellaneous:* Abdominal pain, unspecified pain, vasodilation, myasthenia.

OD Overdose Management: *Symptoms:* Somnolence, impaired consciousness, agitation, confusion, speech difficulties, depression, weakness, myoclonus. *Treatment:* Emesis or gastric lavage, maintain an airway. General supportive treatment.

Drug Interactions
Carbamazepine / ↑ Clearance due to ↑ metabolism
Phenobarbital / ↑ Clearance due to ↑ metabolism
Phenytoin / ↑ Clearance due to ↑ metabolism
Valproate / ↑ Clearance due to ↑ metabolism

EMS CONSIDERATIONS

See also *Nursing Considerations* for *Anticonvulsants, .*
Administration/Storage
1. It is not necessary to modify dose of concomitant anticonvulsant drugs, unless clinically indicated.
2. Dose must be titrated in those taking enzyme-inducing anticonvulsant drugs; consult package insert.
Assessment
1. Document indications for therapy, characteristics of seizures, other agents trialed and outcome.
2. Monitor LFTs; decrease dosage or dosing intervals with dysfunction.

Ticarillin disodium
(tie-kar-SILL-in)
Pregnancy Class: B
Ticar **(Rx)**
Classification: Antibiotic, penicillin

Mechanism of Action: A parenteral, semisynthetic antibiotic with an antibacterial spectrum of activity resembling that of carbenicillin. **Peak plasma levels: IM,** 25–35 mcg/mL after 1 hr; **IV,** 15 min. **t½:** 70 min. Elimination complete after 6 hr.

Uses: Primarily suitable for treatment of gram-negative organisms but also effective for mixed infections. (1) Bacterial septicemia, skin and soft tissue infections, acute and chronic respiratory tract infections caused by susceptible strains of *Pseudomonas aeruginosa, Proteus, Escherichia coli,* and other gram-negative organisms. Combined therapy with gentamicin or tobramycin is sometimes indicated for treatment of *Pseudomonas* infections. (2) GU tract infections (complicated and uncomplicated) caused by the above organisms and by *Enterobacter* and *Streptococcus faecalis.* (3) Anaerobic bacteria causing empyema, anaerobic pneumonitis, lung abscess, bacterial septicemia, peritonitis, intra-abdominal abscess, skin and soft tissue infections, salpingitis, endometritis, pelvic inflammatory disease, pelvic abscess. Ticarcillin may be used in infections in which protective mechanisms are impaired such as during use of oncolytic or immunosuppressive drugs or in patients with acute leukemia.

Precautions: Use with caution in presence of impaired renal function and for patients on restricted salt diets.

Route/Dosage
- **IV Infusion, Direct IV, IM**
    Bacterial septicemia, intra-abdominal infections, skin and soft tissue infections, infections of the female genital system and pelvis, respiratory tract infections.
Adults: 200–300 mg/kg/day by IV infusion in divided doses 4 or 6 hr (3 g q 4 hr or 4 g q 6 hr), depending on the weight and severity of the infection. **Pediatric, less than 40 kg:** 200–300 mg/kg/day by IV infusion q 4 or 6 hr (daily dose should not exceed the adult dose).
    UTIs, uncomplicated.
Adults: 1 g IM or direct IV q 6 hr. **Pediatric, less than 40 kg:** 50–100 mg/kg/day IM or direct IV in divided doses q 6 or 8 hr.
    UTIs, complicated.
Adults: 150–200 mg/kg/day by IV infusion in divided doses q 4 or 6 hr (usual dose is 3 g q.i.d. for a 70-kg patient).
    Neonates with sepsis due to Pseudomonas, Proteus, or E. coli.
Less than 7 days of age and less than 2 kg, 75 mg/kg q 12 hr; **more than 7 days of age and less than 2 kg,** 75 mg/kg q 8 hr; **less than 7 days of age and more than 2 kg,** 75 mg/kg q 8 hr; **more than 7 days of age and more than 2 kg,** 100 mg/kg q 8 hr. Can be given IM or by IV infusion over 10–20 min.

Patients with renal insufficiency should receive a loading dose of 3 g **IV,** and subsequent doses, as follows by C_{CR}. C_{CR} over 60 mL/min: 3 g IV q 4 hr; C_{CR} from 30–60 mL/min: 2 g IV q 4 hr; C_{CR} from 10–30 mL/min: 2 g IV q 8 hr; C_{CR}, less than 10 mL/min: 2 g IV q 12 hr or 1 g IM q 6 hr; C_{CR}, less than 10 mL/min with hepatic dysfunction: 2 g IV q 24 hr or 1 g IM q 12 hr. Patients on peritoneal dialysis: 3 g IV q 12 hr; patients on hemodialysis: 2 g IV q 12 hr and 3 g after each dialysis.

How Supplied: *Powder for injection:* 3 g, 20 g

Side Effects: Additional: Neurotoxicity and neuromuscular excitability, especially in patients with impaired renal function.

Drug Interactions: Additional: Effect of carbenicillin may be enhanced when used in combination with gentamicin or tobramycin for *Pseudomonas* infections.

EMS CONSIDERATIONS
See also *Penicillins.*

------COMBINATION DRUG------

Ticarcillin disodium and Clavulanate potassium

(tie-kar-SILL-in, klav-you-LAN-ate poe-TASS-ee-um)

Pregnancy Class: B
Timentin **(Rx)**
Classification: Antibiotic, penicillin

Mechanism of Action: Contains clavulanic acid, which protects the breakdown of ticarcillin by beta-lactamase enzymes, thus ensuring appropriate blood levels of ticarcillin.

Uses: (1) Septicemia, including bacteremia, due to β–lactamase producing strains of *Klebsiella* sp., *Staphylococcus aureus,* and *Pseudomonas aeruginosa* (and other *Pseudomonas* species). (2) Lower respiratory tract infections due to β–lactamase producing strains of *S. aureus, Haemophilus influenzae,* and *Klebsiella* sp. (3) Bone and joint infections due to β–lactamase producing strains of *S. aureus.* (4) Skin and skin structure infections due to β–lactamase producing strains of *S. aureus, Klebsiella* sp., and *E. coli.* (5) UTIs (complicated and uncomplicated) due to β–lactamase producing strains of *E. coli, Klebsiella* sp., *P. aeruginosa* (and other *Pseudomonas* species), *Citrobacter* sp., *Enterobacter cloacae, Serratia marcescens,* and *S. aureus.* (6) Endometritis due to β–lactamase producing strains of *B. melaninogenicus, Enterobacter* sp. (including *E. cloacae), E. coli, Klebsiella pneumoniae, S. aureus,* and *Staphylococcus epidermidis.* (7) Peritonitis due to β–lactamase producing strains of *E. coli, K. pneumoniae,* and *Bacteroides fragilis* group.

Route/Dosage
• **IV Infusion**
    Systemic and UTIs.
Adults more than 60 kg: 3.1 g (containing 0.1 g clavulanic acid) q 4–6 hr for 10–14 days. **Adults less than 60 kg:** 200–300 mg ticarcillin/kg/day in divided doses q 4–6 hr for 10–14 days.
    Gynecologic infections.

Adults more than 60 kg, moderate infections: 200 mg/kg/day in divided doses q 6 hr; **severe infections:** 300 mg/kg/day in divided doses q 4 hr.
    In renal insufficiency.
Initially, loading dose of 3.1 g ticarcillin and 0.1 g clavulanic acid; **then,** dose based on C_{CR} as follows. C_{CR} over 60 mL/min: 3.1 g q 4 hr; C_{CR} from 30–60 mL/min: 2 g q 4 hr; C_{CR} from 10–30 mL/min: 2 g q 8 hr; C_{CR} less than 10 mL/min: 2 g q 12 hr; C_{CR} less than 10 mL/min with hepatic dysfunction: 2 g q 24 hr. Patients on peritoneal dialysis: 3.1 g q 12 hr; patients on hemodialysis: 2 g q 12 hr and 3.1 g after each dialysis.
How Supplied: See Content

EMS CONSIDERATIONS

See also *Penicillins* and *Ticarcillin disodium.*

Ticlopidine hydrochloride

(tie-KLOH-pih-deen)

Pregnancy Class: B
Ticlid **(Rx)**
Classification: Platelet aggregation inhibitor

Mechanism of Action: Irreversibly inhibits ADP-induced platelet-fibrinogen binding and subsequent platelet-platelet interactions. This results in inhibition of both platelet aggregation and release of platelet granule constituents as well as prolongation of bleeding time.

Uses: To reduce the risk of fatal or nonfatal thrombotic stroke in patients who have manifested precursors of stroke or who have had a completed thrombotic stroke. Due to the risk of neutropenia or agranulocytosis, use should be reserved for patients who are intolerant to aspirin therapy. *Investigational:* Chronic arterial occlusion, coronary artery bypass grafts, intermittent claudication, open heart surgery, primary glomerulonephritis, subarachnoid hemorrhage, sickle cell disease, uremic patients with AV shunts or fistulas.

T

bold italic = life threatening side effect

Contraindications: Use in the presence of neutropenia and thrombocytopenia, hemostatic disorder, or active pathologic bleeding such as bleeding peptic ulcer or intracranial bleeding. Severe liver impairment. Lactation.

Precautions: Use with caution in patients with ulcers (i.e., where there is a propensity for bleeding). Consider reduced dosage in impaired renal function. Geriatric patients may be more sensitive to the effects of the drug. Severe hematological side effects (including thrombotic thrombocytopenic purpura) may occur within a few days of the start of ticlopidine therapy. Safety and effectiveness have not been established in children less than 18 years of age.

Route/Dosage
- **Tablets**
  Reduce risk of thrombotic stroke.
  250 mg b.i.d.

How Supplied: *Tablet:* 250 mg

Side Effects: *Hematologic:* Neutropenia, ***agranulocytosis,*** thrombocytopenia, pancytopenia, thrombotic thrombocytopenia purpura, immune thrombocytopenia, ***hemolytic anemia with reticulocytosis.*** *GI:* Diarrhea, N&V, GI pain, dyspepsia, flatulence, anorexia, GI fullness. *Bleeding complications:* Ecchymosis, hematuria, epistaxis, conjunctival hemorrhage, ***GI bleeding,*** perioperative bleeding, ***intracerebral bleeding (rare).*** *Dermatologic:* Maculopapular or urticarial rash, pruritus, urticaria. *CNS:* Dizziness, headache. *Neuromuscular:* Asthenia, SLE, peripheral neuropathy, arthropathy, myositis. *Miscellaneous:* Tinnitus, pain, allergic pneumonitis, vasculitis, hepatitis, cholestatic jaundice, nephrotic syndrome, hyponatremia, serum sickness.

Drug Interactions
Antacids / ↓ Plasma levels of ticlopidine
Aspirin / Ticlopidine ↑ effect of aspirin on collagen-induced platelet aggregation
Carbamazepine / ↑ Plasma levels of carbamazepine → toxicity

Cimetidine / ↓ Clearance of ticlopidine probably due to ↓ breakdown by liver
Digoxin / Slight ↓ in digoxin plasma levels
Theophylline / ↑ Plasma levels of theophylline due to ↓ clearance

EMS CONSIDERATIONS
None.

Tiludronate disodium
(tye-LOO-droh-nayt)
Pregnancy Class: C
Skelid (Rx)
Classification: Bone growth regulator

Mechanism of Action: Inhibits activity of osteoclasts and decreases bone turnover. Does not interfere with bone mineralization.

Uses: Treatment of Paget's disease where level of serum alkaline phosphatase is at least twice upper limit of normal, in those who are symptomatic, or who are at risk for future complications of disease.

Contraindications: Not recommended for those with C_{CR} less than 30 mL/min.

Precautions: Use with caution during lactation and in those with dysphagia, symptomatic esophageal disease, gastritis, duodenitis, or ulcers. Safety and efficacy have not been determined in children.

Route/Dosage
- **Tablets**
  Paget's disease.

Adults: Single 400 mg dose/day taken with 6 to 8 oz of plain water for period of only 3 months.

How Supplied: *Tablets:* 200 mg

Side Effects: *GI:* Diarrhea, N&V, dyspepsia, flatulence, tooth disorder, abdominal pain, constipation, dry mouth, gastritis. *Body as whole:* Pain, back pain, accidental injury, flu-like symptoms, chest pain, asthenia, syncope, fatigue, flushing. *CNS:* Headache, dizziness, paresthesia, vertigo, anorexia, somnolence, anxiety, nervousness, insomnia. *CV:* Dependent edema, peripheral edema, hypertension, syncope. *Musculoskeletal:* Arthralgia, arthrosis, pathological fracture, involuntary muscle contractions. *Respiratory:* Rhinitis, sinusitis, URTI, coughing, pharyngitis, bronchitis. *Dermatologic:* Rash, skin disorder, pruritus, increased sweating, Stevens-Johnson type syndrome (rare). *Ophthalmic:* Cataract, conjunctivitis, glaucoma. *Miscellaneous:* Hyperparathyroidism, vitamin D deficiency, UTI, infection.

OD **Overdose Management:** *Symptoms:* Hypocalcemia. *Treatment:* Supportive.

Drug Interactions
Antacids, aluminum- or magnesium-containing / ↓ Bioavailability of tiludronate when taken 1 hr before tiludronate
Aspirin / ↓ Bioavailability of tiludronate by 50% when taken 2 hr after tiludronate
Calcium / ↓ Bioavailability of tiludronate when taken at same time
Indomethacin / ↑ Bioavailability of tiludronate by two- to four-fold

EMS CONSIDERATIONS
None.

Timolol maleate
(TIE-moh-lohl)
Pregnancy Class: C
Blocadrin, Timoptic, Eimoptic in Acudose, Timoptic-XE **(Rx)**
Classification: Ophthalmic agent, beta-adrenergic blocking agent

Mechanism of Action: Exerts both beta-1- and beta-2-adrenergic blocking activity. Has minimal sympathomimetic effects, direct myocardial depressant effects, or local anesthetic action.
Onset of Action: 30 min, **Maximum effect:** 1-2 hr.
Duration of Action: 24 hr.
Uses: Tablets: Hypertension (alone or in combination with other antihypertensives such as thiazide diuretics). Within 1–4 weeks of MI to reduce risk of reinfarction. Prophylaxis of migraine. *Investigational:* Ventricu-

lar arrhythmias and tachycardias, essential tremors.
   Ophthalmic solution (Timoptic): Lower IOP in chronic open-angle glaucoma, selected cases of secondary glaucoma, ocular hypertension, aphakic (no lens) patients with glaucoma. *Ophthalmic gel forming solution (Timoptic-XE):* Reduce elevated IOP in glaucoma.
Contraindications: Hypersensitivity to drug. Bronchial asthma or bronchospasm including severe COPD.
Precautions: Use ophthalmic preparation with caution in patients for whom systemic beta-adrenergic blocking agents are contraindicated. Safe use in children not established.

Route/Dosage
• **Tablets**
   Hypertension.
Initial: 10 mg b.i.d. alone or with a diuretic; **maintenance:** 20–40 mg/day (up to 80 mg/day in two doses may be required), depending on BP and HR. If dosage increase is necessary, wait 7 days.
   MI prophylaxis in patients who have survived the acute phase.
10 mg b.i.d.
   Migraine prophylaxis.
Initially: 10 mg b.i.d. **Maintenance:** 20 mg/day given as a single dose; total daily dose may be increased to 30 mg in divided doses or decreased to 10 mg, depending on the response and patient tolerance. If a satisfactory response for migraine prophylaxis is not obtained within 6–8 weeks using the maximum daily dose, discontinue the drug.
   Essential tremor.
10 mg/day.
• **Ophthalmic Solution (Timoptic 0.25% or 0.5%)**
   Glaucoma.
1 gtt of 0.25%–0.50% solution in each eye b.i.d. If the decrease in intraocular pressure is maintained, reduce dose to 1 gtt once a day.
• **Ophthalmic Gel-Forming Solution (Timoptic-XE 0.25% or 0.5%)**
   Glaucoma.

T

---
bold italic = life threatening side effect

1 gtt once daily.

How Supplied: *Gel forming solution:* 0.25%, 0.5%; *Ophthalmic solution:* 0.25%, 0.5%; *Tablet:* 5 mg, 10 mg, 20 mg

Side Effects: *Systemic following use of tablets:* See *Beta-Adrenergic Blocking Agents.*

Following use of ophthalmic product: Few. Occasionally, ocular irritation, local hypersensitivity reactions, slight decrease in resting HR.

Drug Interactions: When used ophthalmically, possible potentiation with systemically administered beta-adrenergic blocking agents.

EMS CONSIDERATIONS

See also *Beta-Adrenergic Blocking Agents* and *Antihypertensive Agents.*

Tioconazole
(tie-oh-KON-ah-zohl)
Pregnancy Class: C
Monistat 1, Vagistat-1, **(Rx) (OTC)**
Classification: Antifungal, vaginal

Mechanism of Action: Antifungal activity thought to be due to alteration of the permeability of the cell membrane of the fungus, causing leakage of essential intracellular compounds.

Uses: *Candida albicans* infections of the vulva and vagina. Also effective against *Torulopsis glabrata.* OTC for recurrent vaginal yeast infections in those who have previously been diagnosed and have the same symptoms again.

Contraindications: Use of a vaginal applicator during pregnancy may be contraindicated.

Precautions: Safety and effectiveness have not been determined during lactation or in children.

Route/Dosage
• **Vaginal Ointment, 6.5%**
One applicator full (about 4.6 g) should be inserted intravaginally at bedtime for 3 days. If needed, the treatment period can be extended to 6 days. Monistat 1 is intended as a one-dose product.

How Supplied: *Ointment:* 6.5%

Side Effects: *GU:* Burning, itching, irritation, vulvar edema and swelling, discharge, vaginal pain, dysuria, dyspareunia, nocturia, desquamation, dryness of vaginal secretions.

EMS CONSIDERATIONS
None.

Tirofiban hydrochloride
(ty-roh-FYE-ban)
Pregnancy Class: B
Aggrastat **(Rx)**
Classification: Antiplatelet drug

Mechanism of Action: Non–peptide antagonist of the platelet glycoprotein (GP) IIb/IIIa receptor, which is the major platelet surface receptor involved in platelet aggregation. Activation of the receptor leads to binding of fibrinogen and von Willebrand's factor to platelets, and thus aggregation. Tirofiban is a reversible antagonist of fibrinogen binding to the GP IIb/IIIa receptor, thus inhibiting platelet aggregation.

Uses: In combination with heparin for acute coronary syndrome ACS), including those being treated medically and those undergoing PTCA or atherectomy.

Contraindications: Active internal bleeding or history of diathesis within the previous 30 days; history of intracranial hemorrhage, intracranial neoplasm, AV malformation, or aneurysm; history of thrombocytopenia following prior use of tirofiban; history of stroke within 30 days or any history of hemorrhagic stroke; major surgical procedure or severe physical trauma within the last month; history, findings, or symptoms suggestive of aortic dissection; severe hypertension (systolic BP greater than 180 mm Hg or diastolic BP greater than 110 mm Hg); concomitant use of another parenteral GP IIb/IIIa inhibitor; acute pericarditis.

Precautions: Use with caution in patients with a platelet count less than 150,000/mm³ in hemorrhagic retinopathy, with other drugs that affect hemostasis (e.g., warfarin). Safety and efficacy in children less than 18 years of age have not been established. Safety when used in combination with thrombolytic drugs has not been determined.

Route/Dosage
• **IV**
Acute coronary syndrome.
Initial: 0.4 mcg/kg/min for 30 min; **then,** 0.1 mg/kg/min. Use half the usual rate in those with severe renal impairment. Consult package insert for the guide to dosage adjustment by weight of the patient.

How Supplied: *Injection:* 50 mcg/mL; *Injection For Solution:* 250 mcg/mL

Side Effects: Most common is bleeding, including intracranial bleeding, retroperitoneal bleeding, major GI and GU bleeding. Female and elderly patients have a higher incidence of bleeding than male or younger patients. *Miscellaneous:* Nausea, fever, headache, bradycardia, coronary artery dissection, dizziness, edema or swelling, leg pain, pelvic pain, vasovagal reaction, sweating.

OD **Overdose Management:** *Symptoms:* Bleeding, including minor mucocutaneous bleeding events and minor bleeding at the site of cardiac catheterization. *Treatment:* Assess clinical condition. Adjust or cease infusion, as appropriate. Can be removed by hemodialysis.

Drug Interactions
Aspirin / ↑ Bleeding
Heparin / ↑ Bleeding
Levothyroxine / ↑ Tirofiban clearance
Omeprazole / ↑ Tirofiban clearance

EMS CONSIDERATIONS
None.

Tizanidine hydrochloride
(tye-ZAN-ih-deen)
Pregnancy Class: C
Zanaflex (Rx)
Classification: Skeletal muscle relaxant, centrally-acting

Mechanism of Action: Acts on central α-2 adrenergic receptors; reduces spasticity by increasing presynaptic inhibition of motor neurons possibly by reducing release of excitatory amino acids. Greatest effects are on polysynaptic pathways. Also may reduce postsynaptic excitatory transmitter activity, decrease the firing rate of noradrenergic locus ceruleas neurons, and inhibit synaptic transmission of nociceptive stimuli in the spinal pathways.
Onset of Action: Peak effect: 1-2 hr.
Duration of Action: 3-6 hr.
Uses: Acute and intermittent management of muscle spasticity.
Contraindications: Use with α-2-adrenergic agonists.
Precautions: Use with caution in renal impairment, in elderly and during laction. Use with extreme caution in hepatic insufficiency. Safety and efficacy have not been determined in children.

Route/Dosage
• **Tablets**
Muscle spasticity.
Initial: 4 mg; **then,** increase dose gradually in 2 to 4 mg steps to optimum effect. Dose can be repeated at 6–8-hr intervals, to maximum of 3 doses/24 hr, not to exceed 36 mg/day. There is no experience with repeated, single, daytime doses greater than 12 mg or total daily doses of 36 mg or more.

How Supplied: *Tablets:* 4 mg
Side Effects: *Note:* Side effects listed are those with a frequency of 0.1% or greater. *CV:* Hypotension, vasodilation, postural hypotension, syncope, migraine, arrhythmia. *GI:* Hepatotoxicity, dry mouth, constipation, pharyngitis, vomiting, abdominal pain, diarrhea, dyspepsia, dysphagia, cholelithiasis, fecal impaction, flatulence, *GI hemorrhage* hepatitis, melena. *CNS:* Dizziness, dyskinesia, nervousness, somnolence, sedation, hallucinations, psychotic-like symptoms, depression, anxiety, paresthesia,

T

tremor, emotional lability, seizures, paralysis, abnormal thinking, vertigo, abnormal dreams, agitation, depersonalization, euphoria, stupor, dysautonomia, neuralgia. *GU:* Urinary frequency, UTI, urinary urgency, cystitis, menorrhagia, pyelonephritis, urinary retention, kidney calculus, enlarged uterine fibroids, vaginal moniliasis, vaginitis. *Hematologic:* Ecchymosis, anemia, leukopenia, leukocytosis. *Musculoskeletal:* Myasthenia, back pain, pathological fracture, arthralgia, arthritis, bursitis. *Respiratory:* Sinusitis, pneumonia, bronchitis, rhinitis. *Dermatologic:* Rash, sweating, skin ulcer, pruritus, dry skin, acne, alopecia, urticaria. *Body as a whole:* Flu syndrome, weight loss, infection, **sepsis, cellulitis, death,** allergic reaction, moniliasis, malaise, asthenia, fever, abscess, edema. *Ophthalmic:* Glaucoma, amblyopia, conjunctivitis, eye pain, optic neuritis, retinal hemorrhage, visual field defect. *Otic:* Ear pain, tinnitus, deafness, otitis media. *Miscellaneous:* Speech disorder.

Drug Interactions
Alcohol / ↑ Side effects of tizanidine; additive CNS depressant effects
Alpha-2-Adrenergic agonists / Additive hypotensive effects
Oral contraceptives / ↓ Clearance of tizanidine

EMS CONSIDERATIONS

See also *Skeletal Muscle Relaxants, Centrally Acting.*

Tobramycin sulfate
(toe-brah-MY-sin)
Pregnancy Class: D (B for ophthalmic use)
Inhalation: TOBI, **Parenteral:** Nebcin, Nebcin Pediatric, **Ophthalmic:** AK-Tob Ophthalmic Solution, Tobrex Ophthalmic Ointment, Tobrex Ophthalmic Solution **(Rx)**
Classification: Antibiotic, aminoglycoside

Mechanism of Action: Similar to gentamicin.
Uses: Systemic: (1) Complicated and recurrent UTIs due to *Pseudo-monas aeruginosa, Proteus, Escherichia coli, Klebsiella, Enterobacter, Serratia, Staphylococcus aureus, Citrobacter,* and *Providencia.* (2) Lower respiratory tract infections due to *P. aeruginosa, Klebsiella, Enterobacter, E. coli, Serratia,* and *S. aureus* (penicillinase– and non–penicillinase producing). (3) Intra-abdominal infections (including peritonitis) due to *E. coli, Klebsiella,* and *Enterobacter.* (4) Septicemia in neonates, children, and adults due to *P. aeruginosa, E. coli,* and *Klebsiella.* (5) Skin, bone, and skin structure infections due to *P. aeruginosa, Proteus, E. coli, Klebsiella, Enterobacter,* and *S. aureus.* (6) Serious CNS infections, including meningitis. Can be used with penicillins or cephalosporins in serious infections when results of susceptibility testing are not yet known.

Ophthalmic: Treat superficial ocular infections due to *Staphylococcus, S. aureus, Streptococcus, S. pneumoniae,* beta-hemolytic streptococci, *Corynebacterium, E. coli, Haemophilus aegyptius, H. ducreyi, H. influenzae, H. parainfluenzae, Klebsiella pneumoniae, Neisseria, N. gonorrhoeae, Proteus, Acinetobacter calcoaceticus, Enterobacter, Enterobacter aerogenes, Serratia marcescens, Moraxella, Pseudomonas aeruginosa,* and *Vibrio.*

Inhalation: Management of lung infections (*P. aeruginosa*) in cystic fibrosis patients.
Contraindications: Ophthalmically to treat dendritic keratitis, vaccinia, varicella, fungal or mycobacterial eye infections, after removal of a corneal foreign body. Lactation.
Precautions: Use with caution in premature infants and neonates. Ophthalmic ointment may retard corneal epithelial healing.

Route/Dosage
• **IM, IV**
Non-life-threatening serious infections.
Adults: 3 mg/kg/day in three equally divided doses q 8 hr.
Life-threatening infections.

Up to 5 mg/kg/day in three or four equal doses. **Pediatric:** Either 2–2.5 mg/kg q 8 hr or 1.5–1.9 mg/kg q 6 hr; **neonates 1 week of age or less:** up to 4 mg/kg/day in two equal doses q 12 hr.

Impaired renal function.

Initially: 1 mg/kg; **then,** maintenance dose calculated according to information supplied by manufacturer.

• **Ophthalmic Ointment (0.3%)**
Acute infections.
0.5-in. ribbon q 3–4 hr until improvement is noted.
Mild to moderate infections.
0.5-in. ribbon b.i.d.–t.i.d.

• **Ophthalmic Solution (0.3%)**
Acute infections.
Initial: 1–2 gtt q 15–30 min until improvement noted; **then,** reduce dosage gradually.
Moderate infections.
1–2 gtt 2–6 times/day.

• **Inhalation Solution**
Pseudomonas aeruginosa in cystic fibrosis.
Dose using a nebulizer b.i.d. for 10–15 min in cycles of 28 days on and then 28 days off. See package insert for detailed instructions for administration.

How Supplied: *Inhalation Solution:* 60 mg/mL; *Injection:* 10 mg/mL, 40 mg/mL; *Powder for injection:* 60 mg, 80 mg, 1.2 g; *Ophthalmic Ointment:* 0.3%; *Ophthalmic Solution:* 0.3%

Side Effects: Additional: *Ophthalmic use:* Transient irritation, burning, stinging, itching, inflammation, angioneurotic edema, urticaria, vensicular and maculopapular dermatitis.

OD Overdose Management: *Symptoms (Ophthalmic Use):* Edema, lid itching, punctate keratitis, erythema, lacrimation.

Drug Interactions: Additional: With carbenicillin or ticarcillin, tobramycin may have an increased effect when used for *Pseudomonas* infections.

EMS CONSIDERATIONS

None.

Tocainide hydrochloride
(toe-KAY-nyd)
Pregnancy Class: C
Tonocard **(Rx)**
Classification: Antiarrhythmic, class IB

Mechanism of Action: Similar to lidocaine. Decreases the excitability of cells in the myocardium by decreasing sodium and potassium conductance. Increases pulmonary and aortic arterial pressure and slightly increases peripheral resistance.

Uses: Life-threatening ventricular arrhythmias, including ventricular tachycardia. Has not been shown to improve survival in patients with ventricular arrhythmias. *Investigational:* Myotonic dystrophy, trigeminal neuralgia.

Contraindications: Allergy to amide-type local anesthetics, second- or third-degree AV block in the absence of artificial ventricular pacemaker. Lactation.

Precautions: Increased risk of death when used in those with non-life-threatening cardiac arrhythmias. Safety and efficacy have not been established in children. Use with caution in patients with impaired renal or hepatic function (dose may have to be decreased). Geriatric patients may have an increased risk of dizziness and hypotension; the dose may have to be reduced in these patients due to age-related impaired renal function.

Route/Dosage

• **Tablets**
Antiarrhythmic.
Adults, individualized, initial: 400 mg q 8 hr, up to a maximum of 2,400 mg/day; **maintenance:** 1,200–1,800 mg/day in divided doses. Total daily dose of 1,200 mg may be adequate in patients with liver or kidney disease.
Myotonic dystrophy.
800–1,200 mg/day.
Trigeminal neuralgia.
20 mg/kg/day in three divided doses.
How Supplied: *Tablet:* 400 mg, 600 mg

T

Side Effects: *CV: **Increased arrhythmias,*** increased ventricular rate (when given for atrial flutter or fibrillation), CHF, tachycardia, hypotension, **conduction disturbances,** bradycardia, chest pain, LV failure, palpitations. *CNS:* Dizziness, vertigo, headache, tremors, confusion, disorientation, hallucinations, ataxia, paresthesias, numbness, nervousness, altered mood, anxiety, incoordination, walking disturbances. *GI:* N&V, anorexia, diarrhea. *Respiratory:* **Pulmonary fibrosis, fibrosing alveolitis,** interstitial pneumonitis, **pulmonary edema,** pneumonia. *Hematologic:* Leukopenia, **agranulocytosis,** hypoplastic anemia, **aplastic anemia,** bone marrow depression, neutropenia, **thrombocytopenia and sequelae as septicemia and septic shock.** *Musculoskeletal:* Arthritis, arthralgia, myalgia. *Dermatologic:* Rash, skin lesion, diaphoresis. *Other:* Blurred vision, visual disturbances, nystagmus, tinnitus, hearing loss, lupus-like syndrome.

OD Overdose Management: *Symptoms:* Initially are CNS symptoms including tremor (see above). GI symptoms may follow (see above). *Treatment:* Gastric lavage and activated charcoal may be useful. In the event of respiratory depression or arrest or seizures, maintain airway and provide artificial ventilation. An IV anticonvulsant (e.g., diazepam, thiopental, thiamylal, pentobarbital, secobarbital) may be required if seizures are persistent.

Drug Interactions
Cimetidine / ↓ Bioavailability of tocainide
Metoprolol / Additive effects on wedge pressure and cardiac index
Rifampin / ↓ Bioavailability of tocainide

EMS CONSIDERATIONS

See also *Antiarrhythmic Agents.*

Tolazamide
(toll-AZ-ah-myd)
Pregnancy Class: C
Tolinase **(Rx)**
Classification: Sulfonylurea, first-generation

Mechanism of Action: Effective in some with a history of coma or ketoacidosis; may be effective in patients who do not respond well to other oral antidiabetics.
Onset of Action: 4-6 hr.
Duration of Action: 12-24 hr.
Contraindications: Additional: Renal glycosuria.

Route/Dosage
• **Tablets**
  Diabetes.
Adults, initial: 100 mg/day if fasting blood sugar is less than 200 mg/100 mL, or 250 mg/day if fasting blood sugar is greater than 200 mg/100 mL. Adjust dose to response, not to exceed 1 g/day. If more than 500 mg/day is required, give in two divided doses, usually before the morning and evening meals.   **Elderly,   malnourished, underweight patients or those not eating properly:** 100 mg once daily with breakfast, adjusting dose by increments of 50 mg/day each week. Doses greater than 1 g/day will probably not improve control.
How Supplied: *Tablet:* 100 mg, 250 mg, 500 mg
Drug Interactions: Additional: Concomitant use of alcohol and tolazamide may → photosensitivity.

EMS CONSIDERATIONS

See also *Antidiabetic Agents, Hypoglycemic Agents.*

Tolbutamide
Tolbutamide sodium
(toll-BYOU-tah-myd)
Pregnancy Class: C
Tolbutamide: Orinase **(Rx)** Tolbutamide sodium: Orinase Diagnostic **(Rx)**
Classification: Sulfonylurea, first-generation

Onset of Action: 1 hr.
Duration of Action: 6-12 hr.
Uses: Additional: Most useful for patients with poor general physical status who should receive a short-acting compound. Tolbutamide sodium is used to diagnose pancreatic islet cell tumors. It causes blood glu-

cose, in the presence of a tumor, to drop quickly after IV administration and remain low for 3 hr.

Route/Dosage
• **Tablets**
Diabetes mellitus.
Adults, initial: 1–2 g/day. Adjust dosage depending on response, up to 3 g/day. **Usual maintenance:** 0.25–3 g/day). A daily dose greater than 2 g is seldom required.
How Supplied: Tolbutamide: *Tablet:* 500 mg; Tolbutamide sodium: *Powder for injection:* 1 g

Side Effects: Additional: Melena (dark, bloody stools) in some patients with a history of peptic ulcer. Relapse or secondary failure may occur a few months after therapy has been started. May cause hyponatremia and a mild goiter.

Drug Interactions: Additional: *Alcohol* / Photosensitivity reactions. *Sulfinpyrazone* / ↑ Effect of tolbutamide due to ↓ breakdown by liver.

EMS CONSIDERATIONS
See also *Antidiabetic Agents, Oral.*

Tolcapone
(TOHL-kah-pohn)
Pregnancy Class: C
Tasmar **(Rx)**
Classification: Antiparkinson drug

Mechanism of Action: Reversible inhibitor of catechol-O-methyltransferase (COMT), resulting in an increase in plasma levodopa. When given with levodopa/carbidopa, plasma levels of levodopa are more sustained, allowing for more constant dopaminergic stimulation of the brain. May also increase side effects of levodopa.
Uses: Adjunct to levodopa and carbidopa for the treatment of idiopathic Parkinson's disease.
Contraindications: Use with a nonselective MAO inhibitor.
Precautions: Use with caution in severe renal or hepatic impairment and during lactation.

Route/Dosage
• **Tablets**
Adjunct for Parkinsonism.
Initial: 100 or 200 mg t.i.d. with or without food, up to a maximum of 600 mg/day. Do not increase the dose to 200 mg t.i.d. in those with moderate to severe liver cirrhosis.
How Supplied: *Tablets:* 100 mg, 200 mg
Side Effects: *GI:* N&V, anorexia, diarrhea, constipation, xerostomia, abdominal pain, dyspepsia, flatulence. *CNS:* Hallucinations, dyskinesias, sleep disorder, dystonia, excessive dreaming, somnolence, confusion, dizziness, headache, syncope, loss of balance, hyperkinesia, paresthesia, hypokinesia, agitation, irritability, mental deficiency, hyperactivity, panic reaction, euphoria, hypertonia. *CV:* Orthostatic hypotension, chest pain, hypotension, chest discomfort. *Respiratory:* URTI, dyspnea, sinus congestion. *Musculoskeletal:* Muscle cramps, stiffness, arthritis, neck pain. *GU:* Hematuria, UTIs, urine discoloration, micturition disorder, uterine tumor. *Dermatologic:* Increased sweating, dermal bleeding, skin tumor, alopecia. *Ophthalmic:* Cataract, eye inflammation. *Body as a whole:* Falling, fatigue, influenza, burning, malaise, fever.

Note: Patients over 75 years of age may develop more hallucinations but less dystonia. Females may develop somnolence more frequently than males.

OD **Overdose Management:** *Symptoms:* Nausea, vomiting, dizziness, possibility of respiratory difficulties. *Treatment:* Hospitalization is advised. Give supportive care.

EMS CONSIDERATIONS
None.

Tolmetin sodium
(TOLL-met-in)
Pregnancy Class: C
Tolectin 200, Tolectin 600, Tolectin DS **(Rx)**

Classification: Nonsteroidal, anti-inflammatory, analgesic

Onset of Action: Anti-Inflammatory effect: within 1 week.
Duration of Action: Anti-Inflammatory effect: 1-2 weeks.
Uses: Acute and chronic treatment of rheumatoid arthritis and osteoarthritis. Juvenile rheumatoid arthritis. *Investigational:* Sunburn.
Precautions: Use with caution during lactation. Dosage has not been determined in children less than 2 years of age.

Route/Dosage —————————
• **Capsules, Tablets**
Rheumatoid arthritis, osteoarthritis.
Adults: 400 mg t.i.d. (one dose on arising and one at bedtime); adjust dosage according to patient response. **Maintenance:** rheumatoid arthritis, 600–1,800 mg/day in three to four divided doses; osteoarthritis, 600–1,600 mg/day in three to four divided doses. Doses larger than 1,800 mg/day for rheumatoid arthritis and osteoarthritis are not recommended.
Juvenile rheumatoid arthritis.
2 years and older, initial: 20 mg/kg/day in three to four divided doses to start; **then,** 15–30 mg/kg/day. Doses higher than 30 mg/kg/day are not recommended. Beneficial effects may not be observed for several days to a week.
How Supplied: *Capsule:* 400 mg; *Tablet:* 200 mg, 600 mg

EMS CONSIDERATIONS

See also *Nonsteroidal Anti-Inflammatory Drugs.*

Tolnaftate
(toll-NAF-tayt)
Absorbine Footcare, Aftate for Athlete's Foot, Aftat for Jock Itch, Genaspor, NP-27, Quinsana Plus, Tinactin, Tinactin for Jock Itch, Ting, Zeasorb-AF **(OTC)**
Classification: Topical antifungal

Mechanism of Action: Exact mechanism not known; is thought to stunt mycelial growth causing a fungicidal effect.
Uses: Tinea pedis, tinea cruris, tinea corporis, and tinea versicolor. Fungal infections of moist skin areas.
Contraindications: Scalp and nail infections. Avoid getting into eyes. Use in children less than 2 years of age.

Route/Dosage —————————
• **Topical: Aerosol Powder, Aerosol Solution, Cream, Ointment, Powder, Solution, Spray Solution**
Apply b.i.d. for 2–3 weeks although treatment for 4–6 weeks may be necessary in some instances.
How Supplied: *Cream:* 1%; *Ointment:* 1%; *Powder:* 1%; *Solution:* 1%; *Spray:* 1%
Side Effects: Mild skin irritation.

EMS CONSIDERATIONS

See also *Anti-Infectives.*

Tolterodine tartrate
(tohl-TER-oh-deen)
Pregnancy Class: C
Detrol **(Rx)**
Classification: Urinary tract drug

Mechanism of Action: Acts as a competitive muscarinic receptor antagonist in the bladder to cause increased bladder control.
Uses: Treat overactive bladder with symptoms of urinary frequency, urgency, or urge incontinence.
Contraindications: Urinary retention, gastric retention, uncontrolled narrow–angle glaucoma, lactation.
Precautions: Use with caution in renal impairment, in bladder outflow obstruction, in GI obstructive disorders (e.g., pyloric stenosis), and in those being treated for narrow–angle glaucoma. Doses greater than 1 mg b.i.d. not to be given to those with significantly decreased hepatic function. Safety and efficacy have not been determined in children.

Route/Dosage —————————
• **Tablets**
Treat overactive bladder.

Initial: 2 mg b.i.d. Dose may be lowered to 1 mg b.i.d. based on individual response and side effects. Adjust dose to 1 mg b.i.d. in those with significantly reduced hepatic funtion or who are currently taking drugs that are inhibitors of cytochrome P450 3A4 (see *Drug Interactions*).

How Supplied: *Tablets:* 1 mg, 2 mg

Side Effects: *GI:* Dry mouth (common), dyspepsia, constipation, abdominal pain, N&V, diarrhea, flatulence. *CNS:* Headache, vertigo, dizziness, somnolence, paresthesia, nervousness. *Respiratory:* URI, bronchitis, coughing, pharyngitis, rhinitis, sinusitis. *Dermatologic:* Rash, erythema, dry skin, pruritus. *GU:* UTI, dysuria, micturition frequency, urinary retention. *Ophthalmic:* Abnormalities with vision, including accommodation. *Musculoskeletal:* Arthralgia, back pain, chest pain. *Miscellaneous:* Fatigue, flu–like symptoms, infection, hypertension, weight gain, fall, fungal infection.

OD Overdose Management: *Symptoms:* Significant anticholinergic symptoms. *Treatment:* Symptomatic. Monitor ECG.

Drug Interactions

Clarithromycin / ↑ Plasma levels of tolterodine due to ↓ break down by liver; do not give doses of tolterodine >1 mg b.i.d.

Erythromycin / ↑ Plasma levels of tolterodine due to ↓ break down by liver; do not give doses of tolterodine >1 mg b.i.d.

Itraconazole / ↑ Plasma levels of tolterodine due to ↓ break down by liver; do not give doses of tolterodine >1 mg b.i.d.

Ketoconazole / ↑ Plasma levels of tolterodine due to ↓ break down by liver; do not give doses of tolterodine >1 mg b.i.d.

Miconazole / ↑ Plasma levels of tolterodine due to ↓ break down by liver; do not give doses of tolterodine >1 mg b.i.d.

EMS CONSIDERATIONS

None.

Topiramate
(toh-PYRE-ah-mayt)
Pregnancy Class: C
Topamax **(Rx)**
Classification: Anticonvulsant, miscellaneous

Mechanism of Action: Precise mechanism not known. The following effects may contribute to the anticonvulsant activity. (1) Action potentials seen repetitively by sustained depolarization of neurons are blocked in a time-dependent manner, suggesting an effect to block sodium channels. (2) Increases the frequency at which GABA activates $GABA_A$ receptors, thus enhancing the ability of GABA to cause a flux of chloride ions into neurons (i.e., enhanced effect of the inhibitory transmitter, $GABA_A$). (3) Antagonizes the ability of kainate to activate the kainate/AMPA subtype of excitatory amino acid aspartate, thus reducing the excitatory effect.

Uses: Adjunct to treat partial onset seizures in adults.

Contraindications: Lactation.

Precautions: Use with caution in impaired hepatic and renal function. Safety and efficacy have not been determined in children.

Route/Dosage
• **Tablets**
   Adjunctive therapy for treatment of partial onset seizures.

Initial: 50 mg/day; **then,** titrate to an effective dose of 400 mg/day in 2 divided doses. Titrate by adding 50 mg each week for eight weeks, until the dose is 400 mg/day. Doses greater than 400 mg/day have not been shown to improve the response. If $C_{CR} < 70$ mL/1.73 m², use one half of the usual adult dose.

How Supplied: *Tablets:* 25 mg, 100 mg, 200 mg.

Side Effects: *Note:* Side effects with an incidence of 0.1% or greater are listed. *CNS:* Psychomotor slowing, including difficulty with concentration and speech or language problems. Somnolence, fatigue, dizziness, atax-

T

ia, nystagmus, paresthesia, nervousness, difficulty with memory, tremor, confusion, depression, abnormal coordination, agitation, mood problems, aggressive reaction, hypoesthesia, apathy, emotional lability, depersonalization, hypokinesia, vertIgo, stupor, *clonic/tonic seizures,* hyperkinesia, hypertonia, insomnia, personality disorder, impotence, hallucinations, euphoria, psychosis, decreased libido, *suicide attempt,* hyporeflexia, neuropathy, migraine, apraxia, hyperesthesia, dyskinesia, hyperreflexia, dysphonia, scotoma, dystonia, coma, encephalopathy, upper motor neuron lesion, paranoid reaction, delusion, paranoia, delirium, abnormal dreaming, neuroses. *GI:* Nausea, dyspepsia, anorexia, abdominal pain, constipation, dry mouth, gingivitis, halitosis, diarrhea, vomiting, fecal incontinence, flatulence, gastroenteritis, gum hyperplasia, hemorrhoids, increased appetite, tooth caries, stomatitis, dysphagia, melena, gastritis, increased saliva, hiccough, gastroesophageal reflux, tongue edema, esophagitis, gall bladder disorder, gingival bleeding. *CV:* Palpitation, hypertension, hypotension, postural hypotension, AV block, bradycardia, bundle branch block, angina pectoris, vasodilation. *Body as a whole:* Asthenia, back pain, chest pain, flu-like symptoms, leg pain, hot flashes, body odor, edema, rigors, fever, malaise, syncope, enlarged abdomen. *Respiratory:* URI, pharyngitis, sinusitis, dyspnea, coughing, bronchitis, asthma, ***bronchospasm, pulmonary embolism.*** *Dermatologic:* Acne, alopecia, dermatitis, nail disorder, folliculitis, dry skin, urticaria, skin discoloration, eczema, photosensitivity reaction, erythematous rash, seborrhea, decreased sweating, abnormal hair texture, facial edema. *GU:* Breast pain, renal stone formation, dysmenorrhea, menstrual disorder, hematuria, intermenstrual bleeding, leukorrhea, menorrhagia, vaginitis, amenorrhea, UTI, micturition frequency, urinary incontinence, dysuria, renal calculus, ejaculation disorder, breast discharge, urinary retention, renal pain, nocturia, albuminuria, polyuria, oliguria. *Musculoskeletal:* Arthralgia, muscle weakness, arthrosis, osteoporosis, myalgia, leg cramps. *Metabolic:* Increased weight, decreased weight, dehydration, xeropthalmia. *Hematologic:* Anemia, leukopenia, lymphadenopathy, eosinophilia, lymphopenia, granulocytopenia, lymphocytosis, thrombocytothemia, purpura, thrombocytopenia. *Dermatologic:* Rash, pruritus, increased sweating, flushing. *Ophthalmic:* Diplopia, abnormal vision, eye pain, conjunctivitis, abnormal accommodation, photophobia, abnormal lacrimation, strabismus, color blindness, myopia, mydriasis, ptosis, visual field defect. *Miscellaneous:* Decreased hearing, epistaxis, taste perversion, tinnitus, taste loss, parosmia, goiter, basal cell carcinoma.

OD **Overdose Management:** *Symptoms:* See side effects. *Treatment:* Gastric lavage or induction of emesis if ingestion is recent. Supportive treatment. Hemodialysis.

Drug Interactions

Alcohol / CNS depression and cognitive and neuropsychiatric side effects

Carbamazepine / ↓ Plasma levels of topiramate

Carbonic anhydrase inhibitors / ↑ Risk of renal stone formation

CNS depressants / CNS depression and cognitive and neuropsychiatric side effects

Oral contraceptives / ↓ Effect of oral contraceptives

Phenytoin / ↓ Plasma levels of topiramate and ↑ plasma levels of phenytoin

Valproic acid / ↓ Plasma levels of both topiramate and valproic acid

EMS CONSIDERATIONS

See also *Anticonvulsant Drugs.*

Toremifene citrate (Fareston)

TOR-em-ih-feen

Pregnancy Class: D

Fareston **(Rx)**
Classification: Antineoplastic, hormone

Mechanism of Action: Antiestrogen that binds to estrogen receptors and may cause estrogenic, antiestrogenic, or both effects, depending on duration of treatment, genders, and endpoint/target organ selected. Antitumor effect is likely due to antiestrogenic effect, i.e., competes for estrogen at receptor and blocks growth-stimulating effects of estrogen in tumor. Well absorbed from GI tract. **Peak plasma levels:** 3 hr. t½, **distribution:** About 4 hr. t½, **elimination:** About 5 days. Extensively metabolized in liver and mainly excreted in feces.

Uses: Metastatic breast cancer in postmenopausal women with positive estrogen-receptor (ER) or ER unknown tumors.

Contraindications: Use with history of thromboembolic disease or in pediatric patients.

Route/Dosage
• **Tablets**
   Metastatic breast cancer.
Adults: 60 mg once daily. Continue until disease progression is observed.
How Supplied: *Tablets:* 60 mg
Side Effects: *CV: **Cardiac failure, MI, pulmonary embolism, CVA,** TIA. GI:* Constipation, nausea. *Hematologic:* Leukopenia, thrombocytopenia. *Dermatologic:* Skin discoloration, dermatitis, alopecia, pruritus. *Ophthalmic:* Cataracts, dry eyes, abnormal visual fields, corneal keratopathy, glaucoma, reversible corneal opacity. *CNS:* Tremor, vertigo, depression. *Miscellaneous:* Dyspnea, paresis, anorexia, asthenia, jaundice, rigors, vaginal bleeding.
Drug Interactions
Carbamazepine / ↓ Blood levels of toremifene due to ↑ breakdown in liver
Clonazepam / ↓ Blood levels of toremifene due to ↑ breakdown in liver

Erythromycin / Inhibition of breakdown of toremifene
Ketoconazole / Inhibition of breakdown of toremifene
Macrolide antibiotics / Inhibition of breakdown of toremifene
Phenobarbital / ↓ Blood levels of toremifene due to ↑ breakdown in liver
Phenytoin / ↓ Blood levels of toremifene due to ↑ breakdown in liver
Warfarin / ↑ PT

EMS CONSIDERATIONS
See also *Nursing Considerations* for *Antineoplastic Agents.*
Assessment
1. Document indications for therapy, characteristics of symptoms, other agents trialed and outcome.
2. Note any history or evidence of thromboembolic disorders.
3. Monitor CBC, calcium, and LFTs.

Torsemide
(TOR-seh-myd)
Pregnancy Class: B
Demadex **(Rx)**
Classification: Loop diuretic

Onset of Action: IV: Within 10 min; **PO:** within 60 min.
Duration of Action: 6-8 hr.
Uses: Congestive heart failure, acute or chronic renal failure, hepatic cirrhosis, hypertension.
Contraindications: Lactation.
Precautions: Patients sensitive to sulfonamides may show allergic reactions to torsemide. Safety and efficacy in children have not been determined.

Route/Dosage
• **Tablets, IV**
   Congestive heart failure.
Adults, initial: 10 or 20 mg once daily.
   Chronic renal failure.
Adults, initial: 20 mg once daily.
   Hepatic cirrhosis.

Adults, initial: 5 or 10 mg once daily given with an aldosterone antagonist or a potassium-sparing diuretic.

Hypertension.

Adults, initial: 5 mg once daily. If this dose does not lead to an adequate decrease in BP within 4–6 weeks, the dose may be increased to 10 mg once daily. If the 10-mg dose is not adequate, an additional antihypertensive agent is added to the treatment regimen.

How Supplied: *Injection:* 10 mg /mL; *Tablet:* 5 mg, 10 mg, 20 mg, 100 mg

Side Effects: *CNS:* Headache, dizziness, asthenia, insomnia, nervousness, syncope. *GI:* Diarrhea, constipation, nausea, dyspepsia, edema, *GI hemorrhage,* rectal bleeding. *CV:* ECG abnormality, chest pain, atrial fibrillation, hypotension, *ventricular tachycardia,* shunt thrombosis. *Respiratory:* Rhinitis, increase in cough. *Musculoskeletal:* Arthralgia, myalgia. *Miscellaneous:* Sore throat, excessive urination, rash.

EMS CONSIDERATIONS

See also *Diuretics, Loop.*

Tramadol hydrochloride
(TRAM-ah-dol)
Pregnancy Class: C
Ultram **(Rx)**
Classification: Analgesic, centrally acting

Mechanism of Action: A centrally acting analgesic not related chemically to opiates. Precise mechanism is not known. It may bind to mu-opioid receptors and inhibit reuptake of norepinephrine and serotonin. The analgesic effect is only partially antagonized by the antagonist naloxone. Causes significantly less respiratory depression than morphine. In contrast to morphine, tramadol does not cause release of histamine. Produces dependence of the mu-opioid type (i.e., like codeine or dextropropoxyphene); however, there is little evidence of abuse. Tolerance occurs but is relatively mild; the withdrawal syndrome is not as severe with other opiates.

Onset of Action: 1 hr. **Peak effect:** 2-3 hr.

Uses: Management of moderate to moderately severe pain.

Contraindications: Hypersensitivity to tramadol. In acute intoxication with alcohol, hypnotics, centrally acting analgesics, opiates, or psychotropic drugs. Use in patients with past or present addiction or opiate dependence or in those with a prior history of allergy to codeine or opiates. Use for obstetric preoperative medication or for postdelivery analgesia in nursing mothers. Use in children less than 16 years of age, as safety and efficacy have not been determined.

Precautions: Use with great caution in those taking MAO inhibitors, as tramadol inhibits norepinephrine and serotonin uptake. Dosage reduction is recommended with impaired hepatic or renal function and in patients over 75 years of age. Use with caution in increased intracranial pressure or head injury, in epilepsy, or in patients with an increased risk for seizures, including head trauma, metabolic disorders, alcohol or drug withdrawal, and CNS infections. Tramadol may complicate the assessment of acute abdominal conditions.

Route/Dosage
• **Tablets**
  Management of pain.

Adults: 50–100 mg q 4–6 hr, as needed, but not to exceed 400 mg/day. For moderate pain, 50 mg, initially, may be adequate, and for severe pain, 100 mg, initially, is often more effective. For patients over 75 years of age, the recommended dose is no more than 300 mg/day in divided doses. In impaired renal function with a C_{CR} less than 30 mL/min, the dosing interval should be increased to 12 hr, with a maximum daily dose of 200 mg. The recommended dose for patients with cirrhosis is 50 mg q 12 hr.

How Supplied: *Tablet:* 50 mg

Side Effects: *CNS:* Dizziness, vertigo, headache, somnolence, CNS stimulation, anxiety, confusion, incoordination, euphoria, nervousness, sleep disorders, *seizures,* paresthesia, cognitive dysfunction, hallucinations, tremor, amnesia, concentration difficulty, abnormal gait, migraine, development of drug dependence. *GI:* Nausea, constipation, vomiting, dyspepsia, dry mouth, diarrhea, abdominal pain, anorexia, flatulence, GI bleeding, hepatitis, stomatitis, dysgeusia. *CV:* Vasodilation, syncope, orthostatic hypotension, tachycardia, abnormal ECG, hypertension, myocardial ischemia, palpitations. *Dermatologic:* Pruritus, sweating, rash, urticaria, vesicles. *Body as a whole:* Asthenia, malaise, allergic reaction, accidental injury, weight loss, *suicidal tendency.* *GU:* Urinary retention, urinary frequency, menopausal symptoms, dysuria, menstrual disorder. *Miscellaneous:* *Anaphylaxis,* visual disturbances, cataracts, deafness, tinnitus, hypertonia, dyspnea.

OD Overdose Management: *Symptoms:* Extension of side effects, especially *respiratory depression and seizures.* *Treatment:* Naloxone will reverse some, but not all, of the symptoms of overdose. General supportive treatment, with special attention to maintenance of adequate respiration. Diazepam or barbiturates may help if seizures occur. Hemodialysis is not helpful.

Drug Interactions
Alcohol / Enhanced respiratory depression
Anesthetics, general / Enhanced respiratory depression
Carbamazepine / ↓ Effect of tramadol due to ↑ metabolism induced by carbamazepine
CNS depressants / Additive CNS depression
MAO Inhibitors / Tramadol may ↑ the risk of seizures in those taking MAO inhibitors
Naloxone / Use of naloxone for tramadol overdose may ↑ risk of seizures.

Quinidine / Quinidine inhibits the isoenzyme that metabolizes tramadol → ↑ levels of tramadol and ↓ levels of M1

EMS CONSIDERATIONS

See also *Narcotic Analgesics.*

Trandolapril
(tran-DOHL-ah-pril)
Pregnancy Class: C (first trimester); D (second and third trimesters)
Mavik **(Rx)**
Classification: Antihypertensive

Onset of Action: 2-4 hr; **Peak effect:** 4-10 hr.
Duration of Action: 24 hr.
Uses: Hypertension, alone or in combination with other antihypertensives such as hydrochlorothiazide. To treat heart failure after MI or ventricular dysfunction after MI.
Contraindications: In those with history of angioedema with ACE inhibitors.
Precautions: Safety and efficacy have not been determined in children.

Route/Dosage
• **Tablets**
Hypertension.
Initial: 1 mg once daily in nonblack patients and 2 mg once daily in black patients. Adjust dosage according to response; usually, adjustments are made at intervals of 1 week. **Maintenance, usual:** 2–4 mg once daily. Those inadequately treated with once-daily dosing can be treated with twice-daily dosing. If BP is still not adequately controlled, diuretic may be added. If C_{CR} is less than 30 mL/min or if there is hepatic cirrhosis, initial dose is 0.5 mg daily.
Heart failure post–MI/Left ventricular dysfunction post–MI.
Initial: 1 mg/day. Then, increase the dose, as tolerated, to a target dose of 4 mg/day. If 4 mg is not tolerated, continue with the highest tolerated dose.

T

---

bold italic = life threatening side effect

How Supplied: *Tablet:* 1 mg, 2 mg, 4 mg.

Side Effects: See also *ACE Inhibitors. Hypersensitivity:* **Angioedema.** *CNS:* Dizziness, headache, fatigue, insomnia, paresthesias, drowsiness, vertigo, anxiety. *GI:* Diarrhea, dyspepsia, gastritis, abdominal pain, vomiting, constipation, pancreatitis. *CV:* Hypotension, bradycardia, chest pain, **cardiogenic shock** , intermittent claudication, stroke. *Respiratory:* Cough, dyspnea, URTI, epistaxis, throat inflammation. *Hepatic:* **Hepatic failure,** including cholestatic jaundice, **fulminant hepatic necrosis, death.** *Dermatologic:* Photosensitivity, pruritus, rash. *GU:* UTI, impotence, decreased libido. *Miscellaneous:* Neutropenia, syncope, myalgia, asthenia, muscle cramps, hypocalemia, intermittent claudication, edema, extremity pain, gout.

Drug Interactions

Diuretics / Excessive hypotensive effects

Diuretics, potassium-sparing: ↑ Risk of hyperkalemia

Lithium / ↑ Risk of lithium toxicity

EMS CONSIDERATIONS

None.

Tranylcypromine sulfate
(tran-ill-SIP-roh-meen)

Pregnancy Class: C

Parnate **(Rx)**

Classification: Antidepressant, monoamine oxidase inhibitor

Mechanism of Action: A MAO inhibitor with a rapid onset of activity. Due to inhibition of MAO, the concentration of epinephrine, norepinephrine, and serotonin increases in storage sites throughout the nervous system. This increase has been alleged to be the basis for the antidepressant effects. No orthostatic hypotensive effect; slight anticholinergic and sedative effects.

Uses: Treatment of major depressive episode without melancholia. Not a first line of therapy; is used when patients have failed to respond to other drug therapy. *Investigational:* Alone or as an adjunct to treat bulimia, obsessive compulsive disorder, and manifestations of psychotic disorders. Also, treatment of social phobia, seasonal affective disorders, adjunct to treat multiple sclerosis, and to treat idiopathic orthostatic hypotension (e.g., Shy-Drager syndrome) refractory to conventional therapy.

Contraindications: Use in those with a confirmed or suspected CV defect or in anyone with CV disease, hypertension, or history of headache. In the presence of pheochromocytoma. History of liver disease or in those with abnormal liver function. Use in combination with a large number of other drugs, especially other MAO inhibitors, tricyclic antidepressants, serotonin-reuptake inhibitors, buspirone, sympathomimetics, meperidine, CNS depressants (e.g., alcohol and narcotics), hypotensive drugs, excessive caffeine, and dextromethorphan (see *Drug Interactions*). Use with tyramine-containing foods (see *Drug Interactions*).

Precautions: Assess benefits versus risks before using during pregnancy and lactation. Use with caution in patients taking antiparkinson drugs, in impaired renal function, in those with seizure disorders, in diabetics, in hyperthyroid patients, and in those taking disulfiram. Geriatric patients may be more sensitive to the drug.

Route/Dosage

• **Tablets**

Major depressive syndrome without melancholia.

Individualize the dose. **Usual effective dose:** 30 mg/day given in divided doses. If there are no signs of improvement in 2 weeks, the dose can be increased by 10 mg/day at intervals of 1 to 3 weeks, up to a maximum of 60 mg/day.

How Supplied: *Tablets:* 10 mg.

Side Effects: *CNS:* Anxiety, agitation, headaches (without elevation of BP), manic symptoms, restlessness, insomnia, weakness, drowsiness, dizziness, significant anorexia. *GI:* Dry mouth, nausea, diarrhea, abdominal pain, constipation. *CV:* Tachycardia, edema, palpitation. *GU:* Impotence, urinary retention, impaired ejaculation. *Musculoskeletal:* Muscle spasm, tremors, myoclonic jerks, numbness, paresthesia. *Hematologic:* Anemia, leukopenia, agranulocytosis, thrombocytopenia. *Miscellaneous:* Blurred vision, chills, impotence, hepatitis, skin rash, impaired water excretion, tinnitus.

OD **Overdose Management:** *Symptoms:* Insomnia, restlessness, anxiety, agitation, mental confusion, incoherence, hypotension, dizziness, weakness, drowsiness, shock, hypertension with severe headache. Rarely, hypertension accompanied by twitching or myoclonic fibrillation of skeletal muscles with **hyperprexia, generalized rigidity, and coma.** The toxic effects may be delayed or prolonged following the last dose of the drug; thus, observe closely for at least a week. *Treatment:* Gastric lavage, if performed early. General supportive measures. Treat hypertensive crisis using phentolamine 5 mg IV. External cooling to treat hyperprexia. Standard measures to treat circulatory shock. Myoclonic effects may be relieved by using barbiturates; however, tranylcypromine may prolong the effects of barbiturates.

Drug Interactions
Alcohol / Possibility of excitation, seizures, delirium, hyperpyrexia, circulatory collapse, coma, death
Anesthetics, general / Hypotensive effect; use together with caution. Phenelzine should be discontinued at least 10 days before elective surgery
Anticholinergic drugs, atropine / MAO inhibitors effect of anticholinergic drugs
Antidepressants, tricyclic / Comcomitant use may result in excitation, sweating, tachycardia, tachypnea, hyperpyrexia, disseminated intravascular coagulation, delirium, tremors, convulsions, death. At least 7-10 days should elapse between discontinuing a MAO inhibitor and initiating a new drug. However,

such combinations have been used together successfully
Antihypertensive drugs / Exaggerated hypotensive effects
Beta-adrenergic blocking drugs / Exaggerated hypotensive effects
Buspirone / Elevated BP
Dextromethorphan / Brief episodes of psychosis or bizarre behavior
Fluoxetine / Possibility of hyperthermia, rigidity, myoclonic movements, death. At least 10 days should elapse between discontinuation of phenelzine and initiation of fluoxetine; and, at least 5 weeks should elapse between discontinuing fluoxetine and beginning phenelzine
MAO Inhibitors / Concomitant use of tranylcypromine with other MAO inhibitors may cause a hypertensive crisis or severe seizures
Meperidine / See *Narcotics*
Narcotics / Possibility of excitation, seizures, delirium, hyperpyrexia, circulatory collapse, coma, death
Selective serotonin reuptake inhibitors /See *Fluoxetine*
Sympathomimetic drugs—amphetamine, cocaine, dopa, ephedrine, epinephrine, metaraminol, methyldopa, methylphenidate, norepinephrine, phenylephrine, phenylpropanolamine. Many OTC cold products, hay fever medications, and nasal decongestants contain one or more of these drugs / All peripheral, metabolic, cardiac, and central effects are potentiated for up to 2 weeks after termination of MAO inhibitor therapy. Symptoms include acute hypertensive crisis with possible intracranial hemorrhage, hyperthermia, coma, and possibly death
Thiazide diuretics / Exaggerated hypotensive effects
Tryptophan / Possibility of behavioral and neurologic effects, including disorientation, confusion, amnesia, delirium, agitation, hypomania, ataxia, myoclonus, hyperreflexia, shivering, ocular oscillation,and Babinski signs

T

Tyramine-rich foods—beer, broad beans, certain cheeses (Brie, cheddar, Camembert, Stilton), Chianti wine, chicken livers, caffeine, cola beverages, figs, licorice, liver, pickled or kippered herring, dry sausage (Genoa salami, hard salami, pepperoni, Lebanon bologna), tea, cream, yogurt, yeast extract, and chocolate / Possible precipitation of hypertensive crisis, including severe headache, hyperension, intracranial hemorrhage, death

EMS CONSIDERATIONS

None.

Trazodone hydrochloride
(TRAYZ-oh-dohn)
Pregnancy Class: C
Desyrel, Desyrel Dividose, Trialodine
(Rx)
Classification: Antidepressant, miscellaneous

Mechanism of Action: A novel antidepressant that does not inhibit MAO and is also devoid of amphetamine-like effects. Response usually occurs after 2 weeks (75% of patients), with the remainder responding after 2–4 weeks. May inhibit serotonin uptake by brain cells, therefore increasing serotonin concentrations in the synapse. May also cause changes in binding of serotonin to receptors. Causes moderate sedative and orthostatic hypotensive effects and slight anticholinergic effects.

Uses: Depression with or without accompanying anxiety. *Investigational:* In combination with tryptophan for treating aggressive behavior. Panic disorder or agoraphobia with panic attacks. Treatment of cocaine withdrawal. Chronic pain including diabetic neuropathy.

Contraindications: During the initial recovery period following MI. Concurrently with electroshock therapy.

Precautions: Use with caution during lactation. Safety and efficacy in children less than 18 years of age have not been established. Geriatric patients are more prone to the sedative and hypotensive effects.

Route/Dosage
• **Tablets**
Antidepressant.
Adults and adolescents, initial: 150 mg/day; **then,** increase by 50 mg/day every 3–4 days to maximum of 400 mg/day in divided doses (outpatients). Inpatients may require up to, but not exceeding, 600 mg/day in divided doses. **Maintenance:** Use lowest effective dose. **Geriatric patients:** 75 mg/day in divided doses; dose can then be increased, as needed and tolerated, at 3- to 4-day intervals.
Treat aggressive behavior.
Trazodone, 50 mg b.i.d., with tryptophan, 500 mg b.i.d. Dosage adjustments may be required to reach a therapeutic response or if side effects develop.
Panic disorder or agoraphobia with panic attacks.
300 mg/day.
How Supplied: *Tablet:* 50 mg, 100 mg, 150 mg, 300 mg

Side Effects: *General:* Dermatitis, edema, blurred vision, constipation, dry mouth, nasal congestion, skeletal muscle aches and pains. *CV:* Hypertension or hypotension, syncope, palpitations, tachycardia, SOB, chest pain. *GI:* Diarrhea, N&V, bad taste in mouth, flatulence. *GU:* Delayed urine flow, priapism, hematuria, increased urinary frequency. *CNS:* Nightmares, confusion, anger, excitement, decreased ability to concentrate, dizziness, disorientation, drowsiness, lightheadedness, fatigue, insomnia, nervousness, impaired memory. Rarely, hallucinations, impaired speech, hypomania. *Other:* Incoordination, tremors, paresthesias, decreased libido, appetite disturbances, red eyes, sweating or clamminess, tinnitus, weight gain or loss, anemia, hypersalivation. Rarely, akathisia, muscle twitching, increased libido, impotence, retrograde ejaculation, early menses, missed periods.

OD Overdose Management: *Symptoms:* ***Respiratory arrest, seizures,*** ECG changes, hypotension, priapism as well as an increase in the incidence and severity of side effects noted above (vomiting and drowsiness are the most common). *Treatment:* Treat symptoms (especially hypotension and sedation). Gastric lavage and forced diuresis to remove the drug from the body.

Drug Interactions

Alcohol / ↑ Depressant effects of alcohol

Antihypertensives / Additive hypotension

Barbiturates / ↑ Depressant effects of barbiturates

Clonidine / Trazodone ↓ effect of clonidine

CNS depressants / ↑ CNS depression

Digoxin / Trazodone may ↑ serum digoxin levels

MAO inhibitors / Initiate therapy cautiously if trazodone is to be used together with MAO inhibitors

Phenytoin / Trazodone may ↑ serum phenytoin levels

EMS CONSIDERATIONS

None.

Tretinoin (Retinoic acid, Vitamin A acid)

(TRET-ih-noyn)

Pregnancy Class: C (Topical products), D (Oral products)

Avita, Renova, Retin-A, Retin-A Micro, Vesanoid **(Rx)**

Classification: Antiacne drug

Mechanism of Action: Topical tretinoin is believed to decrease microcomedone formation by decreasing the cohesiveness of follicular epithelial cells. Also believed to increase mitotic activity and increase turnover of follicular epithelial cells as well as decrease keratin synthesis.

The mechanism of action for PO use in acute promyelocytic leukemia (APL) is not known.

Uses: Dermatologic: A*vita, Retin-A:* Acne vulgaris. *Retin-A* and *Renova:* As an adjunct to comprehensive skin care and sun avoidance to treat fine wrinkles, mottled hyperpigmentation, and roughness of facial skin caused by age and the sun. For those individuals who do not achieve palliation using comprehensive skin care and sun avoidance programs alone. *Investigational (Retin-A):* Treat various forms of skin cancer. Dermatologic conditions including lamellar ichthyosis, mollusca contagiosa, verrucae plantaris, verrucae planae juveniles, ichthyosis vulgaris, bullous congenital ichthyosiform, and pityriasis rubra pilaris. To enhance the percutaneous absorption of topical minoxidil.

Oral: To induce remission in APL. After induction therapy with tretinoin, patients should be given a standard consolidation or maintenance chemotherapy regimen for APL, unless contraindicated.

Contraindications: Eczema, sunburn. Use if inherently sensitive to sunlight or if taking other drugs that increase sensitivity to sunlight. Use of Renova if patient is also taking drugs known to be photosensitizers (e.g., fluoroquinolones, phenothiazines, sulfonamides, tetracyclines, thiazides). Those allergic to parabens (preservative in the gelatin capsules). Use of PO form during lactation. Use around the eyes, mouth, angles of the nose, and mucous membranes.

Precautions: Use with caution during lactation. Safety and effectiveness have not been determined in children. Excessive sunlight and weather extremes (e.g., wind and cold) may be irritating. Use Avita and Renova with caution with concomitant topical medications, medicated or abrasive soaps, shampoos, cleansers, cosmetics with a strong drying effect, permanent wave solutions, electrolysis, hair depilatories or waxes, and products with high concentrations of alcohol, astringents, spices, or lime. Safety and efficacy of Renova have not

T

been determined in children less than 18 years of age, in individuals over the age of 50 years, or in individuals with moderately or heavily pigmented skin. Use of the PO form has resulted in retonic acid-APL syndrome, especially during the first month of treatment. The safety and efficacy of oral tretinoin at doses less than 45 mg/m²/day have not been evaluated in children.

Route/Dosage
- **Cream, Gel, or Liquid**
  Acne vulgaris.
Apply lightly over the affected areas once daily at bedtime. Beneficial effects many not be seen for 2–6 weeks.
- **Cream, 0.025%, 0.05%, 0.1%**
  Palliation for skin conditions.
Apply a pea-sized amount once daily at bedtime, using only enough to lightly cover the entire affected area. Up to 6 months of therapy may be needed before effects are seen.
- **Capsules**
  APL.
Adults: 45 mg/m²/day given as two evenly divided doses. Given until complete remission is obtained. Discontinue 30 days after achieving complete remission or after 90 days of treatment, whichever comes first.

How Supplied: *Cream:* 0.025%, 0.05%, 0.1%; *Gel:* 0.01%, 0.025%, 0.1%; *Liquid:* 0.05%; *Capsules:* 10 mg

Side Effects: Following topical use. *Dermatologic:* Red, edematous, crusted, or blistered skin; hyperpigmentation or hypopigmentation, increased susceptibility to sunlight, erythema, pruritus, burning, dryness. Excessive application will cause redness, peeling, or discomfort with no increase in results.

Following oral use. *Retinoic acid-APL syndrome:* Fever, dyspnea, weight gain, radiographic pulmonary infiltrate, pleural or pericardial effusions. Occasional impaired myocardial contractility and episodic hypotension; possibility of concomitant leukocytosis. *Progressive hypoxemia with possible fatal outcome.* Respir-

atory symptoms, including upper respiratory tract disorders, respiratory insufficiency, pneumonia, rales, expiratory wheezing, lower respiratory tract disorders, bronchial asthma, *pulmonary or larynx edema,* unspecified pulmonary disease. *Pseudotumor cerebri (especially in children):* Papilledema, headache, N&V, visual disturbances. *Typical retinoid toxicity (similar to ingestion of high doses of vitamin A):* Headache, fever, dryness of skin and mucous membranes, bone pain, N&V, rash, mucositis, pruritus, increased sweating, visual disturbances, ocular disorders, alopecia, skin changes, changed visual acuity, bone inflammation, visual field defects. *Body as a whole:* Malaise, shivering, *hemorrhage, DIC,* infections, peripheral edema, pain, chest discomfort, edema, weight increase, anorexia, weight decrease, myalgia, flank pain, cellulitis, facial edema, fluid imbalance, pallor, lymph disorders, acidosis, hypothermia, ascites. *GI:* **GI hemorrhage,** abdominal pain, various GI disorders, diarrhea, constipation, dyspepsia, abdominal distension, hepatosplenomegaly, hepatitis, ulcer, unspecified liver disorders. *CV:* Arrhythmias, flushing, hypotension, hypertension, phlebitis, *cardiac failure, cardiac arrest, stroke,* MI, enlarged heart, heart murmur, ischemia, myocarditis, pericarditis, pulmonary hypertension, secondary cardiomyopathy. *CNS:* Dizziness, paresthesias, anxiety, insomnia, depression, confusion, *cerebral hemorrhage, intracranial hypertension,* agitation, hallucinations, abnormal gait, agnosia, aphasia, asterixis, cerebellar edema, cerebellar disorders, *convulsions, coma,* CNS depression, dysarthria, encephalopathy, facial paralysis, hemiplegia, hyporeflexia, hypotaxia, no light reflex, neurologic reaction, spinal cord disorder, tremor, leg weakness, unconsciousness, dementia, forgetfulness, somnolence, slow speech. *GU:* Renal insufficiency, dysuria, acute renal failure, micturition frequency, renal tubular necrosis, enlarged prostate. *Otic:* Earache, feeling of fullness in the ears, hearing loss, unspecified auricular disorders, irreversible hearing loss. *Other:* Erythema nodosum, basophilia, hyperhistaminemia, Sweet's syndrome, organomegaly, hypercalcemia, pancreatitis, myositis.

Drug Interactions: Concomitant use with sulfur, resorcinol, benzoyl peroxide, or salicylic acid may cause significant skin irritation.

EMS CONSIDERATIONS

None.

Triamcinolone
Triamcinolone acetonide
Triamcinolone diacetate
Triamcinolone hexacetonide

(try-am-SIN-oh-lohn)

Pregnancy Class: C
Triamcinolone: **Dental paste:** Kenalog in Orabase, Oracort, Oralone **(Rx) Tablets:** Aristocort, Atolone, Kenacort **(Rx)** Triamcinolone acetonide: **Inhalation Aerosol:** Azmacort, Nasacort, Nasacort AQ **(Rx) Parenteral:** Kenaject-40, Kenalog-10 and -40, Tac-3 and -40, Triam-A, Triamonide 40, Tri-Kort, Trilog **(Rx) Topical Cream:** Aristocort, Aristocort A, Delta-Tritex, Flutex, Kenac, Kenalog, Kenalog-H, Kenonel, Triacet, Trianide Mild, Trianide Regular, Triderm, Trymex **(Rx)**, **Topical Lotion:** Kenaalog, Kenonel **(Rx) Topical Ointment:** Aristocort, Aristocort A, Kenac, Kenalog, Kenonel, Trymex **Topical Spray:** Nasacort AQ **(Rx)** Triamcinolone diacetatae: **Parenteral:** Amcort, Aristocort Forte, Aristocort Intralesional, Articulose L.A., Kenacort Diacetate, Triam-Forte, Triamolone 40, Trilone, Tristoject **(Rx)** Triamcinolone hexacetonide: Aristospan Intra-Articular, Aristospan Intralesional **(Rx)**
Classification: Corticosteroid, synthetic

Mechanism of Action: More potent than prednisone. Intermediate-acting.

Onset of Action: Several hours.

Duration of Action: One or more weeks.

Uses: Additional: Pulmonary emphysema accompanied by bronchospasm or bronchial edema. Diffuse interstitial pulmonary fibrosis. With diuretics to treat refractory CHF or cirrhosis of the liver with ascites. Multiple sclerosis. Inflammation following dental procedures. Triamcinolone acetonide for PO inhalation is used for maintenance treatment of asthma. Triamcinolone hexacetonide is restricted to intra-articular or intralesional treatment of rheumatoid arthritis and osteoarthritis.

Precautions: Use during pregnancy only if benefits clearly outweigh risks. Use with special caution with decreased renal function or renal disease. Dose must be highly individualized.

Route/Dosage ───────

TRIAMCINOLONE

• **Tablets**

Adrenocortical insufficiency (with mineralocorticoid therapy).
4–12 mg/day.
Acute leukemias (children).
1–2 mg/kg.
Acute leukemia or lymphoma (adults).
16–40 mg/day (up to 100 mg/day may be necessary for leukemia).
Edema.
16–20 mg (up to 48 mg may be required until diuresis occurs).
Tuberculosis meningitis.
32–48 mg/day.
Rheumatic disease, dermatologic disorders, bronchial asthma.
8–16 mg/day.
SLE.
20–32 mg/day.
Allergies.
8–12 mg/day.
Hematologic disorders.
16–60 mg/day.
Ophthalmologic diseases.
12–40 mg daily.
Respiratory diseases.
16–48 mg/day.

TRIAMCINOLONE ACETONIDE

T

- **IM Only (Not for IV Use)**
2.5–60 mg/day, depending on the disease and its severity.
- **Intra-articular,   Intrabursal, Tendon Sheaths**
2.5–5 mg for smaller joints and 5–15 mg for larger joints, although up to 40 mg has been used.
- **Intradermal**
1 mg/injection site (use 3 mg/mL or 10 mg/mL suspension only).
- **Topical: 0.025%, 0.1%, 0.5% Ointment or Cream; 0.025%, 0.1% Lotion; Paste: 0.1%; Aerosol—to deliver 0.2 mg)**
Apply sparingly to affected area b.i.d.–q.i.d. and rub in lightly.
- **Metered Dose Inhaler (Azmacort)**
Adults, usual: 2 inhalations (200 mcg) t.i.d.–q.i.d. or 4 inhalations (400 mcg) b.i.d., not to exceed 1,600 mcg/day. High initial doses (1,200–1,600 mcg/day) may be needed in some patients with severe asthma.
Pediatric, 6–12 years: 1–2 inhalations (100–200 mcg) t.i.d.–q.i.d. or 2–4 inhalations b.i.d., not to exceed 1,200 mcg/day. Use in children less than 6 years of age has not been determined.
- **Intranasal Spray (Nasacort)**
Seasonal and perennial allergic rhinitis.
Adults and children over 12 years of age: 2 sprays (110 mcg) into each nostril once a day (i.e., for a total dose of 220 mcg/day). The dose may be increased to 440 mcg/day given either once daily or q.i.d. (1 spray/nostril).
TRIAMCINOLONE DIACETATE
- **IM Only**
40 mg/week.
- **Intra-articular, Intrasynovial**
5–40 mg.
- **Intralesional, Sublesional**
5–48 mg (no more than 12.5 mg/injection site and 25 mg/lesion).
TRIAMCINOLONE HEXACETONIDE
Not for IV use.
- **Intra-articular**
2–6 mg for small joints and 10–20 mg for large joints.
- **Intralesional/Sublesional**
Up to 0.5 mg/sq. in. of affected area.

How Supplied: Triamcinolone: *Tablet:* 1 mg, 2 mg, 4 mg, 8 mg. Triamcinolone acetonide: *Metered dose inhaler (nasal):* 55 mcg/inh; *Metered dose inhaler (oral)* 100 mcg/inh; *Cream:* 0.025%, 0.1%, 0.5%; *Nasal Spray: Injection:* 3 mg/mL, 10 mg/mL, 40 mg/mL; *Lotion:* 0.025%, 0.1%; *Ointment:* 0.025%, 0.05%, 0.1%, 0.5%; *Paste:* 0.1%, 55 mcg/inh; *Topical Spray:* 0.147 mg/g. Triamcinolone diacetate: *Injection:* 25 mg/mL, 40 mg/mL. Triamcinolone hexacetonide: *Injection:* 5 mg/mL, 20 mg/mL.

Side Effects: Additional: Intra-articular, intrasynovial, or intrabursal administration may cause transient flushing, dizziness, local depigmentation, and rarely, local irritation. Exacerbation of symptoms has also been reported. A marked increase in swelling and pain and further restricted joint movement may indicate septic arthritis. Intradermal injection may cause local vesicular ulceration and persistent scarring. ***Syncope and   anaphylactoid   reactions*** have been reported with triamcinolone regardless of route of administration.

EMS CONSIDERATIONS

See also *Corticosteroids.*

Triamterene
(try-AM-ter-een)
Pregnancy Class: B
Dyrenium **(Rx)**
Classification: Diuretic, potassium-sparing

Mechanism of Action: Acts directly on the distal tubule to promote the excretion of sodium—which is exchanged for potassium or hydrogen ions—bicarbonate, chloride, and fluid.

Onset of Action: 2-4 hr. **Peak effect:** 6-8 hr.

Duration of Action: 7-9 hr.

Uses: Edema due to CHF, hepatic cirrhosis, nephrotic syndrome, steroid therapy, secondary hyperaldosteronism, and idiopathic edema.

May be used alone or with other diuretics. *Investigational:* Prophylaxis and treatment of hypokalemia, adjunct in the treatment of hypertension.

Contraindications: Hypersensitivity to drug, severe or progressive renal insufficiency, severe hepatic disease, anuria, hyperkalemia, hyperuricemia, gout, history of nephrolithiasis. Lactation.

Precautions: Safety and efficacy have not been determined in children.

Route/Dosage —————————

• Capsules.
  Diuretic.

Adults, initial: 100 mg b.i.d. after meals; **maximum daily dose:** 300 mg.

How Supplied: *Capsule:* 50 mg, 100 mg

Side Effects: *Electrolyte:* Hyperkalemia, electrolyte imbalance. *GI:* Nausea, vomiting (may also be indicative of electrolyte imbalance), diarrhea, dry mouth. *CNS:* Dizziness, drowsiness, fatigue, weakness, headache. *Hematologic:* Megaloblastic anemia, thrombocytopenia. *Renal:* Azotemia, interstitial nephritis. *Miscellaneous:* **Anaphylaxis,** photosensitivity, hypokalemia, jaundice, muscle cramps, rash.

OD **Overdose Management:** *Symptoms:* Electrolyte imbalance, especially hyperkalemia. Also, nausea, vomiting, other GI disturbances, weakness, hypotension, reversible acute renal failure. *Treatment:* Immediately induce vomiting or perform gastric lavage. Evaluate electrolyte levels and fluid balance and treat if necessary. Dialysis may be beneficial.

Drug Interactions
Amantadine / ↑ Toxic effects of amantadine due to ↓ renal excretion
Angiotensin-converting enzyme inhibitors / Significant hyperkalemia
Antihypertensives / Potentiated by triamterene

Captopril / ↑ Risk of significant hyperkalemia
Cimetidine / ↑ Bioavailability and ↓ clearance of triamterene
Digitalis / Inhibited by triamterene
Indomethacin / ↑ Risk of nephrotoxicity and acute renal failure
Lithium / ↑ Chance of lithium toxicity due to ↓ renal clearance
Potassium salts / Additive hyperkalemia
Spironolactone / Additive hyperkalemia

EMS CONSIDERATIONS

See also *Diuretics.*

Triamterene and Hydrochlorothiazide Capsules
Triamterene and Hydrochlorothiazide Tablets

(try-AM-teh-reen, hy-droh-klor-oh-THIGH-ah-zyd)

Pregnancy Class: C
Triamterene and Hydrochlorothiazide Capsules: Dyazide **(Rx)** Triamterene and Hydrochlorothiazide Tablets: Dyazide, Maxzide, Maxide-25 MG **(Rx)**

Classification: Diuretic, antihypertensive

Uses: To treat hypertension or edema in patients who manifest hypokalemia on hydrochlorothiazide alone. In patients requiring a diuretic and in whom hypokalemia cannot be risked (i.e., patients with cardiac arrhythmias or those taking digitalis). Usually not the first line of therapy, except for patients in whom hypokalemia should be avoided.

Contraindications: Patients receiving other potassium-sparing drugs such as amiloride and spironolactone. Use in anuria, acute or chronic renal insufficiency, significant renal impairment, preexisting elevated serum potassium.

T

Precautions: Use with caution during lactation. Geriatric patients may be more sensitive to the hypotensive and electrolyte effects of this combination; also, age-related decreases in renal function may require a decrease in dosage.

Route/Dosage
- **Capsules**
  Hypertension or edema.
Adults: Triamterene/hydrochlorothiazide: 37.5 mg/25 mg—1–2 capsules given once daily with monitoring of serum potassium and clinical effect. Triamterene/hydrochlorothiazide: 50 mg/25 mg—1–2 capsules b.i.d. after meals. Some patients may be controlled using 1 capsule every day or every other day. No more than 4 capsules should be taken daily.
- **Tablets**
  Hypertension or edema.
Adults: Triamterene/hydrochlorothiazide: 37.5 mg/25 mg—1–2 tablets/day (determined by individual titration with the components). Or, triamterene/hydrochlorothiazide: 75 mg/50 mg—1 tablet daily.

How Supplied: Capsules. *Diuretic:* Hydrochlorothiazide, 25 or 50 mg. *Diuretic:* Triamterene, 50 or 100 mg. **Tablets.** *Diuretic:* Hydrochlorothiazide, 25 or 50 mg. *Diuretic:* Triamterene, 37.5 or 75 mg. (In Canada the tablets contain 25 mg of hydrochlorothiazide and 50 mg triamterene.)

EMS CONSIDERATIONS
None.

Triazolam
(try-AYZ-oh-lam)
Pregnancy Class: X
Halcion **(C-IV) (Rx)**
Classification: Benzodiazepine sedative-hypnotic

Mechanism of Action: Decreases sleep latency, increases the duration of sleep, and decreases the number of awakenings.
Uses: Insomnia (short-term management, not to exceed 1 month). May be beneficial in preventing or treating transient insomnia from a sudden change in sleep schedule.
Contraindications: Use concomitantly with itraconazole, ketoconazole, nefaxodone. Lactation (may cause sedation and feeding problems in infants).
Precautions: Safety and efficacy in children under 18 years of age not established. Geriatric patients may be more sensitive to the effects of triazolam.

Route/Dosage
- **Tablets**
Adults, initial: 0.25–0.5 mg before bedtime. **Geriatric or debilitated patients, initial:** 0.125 mg; **then,** depending on response, 0.125–0.25 mg before bedtime.
How Supplied: *Tablet:* 0.125 mg, 0.25 mg
Side Effects: *CNS:* Rebound insomnia, anterograde amnesia, headache, ataxia, decreased coordination, "traveler's" amnesia. Psychologic and physical dependence. *GI:* N&V.

EMS CONSIDERATIONS
See also *Tranquilizers, Antimanic Drugs, and Hypnotics.*

Trientine hydrochloride
(TRY-en-teen)
Pregnancy Class: C
Syprine **(Rx)**
Classification: Chelating agent

Mechanism of Action: A chelating agent that binds copper, thus facilitating its excretion from the body.
Uses: Wilson's disease (a metabolic defect resulting in excess copper accumulation) who are intolerant of penicillamine.
Contraindications: Use in cystinuria, rheumatoid arthritis, biliary cirrhosis.
Precautions: Use with caution during lactation. Safety and effectiveness in children have not been determined although the drug has been used in children as young as 6 years of age.

Route/Dosage
- **Capsules**
  Wilson's disease.

Adults, initial: 750 mg/day–1.25 g/day in divided doses b.i.d., t.i.d., or q.i.d.; **then,** may increase to a maximum of 2 g/day. **Children less than 12 years of age, initial:** 500–750 mg/day in divided doses b.i.d., t.i.d., or q.i.d.; **then,** may increase to a maximum of 1.5 g/day.
How Supplied: *Capsule:* 250 mg
Side Effects: Iron deficiency anemia, SLE.

EMS CONSIDERATIONS
None.

Trifluoperazine
(try-flew-oh-PER-ah-zeen)
Pregnancy Class: C
Stelazine **(Rx)**
Classification: Antipsychotic, antiemetic, piperazine-type phenothiazine

Mechanism of Action: Causes a high incidence of extrapyramidal symptoms and antiemetic effects and a low incidence of sedation, orthostatic hypotension, and anticholinergic side effects.
Onset of Action: Maximum therapeutic effect: Usually 2-3 weeks after initiation of therapy.
Uses: To manage psychotic disorders. Suitable for patients with apathy or withdrawal. Short-term treatment of nonpsychotic anxiety (not the drug of choice).
Precautions: Use during pregnancy only when benefits clearly outweigh risks. Dosage has not been established in children less than 6 years of age. Geriatric, emaciated, or debilitated patients usually require a lower initial dose.

Route/Dosage
• **Oral Solution, Tablets**
   Psychotic disorders.
Adults and adolescents, initial: 2–5 mg (base) b.i.d.; **maintenance:** 15–20 mg/day in two or three divided doses. **Pediatric, 6–12 years:** 1 mg (base) 1–2 times/day; adjust dose as required and tolerated.

Anxiety.
Adults and adolescents: 1–2 mg b.i.d, not to exceed 6 mg/day. Not to be given for this purpose longer than 12 weeks.
• **IM**
   Pyschoses.
Adults: 1–2 mg q 4–6 hr, not to exceed 10 mg/day. Switch to PO therapy as soon as possible. **Pediatric:** *Severe symptoms only:* 1 mg 1–2 times/day.
How Supplied: *Injection:* 2 mg/mL; *Tablet:* 1 mg, 2 mg, 5 mg, 10 mg

EMS CONSIDERATIONS
See also *Antipsychotic Agents, Phenothiazines.*

Triflupromazine hydrochloride
(try-flew-PROH-mah-zeen)
Vesprin **(Rx)**
Classification: Antipsychotic, dimethylaminopropyl-type phenothiazine

Mechanism of Action: Produces high incidence of anticholinergic, sedative, and antiemetic effects; moderate extrapyramidal and hypotensive effects.
Uses: Severe N&V. Psychotic disorders (do not use for psychotic disorders with depression).
Contraindications: Use for psychoses in children less than 2.5 years of age.
Precautions: Use during pregnancy only if benefits clearly outweigh risks. Dosage has not been established for children less than 30 months of age. IV use not recommended for children because of hypotension and rapid onset of extrapyramidal side effects. Geriatric, emaciated, or debilitated patients may require a lower initial dose.

Route/Dosage
• **IM**
   Psychoses.
Adults and adolescents: 60 mg up to maximum of 150 mg/day. **Pediatric:**

T

---

bold italic = life threatening side effect

0.2–0.25 mg/kg to maximum of 10 mg/day.

N&V.

Adults and adolescents: 5–15 mg as single dose repeated q 4 hr up to maximum of 60 mg/day (for elderly or debilitated patients: 2.5 mg up to maximum of 15 mg/day). **Pediatric, over 2½ years:** 0.2–0.25 mg/kg up to maximum of 10 mg/day.

• **IV**
  Psychoses.

Adults and adolescents: 1 mg as required, up to a maximum of 3 mg/day.

How Supplied: *Injection:* 10 mg/mL, 20 mg/mL

EMS CONSIDERATIONS

See also *Antipsychotic Agents, Phenothiazines.*

Trifluridine
(try-FLUR-ih-deen)
Pregnancy Class: C
Viroptic **(Rx)**
Classification: Antiviral, ophthalmic

Mechanism of Action: Closely resembles thymidine; inhibits thymidylic phosphorylase and specific DNA polymerases necessary for incorporation of thymidine into viral DNA. Trifluridine, instead of thymidine, is incorporated into viral DNA, resulting in faulty DNA and the ability to infect or reproduce in tissue. Also incorporated into mammalian DNA. Has activity against herpes simplex virus types 1 and 2 and vaccinia virus.

Uses: Primary keratoconjunctivitis and recurrent epithelial keratitis caused by HSV types 1 and 2. Epithelial keratitis resistant to idoxuridine or if ocular toxicity or hypersensitivity to idoxuridine has occurred. Is also indicated for infections resistant to vidarabine.

Contraindications: Hypersensitivity or chemical intolerance to drug.

Precautions: Safe use during pregnancy not established. Use with caution during lactation.

Route/Dosage
• **Solution, 1%**

1 gtt solution q 2 hr onto cornea, up to maximum of 9 gtt/day in each eye during acute stage (presence of corneal ulcer). Following reepithelialization, decrease dosage to 1 gtt/4 hr (or minimum of 5 gtt/day in each eye) for 7 days. Do not use for more than 21 days.

How Supplied: *Ophthalmic Solution:* 1%

Side Effects: *Ophthalmic:* Mild, transient burning or stinging when instilled. Palpebal edema, superficial punctate keratopathy, epithelial keratopathy, hypersensitivity reaction, stomal edema, irritation, eratitis sicca, hyperemia, increased intraocular pressure.

EMS CONSIDERATIONS

See also *Anti-Infectives.*

Trihexyphenidyl hydrochloride
(try-hex-ee-FEN-ih-dill)
Pregnancy Class: C
Artane, Artane Sequels, Trihexy-2 and -5 **(Rx)**
Classification: Antiparkinson agent, anticholinergic

Mechanism of Action: Synthetic anticholinergic, which relieves rigidity but has little effect on tremors. Causes a direct antispasmodic effect on smooth muscle. High incidence of side effects. Small doses cause CNS depression, whereas larger doses may result in CNS excitation.

Onset of Action: PO: 60 min.

Duration of Action: PO: 6-12 hr.

Uses: Adjunct in the treatment of all types of parkinsonism (often used as adjunct with levodopa). Drug-induced extrapyramidal symptoms. Sustained-release medication is for maintenance dosage only.

Contraindications: Additional: Arteriosclerosis and hypersensitivity to drug.

Route/Dosage
• **Elixir, Tablets**

Parkinsonism.
Initial (day 1): 1–2 mg; **then,** increase by 2 mg q 3–5 days until daily dose is 6–10 mg given in divided doses. Some patients may require 12–15 mg/day (especially those with postencephalitic parkinsonism).

Adjunct with levodopa.
Adults: 3–6 mg/day in divided doses.

Drug-induced extrapyramidal reactions.
Initial: 1 mg/day; **then,** increase as needed to total daily dose of 5–15 mg.

How Supplied: *Elixir:* 2 mg/5 mL; *Tablet:* 2 mg, 5 mg

Side Effects: Additional: Serious CNS stimulation (restlessness, insomnia, deliuium, agitation) and psychotic manifestations.

Drug Interactions: Additional: ↑ Effectiveness of levodopa if used together; such combined use not recommended in patients with psychoses.

EMS CONSIDERATIONS

See also *Cholinergic Blocking Agents* and *Antiparkinson Drugs.*

Trimethobenzamide hydrochloride
(try-meth-oh-BENZ-ah-myd)
Pregnancy Class: C
Arrestin, Hymetic, Tebamide, T-Gen, Ticon, Tigan **(Rx)**
Classification: Antiemetic

Mechanism of Action: Related to the antihistamines but with weak antihistaminic properties. Less effective than the phenothiazines but has fewer side effects. Not suitable as sole agent for severe emesis. Can be used PR. Appears to control vomiting by depressing the CTZ in the medulla.
Onset of Action: PO and IM: 10-40 min.
Duration of Action: 3-4 hr after PO and 2-3 hr after IM.
Uses: Nausea and vomiting.
Contraindications: Hypersensitivity to drug, benzocaine, or similar local anesthetics. Use of suppositories for neonates; IM use in children.

Precautions: Use during pregnancy only if benefits outweigh risks. Use with caution during lactation.

Route/Dosage ———————
• **Capsules**
Adults: 250 mg t.i.d.–q.i.d.; **pediatric, 13.6–40.9 kg:** 100–200 mg t.i.d.–q.i.d.
• **Suppositories**
Adults: 200 mg t.i.d.–q.i.d.; **pediatric, under 13.6 kg:** 100 mg t.i.d.–q.i.d.; **13.6–40.9 kg:** 100–200 mg t.i.d.–q.i.d.
• **IM**
Adults only: 200 mg t.i.d.–q.i.d. *IM route not to be used in children.*

How Supplied: *Capsule:* 100 mg, 250 mg; *Injection:* 100 mg/mL; *Suppository:* 100 mg, 200 mg

Side Effects: *CNS:* Depression of mood, disorientation, headache, drowsiness, dizziness, *seizures, coma,* Parkinson-like symptoms. *Other:* Hypersensitivity reactions, hypotension, blood dyscrasias, jaundice, muscle cramps, opisthotonos, blurred vision, diarrhea, allergic skin reactions. *After IM injection:* Pain, burning, stinging, redness at injection site.

Drug Interactions: Concomitant use with atropine-like drugs and CNS depressants including alcohol should be avoided.

EMS CONSIDERATIONS

See also *Antiemetics.*

————*COMBINATION DRUG*————

Trimethoprim and Sulfamethoxazole
(try-METH-oh-prim, sul-fah-meh-THOX-ah-zohl)
Pregnancy Class: C
Bactrim, Bactrim DS, Bactrim IV, Bactrim Pediatric, Cotrim, Cotrim D.S., Cotrim Pediatric, Septra, Septra DS, Septra IV, Sulfatrim **(Rx)**
Classification: Antibacterial

Uses: PO, Parenteral: UTIs due to *Escherichia coli, Klebsiella, Enterobacter, Pseudomonas mirabilis* and *vulgaris,* and *Morganella morganii.* Enteritis due to *Shigella flexneri* or *S.*

T

---

sonnei. Pneumocystis carinii pneumonitis in children and adults. **PO:** Acute otitis media in children due to *Haemophilus influenzae* or *Streptococcus pneumoniae.* Traveler's diarrhea in adults due to *E. coli.* Prophylaxis of *P. carinii* pneumonia in immunocompromised patients (including those with AIDS). Acute exacerbations of chronic bronchitis in adults due to *H. influenzae* or *S. pneumoniae. Investigational:* Cholera, salmonosis, nocardiosis, prophylaxis of recurrent UTIs in women, prophylaxis of neutropenic patients with *P. carinii* infections or leukemia patients to decrease incidence of gram-negative rod bacteremia. Treatment of acute and chronic prostatitis. Decrease chance of urinary and blood bacterial infections in renal transplant patients.

Contraindications: Additional: Infants under 2 months of age. During pregnancy at term. Megaloblastic anemia due to folate deficiency. Lactation.

Precautions: Use with caution in impaired liver or kidney function and in patients with possible folate deficiency. AIDS patients may not tolerate or respond to this product.

Route/Dosage —————————
• **Oral   Suspension,   Double-Strength Tablets, Tablets**
   UTIs, shigellosis, bronchitis, acute otitis media.
Adults: 1 DS tablet, 2 tablets, or 4 teaspoonfuls of suspension q 12 hr for 10–14 days. **Pediatric:** Total daily dose of 8 mg/kg trimethoprim and 40 mg/kg sulfamethoxazole divided equally and given q 12 hr for 10–14 days. (*NOTE:* For shigellosis, give adult or pediatric dose for 5 days.) For patients with impaired renal function the following dosage is recommended: C_{CR} of 15–30 mL/min: one-half the usual regimen and for C_{CR} less than 15 mL/min: use is not recommended.
   Chancroid.
1 DS tablet b.i.d. for at least 7 days (alternate therapy: 4 DS tablets in a single dose).

Pharyngeal gonococcal infection due to penicillinase-producing Neisseria gonorrhoeae.
720 mg trimethoprim and 3,600 mg sulfamethoxazole once daily for 5 days.
   Prophylaxis of P. carinii pneumonia.
Adults: 160 mg trimethoprim and 800 mg sulfamethoxazole q 24 hr. **Children:** 150 mg/m² of trimethoprim and 750 mg/m² sulfamethoxazole daily in equally divided doses b.i.d. on three consecutive days per week. Do not exceed a total daily dose of 320 mg trimethoprim and 1,600 mg sulamethoxazole.
   Treatment of P. carinii pneumonia.
Adults and children: Total daily dose of 15–20 mg/kg trimethoprim and 100 mg/kg sulfamethoxazole divided equally and given q 6 hr for 14–21 days.
   Prophylaxis of P. carinii pneumonia in immunocompromised patients.
1 DS tablet daily.
   Traveler's diarrhea.
Adults, 1 DS tablet q 12 hr for 5 days.
   Prostatitis, acute bacterial.
1 DS tablet b.i.d. until patient is afebrile for 48 hr; treatment may be required for up to 30 days.
   Prostatitis, chronic bacterial.
1 DS tablet b.i.d. for 4–6 weeks.
• **IV**
   UTIs, shigellosis, acute otitis media.
Adults and children: 8–10 mg/kg/day (based on trimethoprim) in two to four divided doses q 6, 8, or 12 hr for up to 14 days for severe UTIs or 5 days for shigellosis.
   Treatment of P. carinii pneumonia
Adults and children: 15–20 mg/kg/day (based on trimethoprim) in 3–4 divided doses q 6–8 hr for up to 14 days.
How Supplied: These products contain the antibacterial agents sulfamethoxazole and trimethoprim. See also *Sulfamethoxazole.*
   Oral Suspension: Sulfamethoxazole, 200 mg and trimethoprim, 40 mg/5 mL.

Tablets: Sulfamethoxazole, 400 mg and trimethoprim, 80 mg/tablet.

Double Strength (DS) Tablets: Sulfamethoxazole, 800 mg and trimethoprim, 160 mg/tablet.

Concentrate for injection: Sulfamethoxazole, 80 mg and trimethoprim, 16 mg/mL.

Drug Interactions: Additional: *Cyclosporine* / ↓ Effect of cyclosporine; ↑ risk of nephrotoxicity.*Dapsone* / ↑ Effect of both dapsone and trimethoprim.*Methotrexate* / ↑ Risk of methotrixate toxicity due to displacement from plasma protein binding sites.*Phenytoin* / ↑ Effect of phenytoin due to ↓ hepatic clearance.*Sulfonylureas* / ↑ Hypoglycemia effect of sulfonylureas.*Thiazide diuretics* / ↑ Risk of thrombocytopenia with purpura in geriatric patients.*Warfarin* / ↑ PT.*Zidovudine* / ↑ Serum levels of AZT due to ↓ renal clearance.

EMS CONSIDERATIONS

See also *Anti-Infectives* and for *Sulfonamides*.

Trimetrexate glucuronate
(try-meh-TREX-ayt gloo-KYOU-roh-nayt)
Pregnancy Class: D
NeuTrexin **(Rx)**
Classification: Miscellaneous anti-infective

Mechanism of Action: Inhibits the enzyme dihydrofolate reductase resulting in interference with thymidylate biosynthesis and inhibition of folate-dependent formyltransferases. This leads to inhibition of purine synthesis and disruption of DNA, RNA, and protein synthesis and ultimately cell death. Must be given with leucovorin to prevent serious or life-threatening complications, including bone marrow suppression, oral and GI mucosal ulceration, and renal and hepatic dysfunction.

Uses: As alternative therapy with concurrent leucovorin for the treatment of moderate to severe *Pneumocystis carinii* pneumonia in immunocompromised patients. Treatment is indicated in patients with AIDS who are intolerant of or refractory to trimethoprim-sulfamethoxazole (TMP/SMZ) therapy or in whom this combination is contraindicated. *Investigational:* Treatment of non-small-cell lung, prostate, or colorectal cancer.

Contraindications: Hypersensitivity to trimetrexate, leucovorin, or methotrexate. Lactation.

Precautions: Use with caution in patients with impaired hematologic, renal, or hepatic function. Safety and efficacy have not been determined for patients less than 18 years of age for use in treating histologically confirmed PCP.

Route/Dosage
• **IV Infusion**
Pneumocystis carinii *pneumonia.*
Adults: 45 mg/m² once daily by IV infusion over 60–90 min. Leucovorin is given IV at a dose of 20 mg/m² over 5–10 min q 6 hr for a total daily dose of 80 mg/m². Leucovorin may also be given orally in four doses of 20 mg/m² spaced equally throughout the day (round the oral dose up to the next higher 25-mg increment).

How Supplied: *Powder for injection:* 25 mg

Side Effects: *GI:* N&V. *Hematologic:* Neutropenia, thrombocytopenia, anemia. *Hepatic:* Hepatic toxicity manifested by increased ALT, AST, alkaline phosphatase, and bilirubin. *Renal:* Increased serum creatinine. *Electrolytes:* Hyponatremia, hypocalcemia.

OD **Overdose Management:** *Symptoms:* Primarily hematologic. *Treatment:* Discontinue trimetrexate and administer leucovorin at a dose of 40 mg/m² q 6 hr for 3 days.

Drug Interactions: Since trimetrexate is metabolized by the P-450 enzyme system in the liver, drugs that stimulate or inhibit this enzyme system may cause drug interactions that may alter plasma levels of trimetrexate (e.g., erythromycin, rifabutin, rifampin).

Acetaminophen / May alter the levels of trimetrexate metabolites

Cimetidine / May ↓ metabolism of trimetrexate

Clotrimazole / ↓ Metabolism of trimetrexate

Ketoconazole / ↓ Metabolism of trimetrexate

Miconazole / ↓ Metabolism of trimetrexate

EMS CONSIDERATIONS

See also *Anti-Infectives.*

Trimipramine maleate
(try-MIP-rah-meen)
Pregnancy Class: C
Surmontil **(Rx)**
Classification: Antidepressant, tricyclic

Mechanism of Action: Causes moderate anticholinergic and orthostatic hypotensive effects and significant sedative effects.

Uses: Treatment of symptoms of depression. PUD. Seems more effective in endogenous depression than in other types of depression.

Contraindications: Use in children less than 12 years of age.

Route/Dosage ——————
• **Capsules**
  Antidepressant.

Adults, outpatients, initial: 75 mg/day in divided doses up to 150 mg/day, but not to exceed 200 mg/day; **maintenance:** 50–150 mg/day. Total dose can be given at bedtime. **Adults, hospitalized, initial:** 100 mg/day in divided doses up to 200 mg/day. If no improvement in 2–3 weeks, increase to 250–300 mg/day. **Adolescent/geriatric patients, initial:** 50 mg/day up to 100 mg/day. Not recommended for children.

How Supplied: *Capsule:* 25 mg, 50 mg, 100 mg

EMS CONSIDERATIONS

See also *Antidepressants, Tricyclic.*

Tripelennamine hydrochloride
(try-pell-EN-ah-meen)
Classification: Antihistamine, ethylenediamine derivative

Mechanism of Action: GI effects more pronounced than other antihistamines. Moderate sedative effects and low to no anticholinergic activity. **Duration:** 4–6 hr.

Contraindications: Use in neonates.

Precautions: Safe use during pregnancy has not been established. Geriatric patients may be more sensitive to the usual adult dose.

Route/Dosage ——————
• **Tablets**

Adults, usual: 25–50 mg q 4–6 hr; as little as 25 mg or as high as 600 mg may be given to control symptoms. **Pediatric:** 5 mg/kg/day or 150 mg/m²/day divided into 4–6 doses, not to exceed 300 mg/day.

• **Extended-Release Tablets**

Adults: 100 mg q 8–12 hr as needed, up to a maximum of 600 mg/day. Do not use sustained-release form in children.

How Supplied: *Tablet:* 25 mg, 50 mg; *Tablet, Extended Release:* 100 mg

Side Effects: Low incidence. Moderate sedation, mild GI distress, paradoxical excitation, hyperirritability.

EMS CONSIDERATIONS

See also *Antihistamines.*

——————COMBINATION DRUG——————
Tylenol with Codeine Elixir or Tablets
(TIE-leh-noll, KOH-deen)
Pregnancy Class: C
(Tablets are C-III and Elixir is C-V) **(Rx)**
Classification: Analgesic

Uses: Tablets: Mild to moderately severe pain. **Elixir:** Mild to moderate pain.

Precautions: Use with caution during lactation. Safety has not been determined in children less than 3 years of age. May be habit-forming due to the codeine component.

Route/Dosage
• **Tablets, Capsules**
Analgesia.
Adults, individualized, usual: 1–2 No. 2 or No. 3 Tablets or No. 3 Capsules q 2–4 hr as needed for pain. Or, 1 No. 4 Tablet or Capsule q 4 hr as required. Maximum 24-hr dose is 360 mg codeine phosphate and 4,000 mg acetaminophen. **Pediatric:** Dosage equivalent to 0.5 mg/kg codeine.
• **Elixir**
Analgesia.
Adults, individualized, usual: 15 mL q 4 hr as needed; **pediatric, 7–12 years:** 10 mL t.i.d.–q.i.d.; **3–6 years:** 5 mL t.i.d.–q.i.d.

How Supplied: *Nonnarcotic analgesic:* Acetaminophen, 300 mg in each tablet, and 120 mg/5 mL elixir. *Narcotic analgesic:* Codeine phosphate, 15 mg (No. 2 Tablets), 30 mg (No. 3 Tablets), 60 mg (No. 4 Tablets), and 12 mg/5 mL (Elixir).

EMS CONSIDERATIONS
See also *Narcotic Analgesics* and *Acetaminophen.*

Urokinase
(your-oh-KYE-nayz)
Pregnancy Class: B
Abbokinase, Abbokinase Open-Cath **(Rx)**
Classification: Thrombolytic agent

Mechanism of Action: Urokinase converts plasminogen to plasmin; plasmin then breaks down fibrin clots and fibrinogen.
Onset of Action: Rapid.
Duration of Action: 12 hr.
Uses: Acute pulmonary thromboembolism. To clear IV catheters that are blocked by fibrin or clotted blood. Coronary artery thrombosis. *Investigational:* Acute arterial thromboembolism, acute arterial thrombosis, to clear arteriovenous cannula.
Contraindications: Active internal bleeding, history of CVA, within 2 months of intracranial or intraspinal surgery or trauma, recent cardiopulmonary resuscitation, intracranial neoplasm, arteriovenous malformation or aneurysm, known bleeding diathesis, severe uncontrolled arterial hypertension. Any condition presenting a risk of hemorrhage, such as recent surgery or biopsies, delivery within 10 days, pregnancy, ulcerative disease. Also hepatic or renal insufficiency, tuberculosis, recent cerebral embolism, thrombosis, hemorrhage, SBE, rheumatic valvular disease, thrombocytopenia.
Precautions: Use in septic thrombophlebitis may be hazardous. Use with caution during lactation. Safe use in children has not been established.

Route/Dosage
• **IV Infusion Only**
Acute pulmonary embolism.
Loading dose: 4,400 IU/kg administered over 10 min at a rate of 90 mL/hr; **maintenance:** 4,400 IU/kg administered continuously at a rate of 15 mL/hr for 12 hr. May be followed by continuous IV heparin infusion to prevent recurrent thrombosis (start only after thrombin time has decreased to less than twice the normal control value).
Coronary artery thrombi.
Initial bolus: Heparin, as a bolus of 2,500–10,000 units **IV; then,** begin infusion of urokinase at a rate of 6,000 IU/min (4 mL/min) for up to 2 hr (average total dose of urokinase may be 500,000 IU). Urokinase should be administered until the artery is opened maximally (15–30 min after initial opening although it has been given for up to 2 hr).
Clear IV catheter.

Instill into the catheter 1–1.8 mL of a solution containing 5,000 IU/mL.

How Supplied: *Powder for injection:* 5000 IU; 9000 IU; 250,000 IU

Side Effects: *CV:* Superficial bleeding, ***severe internal bleeding,*** transient hypotension or hypertension, tachycardia. *Allergic:* Rarely, skin rashes, ***bronchospasm.*** *Other:* Fever, chills, rigors, N&V, dyspnea, cyanosis, back pain, hypoxemia, acidosis.

Drug Interactions: The following drugs increase the chance of bleeding when given concomitantly with urokinase: Anticoagulants, aspirin, heparin, indomethacin, and phenylbutazone.

EMS CONSIDERATIONS

See also *Streptokinase* and *Alteplase, Recombinant.*

Administration/Storage

IV 1. Reconstitute only with sterile water for injection without preservatives. Do not use bacteriostatic water.
2. To reconstitute, roll and tilt the vial but do not shake. Reconstitute immediately before using.
3. Dilute reconstituted urokinase before IV administration in 0.9% NSS or D5W.

Assessment: Monitor ECG.

Ursodiol
(ur-so-DYE-ohl)
Pregnancy Class: B
Actigall, Urso **(Rx)**
Classification: Gall stone solubilizer

Mechanism of Action: Naturally occurring bile acid that inhibits the hepatic synthesis and secretion of cholesterol; it also inhibits intestinal absorption of cholesterol. Acts to solubilize cholesterol in micelles and to cause dispersion of cholesterol as liquid crystals in aqueous media.

Uses: Dissolution of gallstones in patients with radiolucent, noncalcified gallstones (<20 mm) in whom elective surgery would be risky (i.e., systemic disease, advanced age, idiosyncratic reactions to general anesthesia) or in those who refuse surgery. Prevent gallstones in obese patients undergoing rapid weight loss. Primary biliary cirrhosis (Urso).

Contraindications: Patients with calcified cholesterol stones, radiopaque stones, or radiolucent bile pigment stones. Acute cholecystitis, cholangitis, biliary obstruction, gallstone pancreatitis, biliary-gastrointestinal fistula, allergy to bile acids, chronic liver disease. Provide appropriate specifc treatment in those with variceal bleeding, hepatic encephalopathy, ascites, or in need of an urgent liver transplant.

Precautions: Use with caution during lactation. Safety and efficacy have not been determined in children. Safety for use beyond 24 months is not known.

Route/Dosage ———————

• **Capsules**
Gallstones.
Adults: 8–10 mg/kg/day in two or three divided doses, usually with meals.
Prevent gallstones in rapid weight loss in obesity.
Adults: 300 mg b.i.d. during period of weight loss.

• **Tablets**
Primary biliary cirrhosis.
Adults: 13–15 mg/kg/day given in 4 divided doses with food.

How Supplied: *Capsule:* 300 mg; *Tablet:* 250 mg

Side Effects: *GI:* N&V, dyspepsia, metallic taste, abdominal pain, biliary pain, cholecystitis, constipation, stomatitis, flatulence, diarrhea. *Skin:* Pruritus, rash, dry skin, urticaria. *CNS:* Headache, fatigue, anxiety, depression, sleep disorders. *Other:* Sweating, thinning of hair, back pain, arthralgia, myalgia, rhinitis, cough.

OD Overdose Management: *Symptoms:* Diarrhea. *Treatment:* Treat with supportive measures.

Drug Interactions
Antacids, aluminum-containing / ↓ Effect of ursodiol due to ↓ absorption from GI tract
Cholestyramine / ↓ Effect of ursodiol due to ↓ absorption from GI tract
Clofibrate / ↓ Effect of ursodiol by ↑ hepatic cholesterol secretion

U

Colestipol / ↓ Effect of ursodiol due to ↓ absorption from GI tract
Contraceptives, oral / ↓ Effect of ursodiol by ↑ hepatic cholesterol secretion

Estrogens / ↓ Effect of ursodiol by ↑ hepatic cholesterol secretion

EMS CONSIDERATIONS
None.

Valacyclovir hydrochloride
(val-ah-SIGH-kloh-veer)
Pregnancy Class: B
Valtrex **(Rx)**
Classification: Antiviral drug

Mechanism of Action: Rapidly converted to acyclovir, which has inhibitory activity against herpes simplex virus types 1 (HSV-1) and 2 (HSV-2) and varicella-zoster virus. Acts by inhibiting replication of viral DNA by competitive inhibition of viral DNA polymerase, incorporation and termination of the growing viral DNA chain, and inactivation of the viral DNA polymerase.

Uses: Treatment of recurrent episodes of genital herpes in immunocompetent adults. Treatment of herpes zoster in immunocompetent adults. Suppression of genital herpes in adults who have experienced previous outbreaks.

Contraindications: Hypersensitivity or intolerance to acyclovir or valacyclovir. Use in immunocompromised individuals. Lactation.

Precautions: Use with caution in renal impairment or in those taking potentially nephrotoxic drugs. Dosage reduction may be necessary in geriatric patients depending on the renal status. Safety and efficacy have not been determined in children.

Route/Dosage
• **Tablets**
Herpes zoster (shingles).
Adults: 1 g t.i.d. for 7 days. *Dosage with renal impairment:* C_{CR}, 30–49 mL/min: 1 g q 12 hr; C_{CR}, 10–29 mL/

min: 1 g q 24 hr; and, C_{CR}, less than 10 mL/min: 500 mg q 24 hr.
Recurrent genital herpes.
Adults: 500 mg b.i.d. for 5 days. *Dosage with renal impairment:* C_{CR}, 30–49 mL/min: 500 mg q 12 hr; C_{CR}, 10–29 mL/min: 500 mg q 24 hr; and, C_{CR}, less than 10 mL/min: 500 mg q 24 hr.
Suppression of genital herpes.
Adults: 1 g once daily (500 mg once daily for those who have 9 or fewer recurrences per year).

How Supplied: *Tablet:* 500 mg, 1 g
Side Effects: *GI:* N&V, diarrhea, constipation, abdominal pain, anorexia. *CNS:* Headache, dizziness. *Miscellaneous:* Asthenia, precipitation of acyclovir in renal tubules resulting in acute renal failure and anuria.

OD **Overdose Management:** *Symptoms:* Precipitation of acyclovir in renal tubules if the solubility (2.5 mg/mL) is exceeded in the intratubular fluid. *Treatment:* Hemodialysis until renal function is restored. About 33% of acyclovir in the body is removed during a 4-hr hemodialysis session.

Drug Interactions: Administration of cimetidine and/or probenecid decreased the rate, but not the extent, of conversion of valacyclovir to acyclovir. Also, the renal clearance of acyclovir was decreased.

EMS CONSIDERATIONS
See also *Antiviral Drugs.*

Valproic acid
(val-PROH-ick)
Pregnancy Class: D

V

Depakote **(Rx)**
Classification: Anticonvulsant, miscellaneous

Mechanism of Action: The following information also applies to divalproex sodium (Depakote). The precise anticonvulsant action is unknown; may increase brain levels of the neurotransmitter GABA. Other possibilities include acting on postsynaptic receptor sites to mimic or enhance the inhibitory effect of GABA, inhibiting an enzyme that catabolizes GABA, affecting the potassium channel, or directly affecting membrane stability.

Uses: Alone or in combination with other anticonvulsants for treatment of simple and complex absence seizures (petit mal). As an adjunct in multiple seizure patterns that include absence seizures. Alone or as adjunct to treat complex partial seizures that occur either in isolation or in association with other types of seizures. Divalproex sodium delayed release used for the acute treatment of manic episodes in bipolar disorder and for prophylaxis of migraine headaches. *Investigational:* Alone or in combination to treat atypical absence, myoclonic, and grand mal seizures; also, atonic, complex partial, elementary partial, and infantile spasm seizures. Prophylaxis of febrile seizures in children, to treat anxiety disorders/panic attacks, and subchronically to treat minor incontinence after ileoanal anastomosis. Management of anxiety disorders or panic attacks.

Contraindications: Liver disease or dysfunction.

Precautions: Use with caution during lactation. Use with caution in children 2 years of age or less as they are at greater risk for developing fatal hepatotoxicity. Use lower doses in geriatric patients because they may have increased free, unbound valproic acid levels in the serum. Safety and efficacy of divalproex sodium have not been determined for treating acute mania in children less than 18 years of age or for treating migraine in children less than 16 years of age.

Route/Dosage

• **Capsules, Syrup, Enteric-Coated Capsules and Tablets (Divalproex)**

Complex partial seizures.

Adults and children 10 years and older: 10–15 mg/kg/day. Increase by 5–10 mg/kg/week until seizures are controlled or side effects occur, up to a maximum of 60 mg/kg/day. If the total daily dose exceeds 250 mg, divide the dose. Dosage of concomitant anticonvulsant drugs can usually be reduced by about 25% every 2 weeks. Divalproex sodium may be added to the regimen at a dose of 10–15 mg/kg/day; the dose may be increased by 5–10 mg/kg/week to achieve the optimal response (usually less than 60 mg/kg/day).

Simple and complex absence seizures.

Initial: 15 mg/kg/day, increasing at 1-week intervals by 5–10 mg/kg/day until seizures are controlled or side effects occur.

Acute manic episodes in bipolar disorder (use divalproex).

Initial: 250 mg t.i.d.; **then,** increase dose q 2–3 days until a trough serum level of 50 mcg/mL is reached. The maximum dose is 60 mg/kg/day.

Prophylaxis of migraine (divalproex sodium).

250 mg/day b.i.d., although some may require up to 1,000 mg daily.

• **Rectal**

Intractable status epilepticus that has not responded to other treatment.

Adults: 200–1,200 mg q 6 hr rectally with phenytoin and phenobarbital. **Children:** 15–20 mg/kg.

How Supplied: Valproic acid: *Capsule:* 250 mg; *Syrup:* 250 mg/5 mL; Divalproex sodium: *Enteric Coated Capsule:* 125 mg; *Enteric Coated Tablet:* 125 mg, 250 mg, 500 mg

Side Effects: *GI:* (most frequent): N&V, indigestion. Also, abdominal cramps, abdominal pain, dyspepsia, diarrhea, constipation, anorexia with weight loss or increased appetite with weight gain. *CNS:* Sedation, psychosis, depression, emotional upset, aggression, hyperactivity, deterioration of behavior, tremor, headache, dizziness, somnolence, dysarthria, incoordination, coma (rare). *Ophthalmologic:* Nystagmus, diplopia, "spots before eyes." *Hematologic:* Thrombocytopenia, leukopenia, eosinophilia, anemia, bone marrow suppression, relative lymphocytosis, hypofibrinogenemia, myelodysplastic-type syndrome. *Dermatologic:* Transient alopecia, petechiae, erythema multiforme, skin rashes. photosensitivity, pruritus, **Stevens-Johnson syndrome.** *Hepatic:* Hepatotoxicity. Also, minor increases in AST, ALT, LDH, serum bilirubin, and serum alkaline phosphatase values. *Endocrine:* Menstrual irregularities, secondary amenorrhea, breast enlargement, galactorrhea, swelling of parotid gland, abnormal thyroid function tests. *Miscellaneous:* Also asterixis, weakness, asthenia, bruising, hematoma formation, frank hemorrhage, acute pancreatitis, hyperammonemia, hyperglycinemia, hypocarnitinemia, edema of arms and legs, weakness, inappropriate ADH secretion, Fanconi's syndrome (rare and seen mostly in children), lupus erythematosus, fever, enuresis, hearing loss.

OD **Overdose Management:** *Symptoms:* Motor restlessness, asterixis, visual hallucinations, somnolence, heart block, **deep coma.** *Treatment:* Perform gastric lavage if patient is seen early enough (valproic acid is absorbed rapidly). Undertake general supportive measures making sure urinary output is maintained. Naloxone has been used to reverse the CNS depression (however, it could also reverse the anticonvulsant effect). Hemodialysis and hemoperfusion have been used with success.

Drug Interactions
Alcohol / ↑ Incidence of CNS depression
Carbamazepine / Variable changes in levels of carbamazepine with possible loss of seizure control
Charcoal / ↓ Absorption of valproic acid from the GI tract

Chlorpromazine / ↓ Clearance and ↑ t½ of valproic acid → ↑ pharmacologic effects
Cimetidine / ↓ Clearance and ↑ t½ of valproic acid → ↑ pharmacologic effects
Clonazepam / ↑ Chance of absence seizures (petit mal) and ↑ toxicity due to clonazepam
CNS depressants / ↑ Incidence of CNS depression
Diazepam / ↑ Effect of diazepam due to ↓ plasma binding and ↓ metabolism
Erythromycin / ↑ Serum valproic acid levels → valproic acid toxicitiy
Ethosuximide / ↑ Effect of ethosuximide due to ↓ metabolism
Felbamate / ↑ Mean peak valproic acid levels
Lamotrigine / ↓ Valproic acid serum levels and ↑ lamotrigine serum levels (reduce dose of lamotrigine)
Phenobarbital / ↑ Effect of phenobarbital due to ↓ breakdown by liver
Phenytoin / ↑ Effect of phenytoin due to ↓ breakdown by liver or ↓ effect of valproic acid due to ↑ metabolism
Salicylates (aspirin) / ↑ Effect of valproic acid due to ↓ plasma protein binding and ↓ metabolism
Warfarin sodium / ↑ Effect of valproic acid due to ↓ plasma protein binding. Also, additive anticoagulant effect
AZT / ↓ Clearance of AZT in HIV-seropositive patients

EMS CONSIDERATIONS
See also *Anticonvulsants.*

Valsartan (Diovan)
val-SAR-tan
Pregnancy Class: C (1st trimester), D (2nd and 3rd trimesters)
Diovan **(Rx)**
Classification: Antihypertensive, angiotensin II receptor blocker

Mechanism of Action: Angiotensin II receptor blocker specific for AT_1 receptors, which are responsible for

V

cardiovascular effects of angiotensin II. Drug blocks vasoconstrictor and aldosterone-secreting effects of angiotensin II. **Peak plasma levels:** 2–4 hr. Highly bound to plasma proteins. **t½, terminal:** 11–15 hr. Eliminated mostly unchanged in feces (80%) and urine (about 20%).

Uses: Treat hypertension alone or in combination with other antihypertensive drugs.

Contraindications: Lactation.

Route/Dosage
- **Capsules**
  Hypertension.

Adults, initial: 80 mg once daily as monotherapy. **Dose range:** 80–320 mg once daily. If additional antihypertensive effect is needed, dose may be increased to 160 mg or 320 mg once daily or diuretic may be added.

How Supplied: *Capsules:* 80 mg, 160 mg

Side Effects: *CNS:* Headache, dizziness, fatigue, anxiety, insomnia, paresthesia, somnolence. *GI:* Abdominal pain, diarrhea, nausea, constipation, dry mouth, dyspepsia, flatulence. *Respiratory:* URI, cough, rhinitis, sinusitis, pharyngitis, dyspnea. *Body as a whole:* Viral infection, edema, asthenia, allergic reaction. *Musculoskeletal:* Arthralgia, back pain, muscle cramps, myalgia. *Dermatologic:* Pruritus, rash. *Miscellaneous:* Palpitations, vertigo, neutropenia, impotence.

EMS CONSIDERATIONS
None.

Vancomycin hydrochloride
(van-koh-MY-sin)
Pregnancy Class: C, (B for capsules only)
Vancocin, Vancoled **(Rx)**
Classification: Antibiotic, miscellaneous

Mechanism of Action: Appears to bind to bacterial cell wall, arresting its synthesis and lysing the cytoplasmic membrane by a mechanism that is different from that of penicillins and cephalosporins. May also change the permeability of the cytoplasmic membranes of bacteria, thus inhibiting RNA synthesis. Bactericidal for most organisms and bacteriostatic for enterococci.

Uses: PO: Antibiotic-induced pseudomembranous colitis due to *Clostridium difficile.* Staphylococcal enterocolitis. Severe or progressive antibiotic-induced diarrhea caused by *C. difficile* that is not responsive to the causative antibiotic being discontinued; also for debilitated patients.

IV: Severe staphylococcal infections in patients who have not responded to penicillins or cephalosporins, who cannot receive these drugs, or who have resistant infections. Infections include lower respiratory tract infections, bone infections, endocarditis, septicemia, and skin and skin structure infections. Alone or in combination with aminoglycosides to treat endocarditis caused by *Streptococcus viridans* or *S. bovis.* Must combine with an aminoglycoside to treat endocarditis due to *Streptococcus faecalis.* Used with rifampin, an aminoglycoside (or both) to treat early onset prosthetic valve endocarditis caused by *Staphylococcus epidermidis* or other diphtheroids. Prophylaxis of bacterial endocarditis in pencillin-allergic patients who have congenital heart disease or rheumatic or other acquired or valvular heart disease if such patients are undergoing dental or surgical procedures of the upper respiratory tract. The parenteral dosage form may be given PO to treat pseudomembranous colitis or staphylococcal enterocolitis due to *C. difficile.*

Contraindications: Hypersensitivity. Minor infections. Lactation.

Precautions: Use with extreme caution in the presence of impaired renal function or previous hearing loss. Geriatric patients are at a greater risk of developing ototoxicity.

Route/Dosage
- **Capsules, Oral Solution**
Adults: 0.5–2 g/day in three to four divided doses for 7–10 days. Alterna-

tively, 125 mg t.i.d.–q.i.d. for *C. difficile* may be as effective as the 500-mg dosage. **Children:** 40 mg/kg/day in three to four divided doses for 7–10 days, not to exceed 2 g/day. **Neonates:** 10 mg/kg/day in divided doses.

- **IV**

  Severe staphylococcal infections.
  Adults: 500 mg q 6 hr or 1 g q 12 hr. **Children:** 10 mg/kg/6 hr. **Infants and neonates, initial:** 15 mg/kg for one dose; **then,** 10 mg/kg q 12 hr for neonates in the first week of life and q 8 hr thereafter up to 1 month of age.

  Prophylaxis of bacterial endocarditis in dental, oral, or upper respiratory tract procedures in penicillin-allergic patients.
  Adults: 1 g vancomycin over 1 hr plus 1.5 mg/kg gentamicin (IV or IM), not to exceed 80 mg, 1 hr before the procedure. May repeat once, 8 hr after the initial dose. **Children:** 20 mg/kg vancomycin plus 2 mg/kg gentamicin (IV or IM), not to exceed 80 mg, 1 hr before the procedure. May repeat once, 8 hr after the initial dose.

How Supplied: *Capsule:* 125 mg, 250 mg; *Powder for injection:* 500 mg, 1 g, 5 g, 10 g; *Powder for reconstitution:* 250 mg/5 mL, 500 mg/6 mL

Side Effects: Ototoxicity (may lead to deafness; deafness may progress after drug is discontinued), nephrotoxicity (may lead to uremia). *Red-neck syndrome:* Sudden and profound drop in BP with or without a maculopapular rash over the face, neck, upper chest, and extremities. *CV:* Exaggerated hypotension (due to rapid bolus administration), including **shock and possibly cardiac arrest.** *GU:* Renal failure (rare), interstitial nephritis (rare). *Respiratory:* Wheezing, dyspnea. *Dermatologic:* Urticaria, pruritus, macular rashes, exfoliative dermatitis, **Stevens-Johnson syndrome, toxic epidermal necrolysis,** vasculitis. *Allergic:* Drug fever, hypersensitivity, **anaphylaxis.** *At injection site:* Tissue irritation, including pain, tenderness, necrosis, thrombophlebitis. *Miscellane-

ous: Nausea, chills, tinnitus, eosinophilia, neutropenia (reversible), pseudomembranous colitis.

Drug Interactions
Aminoglycosides / ↑ Risk of nephrotoxicity
Anesthetics / Risk of erythema and histamine-like flushing in children
Muscle relaxants, nondepolarizing / ↑ Neuromuscular blockade

EMS CONSIDERATIONS
See also *Anti-Infectives.*

Vasopressin
(vay-so-PRESS-in)
Pregnancy Class: C
Pitressin Synthetic **(Rx)**
Classification: Pituitary (antidiuretic) hormone

Mechanism of Action: Released from the anterior pituitary gland; regulates water conservation by promoting reabsorption of water by increasing the permeability of the collecting ducts in the kidney. Depending on the concentration, the hormone acts on both V_1 and V_2 receptors. Also causes vasoconstriction (pressor effect) of the splanchnic and portal vessels (and to a lesser extent of peripheral, cerebral, pulmonary, and coronary vessels). Also increases the smooth muscular activity of the bladder, GI tract, and uterus.

Uses: Neurogenic (central) diabetes insipidus (ineffective when diabetes insipidus is of renal origin—nephrogenic diabetes insipidus). Relief of postoperative intestinal gaseous distention, to dispel gas shadows in abdominal roentgenography. *Investigational:* Bleeding esophageal varices. May be used as an alternative pressor to epinephrine in the treatment of adult shock-refractory ventricular fibrillation. May also be useful in vasodilatory shock.

Contraindications: Vascular disease, especially when involving coronary arteries; angina pectoris. Chronic nephritis until reasonable

V

---

blood nitrogen levels are attained. Never give the tannate IV.

Precautions: Pediatric and geriatric patients have an increased risk of hyponatremia and water intoxication. Use caution during lactation and in the presence of asthma, epilepsy, migraine, CAD, and CHF.Potent peripheral vasoconstrictor. May provoke cardiac ischemia and angina.

Route/Dosage
- **IM, SC**
  Diabetes insipidus.
  Adults: 5–10 U b.i.d.–t.i.d.; **pediatric:** 2.5–10 U t.i.d.–q.i.d.
  Abdominal distention.
  Adults, initial: 5 U IM; **then,** 10 U IM q 3–4 hr; **pediatric:** individualize the dose (usual: 2.5–5 U).
  Abdominal roentgenography.
  IM, SC: 2 injections of 10 U each 2 hr and ½ hr before X rays are taken.
  Esophageal varices.
  Initial: 0.2 U/min IV or selective IA; **then,** 0.4 U/min if bleeding continues. The maximum recommended dose is 0.9 U/min.
- **Intranasal (Using Injection Solution)**
  Diabetes insipidus.
  Individualize the dose using the injection solution on cotton pledgets, by nasal spray, or by dropper.*Adult Cardiac Arrest:* IV, IO, and ET doses: 40 U IV push X 1.

How Supplied: *Injection:* 20 U/mL.
Side Effects: *GI:* N&V, increased intestinal activity (e.g., belching, cramps, urge to defecate), abdominal cramps, flatus. *Miscellaneous:* Facial pallor, tremor, sweating, *allergic reactions,* vertigo, skin blanching, *bronchoconstriction, anaphylaxis,* "pounding" in head, water intoxication (drowsiness, headache, *coma, convulsions*).

IV use of vasopressin may result in severe vasoconstriction; local tissue necrosis if extravasation occurs. IM use of tannate may cause pain and sterile abscesses at site of injection.

OD Overdose Management: *Symptoms:* Water intoxication. *Treatment:* Withdraw vasopressin until polyuria occurs. If water intoxication is serious, administration of mannitol (i.e., an os-motic diuretic), hypertonic dextrose, or urea alone (or with furosemide) is indicated.

Drug Interactions: Carbamazepine, chlorpropamide, or clofibrate may ↑ antidiuretic effects of vasopressin.

EMS CONSIDERATIONS
None.

Vecuronium bromide
(vh-kyour-OH-nee-um)
Pregnancy Class: C
Norcuron **(Rx)**
Classification: Nondepolarizing neuromuscular blocking agent

Mechanism of Action: Less likely than other agents to cause histamine release. Effects can be antagonized by anticholinesterase drugs.
Onset of Action: 2.5-3 min; **peak effect:** 3-5 min.
Duration of Action: 25-40 min.
Uses: To induce skeletal muscle relaxation during surgery or mechanical ventilation. To facilitate ET intubation. As an adjunct to general anesthesia. *Investigational:* To treat electrically induced seizures or seizures induced by drugs.
Contraindications: Additional: Use in neonated, obesiity. Sensitivity to bromides.
Precautions: Those from 7 weeks to 1 year of age are more sensitive to the effects of vecuronium leading to a recovery time up to 1½ times that for adults. The dose for children aged 1–10 years of age must be individualized and may, in fact, require a somewhat higher initial dose and a slightly more frequent supplemental dosing schedule than adults. Those with myasthenia gravis or Eaton-Lambert syndrome may experience profound effects with small doses of vecuronium. Cardiovascular disease, old age, and edematous states result in increased volume of distribution and thus a delay in onset time—the dose should *not* be increased.

Route/Dosage
- **IV Only**

V

Intubation.

Adults and children over 10 years of age. 0.08–0.1 mg/kg.

For use after succinylcholine-assisted ET intubation.

0.04–0.06 mg/kg for inhalation anesthesia and 0.05–0.06 mg/kg using balanced anesthesia. (*NOTE:* For halothane anesthesia, doses of 0.15–0.28 mg/kg may be given without adverse effects.)

For use during anesthesia with enflurane or isoflurane after steady state established.

0.06–0.085 mg/kg (about 15% less than the usual initial dose).

Supplemental use.

IV only: 0.01–0.015 mg/kg given 25–40 min following the initial dose; **then,** given q 12–15 min as needed.

IV infusion: Initiated after recovery from effects of initial IV dose of 0.08–0.1 mg/kg has started. **Initial:** 0.001 mcg (1 mg)/kg; **then** adjust according to patient response and requirements. Average infusion rate: 0.0008–0.0012 mg/kg/min (0.8–1.2 mcg/kg/min). After steady-state enflurane, isoflurane, and possibly halothane anesthesia has been established: reduce IV infusion by 25%–60%.

How Supplied: *Powder for injection:* 10 mg, 20 mg

Side Effects: Additional: Moderate to severe skeletal muscle weakness, which may require artificial respiration. *Malignant hyperthermia.*

Drug Interactions: Additional: *Bacitracin /* ↑ Muscle relaxation following high IV or IP doses of bacitracin. *Sodium colistimethate /* ↑ Muscle relaxation following high IV or IP doses of sodium colistimethate. *Tetracyclines /* ↑ Muscle relaxation following high IV or IP doses of tetracyclines. *Succinylcholine* ↑ Effect of vecuronium.

EMS CONSIDERATIONS

See also *Neuromuscular Blocking Agents.*

IV **Administration/Storage:** May be mixed with saline, D5W or RL solution.

Interventions

1. Monitor VS and ECG. Drug can cause vagal stimulation resulting in bradycardia, hypotension, and cardiac arrhythmias.

2. Monitor closely for any evidence of malignant hyperthermia, unresponsive tachycardia, jaw spasm, or lack of laryngeal relaxation. Stop infusion and report; temperature elevations are a late sign of this condition.

3. Patient is fully conscious and aware of surroundings and conversations. Drug does not affect pain or anxiety; give analgesics and antianxiety agents as needed.

Venlafaxine hydrochloride
(ven-lah-FAX-een)
Pregnancy Class: C
Effexor, Effexor XR **(Rx)**
Classification: Antidepressant, miscellaneous

Mechanism of Action: Not related chemically to any of the currently available antidepressants. A potent inhibitor of the uptake of neuronal serotonin and norepinephrine in the CNS and a weak inhibitor of the uptake of dopamine. Has no anticholinergic, sedative, or orthostatic hypotensive effects.

Uses: Treatment of depression.

Contraindications: Use with a MAO inhibitor or within 14 days of discontinuation of a MAO inhibitor. Use of alcohol.

Precautions: Use with caution with impaired hepatic or renal function, during lactation, in patients with a history of mania, and in those with diseases or conditions that could affect the hemodynamic responses or metabolism. Although it is possible for a geriatric patient to be more sensitive, dosage adjustment is not necessary. Use for more than 4–6 weeks has not been evaluated.

V

Route/Dosage

• **Tablets**

Depression.

Adults, initial: 75 mg/day given in two or three divided doses. Depending on the response, the dose can be increased to 150–225 mg/day in divided doses. Make dosage increments up to 75 mg/day at intervals of 4 or more days. Severely depressed patients may require 375 mg/day in divided doses. **Maintenance:** Sufficient studies have not been undertaken to determine length of treatment.

• **Capsules, Extended-Release**

Depression.

Adults, initial: 75 mg once daily. Dose can be increased by up to 75 mg no more often than every 4 days, to a maximum of 225 mg/day.

How Supplied: *Capsule, Extended-Release:* 37.5 mg, 75 mg, 150 mg; *Tablet:* 25 mg, 37.5 mg, 50 mg, 75 mg, 100 mg

Side Effects: Side effects with an incidence of 0.1% or greater are listed. *CNS:* Anxiety, nervousness, insomnia, mania, hypomania, **seizures, suicide attempts,** dizziness, somnolence, tremors, abnormal dreams, hypertonia, paresthesia, decreased libido, agitation, confusion, abnormal thinking, depersonalization, depression, twitching, migraine, emotional lability, trismus, vertigo, apathy, ataxia, circumoral paresthesia, CNS stimulation, euphoria, hallucinations, hostility, hyperesthesia, hyperkinesia, hypertonia, hypotonia, incoordination, increased libido, myoclonus, neuralgia, neuropathy, paranoid reaction, psychosis, psychotic depression, sleep disturbance, abnormal speech, stupor, torticollis. *CV:* Sustained increase in BP (hypertension), vasodilation, tachycardia, postural hypotension, angina pectoris, extrasystoles, hypotension, peripheral vascular disorder, syncope, thrombophlebitis, peripheral edema. *GI:* Anorexia, N&V, dry mouth, constipation, diarrhea, dyspepsia, flatulence, dysphagia, eructation, colitis, edema of tongue, esophagitis, gastroenteritis, gastritis, glossitis, gingivitis, hemorrhoids, **rectal hemorrhage,** melena,

stomatitis, stomach ulcer, mouth ulceration. *Body as a whole:* Headache, asthenia, infection, chills, chest pain, trauma, yawn, weight loss, accidental injury, malaise, neck pain, enlarged abdomen, allergic reaction, cyst, facial edema, generalized edema, hangover effect, hernia, intentional injury, neck rigidity, moniliasis, substernal chest pain, pelvic pain, photosensitivity reaction. *Respiratory:* Bronchitis, dyspnea, asthma, chest congestion, epistaxis, hyperventilation, laryngismus, laryngitis, pneumonia, voice alteration. *Dermatologic:* Acne, alopecia, brittle nails, contact dermatitis, dry skin, herpes simplex, herpes zoster, maculopapular rash, urticaria. *Hematologic:* Ecchymosis, anemia, leukocytosis, leukopenia, lymphadenopathy, lymphocytosis, thrombocytopenia, thrombocythemia, abnormal WBCs. *Endocrine:* Hypothyroidism, hyperthyroidism, goiter. *Musculoskeletal:* Arthritis, arthrosis, bone pain, bone spurs, bursitis, joint disorder, myasthenia, tenosynovitis. *Ophthalmic:* Blurred vision, mydriasis, abnormal accommodation, abnormal vision, cataract, conjunctivitis, corneal lesion, diplopia, dry eyes, exophthalmos, eye pain, photophobia, subconjunctival hemorrhage, visual field defect. *GU:* Urinary retention, abnormal ejaculation, impotence, urinary frequency, impaired urination, disturbed orgasm, menstrual disorder, anorgasmia, dysuria, hematuria, metrorrhagia, vaginitis, amenorrhea, kidney calculus, cystitis, leukorrhea, menorrhagia, nocturia, bladder pain, breast pain, kidney pain, polyuria, prostatitis, pyelonephritis, pyuria, urinary incontinence, urinary urgency, enlarged uterine fibroids, **uterine hemorrhage, vaginal hemorrhage,** vaginal moniliasis. *Miscellaneous:* Sweating, tinnitus, taste perversion, thirst, diabetes mellitus, alcohol intolerance, gout, hypoglycemic reaction, hemochromatosis, ear pain, otitis media.

Withdrawal syndrome: Anxiety, agitation, tremors, vertigo, headache, nausea, tachycardia, tinnitus, akathisia.

OD **Overdose Management:** *Symptoms:* Extensions of side effects, especially somnolence. Other symptoms include prolongation of QTc, mild sinus tachycardia, and **seizures.** *Treatment:* General supportive measures; treat symptoms. Ensure an adequate airway, oxygenation, and ventilation. Monitor cardiac rhythm and VS. Activated charcoal, induction of emesis, or gastric lavage may be helpful.

Drug Interactions

Cimetidine / ↓ First-pass metabolism of venlafaxine

MAO inhibitors / Serious and possibly fatal reaction, including hyperthermia, rigidity, myoclonus, autonomic instability with rapid changes in VS, extreme agitation, coma

---

EMS CONSIDERATIONS

None.

Verapamil
(ver-AP-ah-mil)

Pregnancy Class: C

Calan, Calan SR, Covera HS, Isoptin, Isoptin SR, Verelan **(Rx)**

Classification: Calcium channel blocking agent

Mechanism of Action: Slows AV conduction and prolongs effective refractory period. IV doses may slightly increase LV filling pressure. Moderately decreases myocardial contractility and peripheral vascular resistance. Worsening of heart failure may result if verapamil is given to patients with moderate to severe cardiac dysfunction.

Onset of Action: PO: 30 min; **IV:** 3-5 min.

Duration of Action: PO: 8-10 hr (24 hr for extended-release). **IV:** 10-20 min for hemodynamic effect and 2 hr for antiarrhythmic effect.

Uses: PO: Angina pectoris due to coronary artery spasm (Prinzmetal's variant), chronic stable angina including angina due to increased effort, unstable angina (preinfarction, crescendo). With digitalis to control rapid ventricular rate at rest and during stress in chronic atrial flutter or atrial fibrillation. Prophylaxis of repetitive paroxysmal supraventricular tachycardia. Essential hypertension. Sustained-release tablets are used to treat essential hypertension (Step I therapy). **IV:** Supraventricular tachyarrhythmias. Atrial flutter or fibrillation *Investigational:* PO for prophylaxis of migraine, manic depression (alternate therapy), exercise-induced asthma, recumbent nocturnal leg cramps, hypertrophic cardiomyopathy, cluster headaches.

Contraindications: Severe hypotension, second- or third-degree AV block, cardiogenic shock, severe CHF, sick sinus syndrome (unless patient has artificial pacemaker), severe LV dysfunction. Cardiogenic shock and severe CHF unless secondary to SVT that can be treated with verapamil. Lactation. Use of verapamil, IV, with beta-adrenergic blocking agents (as both depress myocardial contractility and AV conduction). Ventricular tachycardia.

Precautions: Infants less than 6 months of age may not respond to verapamil. Use with caution in hypertrophic cardiomyopathy, impaired hepatic and renal function, and in the elderly.

Route/Dosage ——————
• **Tablets**
Angina at rest and chronic stable angina.
Individualized. Adults, initial: 80–120 mg t.i.d. (40 mg t.i.d. if patient is sensitive to verapamil); **then,** increase dose to total of 240–480 mg/day. Covera HS is given once daily at bedtime in doses of either 180 or 240 mg.
Arrhythmias.
Dosage range in digitalized patients with chronic atrial fibrillation: 240–320 mg/day in divided doses t.i.d.–q.i.d. For prophylaxis of nondigitalized patients: 240–480 mg/day in divided doses t.i.d.–q.i.d. Maximum effects are seen within 48 hr.
Essential hypertension.

V

Initial, when used alone: 80 mg t.i.d. Doses up to 360 mg daily may be used. Effects are seen in the first week of therapy. In the elderly or in people of small stature, initial dose should be 40 mg t.i.d.

• **Extended-Release Capsules and Tablets**

Essential hypertension.

Initial: 240 mg/day in the a.m (120 mg/day in the elderly or people of small stature). If response is inadequate, increase dose to 240 mg in the a.m. and 120 mg in the evening and then 240 mg q 12 hr. Covera HS is given once daily at bedtime in doses of either 180 or 240 mg.

• **IV, Slow**

Supraventricular tachyarrhythmias.

Adults, initial: 5–10 mg (0.075–0.15 mg/kg) given over 2 min (over 3 min in older patients); **then,** 10 mg (0.15 mg/kg) 30 min later if response is not adequate. **Infants, up to 1 year:** 0.1–0.2 mg/kg (0.75–2 mg) given as an IV bolus over 2 min; **1–15 years:** 0.1–0.3 mg/kg (2–5 mg, not to exceed 5 mg total dose) over 2 min. If response to initial dose is inadequate, it may be repeated after 30 min, but not more than a total of 10 mg should be given to patients from 1 to 15 years of age.

How Supplied: *Capsule, extended release:* 240 mg; *Injection:* 2.5 mg/mL; *Tablet:* 40 mg, 80 mg, 120 mg; *Tablet, extended release:* 120 mg, 180 mg, 240 mg

Side Effects: *CV:* CHF, bradycardia, *AV block, asystole,* premature ventricular contractions and tachycardia (after IV use), peripheral and pulmonary edema, hypotension, syncope, palpitations, AV dissociation, *MI, CVA. GI:* Nausea, constipation, abdominal discomfort or cramps, dyspepsia, diarrhea, dry mouth. *CNS:* Dizziness, headache, sleep disturbances, depression, amnesia, paranoia, psychoses, hallucinations, jitteriness, confusion, drowsiness, vertigo. IV verapamil may increase intracranial pressure in patients with supratentorial tumors at the time of induction of anesthesia. *Dermatologic:*

Rash, dermatitis, alopecia, urticaria, pruritus, erythema multiforme, *Stevens-Johnson syndrome. Respiratory:* Nasal or chest congestion, dyspnea, SOB, wheezing. *Musculoskeletal:* Paresthesia, asthenia, muscle cramps or inflammation, decreased neuromuscular transmission in Duchenne's muscular dystrophy. *Other:* Blurred vision, equilibrium disturbances, sexual difficulties, spotty menstruation, sweating, rotary nystagmus, flushing, gingival hyperplasia, polyuria, nocturia, gynecomastia, claudication, hyperkeratosis, purpura, petechiae, bruising, hematomas, tachyphylaxis.

OD **Overdose Management:** *Symptoms:* Extension of side effects. *Treatment:* Beta-adrenergics, IV calcium, vasopressors, pacing, and resuscitation.

EMS CONSIDERATIONS

See also *Calcium Channel Blocking Agents.*

Vidarabine

(vye-DAIR-ah-been)
Pregnancy Class: C
Vira-A **(Rx)**
Classification: Antiviral

Mechanism of Action: Phosphorylated in the cell to arabinosyl adenosine monophosphate (ara-AMP) or the triphosphate (ara-ATP). These compounds cause inhibition of viral DNA polymerase, inhibition of virus-induced ribonucleotide reductase. The drug may also incorporate into the viral DNA molecule leading to chain termination. Due to low solubility, systemic absorption is not expected to occur after ophthalmic use.

Uses: Acute keratoconjunctivitis and recurrent epithelial keratitis caused by HSV types 1 and 2. Superficial keratitis caused by HSV that is resistant to idoxuridine or when toxic or hypersensitivity reactions have resulted from idoxuridine. It is more effective than idoxuridine for deep recurrent infections.

Contraindications: Hypersensitivity to drug. Concomitant use of corticosteroids usually contraindicated. Use in presence of sterile trophic ulcers.

Route/Dosage ————————
• **Ophthalmic Ointment, 3%**
½ in. applied to lower conjunctival sac 5 times/day at 3-hr intervals. Continue therapy for 7 days after complete reepithelialization but at reduced dosage (e.g., b.i.d.). If there are no signs of improvement after 7 days or if complete reepithelialization has not occurred within 21 days, consider other therapy.

How Supplied: *Ophthalmic ointment:* 3%
Side Effects: Photophobia, lacrimation, conjunctival infection, foreign body sensation, temporal visual haze, burning, irritation, superficial punctate keratitis, pain, punctal occlusion, sensitivity to bright light.
OD Overdose Management: [0]
Drug Interactions: [0]

EMS CONSIDERATIONS
See also *Anti-Infectives.*

Warfarin sodium
(WAR-far-in)
Pregnancy Class: X
Coumadin **(Rx)**
Classification: Anticoagulant

Mechanism of Action: Interferes with synthesis of vitamin K–dependent clotting factors resulting in depletion of clotting factors II, VII, IX, and X. Has no direct effect on an established thrombus although therapy may prevent further extension of a formed clot as well as secondary thromboembolic problems.
Onset of Action: Peak activity: 1.5-3 days.
Duration of Action: 2-5 days.
Uses: Prophylaxis and treatment of venous thrombosis and its extension. Prophylaxis and treatment of atrial fibrillation with embolization. Prophylaxis and treatment of pulmonary embolism. Prophylaxis and treatment of thromboembolic complications associated with atrial fibrillation. *Investigational:* Adjunct to treat small cell carcinoma of the lung with chemotherapy and radiation. Prophylaxis of recurrent transient ischemic attacks and to reduce the risk of recurrent MI. In combination with aspirin to reduce risk of a second MI.

Contraindications: Additional: Lactation. IM use. Use of a large loading dose (30 mg) is not recommended due to increased risk of hemorrhage and lack of more rapid protection.
Precautions: Geriatric patients may be more sensitive. Anticoagulant use in the following patients leads to increased risk: trauma, infection, renal insufficiency, sprue, vitamin K deficiency, severe to moderate hypertension, polycythemia vera, severe allergic disorders, vasculitis, indwelling catheters, severe diabetes, anaphylactic disorders, surgery or trauma resulting in large exposed raw surfaces. Use with caution in impaired hepatic and renal function. Safety and efficacy have not been determined in children less than 18 years of age. Careful monitoring and dosage regulation are required during dentistry and surgery.

Route/Dosage ————————
• **Tablets, IV**
  Induction.
Adults, initial: 5–10 mg/day for 2–4 days; **then,** adjust dose based on prothrombin or INR determinations. A lower dose should be used in geriatric or debilitated patients or patients with increased sensitivity.

W

bold italic = life threatening side effect

Dosage has not been established for children.

Maintenance.
Adults: 2–10 mg/day, based on prothrombin or INR.
Prevent blood clots with prosthetic heart valve replacement.
2–5 mg daily.

How Supplied: *Powder for injection:* 5 mg; *Tablet:* 1 mg, 2 mg, 2.5 mg, 4 mg, 5 mg, 6 mg, 7.5 mg, 10 mg

Side Effects: *CV: Hemorrhage* is the main side effect and may occur from any tissue or organ. Symptoms of hemorrhage include headache, paralysis; pain in the joints, abdomen, or chest; difficulty in breathing or swallowing; SOB, unexplained swelling or shock. *GI:* N&V, diarrhea, sore mouth, mouth ulcers, anorexia, abdominal cramping, paralytic ileus, intestinal obstruction (due to intramural or submucosal hemorrhage). *Hepatic:* Hepatotoxicity, cholestatic jaundice. *Dermatologic:* Dermatitis, exfoliative dermatitis, urticaria, alopecia, necrosis or gangrene of the skin and other tissues (due to protein C deficiency). *Miscellaneous:* Pyrexia, red-orange urine, priapism, leukopenia, systemic cholesterol microembolization ("purple toes" syndrome), hypersensitivity reactions, compressive neuropathy secondary to hemorrhage adjacent to a nerve (rare).

OD Overdose Management: *Symptoms:* Early symptoms include melena, petechiae, microscopic hematuria, oozing from superficial injuries (e.g., nicks from shaving, excessive bruising, bleeding from gums after teeth brushing), excessive menstrual bleeding. *Treatment:* Discontinue therapy. Administer oral or parenteral phytonadione (e.g., 2.5–10 mg PO or 5–25 mg parenterally). In emergency situations, 200–250 mL fresh frozen plasma or commercial factor IX complex. Fresh whole blood may be needed in patients unresponsive to phytonadione.

Drug Interactions: Warfarin is responsible for more adverse drug interactions than any other group. Patients on anticoagulant therapy must be monitored carefully each time a drug is added or withdrawn. Monitoring usually involves determination of PT. In general, a lengthened PT means potentiation of the anticoagulant. Since potentiation may mean hemorrhages, a lengthened PT warrants **reduction of the dosage of the anticoagulant.** However, the anticoagulant dosage must again be increased when the second drug is discontinued. A shortened PT means inhibition of the anticoagulant and may require an increase in dosage.

Acetaminophen / ↑ Anticoagulant effect
Alcohol, ethyl / Chronic alcohol use ↓ effect of warfarin
Aminoglutethimide / ↓ Effect of warfarin due to ↑ breakdown by liver
Aminoglycoside antibiotics / ↑ Effect of warfarin due to interference with vitamin K
Amiodarone / ↑ Effect of warfarin due to ↓ breakdown by liver
Androgens / ↑ Effect of warfarin
Ascorbic acid / ↓ Effect of warfarin by unknown mechanism
Barbiturates / ↓ Effect of warfarin due to ↑ breakdown by liver
Beta-adrenergic blockers / ↑ Effect of wafarin
Carbamazepine / ↓ Effect of warfarin due to ↑ breakdown by liver
Cephalosporins / ↑ Effect of warfarin due to effects on platelet function
Chloral hydrate / ↑ Effect of warfarin due to ↓ binding to plasma proteins
Chloramphenicol / ↑ Effect of warfarin due to ↓ breakdown by liver
Cholestyramine / ↓ Anticoagulant effect due to binding in and ↓ absorption from GI tract
Cimetidine / ↑ Anticoagulant effect due to ↓ breakdown by liver
Clofibrate / ↑ Anticoagulant effect
Contraceptives, oral / ↓ Anticoagulant effect by ↑ activity of certain clotting factors (VII and X); rarely, the opposite effect of ↑ risk of thromboembolism
Contrast media containing iodine / ↑ Effect of warfarin by ↑ PT

Corticosteroids / ↑ Effect of warfarin; also ↑ risk of GI bleeding due to ulcerogenic effect of steroids

Cyclophosphamide / ↑ Anticoagulant effect

Dextrothyroxine / ↑ Effect of warfarin

Dicloxacillin / ↓ Effect of warfarin

Diflunisal / ↑ Anticoagulant effect and ↑ risk of bleeding due to effect on platelet function and GI irritation

Disulfiram / ↑ Effect of warfarin

Erythromycin / ↑ Effect of warfarin

Estrogens / ↓ Anticoagulant response by ↑ activity of certain clotting factors; rarely, the opposite effect of ↑ risk of thromboembolism

Ethchlorvynol / ↓ Effect of warfarin

Etretinate / ↓ Effect of warfarin due to ↑ breakdown by liver

Fluconazole / ↑ Effect of warfarin

Gemfibrozil / ↑ Effect of warfarin

Glucagon / ↑ Effect of warfarin

Glutethimide / ↓ Effect of warfarin due to ↑ breakdown by liver

Griseofulvin / ↓ Effect of warfarin

Hydantoins / ↑ Effect of warfarin; also, ↑ hydantoin serum levels

Hypoglycemics, oral / ↑ Effect of warfarin due to ↓ plasma protein binding; also, ↑ effect of sulfonylureas

Ifosfamide / ↑ Effect of warfarin due to ↓ breakdown by liver and displacement from protein binding sites

Indomethacin / ↑ Effect of warfarin by an effect on platelet function; also, indomethacin is ulcerogenic cause GI hemorrhage

Isoniazid / ↑ Effect of warfarin

Ketoconazole / ↑ Effect of warfarin

Loop diuretics / ↑ Effect of warfarin by displacement from protein binding sites

Lovastatin / ↑ Effect of warfarin due to ↓ breakdown by liver

Metronidazole / ↑ Effect of warfarin due to ↓ breakdown by liver

Miconazole / ↑ Effect of warfarin

Mineral oil / ↑ Hypoprothrombinemia by ↓ absorption of vitamin K from GI tract; also mineral oil may

↓ absorption of warfarin from GI tract

Moricizine / ↑ Effect of warfarin

Nafcillin / ↓ Effect of warfarin

Nalidixic acid / ↑ Effect of warfarin due to displacement from protein binding sites

Nonsteroidal anti-inflammatory agents / ↑ Effect of warfarin and ↑ risk of bleeding due to effects on platelet function and GI irritation

Omeprazole / ↑ Effect of warfarin due to ↓ breakdown by liver

Penicillins / ↑ Effect of warfarin and ↑ risk of bleeding due to effects on platelet function

Phenylbutazone / ↑ Effect of warfarin due to ↓ breakdown by liver and ↑ displacement from protein binding sites

Propafenone / ↑ Effect of wafarin due to ↓ breakdown by liver

Propoxyphene / ↑ Effect of warfarin

Quinidine, quinine / ↑ Effect of warfarin due to ↓ breakdown by liver

Quinolones / ↑ Effect of warfarin

Rifampin / ↓ Anticoagulant effect due to ↑ breakdown by liver

Salicylates / ↑ Effect of warfarin and ↑ risk of bleeding due to effect on platelet function and GI irritation

Spironolactone / ↓ Effect of warfarin due to hemoconcentration of clotting factors due to diuresis

Streptokinase / ↑ Effect of warfarin

Sucralfate / ↓ Effect of warfarin

Sulfamethoxazole and Trimethoprim / ↑ Effect of warfarin due to ↓ breakdown by liver

Sulfinpyrazone / ↑ Anticoagulant effect due to ↓ breakdown by liver and inhibition of platelet aggregation

Sulfonamides / ↑ Effect of sulfonamides

Sulindac / ↑ Effect of warfarin

Tamoxifen / ↑ Effect of warfarin

Tetracyclines / ↑ Effect of warfarin due to interference with vitamin K

Thiazide diuretics / ↓ Effect of warfarin due to hemoconcentration of clotting factors

W

Thioamines / ↑ Effect of warfarin
Thiopurines / ↓ Effect of warfarin due to ↑ synthesis or activation of prothrombin
Thyroid hormones / ↑ Anticoagulant effect
Trazodone / ↓ Effect of warfarin
Thiazide diuretics / ↓ Effect of warfarin due to hemoconcentration of clotting factors due to diuresis
Troglitazone / Possible ↑ effect of warfarin due to ↓ breakdown by liver or displacement from plasma proteins
Urokinase / ↑ Effect of warfarin
Vitamin E / ↑ Effect of warfarin due to interference with vitamin K
Vitamin K / ↓ Effect of warfarin

EMS CONSIDERATIONS

See also *Anticoagulants*.

Z

Zafirlukast
(zah-FIR-loo-kast)
Pregnancy Class: B
Accolate **(Rx)**
Classification: Antiasthmatic

Mechanism of Action: A selective and competitive antagonist of leukotriene receptors D_4 and E_4, which are components of slow-reacting substance of anaphylaxis. It is believed that cysteinyl leukotriene occupation of receptors causes asthma, including airway edema, smooth muscle constriction, and altered cellular activity associated with the inflammatory process. Zafirlukast inhibits bronchoconstriction caused by sulfur dioxide and cold air in patients with asthma. It also attenuates the early- and late-phase reaction in asthmatics caused by inhalation of antigens such as grass, cat dander, ragweed, and mixed antigens.

Uses: Prophylaxis and chronic treatment of asthma in adults and children 12 years of age and older.

Contraindications: Use to terminate an acute asthma attack, including status asthmaticus. Lactation.

Precautions: The clearance is reduced in patients 65 years of age and older. Safety and efficacy have not been determined in children less than 12 years of age.

Route/Dosage
• **Tablets**
Asthma.

Adults and children aged 12 and older: 20 mg b.i.d.

How Supplied: *Tablet:* 20 mg

Side Effects: *GI:* N&V, diarrhea, abdominal pain, dyspepsia. *CNS:* Headache, dizziness. *Hepatic:* Rarely, symptomatic hepatitis and hyperbilirubinemia. *Hypersensitivity reactions:* Urticaria, angioedema, rashes (with and without blistering). *Miscellaneous:* Infection, generalized pain, asthenia, accidental injury, myalgia, fever, back pain, systemic eosinophilia with vasculitis consistent with Churg-Strauss syndrome.

Drug Interactions
Aspirin / ↑ Plasma levels of zafirlukast
Erythromycin / ↓ Plasma levels of zafirlukast
Terfenadine / ↓ Plasma levels of zafirlukast
Theophylline / ↓ Plasma levels of zafirlukast
Warfarin / Significant ↑ PT

EMS CONSIDERATIONS

None.

Zalcitabine (Dideoxycytidine, ddC)
(zal-SIGH-tah-been)
Pregnancy Class: C
Hivid **(Rx)**
Classification: Antiviral

Mechanism of Action: Converted in cells to the active metabolite, dideoxycytidine 5'-triphosphate (ddCTP), by cellular enzymes. ddCTP serves as an alternative substrate to deoxycytidine triphosphate for HIV-reverse transcriptase, thereby inhibiting the in vitro replication of HIV-1 and inhibiting viral DNA synthesis. The incorporation of ddCTP into the growing DNA chain leads to premature chain termination. ddCTP serves as a competitive inhibitor of the natural substrate for deoxycytidine triphosphate for the active site of the viral reverse transcriptase, which further inhibits viral DNA synthesis.

Uses: In combination with AZT in advanced HIV infections (CD_4 cell count of 300/mm³ or less and who have shown significant clinical or immunologic deterioration). Alone for HIV-infected adults with advanced disease who are intolerant to AZT or where the disease has progressed while taking AZT.

Contraindications: Hypersensitivity. Use in moderate or severe peripheral neuropathy or with drugs that have the potential to cause peripheral neuropathy (see *Drug Interactions*). Concomitant use with didanosine. Lactation.

Precautions: Use with extreme caution in patients with low CD_4 cell counts (< 50/mm³). Use with caution in patients with a history of pancreatitis or known risk factors for the development of pancreatitis. Patients with a C_{CR} less than 55 mL/min may be at a greater risk for toxicity due to decreased clearance. Patients may continue to develop opportunistic infections and other complications of HIV infection. Safety and efficacy have not been determined in HIV-infected children less than 13 years of age.

Route/Dosage
• **Tablets**
In combination with AZT in advanced HIV infection.
Adults: 0.75 mg given at the same time with 200 mg AZT q 8 hr for a total daily dose of 2.25 mg zalcitabine and 600 mg AZT.

Alone in advanced HIV infection. 0.75 mg q 8 hr (2.25 mg/day).
How Supplied: *Tablet:* 0.375 mg, 0.75 mg

Side Effects: The incidence of certain side effects is dependent on the duration of use and the dose of the drug. *Neurologic:* Peripheral neuropathy (may be severe) characterized by numbness and burning dysesthesia involving the distal extremities; this may be followed by sharp shooting pains or severe continuous burning pain if the drug is not withdrawn. The neuropathy may progress to severe pain requiring narcotic analgesics and may be irreversible. *GI: Fatal pancreatitis* when given alone or with AZT. Esophageal ulcers, oral ulcers, nausea, dysphagia, anorexia, abdominal pain, vomiting, constipation, ulcerative stomatitis, aphthous stomatitis, diarrhea, dry mouth, dyspepsia, glossitis, *rectal hemorrhage,* hemorrhoids, enlarged abdomen, gum disorders, flatulence, anorexia, tongue ulceration, dysphagia, eructation, gastritis, *GI hemorrhage,* left quadrant pain, salivary gland enlargement, esophageal pain, esophagitis, rectal ulcers, melena, painful swallowing, mouth lesion, acute pharyngitis, abdominal bloating or cramps, anal/rectal pain, colitis, dental abscess, epigastric pain, gagging with pills, gingivitis, heartburn, *hemorrhagic pancreatitis,* increased salivation, odynophagia, painful sore gums, rectal mass, sore tongue, sore throat, tongue disorder, toothache, unformed/loose stools. *Dermatologic:* Rash (including erythematous, maculopapular, follicular), pruritus, night sweats, dermatitis, skin lesions, acne, alopecia, bullous eruptions, increased sweating, urticaria, hot flashes, lip blister or lesions, carbuncle/furuncle, cellulitis, dry skin, dry rash desquamation, exfoliative dermatitis, finger inflammation, impetigo, infection, itchy rash, moniliasis, mucocutaneous/skin disorder, nail disorder, photosensitivity, skin fissure, skin ulcer. *CNS:* Headache, dizzi-

bold italic = life threatening side effect

Z

ness, seizures, ataxia, abnormal coordination, Bell's palsy, dysphonia, hyperkinesia, hypokinesia, migraine, neuralgia, neuritis, stupor, aphasia, decreased neurologic function, disequilibrium, facial nerve palsy, focal motor seizures, memory loss, paralysis, speech disorder, *status epilepticus,* tremor, vertigo, hypertonia, hand tremor, twitching, confusion, impaired concentration, insomnia, agitation, depersonalization, hallucinations, emotional lability, nervousness, anxiety, depression, euphoria, manic reaction, dementia, amnesia, somnolence, abnormal thinking, crying, loss of memory, decreased concentration, acute psychotic disorder, acute stress reaction, decreased motivation, decreased sexual desire, mood swings, paranoid states, *suicide attempt. Respiratory:* Coughing, dyspnea, respiratory distress, rales/rhonchi, nasal discharge, flu-like symptoms, cyanosis, acute nasopharyngitis, chest congestion, dry nasal mucosa, hemoptysis, sinus congestion, sinus pain, sinusitis, wheezing. *Musculoskeletal:* Myalgia, arthralgia, arthritis, arthropathy, cold extremities, leg cramps, myositis, joint pain or inflammation, weakness in leg muscle, generalized muscle weakness, back pain, backache, bone aches and pains, bursitis, pain in extremities, joint swelling, muscle disorder, muscle stiffness, muscle cramps, arthrosis, myopathy, neck pain, rib pain, stiff neck. *Hepatic:* Exacerbation of hepatic dysfunction, especially in those with preexisting liver disease or with a history of alcohol abuse. Abnormal hepatic function, hepatitis, jaundice, hepatocellular damage, hepatomegaly with steatosis, cholecystitis. *CV:* **Cardiomyopathy,** CHF, abnormal cardiac movement arrhythmia, atrial fibrillation, *cardiac failure,* cardiac dysrhythmias, heart racing, hypertension, palpitations, **subarachnoid hemorrhage,** syncope, tachycardia, ventricular ectopy, epistaxis. *Hematologic:* Anemia, leukopenia, thrombocytopenia, alteration of absolute neutrophil count, granulocytosis, eosinophilia, neutropenia,

hemoglobinemia, neutrophilia, platelet alteration, purpura, thrombus, unspecified hematologic toxicity, alteration of WBCs. *Hypersensitivity:* Urticaria, **anaphylaxis** (rare). *Endocrine:* Diabetes mellitus, gout, hot flushes, hypoglycemia, hyperglycemia, hypocalcemia, hypophosphatemia, hypernatremia, hyponatremia, hypomagnesemia, hyperkalemia, hypokalemia, hyperlipidemia, polydipsia. *GU:* Dysuria, toxic nephropathy, polyuria, renal calculi, **acute renal failure,** hyperuricemia, increased frequency of micturition, abnormal renal function, renal cyst, albuminuria, bladder pain, genital lesion/ulcer, nocturia, painful/sore penis, penile edema, testicular swelling, urinary retention, vaginal itch/ulcer/pain, vaginal/cervix disorder. *Ophthalmologic:* Abnormal vision, burning or itching eyes, xerophthalmia, eye pain or abnormality, blurred or decreased vision, eye inflammation/irritation, eye redness/hemorrhage, increased tears, mucopurulent conjunctivitis, photophobia, dry eyes, unequal sized pupils, yellow sclera. *Otic:* Ear pain/blockage, fluid in ears, hearing loss, tinnitus. *Body as a whole:* Fatigue, fever, rigors, chest pain or tightness, weight decrease, pain, malaise, asthenia, generalized edema, general debilitation, chills, difficulty moving, facial pain or swelling, flank pain, flushing, pelvic/groin pain. *Miscellaneous:* Lymphadenopathy, taste perversion, decreased taste, parosmia, lactic acidosis.

Drug Interactions: The following drugs have the potential to cause peripheral neuropathy and should probably not be used concomitantly with zalcitabine: chloramphenicol, cisplatin, dapsone, disulfiram, ethionamide, glutethimide, gold, hydralazine, iodoquinol, isoniazid, metronidazole, nitrofurantoin, phenytoin, ribavirin, vincristine. Drugs such as amphotericin, foscarnet, and aminoglycosides may increase the risk of peripheral neuropathy by interfering with the renal clearance of zalcitabine, thus increasing plasma levels.

Antacids (Mg/Al-containing) / ↓ Absorption of zalcitabine
Cimetidine / ↓ Elimination of zalcitabine by ↓ renal tubular secretion
Pentamidine / ↑ Risk of fulminant pancreatitis
Probenecid / ↓ Elimination of zalcitabine by ↓ renal tubular secretion

EMS CONSIDERATIONS
None.

Zaleplon
ZAL-leh-plon
Pregnancy Class: C
Sonata (Rx)
Classification: Hypnotic

Mechanism of Action: Nonbenzodiazepine hypnotic. However, it interacts with the GABA-benzodiazepine receptor complex. It binds selectively to the brain omega-1 receptor located on the alpha subunit of $GABA_A$ receptor complex and potentiates t-butyl-bicyclophosphorothionate (TBPS) binding. Although it decreases the time to sleep, it does not increase total sleep time or decrease the number of awakenings.

Uses: Short-term treatment of insomnia.

Contraindications: Use with alcohol, severe hepatic impairment, or during lactation.

Precautions: Use with caution in diseases or conditions that could affect metabolism or hemodynamic responses, in patients with compromised respiratory function, or in patients showing signs or symptoms of depression. Abuse potential is similar to benzodiazepine and benzodiazepine-like hypnotics. The products contain tartrazine (FD&C yellow #5) which may cause an allergic-type reaction, especially in those with aspirin hypersensitivity. May cause amnesia and dependence.

Route/Dosage
• **Capsules**
  Insomnia.
Adults, nonelderly: 10 mg for no more than 7–10 days. Consider 20 mg for the occasional patient who does not benefit from the lower dose. Do not exceed a dose of 20 mg. **Mild to moderate hepatic impairment, elderly patients, or low-weight individuals:** 5 mg, not to exceed 10 mg..

How Supplied: *Capsules:* 5 mg, 10 mg

Side Effects: Listed are side effects with an incidence of 0.1% or greater.
CNS: Dizziness, amnesia, somnolence, anxiety, paresthesia, depersonalization, hypesthesia, tremor, hallucinations, vertigo, depression, hypertonia, nervousness, abnormal thinking/concentration, abnormal gait, agitation, apathy, ataxia, circumoral paresthesia, confusion, emotional lability, euphoria, hyperesthesia, hyperkinesia, hypotonia, incoordination, insomnia, decreased libido, neuralgia, nystagmus.
GI: Nausea, dyspepsia, anorexia, colitis, constipation, dry mouth, eructation, esophagitis, flatulence, gastritis, gastroenteritis, gingivitis, glossitis, increased appetite, melena, mouth ulceration, rectal hemorrhage, stomatitis.
CV: Migraine, angina pectoris, bundle branch block, hypertension, hypotension, palpitation, syncope, tachycardia, vasodilation, ventricular extrasystoles. *Dermatologic:* Pruritus, rash, acne, alopecia, contact dermatitis, dry skin, eczema, maculopapular rash, skin hypertrophy, sweating, urticaria, vesiculobullous rash. *GU:* Bladder pain, breast pain, cystitis, decreased urine stream, dysuria, hematuria, impotence, kidney calculus, kidney pain, menorrhagia, metorrhagia, urinary frequency, urinary incontinence, urinary urgency, vaginitis, dysmenorrhea. *Respiratory:* Bronchitis, asthma, dyspnea, laryngitis, pneumonia, snoring, voice alteration. *Musculoskeletal:* Arthritis, arthrosis, bursitis, joint disorder (swelling, stiffness, pain), myasthenia, tenosynovitis. *Hematologic:* Anemia, ecchymosis, lymphadenopathy. *Metabolic:* Edema, gout, hypercholesterolemia, thirst, weight gain. *Ophthalmic:* Eye pain, abnormal vision, conjunctivitis,

---

bold italic = life threatening side effect

Z

diplopia, dry eyes, photophobia, watery eyes. *Otic:* Ear pain, hyperacusis, tinnitus. *Body as a whole:* Headache, asthenia, myalgia, fever, malaise, chills, generalized edema. *Miscellaneous:* Abdominal pain, photosensitivity, peripheral edema, epistaxis, back pain, chest pain, substernal chest pain, face edema, hangover effect, neck rigidity, parosmia.

Drug Interactions
Cimetidine / Significantly ↑ zaleplon serum levels
CNS depressants (anticonvulsants, antihistamines, ethanol) / Additive CNS depression
Rifampin / Significantly ↓ zaleplon serum levels

EMS CONSIDERATIONS
None.

Zanamivir
zah-NAM-ih-vir
Pregnancy Class: B
Relenza **(Rx)**
Classification: Antiviral drug

Mechanism of Action: Selectively inhibits influenza virus neuraminidase. The enzyme allows virus release from infected cells, prevents virus aggregation, and possibly decreases virus inactivation by respiratory mucus. Zanamivir may alter virus particle aggregation and release. There is the possibility of emergence of resistance.

Uses: Treatment of uncomplicated acute illness due to influenza virus A and B (limited) in adults and adolescents (12 years and older) who have been symptomatic for 2 or less days. *Note:* There is no evidence that zanamivir is effective in any illness caused by agents other than influenza virus A and B.

Precautions: Use with caution during lactation. It is possible the elderly may be more sensitive to effects of the drug. Safety and efficacy have not been determined in children less than 12 years of age, in patients with underlying chronic pulmonary disease, for prophylactic use to prevent influenza (patients should still take annual flu vaccinations), or in those with high-risk underlying medical conditions.

Route/Dosage
• **Powder for oral inhalation**
Influenza treatment.
Adults and children over 12 years: 2 inhalations (one 5-mg blister per inhalation for a total dose of 10 mg) b.i.d. for 5 days. Two doses are taken on the first day of treatment whenever possible, provided there is 2 or more hr between doses. On subsequent days, doses are taken about 12 hr apart (i.e., morning and evening) at about the same time each day. Safety and efficacy of repeated treatment courses have not been studied.

How Supplied: *Powder for Inhalation, Blisters:* 5 mg

Side Effects: *GI:* Diarrhea, N&V. *Respiratory:* Nasal signs and symptoms, bronchitis, cough, sinusitis, infections of the ear, nose, and throat. *Miscellaneous:* Dizziness, headache, malaise, fatigue, fever, abdominal pain, myalgia, arthralgia, urticaria.

EMS CONSIDERATIONS
None.

Zidovudine (Azidothymidine, AZT)
(zye-DOH-vyou-deen, ah-zee-doh-THIGH-mih-deen)
Pregnancy Class: C
Retrovir **(Rx)**
Classification: Antiviral

Mechanism of Action: The active form of the drug is AZT triphosphate, which is derived from AZT by cellular enzymes. AZT triphosphate competes with thymidine triphosphate (the natural substrate) for incorporation into growing chains of viral DNA by retroviral reverse transcriptase. Once incorporated, AZT triphosphate causes premature termination of the growth of the DNA chain. Low concentrations of AZT also inhibit the activity of *Shigella, Klebsiella, Salmonella, Enterobacter, Escherichia coli,* and *Citrobacter,* although resistance develops rapidly.

Uses: PO: Initial treatment of HIV-infected adults who have a CD_4 cell count of 500/mm³ or less. Superior to either didanosine or zalcitabine monotherapy for initial treatment of HIV-infected patients who have not had previous antiretroviral therapy. To prevent HIV transmission from pregnant women to their fetuses. For HIV-infected children over 3 months of age who have HIV-related symptoms or are asymptomatic with abnormal laboratory values indicating significant immunosuppression. In combination with zalcitabine in selected patients with advanced HIV disease (CD_4 cell count of 300 cells/mm³ or less).

IV: Selected adults with symptomatic HIV infections who have a history of confirmed *Pneumocystis carinii* pneumonia or an absolute CD_4 (T_4 helper/inducer) lymphocyte count of less than 200 cells/mm³ in the peripheral blood prior to therapy.

Contraindications: Allergy to AZT or its components. Lactation.

Precautions: Use with caution in patients who have a hemoglobin level of less than 9.5 g/dL or a granulocyte count less than 1,000/mm³. AZT is not a cure for HIV; thus, patients may continue to acquire opportunistic infections and other illnesses associated with ARC or HIV. AZT has not been shown to reduce the risk of HIV transmission to others through sexual contact or blood contamination.

Route/Dosage

• **Capsules, Syrup**

Symptomatic HIV infections.

Adults: 100 mg (one 100-mg capsule or 10 mL syrup) q 4 hr around the clock (i.e., total of 600 mg daily).

Asymptomatic HIV infections.

Adults: 100 mg q 4 hr while awake (500 mg/day); **Pediatric, 3 months– 12 years, initial:** 180 mg/m² q 6 hr

(720 mg/m²/day, not to exceed 200 mg q 6 hr).

Prevent transmission of HIV from mothers to their fetuses (after week 14 of pregnancy).

Maternal dosing: 100 mg 5 times a day until the start of labor. During labor and delivery, AZT IV at 2 mg/kg over 1 hr followed by continuous IV infusion of 1 mg/kg/hr until clamping of the umbilical cord. **Infant dosing:** 2 mg/kg PO q 6 hr beginning within 12 hr after birth and continuing through 6 weeks of age. Infants unable to take the drug PO may be given AZT IV at 1.5 mg/kg, infused over 30 min q 6 hr.

In combination with zalcitabine.
Zidovudine, 200 mg, with zalcitabine, 0.75 mg, q 8 hr.

• **IV**

1–2 mg/kg infused over 1 hr. The IV dose is given q 4 hr around the clock only until PO therapy can be instituted. Dosage adjustment may be necessary due to hematologic toxicity.

How Supplied: *Capsule:* 100 mg; *Injection:* 10 mg/mL; *Syrup:* 50 mg/5 mL; *Tablet:* 300 mg

Side Effects: Adults. *Hematologic:* Anemia (severe), granulocytopenia. *Body as a whole:* Headache, asthenia, fever, diaphoresis, malaise, body odor, chills, edema of the lip, flu-like syndrome, hyperalgesia, abdominal/chest/back pain, lymphadenopathy. *GI:* Nausea, GI pain, diarrhea, anorexia, vomiting, dyspepsia, constipation, dysphagia, edema of the tongue, eructation, flatulence, bleeding gums, mouth ulcers, ***rectal hemorrhage.*** *CNS:* Somnolence, dizziness, paresthesia, insomnia, anxiety, confusion, emotional lability, depression, nervousness, vertigo, loss of mental acuity. *CV:* Vasodilation, syncope, vasculitis (rare). *Musculoskeletal:* Myalgia, myopathy, myositis, arthralgia, tremor, twitch, muscle spasm. *Respiratory:* Dyspnea, cough, epistaxis, rhinitis, pharyngitis, sinusitis, hoarseness. *Dermatologic:* Rash, pruritus, urticaria, acne, pigmentation changes of the skin and nails. *GU:*

---

bold italic = life threatening side effect

Dysuria, polyuria, urinary hesitancy or frequency. *Other:* Amblyopia, hearing loss, photophobia, **severe hepatomegaly with steatosis,** lactic acidosis, change in taste perception, hepatitis, pancreatitis, hypersensitivity reactions, including **anaphylaxis,** hyperbilirubinemia (rare), **seizures.**

Children. The following side effects have been observed in children, although any of the side effects reported for adults can also occur in children. *Body as a whole:* Granulocytopenia, anemia, fever, headache, phlebitis, bacteremia. *GI:* N&V, abdominal pain, diarrhea, weight loss. *CNS:* Decreased reflexes, nervousness, irritability, insomnia, **seizures.** *CV:* Abnormalities in ECG, left ventricular dilation, CHF, generalized edema, **cardiomyopathy,** S_3 gallop. *GU:* Hematuria, viral cystitis

OD Overdose Management: *Symptoms:* N&V. Transient hematologic changes. Headache, dizziness, drowsiness, confusion, lethargy. *Treatment:* Treat symptoms. Hemodialysis will enhance the excretion of the primary metabolite of AZT.

Drug Interactions
Acetaminophen / ↑ Risk of granulocytopenia
Adriamycin / ↑ Risk of cytotoxicity, nephrotoxicity, or hematologic toxicity
Dapsone / ↑ Risk of cytotoxicity, nephrotoxicity, or hematologic toxicity
Flucytosine / ↑ Risk of cytotoxicity, nephrotoxicity, or hematologic toxicity
Fluconazole / ↑ Levels of AZT
Ganciclovir / ↑ Risk of hematologic toxicity
Interferon alfa / ↑ Risk of hematologic toxicity
Interferon beta-1b / ↑ Serum levels of AZT
Phenytoin / Levels of phenytoin may ↑, ↓, or remain unchanged; also, ↓ excretion of AZT
Probenecid / ↓ Biotransformation or renal excretion of AZT → flu-like symptoms, including myalgia, malaise or fever, and maculopapular rash
Rifampin / ↓ Levels of AZT
Trimethoprim / ↑ Serum levels of AZT
Vinblastine / ↑ Risk of cytotoxicity, nephrotoxicity, or hematologic toxicity
Vincristine / ↑ Risk of cytotoxicity, nephrotoxicity, or hematologic toxicity

EMS CONSIDERATIONS
See also *Anti-Infectives.*

Zileuton
(zye-LOO-ton)
Pregnancy Class: C
Zyflo **(Rx)**
Classification: Antiasthmatic, leukotriene receptor inhibitor

Mechanism of Action: Specific inhibitor of 5-lipoxygenase; thus, inhibits the formation of leukotrienes. Leukotrienes are substances that induce various biological effects including aggregation of neutrophils and monocytes, leukocyte adhesion, increase of neutrophil and eosinophil migration, increased capillary permeability, and contraction of smooth muscle. These effects of leukotrienes contribute to edema, secretion of mucus, inflammation, and bronchoconstriction in asthmatic patients. By inhibiting leukotriene formation, zileuton reduces bronchoconstriction due to cold air challenge in asthmatics.

Uses: Prophylaxis and chronic treatment of asthma in adults and children over 12 years of age.

Contraindications: Active liver disease or transaminase elevations greater than or equal to three times the upper limit of normal. Hypersensitivity. Treatment of bronchoconstriction in acute asthma attacks, including status asthmaticus. Lactation.

Precautions: Use with caution in patients who ingest large quantities of alcohol or who have a past history of liver disease. Safety and efficacy have not been determined in children less than 12 years of age.

Z

Route/Dosage —————————————
• **Tablets**
Symptomatic treatment of asthma.
Adults and children over 12 years of age: 600 mg q.i.d.
How Supplied: *Tablets:* 600 mg.
Side Effects: *GI:* Dyspepsia, N&V constipation, flatulence. *CNS:* Headache, dizziness, insomnia, malaise, nervousness, somnolence. *Body as a whole:* Unspecified pain, abdominal pain, chest pain, asthenia, accidental injury, fever. *Musculoskeletal:* Myalgia, arthralgia, neck pain/rigidity. *GU:* UTI, vaginitis. *Miscellaneous:* Conjunctivitis, hypertonia, lymphadenopathy, pruritus.
Drug Interactions
Propranolol / ↑ Effect of propranolol
Terfenadine / ↑ Effect of terfenadine due to ↓ clearance
Theophylline / Doubling of serum theophylline levels → ↑ effect
Warfarin / ↑ Prothrombin time

EMS CONSIDERATIONS
None.

Zolmitriptan
(zohl-mih-TRIP-tin)
Pregnancy Class: C
Zomig **(Rx)**
Classification: Antimigraine drug

Mechanism of Action: Binds to serotonin 5-HT$_{1B/1D}$ receptors on intracranial blood vessels and in sensory nerves of trigeminal system. This results in cranial vessel constriction and inhibition of pro-inflammatory neuropeptide release.
Uses: Treatment of acute migraine in adults with or without aura. Use only when there is clear diagnosis of migraine.
Contraindications: Prophylaxis of migraine or management of hemiplegic or basilar migraine. Use in angina pectoris, history of MI, documented or silent ischemia, ischemic heart disease, coronary artery vasospasm (including Prinzmetal's variant angina), other significant underlying CV disease. Also use in uncontrolled hypertension, within 24 hr of treatment with another serotonin HT$_1$ agonist or an ergotamine-containing or ergot-type drug (e.g., dihydroergotamine, methysergide). Concurrent use with MAO inhibitor or within 2 weeks of discontinuing MAO A inhibitor.
Precautions: Use with caution in liver disease and during lactation. A significant increase in BP may occur in those with moderate-to-severe hepatic impairment. Safety and efficacy have not been determined for cluster headache.

Route/Dosage —————————————
• **Tablets**
Migraine headaches.
Adults, initial: 2.5 mg or lower. Dose of 5 mg may be required. If headache returns, repeat dose after 2 hr, not to exceed 10 mg in 24-hr period.
How Supplied: *Tablets:* 2.5 mg, 5 mg
Side Effects: *GI:* Dry mouth, dyspepsia, dysphagia, nausea, increased appetite, tongue edema, esophagitis, gastroenteritis, abnormal liver function, thirst. *CV:* Palpitations, arrhythmias, hypertension, syncope. *Atypical sensations:* Hypesthesia, paresthesia, warm/cold sensation. *CNS:* Dizziness, somnolence, vertigo, agitation, anxiety, depression, emotional lability, insomnia. *Pain pressure sensations:* Chest pain, tightness, pressure and/or heaviness. Pain, tightness, or heaviness in the neck, throat, or jaw. Heaviness, pressure, tightness other than in the chest or neck. *Musculoskeletal:* Myalgia, myasthenia, back pain, leg cramps, tenosynovitis. *Respiratory:* Bronchitis, **bronchospasm,** epistaxis, hiccup, laryngitis, yawn. *Dermatologic:* Sweating, pruritus, rash, urticaria, ecchymosis, photosensitivity. *GU:* Hematuria, cystitis, polyuria, urinary frequency or urgency. *Body as a whole:* Asthenia, allergic reaction, chills, facial edema, edema, fever,

Z

malaise. *Miscellaneous:* Dry eye, eye pain, hyperacusis, ear pain, parosmia, tinnitus.

Drug Interactions

Cimetidine / Half life of zolmitriptan is doubled

Ergot-containing drugs / Prolonged vasospastic reactions

MAO Inhibitors / ↑ Levels of zolmitriptan

Oral contraceptives / ↑ Plasma levels of zolmitriptan

Selective serotonin reuptake inhibitors / Rarely, weakness, hyperreflexia, and incoordination

---

EMS CONSIDERATIONS

None.

Zolpidem tartrate

(ZOL-pih-dem)

Pregnancy Class: B

Amblen (Rx) (C-IV)

Classification: Nonbarbiturate, non-benzodiazepine sedative-hypnotic

Mechanism of Action: May act by subunit modulation of the GABA receptor chloride channel macromolecular complex resulting in sedative, anticonvulsant, anxiolytic, and myorelaxant properties. Although unrelated chemically to the benzodiazepines or barbiturates, it interacts with a GABA-benzodiazepine receptor complex and shares some of the pharmacologic effects of the benzodiazepines. Specifically, it binds the omega-1 receptor preferentially. No evidence of residual next-day effects or rebound insomnia at usual doses; little evidence for memory impairment. Sleep time spent in stage 3 to 4 (deep sleep) was comparable to placebo with only inconsistent, minor changes in REM sleep at recommended doses.

Uses: Short-term treatment of insomnia.

Contraindications: Lactation.

Precautions: Use with caution and at reduced dosage in patients with impaaired hepatic function, in compromised respiratory function, in those with impaired renal function, and in patients with S&S of depression. Impaired motor or cognitive performance after repeated use or unusual sensitivity to hypnotic drugs may be noted in geriatric or debilitated patients. Closely observe individuals with a history of dependence on or abuse of drugs or alcohol. Safety and efficacy have not been determined in children less than 18 years of age.

Route/Dosage —————

• **Tablets**

Hypnotic.

Adults, individualized, usual: 10 mg just before bedtime. In hepatic insufficiency, use an initial dose of 5 mg.

How Supplied: *Tablet:* 5 mg, 10 mg

Side Effects: *Symptoms of withdrawal:* Although there is no clear evidence of a withdrawal syndrome, the following symptoms were noted with zolpidem following placebo substitution: fatigue, nausea, flushing, lightheadedness, uncontrolled crying, emesis, stomach cramps, panic attack, nervousness, abdominal discomfort.

The most common side effects following use for up to 10 nights included drowsiness, dizziness, and diarrhea. The side effects listed in the following are for an incidence of 1% or greater. *CNS:* Headache, drowsiness, dizziness, lethargy, drugged feeling, lightheadedness, depression, abnormal dreams, amnesia, anxiety, nervousness, sleep disorder, ataxia, confusion, euphoria, insomnia, vertigo. *GI:* Nausea, diarrhea, dyspepsia, abdominal pain, constipation, anorexia, vomiting. *Musculoskeletal:* Myalgia, arthralgia. *Respiratory:* URI, sinusitis, pharyngitis, rhinitis. *Body as a whole:* Allergy, back pain, flu-like symptoms, chest pain, fatigue. *Ophthalmologic:* Diplopia, abnormal vision. *Miscellaneous:* Rash, UTI, palpitations, dry mouth, infection.

OD **Overdose Management:** *Symptoms:* Symptoms ranging from somnolence to light coma. Rarely, CV and respiratory compromise. *Treatment:* Gastric lavage if appropriate. General symptomatic and supportive measures. IV fluids as needed. Flumazenil may be effective in reversing CNS depression. Monitor hypotension and CNS depression and treat appropriately. Sedative drugs should not be used, even if excitation occurs. Zolpidem is not dialyzable.

Drug Interactions: Additive CNS depressant effects are possible when combined with alcohol and other drugs with CNS depressant effects.

EMS CONSIDERATIONS

None.

APPENDIX 1
Controlled Substances in the United States and Canada

Controlled Substances Act—United States

The U.S. Federal Controlled Substances Act of 1970 placed drugs controlled by the Act into five categories or schedules based on their potential to cause psychologic and/or physical dependence as well as on their potential for abuse. The schedules are defined as follows:

Schedule (C-I): Includes substances for which there is a high abuse potential and no current approved medical use (e.g., heroin, marijuana, LSD, other hallucinogens, certain opiates and opium derivatives).

Schedule (C-II): Includes drugs that have a high abuse potential and a high ability to produce physical and/or psychologic dependence and for which there is a current approved or acceptable medical use.

Schedule (C-III): Includes drugs for which there is less potential for abuse than drugs in Schedule II and for which there is a current approved medical use. Certain drugs in this category are preparations containing limited quantities of codeine. Also, anabolic steroids are classified in Schedule III.

Schedule (C-IV): Includes drugs for which there is a relatively low abuse potential and for which there is a current approved medical use.

Schedule (C-V): Drugs in this category consist mainly of preparations containing limited amounts of certain narcotic drugs for use as antitussives and antidiarrheals. Federal law provides that limited quantities of these drugs (e.g., codeine) may be bought without a prescription by an individual at least 18 years of age. The product must be purchased from a pharmacist who must keep appropriate records. However, state laws vary, and in many states such products require a prescription.

Controlled Substances—Canada

In Canada, narcotics are governed by the Narcotics Control regulations and are designated by the letter N. Drugs that are considered subject to abuse, have an approved medical use, and are not narcotics are designated by the letter C.

Generally prescriptions for Schedule II (high-abuse-potential) drugs cannot be transmitted over the phone and they cannot be refilled. Prescriptions for Schedule III, IV, and V drugs may be refilled up to five times within 6 months. Schedule II drugs are not necessarily "stronger" than drugs in Schedules III, IV, or V; Schedule II drugs are classified as such due to their high abuse potential.

APPENDIX 2

Elements of a Prescription

In order to safely communicate the exact elements desired on a prescription, the following items should be addressed:

A. The prescriber: Name, address, phone number, and associated practice/speciality

B. The client: Name, age, address and social security number

C. The prescription itself: Name of the medication (generic or trade); quantity to be dispensed (e.g., tablets or capsules, 1 vial, 1 tube, volume of liquid); the strength of the medication (e.g., 125-mg tablets, 250 mg/5 mL, 80mg/1 mL, 10%); and directions for use (e.g., 1 tablet po t.i.d.; 2 gtt to each eye q.i.d.; 1 teaspoonful po q 8 hr for 10 days; apply a thin film to lesions b.i.d. for 14 days)

D. Other elements: Date prescription is written, signature of the provider, number of refills; provider number: state license number and Drug Enforcement Agency (DEA) number (when applicable); and brand-product-only indication (when applicable)

A typical prescription is depicted as follows:

A.   **Julia Bryan, MSN, RN, CPNP**
Pediatric Associates
1611 Kirkwood Highway
Wilmington, DE 19805
302-645-8261

Date: July 10, 2001

B.   For: **Kathryn Woods, Age 8**
27 East Parkway
Lewes, DE 19958
123-555-1234

C.   Rx   **Amoxicillin susp. 250 mg/5 mL**
Disp. 150 mL
Sig: 1 teaspoon PO q 8 hr x 10 days

D.   Refills : 0

Provider signature
Provider/State license number

Interpretation of prescription: The above prescription is written by Pediatric Nurse Practitioner Julia Bryan for Kathryn Woods and is for amoxicillin suspension. The concentration desired is 250 mg/5 mL. The directions for taking the medication are 1 teaspoon (i.e., 5 mL) by mouth every 8 hr for 10 days. The prescriber wants 150 mL dispensed and there are no refills allowed.

APPENDIX 3
Pregnancy Categories: FDA Assigned

The U.S. Food and Drug Administration's use-in-pregnancy rating system weighs the degree to which available information has ruled out risk to the fetus against the drug's potential benefit to the patient. The ratings, and their interpretation, are as follows:

Category	Interpetation
A	**CONTROLLED STUDIES SHOW NO RISK.** Adequate, well-controlled studies in pregnant women have failed to demonstrate a risk to the fetus in any trimester of pregnancy.
B	**NO EVIDENCE OF RISK IN HUMANS.** Adequate, well-controlled studies in pregnant women have not shown increased risk of fetal abnormalities despite adverse findings in animals, or, in the absence of adequate human studies, animal studies show no fetal risk. The chance of fetal harm is remote, but remains a possibility.
C	**RISK CANNOT BE RULED OUT.** Adequate, well-controlled human studies are lacking, and animal studies have shown a risk to the fetus or are lacking as well. There is a chance of fetal harm if the drug is administered during pregnancy; but the potential benefits may outweigh the potential risk.
D	**POSITIVE EVIDENCE OF RISK.** Studies in humans, or investigational or post-marketing data, have demonstrated fetal risk. Nevertheless, potential benefits from the use of the drug may outweigh the potential risk. For example, the drug may be acceptable if needed in a life-threatening situation or serious disease for which safer drugs cannot be used or are ineffective.
X	**CONTRAINDICATED IN PREGNANCY.** Studies in animals or humans, or investigational or post-marketing reports, have demonstrated positive evidence of fetal abnormalities or risk which clearly outweighs any possible benefit to the patient.

APPENDIX 4

Nomogram for Estimating Body Surface Area

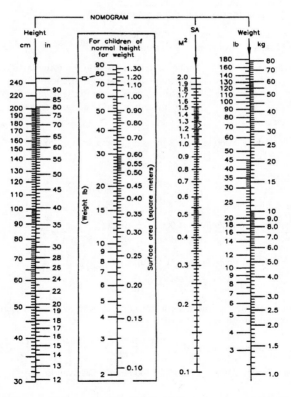

NOMOGRAM

Directions for use: (1) Determine client height. (2) Determine client weight. (3) Draw a straight line to connect the height and weight. Where the line intersects on the surface area line is the derived body surface area (M²).

Reprinted with permission from Behrman, R. E., Kliegman, R., and Arvin, A. M., eds. *Nelson Textbook of Pediatrics,* 15th ed. (Philadelphia: W. B. Saunders Company, 1996).

APPENDIX 5
Easy Formulas for IV Rate Calculation

In order to calculate the continuous drip rate for an IV infusion, the following information is necessary:

    a. amount of solution to be infused
    b. time for infusion to be administered
    c. *drop factor (found in the tubing package)

$$\frac{\text{Total volume to be infused}}{\text{Total hours for infusion}} \times \frac{\text{*drop factor}}{60 \text{ min/hr}} = \text{gtt/min}$$

    *If drop factor is: 60 gtt/min, then use 1 in the formula
                                    10 gtt/min, then use ⅙ in the formula
                                    15 gtt/min, then use ¼ in the formula
                                    20 gtt/min, then use ⅓ in the formula

This gives you $\frac{\text{gtt}}{\text{min}}$.

Example: Infuse 1,000 cc over 8 hr using tubing with a drop factor of 10 gtt/min.

$$\frac{1,000 \text{ cc}}{8 \text{ hr}} \times \frac{1}{6} = 20.8 \text{ or } 21 \ \frac{\text{gtt}}{\text{min}}$$

Complete equation is:

$$\frac{1,000 \text{ cc}}{8 \text{ hr}} \times \frac{10 \text{ gtt/min}}{60 \text{ min/1 hr}} = \frac{1,000 \text{ cc}}{8 \text{ hr}} \times \frac{10 \text{ gtt}}{\text{cc}} \times \frac{1 \text{hr}}{60 \text{ min}} = 21 \ \frac{\text{gtt}}{\text{min}}$$

To get $\frac{\text{cc}}{\text{hr}}$ invert drop factor and multiply by $\frac{\text{gtt}}{\text{min}}$, or:

$$\frac{6}{1} \times 21 \ \frac{\text{gtt}}{\text{min}} = 126 \ \frac{\text{cc}}{\text{hr}}$$

When administering intermittent infusions, as with antibiotic therapy, use the following formula:

$$\text{Total volume to be infused} \div \frac{\text{minutes to administer}}{60 \text{ min/hr}} = \frac{\text{mL}}{\text{hr}}$$

Example: Administer 3 g Zosyn in 100 cc of D5W over 45 min

$$100 \div \frac{45}{60} \text{ (invert to multiply)}$$

or

$$100 \times \frac{60}{45} = 133.3 \text{ or } 134 \ \frac{\text{mL}}{\text{hr}}$$

APPENDIX 6
Tables of Weights and Measures

Weights	Exact Equivalents	Approximate Equivalents
1 ounce (oz)	28.35 g	30 g
1 pound (lb)	453.6 g	454 g
1 gram (g)	0.0353 oz	0.035 oz
1 kilogram (kg)	2.205 lb	2.2 lb

Fluid Measures

1 teaspoon (t)		5 mL
1 tablespoon (T)	3 tsp	15 mL (½ fl oz)
1 fluid ounce (fl oz)	29.57 mL	30 mL
1 pint (16 fl oz)	473.0 mL	473 mL
1 quart (32 fl oz)	946 mL	945 mL
1 gallon (128 fl oz)	3.785 L	3.8 L
1 milliliter (mL)	0.0352 fl oz (Imperial)	0.0345 fl oz
1 liter (L)	2.11 pt	2 pt

Lengths

1 inch (in)	2.54 cm	2.5 cm
1 foot (ft)	30.48 cm	30.0 cm
1 yard (yd)	0.914 m	0.9 m
1 centimeter (cm)	0.3937 in	
1 meter (m)	39.4 in	

Approximate Conversions to Metric Measures

To Convert	To	Multiply By
Inches	Centimeters	2.54
Feet	Centimeters	30.48
Grains	Grams	0.065
Ounces	Grams	28.35
Pounds	Kilograms	0.45
Teaspoons, Medical	Milliliters	5.0
Tablespoons	Milliliters	15.0
Fluid ounces	Milliliters	29.57
Cups	Liters	0.24
Pints	Liters	0.47
Quarts	Liters	0.95
Gallons	Liters	3.8

Approximate Conversions to Metric Measures

To Convert	To	Multiply By
Millimeters	Inches	0.039
Centimeters	Inches	0.39
Grams	Grains	15.432
Kilograms	Pounds	2.2
Milliliters	Fluid ounces	0.034
Liters	Pints	2.1
Liters	Quarts	1.06
Liters	Gallons	0.26
Deg. Fahrenheit	Deg. Celsius	5/9 (after subtracting 32)
Deg. Celsius	Deg. Fahrenheit	9/5 (then add 32)

Index

Boldface = generic drug names
Italics = therapeutic drug class

Regular type = trade names
CAPITALS = combination drugs

Boldface = generic drug names
Italics = therapeutic drug class

Regular type = trade names
CAPITALS = combination drugs

Boldface = generic drug names
Italics = therapeutic drug class

Regular type = trade names
CAPITALS = combination drugs

Boldface = generic drug names
Italics = therapeutic drug class

Regular type = trade names
CAPITALS = combination drugs

Boldface = generic drug names
Italics = therapeutic drug class

Regular type = trade names
CAPITALS = combination drugs

Boldface = generic drug names
Italics = therapeutic drug class

Regular type = trade names
CAPITALS = combination drugs

Boldface = generic drug names
Italics = therapeutic drug class

Regular type = trade names
CAPITALS = combination drugs

Boldface = generic drug names
Italics = therapeutic drug class

Regular type = trade names
CAPITALS = combination drugs

Boldface = generic drug names
Italics = therapeutic drug class

Regular type = trade names
CAPITALS = combination drugs

Intron A **(Interferon alfa-2b recombinant)**, 443
Intropin **(Dopamine hydrochloride)**, 322
Invirase **(Saquinavir mesylate)**, 711
Ipecac syrup (PMS Ipecac Syrup), **450**
Ipratropium bromide (Atrovent), **451**
Ipratropium bromide and Albuterol sulfate (Combivent), **452**
Irbesartan (Avapro), **453**
Ircon **(Ferrous fumarate)**, 366
Ismelin Sulfate **(Guanethidine monosulfate)**, 410
ISMO **(Isosorbide mononitrate, oral)**, 459
Isodorbide dinitrate tablets, **458**
Isoetharine hydrochloride, **454**
Isoniazid, **454**
Isonicotinic acid hydrazide, **454**
Isophane insulin suspension, **456**
Isophane insulin suspension and insulin injection, **456**
Isoproterenol hydrochloride (Isuprel), **456**
Isoproterenol sulfate (Medihaler-Iso), **456**
Isoptin **(Verapamil)**, 805
Isoptin SR **(Verapamil)**, 805
Isopto Atropine Ophthalmic **(Atropine sulfate)**, 162
Isopto Carpine **(Pilocarpine hydrochloride)**, 643
Isopto Hyoscine Ophthalmic **(Scopolamine hydrobromide)**, 714
Isopto-Cetamide **(Sulfacetamide sodium)**, 737
Isordil **(Isosorbide dinitrate sublingual tablets)**, 458
Isordil Tembids **(Isosorbide dinitrate extended-release capsules)**, 458
Isordil Titradose **(Isodorbide dinitrate tablets)**, 458
Isosorbide dinitrate chewable tablets, **458**
Isosorbide dinitrate extended-release capsules, **458**
Isosorbide dinitrate extended-release tablets (Cedocard-SR), **458**
Isosorbide dinitrate sublingual tablets (Isordil), **458**
Isosorbide mononitrate, oral (ISMO), **459**
Isotretinoin (Accutane), **460**
Isradipine (DynaCirc), **461**
I-Sulfacet **(Sulfacetamide sodium)**, 737
Isuprel **(Isoproterenol hydrochloride)**, 456
Isuprel Mistometer **(Isoproterenol hydrochloride)**, 456

Itraconazole (Sporanox), **461**
Iveegam **(Immune globulin IV)**, 434
Ivermectin (Stromectol), **463**

Jenest-28, 89
Junior Strength Feverall **(Acetaminophen)**, 115
Junior Strength Motrin Caplets **(Ibuprofen)**, 428

K + Care ET **(Potassium bicarbonate)**, 652
K + Care ET **(Potassium bicarbonate and Citric acid)**, 652
K+ Care **(Potassium Chloride)**, 652
K+ 10 **(Potassium Chloride)**, 652
Kabikinase **(Streptokinase)**, 732
Kadian **(Morphine sulfate)**, 557
Kalcinate **(Calcium gluconate)**, 201
Kanamycin sulfate (Kantrex), **464**
Kantrex **(Kanamycin sulfate)**, 464
Kaochlor 10% Liquid **(Potassium Chloride)**, 652
Kaon **(Potassium gluconate)**, 652
Kaon-Cl **(Potassium Chloride)**, 652
Kaon-Cl-10 **(Potassium Chloride)**, 652
Kaopectate II Caplets **(Loperamide hydrochloride)**, 497
Kay Ciel **(Potassium Chloride)**, 652
Kaybovite-1000 **(Cyanocobalamin)**, 273
Kayexalate **(Sodium polystyrene sulfonate)**, 725
Kaylixir **(Potassium gluconate)**, 652
K-Dur 10 and 20 **(Potassium Chloride)**, 652
Keflex **(Cephalexin monohydrate)**, 228
Keftab **(Cephalexin hydrochloride monohydrate)**, 228
Kefurox **(Cefuroxime sodium)**, 225
Kefzol **(Cefazolin sodium)**, 214
Kenac **(Triamcinolone acetonide)**, 785
Kenacort **(Triamcinolone)**, 785
Kenacort Diacetate **(Triamcinolone diacetatae)**, 785
Kenaject-40 **(Triamcinolone acetonide)**, 785
Kenalog **(Triamcinolone acetonide)**, 785
Kenalog in Orabase **(Triamcinolone)**, 785
Kenalog-H **(Triamcinolone acetonide)**, 785
Kenalog-10 and -40 **(Triamcinolone acetonide)**, 785
Kenonel **(Triamcinolone acetonide)**, 785
Keppra **(Levetiracetam)**, 481

Boldface = generic drug names
Italics = therapeutic drug class
Regular type = trade names
CAPITALS = combination drugs

Boldface = generic drug names
Italics = therapeutic drug class

Regular type = trade names
CAPITALS = combination drugs

Boldface = generic drug names
Italics = therapeutic drug class

Regular type = trade names
CAPITALS = combination drugs

Boldface = generic drug names
Italics = therapeutic drug class

Regular type = trade names
CAPITALS = combination drugs

Boldface = generic drug names
Italics = therapeutic drug class

Regular type = trade names
CAPITALS = combination drugs

Boldface = generic drug names
Italics = therapeutic drug class

Regular type = trade names
CAPITALS = combination drugs

Boldface = generic drug names
Italics = therapeutic drug class

Regular type = trade names
CAPITALS = combination drugs

Boldface = generic drug names
Italics = therapeutic drug class

Regular type = trade names
CAPITALS = combination drugs
